VOLUME 89 - JULY-AUGUST, 1980
No. 4, Part 1 (Issued in 5 Parts)

THE ANNALS OF OTOLOGY RHINOLOGY & LARYNGOLOGY

ANNALS OF HEAD & NECK MEDICINE & SURGERY

Tympanosclerosis. A Theory of Pathogenesis.
M. Schiff, MD, J.F. Poliquin, MD,
A. Catanzaro, MD, A.F. Ryan, PhD.
Supplement 70

Myringoplasty. A Review of 472 Cases.
J.L. Sheehy, MD, R.G. Anderson, MD

Congenital Malformations of the Ear. Analysis of 94 Operations.
R. Jahrsdoerfer, MD

Characteristics of Capillary Permeability in Nasal Mucosa.
K. Watanabe, MD, Y. Saito, MD,
I. Watanabe, MD, V. Mizuhira, MD

Thyroid Disease: A Guide for the Head and Neck Surgeon.
R. M. Bumsted, MD. Supplement 72

Care of the Montgomery Silicone Tracheal T-Tube.
W.W. Montgomery, MD. Supplement 73

ANNALS PUBLISHING COMPANY
SAINT LOUIS, MISSOURI 63108

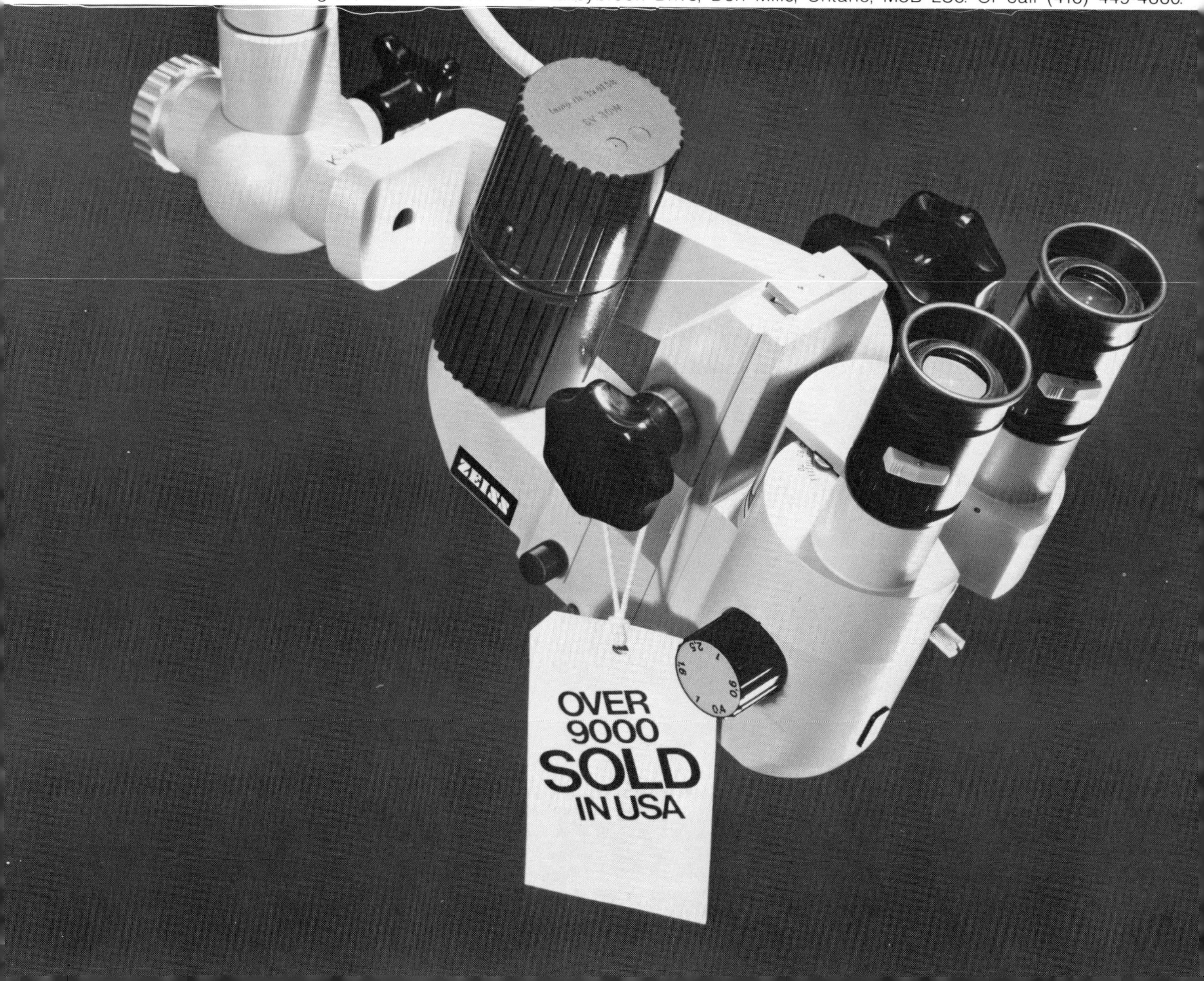

ZEISS
OVER
9000
SOLD
IN USA

ANNALS OF OTOLOGY, RHINOLOGY AND LARYNGOLOGY
ANNALS OF HEAD AND NECK MEDICINE AND SURGERY
VOL. 89 JULY-AUGUST 1980 NO. 4

CONTENTS

Tympanosclerosis. A Theory of Pathogenesis. M. Schiff, MD, J. F. Poliquin, MD, A. Catanzaro, MD, A. F. Ryan, PhD . . . . Supplement 70

Brainstem Auditory Evoked Potentials for Detection of Retrocochlear Pathology. S. E. Kinney, MD, R. H. Nodar, MD 291

Acoustic Reflex Latency Test in the Evaluation of Nontumor Patients with Abnormal Brainstem Latencies. J. D. Clemis, MD, C. N. Sarno, MD 296

Plasticity of the Developing Auditory System. R. J. Ruben, MD, I. Rapin, MD 303

Intramembranous and Mesotympanic Cholesteatomas Associated with an Intact Tympanic Membrane in Children. S. M. Sobel, MD, T. J. Reichert, MD, K. D. Faw, MD, M. H. Stroud, MD, G. J. Spector, MD, J. H. Ogura, MD 312

Labyrinthectomy versus Middle Fossa Vestibular Nerve Section in Menière's Disease. A Critical Evaluation of Relief of Vertigo. M. E. Glasscock III, MD, FACS, G. B. Hughes, MD, W. E. Davis, MD, FACS, C. G. Jackson, MD 318

Attachment of the Tectorial Membrane Revealed by Scanning Electron Microscope. M. Lawrence, PhD, P. A. Burgio, MA 325

Myringoplasty. A Review of 472 Cases. J. L. Sheehy, MD, R. G. Anderson, MD 331

Cochlear Fluid Balance. A Clinical/Research Overview. A. J. Duvall III, MD, P. A. Santi, PhD, M. J. Hukee 335

Sickle Cell Anemia and Hearing. E. M. Friedman, MD, G. R. Herer, PhD, N. L. C. Luban, MD, I. Williams, PNP . . 342

Congenital Malformations of the Ear. Analysis of 94 Operations. R. Jahrsdoerfer, MD 348

Acute Cochlear Disorders: The Combination of Hearing Loss, Recruitment, Poor Speech Discrimination, and Tinnitus. J. Tonndorf, MD 353

Immunopathological Study of the Larynx. IgA Distribution and Secretory Activity. T. Nakashima, MD, S. Komiyama, MD, K. Makishima, MD, K. Takeda, MD, I. Hiroto, MD 359

Comparative Preoperative Evaluation of Eustachian Tube Function in Pathological Ears. H. Virtanen, MD, T. Palva, MD, T. Jauhiainen, MD 366

Vestibular and Oculomotor Abnormalities in Vertebrobasilar Insufficiency. J. Corvera, MD, L. D. Benitez, MD, G. Lopez-Rios, MD, M. T. Rabiela, MD 370

Characteristics of Capillary Permeability in Nasal Mucosa. K. Watanabe, MD, Y. Saito, MD, I. Watanabe, MD, V. Mizuhira, MD 377

Grand Rounds — Albany Medical Center. Septic Osteoradionecrosis of the Mandible. S. S. Parulekar, MD, MS, FRCS, D. F. Paonessa, MD 383

The Eye-Tracking Test. Y. Umeda, MD . . . . Supplement 71

Thyroid Disease: A Guide for the Head and Neck Surgeon. R. M. Bumsted, MD . . . . Supplement 72

Manual for Care of the Montgomery Silicone Tracheal T-Tube. W. W. Montgomery, MD . . . . Supplement 73

Letters to the Editor 388

Book Reviews 389

Abstracts from National and International Journals 390

Index to Advertisers xxiv

ANNALS OF OTOLOGY, RHINOLOGY AND LARYNGOLOGY
ANNALS OF HEAD AND NECK MEDICINE AND SURGERY
VOL. 89 SEPTEMBER-OCTOBER 1980 NO. 5

CONTENTS

Chevalier Jackson Lecture. Esophageal Stenosis in Children. F. Aprigliano, MD 391

Etiology of Stridor in the Neonate, Infant and Child. L. D. Holinger, MD 397

Innominate Artery Compression of the Trachea in Infants with Reflex Apnea. J. M. Ardito, MD, R. H. Ossoff, DMD, MD, G. F. Tucker, Jr., MD, S. Y. DeLeon, MD 401

Congenital Tracheal Diverticulum. A Case Report. S. Frenkiel, MD, FRCS (C), I. K. Assimes, MD, J. K. Rosales, MD, FRCP(C) 406

Internal Laryngocele and Saccular Cysts in Children. J. O. Donegan, MD, J. L. Strife, MD, A. B. Seid, MD, R. T. Cotton, MD, J. S. Dunbar, MD 409

Pediatric Flexible Bronchoscopy. R. E. Wood, PhD, MD, J. M. Sherman, MD 414

Acute Upper Airway Obstruction in Infants and Children. Evaluation by the Fiberoptic Bronchoscope. P. A. Vauthy, MD, R. Reddy, MD 417

Hemoptysis in Children. L. W. C. Tom, MD, R. A. Weisman, MD, S. D. Handler, MD 419

Carcinoid and Mucoepidermoid Carcinoma of Bronchus in Children. J. C. McDougall, MD, A. Gorenstein, DDS, MD, K. Unni, MD, E. J. O'Connell, MD 425

Epidermolysis Bullosa Dystrophica of the Larynx and Trachea. Acute Airway Obstruction. J. W. Thompson, MD, A. R. Ahmed, MD, J. P. Dudley, MD 428

Upper Airway Obstruction in Infectious Mononucleosis. J. A. Wolfe, MD, L. D. Rowe, MD 430

Foreign Bodies in the Larynx and Tracheobronchial Tree in Children. A Review of 225 Cases. B. F. Rothmann, MD, C. R. Boeckman, MD 434

Foreign Bodies in the Airway. Five-Year Retrospective Study with Special Reference to Management. S. R. Cohen, MD, W. I. Herbert, MD, G. B. Lewis, Jr., MD, K. A. Geller, MD 437

Endoscopy and Biopsy in Gastroesophageal Reflux in Infants and Children. B. Benjamin, FRACS, D. Pohl, MB, BS, P. M. Bale, FRCPA 443

The Cricopharyngeus in the Neonate. T. J. Reichert, MD, K. D. Faw, MD 446

High Incidence of Pulmonary Symptoms in Infants Evaluated for Esophageal Disease. F. C. Rothstein, MD, T. C. Halpin, MD 450

Laryngeal Stenosis from Endotracheal Intubation. A Review of 58 Cases. D. B. Hawkins, MD, W. M. Luxford, MD . 454

Prolonged Orotracheal Intubation in the Newborn. G. H. Conner, MD, M. J. Bushey, MD, M. J. Maisels, MD, BCh . 459

Laryngeal Regulation of Airway Resistance. II. Pulmonary Receptor Reflexes. T. V. McCaffrey, MD, E. B. Kern, MD 462

Relationship Between Condylomata and Laryngeal Papillomata. Clinical and Molecular Virological Evidence. C. A. Quick, MD, S. L. Watts, PhD, R. A. Krzyzek, PhD, A. J. Faras, PhD 467

Topical Chemotherapy of Recurrent Respiratory Papillomatosis. A Preliminary Report. H. G. Smith, MD, G. B. Healy, MD, C. W. Vaughan, MD, M. S. Strong, MD 472

Experimental Otitis Media Following Middle Ear Inoculation of Nonviable *Streptococcus pneumoniae*. S. H. Lowell, MD, PhD, S. K. Juhn, MD, G. S. Giebink, MD 479

Childhood Communication Disorders: Present Status and Future Priorities. .... Supplement 74

X-Ray of the Month. Pituitary Adenoma Presenting as a Sphenoid Sinus Lesion. J. M. Davis, MD, A. L. Weber, MD 483

Book Reviews 485

Books Received 487

Abstracts 488

Index to Advertisers xxvi

ANNALS OF OTOLOGY, RHINOLOGY AND LARYNGOLOGY
ANNALS OF HEAD AND NECK MEDICINE AND SURGERY
VOL. 89 NOVEMBER-DECEMBER 1980 NO. 6

CONTENTS

Sixth Daniel C. Baker, Jr. Memorial Lecture. Induction of Cancer by DNA Viruses. J.D. Watson, PhD 489

Papilloma of the Larynx and Tracheobronchial Tree in Children. A Retrospective Study. S.R. Cohen, MD, K.A. Geller, MD, S. Seltzer, MD, J.W. Thompson, MD 497

Double-Barreled (Diversionary) Tracheostomy in the Management of Juvenile Laryngeal Papillomatosis. H.M. Tucker, MD 504

Management of the Extubation Problem in the Premature Child. Anterior Cricoid Split as an Alternative to Tracheotomy. R.T. Cotton, MD, A.B. Seid, MD 508

Acquired Stenosis of the Upper Airway in Neonates. An Increasing Problem. M.J. Papsidero, MD, N.R.T. Pashley, MB, FRCS(C) 512

Long-Term Stenting for Laryngotracheal Stenosis. D.E. Schuller, MD 515

Silicone Tracheal Cannula. W.W. Montgomery, MD 521

An Endoscopic Technique for Restoration of Voice after Laryngectomy. M.I. Singer, MD, E.D. Blom, PhD 529

Neoglottic Reconstruction Following Total Laryngectomy. A Reappraisal. B. Leipzig, MD 534

Laryngology and the Numbers Game. F.E. Lucente, MD 538

Vocal Cord Positioning by Selective Denervation. Old Territory Revisited. C.T. Sasaki, MD, M. Horiuchi, MD, T. Ikari, MD, J.A. Kirchner, MD 541

A Simple Method of Laryngeal Photography through the Operating Microscope. "Macrolens Technique." E. Yanagisawa, MD, D.E. Eibling, MD, M. Suzuki, MD 547

Evolution of the Clinically Negative Neck. E.M. Skolnik, MD, A.H. Katz, MD, S.P. Becker, MD, R. Mantravadi, MD, S. Stal, MD 551

Extended Partial Laryngectomy. D.G. Sessions, MD 556

Acute Cricoarytenoid Arthritis: Local Periarticular Steroid Injection. G.T. Simpson II, MD, MPH, A. Javaheri, MD, P. Janfaza, MD 558

Blastomycosis of the Larynx. J.Y. Suen, MD, S.J. Wetmore, MD, W.J. Wetzel, MD, R.D. Craig, MD 563

Conserative Surgical Treatment of Chondrosarcoma of the Larynx. R.W. Cantrell, MD, J.F. Reibel, MD, R.A. Jahrsdoerfer, MD, M.E. Johns, MD 567

Airway Obstruction in a Hemophiliac Child. J.F. Stanievich, MD, G. Marshak, MD, S.E. Stool, MD 572

Candida Laryngitis in Chronic Mucocutaneous Candidiasis. Its Association with *Candida* Esophagitis. J.P. Dudley, MD, R. Kobayashi, MD, H.M. Rosenblatt, MD, W.J. Byrne, MD, M.E. Ament, MD, E.R. Stiehm, MD 574

Repair of Supraglottic Laryngeal Stenosis with Postcricoid Involvement. A Case Report. P.J. Doyle, MD 576

Retrospective Comparison of Conservative and Radical Neck Dissection in Laryngeal Cancer. R. Molinari, MD, G. Cantu, MD, F. Chiesa, MD, C. Grandi, MD 578

Destruction and Regeneration of Jawbone after Cryogenic Application. An Experimental Study. R. Kuylenstierna, MD, P-G. Lundquist, MD, A. Nathanson, MD 582

Otolaryngology and Medicine Today in the People's Republic of China. B.F. McCabe, MD 590

ENG of the Month. Pacemaker Artifact on ENG Tracing. W.R. Wilson, MD 591

Electrocochleography and Auditory Brainstem Electric Responses in Patients with Pontine Angle Tumors. J.J. Eggermont, PhD, M. Don, PhD, D.E. Brackmann, MD .... Supplement 75

Menière's Disease and Endolymphatic Hydrops. Clinical-Histopathological Correlations. B.G. Fraysse, MD, A. Alonso, MD, W.F. House, MD.
Computer-Aided and Graphic Reconstruction of the Human Endolymphatic Duct and Sac. A Method for Comparing Menière's and Non-Menière's Disease Cases. J-C. M. Antunez, MD, F.R. Galey, PhD, F.H. Linthicum, MD, G.D. McCann, PhD .... Supplement 76

Aminoglycoside Ototoxicity Following Middle Ear Injection. M.D. Rudnick, PhD, I.A. Ginsberg, MD, P.S. Huber, MS .... Supplement 77

Book Reviews 592

Books Received 592

An Appreciation 593

Author Index 594

Subject Index 597

Statement of Ownership 605

Index to Advertisers xxvii

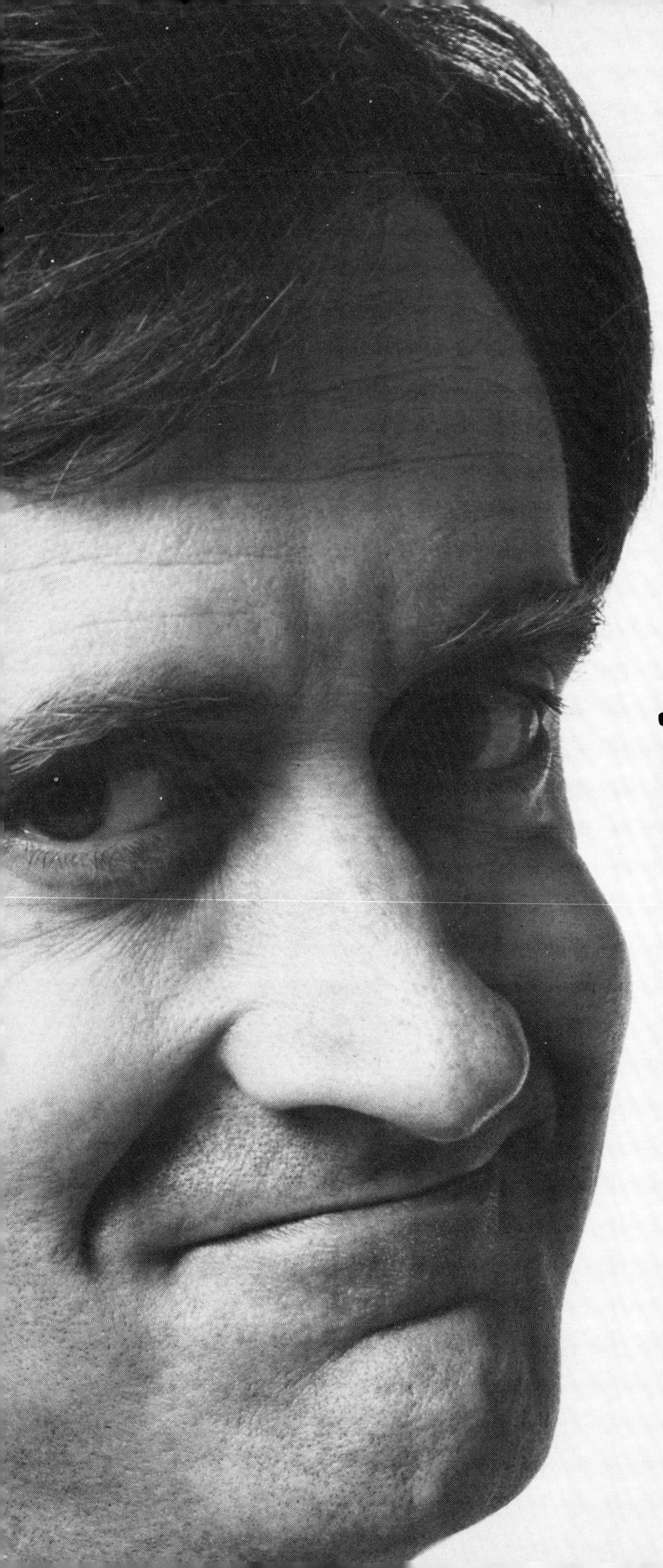

BRAINSTEM AUDITORY EVOKED POTENTIALS FOR DETECTION OF RETROCOCHLEAR PATHOLOGY

SAM E. KINNEY, MD

RICHARD H. NODAR, MD

CLEVELAND, OHIO

Since May 1976 the techniques of brainstem auditory evoked potential (BAEP) testing have been used as a clinical tool in evaluating patients with neurotologic disease in the Department of Otolaryngology and Communicative Disorders at the Cleveland Clinic Foundation. A total of 676 patients was tested using this technique and included patients with primary otologic complaints as well as patients with neurologic disorders. Patients were evaluated with suspected multiple sclerosis, for threshold assessment, children at risk for possible sudden infant death syndrome, brainstem gliomas, systemic neurologic or metabolic disorders, and the final group of 408 patients or 60% were tested for suspected eighth nerve lesions. In the group of patients studied for detection of an eighth nerve lesion, the BAEP test was extremely useful if the result was found to be normal, for at the time of this report, no patient with an eighth nerve lesion, such as an acoustic neuroma, had a normal BAEP test result. However, abnormal results in the BAEP test were found in approximately 34% of patients who underwent Pantopaque® myelography for definitive detection of an eighth nerve lesion in which the myelogram was normal. This unusually high false-positive rate is thought to be the result of testing a different patient population than those that have previously been reported in the literature. There still may be some eighth nerve pathology present; however, the results of the BAEP test which have been suggestive of an eighth nerve lesion remain unexplained at this time. The BAEP test is a very important part of the evaluation of patients with neurotologic disease; however, it is not sufficiently understood to eliminate the need for a complete work-up in patients suspected to have a retrocochlear lesion.

INTRODUCTION

Since May 1976 the techniques of brainstem auditory evoked potential (BAEP) testing have been used as a clinical tool in the evaluation of patients with neurotologic disease in the Department of Otolaryngology and Communicative Disorders at the Cleveland Clinic Foundation. The patient population has included patients with primary otologic complaints as well as patients with neurologic disorders. The BAEP technique has been employed to evaluate patients who have suspected lesions involving the acoustic branch of the eighth nerve, such as an acoustic tumor in the internal auditory canal or cerebellopontine angle. Although it is believed that this technique is useful in evaluating patients for potential retrocochlear pathology, the authors were concerned that the test was not as specific for detecting acoustic tumors as had been reported by other authors. Specifically, BAEP test results identified a larger percentage of patients with abnormal BAEP recordings who were not found to have a specific eighth nerve lesion, such as an acoustic neuroma. Therefore, it was decided to review the entire series of patients tested with BAEP in order to evaluate its usefulness for detecting retrocochlear pathology in our clinical setting.

This paper will 1) discuss the entire population of patients that have been tested, 2) break these patients down into categories of known neurologic disease, 3) give particular examples of the test results for specific neurologic problems, 4) evaluate results in patients for whom the test was used to detect an acoustic tumor, 5) compare the test for accuracy with other modalities of evaluation of potential acoustic tumor patients, 6) evaluate the accuracy of BAEP testing as a screening tool for the detection of acoustic tumors, and finally, 7) discuss the relationship between BAEP and the need for other diagnostic tests in what presently is a rather extensive and costly evaluation for this problem.

METHODS

The patient population included 676 patients tested with BAEP techniques between May 1976 and December 1979 in the Department of Otolaryngology and Communicative Disorders at the Cleveland Clinic Foundation. The data were collected and analyzed on a clinical computer of average transients (Nicolet CA-1000). Stimuli consisted of 2,000 100 msec clicks presented at an interval of 11.1 per second. The stimuli were presented at 65 dB above threshold (SL) whenever the hearing in the test ear would allow this level. In instances where the hearing loss was sufficiently great that the SL was less than 65 dB, an appropriate correction was made in the latency determinations based on normative data collected in our own clinic and also as noted by Starr and Achor.[1] Low and high band pass filters were set to allow frequency analysis from 150 to 3,000 Hz. The analysis window was set at 10 msec and the sensitivity was set at $\pm 625\ \mu V$. Each ear was tested twice.

The BAEP test results were then assessed on the basis of the seven criteria previously outlined by Nodar et al.[2] These include: 1) peak latency, 2) intrapeak latency, 3) interpeak latency, 4) response stability, 5) amplitude, 6) wave shape, and 7) peak presence. When looking at the acoustic tumor-suspect patient, we specifically evaluated the BAEP using the criterion as outlined by Selters and Brackmann,[3] ie, the absolute latency of the Jewett wave V compared to the same peak for the opposite ear. The ad-

From the Department of Otolaryngology and Communicative Disorders, Cleveland Clinic Foundation, Cleveland, Ohio.

Presented at the meeting of the American Otological Society, Inc., Palm Beach, Florida, April 13-14, 1980.

REPRINTS — Sam E. Kinney, MD, Cleveland Clinic Foundation, 9500 Euclid Avenue, Cleveland, OH 44106.

TABLE 1. DISTRIBUTION OF TOTAL POPULATION TESTED WITH BAEP (N = 676)

Multiple sclerosis	61
Threshold assessment	73
Sleep apnea	37
Brainstem gliomas	9
Systemic neurologic or metabolic disorder	88
Retrocochlear pathology	408

TABLE 2. DISTRIBUTION OF PATIENT POPULATION TESTED WITH BAEP SUSPECTED TO HAVE AN EIGHTH NERVE LESION (N = 408)

Normal BAEP	265
Abnormal BAEP — no myelogram	92
Abnormal BAEP — normal hearing, no myelogram	10
Abnormal BAEP — myelogram, no tumor	13
Abnormal BAEP — CT scan, tumor present	20
Abnormal BAEP — myelogram, tumor present	8

justed Jewett wave V criteria as outlined by Selters and Brackmann[3] were used on the hearing in the test ear at 4,000 Hz. If the hearing loss in the test ear at 4,000 Hz was above 50 dB, 0.1 msec was subtracted from the absolute Jewett wave V response and an additional 0.1 msec was subtracted for each additional 10 dB or fraction thereof.

Posterior fossa myelography is considered the most definitive test for an acoustic neuroma if the CT scan is negative. The decision to recommend Pantopaque myelography to a patient in our office is determined by the following criteria: the patient presents with a history of unilateral hearing loss, unilateral tinnitus, or dizziness and is placed into a category of a possible acoustic tumor suspect. The patient has a complete basic audiogram performed including pure tone air and bone conduction, speech discrimination, and tympanometry including reflex decay testing whenever technically possible. The patient then undergoes electronystagmography, x-rays of internal auditory canals, and special audiometric tests. Based on the results of this initial evaluation, the patient then may have BAEP testing. All patients who have evidence of an enlarged internal auditory canal by x-ray continue further with the acoustic tumor evaluation. If the BAEP test is normal, the patient may not be tested with posterior fossa myelography and is asked to return for further audiometric testing in approximately four to six months. If there has been continued progression of hearing loss, the patient then proceeds with a CT scan and posterior fossa myelography. If the BAEP test is abnormal and there is one other portion of the work-up that suggests an acoustic neuroma, a CT scan and posterior fossa myelography is recommended.

In some patients suspected to have an acoustic tumor, the hearing in the involved ear was inadequate to perform BAEP testing; however, the test was completed on the opposite ear for the purpose of detecting contralateral effects on BAEP testing due to distortion of the brainstem by a large cerebellopontine angle tumor, as outlined by Nodar and Kinney.[4]

A review of the patients tested with BAEP indicated that a number were found to have a suspicious or abnormal test result; however, the remainder of the neurotologic evaluation did not support a possible eighth nerve tumor and the evaluation did not continue. These patients did not have a CT scan and/or posterior fossa myelography. This group of patients will not be listed as false-positives in our series. We will determine our false-positive rate based only on whether or not a tumor was confirmed by CT scan or posterior fossa myelography.

RESULTS

In our total patient population 61 patients were tested who were being evaluated for neurologic complaints suggestive of multiple sclerosis (Table 1). These patients were seen retrospectively after the diagnosis of multiple sclerosis had been made. We will discuss the findings in these patients later; however, at this point, BAEP testing is not the sole determinant in the diagnosis of multiple sclerosis. The patient population also included 73 patients seen for threshold assessment; 20 patients were tested under general anesthesia in the operating room because of inability of the patients to be tested under sedation in the outpatient office; a small number of patients in this group were tested for the purpose of confirming a clinical diagnosis of pseudohypoacusis; 37 patients tested were diagnosed at risk for sudden infant death syndrome (SIDS); 9 children were tested for the purpose of localizing brainstem gliomas as reported by Nodar et al;[2] 88 patients were tested because of systemic neurologic or metabolic disorders; 408 patients were tested in this series specifically for the purpose of identifying a possible retrocochlear lesion (Table 2). In this group of 408, 265 were felt to have normal BAEP test results. This represents 60% of the entire patient population. For 143 patients an abnormality was found on the BAEP test based on the seven criteria outlined by Nodar et al.[2] When the correction factor for hearing loss at 4,000 Hz, as proposed by Selters and Brackmann,[3] was applied, or because there was insufficient evidence in the remainder of the tumor work-up, 92 of the 143 patients did not proceed to CT scan and/or posterior fossa myelography. Of the remaining 51 patients, 10 patients had an abnormal BAEP test using the interaural peak latency delay criteria of 0.2 msec, but because they had audiograms showing normal pure tone sensitivities and speech discrimination in both ears, they did not progress further to Pantopaque myelography. Twenty patients were found to have positive BAEP tests and were later confirmed to have an acoustic tumor by CT scan; 8 patients with positive BAEP were found to have a tumor by Pantopaque myelography; 15 additional patients with confirmed acoustic tumors did not have BAEP tests performed either because of inadequate hearing in the involved ear or the diagnosis of an acoustic tumor based on a positive CT scan prior to the time that the patient was referred to our department. There were 13 patients who had a positive BAEP test result who had normal Pantopaque myelography. (This was out of a series of 51 patients who underwent Pantopaque myelography for investigation of the internal auditory canals.)

A review of the entire series of patients who underwent Pantopaque myelography (N = 51) revealed that 13 patients did not receive BAEP testing on the basis of an enlarged internal auditory canal, retrocochlear audiometric findings, or positive findings in electronystagmography. Of the remaining 38 patients who had BAEP testing and a Panto-

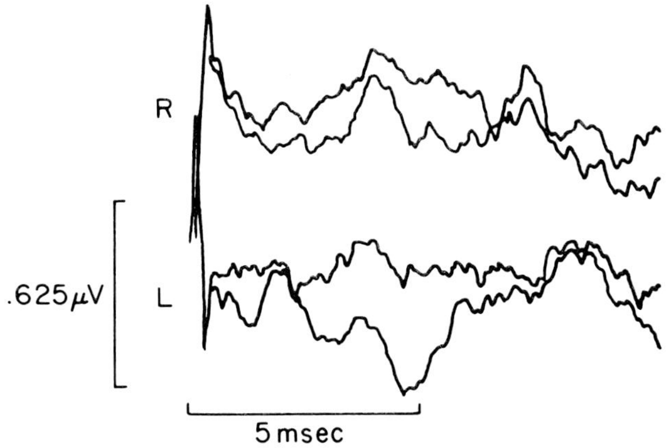

Fig. 1. The BAEP result from a patient with multiple sclerosis. The patient has a normal pure tone and speech discrimination audiogram. Note that on repeat testing there is poor response stability.

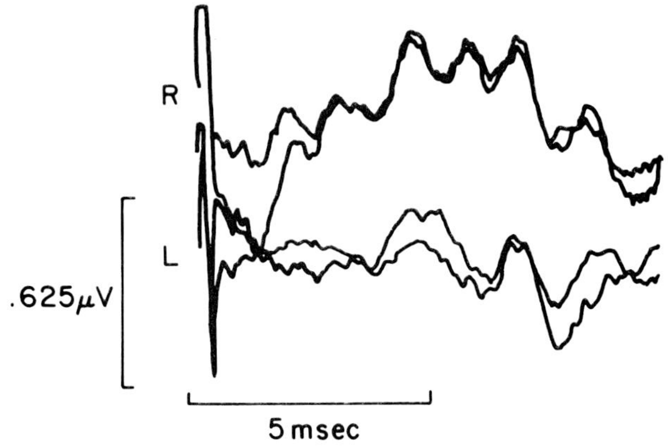

Fig. 2. The BAEP result from a child felt to be at risk for sudden infant death syndrome. Note abnormality of Jewett waves II and III in the left ear; however, the latencies of Jewett wave V are normal in both ears. This suggests an abnormality in the low brainstem left with normal hearing.

paque myelogram, 13 had positive BAEP results based on the Selters and Brackmann[3] criteria and were found to have a normal internal auditory canal Pantopaque myelogram. This represents a false-positive rate for tumor of 34% in patients undergoing Pantopaque myelography. We have yet to identify a patient with an acoustic tumor who had a normal BAEP test result. Thus, the false-negative rate in our series remains at 0%. In the entire series of 51 patients we identified eight patients with acoustic tumors, a 15.7% positive rate on identifying acoustic tumors by Pantopaque myelography.

DISCUSSION

The purpose of this paper is to assess clinical experience over a period of 3 1/2 years using BAEP testing to evaluate patients for potential retrocochlear pathology. In this series 61 patients were evaluated because of the clinical diagnosis of multiple sclerosis. Robinson and Rudge,[5] report a significantly high correlation between abnormal findings in the BAEP of patients with multiple sclerosis. One finding is that of a rather significant decrease in the response stability of the BAEP result (Fig. 1).

Over 10% of the patients reported in this series received BAEP testing for the purpose of determining auditory thresholds. Although the technique generally tells us more about the auditory threshold at 4,000 Hz and above, it has been an extremely useful clinical tool, particularly in patients who are unable to cooperate for an adequate behavioral threshold. We have found patients who have a profound sensorineural hearing loss, and in some instances we were able to determine that the hearing threshold was considerably better in one ear, thus allowing us to make an accurate decisison on which ear to place a hearing aid. A number of patients were evaluated because of suspected pseudohypoacusis. Using BAEP, we were able to establish physiologic thresholds.

The application of BAEP testing in the area of the SIDS may represent one of the most significant developments of this test procedure.[6] There appears to be a predictable maturation of brainstem auditory evoked potentials in newborn infants.[7] Infants with sleep apnea have been found to demonstrate abnormal BAEP results well beyond the range of what would be considered normal based on maturation of the newborn infant brainstem (Fig. 2).

Finally, BAEP testing has been extremely useful localizing central brainstem lesions, such as brainstem gliomas in children.[2]

The purpose of this report is to review BAEP testing at Cleveland Clinic for the identification of retrocochlear lesions involving the eighth nerve. Selters and Brackmann[3] reported their false-positive rate to be 8% in the detection of acoustic tumors in 276 patients with unilateral hearing loss. They also noted a false-negative rate of 2.3% in patients with confirmed acoustic tumors. Glasscock et al[8] reported BAEP testing to be 98% effective in determining site of lesion pathology; they also reported a false-negative rate of approximately 2%. In this study, a significantly higher false-positive rate was found which has significantly influenced the application of BAEP testing in the evaluation of patients for potential acoustic neuromas. Figure 3 shows the type of BAEP result listed as false-positive in our series. To date, we have not identified a patient with an acoustic tumor which was not predictable using the BAEP test procedure. An example of a patient with a strong suspicion for an acoustic tumor with a normal BAEP is shown in Figure 4. An attempt to determine the reason for this apparent high false-positive rate led to the observation that we had not been compulsive in using the BAEP test in all patients with suspected retrocochlear pathology. Further, the results of the BAEP test were ignored in our total evaluation based on an in-

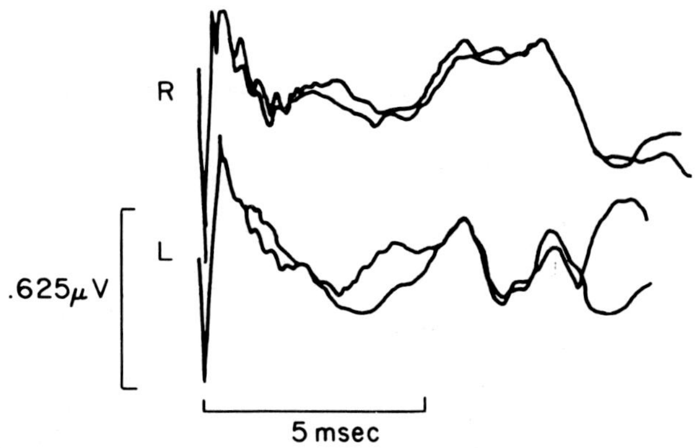

Fig. 3. The BAEP result of a patient with symptoms suggestive of Menière's disease in his right ear and a negative myelogram. Note marked abnormality and prolonged latency of Jewett wave V in the right ear. This finding remains unexplained and is a false-positive result in our series.

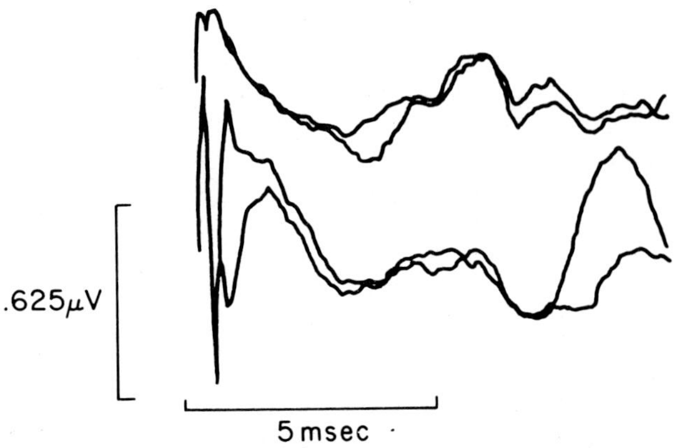

Fig. 4. The BAEP result in a patient with unilateral hearing loss and a wide internal auditory canal by x-ray. The myelogram showed filling of both internal canals. Note that the interpeak latency of Jewett wave V was not prolonged. The normal BAEP predicted that there was no eighth nerve lesion.

ordinate number of patients with markedly positive BAEP results who were found to have normal Pantopaque myelograms of the internal acoustic meatus. The test procedure had not been performed on every patient because of the cost and time scheduling pressures involved. Therefore, there is a relatively small sample size which may account for an abnormally high false-positive rate for acoustic tumors.

An examination of the series of patients reported by Glasscock et al[8] reveals that their patients had a pure tone hearing loss that ranged from 11.5 to 75 dB with a mean hearing loss of 56 dB in the suspect ear. Selters and Brackmann[3] state that all of the 276 patients included in the group demonstrating an 8% false-positive rate had a unilateral hearing loss. In the present study, BAEP tests were performed on a large number of patients with normal pure tone thresholds and speech discrimination scores who had abnormal findings on their BAEP results. Ten patients had a unilateral abnormal finding of the latency of the Jewett wave V suggestive of an eighth nerve lesion who otherwise had a completely normal retrocochlear evaluation including normal pure tone, speech, and reflex decay testing, normal x-rays of the internal auditory canals, and normal electronystagmography.

The series reported by Selters and Brackmann[3] and Glasscock[8] appear to be patient populations with a fairly strong suspicion for eighth nerve lesions. However, the patient population, seen at the Cleveland Clinic Foundation includes patients with a broad spectrum of disorders who are undergoing BAEP testing for reasons other than unilateral hearing loss. Consequently, we are encountering a greater number of unexplained abnormal BAEP findings.

In the series of confirmed acoustic tumor patients, nearly 50% had BAEP results which were not a significant factor in arriving at the diagnosis. A possible explanation of this is that the series of tumor patients is heavily weighted for large tumor patients, ie, more than 50% had tumors larger than 2 cm when the patient presented. In many of the patients, the hearing was sufficiently poor to make the BAEP test not of value; however, results were similar to those described by Selters and Brackmann[3] in the large tumor series. In an earlier study, the authors reported on 13 patients with abnormal BAEP results contralateral to the side involved. In all of these patients, the tumors were larger than 2 cm, suggesting that the BAEP test may be useful in assessing brainstem compression by a cerebellopontine angle lesion. However, it is important to note that abnormal findings contralateral to the suspected ear may represent the presence of an eighth nerve lesion in the contralateral ear.

SUMMARY

Results of this review of 3 1/2 years' experience using the BAEP test to detect retrocochlear pathology indicate that the technique is useful in the evaluation of patients with suspected brainstem pathology, including patients with multiple sclerosis, sleep apnea, and patients with space-occupying lesions of the brainstem. The test is also useful in the evaluation of patients for whom we could not otherwise obtain reliable behavioral auditory thresholds including patients with pseudohypoacusis.

The accuracy of this test in detecting eighth nerve lesions, specifically the acoustic neuroma, has been somewhat different than previously reported in the literature. The data suggest a fairly high false-positive rate in the neighborhood of 34% in detecting lesions involving the eighth nerve. This may be partially a function of inadequate sample size, but also may be influenced by the differences in patient populations undergoing the BAEP test. No patient in this series with normal BAEP test results was found to have a cerebellopontine angle or eighth nerve tumor. This alone has made the test extremely useful, for if the patient's BAEP test result is normal, we can feel quite comfortable that we have not overlooked an eighth nerve tumor.

In conclusion, BAEP testing is an extremely useful clinical tool in a neurotologic practice; however, its specificity for identifying eighth nerve lesions does not eliminate the need for a complete evaluation including audiologic testing with tympanometry and reflex decay testing, radiographic evaluation of the internal auditory canals, and an evaluation of the vestibular system.

REFERENCES

1. Starr A, Achor LJ. Auditory brainstem responses in neurological disease. Arch Neurol 1975; 32:761-8.

2. Nodar RH, Hahn J, Levine HL. Brainstem auditory evoked potentials in determining site of lesion of brainstem gliomas in children. Laryngoscope 1980; 40:258-65.

3. Selters WA, Brackmann DE. Brainstem electric response audiometry in acoustic tumor detection. In: House WF, Luetje CM, eds. Acoustic tumors: diagnosis. Baltimore: University Park Press, 1979:225-35.

4. Nodar RH, Kinney SE. The contralateral effects of large tumors on brainstem auditory evoked potentials. Laryngoscope (in press).

5. Robinson K, Rudge P. Auditory evoked responses in multiple sclerosis. Lancet 1975; 1:1164-6.

6. Orlowski JP, Nodar RH, Lonsdale D. Abnormal brainstem auditory evoked potentials in infants with threatened sudden infant death syndrome. Cleve Clin Q 1979; 46:77-81.

7. Starr A, Amlie RN, Martin WH, Sanders S. Development of auditory function in newborn infants revealed by auditory brainstem potentials. Pediatrics 1977; 60:831-9.

8. Glasscock ME, Jackson CG, Josey AF, Dickins JRE, Wiet RJ. Brainstem evoked response audiometry in a clinical practice. Laryngoscope 1979; 89:1021-35.

≈

NINCDS NOTES*

NEW PROGRAM DIRECTOR NAMED FOR COMMUNICATIVE DISORDERS

Dr. Ralph F. Naunton has been named director of the Communicative Disorders Program, National Institute of Neurological and Communicative Disorders and Stroke. In this post he will oversee a $28 million program of extramural grants and contracts to support research on speech, language, and hearing disorders, their medical and surgical treatment, and approaches to rehabilitation. Dr. Naunton received B.S. and M.B. degrees in 1945 from the University of London and served his residency in ear, nose, and throat medicine and surgery at University College Hospital, London. He is certified by the American Board of Ophthalmology and Otolaryngology and has a similar certification in audiology from the American Speech and Hearing Association.

*This column is prepared monthly by the Office of Scientific and Health Reports, National Institute of Neurological and Communicative Disorders and Stroke. For further information, write or call Carolyn Holstein, NINCDS/OSHR, NIH Bldg. 31, Room 8A-16, Bethesda, MD 20014. (301) 496-5751.

Ann Otol 89:1980

ACOUSTIC REFLEX LATENCY TEST IN THE EVALUATION OF NONTUMOR PATIENTS WITH ABNORMAL BRAINSTEM LATENCIES

JACK D. CLEMIS, MD CYNTHIA N. SARNO, MA

CHICAGO, ILLINOIS

The acoustic reflex latency test (ARLT), an indirect measure of neural conduction time utilizing the electroimpedance method, was used to evaluate 43 highly suspect, nontumor patients who demonstrated abnormal latency results on brainstem electric response audiometry (BERA), false-positive for tumor. Normative values and criteria for tumor-positive ARLT results were established on a control group using a second generation test unit, comprised of dual impedance bridges and a digital signal averager, designed especially to perform the ARLT. When cut-off criteria for both absolute reflex latency and interaural latency difference (ILD) values were applied to this BERA false positive population, the ARLT correctly identified 93% of patients as having end-organ lesions. Differences in ARLT and BERA test results are attributed to differences in 1) method of measurement, 2) characteristics of the eliciting signal, and 3) generation of the response. These factors are discussed as sources of variability. Both ARLT and BERA are recommended as tandem procedures when screening for acoustic or angle tumors.

INTRODUCTION

The otologic focus on acoustic tumors initiated by William House in the early 1960s has resulted in the evolution of an armamentarium of diagnostic tools, so finely developed that it is now possible to identify tumors as small as a few millimeters in size. While most techniques are noninvasive, certain radiographic studies remain invasive with some degree of associated risk. Definitive presurgical diagnosis is still radiographic. It is, therefore, important to temper radiographic referrals with a careful neurotologic evaluation including high quality, highly efficient screening techniques. Two of the newer techniques that seem to satisfy these requirements include brainstem electric response audiometry (BERA) and acoustic reflex latency test (ARLT).[1]

Over the past decade, the auditory brainstem response has evolved to become an important clinical diagnostic technique for tumor diagnosis. The high true-positive and low false-negative rate of BERA in patients with surgically confirmed neuromas has been well documented and makes it the most effective audiometric test for tumor diagnosis to date. BERA indicators of retrocochlear disease include the abnormal test findings of: 1) increased wave V latency, 2) increased wave I-V or III-V interval, 3) increased wave V interaural latency difference (ILD), 4) absent wave V in the presence of auditory sensitivity of 70 dB HL or better, and 5) a significant discrepancy between behavioral and wave V thresholds when pseudohypoacusis has been ruled out. In the patient with a lesion affecting the eighth nerve or lower brainstem, it is likely one or more of these abnormal indicators will be present, when thresholds permit. An apparent disadvantage of BERA is a reportedly high false-positive rate which ranges from a conservative 12%[2] to less optimistic estimates of 22%[3] and 30%.[4,5] In nontumor cases, the finding of an abnormal delay in brainstem response latency (false-positive for tumor) is felt to be due to audiometric configuration, particularly in cases of precipitous, severe, high frequency hearing loss.[2,3,6,7]

More recently, the ARLT has been applied to tumor diagnosis.[1] It provides an indirect measure of seventh and eighth nerve function based on changes in the acoustic impedance of the middle ear. Nerve tracts and nuclei in the afferent portion of this polysynaptic reflex arc coincide with some of the proposed generator sites of the brainstem response (Fig. 1). These include the eighth nerve, the cochlear nucleus, and the superior olivary complex. At this point, similarities in pathways end. The acoustic reflex arc decussates to send contralateral fiber tracts across the brainstem, then both the ipsilateral and contralateral tracts continue their descent to the facial nerve nuclei. The efferent pathway includes the facial nerve and the nerve to stapedius. The end result is the closing of an auditory feedback loop completed by bilateral contraction of the middle ear muscles.

Acoustic reflex latency, defined as the time interval between the onset of the stimulus and the onset of the middle ear muscle contraction, appears to be of more diagnostic value for tumor detection than other reflex parameters including reflex decay and elevated reflex threshold.[8,9] Latency of the acoustic reflex has been shown to be a sensitive test of tumor

From the Department of Otolaryngology and Maxillofacial Surgery, Northwestern University Medical School, and the American Hearing Research Foundation, Chicago, Illinois. Supported in part by the American Hearing Research Foundation, Kiwanis International Foundation, and Mercy Hospital and Medical Center, Chicago, Illinois.

Presented at the meeting of the American Otological Society, Inc., Palm Beach, Florida, April 13-14, 1980.

REPRINTS — Jack D. Clemis, MD, American Hearing Research Foundation, 55 East Washington Street, Chicago, IL 60602.

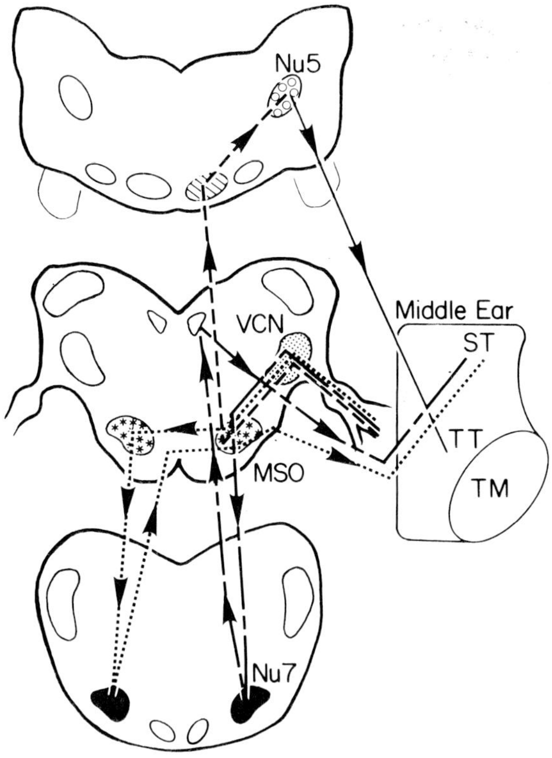

Fig. 1. Schematic drawing of the brainstem pathways for the middle ear muscle reflex. Both ipsilateral and contralateral stapedius pathways are shown. ST - Stapedius muscle; TT - Tensor tympani muscle; TM - Tympanic membrane; VCN - Ventral cochlear nucleus; MSO -Medial superior olive; Nu7 - Facial nerve motor nucleus; Nu5 - Trigeminal motor nucleus. (Adapted from Borg E. On the neuronal organization of the acoustic middle ear reflex. A physiological and anatomical study. Brain Res 1973; 49:101-23.)

detection based on: 1) the investigations of the effect of simulated acoustic tumor in animals;[8] 2) the finding of normal latencies in a normal control group;[1] 3) the finding of abnormal latency in a group of patients with surgically confirmed acoustic tumor;[1,9] and 4) the finding of normal latency in a nontumor group of patients with sensorineural hearing loss of variable etiology.[1] The ARLT is considered abnormal when the absolute latency and/or the ILD values exceed the cut-off criteria for contralateral and/or ipsilateral measurements at 1,000 and/or 2,000 Hz.

The goal of this study is to compare and contrast BERA and ARLT as applied to acoustic and angle tumor diagnosis and to try to assess more objectively the current role of ARLT in tumor diagnosis. With this goal in mind, an investigation was undertaken to determine if those nontumor patients who had manifested abnormal BERA results (false-positive for tumor) could be correctly identified as nontumor by the ARLT.

METHODS

Subjects. The study included two groups: 1) a control group of 25 volunteers with normal auditory sensitivity, normal tympanograms and no past otologic complaints, and 2) a special experimental population consisting of 43 acoustic tumor-suspect patients who exhibited abnormal findings on BERA (tumor-positive in accordance with the Selters and Brackmann criteria[2]) and in whom acoustic or angle tumors were ultimately ruled out. Symptoms characterizing this population include 1) hearing loss (asymmetric, progressive, fluctuant or sudden), 2) disequilibrium, dizziness or vertigo, 3) tinnitus, and 4) fullness or pressure in the ear (most frequently in combination). Audiometric signs include: 1) asymmetric sensorineural hearing loss, 2) disproportionate reduction in speech discrimination score, 3) abnormal tone decay, 4) acoustic reflex decay or elevation in reflex threshold, 5) abnormal BERA findings. Many or most of these findings were in combination. Vestibular function tests were restricted to caloric studies and usually demonstrated a reduced vestibular response (RVR) in the involved ear. The BERA test results were labeled false-positive for tumor subsequent to definitive x-ray examination including polytomography, computerized axial tomography (CAT) scan and/or posterior fossa myelography.

Apparatus. Two standard electroacoustic impedance bridges (Amplaid 702) were modified to perform either individual or simultaneous tympanograms and acoustic reflex measurements. Switching arrangements permitted the units to function either in the standard or in the modified mode. The stimulus tone initially generated by the dual tympanometers was routed to an output jack on the front panel of each unit. The stimulus tone was gaited by means of an electronic switch (Coulbourn model S84-04) which was in turn controlled by two one-shot timers (Coulbourn model S52-53), thereby relinquishing all internal signal timing control. The output of the electronic switch was then split and returned to an input jack on the front panel of each electroacoustic impedance bridge. The shared acoustic signal was amplified and attenuated by the standard intensity control on each unit. Use of these controls limited attenuation to 5 dB increments. All probe and stimulus levels were matched within better than ± 1 dB by standard calibration procedures. Level and frequency were calibrated according to the manufacturer's specifications for the Amplaid units.

Two separate output modes from each meter were employed. To perform routine tympanograms, the output of each system was routed through calibration potentiometers into a standard X-Y plotter (Hewlett-Packard model 7010B). To perform acoustic reflex measurements, the "scope" output from each meter was fed to separate input channels of a dual-channel signal averager (Tracor-Northern model 570A). Output of the signal averager was connected to the plotter to obtain permanent record of the reflex response. Daily calibration and monitoring of the reflex-eliciting stimulus was facilitated by means of a separate oscilloscope mounted above the equipment rack (Tektronix T912). A standard head band was modified to accommodate two probe-tip assemblies, each presenting a 220 Hz probe tone. This arrangement permitted stimuli for both ipsilateral and contralateral measurements to be presented through like transducers as opposed to the standard earphone versus probe-tip method of measurement.

Procedures. All control subjects were required to pass a screening procedure performed on this apparatus to confirm normal hearing sensitivity for the ARLT test stimulus. A 300 msec tone with 5 msec rise/fall times was presented through the probe-assembly speaker at 20 dB HL for the test frequencies 500 to 4,000 Hz. In the experimental group, audiometric thresholds were established with standard clinical procedures for the frequency range 250 to 8,000 Hz (reference ANSI, 1969). Only those subjects with no air-bone gap, ie, pure sensorineural losses, were included in order to eliminate latency delay caused by a conductive component. In both groups, ipsilateral and contalateral acoustic reflex thresholds were established for the test signal at frequencies of 2,000 and 1,000 Hz. Reflex threshold was taken as a time-locked needle deflection in response to the eliciting signal as seen on the balance meter. In cases where a deflection was in question, the reflex threshold was taken as the first change from baseline impedance in a positive direction as seen on the oscilloscope of the signal averager.

To perform the ARLT, ipsilateral and contralateral test stimuli were presented at 10 dB above the established reflex threshold. Each measurement represented the averaged response from four signal presentations. An interstimulus interval of 5 seconds was used to minimize any reflex adaptation effects. Reflex latency was calculated by use of the address select cursor and the count digital display of the signal averager. In this manner, an increase from baseline impedance could be detected to within 1 msec. Reflex responses were written out on the X-Y plotter for permanent record. The entire test procedure takes approximately one-half hour per patient.

RESULTS

Control Group. It was first necessary to reestablish normal values utilizing the second generation test equipment. Acoustic reflex latency measurements were analyzed for a) frequency effects (1,000 and 2,000 Hz) and b) ear effects (ipsilateral and contralateral). To determine the effect of stimulus frequency, independent *t*-tests were performed on measurements of like ears at each frequency, ie, ipsilateral 1,000 Hz/ipsilateral 2,000 Hz, contralateral 1,000 Hz/contralateral 2,000 Hz. Results revealed no significant difference at the 0.1 level. To determine ear effects, *t*-tests were performed between measurements of like frequencies/different ear, ie, ipsilateral 1,000 Hz/contralateral 1,000 Hz, etc. Results revealed no significant difference at the 0.05 level. Based on these findings, data were collapsed to compute a mean absolute latency for the control group. Averaging all four measurements resulted in a mean absolute latency of 95 msec, with a standard deviation of 24.5 msec. This value is in excellent agreement with the mean latency values for the normal group reported in our previous investigation.[1] However, the frequency effect found in our earlier study did not occur in the present investigation. This may have been due to the difference in transducers utilized in the former (earphone) and the present (probe-assembly) study for delivery of the contralateral stimulus.

A mean ILD was then computed utilizing differences between like measurements for all four conditions. This resulted in a mean ILD of 14.7 msec with a standard deviation of 10.4 msec.

The criteria for abnormal latency for both absolute and ILD measures were derived from the mean latency plus two standard deviations. The resultant cut-off values were 144 and 36 msec respectively. These values are in good agreement with the 2,000 Hz absolute latency and the average of the 1,000 and 2,000 Hz ILD values reported in the previous study.[1] The difference in normal cut-off values, mean latency plus two standard deviations, between studies represents patient variability only, as reflected in the standard deviation. Mean latency values are constant. It is felt that when large numbers of patients have been tested with the ARLT, the standard deviation will stabilize resulting in uniform cut-off criteria. Until this occurs, caution should be exercised in application of any one cut-off value.

Experimental Group. To determine any significant difference in absolute latencies between the control and the experimental group, a *t*-test was administered for all conditions between populations. Results revealed no significant difference at the 0.1 level. These results are comparable to those of the heterogeneous group of patients from our earlier study with sensorineural hearing loss of variable etiology in which tumor had been ruled out. The above criteria established from the control group were applied to the absolute latency and ILD measurements in the experimental group. No response could be obtained from 13 of 43 (30%) patients in this group. In those patients with reliable latencies, 28 or 93% fell within normal limits (WNL) at both test frequencies and two patients fell outside normal limits (ONL). In these two cases, one patient was delayed beyond the absolute cut-off value by 4 msec but had a normal ILD; the second patient was both delayed beyond the absolute cut-off value by 52 msec and had an abnormal ILD.

The ILD criterion derived from the control group was applied to the experimental group. In 15 of 43 (35%) patients, no ILD could be obtained. Of the 28 patients with bilateral measurements, 25 (89%) had an ILD WNL at both test frequencies, and 3 had an ILD outside the normal range. In two of these three patients, the absolute latencies were WNL at both frequencies. In the patient with the greatest ILD, absolute latency at 1,000 Hz fell WNL but fell ONL at 2,000 Hz.

DISCUSSION

An examination of our data reveals two outstanding characteristics that differentiate BERA from ARLT response in this nontumor group: 1) a wave V latency delay and abnormal ILD in the presence of elevated high frequency thresholds, and 2) "recruiting-like" latency/intensity function. If the brainstem response is influenced by audiometric configuration, why is the acoustic reflex latency not similarly influenced, and does a similar recruiting-like phenomenon play a role in the ARLT results? To answer these questions, the following discussion compares 1) the method of measurement of ARLT and BERA and the effect of high frequency loss on each method, and 2) the recruiting-type latency/intensity function seen in patients with end-organ disease.

Method of Measurement. The ARLT, utilizing the electroacoustic impedance method, is an indirect measurement totally dependent on the movement of the tympanic membrane in response to the contraction of the stapedius muscle. The magnitude

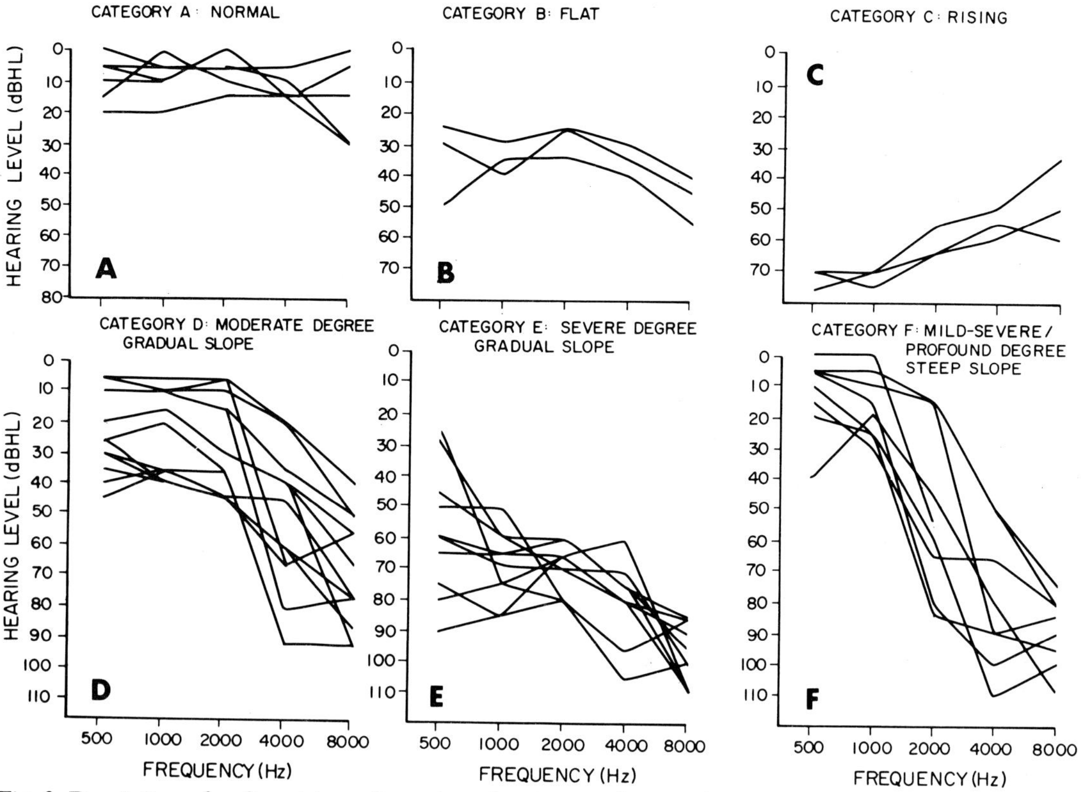

Fig. 2. Descriptions of audiometric configurations of patients in the special experimental group demonstrating abnormal BERA results. A) Normal - Hearing thresholds 0 to 30 dB HL from 500 to 8,000 Hz. B) Flat - 1,000 and 4,000 Hz threshold within 5 dB of one another. No precipitous drop in 8,000 Hz threshold. C) Rising - 4,000 or 8,000 Hz threshold 20 dB or more poorer than 1,000 Hz threshold. D) Moderate degree: Gradual slope - 2,000 Hz threshold less than 50 dB HL; 8,000 Hz threshold greater than 50 dB HL. E) Severe degree: Gradual slope - 1,000 Hz threshold greater than 30 dB HL, 2,000 Hz and 4,000 Hz thresholds greater than 50 dB HL. F) Mild-Severe/Profound degree: Steep slope - 1,000 Hz threshold less than 50 dB HL, 4,000 Hz threshold greater than 50 dB HL.

of static acoustic impedance at the eardrum and the cochlear microphonic (CM) sensitivity curve are almost identical in the frequency range between 400 and 4,000 Hz.[10] At the round window CM is proportional to pressure at the oval window and input admittance is the valid measure of the output of the middle ear up to 4,000 Hz. Above 4,000 Hz, changes in the acoustic impedance and CM sensitivity become disproportionate, with as much as a 15 dB lag in acoustic impedance values by 8,000 Hz. This "deviation from proportionality" is felt to be due to mechanical properties of the middle ear system. Therefore, the ARLT, utilizing the electroacoustic impedance method, is an accurate indicator of cochlear response only in a limited frequency range up to 4,000 Hz. The acoustic reflex is a low frequency feedback loop with an afferent and efferent limb. Afferent excitation is maximal below 2,000 Hz, resulting in a stapedius contraction which is not vigorous and most stable when elicited by stimuli in this range.[11] The resultant effect of the reflex is on suprathreshold sound transmission to the cochlea in the same frequency range. Test signals for ARLT are in the low to midfrequency range, 1,000 and 2,000 Hz.

In the normal ear or the ear with a flat audiometric configuration, ARLT and BERA responses originate from different frequency regions within the cochlea. The brainstem response is felt to come from more basal portions of the cochlea and the best information is obtained with a click. Most of the explanations for BERA false-positive responses hinge around loss of acuity in the high frequency region. Some investigators claim a linear relationship between the wave V latency and the 8,000 Hz threshold.[3] In the case of high frequency hearing loss, the hair cells in the basal portion of the cochlea may be damaged or absent.[7] Under these conditions neural firing will not be initiated until intact receptor cells in a more apical portion along the basilar membrane have been stimulated resulting in a "cochlear delay" in latency. This theory has been used to explain the cochlear delay which clinically manifests as a false-positive for tumor. However, high frequency hearing loss and the cochlear delay theory cannot explain all BERA false-positive results (Fig. 2 A-F). To illustrate this point, pure tone configurations of the patients with BERA false-positive results are classified by slope and degree of loss and displayed on these composite audiograms. It may be seen that not all patients display a precipitous, high frequency loss. In cases of high frequency loss, the actual region of excitation in the cochlea from which the ARLT and BERA responses are now generated may be quite similar. To com-

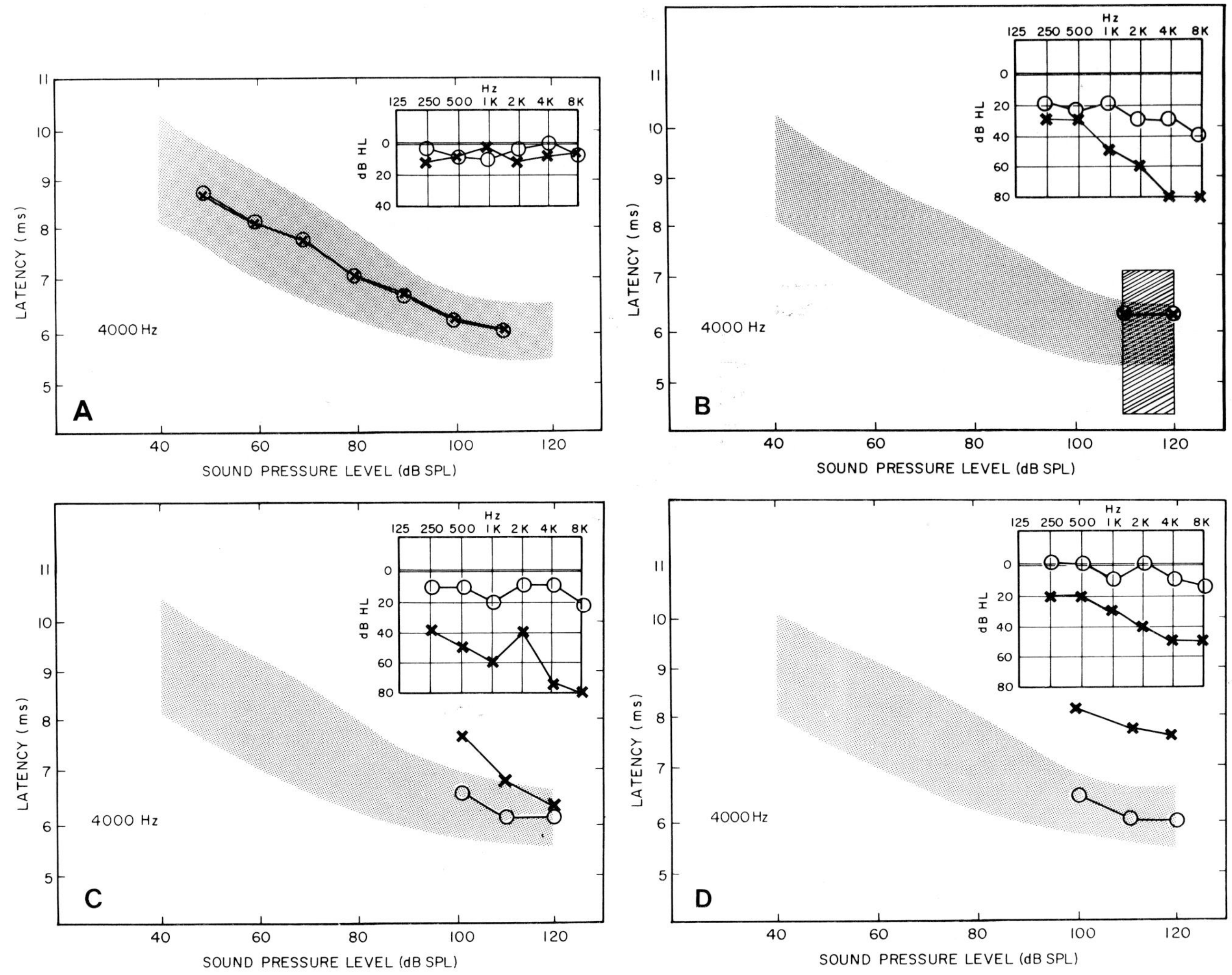

Fig. 3. A) Normal latency/intensity function. Wave V latencies elicited with a 2 msec, 4,000 Hz tone burst, plotted on a template derived from the normative group mean and 2 standard deviations. B) Normal latency/intensity function in ear with sensory hearing loss. Both wave V latencies and ILD are equal and within normal limits bilaterally. Hatched area indicated limited response range due to hearing loss. C) "Recruiting-like" latency/intensity function in ear with Menière's disease. Wave V latencies are delayed at lower intensity levels but "recruit" to normal limits at 120 dB SPL. D) "Nonrecruiting-like" latency/intensity function in ear with acoustic neuroma. Wave V latencies fail to "recruit" to normal limits and remain delayed even at most intense stimulus levels.

pensate for cochlear delay, a correction factor based on the 4,000 Hz audiometric threshold has been derived and utilized by Selters and Brackmann as a compromise value in an effort to reduce the false-positive rate without increasing the false-negative rate.[2] It has been pointed out, however, that such a correction factor should depend on the validity of the generator sites and not on the integrity of the peripheral end-organ.[6] The audiometric threshold is a direct manifestation of cochlear function. Conversely, wave V in a composite response involving multiple generator sites, possibly even at the cortical level.[12] To correct for one in order to interpret the other is incorrect. Up to this point in time, however, this compromise has been a worthwhile, working manipulation of the cut-off criteria.

Recruiting-Type Latency/Intensity Function. The Menière's group accounted for 46% of the abnormal ILD measures and 52% of the abnormal wave V latencies in an investigation of abnormal BERA results in nontumor patients (false-positive for tumor). In a study of Menière's patients tested with ARLT,[1] the false-positive rate was shown to be as low as 4.6% using absolute latency and 0% using the ILD. On the ARLT, abnormal growth of reflex amplitude, a likely correlate of abnormal loudness growth, was observed to coincide with significantly shorter reflex latencies in this group of Menière's patients. These findings suggest the presence of a recruiting-type latency/intensity function with ARLT; not an unlikely suggestion in view of the theory that the acoustic reflex is loudness governed. Latency is inversely proportional to stimulus intensity. Figure 3A represents the normal latency/intensity function curve plotted an a template derived from our normative data for BERA latency values. In the recruiting ear, the inverse relationship is maintained, but the slope of the function is steeper (Fig. 3C). At lower intensity levels, the wave V latencies in the damaged ear are delayed beyond those of the good ear, often falling outside the normal range. As the level of the stimulus is increased, the latency rapidly decreases or "recruits" to latencies within the normal range. The appearance of this recruiting-type latency/intensity function almost always signifies cochlear lesion, but not all cochlear lesions demonstrate this pattern (Fig. 3B). It is most consistent in Menière's patients.

Recruitment, defined behaviorally as an abnormally rapid growth in loudness, is commonly seen in ears with end-organ lesions. In electrocochleography, a physiological correlate of loudness recruitment has been proposed based on the dependency of the compound action potential (AP) waveform, amplitude, and latency on the signal intensity.[13] In subjects with Menière's disease, AP latencies were shorter than those of the normal ears for a given hearing level. It was concluded that the latency criterion with the presence of recruitment is actually a threshold criterion in the ear with cochlear lesion.

This recruiting-type function has yet to be seen in ears with acoustic neuroma (Fig. 3D). In these ears, increases in stimulus level fail to result in abnormally rapid decreases in latency. The latency/intensity curve characterizing both conductive and retrocochlear lesions is elevated well beyond the normal range, usually remaining parallel to the slope of the normal latency/intensity curve.

Some of the patients who did not show the recruiting-type latency/intensity function on BERA did demonstrate recruitment-like reflex patterns on ARLT. This may be due to differences in the level of the test stimulus and its relationship to the recruitment phenomenon.

A 300 msec signal has been specifically selected as the ARLT stimulus because its perceptible intensity is equivalent to that of a continuous tone. The maximum signal output available from our equipment, as in most standard acoustic impedance bridges, is in the order of 120 dB HL.

A common signal utilized in BERA is a click. The instantaneous rise/fall results in the synchronous neural excitation required to elicit the brainstem response. In this present study, a 2 msec tone burst was used as a test signal. Due to the brief signal duration and the effect of temporal integration, the maximum available output of the BERA stimulus is only in the order of 95 to 100 dB HL. Therefore, a difference in the ARLT and BERA signal duration results in a 20 to 30 dB difference in available stimulus intensity.

A minimum of three points at consecutive intensity levels is needed to obtain a valid BERA latency/intensity function. However, the response range for BERA is often limited on the lower end by the patient's elevated hearing threshold and on the upper end by the maximum available sound pressure level. It seems likely that those nontumor patients who had normal results on ARLT and who did not exhibit recruitment on BERA might have recruited if hearing loss did not prevent deriving an adequate latency/intensity function or higher signal intensity level was available to reach a point at which recruitment occurs.

CONCLUSIONS

The ARLT and BERA are both objective, indirect measures of neural conduction time. Gross similarities appear to exist in the neuronal organization of the initial segments of the pathways generating the acoustic reflex and the brainstem response. However, beyond a certain critical point, possibly at the level of the superior olive, pathways become disparate. The difference in ARLT and BERA test results seen in this population of nontumor patients (BERA false-positives) is felt to be due to differences in 1) the method of measurement, 2) the characteristics of the eliciting signal which deal mainly with cochlear mechanics, and 3) the generation of the response, which encompasses the above-mentioned disparity in neural pathways.

Due to the high efficiency rate of both ARLT and BERA as screening tests in tumor diagnosis, we recommend both tests be used in tandem. The ARLT is less expensive and less complicated than BERA and has been shown to correctly identify most (93%) nontumor patients with tumor-positive BERA results. For these reasons, in those patients whose hearing loss does not preclude ARLT, we suggest that ARLT precede BERA. While we consider ARLT to be a useful clinical tool, we feel wider clinical investigation of this test is required.

When screening for acoustic or angle tumor with BERA and an abnormal latency is identified, a latency/intensity function should then be plotted to determine the presence of a recruiting-type pattern. The presence of this pattern generally indicates end-organ dysfunction.

ACKNOWLEDGMENT — The authors wish to thank Therese McGee, PhD, for her contribution to this paper, and William Ballad, MA, for his assistance in designing and constructing the equipment used in this project.

REFERENCES

1. Clemis JD, Sarno CN. The acoustic reflex latency test: clinical application. Laryngoscope (in press).

2. Selters WA, Brackmann DE. Acoustic tumor detection with brainstem electric response audiometry. Arch Otolaryngol 1977; 103:181-7.

3. Coats AC, Martin JL. Human auditory nerve action po-

tentials and brainstem evoked responses. Arch Otolaryngol 1977; 103:605-22.

4. Clemis JD, Mitchell C. Electrocochleography and brainstem responses used in the diagnosis of acoustic tumors. J Otolaryngol 1977; 6:447-59.

5. Clemis JD, McGee T. Brainstem electric response audiometry in the differential diagnosis of acoustic tumors. Laryngoscope 1979; 89:1-12.

6. Eggermont JJ, Don M, Brackmann DE. Electrocochleography and brainsten electric responses in patients with pontine angle tumors. Ann Otol Rhinol Laryngol (in press).

7. McGee TJ, Clemis JD. Audiogram derivation with brainstem electric response. Presented at the Sixth Symposium of the International ERA Study Group, Santa Barbara, California, 1979.

8. Mangham CA, Miller JM. A case for further quantification of the stapedius reflex. Arch Otolaryngol 1979; 105:593-6.

9. Mangham CA, Lindeman RC, Dawson WR. Stapedius reflex quantification in acoustic tumor patients. Presented at the Western Section Meeting of the Triological Society, Scottsdale, Arizona, January 1979.

10. Møller AR. An experimental study of the acoustic impedance of the middle ear and its transmission properties. Acta Otolaryngol (Stockh) 1965; 60:129-49.

11. Anderson SD. Intratympanic muscles. In: Hinchcliffe R, Harrison D, eds. Scientific foundations of otolaryngology. Chicago: William Heineman, 1976:257-80.

12. Kiang NYS. Foundation for clinical interpretations of auditory "brainstem" recordings. Presented at the Annual Meeting of the American Speech-Language-Hearing Association, Atlanta, November 1979.

13. Eggermont JJ. Electrocochleography and recruitment. Ann Otol Rhinol Laryngol 1977; 86:138-49.

≈

XVII CONGRESS OF PAN AMERICAN ASSOCIATION OF OTOLARYNGOLOGY AND BRONCHOESOPHAGOLOGY

The XVII Congress of the Pan American Association of Otolaryngology and Bronchoesophagology will take place in Santiago, Chile December 7-10, 1980. For further information contact: General Secretary Dr. Jorge Otte, Avenida Vitacura 2653, Santiago, Chile.

PLASTICITY OF THE DEVELOPING AUDITORY SYSTEM

R. J. RUBEN, MD ISABELLE RAPIN, MD
NEW YORK, NEW YORK

Anatomical, physiological and behavioral data indicate that the auditory system matures from the periphery centrally, ie, centripetally. There is now information which shows that the developing auditory system can be modified by anatomical changes which have their greatest effect during early development. Anatomical, physiological and behavioral changes can also be brought about by the quality of the auditory stimuli which the auditory system experiences. Evidence for the plasticity of the developing auditory system has come from studies of a number of different species. The plasticity of the auditory system is of theoretical and clinical significance.

INTRODUCTION

The developing auditory system, like the visual system, is able to be modified by anatomical alteration and variations of acoustic stimuli. This biological characteristic is called plasticity. Audition is dependent on the development of a normal anatomic transformer (middle ear) and transducer (inner ear); a central nervous system and its auditory afferent and efferent connections; and, in birds and mammals, exposure to appropriate auditory stimuli which is an essential component of the normal development of audition. Failure either in the formation of any structural part or in the exposure to sound stimuli will result in deviant auditory function. There are at least three types of developmental errors of exposure to sound which can result in abnormal audition: in the quality, the quantity, and the timing of the sound stimuli to which the developing organism is exposed.

This paper will summarize the known anatomical, physiological and biological aspects of the development of audition. Anatomical, physiological and behavioral evidence for the plasticity of the auditory system will be presented. The consequences of intervention in terms of hearing loss become apparent.

ANATOMIC DEVELOPMENT

The basic histological outline of the anatomic development of the ear has been known since the last half of the 19th century.[1,2] More recently Bast and Anson,[3] Bredberg[4] and Sher[5] have refined these original observations. The general outline of the development of the mammalian cochlea is the initial formation of an otic placode on the dorsolateral anterior aspect of the head region of the embryo. The placode invaginates to form an otic cup and this process continues until an otic cyst is formed. Studies by Li et al[6] have shown in the mouse that the cells of the otocyst that have formed the ventral portion will become the cochlea. The otocyst then begins to take on the shape of the mature labyrinth and in man is anatomically mature at approximately the fifth or sixth month of fetal life.

The epithelium of the cochlea, the organ of Corti, consists of a number of different cell types, some of which are primary receptor cells, the hair cells, and others which are supporting cells, eg, Hensen's cells and Deiters' cells. These cells have been found to be end state cells[7] in that in the mature animal there is no increase or replacement of these cells. In the mouse these cells undergo their terminal mitosis during the 13th and 14th day of gestation. There are no comparable data for man but, while extrapolation from mouse to man is imperfect, it can be surmised that the cells which comprise the organ of Corti in man probably undergo their terminal mitosis by the end of the second month of fetal life. Thus the receptor cells which serve to transduce sound are laid down early in fetal life and must serve the organism until death. Any loss of these cells, either during fetal life or postpartum, will result in a loss of hearing.

The histological differentiation of these cells occurs at various time periods after they have undergone their terminal mitosis. The pattern of differentiation appears to start near the base of the cochlea and spreads apically with the cells of the apex differentiating last. The inner hair cells differentiate before the outer hair cells.

The patterns of development of innervation of the inner and outer hair cells in the kitten[8] reveal that initially the inner hair cells are innervated by both afferents and efferents with very little afferent innervation of the outer hair cells. As the kitten matured there was an increase in afferent and efferent innervation of the outer hair cells with a decreased efferent innervation of the inner hair

From the Departments of Otolaryngology and Neurology, Albert Einstein College of Medicine of Yeshiva University, and Montefiore Hospital and Medical Center, New York, New York. This work is supported by NIH grants No. 5R01NSOA365-12CMS and No. GM-19100, Deafness Research Foundation, National Foundation — March of Dimes No. 1372 and No.6-234, C.H.E.A.R. and the Manheimer Fund.

Presented at the meeting of the American Otological Society, Inc., Palm Beach, Florida, April 13-14, 1980.

REPRINTS — R. J. Ruben, MD, Albert Einstein College of Medicine, 1300 Morris Park Avenue, Bronx, NY 10461.

cells. The process of innervation of the inner hair cells coincides in time with the first physiological and behavioral responses to sound.[9]

The mechanisms which control the process of differentiation from the otic placode to the mature cochlea are now being defined.[10] It would appear that in the mouse the neural tube and the cephalic mesenchyme are essential for the development of the early otocyst. The neural tube is needed first and is gradually supplanted by the action of the cephalic and then the periotic mesenchyme. Deol, who has studied a number of mutant mice, demonstrated that abnormalities of the developing neural tube will result in abnormalities of the structure of the inner ear.[11] Organ culture studies indicate that an abnormally programmed neural tube can transmit an abnormal message to a normal mouse otocyst. The converse also appears to occur in that a normal neural tube can correct abnormalities in an abnormal otocyst.*

Many questions remain to be answered at the tissue and cellular level concerning the development of the mammalian inner ear. Among those questions pertinent to an understanding of audition are the factors controlling the peripheral innervation of the cochlea. Studies have shown that peripheral innervation is not necessary for the development of the sensory structures of the otocyst and do not appear to be necessary for the maintenance of the sensory structures in the adult.[12,13] The control factors that cause each nerve fiber to connect with specific hair cells and to a specific cell in the cochlear nucleus complex are being studied. Experiments in which one statoacoustic ganglion complex is placed between two growing otocysts have been carried out in our laboratory and our preliminary results show that nerve fibers will grow to both otocysts. There are, as expected, mechanisms which control this neuronal specificity. In what way these patterns of growth occur and how they are regulated are, at the present time, unknown.

It is known that in the cat the pattern of peripheral innervation is not completed until after the advent of physiologic and behavioral evidence of hearing. Whether or not the same is true of central connections is not entirely known. Mlonyeni[14] states that in the mouse the number of differentiated neurons in the ventral part of the cochlear nucleus reaches adult values at the 11th postpartum day, but in the dorsal portion not until the 16th day. Webster and Webster[15] showed that the neurons of the brainstem auditory nuclei achieve adult size of their soma by the 12th postpartum day. There is no information concerning the formation of synapses or the development of dendritic arborization in the central nuclei.

Thus it would appear that the ear in mammals may not be committed to a fixed pattern of peripheral innervation until after it is functional, which leaves the possibility of environmental sound causing a change in the neural pattern of auditory input. It is also known that the primary auditory nuclei of the cochlear nucleus complex in the mouse show evidence of maturation of cell and soma size during the period of postfunctional development. Thus there may also be changes in the pattern of brainstem innervation during environmental exposure to sound.

There are a number of studies that show that there is anatomical plasticity in both the developing and mature auditory central nervous system.[16] The first of these studies was by Levi-Montalcini[17] and was later expanded by Parks.[18] The studies consisted of removing the otocyst of the developing chick unilaterally, allowing the embryo to continue to develop. The central auditory nucleus system of embryologically deafferentated chicks was examined and found to have, on the ablated side, anatomical differences in the primary auditory nuclei. These differences were a decrease in the size of the nuclei and in the number of cells composing the nuclei, alteration in shape of the nuclear mass, and a different position of the primary auditory nuclei within the brainstem. These studies have shown that in the developing chick the auditory afferents exert control over the development of the primary portion of the central auditory nervous system.

Experiments assessing the effects of destruction of the mature cochlea and its afferents show that there is degeneration in both primary and secondary central auditory nuclei.[16] Van den Pol et al[19] stated that in the posthatched chick there is degeneration in secondary and tertiary auditory nuclei after removal of the inner ear. In a series of studies Gulley et al[20] found significant changes in the presynaptic and postsynaptic organelles of the primary (anteroventral cochlear nucleus) brainstem auditory nuclei in the waltzing guinea pig, an autosomal dominant mutant guinea pig in which there is primary hair cell degeneration with a minimal amount of neural degeneration.

Several experiments have been carried out to explore the possibility that degeneration in central auditory nuclei may result from a diminution of auditory stimulation without disruption of the transducer or primary afferents. Coleman and O'Connor[21] removed the middle ear ossicles from rat pups and found a decrease in the size of the spherical cells in the anteroventral cochlear nucleus. The effect was only noted in the monaural preparations and not in animals who had the ossicles removed in both ears (these data are congruent with the physiological data of Clopton and Silverman[22] — see Electrophysiologic Development). Webster and Webster[15,23,24] found that in young mice sound deprivation or occlusion of the

*Van De Water TR. Personal communication.

middle ear resulted in a statistically significant decrease in the size of various cell groups in primary and secondary central auditory nuclei. The Websters also noted that the effect could not be reversed by exposure to auditory stimuli after a period of deprivation.

This information shows that the central and peripheral auditory systems exert reciprocal control over each other. Early in embryonic life the major inducer for the inner ear is the developing rhombencephalon. As the inner ear matures its input is necessary for the developmental organization of at least part of the central auditory nervous system. As the organism develops further, to a state at which the peripheral auditory system is functional, input from this system appears to be necessary for the control of maturation and innervation of portions of the central auditory system. In the mouse and the rat it is apparent that sensory input will affect the anatomical configuration of the auditory central nervous system.

Studies of human material in this area are difficult to do because of many confounding variables. Studies of the brains of patients with deafness are being undertaken but one must be sure that the peripheral lesion occurred before the central lesion as would be the case in postnatally acquired deafness. In other cases, eg, rubella embryopathy or Waardenburg's syndrome, the same teratogen may have effected both sites independently. There are some data[25] that correlate the effects of anencephaly, a massive anomaly of the skull and brain, with abnormal formation of the inner ear. Our own clinical experience indicates that severe central nervous system malformations other than anencephaly may be associated with normal inner ears at least as assessed by x-ray or auditory evoked potential testing. Minor abnormalities of the bony structure of the inner ear have also been found in infants without obvious CNS malformation.

ELECTROPHYSIOLOGIC DEVELOPMENT

The electrophysiological development of the cochlea and the eighth nerve has been studied in a number of mammals including the mouse,[26,27] rat,[28] opossum,[29-31] rabbit,[32] cat,[9,33,34] chick,[35] and gerbil.[36] These studies found that functional development of hair cells, as measured by the cochlear microphonic, appears to start near the base and extend to the remainder of the base and to the apex of the cochlea. There is both an increasing sensitivity and an increase in the range of frequency to which they respond. These physiological changes parallel the anatomical changes in the organ of Corti,[37] although no one specific change in the organ of Corti has been found to be responsible for reactivity of the hair cells. The two DC potentials, the summating potential and the endocochlear potential, have been shown to develop in conjunction with the development of the cochlear microphonic.[32] The ability of the eighth nerve to transmit messages from the cochlea parallels cochlear development.[35]

Pujol[9] has shown that the various auditory centers of the central nervous system, including the cochlear nucleus, inferior colliculus, medial geniculate body, and auditory cortex, have a centripetal pattern of maturation. Studies of the latency of auditory evoked responses indicate that the maturation proceeds from the periphery to the cortex. Pujol[9] also examined other physiological patterns of cell reactivity. He recorded from single units within the cochlear nucleus, inferior colliculus and medial geniculate body in the developing kitten. He found that initially cells in the central auditory nuclei are capable of "on" responses. They then developed rhythmic responses which are followed by the mature pattern of firing throughout stimulation. He also examined the development of inhibitory mechanisms. His tentative conclusion is that they make their appearance first in the inferior colliculus and medial geniculate body. Their onset is relatively late in the maturational process.

Aitken and Moore[38] showed that at first the tuning curves of single units in the pericentral portion of the cochlear nucleus of the kitten are broader than those of cells in its central portion. The threshold of these units drops from 100 dB at the sixth to 11th day of life to near 40 dB in the adult. This marked drop in threshold occurs from the 11th to the 21st postpartum day and tonotopic organization of the central nucleus of the inferior colliculus is observable by the 11th day. The investigators felt that some of these findings could be accounted for by anatomic maturation of the central nervous system. Several observers[39,40] have found that the central nervous system may be capable of processing auditory information before the cochlea matures. These investigations included a series of studies in which developing animals, cats and rats, had their medial geniculate bodies stimulated electrically before there was evidence of hearing based on the ability to record evoked potentials from the eighth nerve. They were able to evoke potentials within the cortex by electrical stimulation of the medial geniculate. The conclusion from these studies is that the central auditory system is capable of transmitting information before the end-organ and eighth nerve are able to transmit it to the central nervous system.

Electrophysiological studies of the development of audition have been carried out[41-44] in both premature and term infants by recording brainstem and cortical auditory evoked potentials. Starr et al[44] found a decrease in latency and an increase in amplitude of brainstem potential with age. The largest shift occurred at 34 weeks gestational age. Waveforms recorded by the brainstem auditory evoked potential technique are felt to represent the evoked responses from the various auditory relays. The first wave was thought to originate from the eighth nerve and the fifth wave from the region of the inferior colliculus. Wave I, purportedly from the eighth nerve, has been observed to mature earlier, at approximately five to seven months depending on the stimulus used[45,46] than wave V, which is more central. It would appear that in man, as well as in the rodent species studied, there is a peripheral-to-central pattern of physiological development. However, Graziani et al[47] and Starr et al[44] also noted that a cortical response could be recorded in infants less than 28 weeks gestational age, at a time when the same sound stimulus did not elicit a recordable brainstem auditory evoked potential.[44] This discrepancy may be a reflection of the small amplitude of waves generated by the brainstem because of poorly synchronized firing or of some other factor in the organization of the developing central auditory nervous system in man.

The maturation of the electrophysiological response in man appears to be dependent upon the anatomical maturation of the inner ear.[4] Keith[48] examined the possibility that the middle ear may be responsible for decreased sensitivity of auditory acuity in newborns. He found that term infants 2½ to 20 hours after birth had normally functioning middle ears when assessed by measures of middle ear compliance, tympanometry and middle ear pressure. The electrophysiologic data suggests that the term infant has anatomically mature middle and inner ears and that the maturation of the remainder of the auditory system takes place over the next 18 months.

Auditory deprivation has been shown in animals to have electrophysiologic consequences both in the periphery and centrally. In two strains of mice with genetically determined progressive inner ear deafness, recordings of the cochlear microphonic and eighth nerve action potential[27,49-51] demonstrated increased sensitivity and narrowing of the frequency range at the level of the inferior colliculus. Batkin et al[52] showed that rats deprived for eight months had a 29 dB increase in threshold when tested by auditory evoked potentials.

The consequences of unilateral auditory deprivation have been studied in the rat.[22,53] There is a decrease in the number of units in the inferior colliculus that respond when the deprived ear is stimulated. The normal inhibition that occurs when sound is presented binaurally does not occur in animals who had sustained unilateral deprivation. This effect was not present when the deprivation had been binaural. Deprivation had to occur between the 10th and 60th day after birth in order to produce these effects; there was no effect if deprivation occurred later than the 60th postpartum day.

The pattern of sound stimulation experienced by young rats during the first four months of life was found to influence the pattern of response at the collicular level.[28] The firing rate of single units in the inferior colliculus increased selectively when stimulated with a familiar sound pattern compared to their firing rate with a novel sound pattern. This evidence indicates that in the rat the responsiveness of cells at the level of the inferior colliculus can be modified by auditory experience.

The electrophysiological patterns of auditory development have just started to be outlined in various species. As a general principle they appear to mature centripetally, starting from the periphery and occurring last at the cortical level. Thus far, most of the investigators have examined sensitivity and frequency selectivity and only one study has looked at the development of integrative function in the auditory system. The physiological effects of loss of the peripheral system are not well known.

The physiology of the auditory system is modified by environmental sound, judging by the deprivation studies and the one study[28] in which there was modification of the reactivity of units based on their previous pattern of sound exposure. Both the anatomical and physiological studies thus indicate that deprivation appears to be effective in the rodent only during the immediate postpartum period. Whether these findings apply to man is not known, but one would be surprised if the same were not true for man since his central nervous system also continues to develop after birth. Plasticity is likely to play a more important role for the premature than the term infant because of greater immaturity of the central nervous system. The extent to which sound controls the development of the auditory system is unknown except for the changes in sensitivity to loudness and loss of binaural interaction just described and the one experiment showing modification of the sensitivity of single units in response to changes in sound patterns.

BEHAVIORAL DEVELOPMENT

Study of the behavioral correlates of auditory development is limited by the methodologies available to assess this behavior. It is particularly difficult when working with immature organisms, be they birds, rats, mice or children. Many kinds of measurements have been used to attempt to correlate the organism's response to a particular stimulus. Some studies have relied on performed behavioral patterns occurring in response to sound.

The ontogeny of behavioral responses to sound correlate well with the physiologic data.[54-56] Ehret's studies[54,55] in the mouse show that even after physiological and anatomical maturation of the ear and eighth nerve are complete, threshold for pure tones and masked threshold continue to decrease. These findings were attributed to the late maturation of the central auditory system in this species. The data imply that final maturation of audition in the mouse may be dependent upon central mechanisms and that these maturational processes are centripetal. This is in agreement with the known anatomical and physiological information obtained from this and other species.

The development of behavioral responses to sound in man appears to occur as early as the 20th fetal week.[57,58] That the premature infant will respond behaviorally to sound has also been well documented. There is little information concerning the frequency range, loudness and difference limens of the premature infant's responses to sound.

The term infant responds to a variety of auditory stimuli, depending upon his level of arousal, the repetition rate and the character of the stimulus. Threshold for behavioral responses to sound decreases during the first two to three years of life. These changes and other factors must be taken into account before making any statement about an absolute behavioral threshold in the infant.

Ability to discriminate among speech sounds occurs early in the normal human infant. Kuhl[59] states that one to three-month-old infants can discriminate all of the speech sounds which are phonologically relevant in the English language. Skinner[60] has summarized available information concerning infants' perception of speech sounds. At two weeks of age the infant can recognize the overall rhythmic pattern of speech. The ability to discriminate between a statement and a question which used the same words but a different intonational pattern is apparent at eight months of age. Menyuk[61] discussed another aspect of the development of audition. This is the more complex interaction between the perception and mechanisms of speech production, that is between hearing and vocalization. This can be measured by studying the effects of delayed auditory feedback. In the adult, delaying the auditory feedback of an individual's voice will slow the rate of his speech. This effect was reported not to be seen in children at one year, nine months of age. It began at two years, four months of age, and was similar to the adult response at four years of age. This may indicate that the complex operations required for central auditory processing may take a number of years to be fully developed in man.

The nature of environmental sound to which the developing organism is exposed seems to determine, in part, its eventual auditory capabilities. Most of the studies have used various types of sensory deprivation. Gottlieb[62] showed that if a duckling is deprived of its own voice immediately before hatching it will not be able to discriminate its mother's call as would ducklings who were not deprived of the auditory stimulation of their own cries. Further experiments showed that the deficit involves a decrease in the ability to attend to the high frequency component of the maternal call. Exposure to other sounds in the high frequency range compensates in part for the deprivation. The effect persists up to 65 hours after hatching.

Kerr et al[63] plugged the ears of prehatched 18 1/2-day-old chick embryos. This resulted in a 40 dB attenuation of sound which was maintained to the third or fourth day posthatching. It was found that the ability of the deprived chicks to discriminate among auditory stimuli was decreased when compared to normal.

One of the earliest studies on the behavioral effects of auditory deprivation in animals was carried out by Wolf[64] in the rat. He raised rats with either visual or auditory deprivation. Animals deprived of auditory stimulation did better in competing for food when visual cues were used than with auditory cues. Animals raised with visual deprivation did better in food competition tasks when attending to auditory stimuli than to visual stimuli.

Tees[65] noted that rats who underwent auditory deprivation after birth took longer to discriminate between patterns, and discriminations were poorer than in normal rats. He felt that auditory deprivation damaged the development of auditory acuity in these animals. Thus it would appear that in the rat ability to process auditory patterns is dependent to some degree on sensory input.

The effect of auditory trauma producing hearing loss has been investigated in certain strains of mice.[66] It appears that a partial loss of peripheral auditory function during the early postpartum period in these mice increases the responsiveness of the central auditory nervous system since later exposure to noise will result in epileptic seizures. "Disuse supersensitivity" has been hypothesized to account for this effect. Henry and Haythorn[67] studied this problem by comparing mice with a genetic hearing loss to mice with experimentally produced conductive hearing loss. They found that they could induce audiogenic seizures in both groups of animals. This evidence gives further support to the occurrence of disuse supersensitivity during early periods of development. These studies of priming for audiogenic seizures provide evidence of the ability of environmental sound to alter the behavioral responsiveness of the central nervous system.

Studies of the behavioral effects of the acoustic environment in maturing infants have followed several lines of evidence. Perhaps the most obvious was to investigate the behavioral consequences of congenital hearing loss.[68] The effects of severe to profound sensorineural hearing loss on the individual are pleomorphic. Most congenitally deaf individuals exhibit substantial deficits in linguistic skills and are subjected to profound experiential deprivation.[69] They are deficient economically and socially.[70] The well-known difference between the consequences of severe to profound deafness acquired early in life, before the age of two, compared to deafness acquired later in life can be attributed to the better linguistic ability of this latter group.[68,70,71]

The effect in man of auditory deprivation unassociated with loss of end-organ function has also been examined. Perhaps the earliest study was reported by Herodotus.[72] He reports that Pharaoh Psammetichus had two infants raised in total isolation from human speech. The infants were nursed by goats. Their first recorded utterance, at the age of two, was "becos," which Itard[73] conjectures was an imitation of the bleeting of the goat.

There have been other children whom circumstances caused to be raised with little or minimal exposure to speech. The best known are the boy Victor[74] and the girl Genie.[75] There are many confounding variables in both these cases, such as the possibility of mental retardation and the lack of complete history as to when they were isolated from speech. Both children, as far as can be ascertained, could hear normally. The children had no language when they were first brought to professional attention. Victor did not develop speech but was able to communicate, to a modest extent, by gesture. Genie did develop some rudiments of spoken language but, at the time of the report, her language was still grossly immature. These cases underscore that prolonged exposure to spoken language at the critical age is required for normal language acquisition.

There are a large number of infants who, because of otitis media, have undergone a modest amount of auditory deprivation during their first few years of life. Many studies attempted to show that children who had otitis media suffered a cognitive deficit as a direct or indirect consequence of deficient linguistic skills secondary to their auditory deprivation.[76] All of these studies suffer from various difficulties in their design. Some use esoteric groups, eg, Australian aborigines. They may not provide information on the extent or the duration of the hearing loss, include normal controls, or indicate the child's hearing level at the time of testing. Nevertheless, when the entire body of data is considered, there would appear to be a correlation between modest auditory deprivation during the first two years of life and a deficit in linguistically determined cognitive function during later childhood and adolescence. Whether or not these effects are permanent and invariably present is not known.

One of the earliest clinical descriptions of the effects of middle ear effusion is that of a seven-year-old who had middle ear infections up to the age of three.[77] Clinical examination of this boy at age seven, when his hearing was normal, showed him to be behaving like a hearing-impaired child. He had difficulty localizing sound and determining where background sounds came from; words were not discriminated clearly; his fund of general knowledge was impoverished; he could not find words to express his thoughts; he had difficulty with tasks requiring abstraction and conceptualization; he could not understand what was expected of him in social situations and he did not understand other peoples' social behavior. There was a delay between his being asked a question and his answer, as if he were thinking over the question. How much of these effects were due to the hearing loss before the age of three and what the role of other intrinsic and extrinsic factors was is not known.

Needleman[78] examined the speech and language development between ages three and eight in a small group of children in whom otitis media had been documented before age 18 months and had persisted for at least two years. She found that children who had had otitis media did significantly worse in word articulation, articulation of connected speech, and in the use of word endings than normals. While the study group was small and long-term effects were not known, there were clear deficiencies in the children's ability to discriminate some types of speech sounds.

Available studies of the impact of auditory deprivation have shown that there is a correlation between the anatomical and physiological effects of deprivation and its behavioral consequences. Behavioral effects of auditory deprivation, whether partial or total, appear to be significant in the species examined. They impair the ability of the organism to make fine discriminations and, in the case of man, jeopardize the child's linguistic development. The impact of this impairment is not only cognitive, but also social and psychological.

SUMMARY AND CONCLUSIONS

Plasticity of the auditory system is one of the dominant theoretical issues in the development of audition. There is evidence indicating that early in embryonic life the central nervous system plays a major role for the orderly development of the inner ear. The developing inner ear in turn appears to control the anatomical formation of the central auditory nervous system. As the animal matures, auditory stimulation governs the physiological, behavioral and auditory abilities of the organism. The effects of environmental sound in shaping the organism's ability to hear appear to occur before the central auditory nervous system matures. Available information would indicate that the maturation of the auditory system is centripetal, proceeding from the inner ear to the auditory cortex. Environmental sound would appear to have its greatest effect in shaping auditory ability from the time the inner ear and eighth nerve first become functional to the time when maturation of the central nervous system is achieved. Major theoretical questions to be answered are the extent to which environmental sounds are able to shape the developing auditory system, and the long-term effects of various acoustical environments on the organism's auditory ability.

These problems are of importance to the prevention and care of auditory disease. The issue is clearest for the child who is born with a significant hearing loss. All available information suggests that the infant should be placed in as near a normal hearing environment as possible, as early as possible. In most cases this would mandate the use of hearing aids. But even with hearing aids the child's acoustic environment is abnormal. Other interventions must be developed to mitigate these deficits.

Another problem, which affects a population much larger than those with severe to profound hearing loss, is what, if anything, should be done to normalize the auditory environment experienced by the many young infants and children with modest intermittent fluctuating hearing losses due to persistent middle ear effusion. The answer to this question is not as clear as the answer for the severely to profoundly deaf. The evidence in man would indicate that diminution of sound stimulation during maturation of the central nervous system does result in aberrant auditory function. The significance and sequelae of these abnormalities are not known. They are probably dependent not only upon the extent and duration of the auditory impairment, but also on numerous other intrinsic (genetic) and extrinsic (environmental) factors. The answers to these questions are important because there is evidence to suggest that these effects may be significant to the total function of a person, especially in a society which is based, to a large extent, on auditory communication and auditory-based language skills.

REFERENCES

1. Boettcher A. Uber Entwicklung und Bau des Gehorlabyrinths. Dresden: Blockmann, Soba and Schultze, 1869.
2. Retzius MG. Das Gehororgan der Wirbelthiere. 2 vols. Stockholm: Samson and Wallin, 1881 and 1884.
3. Bast TH, Anson BJ. The temporal bone and the ear. Springfield: Charles C. Thomas, 1949.
4. Bredberg G. Cellular pattern of nerve supply of the human organ of Corti. Acta Otolaryngol (Stockh) 1968; Suppl 236.
5. Sher AE. The embryonic and post-natal development of the inner ear of the mouse. Acta Otolaryngol (Stockh) 1971; Suppl 285.
6. Li CW, Van De Water TR, Ruben RJ. The fate mapping of the 11th and 12th day mouse otocyst: an in vitro study of the sites of origin of embryonic inner ear sensory structures. J Morphol 1978; 157:249-68.
7. Ruben RJ. Development of the inner ear of the mouse: a radioautographic study of terminal mitoses. Acta Otolaryngol (Stockh) 1967; Suppl 220.
8. Pujol R, Carlier E, Devigne C. Different patterns of cochlear innervation during the development of the kitten. J Comp Neurol 1978; 177:529-36.
9. Pujol R. Development of toneburst responses along the auditory pathway in the cat. Acta Otolaryngol (Stockh) 1972; 74:383-91.
10. Van De Water TR, Li CW, Ruben RJ, Shea CA. Ontogenic aspects of mammalian inner ear development. In: Gorlin R, Ruben RJ, Schuknecht H, eds. Symposium on the ear. NFMD, Birth Defects: Original Article Series (in press).
11. Deol MS. Deficiencies of the inner ear in the mouse and their origin. Colloques Internationaux C.N.R.S., Mechanisms of the embryogenesis of the organs of vertebrate embryos. 1978; 266:163-77.
12. Van De Water TR. Effects of removal of the statoacoustic ganglion upon the growing otocyst. Ann Otol Rhinol Laryngol 1976; 85 Suppl 33.
13. Ruben RJ, Hudson W, Chiong A. Anatomical and physiological effects of chronic section of the eighth nerve in cat. Acta Otolaryngol (Stockh) 1963; 55:473-84.
14. Mlonyeni M. The late stages of the development of the primary cochlear nuclei in mice. Brain Res 1967; 4:334-44.
15. Webster DB, Webster M. Mouse brainstem auditory nuclei development. Ann Otol Rhinol Laryngol 1980; 89 Suppl 68:254-6.
16. Ruben RJ. A review of transneuronal changes of the auditory central nervous system as a consequence of auditory defects. Internatl J Pediatr Otorhinolaryngol 1980; 1:269-77.
17. Levi-Montalcini R. Development of the acousticovestibular centers of the chick embryo in absence of the afferent root fibers and of descending fiber tracts. J Comp Neurol 1949; 91:209-42.
18. Parks TN. Afferent influences of the development of the brainstem auditory nuclei of the chicken: otocyst ablation. J Comp Neurol 1979; 183:665-77.
19. Van den Pol AN, Kliot M, Kuritzken R. Responses of second and third order auditory neurons to deafferentation. Soc Neurosci Abstr 1979; 5:31.
20. Gulley RL, Wenthold RJ, Neises GR. Changes in synapses of spiral ganglion cells in the rostral anteroventral cochlear nucleus of the waltzing guinea pig following hair cell loss. Brain Res 1978; 158:279-94.
21. Coleman JR, O'Connor P. Effects of monaural and binaural sound deprivation on cell development in the anteroventral cochlear nucleus of rats. Exp Neurol 1979; 64:553-66.
22. Clopton BM, Silverman MS. Plasticity of binaural interaction: II. Critical period and changes in midline response. J Neurophysiol 1977; 40:1275-80.
23. Webster DB, Webster M. Neonatal sound deprivation affects brainstem auditory nuclei. Arch Otolaryngol 1977; 103:392-6.
24. Webster DB, Webster M. Effects of neonatal conductive hearing loss on brain stem auditory nuclei. Ann Otol Rhinol Laryngol 1979; 88:684-8.
25. Marx H. Die Missbildungen des Ohres. In: Henke F, Lubarsch O, eds. Handbuch der Speziellen Pathologischen Anatomie und Histologie Gehororgan. Berlin: Springer, 1925: 609-729.
26. Alford BR, Ruben RJ. Physiological, behavioral and anatomical correlates of the development of hearing in the mouse. Ann Otol Rhinol Laryngol 1963; 72:237-47.
27. Mikaelian D, Ruben R. Development of hearing in the normal CBA/J mouse. Acta Otolaryngol (Stockh) 1965; 59:451-61.
28. Clopton BM, Winfield JA. Effects of early exposure to pat-

tern sound on unit activity in rat inferior colliculus. J Neurophysiol 1976; 39:1081-9.

29. Larsell O, McCrady E Jr, Zimmerman AA. Morphology of functional development of the membraneous labyrinth of the opossum. J Comp Neurol 1935; 63:95-119.

30. McCrady E Jr, Wever EG, Gray CW. Development of hearing in the opossum. J Exp Zool 1937; 75:503-15.

31. McCrady E Jr, Wever EG, Gray CW. Further investigation in the development of hearing in the opossum. J Comp Psychol 1940; 30:17-21.

32. Anggard L. An electrophysiological study in the development of cochlear function in the rabbit. Acta Otolaryngol (Stockh) 1965; Suppl 203:5-66.

33. Brugge JR, Javel E, Kitzes LM. Signs of functional maturation of peripheral auditory system in discharge patterns of neurons in anteroventral cochlear nucleus of kitten. J Neurophysiol 1978; 41:1557-79.

34. Mair IWS, Elverland HH, Laukli E. Development of early auditory evoked responses in the cat. Audiology 1978; 17:469-88.

35. Konishi M. Development of auditory responses in avian embryos. Proc Natl Acad Sci USA 1970; 70:1975.

36. Finck A, Schenck C, Hartman AF. Development of cochlear function in the neonate Mongolian gerbil (Meriones unguiculatus). J Comp Physiol Psychol 1972; 78:375-80.

37. Pujol R, Hilding D. Anatomy and physiology of the onset of auditory function. Acta Otolaryngol (Stockh) 1973; 76:1-10.

38. Aitkin LM, Moore DR. Inferior colliculus: II. Development of tuning characteristics and tonotopic organization in central nucleus of the neonatal cat. J Neurophysiol 1975; 38:1208-16.

39. Hassmannova J, Myslivecek J. Maturation of the primary cortical response to stimulation of the medial geniculate body. Electroencephalogr Clin Neurophysiol 1967; 22:547-55.

40. Marty R, Thomas J. Response electro-corticale a la stimulation de merf cochleaire chez le chat nouveau-ne. J Physiol (Paris) 1963; 55:165-6.

41. Ohlrich G, Barnet A, Weiss I, Shanks T. Auditory evoked potential development in early childhood: a longitudinal study. Electroencephalogr Clin Neurophysiol 1978; 44:411-23.

42. Schulman-Galambos C, Galambos R. Brainstem auditory evoked potentials in the premature infant. J Speech Hear Res 1975; 18:456-65.

43. Schulman-Galambos C, Galambos R. Brainstem evoked response audiometry in newborn hearing screening. Arch Otolaryngol 1979; 105:86-90.

44. Starr A, Amlie RN, Martin WH, Sanders S. Development of auditory function in newborn infants revealed by auditory brainstem potentials. Pediatrics 1977; 60:831-9.

45. Hekox K. Human brainstem evoked potentials: acoustical pathological and developmental dependencies, thesis. University of California, San Diego, 1975.

46. Salamy A, McKean CM, Buda FB. Maturational changes in auditory transmission as reflected in human brainstem potentials. Brain Res 1975; 96:361-6.

47. Graziani LJ, Weitzman ED, Velasco MSA. Neurologic maturation and auditory evoked responses in low birth weight infants. Pediatrics 1968; 41:483-94.

48. Keith RW. Middle ear function in neonates. Arch Otolaryngol 1975; 101:376-9.

49. Henry KR, Kepkowski CM. Evoked potential correlates which note a progressive hearing loss: age related changes from the ear to the inferior colliculus of the C-57BL/6 and CBA/J mice. Acta Otolaryngol (Stockh) 1978; 86:366-74.

50. Mikaelian D, Alford B, Ruben RJ. Cochlear potentials and VIII nerve action potentials in normal and genetically deaf mice. Ann Otol Rhinol Laryngol 1965; 74:146-58.

51. Mikaelian DO, Ruben RJ. Hearing degeneration in the shaker I mouse. Arch Otolaryngol 1964; 84:418-30.

52. Batkin S, Groth H, Watson JR, Ansbery M. Effects of auditory deprivation on the development of the auditory sensitivity in albino rats. Electroencephalogr Clin Neurophysiol 1970; 28:351-9.

53. Silverman MS, Clopton BM. Plasticity of binaural interaction: I. Effect of early auditory deprivation. J Neurophysiol 1977; 40:1266-74.

54. Ehret G. Development of absolute auditory thresholds from the house mouse (Mus musculus). J Am Audiol Soc 1976; 1:179-84.

55. Ehret G. Postnatal development of the acoustical system of the house mouse in light of developing masked thresholds. J Acoustic Soc Am 1977; 62:143-8.

56. Warfield D, Ruben RJ, Mikaelian DO. Behavior measurements of pure tone thresholds in normal CBA/J mice. J Audiol Res 1968; 8:459-68.

57. Eisenbert RB. Auditory competence in early life, roots of communicative behavior. Baltimore: University Park Press, 1976.

58. Northern JL, Downs MP. Hearing in children. Baltimore: Williams and Wilkins Co, 1974.

59. Kuhl PK. Speech perception in early infancy: the acquisition of speech sound categories. In: Hirsch SK, Eldridge DH, Hirsch IJ, Silverman SR, eds. Hearing and Davis: essays honoring Hallowell Davis. St. Louis: Washington University Press, 1976:265-76.

60. Skinner MW. The hearing of speech during language acquisition. Otolaryngol Clin North Am 1978; 11:631-50.

61. Menyuk P. Effect of hearing loss on language acquisition in the babbling stage. In: Jaffe B, ed. Hearing loss in children. Baltimore: University Park Press, 1977:621-9.

62. Gottlieb G. Early development of species specific auditory perception in birds. In: Gottlieb G, ed. Studies in the development of behavior and the nervous system: III. Neural and behavioral specificity. New York: Academic Press, 1976:237-80.

63. Kerr LM, Ostapoff EN, Rubel EW. The influence of acoustic experience on the otology of frequency generalization gradients in the chicken. J Exp Psychol [Anim Behav] (in press).

64. Wolf A. The dynamics of selective inhibition of specific function in neurosis. Psychosom Med 1943; 5:27-38.

65. Tees R. The effect of early auditory restrictions in the rats on adult pattern discrimination. J Comp Physiol Psychol 1967; 63:389-93.

66. Saunders JC, Bock GR. Influence of early auditory trauma on auditory development. In: Gottlieb G, ed. Studies of behavior in the nervous system: early influences. New York: Academic Press, 1978:249-87.

67. Henry KR, Haythorn M. Auditory similarities associated with genetic and experimental acoustic deprivation. J Comp Physiol Psychol 1975; 89:213-8.

68. Rapin I. Effects of early blindness and deafness on cognition. Res Publ Assoc Res Nerv Ment Dis 1979; 57:189-245.

69. Conrad R. The deaf school child. London: Harper and Row, 1979.

70. Schien JD, Delk MT Jr. The deaf population of the United States. Silver Spring: National Association for the Deaf, 1974.

71. Leininberg E. Biological foundation of language. New York: John Wiley and Sons, 1967.

72. Herodotus. History. Rawlinson G, Komorff N, trans-eds. New York: Turdo Publishing Co, 1946:81f.

73. Itard JMC. Traite des maladies de l'oreille et de l'audition. Paris: Meguignon-Marvis, 1821.

74. Lane H. The wild boy of Aveyron. Cambridge: Harvard University Press, 1976.

75. Curtiss S. Genie, a psycholinguistic study of a modern day "wild child." New York: Academic Press, 1977.

76. Rapin I. Conductive hearing loss effects on children's language and scholastic skills. In: Hanson D, Ulvestad RF, eds. Otitis media and child development: speech, language and education. Ann Otol Rhinol Laryngol 1979; 88 Suppl 60:3-12.

77. Eisen NH. Some effects of early sensory deprivation on later behavior: the quondam hard of hearing child. J Abnorm Soc Psychol 1962; 65:338-42.

78. Needleman H. Effects of hearing loss from early recurrent otitis media on speech and language development. In: Jaffe B, ed. Hearing loss in children. Baltimore: University Park Press, 1977:640-9.

≈

GUIDELINES FOR GRANTS
TRUSTEES OF THE RESEARCH FUND OF THE AMERICAN OTOLOGICAL SOCIETY, INC.

The members of the Board of Trustees of the Research Fund of the American Otological Society have determined guidelines for making grants from the Fund. The following is the formulation of policy.

Grants will be given in the area of otosclerosis: its diagnosis and management, the possible causes and underlying conditions, and an understanding of the disorder that may lead eventually to its prevention or cure.

The present lack of understanding of the disorder and the absence of similar conditions in other animals makes research in this field difficult. A direct approach to the disease may or may not be feasible; therefore, a sound strategy would be to use other approaches, such as the investigation of bone development, growth and repair under various conditions, and the study of other diseases that may be similar to otosclerosis. It is possible that investigations which may seem initially remote from otosclerosis may provide information which will eventually lead to a substantive further understanding of the disease process which underlies otosclerosis. The applicant should describe correlations between proposed research with the clinical pathological entity of otosclerosis.

The policy is to aid and encourage research in the immediate field of otosclerosis and also in adjoining fields, if, in the opinion of the Board, there is a substantial promise that results obtained will be of assistance in the ways indicated, and may lead to the attainment of the objective of the further understanding of otosclerosis.

Applications for a research grant from the Research Fund of the American Otological Society may be obtained from the Office of the Secretary-Treasurer of the Research Fund of the American Otological Society. Write to Robert J. Ruben, M.D., Secretary-Treasurer, Department of Otolaryngology, Albert Einstein College of Medicine, 1300 Morris Park Avenue, Bronx, New York 10461; (212) 430-3036.

All grant requests must be submitted by January 31, 1981.

INTRAMEMBRANOUS AND MESOTYMPANIC CHOLESTEATOMAS ASSOCIATED WITH AN INTACT TYMPANIC MEMBRANE IN CHILDREN

STEVEN M. SOBOL, MD
CLEVELAND, OHIO

TIMOTHY J. REICHERT, MD
ST. LOUIS, MISSOURI

KENNETH D. FAW, MD
ST. LOUIS, MISSOURI

MALCOLM H. STROUD, MD

GERSHON J. SPECTOR, MD
ST. LOUIS, MISSOURI

JOSEPH H. OGURA, MD

A series of 15 intramembranous (IMTC) and mesotympanic (MTC) cholesteatomas associated with intact tympanic membranes in children is presented. Clinical observations, audiometric and radiographic data, and surgical findings are correlated. A history of recurrent otitis media was obtained in 85% (13/15) of the cases, differentiating them from the usual congenital cholesteatomas. The possibility that many of these are indeed "acquired" lesions is emphasized. Hypothetical pathogenetic mechanisms are discussed. The basal cell papillary proliferation theory is considered the most attractive explanation of the development of both IMTCs and MTCs. The need for careful, prolonged, follow-up otoscopic examination of children with recurrent otitis media is stressed, if more of these lesions are to be recognized early.

Primary cholesteatoma associated with an intact tympanic membrane remains a relatively rare entity. Most cases published to date have been classified as congenital, rather than acquired. Derlacki[1] defined congenital cholesteatomas as: 1) developing behind an intact tympanic membrane; 2) occurring without previous history of aural infections; and 3) arising from embryonal inclusion of squamous epithelium within the middle ear.

Convincing evidence that many of the congenital cases reported to date were not associated with prior otologic infection is difficult to obtain. While the concept of an "acquired" cholesteatoma *behind* an intact tympanic membrane is not new, there is a paucity of well-documented cases. Moreover, primary intramembranous keratomas (ie, *within* the drum) not resulting from implantation are even less common. Ruedi,[2] Nager,[3] and others [4,5] have discussed the development of *acquired* cholesteatomas with intact tympanic membranes, thus raising suspicion that some "congenital" cholesteatomas are indeed "acquired" lesions.

Five patients with intramembranous tympanic cholesteatomas (IMTC) and ten with mesotympanic cholesteatomas (MTC) occurring in association with intact tympanic membranes are presented. Their histories, especially related to previous infections, and findings upon evaluation and at surgery are described. Clinical observations, as they may relate to pathogenesis, as well as suggestions for identification and treatment are presented.

METHODS

The records of 15 patients, 12 seen at St. Louis Children's Hospital from December 1977 to March 1980 and three seen at Barnes Hospital, were reviewed. Clinical, audiometric, radiographic, and surgical data were reviewed. Records from primary care physicians were consulted to accurately determine the frequency of otitis media in the involved ear.

CLINICAL DATA

The clinical data for the patients with IMTC and MTC are summarized in Tables 1 and 2 respectively.

Age and Sex. In the group of patients with IMTC, the average age was approximately one year, seven months. This was significantly younger than the group of children with MTC, whose ages ranged from 17 months to eight years.

Previous Infections. Only one patient with an IMTC had no available history from the pediatrician, but the incidence of previous otitis media in the involved ears of the other children ranged from one to four. The parents of all patients with IMTCs also denied any previous history of otorrhea. Of our ten children with MTCs, eight had a history of documented recurrent otitis media. Records of their pediatricians disclosed an average of six bouts of otitis

TABLE 1. SUMMARY OF CLINICAL OBSERVATIONS IN CHILDREN WITH INTRAMEMBRANOUS CHOLESTEATOMAS

TM Site	*Appearance*	*Age (mo)*	*Sex*	*History of Recurrent OM*	*No. of Documented Bouts OM*
Mult.	Uni.	6	F	Yes	2
P	Uni.	13	M	Yes	3
PI	Uni.	16	M	Yes	?
PI	Uni.	27	F	Yes	4
I	Uni.	36	M	Yes	1

OM - Otitis media; TM - Tympanic membrane; ? - Unknown; Uni. - Unilocular; Mult. - Multiple; P - Posterior; I - Inferior; PI - Posteroinferior.

From the Department of Otolaryngology, Washington University School of Medicine, and the Division of Pediatric Otolaryngology, St. Louis Children's Hospital, St. Louis, Missouri.

Presented at the meeting of the American Otological Society, Inc., Palm Beach, Florida, April 13-14, 1980.

REPRINTS — Steven M. Sobol, MD, Department of Otolaryngology, Washington University School of Medicine, 517 S. Euclid Ave., St. Louis, MO 63110.

TABLE 2. SUMMARY OF HISTORIES AND AUDIOLOGIC, RADIOGRAPHIC AND SURGICAL DATA IN CHILDREN WITH MESOTYMPANIC CHOLESTEATOMAS

Site	*Appearance*	*Age/Sex*	*History of OM*	*No. of Documented Bouts OM*	*Pure Tone Average*	*T-Gram Type*	*Polytomes*	*Adherence to TM*	*Ossic Erosion*
Anterior	Uni.	19 mo/M	+	?	ND	ND	ND	+	–
Anterior	Uni.	3 yr/F	+	7	10 dB	A	Normal	–	–
Anterior	Uni.	4 yr/F	–	0	ND	A		–	–
Anterior	Multi.	4 yr/F	–	0	20 dB	ND	Normal	?	–
Posterior	Multi.	17 mo/M	+	3	ND	ND	Normal	–	–
Posterior	Multi.	5 yr/M	+	6	35 dB	B	ND	+	Incus
Subtotal*	Multi.	5 yr/M	+	9	20 dB	B	Clouding	+	–
Subtotal	Multi.	5 yr/M	+	7	15 dB	A	Normal	–	–
Subtotal	Multi.	6 yr/F	+	6	25 dB	B	ND	+	Incus
Subtotal	Multi.	8 yr/F	+	?	15 dB	A	ND	?	I-S joint

*Subtotal - Occupying almost the entire mesotympanum.
OM - Otitis media;TM - Tympanic membrane; ND - Not done; I-S - Incudostapedial; ? - Unknown; Uni. - Unilocular; Multi. - Multilocular.

media in the involved ears. Documentation was unavailable on two children.

Audiologic Findings. None of the five patients with IMTC would cooperate to allow tympanometry or pure tone audiometry. The ten patients with MTC had no initial complaints of hearing loss when originally seen. Seven children had preoperative audiometry. Three were found to have mild hearing losses (≤15 dB) and four had losses ≥20 dB. Four had type A tympanograms and three with obvious middle ear effusions on physical examination had type B tympanograms. Acoustic reflexes were normal in three of the four type A patterns; in one, the reflex was absent. Incudostapedial joint erosion was found at surgery in that patient.

Radiologic Findings. No patients with IMTC had polytomography. Five patients with MTC had polytomography, which revealed no bony abnormalities. In one patient, clouding of the mesotympanum and mastoid air cells was noted.

Surgical Findings. Three IMTCs clearly involved the posterior aspect of the pars tensa. One patient had multiple keratomas (Fig. 1) while the others had single keratomas (Fig. 2). The integrity of the fibrous layer of the tympanic membrane (TM) was at least partially intact with all the IMTCs. Of the patients with MTCs, four were found in the anterior mesotympanum. These were usually well circumscribed unilocular cysts (3/4). A photograph of an anterior MTC is seen in Figure 3. The multiloculated cysts were found more often in the posterior mesotympanum or subtotally filling the mesotympanum. A photograph of a posterior MTC is seen in Figure 4. In half (3/6) of these latter types, incus erosion was found. In four cases, the cholesteatoma was intimately adherent to the medial surface of the drum.

Management and Outcome. Three of the four cases of IMTC had simple removal of the superficial surface of the tympanic membrane with enucleation of the cyst. One patient had a complete excision of that area of the TM containing the cholesteatoma and repair of the resultant perforation with an underlay fascia graft. Those patients with MTCs underwent transcanal tympanotomy with ossicular reconstruction in three cases, while one patient required a modified radical mastoidectomy in order to remove more extensive disease. One patient had a recurrence of an anterior mesotympanic cyst one year after initial excision. Residual disease localized to the stapes suprastructure was identified at a "second look" procedure in the patient who had a modified radical mastoidectomy.

DISCUSSION

Although cholesteatomas associated with an intact tympanic membrane have been known to exist for some time, their actual incidence is not established. In a recent report, House and Sheehy[6] reported on 41 cases from the Otologic Medical Group, and noted that they represented 3.7% of their total number of cholesteatoma cases from 1964-1975. Not unlike most, these authors classified the majority of the lesions as congenital. Only a few descriptive reports of primary "acquired" intramembranous or mesotympanic cholesteatomas with an intact TM may be found in the literature.

Concerning IMTC, Teed[7] in 1936 cited a series of reports of primary cholesteatomas of the tympanic membrane, the earliest of which was described by Hinton in 1863,[8] as a "sebaceous tumor . . . on the external surface of the membrana tympani." In 1883, Politzer[9] described globular pearly growths on the left tympanic membrane of a youngster which had developed in the course of chronic inflammation. Subsequently, he recognized the presence of squamous debri within these cysts, and suggested they could disappear spontaneously.[10]

More recently, Smith and Moran[11] in 1977 described three cases of presumably primary ac-

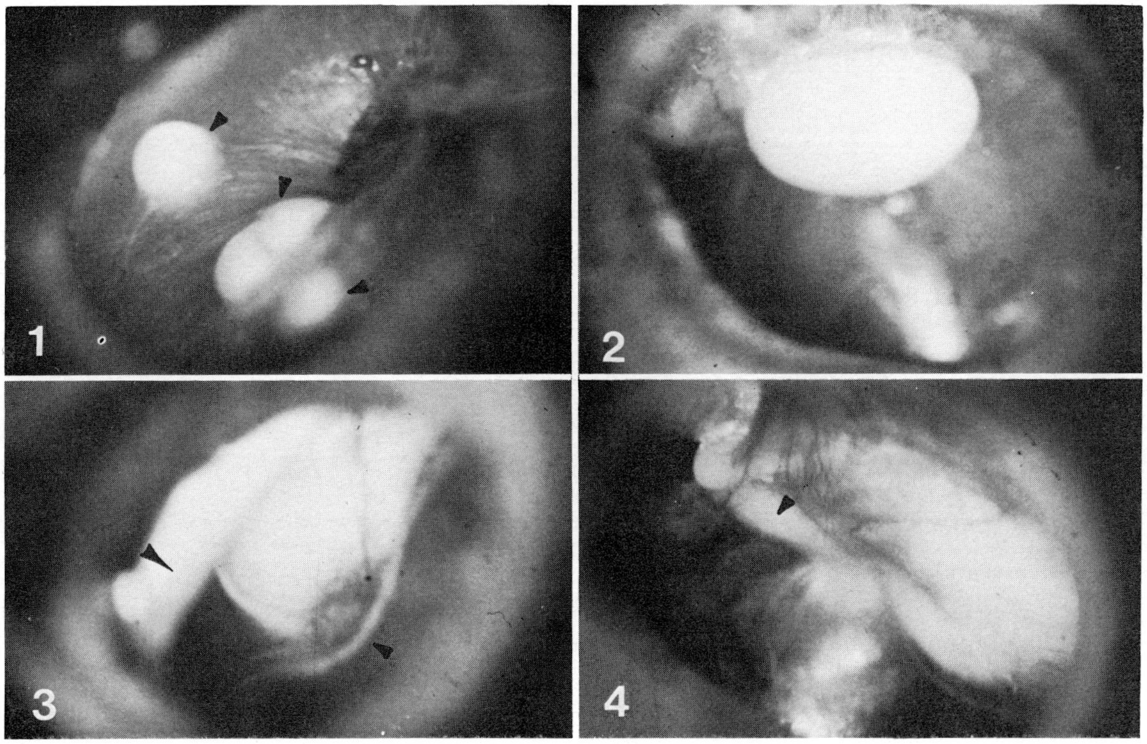

Fig. 1. Multiple intramembranous keratomas within the pars tensa (arrows).

Fig. 2. Solitary unilocular intramembranous keratoma overlying the malleus and superior pars tensa.

Fig. 3. Anterior mesotympanic cholesteatoma. Large arrow - Anterior canal wall; Small arrow - Umbo.

Fig. 4. Posterior mesotympanic cholesteatoma. Arrow - Malleus.

quired IMTCs in children with histories of one or more bouts of otitis media and no prior otologic surgery. They speculated that the basal cell proliferation theory best explained the tendency of these intramembranous keratomas to invade the fibrous layer of the drum.

Concerning mesotympanic lesions, Curtis[12] recently published a comprehensive review of the 43 congenital middle ear cholesteatomas reported to date, including the 23 cases described by Derlacki.[1] Although his analysis included a detailed clinicopathologic description of this disease, the possibility that some of these cases might have been "acquired" was not suggested. House and Sheehy felt that the question of "congenital" versus "acquired" was moot, suggesting that simply being alert to the diagnosis of cholesteatoma behind an intact TM was sufficient.

PATHOGENESIS

Although the etiology, pathogenesis and nomenclature of cholesteatoma has been extensively discussed and debated, a consensus has not been achieved. The central issue concerning the pathogenesis of cholesteatomas in association with an intact TM lies in determining whether they are congenital or acquired. Most of the intramembranous and mesotympanic cholesteatomas in this report (14/16) share two distinguishing features: 1) the presence of an intact tympanic membrane; 2) a documented history of repeated otologic infection.

It is generally agreed that true congenital cholesteatomas arise from preexisting embryonal epithelial rests or pleuripotential tissue which changes to squamous epithelium and retains the ability to keratinize and form epidermal cysts under appropriate conditions.[1] While few doubt the possibility of occult ectodermal rests within the entodermally derived middle ear mucosa, most agree that the microenvironmental condition necessary to stimulate these to form cholesteatomas is difficult to define. As initially postulated by Körner[13] and popularized by Derlacki,[1] the key to the diagnosis of a "congenital" cholesteatoma is the absence of a history of local trauma or infection. Therefore, while a congenital origin of many of the intramembranous or mesotympanic cholesteatomas in this report cannot be entirely disregarded, its likelihood is reduced. Since most of our patients had a history of repeated ear infections, it seems likely that *inflammation* relates to their pathogenesis.

Sadé[14] supports the theory of mucosal squamous metaplasia first emphasized by Wendt[15] in 1873, and subsequently repopularized by Tumarkin.[16] According to this theory, acquired cholesteatomas form as a result of keratinizing squamous metaplasia of epitympanic and mesotympanic mucosa. Interaction with local connective tissue resulting from recurrent inflammation leads to the formation of attic or mesotympanic cholesteatomas. Ultimately, as these cholesteatomas enlarge, they communicate with the external ear canal by fistulization resulting from gradual growth and erosion.

To support this concept, Sadé and Weinberg[17] have shown that as high as 60% of chronic ears have foci of stratified squamous mucosal metaplasia in various degrees. Other investigators have confirmed the occurrence of squamous metaplasia, but few have demonstrated active keratinization. While good experimental evidence supports the concept of mucosal metaplasia, less data are available to confirm the ability of this transformed mucosa to develop into active cholesteatoma.

The bulk of available clinical, experimental, and histopathologic evidence suggests that most acquired cholesteatomas are derived from the aberrant inward migration of keratinizing squamous epithelium of the drum or canal skin. The migration theory which best explains the development of cholesteatomas associated with an intact drum is that of basal cell papillary proliferation.

Lange[18] in 1925 furnished histopathological evidence of ingrowing prickle cells in the epithelium of Shrapnell's membrane in the absence of an attic retraction pocket. More recent work of Ojala and Saxen[19] and Ruedi[20] showed the presence of proliferative drum basal cells penetrating the subepithelial connective tissue in response to irritating stimuli. Ruedi claimed that the basal cells in the stratum germinativum maintained the potential for downward proliferative growth into underlying connective tissues in response to inflammation.

To test this concept experimentally, Ruedi[2] applied an irritative mixture of talc and fibrin to the medial surface of an intact TM in guinea pigs. After two to three weeks, active invasion of the drum epidermal basal cells occurred, ultimately penetrating the basement membrane and proliferating into columns of desquamating squamous epithelium within the newly formed granulation tissue. Typical cholesteatomatous masses were thus formed behind an intact drum.

Similarily, studies by Abramson and his coworkers[21] have confirmed the ability of drum epidermis to migrate and form cholesteatomas even in the absence of a perforation. Their observations suggest that with persistent inflammation, migrating drum eithelium will penetrate the basement membrane and lamina propria. Nager[3] claimed that although the pars flaccida and posterosuperior TM were the predelective sites for this process to occur, focal central papillary-basal cell proliferation within the pars tensa could also occur, provided the local inflammatory conditions were present.

The specific mechanics of this process are derived from the physiology of dermal-epithelial interaction. Local patterns of epithelial differentiation, spatial orientation and cellular growth have been shown experimentally to be largely influenced by epithelial-mesenchymal interactions. The precise nature of these mesenchymal clues is, however, somewhat of a mystery but would appear to be tissue specific. Inhibitory mechanisms normally active in other mesenchymal-epithelial interfaces may not exist or fail to prevent the proliferation of keratinizing drum basal cells under the influence of inflammation. Examining these growth patterns more closely, Lim and his associates[22] using phase contrast and electron microscopy observed numerous fine fibrils attached to basal cells serving as a guide to epidermal advancement. Epidermal migration follows this fibrillar orientation, ultimately disrupting the basal lamina and basement membrane, and invading the underlying connective tissue stroma. The local microchemical environment determines the degree of invasion and the tendency toward epidermal cyst formation and active growth. It would appear that the provocative impulse for active proliferation and migration is inflammation.

A still unsettled issue concerns the precise nature of the underlying inflammatory process. As suggested by Lim et al, at times this localized inflammatory reaction must persist in the absence of generalized middle ear infection. Perhaps the advancing edge of the keratinizing epithelium serves as its own stimulus for continued inflammation, thus producing the necessary vicious cycle for the development of cholesteatoma.

Upon reviewing these cases, almost all the children had histories of multiple bouts of otitis media. In applying the previously discussed theoretical concepts, it is reasonable to assume repeated bouts of middle ear infection stimulated active basal cell ingrowth and proliferation of tympanic membrane epithelium. Those occurring within the drum (IMTC) may have resulted from a primary focus within the fibrous layer of the TM, while those occurring within the mesotympanum (MTC) may have resulted from more diffuse middle ear inflammation. The degree of secondary inflammation around the desquamated material would likely determine the degree of active growth and erosion. This process is schematically represented in Figure 5. The time required to develop these cholesteatomas is not known, but it undoubtedly varies with the severity of disease. That most occurred in young children suggests that the process may occur rapidly, given the necessary local environment.

The other theories offered to explain cholesteatomas associated with an intact TM, namely a) con-

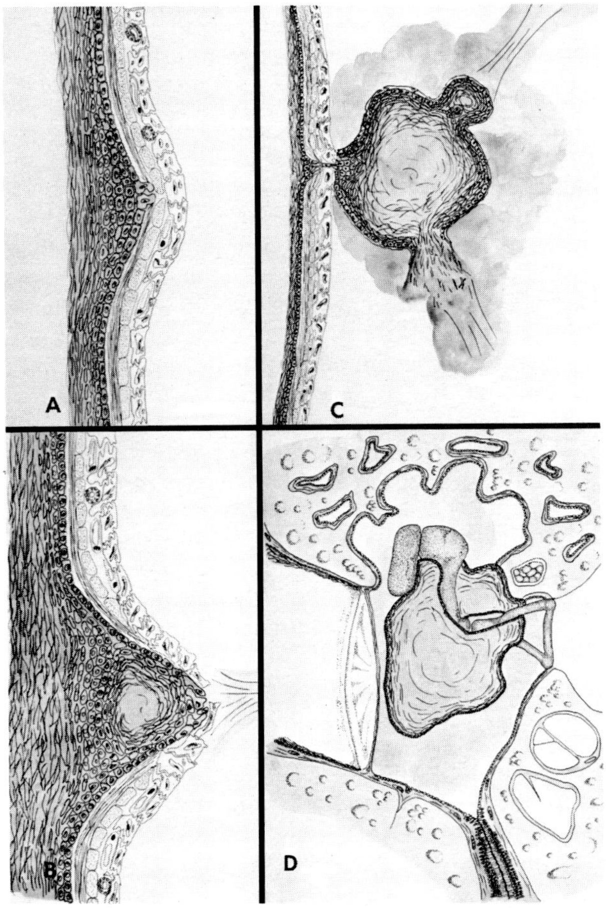

Fig. 5. Schematic representation of events during basal cell papillary proliferation leading to the formation of IMTC or MTC. Initial conelike proliferation A) of prickle cells; B) coalescing into an intramembranous keratoma; C) penetrating through TM into ME space, with continued growth or rupture; D) encasing ossicles.

genital, b) migration through a microperforation, and c) mucosal metaplasia, are less likely explanations for most of the cholesteatomas in his report.

Only two patients had no history of otitis media, which would fulfill Derlacki's criteria for a congenital cholesteatoma. However, while recurrent infections would make the congenital theory less attractive, the possibility of infection acting as the provocative impulse to the growth of dormant epithelial rests (Fig. 6) must be considered.

The possibility of epithelium migrating through an undetected and healed perforation cannot be entirely disregarded. However, none of the patients had a history of otorrhea and most had frequent examinations by their pediatricians with no observation of perforation.

Last, the fact that all the lesions arose within the drum or mesotympanum, and none was found in the attic or mastoid, would speak against mucosal metaplasia as the origin of these cholesteatomas. Moreover, that four lesions were clearly attached to the TM, but separated from the promontory mucosa, would further support the notion of the development of these lesions from tympanic membrane epithelium.

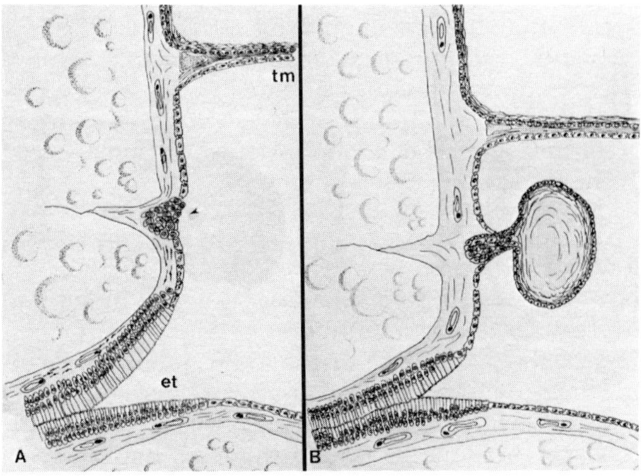

Fig. 6. Schematic representation showing a focus of pleuripotential cells within the middle ear cleft (A) evolving into a MTC (B) presumably provoked by an inflammatory stimulus.

CLINICAL EVALUATION AND MANAGEMENT

Our observations are in general agreement with those of Curtis.[12] Small, unilocular, localized mesotympanic cysts tend to occur in younger children whereas those with more extensive mesotympanic involvement tend to be a few years older.

The diagnosis of either IMTC or MTC is made primarily by pneumo-otoscopy. Generally, a whitish mass is seen within or behind a translucent TM. The mass may bulge, and its contours may be accentuated by pneumatization. IMTCs tend to be more circumscribed and move with the TM on pneumatization.

Although associated attic retraction was noted in one quarter of the patients reviewed by Curtis, none of our patients displayed this finding. Otitis media with effusion may accompany this disease, and obscure the diagnosis.

Children in our series did not complain of hearing loss, although pure tone thresholds were elevated in five cases. Tympanometry, although helpful in identifying associated middle ear effusions, did not seem to be of value in correctly identifying the presence of cholesteatoma.

Similarly, radiological evaluation was not helpful in that bony erosion was not seen on any of the polytomes obtained. Nevertheless, as suggested by Derlacki[1] and Curtis,[12] polytomography may be important in identifying disease extending into the mastoid or intracranially. Such information would, of course, be helpful preoperatively.

The surgical approach to this disease is foremost to effect cure. The patient should be prepared for a possible open or closed tympanomastoid procedure. The surgeon may be assisted in his approach by knowing that the posterior MTCs have a high incidence of ossicular erosion.

This series of patients is too small and the follow-up too short to ascertain the natural history of these cholesteatomas and the effectiveness of the various mastoidectomy procedures used to treat them. The philosophy of treatment has been to remove localized mesotympanic disease which shells out easily without necessarily performing a mastoid procedure. In those cases where the matrix has to be dissected from hyperplastic or metaplastic diseased mucosa, the danger of incomplete removal of entrapped keratinizing epithelium, which is presumably capable of developing into a recurrent cholesteatoma pearl, would preclude the use of immediate ossicular reconstruction. Second-look procedures are planned for these patients. Careful, frequent, and prolonged follow-up for four to five years is imperative to detect recurrent disease.

Derlacki[1] reported six recurrent cholesteatomas in his series, which occurred from 5 to 42 months after surgery. House and Sheehy[6] managed 97% of these cases with intact canal wall tympanomastoidectomy. In the 60% who underwent a planned second stage procedure, residual disease was encountered in 32%

In conclusion, although Nager[23] claimed that these lesions were so rare "as to lose all practical importance in diagnosis and therapy," it is our belief that cholesteatomas behind an intact tympanic membrane may be more common than is generally recognized. Careful follow-up examination of children with recurrent otitis media is mandatory if such delayed sequelae are to be discovered. Moreover, more scrutiny in the labelling of "congenital" cholesteatoma might reveal more of these to be "acquired" lesions. To gain more insight into the pathogenesis of such lesions, closer operative and histologic examination at the time of surgery of the mucosal tissues attached to and surrounding these cholesteatomas is necessary.

SUMMARY

"Acquired" intramembranous and mesotympanic cholesteatomas associated with an intact tympanic membrane are probably more common than the literature would indicate. Careful follow-up and microscopic examination of children with a history of recurrent bouts of otitis media are necessary if more of these are to be discovered. We believe that their pathogenesis can best be explained by the basal cell proliferation theory of acquired cholesteatoma development, the provocative impulse being the inflammatory process. Closer scrutiny of lesions now classified as congenital cholesteatomas may reveal some of these to be indeed acquired lesions.

REFERENCES

1. Derlacki EL. Congenital cholesteatoma of the middle ear and mastoid: a third report. Arch Otolaryngol 1973; 97:177-82.

2. Ruedi L. Middle ear cholesteatoma. Acta Otolaryngol (Stockh) 1979; Suppl 361:6-26.

3. Nager G. Cholesteatoma of the middle ear: pathogenesis and surgical indication. In: McCabe B, Sadé J, Abramson M, eds. Cholesteatoma: first international conference. Birmingham: Aesculapius, 1977.

4. Buckingham RA. Etiology of a middle ear cholesteatoma: Kodachrome study of pathogenesis. Ann Otol Rhinol Laryngol 1968; 77:1054-9.

5. Juers AL. Cholesteatoma genesis: clinical observations. Arch Otolaryngol 1965; 81:5-8.

6. House J, Sheehy J. Cholesteatoma with intact tympanic membrane: a report of 41 cases. Laryngoscope 1980; 90:70-5.

7. Teed R. Cholesteatoma verum tympani: its relationship to the first epibranchial placode. Arch Otolaryngol 1936; 24:455-74.

8. Hinton J. Sebaceous tumor within the tympanum originating on the external surface of the membrana tympani. Guy's Hosp Rep 1863; 9:264.

9. Politzer A. A textbook of diseases of the ear and adjacent organs. Cassell JP, trans-ed. Philadelphia: Lea's Son and Co, 1883.

10. Politzer A. Das Cholesteatom des Gehorogans von anatomischen and klinischen Standpunlite. Wien Med Wochenschr 1891; 41:8-12.

11. Smith R, Moran W. Tympanic membrane keratoma in children with no prior otologic surgery. Laryngoscope 1977; 87:237-45.

12. Curtis A. Congenital middle ear cholesteatoma: two unusual cases and a review of the literature. Laryngoscope 1979; 89:1159-65.

13. Korner O. Die Eitrigen Erkrankungen des Schlafenbeins. Wiesbaden 1899. Ein Cholesteatoma verum in der hinteren Schadelgrube. Z Ohrenheilkd Krankheiten Luftwege 1900; 37:352.

14. Sadé J. Pathogenesis of cholesteatoma: the metaplasia theory. In: McCabe B, Sadé J, Abramson M, eds. Cholesteatoma: first international conference. Birmingham: Aesculapius, 1977.

15. Wendt H. Desquamative entzundung des mitelhors ("Cholesteatom des Felsen beins" der Autoren). Arch Heilkd (Leipzig) 1873; 14:428-551.

16. Tumarkin A. A contribution to the study of middle ear suppuration with special reference to the pathogeny and treatment of cholesteatoma. J Laryngol Otol 1938; 53:685-709.

17. Sade J. Weinberg J. Mucus production in the chemically infected middle ear. Ann Otol Rhinol Laryngol 1969; 78:148-55.

18. Lange W. Uber die Entstehung der mittelohr-Cholesteatome. Z Hals Nasen Ohrenheilkd 1925; 11:250-7.

19. Ojala L, Saxen A. Pathogenesis of middle ear cholesteatoma arising from Schrapnell's membrane. Acta Otolaryngol (Stockh) 1952; Suppl 100:53-4.

20. Ruedi L. Cholesteatoma formation in the middle ear in animal experiments. Acta Otolaryngol (Stockh) 1959; 50:233-44.

21. Abramson M, Gantz B, Asarch R, Litton W. Cholesteatoma pathogenesis: evidence for the migration theory. In: McCabe B, Sadé J, Abramson M, eds. Cholesteatoma: first international conference. Birmingham: Aesculapius, 1977:176-86.

22. Lim D, Birck H, Saunders W. Aural cholesteatoma and epidermization: a fine morphological study. In: McCabe B, Sadé J, Abramson M, eds. Cholesteatoma: first international conference. Birmingham: Aesculapius, 1977:233-52.

23. Nager FR. The cholesteatoma of the middle ear — its etiology, pathogenesis, diagnosis and therapy. Ann Otol Rhinol Laryngol 1925; 34:1249-58.

Ann Otol 89:1980

LABYRINTHECTOMY VERSUS MIDDLE FOSSA VESTIBULAR NERVE SECTION IN MENIÈRE'S DISEASE

A CRITICAL EVALUATION OF RELIEF OF VERTIGO

MICHAEL E. GLASSCOCK III, MD, FACS
NASHVILLE, TENNESSEE

GORDON B. HUGHES, MD
NASHVILLE, TENNESSEE

WILLIAM E. DAVIS, MD, FACS
COLUMBIA, MISSOURI

C. GARY JACKSON, MD
NASHVILLE, TENNESSEE

Labyrinthectomy has been used for years in the surgical management of Menière's disease for the control of vertigo. The effects of this procedure are predictable and satisfying but residual hearing is sacrificed. With the advent of the middle fossa section of the vestibular nerve, it soon became apparent that it was possible to obtain relief from vertigo and at the same time preserve residual hearing. How do the two procedures actually compare as far as relief of vertigo, postsurgical ataxia, and recovery periods? The purpose of this paper is to evaluate the two procedures in regard to these three parameters. A series of middle fossa operations is compared to one in which the patients received a labyrinthectomy. Results and complications in both groups are covered in detail.

At one time the only procedures available for the surgical management of Menière's disease were the labyrinthectomy[1] and the suboccipital section of the vestibular nerve.[2] The patient with servicable hearing lost all auditory function at the time of surgery with labyrinthectomy and most of the time with nerve section. The past 15 years has witnessed an upsurge of interest in operations to eliminate vertigo but at the same time preserve residual hearing. Few if any of these surgical procedures could relieve vertigo with the predictable regularity of a labyrinthectomy. The introduction of the middle fossa vestibular nerve section has been heralded as a method of preserving hearing and yet controlling vertigo at the same rate as the standard labyrinthectomy. The purpose of this paper is to review the criteria for surgical intervention in Menière's disease and to compare the functional results of these two operations as they relate to control of vertigo, postsurgical ataxia and recovery period. Results and complications for both operations are covered in detail.

NATURAL COURSE OF MENIÈRE'S DISEASE

The classic triad of Menière's disease has been well established and the diagnosis is basically one that can be made by history alone. The individual complains of a fluctuating hearing loss, tinnitus, and episodic attacks of vertigo associated with nausea and vomiting. A fourth symptom, fullness or pressure in the involved ear, is experienced by a majority of patients.

There are two aberrant forms of Menière's disease in which the individual does not exhibit the full triad. Cochlear hydrops is the term employed when the patient experiences fluctuating hearing loss, tinnitus, and fullness but no vertigo, while vestibular Menière's disease is used to describe those individuals who have the typical episodic attacks of vertigo but no cochlear symptoms. In reality, all three forms of the disease seem to represent a basic underlying process of endolymphatic hydrops. Given enough time, those patients with pure cochlear symptoms usually develop the full triad. The same holds true for those individuals with vestibular Menière's disease. The basis for the variation in severity of the process is not well understood because the etiology of endolymphatic hydrops itself has not been established. From clinical observation, however, it is possible to establish a series of stages through which the average patient progresses.

Regardless of which form of the disease the individual may experience, characteristically there are remissions and exacerbations. Early in the process, the attacks are usually spread out over a period of several weeks or months and the hearing returns to normal after each event. If the hydrops is not kept under control, the disease progresses and the symptoms become more frequent. The hearing does not return after the episode and the individual is left with a permanent, low frequency hearing loss. The sensation of fullness or pressure becomes constant as does the tinnitus. The hearing may continue to fluctuate with each exacerbation but usually only returns to the preattack level. At this stage of the disease the individual has some warning (aura) prior to the episode.

From the Otology Group and from the Department of Surgery (Otology and Neurotology), Vanderbilt University School of Medicine, Nashville, Tennessee; and from the Department of Surgery, University of Missouri, Columbia, Missouri.

Presented at the meeting of the American Otological Society, Inc., Palm Beach, Florida, April 13-14, 1980.

REPRINTS — Michael E. Glasscock III, MD, 118 State Street, Nashville, TN 37203.

With time the hearing gradually decreases (both pure tone and speech discrimination) and the patient enters a period in which there is no warning before the attack. House[3] refers to this as the uncompensated stage of Menière's disease. From this point on, the disease may progress in one of two ways, either the patient has almost constant unsteadiness and frequent attacks of vertigo or may become symptom free. In either case the hearing is, in most cases, essentially destroyed. Fortunately, Menière's disease in the majority of instances, is a unilateral entity. One must be cognizant of the fact, however, that some individuals may develop bilateral symptoms.

It is important to understand these stages of Menière's disease because the treatment varies depending upon where the individual is in this cycle when he seeks medical advice. The status of the better or only hearing ear plays an important role in the decision-making process of therapy.

DIAGNOSIS

Because Menière's disease is associated with a unilateral sensorineural hearing loss, one must not rely on the history alone to establish the diagnosis. A full neurotologic workup[4] must be performed to rule out the possibility of a cerebellopontine angle lesion. This should include a history and physical, pure tone air and bone conduction audiogram with speech scores, vestibular studies, and x-rays of the petrous pyramid.

There are several specific audiometric studies that are helpful in confirming the presence of hydrops. These include tests such as the ABLB,[5] SISI scores,[6] BERA,[7] impedance audiometry,[8] and glycerol test.[9] The glycerol test is particularly helpful when the hearing (pure tone and/or discrimination) can be made to fluctuate.

TREATMENT

The treatment of Menière's disease is either medical or surgical depending upon which stage the individual is in when first seen and whether he has undergone an adequate medical trial.

Medical. Assuming that the underlying histopathology of Menière's disease is a hydrops of the endolymphatic system, it would seem logical to base the medical management on salt restriction in the diet coupled with a systemic diuretic. Jackson et al[10] have reported a large series of patients managed in this manner with a success rate of 75-80%. When considering the results of any therapy (medical or surgical) it is important to use the same parameters for judging success. Control of vertigo alone is not considered adequate; the hearing must be stabilized as well. The tinnitus and sensation of fullness should at least be diminished.

In addition to salt restriction and diuretics it may be necessary to use labyrinthine sedatives from time to time to control the vertigo. A combination of diazepam and glycopyrrolate has been found to be very effective in most individuals. While they are experiencing frequent attacks they are kept on this combination for one to two months. Once their symptoms are under control the drugs are discontinued and used only as needed. Salt restriction must be a lifetime commitment.

Surgical. Surgical intervention is only considered when the patient is declared a medical failure. There are numerous operative procedures available for the control of Menière's disease. It is not within the scope of this paper to review these. Instead we would like to describe the criteria used in selecting any one of the three operations commonly employed at the Otology Group. The three surgical procedures used are the endolymphatic shunt with the Arenberg valve,[11] the middle fossa total vestibular nerve section,[12] and the translabyrinthine labyrinthectomy.[1] The criteria for deciding which operation to recommend depend on several factors including frequency of attacks and the status of hearing in the involved ear as well as the opposite ear. For example, if the patient had the disease in his only hearing ear, one would not consider a labyrinthectomy (destructive procedure). Should surgery be contemplated at all, it would have to be an operation in which the hearing would usually be spared (conservative procedure).

At the Otology Group the endolymphatic sac procedure is reserved for those individuals who are in the early stages of the disease process. Their hearing may still be fluctuating and between attacks they are symptom free. This operation is also advised in bilateral cases and occasionally in only hearing ears when it is apparent that, left unchecked, the disease will destroy the hearing. The middle fossa nerve section is advised in shunt failure cases when the hearing is still serviceable (arbitrarily set at 50 dB and 80% speech discrimination score). In some instances a nerve section might be recommended instead of a shunt if the individual's hearing was not fluctuating (negative glycerol test) and he was experiencing severe bouts of episodic vertigo. When the hearing loss reaches an unserviceable range and the disease is unilateral, a translabyrinthine labyrinthectomy is advised.

SURGICAL TECHNIQUE

Both the endolymphatic sac and middle fossa vestibular nerve section procedures have been described in detail elsewhere[11,12] and therefore will not be discussed here.

Translabyrinthine Labyrinthectomy. The purpose of this procedure is to totally remove the neuroepithelium of the vestibular end-organ. The pa-

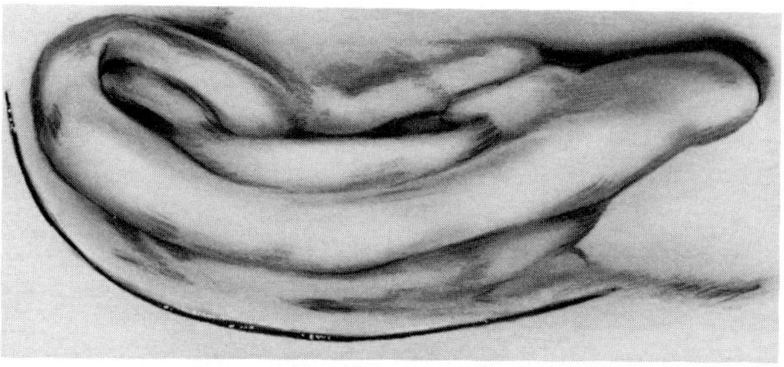

Fig. 1. A standard postauricular incision is used to expose the mastoid process.

tient is placed in the supine position with the involved ear up. After a standard preparation and drape, a postauricular incision is made (Fig. 1). Using a high speed air drill and suction irrigation a simple mastoidectomy is performed outlining the three semicircular canals, the sigmoid sinus, sinodural angle and posterior ear canal wall (Fig. 2). The course of the facial nerve is determined by uncapping its sheath from the horizontal canal to the digastric ridge. Next, the three semicircular canals are opened (Fig. 3) to expose their membranous conterparts. The dissection is carried under the facial nerve to open the vestibule (Fig. 4). Once this has been accomplished, the membranous labyrinth is completely removed, including the neuroepithelium of all three ampulae, the utricle and saccule.

In those individuals complaining of severe tinnitus, the operation may be extended at this point to include section of the superior and inferior divisions of the vestibular nerve as well as the cochlear nerve. To do so one must outline the internal auditory canal (IAC) by removing all the bone superior, posterior, and inferior to the canal. Opening the dura of the canal allows the surgeon to identify Bill's bar[12] and the facial nerve. With a long right-angle pick the operator avulses the other three nerves filling the IAC (Fig. 5). These nerves are severed with

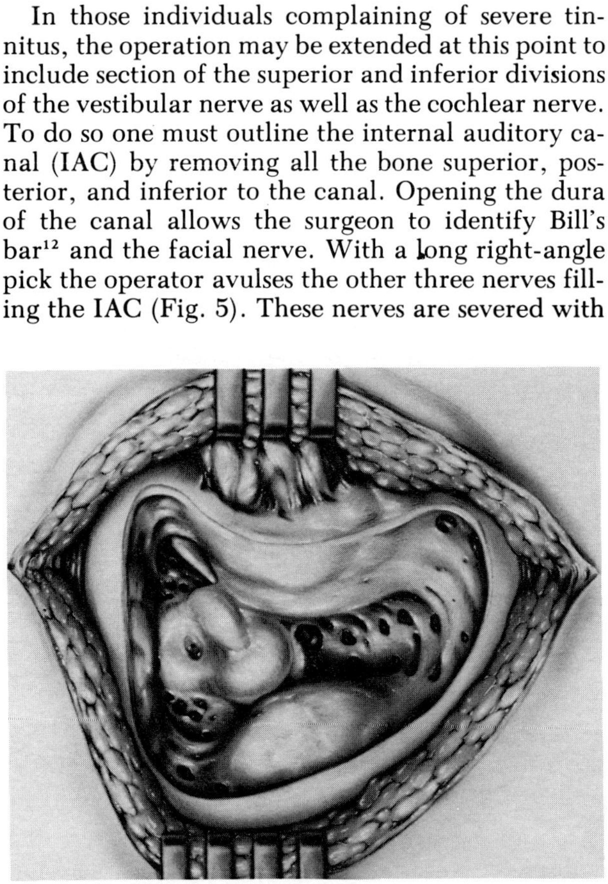

Fig. 2. A simple mastoidectomy is completed and the three semicircular canals are exposed.

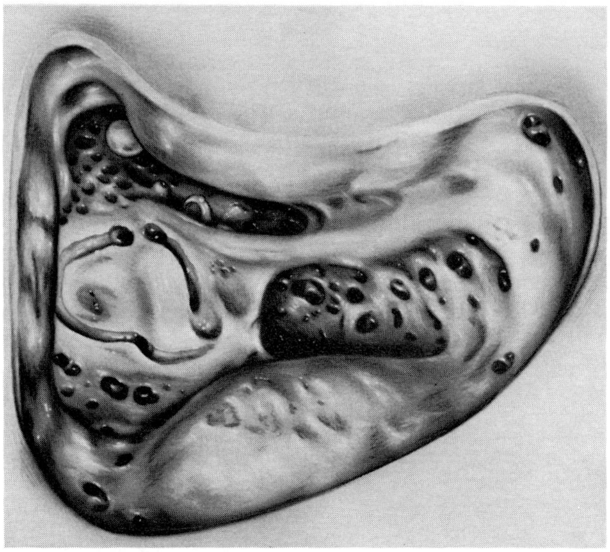

Fig. 3. Note that all three canals have been opened, exposing their membranous portions.

microscissors (medial to Scarpa's ganglion on the vestibular nerves) and their blood vessels cauterized with a bipolar cautery. Abdominal fat is placed into the mastoid to prevent postoperative cerebrospinal fluid leak. The incision is closed with interrupted subcutaneous sutures and a disposable mastoid dressing is applied.

CASE MATERIAL

This study spans a time frame from January 1970 to December 31, 1978; therefore all patients have had at least 15 months follow-up and in some cases as much as nine years. There were 1,143 individuals with Menière's disease seen at the Otology Group during this nine-year period. Of these, 55 total vestibular nerve sections are being reported. There were 25 males and 30 females in the middle fossa groups. In the labyrinthectomy series

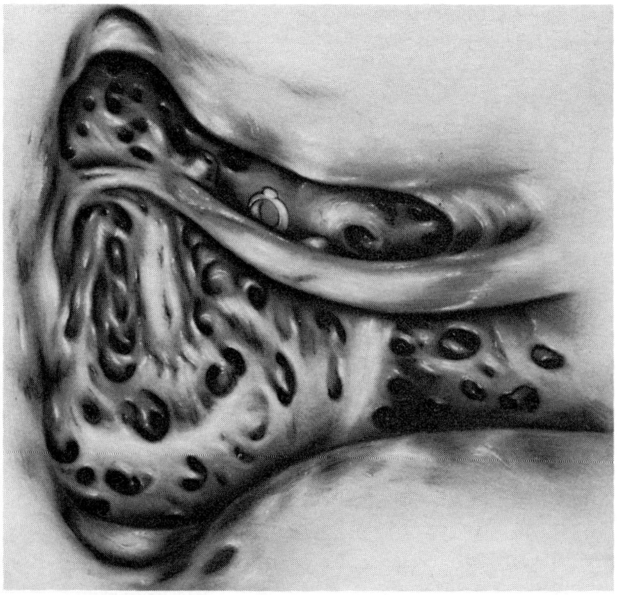

Fig. 4. All of the neuroepithelium of the labyrinth has been removed, completely denervating the vestibular endorgan.

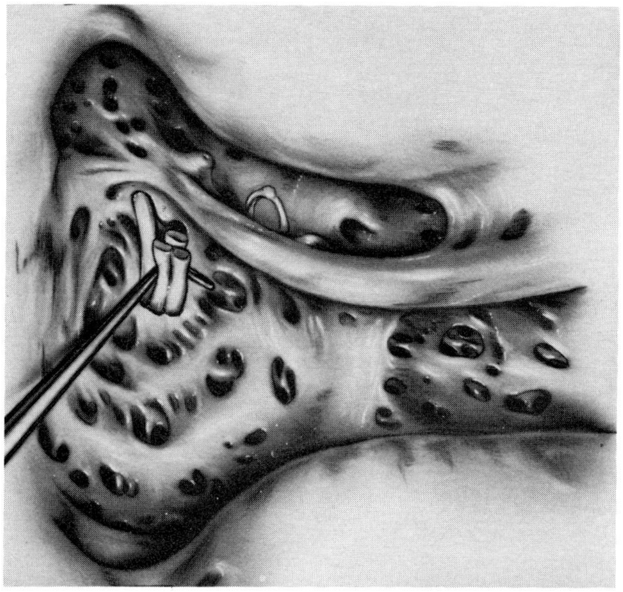

Fig. 5. Those patients complaining of severe vertigo may receive some relief by section of the cochlear nerve. Note a right-angle hook being used to sever the cochlear nerve and the superior and inferior branches of the vestibular nerve. The facial nerve is seen to the left of the surgeon's instrument.

there were 38 females and 33 males. The mean age of the first group was 44 years and the second 51 years. Of special interest is the fact that only two individuals over 60 underwent a middle fossa procedure while 19 patients in their 60s had a translabyrinthine labyrinthectomy. In the middle fossa group 14 of the patients were endolymphatic sac surgery failures, and five had undergone medical management at the Otology Group without success. The remaining 36 cases were either medical or surgical failures who had been referred specifically for further surgical management. All of the labyrinthectomy series were medical failures. Two had experienced previous oval window labyrinthectomies, 2 had undergone middle fossa superior vestibular nerve section and 12 were endolymphatic shunt failures. When initially seen all patients had unilateral classic Menière's disease.

RESULTS AND COMPLICATIONS

Every individual in this study underwent a thorough neurotological evaluation prior to therapy. Results are reported according to AAOO standards[13] using the class A, B, C, and D definitions for control of vertigo and stabilization of hearing. Class A suggests that the hearing improved and that the vertigo was controlled. Class B implies that the vertigo was improved and that the hearing remained stable. Class C states that the vertigo was controlled but that the hearing was made worse. Failure to control hearing or vertigo would place the individual in class D.

Most patients undergoing a middle fossa procedure had serviceable hearing (30 dB HL speech reception threshold and 80% speech discrimination score) in the involved ear at the time of surgery. Those individuals subjected to a translabyrinthine labyrinthectomy were in a "burned out" stage of Menière's disease and did not have serviceable hearing. Results and complications in both series were tabulated by an independent observer and not the surgeon.

Middle Fossa Vestibular Nerve Section (Superior and Inferior). Of the 55 patients in this series 53 were relieved of their vertigo (96%). Seven fell into the class A group (13%), 33 in class B (60%), and 13 in class C (23%). The hearing was stabilized or improved in 40 of the 55 individuals (73%). There were four dead ears (7%). In the 55 patients who underwent a middle fossa vestibular nerve section only 31 had a record that would indicate whether they had tinnitus and if it was improved or not. Of these 31, 18 (52%) had relief of their symptoms. The records were also incomplete concerning the sensation of pressure in the involved ear; however, 29 of 36 (80%) patients did state that the pressure was improved following surgery.

Complications following an intracranial procedure can be serious. There is always the possibility of extradural or subdural hematoma with resulting hemiparesis. Trauma to the temporal lobe can cause edema of the brain followed by expressive aphasia. There were no serious complications in this group. One individual developed a subdural hematoma (1.8%) during the operative procedure when the surgeon placed a suture through the dura to pull it up against the bone of the skull. In doing so an artery on the temporal lobe was injured with the cutting needle. The complication was recognized as the muscle layer was being closed. The dura was opened, the blood clot evacuated and the blood vessel cauterized with the bipolar. The individual did not develop any neurological deficit. There were two (3.6%) transient facial weaknesses that returned to normal within two weeks. Four patients (7.2%) experienced dead ears in the postoperative period. There were three wound infections (5.4%) and no CSF leaks. Eight individuals (14%) continued to experience unsteadiness in the postoperative period and never fully compensated for the loss of their vestibular function.

Translabyrinthine Labyrinthectomy. Of the 71 patients in this series 66 were relieved of their vertigo (93%). By definition none of this group could fall into either class A or B because the residual hearing was destroyed at surgery. Therefore, all 66 cases were placed in class C. Those patients not improved by surgery[5] were put into the class D category. A similar problem of record keeping occurred in the labyrinthectomy series concerning tinnitus and pressure. Twenty-three of 32 cases (72%) did have improvement in their tinnitus whereas 18 of 21 (85%) had relief of the pressure sensation. Only pure translabyrinthine labyrinthectomies are reported here. Those individuals having cochlear and vestibular nerve sections have been excluded. Of some significance is the fact that 25% of these labyrinthectomy patients continued to have unsteadiness in the postoperative period.

Complications in this group were limited to two wound infections. This is understandable considering that hearing is not a factor, that the subarachnoid space is not violated and the facial nerve is not exposed in an area where it is not covered by a thick sheath. This is a transmastoid procedure so there are none of the potential complications one would associate with an intracranial operation.

DISCUSSION

In the past ten years a large number of patients with Menière's disease have been seen at the Otology Group. Working closely with these individuals and observing their disease in all its stages has lead the authors to establish a series of criteria for medical management and surgical intervention.

At the initial visit it is extremely important to reassure the patient and explain that symptoms can be brought under control either by medical means or by one of several operations that are available. An important part of the treatment of individuals with Menière's disease is to make them feel their physician is compassionate and understands the symptoms they have been experiencing. Just the simple statement "I feel that it is possible to control your dizzy spells" is of tremendous psychological value. Once the patient's confidence has been gained, it is important to explain the disease in simple terms so that the rationale for treatment will be understood.

There is, of course, a great deal of disagreement as to the proper medical management of Menière's disease, but the authors continue to be amazed at the number of patients seen at the Otology Group who have simply had no attempt at medical control. It has been the authors' experience that 75% of these individuals will benefit from salt restriction and diuretics alone.[10] When Menière's patients become refractory to these measures they should be offered some type of surgical procedure depending upon what stage of the disease they are in when they become medical failures.

For years the only operation available was the labyrinthectomy procedure and the less frequently employed suboccipital vestibular nerve section. The labyrinthectomy operation destroys the residual hearing but has always been considered a good method of controlling vertigo. This therapy was not recommended until the patient was incapacitated by vertigo because few surgeons were willing to destroy an ear with serviceable hearing. While hearing could be preserved in some instances of suboccipital vestibular nerve section, by and large this was not the case. The early work of House,[14] Wolfson et al,[15] Fick,[16] Arslan,[17] and others were attempts to control the vertigo surgically without destroying the hearing. This led to earlier surgical intervention and in some cases success in management of the disease.

TABLE 1. POSTOPERATIVE SYMPTOMS IN MIDDLE FOSSA VESTIBULAR NERVES SECTION PATIENTS

Age (yr)	20-29	30-39	40-49	50-59	≥ 60
Total patients	6	11	21	15	2
Unsteady patients	0	0	3	4	1

Over the years the endolymphatic shunt procedure has become popular and is being used more frequently and earlier in the course of the disease in an attempt to control the hearing fluctuations. Glasscock et al[18] and House[13] have found the success rate for this procedure to be about 65%. Based upon these figures this procedure probably should be offered a patient as a first choice because its morbidity is low.

When the individual is a shunt failure or when hearing is serviceable but not fluctuating, and vertigo is severe, a middle fossa vestibular nerve section (MF) would seem a logical choice. At the beginning of this study the authors wanted to compare this procedure to the translabyrinthine labyrinthectomy (TL) with regard to the complete control of vertigo, the postoperative recovery period, and residual ataxia. By simple logic, it would seem reasonable to assume that these factors should be essentially the same, the reason being that when a total vestibular nerve section is performed the vestibular end-organ is completely denervated just as in a labyrinthectomy. While this seemed reasonable, the authors had never compared the two procedures according to these parameters.

There was no difference between the operations in the control of vertigo (MF 96%, TL 93%). The authors had assumed that the postoperative recovery period would be essentially the same and that this would depend upon two factors: age of the patient at the time of surgery and the amount of remaining vestibular function. This was not necessarily the case. Table 1 shows a breakdown according to age groups for the middle fossa cases and Table 2 depicts the labyrinthectomy patients. It is interesting to note that the MF patients had residual ataxia in 14% of the cases while 25% of the labyrinthectomy group continued to have balance problems. At first glance it might seem that this was a significant difference and that perhaps it was the removal of Scarpa's ganglion that made the difference. This might be partly true, but Tables 1 and 2 show that the labyrinthectomy group contained 19 patients over 60 years of age as compared to only 2 in the MF series. Certainly there is no question that

TABLE 2. POSTOPERATIVE SYMPTOMS IN TRANSLABYRINTHINE LABYRINTHECTOMY PATIENTS

Age (yr)	20-29	30-39	40-49	50-59	≥ 60
Total patients	3	8	20	21	19
Unsteady patients	0	1	5	7	4

TABLE 3. IPSILATERAL CALORIC FUNCTION VS POSTOPERATIVE DAYS IN HOSPITAL IN TL PATIENTS (N = 71)

Caloric	*Days*
Normal	6.1
Reduced	5.7
Absent	5.0

TL - Translabyrinthine labyrinthectomy.

TABLE 4. IPSILATERAL CALORIC FUNCTION VS POSTOPERATIVE DAYS IN HOSPITAL IN MF PATIENTS (N = 55)

Caloric	*Days*
Normal	9.2
Reduced	8.0
Absent	8.7

MF - Middle fossa vestibular nerve section.

patients in the older age range (60 +) do not compensate for the loss of one vestibular apparatus as well as younger individuals. There are several reasons for this. Most of these patients have failing vision and/or arthritis which deprive them of two important aspects of their general equilibrium.

One reason for a larger number of individuals over 60 in the labyrinthectomy group is that these patients have had their disease longer and therefore have a tendency to be in a burned-out stage. A second reason is that the surgeon involved has been reluctant to perform an intracranial procedure in older individuals because of the technical difficulties encountered at surgery. These patients have thin dura that is easily torn, difficult to elevate, and which bleeds excessively. The risks of intracranial complications, therefore, increase in the over-60 age group.

Fisch[19] has implied that the nerve section patients accommodate more readily than the labyrinthectomized individuals but this has not been the authors' experience. If two individuals have approximately the same residual vestibular function and are of compatible ages, the authors feel the recovery time is identical for vestibular nerve section and labyrinthectomized patients. The usual patient is quite miserable for approximately three days following surgery. When lying still they experience very little difficulty but upon moving their head, will become nauseated and in many instances quite vertiginous. By the fourth day, they feel much improved and can usually sit up in bed and take fluids by mouth. From this point on improvement comes daily, so that each day they feel better than the previous one. At the end of one week almost all individuals are able to be discharged from the hospital. Usually they remain somewhat unsteady and may need to brace themselves when walking by holding on to furniture or the walls. By three weeks, most have regained their balance sufficiently to perform routine daily tasks.

The authors had felt that hospital stay would be directly related to the amount of caloric function at the time of surgery. In analyzing the caloric function versus postoperative days in the hospital there appeared to be little difference (Tables 3 and 4).

While 93 and 96% relief of vertigo must be considered quite satisfactory, how can one account for those individuals who continued to have difficulty? Given the fact that they did not develop bilateral disease and if the symptoms were indeed coming from the vestibular end-organ, denervation either by nerve section or destruction should render every individual symptom free. Accepting the fact that it is seldom possible to alleviate symptoms in any patient 100% of the time, this particular question remains a mystery. Perhaps in association with Menière's the individual had a second disease process such as multiple sclerosis. Discounting this circumstance, one must consider the possibility of some central problem related to the long duration of time the individual experienced a defective labyrinth. There may be some poorly understood process in the vestibular nuclei of the brainstem that occurs as a result of misinformation from the malfunctioning neuroepithelium of the vestibular end-organ affected by Menière's disease.

There is no question that both the middle fossa nerve section and the labyrinthectomy procedures are effective in controlling the symptom of vertigo in Menière's disease. Their indications are different based upon the amount of residual hearing present at the time of surgery. Menière's patients in the burned-out stage, if they are to undergo surgery, should definitely have a labyrinthectomy. The authors continue to see individuals who are incapacitated by their disease and refractory to medical management, yet a straightforward destructive procedure has never been suggested to them as a solution to their problem. When they are finally operated upon they are extremely grateful individuals and their whole outlook on life changes. Much the same can be said of candidates for vestibular nerve section, as these patients are extremely happy after surgery. Most no longer experience any vertigo, their hearing stabilizes and they can lead more normal lives.

This study has proven to the authors that the success rate for the control of vertigo is essentially the same for middle fossa vestibular nerve section and translabyrinthine labyrinthectomy. The recovery periods and probably the persistent unsteadiness rates are essentially the same. For this reason the authors feel quite strongly that labyrinthectomy should not be offered to a patient with serviceable hearing unless there is some extenuating circumstance to preclude a middle fossa vestibular nerve section. The authors have seen several patients who had undergone a labyrinthectomy elsewhere when they had serviceable hearing in the involved ear. Several years later they developed Menière's disease in their only hearing ear. When recommending the initial surgery it is extremely important to keep in mind that bilateral disease does occur. If a patient has serviceable hearing, the operation should be one in which the hearing is spared the majority of the time.

When a patient presents with bilateral disease the authors do not recommend unilateral or bilateral middle fossa vestibular nerve section. In these cases it is much better to treat the patient with streptomycin injections as described by Singleton and Schuknecht[20] as the vestibular function can be ablated bilaterally with the preservation of residual hearing.

Because of all these factors, it is extremely important for the surgeon to study each patient carefully, take into consideration his occupation, his emotional status and the hearing in his involved and opposite ear before making a decision as to what type of surgical procedure to recommend. Above all, the patient must not be made to continue to suffer the consequence of his disease without aggressive medical and/or surgical management by his physician.

REFERENCES

1. Pulec JL. Labyrinthectomy: indications, technique and results. Laryngoscope 1974; 84:1552-73.

2. Dandy WE. The surgical treatment of Meniere's disease. Surg Gynecol Obstet 1941; 72:421-5.

3. House WF. Cryosurgical treatment of Meniere's disease. Arch Otolaryngol 1966; 84:616-29.

4. Glasscock ME. Evaluation of the neurotologic patient. Trans Pac Coast Otoophthalmol Soc 1969; 50:341-50.

5. Fowler EP. The diagnosis of diseases of the neural mechanism of hearing by the aid of sounds well above threshold. Trans Am Otol Soc 1937; 27:207-19.

6. Jerger J. DL difference test: improved method for clinical measurement of recruitment. Arch Otolaryngol 1953; 57: 490-500.

7. Glasscock ME, Jackson CJ, Josey AF, Dicking JR, Wiet JR. Brain stem evoked response audiometry in a clinical practice. Laryngoscope 1979; 89:1021-34.

8. Jerger J. Diagnostic use of impedance measures. In: Jerger J, ed. Handbook of clinical impedance audiometry. New York: American, 1975:149-74.

9. Klockhoff I, Lindblom U. Glycerol test and diuretics in Meniere's disease. Otolaryngol Clin North Am 1968;541-9.

10. Jackson CG, Glasscock ME III, Davis WE, Hughes GB, Sismanis A. The medical management of Meniere's disease. Ann Otol Rhinol Laryngol (in press).

11. Arenberg IK, Stahle J, Glasscock ME III, Shambaugh EG Jr. Endolymphatic sac valve implant surgery I. Technique. Laryngoscope 1979; 89 Suppl 17.

12. Glasscock ME, Miller GW. Middle fossa vestibular nerve section in the management of Meniere's disease. Laryngoscope 1977; 87:529-41.

13. Committee on Hearing and Equilibrium. Report of the subcommittee on equilibrium and its measurement. Trans Am Acad Ophthalmol Otolaryngol 1972; 76:1462-4.

14. House WF. Subarachnoid shunt for drainage of endolymphatic hydrops. Laryngoscope 1962; 72:713-29.

15. Wolfson RJ, Cutt RA, Myers D. Cryosurgery of the labyrinth: preliminary report of a new surgical procedure. Laryngoscope 1966; 76:733-57.

16. Fick IA. Sacculotomy. Otolaryngol Clin North Am 1968;625-35.

17. Arslan M. Treatment of Meniere's syndrome by direct application of ultrasound waves to the vestibular system. Proceedings of the international congress of otolaryngology. Amsterdam, 1953:429-36.

18. Glasscock ME, Miller GW, Drake FD, Kanok MM. Surgical management of Meniere's disease with endolymphatic subarachnoid shunts: a five-year study. Laryngosocpe 1977; 87:1668-75.

19. Fisch U. Vestibular and cochlear neurectomy. Trans Am Acad Ophthalmol Otolaryngol 1974; 78:252-5.

20. Singleton EF, Schuknecht HF. Streptomycin sulfate in the management of Meniere's disease. Otolaryngol Clin North Am 1968; 531-9.

Ann Otol 89:1980

ATTACHMENT OF THE TECTORIAL MEMBRANE REVEALED BY SCANNING ELECTRON MICROSCOPE

MERLE LAWRENCE, PhD

PAUL A. BURGIO, MA

ANN ARBOR, MICHIGAN

Our present-day descriptions of the causes of many forms of sensorineural deafness are based on what is known about the morphology of the organ of Corti. Unfortunately, this information is still woefully inadequate for a complete interpretation of normal events within this structure. Nevertheless there has been no shortage of theories based, in part at least, on assumptions of what the unknown morphology might be. One of the least understood structures is the tectorial membrane, for which the extent and position have had many descriptions. A review of these reveals that the observations vary with the techniques used, and different techniques have various effects on the sticky gel of the tectorial membrane which is reported to be 90% water. Here is described a technique whereby the bulk frozen-hydrated tectorial membrane is viewed by scanning electron microscopy. In its natural living state the tectorial membrane is sealed to the Hensen's cells, protecting the reticular lamina from endolymph.

The pathology of many forms of sensorineural deafness will never be understood until we know much more about the organ of Corti than we now know. Temporary threshold shifts resulting from loud sounds, tinnitus, and fluctuant hearing loss are examples of auditory phenomena for which there is no explanation. Certainly one of the most obvious reasons for our inability to fathom the altered physiology is our lack of even the basic morphology of the organ of Corti, and the main reason for this lies in the difficulty of approaching the inner ear for study without altering it in some way.

In general, the action of the organ of Corti has been described in mostly mechanical terms. The popular notion is that the organ of Corti moves up and down on the basilar membrane and that the tectorial membrane pulls on the stereocilia of the sensory cells, somehow producing a stimulus to the nerve endings. Theory has it that increased fluid pressure resulting from the hydrops of Menière's disease alters this process, and that too violent a motion produces a depletion of necessary metabolic elements producing a temporary threshold shift.

But for many decades the exact extent and position of the tectorial membrane has had many descriptions, and theories of operation have depended upon which observation is considered valid. For the most part, each conclusion has depended upon the technique used to make the study.

Interestingly, this problem has produced much conflicting evidence which makes it difficult to resolve. When Hilding published his paper in 1952[1] on the origin and insertion of the tectorial membrane, he mentioned that not only has this topic been the subject of study and speculation for many years, but also resolving the problem is one of paramount importance if one is to understand the physiology and pathology of hearing.

Hilding reported that the insertion of the tectorial membrane in his specimens was firm enough to lift and rotate the entire organ of Corti and basilar membrane during attempts to remove it. As he described it this insertion is quite complex, consisting of four planes which are fused together (Fig. 1A). One is a continuous membrane which extends inward from the slope of Hensen's cells across the top of the organ of Corti. Above this there is a marginal membrane or net extending from the thicker portion of the tectorial membrane over the top of Hensen's cells to their base. The *Randfasernetz* of Held[2] is a torn remnant of this. He also describes long tongue-like processes of cement substance attached to the undersurface of the tectorial membrane and extending to its outer slope (Hensen's cells). Hensen's stripe is reported to be attached to the border cell supporting the inner hair cell.

Corti[3] in 1851 had said of the tectorial membrane, "Beyond the external limit [hair cells] the same membrane [tectorial membrane] extends over the pectinate zone which follows, and nearly covers three rows of epithelial cells." In a footnote he explains these epithelial cells as being close together and in contact with each other which describes Hensen's cells.

Tonndorf et al,[4] in experiments using various stains in living animals, found the tectorial membrane adhering tightly to Hensen's cells, confirming Hilding and the even earlier observations of de Vries[5] who froze fresh temporal bones in liquid air

From the Kresge Hearing Research Institute, Department of Otorhinolaryngology, University of Michigan Medical School, Ann Arbor, Michigan. This research was supported by PHS grants NS-11731 and NS-05785.

Presented at the meeting of the American Otological Society, Inc., Palm Beach, Florida, April 13-14, 1980.

REPRINTS — Merle Lawrence, PhD, Kresge Hearing Research Institute, Department of Otorhinolaryngology, University of Michigan Medical School, 1301 E. Ann Street, Ann Arbor, MI 48109.

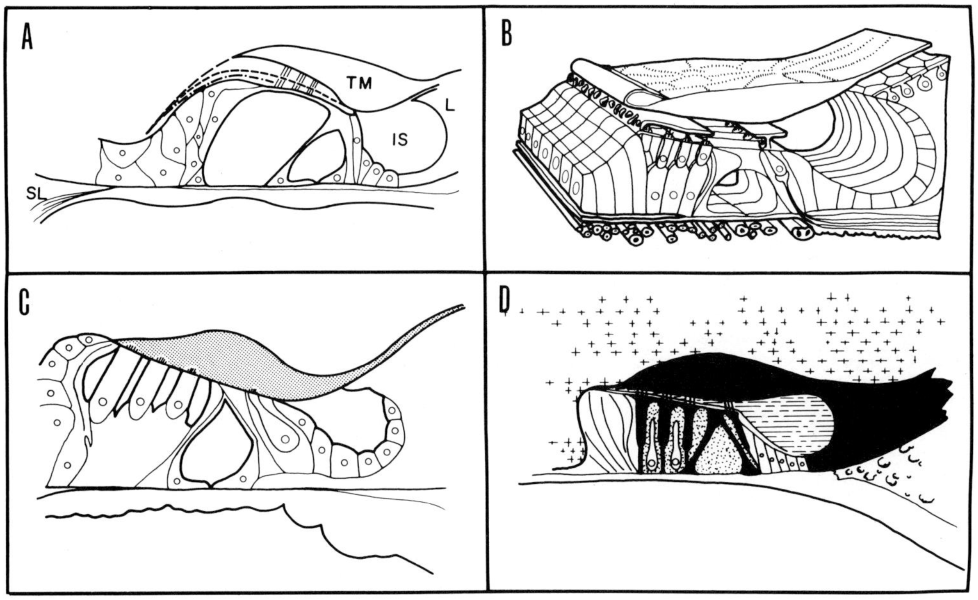

Fig. 1. Various existing descriptions of tectorial membrane attachment. A) Hilding, B) Lim, C) Ross, and D) Rauch. TM - Tympanic membrane; L - Spiral limbus; IS - Inner sulcus.

and then broke them into fragments to make his observations. It is interesting that Tonndorf used, among many other stains, Janus green B, the same as that used by Békésy[6] to facilitate observation of the tectorial membrane. This stain, when applied to the scala media surface, provides an impressive view of the tectorial membrane, but it soon causes the seal at Hensen's cells to break.

With the advent of new techniques, different concepts of the tectorial membrane have developed. Lim[7] prepared the temporal bones of various animals for scanning and transmission electron microscopy and gave a very thorough study of the tectorial membrane (Fig. 1B). He describes the "outer" margin of the tectorial membrane as being formed by a marginal net anchored to the phalanges of the outermost row of Deiters' cells, Hensen's cells, or both. This marginal complex appeared as "finger-like processes or ladder-like bands which would allow the passage of endolymph."

In a rather extensive investigation, Ross[8] employed several different techniques in a study of the tectorial membrane of the rat (Fig. 1C). Her description is somewhat different from the rest but still consistent with the view that endolymph does not flow beneath the tectorial membrane. Her method of study has revealed the membrane as attached to the reticular lamina and to the hair tips of the outer hair cells. It is attached to the inner hair cells enclosing the hairs. Tiny fluid compartments may exist beneath the tectorial membrane, around the hairs of the inner cells.

Rauch,[9] following a biochemical analysis of the fluids within the spaces of the organ of Corti obtained by separating the frozen areas, concluded that the tectorial membrane is sealed and that it forms a closed space with the reticular lamina such that the fluid within the inner sulcus and subtectorial space has its own unique chemical constituency (Fig. 1D).

Another approach to the question of whether or not the tectorial membrane is sealed against endolymph is to compare the chemical composition of the fluid in the subtectorial space with that of endolymph. Rauch made this comparison and concluded that these fluids are different. Use of x-ray microanalysis makes possible the determination of element concentration by electron probe.

Utilizing this method, Ross's studies were interpreted as showing the tectorial membrane having an ionic composition different from both endolymph and perilymph, a conclusion similar to that of Rauch.

On the other hand, Flock,[10] using similar methods, found high potassium content in endolymph and in the tectorial membrane indicating that the tectorial membrane is not a barrier and that the hair-bearing ends of the hair cells are exposed to endolymph.

Why is there such a difference in the conclusions reached from these various studies? There are many more studies of the tectorial membrane than those reported here, and in reviewing them it becomes apparent that the observations vary in accordance with the technique used. As Lindeman et al[11] have pointed out, an obvious reason is the technical difficulty of preserving the tectorial membrane in its normal form and position during preparation for study. All processes of chemical fixation and embedding alter the shape and attachment of the tectorial membrane. Conventional histology with cel-

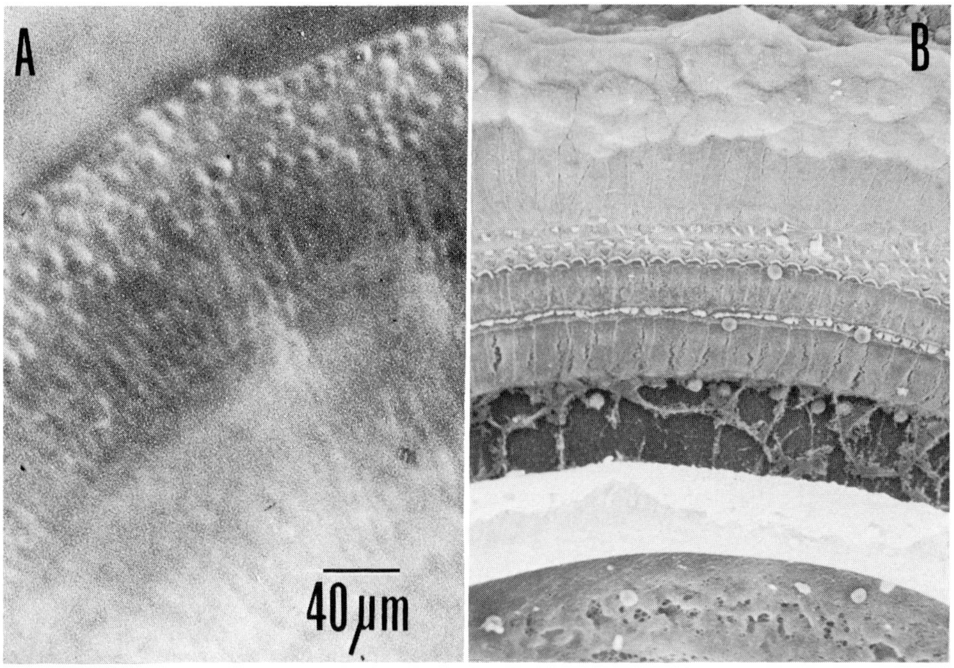

Fig. 2. A view of the organ of Corti from "above." A) In the apical turn of the living guinea pig the tectorial membrane is seen as an almost transparent structure but striations can be seen passing over the hair cells and on to Hensen's cells. B) For orientation and comparison the organ of Corti stripped of the tectorial membrane is shown in comparable magnification by scanning electron microscopy. Preparations made by Paul Burgio.

loidin embedding almost always shows the tectorial membrane detached and floating free above the organ of Corti. Methods of preparation for scanning electron microscopy are bound to be equally devastating.

The component of greatest quantity in any biological material is water, reported to be 70 to 80% of the total weight. The tectorial membrane is described as a gel with more than 90% water in its "solid" constitution[12] and as having a unique ionic content. The shape and attachment of this membrane are considerably altered by hydration-dehydration changes, thus it is extremely sensitive and subject to change by any method of histological processing. All of the reports referred to here that have involved examining the tectorial membrane in its natural living state report it sealed and extending over Hensen's cells.[1,3-5,9,12] Measures[13,14] of the electric DC potentials in the various fluid spaces of the organ of Corti have also indicated this seal, and Naftalin[15] has discussed the theoretical implications.

All of the reports that have used a fixative, and except for Ross,[8] have presented pictures with the tectorial membrane unattached and a free-flow of endolymph around it.[7,10,11]

Because the position of the tectorial membrane in vivo is almost impossible to picture, a technique has been needed that can demonstrate the normal condition without changing the original structural relationships (Fig. 2). Since water plays an important role in maintaining the structure and function of the tectorial membrane its removal most certainly will produce changes in the membrane's morphology. Fixation for histology and conventional preparation for electron microscopy require dehydration. Unfortunately, because of the high vacuum employed, observing hydrated specimens in the electron microscope has been difficult. Freezing techniques have been used but maintenance of temperature and avoidance of dehydration have been a problem.

Burgio,[16] as part of his doctoral dissertation, has successfully developed a method whereby the hydrated unaltered organ of Corti and tectorial membrane can be observed on a cold stage by scanning electron microscopy. This has made possible accurate determination of the morphology of the structure as well as permitting exact electron probe microanalysis of ionic content of the various fluid spaces.

METHODS

A complete description of the method used is in Burgio's thesis.[16] Here we report only a short summary.

In these preparations guinea pigs and gerbils have been used. The animals are anesthetized and prepared as usual for surgery. After exposure through a ventral approach in the living animal the cochlea is quenched in Freon® -22 cooled by liquid nitrogen at − 190 C. From this point on, the specimen is maintained in a liquid nitrogen bath until it is transported to the cold stage. The cochlea is removed by saw cuts and prepared for placement in a unique specially designed holder.

The specimen is shaped to fit into the holder with the surfaces fine polished and with aluminum foil under the specimen to assure good thermal conduction between specimen and holder. This tissue is secured in the receptacle of the holder and the view-

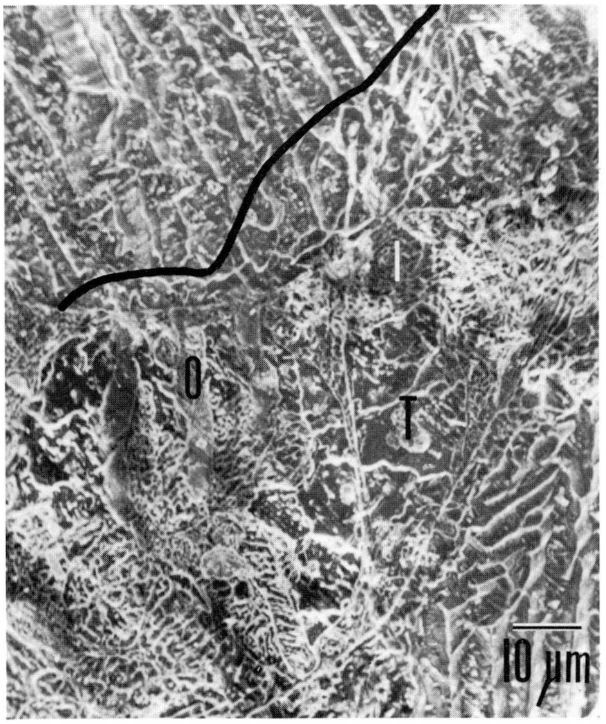

Fig. 3. The organ of Corti and tectorial membrane in the bulk frozen-hydrated state as seen through the scanning electron microscope. The inserted dark line marks the endolymphatic border of the tectorial membrane. The arch and hair cells can be seen. O - Outer hair cells; I - Inner hair cells; T - Tunnel.

ing surface prepared under a dissecting microscope. It is essential that all preparation be done well below the surface of the liquid nitrogen and that the cutting tool be cooled to the same temperature.

The viewing surface on the specimen is prepared by a cutting tool which was chosen to assure that the viewing surface is flat and smooth and is in the same plane as the surface of the specimen holder. The holder was designed to maintain the specimen at cryogenic temperature, and thereby prevent the generation of artifacts when transferring the specimen from the liquid nitrogen bath to the cold stage in the scanning electron microscope.

The specimen temperature upon arrival at the cold stage is about − 185 C and hydration has been maintained. The polished flat surface of interest is normal to the electron beam when the holder is placed on the cold stage, so the goniometer can be used to adjust the take-off angle for maximum collection efficiency. The specimen was viewed in a JSM U-3 scanning electron microscope and specimen temperature was maintained by a Joule-Thompson refrigerator. A cryo-tip panel (Air Products) was used to regulate the pressure of nitrogen gas feeding the refrigerator thus controlling the temperature of the specimen.

RESULTS

When first viewed, the prepared surface of the frozen-hydrated specimen appears featureless. As water sublimates off with slightly rising temperature more morphological detail is revealed. At a very early stage of this process the fine structures of the organ of Corti can be seen with minimal distortion due to dehydration.

Figure 3 shows the bulk frozen-hydrated specimen with minimal surface water sublimated. In this figure details of the tectorial membrane are outlined. In Figure 4A the same picture is shown without an outline. This specimen has been cut through at a slight angle as evidenced by the section through two outer hair cells. This angle of cut also gives the basilar membrane an uneven appearance.

The tectorial membrane thickens immediately upon leaving the limbus and makes contact with the supporting cell around the inner hair cell. This is the region of Hensen's stripe and is the region of greatest thickness of the membrane. Directly above the row of outer hair cells the membrane reduces down to a very thin membrane. This is not a porous net but a continuous solid membrane which on dehydration breaks free from its attachment to Hensen's cells and shrinks unevenly giving the appearance of a net — the *Randfasernetz* of Held. In the normal position this thin portion of the tectorial membrane extends over Hensen's cells after its attachment, just as described by Hilding. Lim[7] in his paper shows a view of the undersurface of the tectorial membrane by scanning electron microscopy. His picture fits perfectly with what we have just described, showing Hensen's stripe for attachment at the inner hair cell and the outer hair cell hair imprints just at the edge of tectorial membrane thinning to show remnants of the thin extension after being broken free from Hensen's cells by dehydration.

With slightly rising temperature and minimal further sublimation (Fig. 4B), the tectorial membrane thins somewhat and shrinks in its long dimension breaking the attachment to Hensen's cells. The last portion to break free from the reticular lamina is Hensen's stripe. Figure 4 B, C, and D show progressive steps of these changes. As sublimation continues the features of the organ of Corti become more readily distinguishable. In Figure 4C the tectorial membrane has become completely separated from the organ of Corti.

CONCLUSIONS

The picture that results from this study is that the tectorial membrane normally lies close to the reticular lamina from the inner hair cell supporting cell to the outermost hair cell where the membrane thins down to attach to and extend over the Hensen's cells. Much support for this observation has recently come from other studies. Kohllöffel,[17] reporting for several species of animals (sheep, cow, pig, guinea pig, golden hamster, and mole), describes that in all of these there were preparations where the tectorial membrane is attached to the organ of Corti. "The attachment was firm so that teasing the tectorial membrane deformed the organ of Corti and teasing the organ of Corti deformed the tectorial membrane."[17]

Kronester-Frei[18,19] has developed a preparation

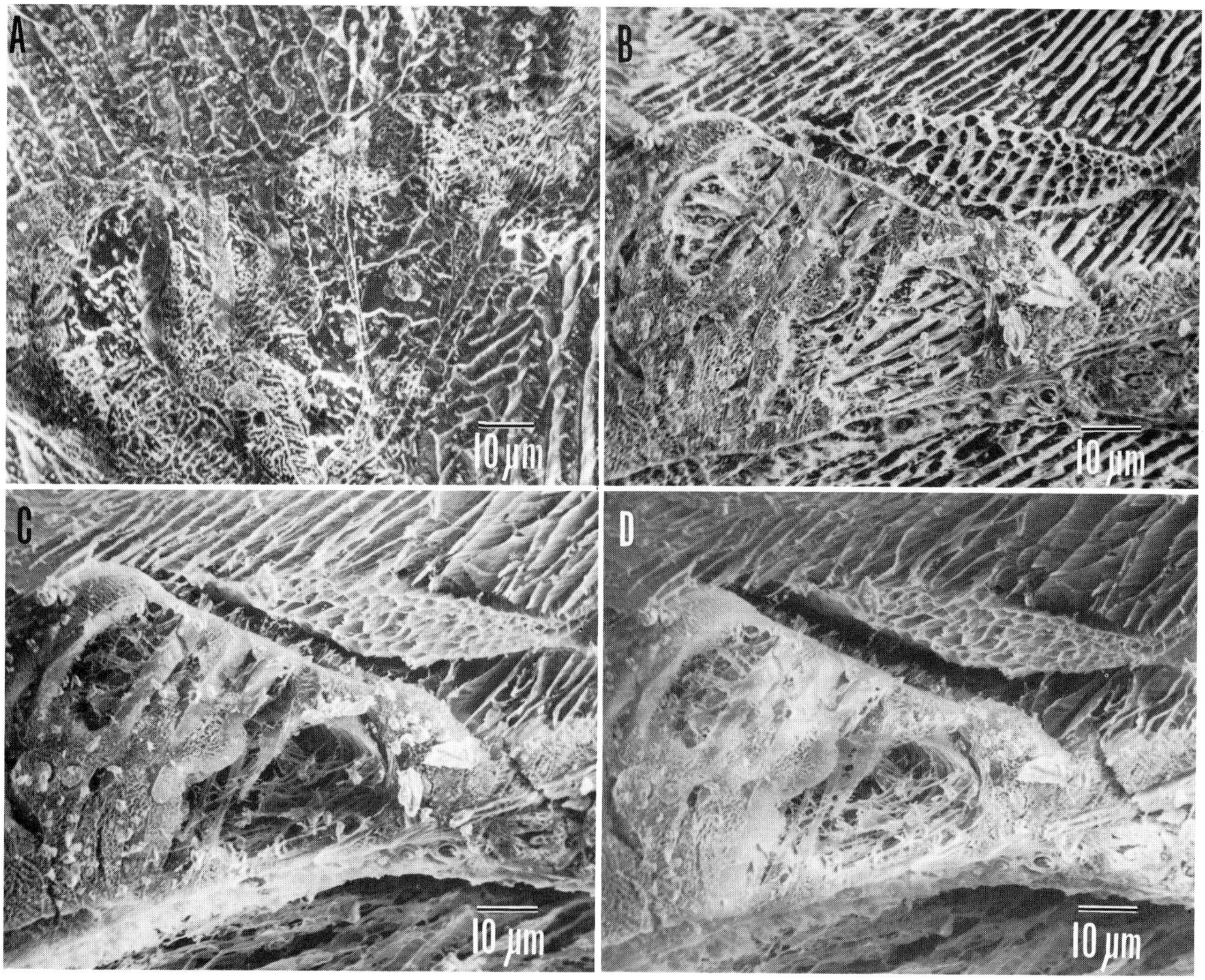

Fig. 4. The appearance and position of the tectorial membrane as the ice crystals sublimate with slight rise in temperature. A) Same view as Fig. 2 with minimal sublimation; temperature −85 C; B) 10 minutes after A, temperature −75 C; C) 30 minutes after A, temperature −50 C; D) 45 minutes after A, temperature −35 C.

making it possible to study the unfixed tectorial membrane in its normal position in relation to the cochlea and with in vivo-like ionic condition. Under normal conditions she observed that "the marginal zone lies in close contact with the organ of Corti" so that the subtectorial space is sealed from the endolymph. She reports further that a change in the ionic content of endolymph, by such a solution as perilymph, changes its hydration state and size. The membrane shrinks and detaches from the organ of Corti.

These observations have provided us with an answer to a puzzling paradox. It is now well established that the fluid spaces of the organ of Corti are filled with so-called Cortilymph which is a special variation of perilymph produced by the spiral capillaries of the osseous spiral lamina. It is also well documented that if Reissner's membrane is broken and perilymph enters the scala media, the hair cells degenerate. Why should perilymph from one direction destroy the hair cells while from the other it does not?

Now we know, from Kronester-Frei's work, that the change in ionic content of the endolymph causes the protecting tectorial membrane to shrink and detach allowing the high potassium of the endolymph to enter the subtectorial space and affect the hair cells.

This also suggests an explanation for those auditory phenomena for which we have had, until now, no explanation. Any slight change in the ionic content of endolymph changes the normal attachment of the tectorial membrane, allowing an abnormal ionic fluid to bathe the cuticular plate of the hair cells. This need not be permanent because the tectorial membrane, constantly being regenerated by the spiral limbus, can repair itself. Temporary threshold shifts, tinnitus, and fluctuating hearing loss could be produced this way.

Aside from faulty absorption of endolymph by

the endolymphatic sac, a hydrops could be produced by osmotic changes in the endolymph-perilymph condition, and the changed chemical composition of endolymph producing this might well affect both the auditory and nonauditory labyrinth.

REFERENCES

1. Hilding AC. Studies on the otic labyrinth: on the origin and insertion of the tectorial membrane. Ann Otol Rhinol Laryngol 1952; 61:354-70.

2. Held H. Die Cochlea der Säuger und der Vögel, ihre Entwicklung und ihr Bau. In: Bethe A. Handbuch der normalen und pathologischen Physiologie: II. Receptionsorgane. Berlin: Springer, 1926:476-534.

3. Corti A. Recherches sur l'organe de l'ouie des mammifères. Z Wiss Zool 1851; 3:109-69.

4. Tonndorf J, Duvall AJ, Reneau JP. Permeability of intracochlear membranes to various vital stains. Ann Otol Rhinol Laryngol 1962; 71:801-41.

5. deVries HL. Struktur und Lage der Tektorialmembran in der Schnecke, untersucht mit neueren Hilfsmitteln. Acta Otolaryngol (Stockh) 1949; 37:334-8.

6. von Békésy G. Experiments in hearing. New York: McGraw-Hill, 1960:488.

7. Lim DJ. Fine morphology of the tectorial membrane. Arch Otolaryngol 1972; 96:199-215.

8. Ross MD. The tectorial membrane of the rat. Am J Anat 1974; 139:449-81.

9. Rauch S. Entstehung, Transport und Resorption der Innenohrflüssigkeiten. In: Rauch S. Biochemie des Hörogans. Stuttgart: Thieme, 1964:278.

10. Flock Å. Electron probe determination of relative ion distribution in the inner ear. Acta Otolaryngol (Stockh) 1977; 83:239-44.

11. Lindeman HH, Ades HW, Bredberg G, Engström H. The sensory hairs and the tectorial membrane in the development of the cat's organ of Corti. Acta Otolaryngol (Stockh) 1971; 72:229-42.

12. Naftalin L, Harrison MS, Stephens A. The character of the tectorial membrane. J Laryngol Otol 1964; 78:1061-78.

13. Lawrence M, Nuttall AL, Clapper MD. Electrical potentials and fluid boundaries within the organ of Corti. J Acoust Soc Am 1974; 55:122-38.

14. Tanaka Y, Asanuma A, Yanagisawa K, Katsuki Y. DC potential and distribution of the cochlear microphonic potential. Audiol Jpn 1975; 18:241-5 (in Japanese).

15. Naftalin L. The peripheral hearing mechanism: new biophysical concepts for transduction of the acoustic signal to an electrochemical event. Physiol Chem Phys 1977; 9:337-82.

16. Burgio PA. The distribution of ions in the fluid spaces of the organ of Corti. Thesis, University of Michigan, Ann Arbor, 1980.

17. Kohllöffel LUE. On the connection membrana Corti — organ of Corti. Institut National de la Santé et de la. Recherche Mèdicale, 1977:15-24.

18. Kronester-Frei A. Localization of the marginal zone of the tectorial membrane in situ, unfixed, and with in-vivo-like ionic milieu. Arch Otorhinolaryngol 1979; 224:3-9.

19. Kronester-Frei A. The effect of changes in endolymphatic ion concentrations on the tectorial membrane. Hear Res 1979; 1:81-94.

≈

SECOND INTERNATIONAL CONFERENCE ON CHOLESTEATOMA AND MASTOID SURGERY

The Second International Conference on Cholesteatoma and Mastoid Surgery will be held March 22-27, 1981 in Tel-Aviv, Israel under the auspices of Tel-Aviv University and Weizmann Institute of Science. For further information contact: Professor J. Sade, P. O. Box 16271, Tel-Aviv, Israel. Telex: 342272 (Kenes) Tel-Aviv.

MYRINGOPLASTY

A REVIEW OF 472 CASES

JAMES L. SHEEHY, MD
LOS ANGELES, CALIFORNIA

ROBERT G. ANDERSON, MD
DALLAS, TEXAS

We reviewed the records of 472 patients who had undergone myringoplasty during an 11-year period at the Otologic Medical Group. There was a statistically significant relationship between the size of the perforation and the degree of hearing impairment, but no relationship between the degree of impairment and the complaint of tinnitus. The majority of operations were performed using the lateral surface fascia grafting technique. Those 168 operations performed postauricularly were successful in closing the tympanic membrane perforation in over 97% of the cases and in reducing the conductive deficit to 10 dB or less in 88%. There were no total sensorineural impairments, although 3% of the patients developed a high tone sensorineural impairment. Blunting in the anterior sulcus and lateral healing of the graft were very uncommon. Canal skin was used as a graft in 16% of the patients. The graft take results and hearing results were less favorable than with fascia.

Patients undergoing myringoplasty are an ideal group to study to determine the effect of a tympanic membrane perforation on the hearing mechanism and to evaluate the effectiveness of tympanic membrane grafting techniques. This is a review of 472 primary myringoplasty operations performed at the Otologic Medical Group over an 11-year period.

DEFINITION

Myringoplasty is an operation in which the reconstructive procedure is limited to repair of a tympanic membrane perforation.[1] Implicit in the definition is that the ossicular chain is intact and mobile and that there is no middle ear disease such as infected mucosa or ingrowth of skin. Exploration of the middle ear and ossicular chain is a routine part of most myringoplasty operations.

We reviewed the charts of all patients at the Otologic Medical Group who had had a myringoplasty performed during the years 1967-1977. There were 545 operations of which 472 were primary procedures. These 472 myringoplasties represent 10% of the primary operations performed during the 11 years on patients with tympanic membrane perforations. We did not contact patients for additional follow-up. All had early follow-up information but only 50% had been observed for one year or more (Table 1).

TABLE 1. LENGTH OF FOLLOW-UP IN CASES WITH INITIAL GRAFT TAKE

Length of Follow-Up (mo)	%
≥ 2	100
≥ 6	82
≥ 12	51
≥ 24	32

PREOPERATIVE INFORMATION

Age. We do not usually recommend elective tympanic membrane grafting on patients under the age of seven because of the possibility of postoperative middle ear effusion or patient management problems. There were, however, three 6-year-olds, four 5-year-olds and one child of 4 years in this series. All but one had had a recurrent discharge problem without any evidence of serous effusion in the opposite ear. Of the total myringoplasties performed, 88% were on patients 16 years of age or older (Table 2).

TABLE 2. PRIMARY CASES BY AGE (N = 472)

Age of Patients (yr)	%
≤ 6 (8 cases)	2
≤ 15	12
≥ 16	88
≥ 70 (13 cases)	3

Etiology. The majority of patients stated that their problem was the result of infection (Table 3). Slag injuries were uncommon in this study because injuries of this type usually result in a middle ear problem which takes them out of the category of myringoplasty despite an intact and mobile ossicular chain.

Duration of Disease. The few patients with slag injuries and those with traumatic perforations usually sought operative treatment within a year of injury. The majority of those whose disease was the

TABLE 3. FIRST EAR ONLY (N = 446)

Etiology of Perforation	%
Chronic otitis media	78
Trauma	19
Slag injury	3

From the Otologic Medical Group, Inc., Los Angeles, California. Supported by funds from the Ear Research Institute, Los Angeles, California.
Presented at the meeting of the American Otological Society, Inc., Palm Beach, Florida, April 13-14, 1980.
REPRINTS — James L. Sheehy, MD, 2122 West Third Street, Los Angeles, CA 90057.

TABLE 4. PRIMARY CASES, 1967-1977 (N = 472)

Graft Material	%
Fascia	71
Canal skin	16
Other*	13

*Fascia combined with canal skin; perichondrium; homograft.

result of infection delayed surgery for five years or more.

Tinnitus. Myringoplasty cases are an ideal group to evaluate tinnitus in relationship to the degree of hearing impairment. Theoretically there is no disease other than the perforation of the tympanic membrane. A statement in regard to tinnitus was found in 85% of the records examined. Tinnitus was present in 90% of the small number of slag injuries and 55% of the remainder.

We expected to find that patients with a 20 dB or more conductive deficit would be more likely to notice tinnitus than those with an impairment of 10 dB or less. Furthermore, we expected that those with some degree of sensorineural impairment would be more likely to notice tinnitus. We were not able to prove either of these assumptions. In fact, those with a minimal impairment were more likely to notice tinnitus, but the difference did not prove to be statistically significant.

Size of Perforation. We were interested in determining whether there was relationship between the size of the perforation and the degree of conductive impairment. Thirteen (60%) of 22 large perforations (more than 75% of the drumhead) were associated with a conductive impariment of 21 dB or more, and the mean impairment was 21 dB. Two patients (10%), however, had an impairment of 10 dB or less. There were 166 small perforations (quadrant size), and 55% of these patients had an impairment of 10 dB or less, with a mean of 13 dB. (Anteriorly located perforations were associated with this minimal gap three fourths of the time.) Eighteen patients (10%), however, had an impairment of 21 dB or more. The majority of perforations (224) were of medium size and 70% of these patients had an impairment greater than 10 dB (mean of 17 dB). The difference between impairments in the small and the large perforations was statistically significant ($X^2 = 74.3$, $P = 0.001$). Differences between small and medium, and medium and large perforations were not statistically significant.

GRAFTING TECHNIQUE

The 472 operations were performed by 14 otologists, six of whom are present members of the Group. These six performed 55% of the procedures. The lateral grafting technique was used in all but 12 cases. The majority of operations were with fascia, but a significant number were performed with canal skin or a combination of canal skin and fascia (Table 4).

TABLE 5. HEALING PROBLEMS IN FASCIA GRAFT CASES

Healing Problems	%
Temporary canal stenosis	1.3
Anterior blunting	1.3
Lateral healing	0.7
Persistent epithelitis of membrane	1.3

Canal Skin. We used the canal skin grafting technique frequently in the 1960s.[2] One member of our Group still prefers canal skin for closing a small perforation.

Fascia. We have described in detail the lateral surface fascia grafting technique using autograft fascia, dehydrating and rehydrating it before use.[3] This technique involves removal of canal skin, removal of the anterior canal bulge, lateral grafting with fasica placed under the malleus handle and replacement of canal skin. All but two in our Group use a postauricular approach with this technique. The 168 operations performed postauricularly will be reported separately throughout the paper as a selected group of cases.

Lateral surface grafting has come under considerable criticism. Experienced otologists who are advocates of either the lateral (onlay) or medial (underlay) grafting techniques appear to obtain almost identical results. But those not experienced have had more difficulty with the lateral surface technique, and it is indeed more difficult for the novice.

The novice will find that the medial surface technique is less difficult and is not associated with the healing problems which occur occasionally when using the lateral surface technique. He may also have a lower rate of graft take until he obtains proficiency with the technique.[3] In contrast, the lateral surface technique, although more difficult for the novice to master, will give him greater exposure and a higher graft take rate. But healing problems, particularly blunting in the anterior sulcus and lateral healing of the graft, may occur until the technique is mastered. That these problems have not been frequent in our hands is obvious from Table 5.

RESULTS OF SURGERY

We would like to report that almost all patients had a successful graft take and a postoperative conductive deficit of 10 dB or less. This was not the case unless we look only at those 31% operated on with the recommended technique: postauricular approach,

TABLE 6. GRAFT FAILURE IN PRIMARY CASES WITH 6 MONTHS OR MORE FOLLOW-UP

	All Cases (N = 387)	*Canal Skin (N = 64)*	*Fascia (N = 273)*	*Fascia (Selected Group) (N = 153)*
Graft failure	12.1%	15.6%	9.5%	2.6%
≤6 mo	9.0%	10.9%	7.7%	2.0%
Late	3.1%	4.7%	1.8%	0.6%

TABLE 7. POSTOPERATIVE CONDUCTIVE DEFICIT IN SUCCESSFULLY GRAFTED CASES WITH 6 MONTHS OR MORE FOLLOW-UP

Postoperative Conductive Deficit (dB)	*All Cases (N = 340)*	*Canal Skin (N = 54)*	*Fascia (Selected Group) (N = 149)*
≤ 5	58%	53%	69%
≤ 10	79%	68%	88%
≤ 15	93%	93%	96%
≤ 20	96%	98%	97%

fascia graft only, always placed under the malleus handle. This group is referred to as the selected group (Tables 6 and 7).

Graft Failure. The selected group fascia graft failure rate was less than 3% (Table 6). The overall failure rate in primary cases with six months or more follow-up was unacceptably high: 9%. A small but significant number of cases failed later. The canal skin graft results were less favorable than the fascia graft results, a not unanticipated finding.[4] In recent years this technique has been used by one of our Group only in small inferior perforations and the initial graft take rate has been comparable to the fascia.

Healing Problems. Many advocates of the undersurface technique comment that one of the major reasons for using that technique is to avoid the healing problems encountered with lateral surface grafting: anterior blunting and lateral healing. Having used the lateral surface grafting technique almost exclusively since 1955, members or our Group became experts on these problems and how to prevent them: always remove the anterior canal wall bulge, never place the fascia on the anterior canal wall and always place the fascia under the malleus handle (or under the lateral epitympanic wall when the malleus is absent).[3] Healing problems still occur at times but in less than 2% of the cases (Table 5).

Hearing Results. We determine the postoperative conductive deficit by comparing the postoperative air conduction level (averaged at 500, 1,000 and 2,000 Hz) with the best bone conduction (BC) level (averaged at the same frequencies) obtained at any time, and in most cases this is a postoperative BC level. We believe that using the best BC level gives a truer picture of the mechanical efficiency of the reconstruction than does computing the gap closure based entirely on the preoperative BC which may be influenced, particularly in unilateral cases, by the affect of masking.

One would expect a successful myringoplasty to have a perfect hearing result: a postoperative deficit of 5 dB or less. This was not the case (Table 7). Overall less than two thirds are within 5 dB and only 80% are within 10 dB. The selected group of fascia graft cases heard better, but not by much. An easy and immediate explanation of this is the commonly stated (and to a certain extent true) statement that laterally grafted drums are thicker. But canal skin grafted drums tend to be very thin and the results were not better in this small group of cases (Table 7). The most likely explanation for this lack of complete success from a hearing standpoint is that in most cases of chronic otitis media, even though the ossicular chain may appear normal, there is some factor of scar tissue which prevents total restoration of hearing. The findings in Table 8 tend to substantiate this possibility: the larger the preoperative conductive deficit, the less likely the patient is to obtain an ideal hearing result. This points out the difficulty the surgeon may have in assessing whether the ossicular chain movement is normal.

TABLE 8. POSTOPERATIVE CONDUCTIVE DEFICIT COMPARED TO PREOPERATIVE DEFICIT IN PRIMARY CASES WITH ONE OR MORE YEAR FOLLOW-UP AND INTACT TYMPANIC MEMBRANE

Postoperative Conductive Deficit (dB) (N = 276)	*Preoperative Conductive Deficit (N = 472)* ≤ *10 dB (35%)*	≤ *20 dB (76%)*	*21-30 dB (20%)*	≥ *31 dB (4%)*
≤ 5	66%	62%	46%	42%
≤ 10	87%	82%	81%	58%
≤ 15	97%	94%	94%	92%
≥ 16	3%	6%	6%	8%

Sensorineural Hearing Impairment. There were no dead ears or serious sensorineural impairments in this group of 472 myringoplasty operations. A loss of BC of 10 dB or more at 2 kHz or 4 kHz or both occurred in 3% of the cases. In 1.3% of the primary cases this high tone loss resulted in a 15 to 20 dB loss of BC averaged in the three frequencies. It would be reasonable to speculate that this sensorineural impairment was due to trauma to the ossicular chain, perhaps due to the drill which we use routinely in the fascia graft technique.

Traumatic Perforations. There was no clinically significant difference in the graft take results in the traumatic perforation or slag injury cases when compared to the other cases.

Tympanosclerosis. Some have said that the presence of tympanosclerosis in the membrane is a bad prognostic sign in regard to graft take. In the selected group of fascia graft cases there was no difference between the graft take results in cases with and without tympanosclerosis in the membrane. We routinely remove plaques of tympanosclerosis in the membrane before grafting, however.

Postoperative Serous Effusion. We do not perform eustachian tube function tests preoperatively. Of significance in light of this is that middle ear effusion was detected postoperatively in only one case, and that was an adult.

COMMENTS

Tinnitus. The only big surprise in this study was the lack of any apparent relationship between the complaint of tinnitus and the degree of conductive hearing impairment. Unfortunately we were not able to draw any conclusions in regard to relief of tinnitus following successful surgery because this information was not recorded in the chart.

Graft Take. We were not pleased with the overall graft take results but are not too surprised at the findings. Canal skin grafts which were used in all cases 20 years ago have an unacceptably high failure rate in large perforations and a significant late failure rate. In recent years those in our Group who prefer this technique and its transcanal approach have limited the technique to smaller perforations in dry ears, a situation in which the failure rate is lower.

The 7.7% early failure rate with fascia in myringoplasty was higher than anticipated. We had known from yearly audits of short-term results over the last 15 years that myringoplasty cases fared worse than our tympanoplasty with mastoidectomy cases and have had no good explanation for this difference. The higher than anticipated failure rate here turned out to be due to technique differences among various members of the Group. Those who used a postauricular approach had an early failure rate (2%) which we believe is acceptable. The hearing results also were better in this selected group of cases.

Afterthoughts. What have members of our Group learned from this study? Except under unusual circumstances lateral surface fascia grafting should be performed through a postauricular approach. The canal skin grafting technique does not produce as satisfactory results as had been assumed by some of our Group and this technique should be limited to closure of small perforations. We may continue to counsel patients contemplating myringoplasty that the graft take rate is over 90%, that hearing improvement may be noted in 70-80% (of those whose preoperative deficit is more than 10 dB), that 2-3% may have worse hearing following surgery and that the likelihood of a total loss of hearing following surgery is very remote.

CONCLUSIONS

1. The graft failure rate in myringoplasty may vary considerably with the surgeon's technique. Lateral surface fascia grafting through a postauricular approach was successful in over 97% of the cases.

2. The incidence of healing problems (blunting, lateral healing) with lateral surface fascia grafting is low.

3. Despite a successful grafting procedure up to 20% of patients may maintain a residual conductive deficit of 11 dB or more and this is more likely to occur in patients whose preoperative conductive deficit is over 30 dB.

4. The incidence of high tone sensorineural hearing impairment was 3%. Severe sensorineural impairment did not occur.

REFERENCES

1. Committee on Conservation of Hearing of the American Academy of Ophthalmology and Otolaryngology. Standard classification for surgery of chronic ear infection. Arch Otolaryngol 1965; 81:204-5.

2. House WF, Sheehy JL. Myringoplasty. Use of ear canal skin compared with other techniques. Arch Otolaryngol 1961; 73:407-15.

3. Sheehy JL. Surgery of chronic otitis media. In: English G, ed. Otolaryngology. Hagerstown: Harper and Row, 1977.

4. Sheehy JL, Glasscock ME. Tympanic membrane grafting with temporalis fascia. Arch Otolaryngol 1967; 86:391-402.

COCHLEAR FLUID BALANCE
A CLINICAL/RESEARCH OVERVIEW

ARNDT J. DUVALL III, MD

PETER A. SANTI, PhD

MARGARET J. HUKEE

MINNEAPOLIS, MINNESOTA

Stria edema, and in some cases atrophy, follows osmotic agents, loop-inhibiting diuretics, acoustic trauma, and rupture of Reissner's membrane. All have in common an imbalance of fluid and electrolytes in the cochlear duct. The glycerol test causes temporary improvement in hearing in Menière's disease. Glycerol causes stria edema and collapse of Reissner's membrane in the chinchilla. Stria edema, as well as stria atrophy, are found in Menière's disease. Metabolic manipulation of the stria might be the best approach in the search for successful treatment of Menière's disease.

The stria vascularis appears to be important for the regulation of the fluid and electrolyte balance of the endolymph, perhaps as the kidney regulates the fluid and electrolytes in the whole extracellular fluid volume. Stria marginal cells are characterized by numerous basal cell processes that contain large numbers of mitrochondria, and large amounts of Na^+-K^+-adenosine triphosphatase (ATPase).[1] Contraluminal surfaces of proximal convoluted and distal tubules in the kidney have a similar morphology and enzyme content.[2] Large surface area, ample supplies of adenosine triphosphate (ATP) and large amounts of Na^+-K^+-ATPase in both cell types, suggest a contraluminal site for an active ion transport pump.

The stria vascularis is in contact with the endolymph at the marginal cell surface, and with a perilymphatic tissue (the spiral ligament) at the basal cell surface. A protein, horseradish peroxidase (HRP), introduced into the cerebrospinal fluid diffuses through the perilymphatic tissues, but does not enter the stria through the basal cell layer.[3] When HRP is introduced intravenously, it leaves the stria vessels and remains within the stria.[4] Jahnke[5] concluded from freeze fracture studies that the marginal cell tight junctions are "intermediate to tight," whereas the basal cells are sealed from the perilymphatic tissues of the spiral ligament by numerous "very tight" junctions.[5] This suggests that the stria is isolated from its surrounding tissues except for its vascular bed and perhaps the endolymph.

In the kidney proximal tubule, an intercellular pathway that is permeable to water and ions can be demonstrated from the tubular lumen, through the tight junctions and intercellular spaces, and through the basement membrane to the vessels.[6] The tight junctions between proximal tubule cells are freely permeable to ionic and colloidal lanthanum[7] and are thought also to allow the passage of NaCl and water.[6] Freeze fracture studies of these "leaky" tight junctions show that they are joined by a single junctional strand.[2]

The leaky tight junctions between proximal tubule cells have been widened following mannitol.[8] Tight junctions (five to ten strands) have been ruptured by hypertonic urea, mannitol, and glycerol in the epithelium of the toad bladder.[9] Ultrastructurally clear "bubbles" are found within these junctions,[9] and freeze fracture studies confirmed that these bubbles ultimately are accompanied by disruption of the junctional connecting strands.[10] In addition, these junctions allow passage of barium sulfate.[9] In the stria vessel endothelial cells, similar bubbles associated with the tight junctions have been frequently found ten minutes after intravenous glycerol (Fig. 1, inserts A and B). Tight junctions between stria marginal cells and between endothelial cells are frequently widened after intravenous glycerol administration (Fig. 2). While we suspect that these junctions are open, confirmation will require the use of tracers and freeze fracture techniques.

Extensive intercellular expansion between kidney proximal tubule cells has been demonstrated during osmotic diuresis induced by glucose.[11] Mannitol, also an osmotic agent, causes diuresis by inhibiting fluid reabsorption in the kidney proximal tubules.[12] Large dosages of mannitol cause vacuolization of proximal tubule cells and a widening of the intercellular spaces.[13] Mannitol also causes fluid accumulation (edema) in the stria intercellular spaces.[14] Therefore, in both kidney and stria, permeable tight junctions and widened intercel-

From the Department of Otolaryngology, University of Minnesota, Minneapolis, Minnesota. This research was supported by NINCDS grants NS12125 and NSO4615.

Presented at the meeting of the American Otological Society, Inc., Palm Beach, Florida, April 13-14, 1980.

REPRINTS — Arndt J. Duvall III, MD, Department of Otolaryngology, Box 478 Mayo Building, University of Minnesota Medical School, Minneapolis, MN 55455.

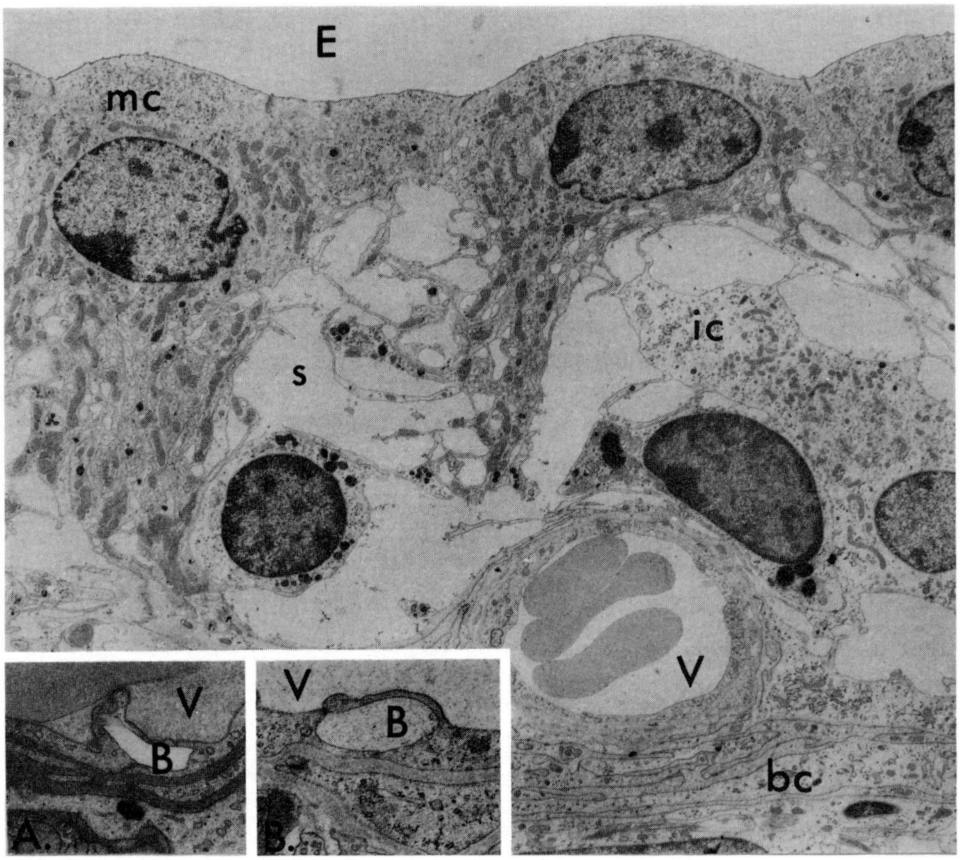

Fig. 1. Stria from chinchilla sacrificed three hours after 6 gm/kg IV glycerol. Stria edema (s) is marked, and marginal cells (mc) are scalloped. ic - Intermediate cell; V - Stria vessel; bc - Basal cells; E - Endolymph. (x4,300). Insert A. Ten minute sacrifice; 6 gm/kg IV glycerol. Stria vessel endothelial cell with junctional "bubble" (B) associated with the tight junction. V -Vessel lumen (x15,700). Insert B. Three hour sacrifice; 6 gm/kg IV glycerol. Stria vessel endothelial cell with junctional "bubble" (B). V - Vessel lumen (x15,300).

lular spaces suggest that osmotic agents alter fluid transport through an intercellular pathway.

Stria vessels are more permeable to protein than other vessels in the cochlear duct[4] and probably allow for the passage of mannitol into the intercellular spaces of the stria. After mannitol administration, expansion of these spaces is the first morphological alteration (Fig. 3A). The molecular size of mannitol (8.6 A diameter) is larger than plasma membrane pores (8.0 A diameter).[15] This is thought to limit mannitol diffusion into cells. Thus, the initial effect of mannitol is to raise the osmolarity of the intercellular space, drawing fluid from the endolymph and/or stria cells. Condensed marginal cell cytoplasm suggests that fluid is drawn from marginal cells (Fig. 3B). However, an overall increase in stria thickness indicates that intercellular fluid must be derived at least partially from outside the stria. Scalloping of the endolymphatic surface takes place after stria edema is extensive, and stria thickness is increased. This scalloping may simply be due to increased fluid pressure within the stria causing the marginal cells to bulge into the endolymphatic space.

While the expansion of the intercellular spaces appears to be the initial event after mannitol, the expansion of marginal cells occurs first after glycerol. Thirty seconds following completion of an intravenous infusion of glycerol in the chinchilla, vacuolization and massive swelling of the apical portion of the stria marginal cell is evident (Fig. 4). This cell swelling is accompanied by only a slight intercellular spacing. Ten minutes after glycerol, moderate intercellular edema is evident and the swelling at the endolymphatic surface of the marginal cells has subsided. Thirty minutes after glycerol, stria edema is marked and the endolymphatic surface of the marginal cells appears normal. Stria edema is still extensive and the marginal cell surface is scalloped three hours after glycerol administration (Fig. 1). Widened junctions are present between vessel endothelial cells at 30 seconds and 10 minutes, and between marginal cells 10 minutes and 3 hours after glycerol (Fig. 2).

The glycerol molecule is smaller (6.2 A diameter) than the plasma membrane pores (8.0 A diameter)[15] and may readily diffuse into the cell. Stria pathology suggests that glycerol enters the stria marginal cells, raising their osmolarity, causing the cell to absorb fluid from the endolymph. When the stria cells have become hypotonic relative to the intercellular

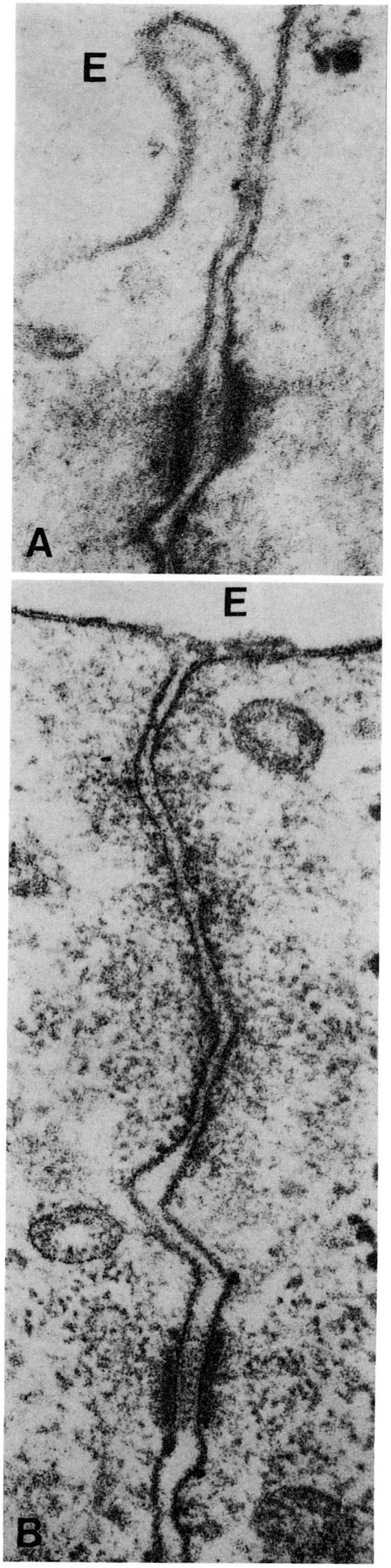

Fig. 2. A) Ten minute sacrifice; 6 gm/kg IV glycerol. Stria marginal cell tight junction appears widened. E - Endolymph. (x121,300). B) Three hour sacrifice; 6 gm/kg IV glycerol. Marginal cell tight junction appears widened. E -Endolymph (x116,100).

spaces, cellular fluid is drawn into these spaces, demonstrating a transcellular pathway for osmotic fluid transport to the stria vessels.

The glycerol test has been used to diagnose endolymphatic hydrops. Klockhoff and Lindblom[16] reported that 1.5 gm/kg glycerol taken orally often results in temporary hearing improvement two to three hours after administration. Angelborg and colleagues[17] found that urea, but not mannitol,[18] also improves hearing. They reported that intravenous glycerol[19] and urea[18] reduce cochlear pressure in guinea pigs while mannitol does not. Preliminary findings show that intravenous glycerol in the chinchilla causes an almost immediate collapse of Reissner's membrane (Fig. 5). These cochleae were fixed by immersion with no perfusion in order to avoid disturbance of cochlear partitions. There was no collapse of Reissner's membrane in saline control animals. This collapse induced by glycerol occurs at the same time as the massive swelling and vacuolization of the marginal cells, suggesting that endolymph volume may be reduced by fluid absorption into the stria marginal cells and transported out of the stria through the vessels. We have not found collapse of Reissner's membrane after intravenous mannitol. Perhaps a significant transcellular transport route is necessary to quickly reduce endolymph volume. Such could explain Angelborg's[18] lack of hearing improvement in patients and absence of cochlear fluid pressure reduction in animals following mannitol.

While the administration of an osmotic overload to the stria is effective in producing temporary stria edema, other mechanisms may also be implicated. Temporary stria edema is present after ethacrynic acid administration and is thought to be a result of enzyme inhibition. The presence of adenylate cyclase (ACase) has been demonstrated in the stria vascularis;[20] ACase is a magnesium-dependent ATPase that converts ATP to cyclic adenosine monophosphate (AMP), liberating energy. Cyclic AMP (cAMP) levels in the cell are thought to regulate electrolyte and fluid transport in some tissues.[21] In the kidney, ethacrynic acid inhibits the activity of plasma membrane ACase,[22] and decreases the reabsorption of sodium chloride and water in the kidney tubules.[23] The inhibition of ACase activity by ethacrynic acid has also been shown in the stria.[24,25]

While the inhibition of stria ACase activity after ethacrynic acid may be a factor in the formation of stria edema, a possible reduction of endolymph volume has not been investigated after ethacrynic acid. ACase activity is stimulated in the intestine by cholera toxin, and massive intestinal secretion (diarrhea) is thought to be a result of cAMP elevation.[26] Feldman and Brusilow[27] injected active cholera toxin into the scala media and reported a significant increase in endolymph volume. If the stimulation of ACase activity by cholera toxin increases the en-

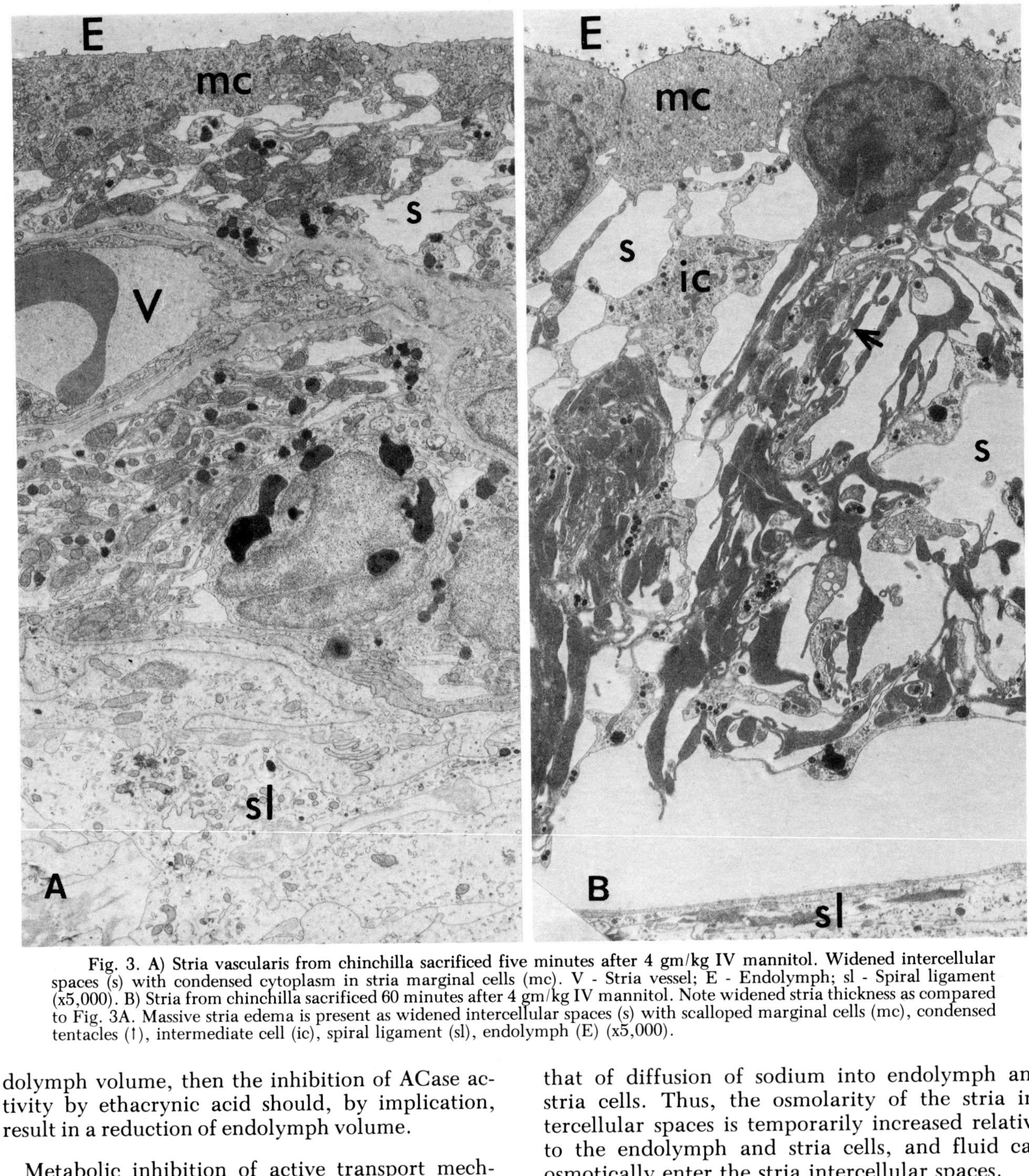

Fig. 3. A) Stria vascularis from chinchilla sacrificed five minutes after 4 gm/kg IV mannitol. Widened intercellular spaces (s) with condensed cytoplasm in stria marginal cells (mc). V - Stria vessel; E - Endolymph; sl - Spiral ligament (x5,000). B) Stria from chinchilla sacrificed 60 minutes after 4 gm/kg IV mannitol. Note widened stria thickness as compared to Fig. 3A. Massive stria edema is present as widened intercellular spaces (s) with scalloped marginal cells (mc), condensed tentacles (↑), intermediate cell (ic), spiral ligament (sl), endolymph (E) (x5,000).

dolymph volume, then the inhibition of ACase activity by ethacrynic acid should, by implication, result in a reduction of endolymph volume.

Metabolic inhibition of active transport mechanisms may allow intercellular sodium to enter the stria cells and endolymph, and allow potassium to enter the stria intercellular spaces from the stria cells and endolymph. The effective diameter of the ion influences its diffusion rate through the cell membrane. Hydrated potassium is 30% smaller than hydrated sodium and diffuses out of the nerve cell 100 times faster than sodium can enter the cell.[15] Therefore, if we assume by extrapolation that an analogous situation exists in the stria, inhibition of ion transport will lead to a diffusion of potassium into the intercellular spaces at a rate faster than that of diffusion of sodium into endolymph and stria cells. Thus, the osmolarity of the stria intercellular spaces is temporarily increased relative to the endolymph and stria cells, and fluid can osmotically enter the stria intercellular spaces.

Ethacrynic acid inhibits the active reabsorption of sodium chloride in the kidney, resulting in increased urine excretion. If one assumes that the drug acts in an analogous way upon a sodium chloride pump at the base of the stria cell, one would expect this to lead to a retention of sodium chloride which should manifest itself anatomically as swelling of the stria cells. In reality, however, the stria marginal and intermediate cells are shrunken during the stria edema after ethacrynic acid,[28,29] indicating a fluid movement out of the stria cells. A

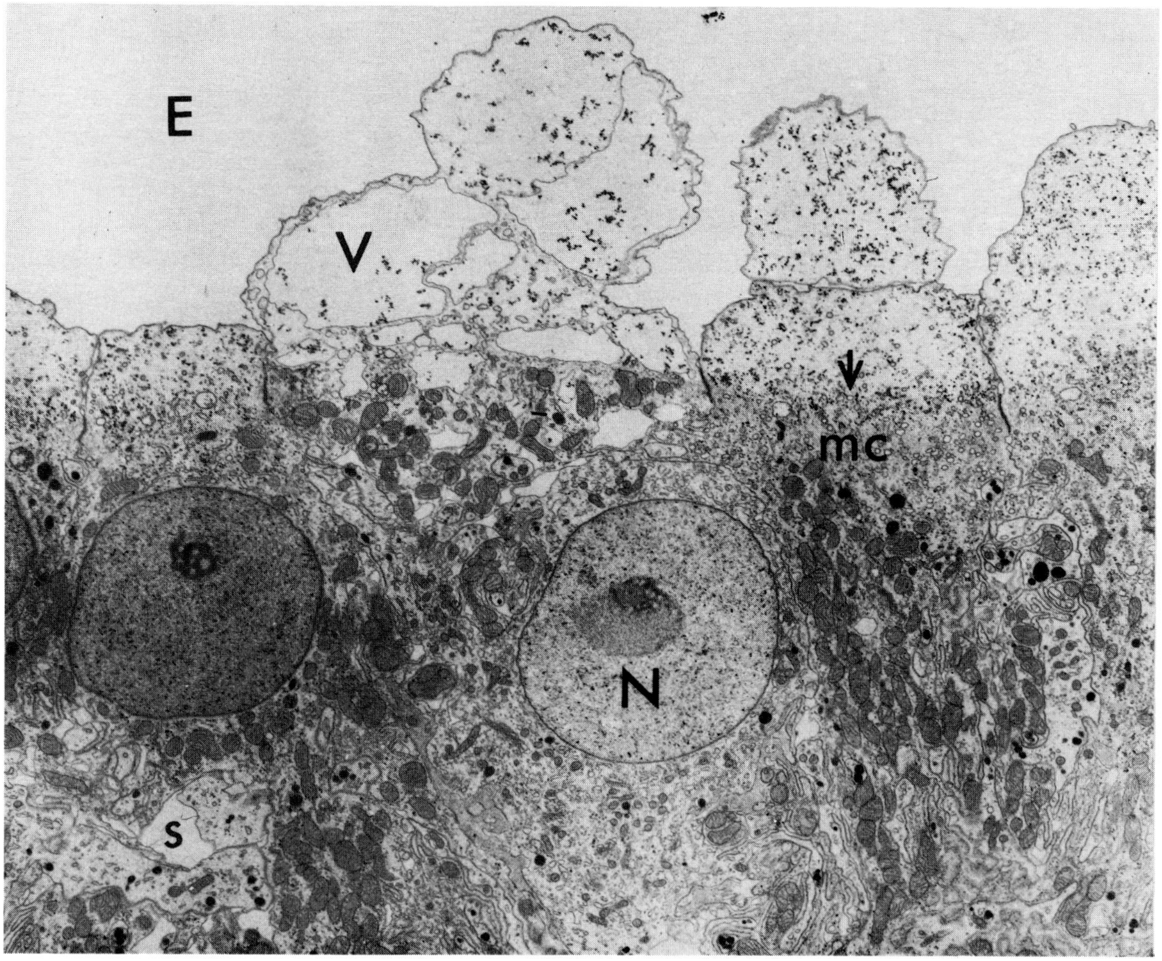

Fig. 4. Stria from chinchilla sacrificed 30 seconds after 6 gm/kg IV glycerol. Stria edema is slight (s), but there is massive swelling of the apical portion of the marginal cell (mc) and vacuole formation (V). N - Nucleus; ↓ - Stratification of marginal cell cytoplasm at the level of the tight junction. E - Endolymph (x4,200).

mechanism that would increase the osmolarity of the intercellular spaces would seem a more logical explanation than inhibition of NaCl transport from the cell.

Stria edema after ethacrynic acid may be a result of directly inhibiting a stria potassium pump,[30] allowing diffusion of potassium out of the endolymph and sodium into the endolymph. A change of ion concentration in the endolymph, decrease in the endolymphatic potential, and stria edema have all been demonstrated after ethacrynic acid.[31] Ethacrynic acid inhibits ACase activity in the stria.[24] A potassium pump maintaining a positive potential that is associated with ACase activity has been demonstrated in the salivary gland of the blowfly (*Calliphora erythrocephala*).[32] When ACase activity is stimulated by 5-hydroxytryptamine (serotonin), an active secretion of KCl into the gland lumen is accompanied by the elevation of intracellular cAMP levels. Normally, a positive potential is maintained in the gland lumen, and this potential is increased when cAMP levels are increased.[32] A similar potassium pump may be used in the stria to maintain the positive endolymphatic potential. The ultrastructural localization of ACase activity on the stria marginal cell endolymphatic surface might indicate that an active potassium pump at this site is regulated by ACase activity. Preliminary results show that ACase activity is concentrated along this endolymphatic surface (Fig. 6).

Diuretics are not the only cause of stria edema. Edema occurs after many diverse stimuli that have in common an interruption of the cochlear duct allowing endolymph and perilymph intermixing. When Reissner's membrane is damaged by mechanical tearing,[33] acoustic overstimulation,[34] or atoxyl poisoning,[35] stria edema is the common pathology. Stria edema also follows an acoustic insult of 123 dB for 15 minutes (two octave band) that tears the organ of Corti from the basilar membrane. This removes the only effective barrier at this site to endolymph-perilymph exchange,[36] since the basilar membrane is freely permeable to even a protein.[3] Stria edema after one such acoustic insult is reversible because the basilar membrane is soon covered by a layer of epithelial cells. Less stria edema follows a repeat of this acoustic insult 28 days later, presumably because the epithelial cells that cover

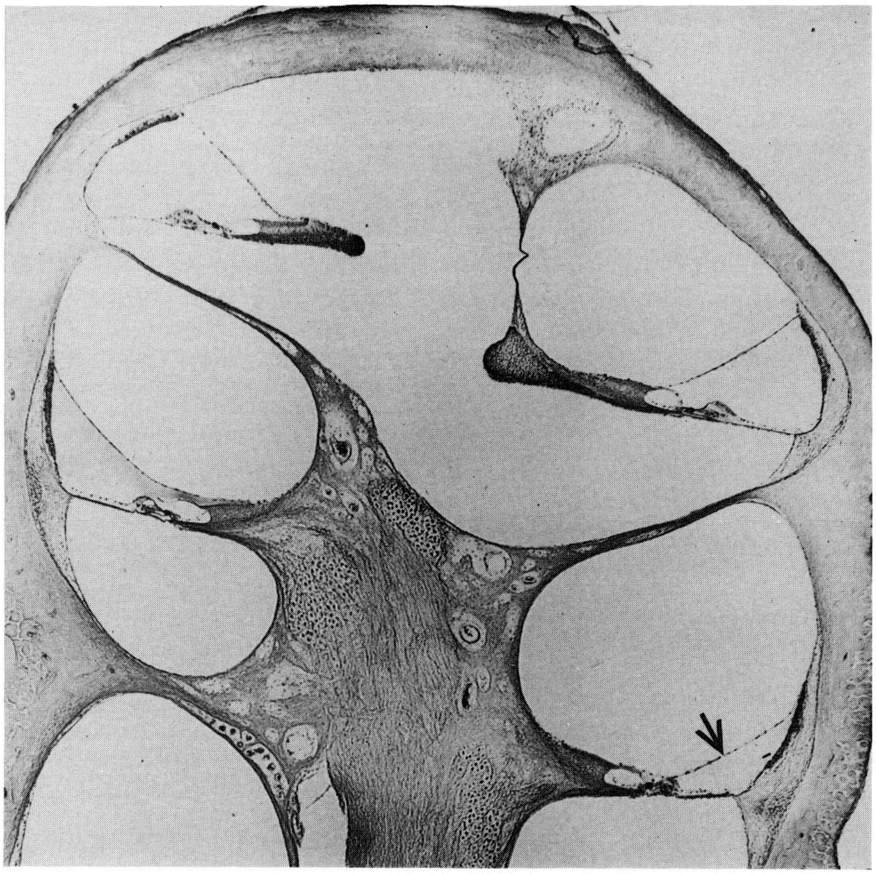

Fig. 5. Midmodiolar cochlear section from chinchilla sacrificed 30 seconds after 6 gm/kg IV glycerol. ↑ - Collapsed Reissner's membrane (x60).

the basilar membrane after the first insult are resistant to separation from the basilar membrane. Therefore less endolymph-perilymph exchange occurs.[36]

After the mechanical[33] and acoustic rupture[34] of Reissner's membrane, stria edema is followed by stria atrophy. This suggests that the endolymph-perilymph exchange in these situations is prolonged or too extensive for the stria to return the sodium-potassium concentrations in endolymph to normal values. Thus, when the stria overload is too great, stria edema may progress to atrophy. Stria atrophy is found in temporal bones with endolymphatic hydrops.[37,38] In ultrastructural studies of human strias obtained at labyrinthectomy, Kimura and Schuknecht[39] found stria edema and scalloping of the marginal cell surface in portions of the stria that were minimally atrophic. Thus, in Menière's disease, as well as in animal experiments, stria edema appears to indicate overload that is temporary, while atrophy indicates overload that is overwhelming and irreversible.

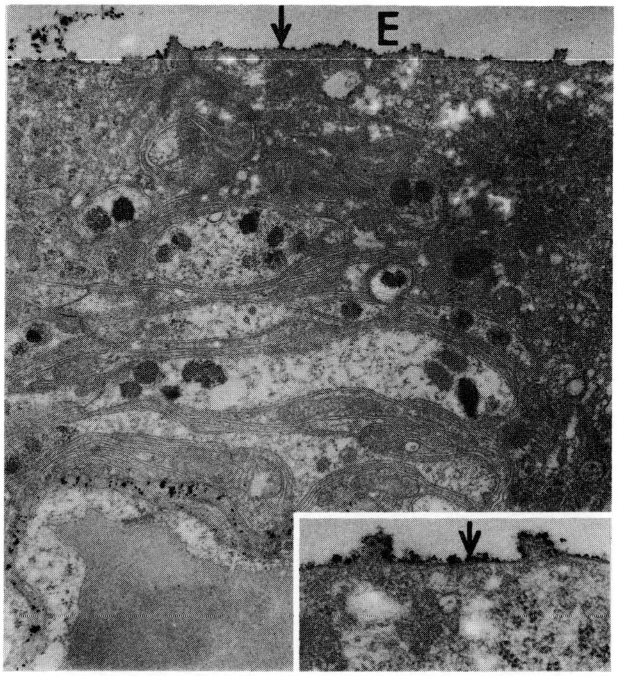

Fig. 6. Stria of normal chinchilla incubated with substrate 5′-adenyl-imidodiphosphate. Lead precipitate on endolymphatic surface (↓) and in stria vessel basal lamina denotes adenylate cyclase activity in the stria (x15,800). Insert - Higher magnification of endolymphatic surface (↓) (x38,900).

CONCLUSIONS

Various stria vascularis pathologies indicate that the stria is important for endolymph maintenance. Kidney tubules and the stria vascularis demonstrate many anatomic and enzymatic similarities. Edema is a common manifestation of overload in both tissues. In addition, the stria edema following osmotic overload is accompanied by Reissner's membrane collapse. This provides a logical explanation for the temporary hearing improvement that follows the ingestion of glycerol in early Menière's disease. Failure to respond to glycerol in long-standing Menière's disease might be explained by stria exhaustion as indicated by stria atrophy. Edema without significant atrophy probably indicates an ability of the stria to still respond to overload.

ACKNOWLEDGMENTS — We thank Dr. Robert L. Vernier, Pediatric Nephrologist, for his advice on the kidney portions, and Alice M. Harju-Ressler, Marilyn T. Matheny and Sherry Lamey for their technical assistance.

REFERENCES

1. Kerr TP, Ross MD, Ernst SA. Cellular localization of transport ATPase in the lateral wall of the cochlear duct: a reassessment. Association for Reseach in Otolaryngology. Abstracts of the Third Midwinter Research Meeting, Columbus, Ohio, 1980; 10:8.
2. Tisher CC. Anatomy of the kidney. In: Brenner BM, Rector FC Jr, eds. The kidney. Vol 1. Philadelphia: WB Saunders Co, 1976.
3. Duvall AJ, Sutherland CR. Cochlear transport of horseradish peroxidase. Ann Otol Rhinol Laryngol 1972; 81:705-14.
4. Duvall AJ, Quick CA, Sutherland CR. Horseradish peroxidase in the lateral cochlear wall. Arch Otolaryngol 1971; 93:304-16.
5. Jahnke K. The fine structure of freeze-fractured intercellular junctions in the guinea pig inner ear. Acta Otolaryngol (Stockh) 1975; Suppl 336.
6. Burg MB, Orloff J. Perfusion of isolated renal tubules. In: Orloff J, Berlinger RW, eds. Handbook of physiology — renal physiology. Washington: American Physiology Society, 1973:145-59.
7. Tisher CC, Yarger WE. Lanthanum permeability of the tight junction (zonula occludens) in the renal tubule of the rat. Kidney Int 1973; 3:238-50.
8. Rawlins FA, Gonzáles E, Pérez-González M, Wittemburg G. Effect of transtubular osmotic gradients on the paracellular pathway in toad kidney proximal tubule: electron microscopic observations. Pfluegers Arch 1975; 353:287-302.
9. Wade JB, Revel JP, DiScala VA. Effect of osmotic gradients on intercellular junctions of the toad bladder. Am J Physiol 1973; 224:407-15.
10. Wade JB, Karnovsky MJ. Fracture faces of osmotically disrupted zonulae occludentes. J Cell Biol 1974; 62:344-50.
11. Latta H, Bencosme SA, Knigge KM, Madden SC. Extracellular compartments in renal tubules associated with polyuria from glucose imbibation. Lab Invest 1962; 11:569-79.
12. Gennari JF, Kassirer JP. Osmotic diuresis. N Engl J Med 1974; 291:714-20.
13. DiScala VA, Mautner W, Cohen JA, Levitt MF, Churg J, Yunis SL. Tubular alterations produced by osmotic diuresis with mannitol. Ann Int Med 1965; 63:767-75.
14. Duvall AJ, Hukee MJ, Santi PA. Mannitol-induced stria vascularis edema. Arch Otolaryngol (in press).
15. Guyton AC. Textbook of medical physiology. Philadelphia: WB Saunders Co, 1976:44.
16. Klockhoff I, Lindblom U. Glycerol test in Meniere's disease. Acta Otolaryngol (Stockh) 1967; Suppl 224:449-51.
17. Angelborg C, Klockhoff I, Stahle J. Urea and hearing in patients with Meniere's disease. Scand Audiol 1977; 6:143-6.
18. Angelborg C. Mechanism of threshold shift with glycerin and other hyperosmolar solutions. Presented at Sixth Shambaugh International Workshop on Otomicrosurgery and Third Shea Fluctuant Hearing Loss Symposium, Chicago, March 1980.
19. Angelborg C, Agerup B. Glycerol effects on the perilymphatic and cerebro-spinal fluid pressure. Acta Otolaryngol (Stockh) 1975; 79:81-7.
20. Ahlstrom P, Thalmann I, Thalmann R. Cyclic AMP and adenylate cyclase in the inner ear. Laryngoscope 1975; 85:1241-58.
21. Strewler GJ, Orloff J. Role of cyclic nucleotides in the transport of water and electrolytes. Adv Cyclic Nucleotide Res 1977; 8:311-61.
22. Dawborn JK, Macneil S, Martin TJ. Diuretics and the renal adenylate cyclase system. Br J Pharmacol 1977; 61:657-67.
23. Burg MB, Green N. Effect of ethacrymic acid on the thick ascending limb of Henle's loop. Kidney Int 1973; 4:301-8.
24. Paloheimo S, Thalmann R. Influence of "loop" diuretics upon $Na^{+}K^{+}$-ATPase and adenylate cyclase of the stria vascularis. Arch Otorhinolaryngol 1977; 217:347-59.
25. Tran-ba-hui P, Servin F, Ohresser M, Kuntziger H. Characteristics and stimulation tests of adenyl cyclase in guinea pig stria vascularis. In: Portmann M, Aran JM, eds. Inner ear biology. Paris: I.N.S.E.R.M. 1977:223-4.
26. Hynie S, Sharp GWG. The effect of cholera toxin on intestinal adenyl cyclase. Adv Cyclic Nucleotide Res 1972; 1:163-74.
27. Feldman AM, Brusilow SW. Effects of cholera toxin on cochlear endolymph production: model for endolymphatic hydrops. Proc Natl Acad Sci USA 1976; 73:1761-4.
28. Quick CA, Duvall AJ. Early changes in the cochlear duct from ethacrynic acid: an electronmicroscopic evaluation. Laryngoscope 1970; 80:954-65.
29. Brummett R, Smith CA, Ueno Y, Cameron S, Richter R. The delayed effects of ethacrynic acid on the stria vascularis of the guinea pig. Acta Otolaryngol (Stockh) 1977; 83:98-112.
30. Sellick PM, Johnstone BM. Production and role of inner ear fluids. Prog Neurobiol 1975; 5:337-62.
31. Bosher SK, Smith CA, Warren RL. The effects of ethacrynic acid upon the cochlear endolymph and stria vascularis. Acta Otolaryngol (Stockh) 1973; 75:184-91.
32. Berridge MJ. The interaction of cyclic nucleotides and calcium in the control of cellular activity. Adv Cyclic Nucleotide Res 1975; 6:1-98.
33. Duvall AJ. Ultrastructure of the lateral cochlear wall following intermixing of fluids. Ann Otol Rhinol Laryngol 1968; 77:317-22.
34. Lawrence M, Yantis PA. Individual differences in functional recovery and structural repair following overstimulation of the guinea pig ear. Ann Otol Rhinol Laryngol 1957; 66:595-621.
35. Anniko M, Wersäll J. Damage to the stria vascularis in the guinea pig by acute atoxyl intoxication. Acta Otolaryngol (Stockh) 1975; 80:167-79.
36. Santi PA, Duvall AJ. Stria vascularis pathology and recovery following noise exposure. Otolaryngology 1978; 84:354-61.
37. Friedmann I. Pathology of the ear. Oxford: Blackwell Scientific Publications, 1974:476.
38. Schuknecht HF, Watanuki K, Takahashi T, et al. Atrophy of the stria vascularis, a common cause for hearing loss. Laryngoscope 1974; 84:1777-821.
39. Kimura RS, Schuknecht HF. The ultrastructure of the human stria vascularis. Acta Otolaryngol (Stockh) 1970; 70:301-18.

Ann Otol 89:1980

SICKLE CELL ANEMIA AND HEARING

ELLEN M. FRIEDMAN, MD
BOSTON, MASSACHUSETTS
NAOMI L. C. LUBAN, MD
WASHINGTON, D.C.
GILBERT R. HERER, PhD
WASHINGTON, D.C.
IOLA WILLIAMS, PNP
WASHINGTON, D.C.

The present investigation examined the effects of sickle cell anemia on threshold hearing. The study included 43 homozygous sickle cell anemia patients, ages 7-18 years, and 23 age-matched controls with documented normal hemoglobin. Both the study and control groups received otologic and audiologic examinations. Bilaterally normal hearing was found in 88% of the sickle cell subjects. Unilateral or bilateral mild high frequency sensorineural hearing loss was demonstrated in 12% (5 of 43). The control subjects revealed no hearing loss. The sickle cell group, therefore, exhibited a higher than usual incidence of hearing loss. Further, three of the five subjects with hearing loss evidenced central nervous system involvement, resulting in a probability of < 0.025 that this relation might occur by chance. Periodic hearing evaluations of children with sickle cell anemia should be performed to identify those with auditory complications and those who possibly may have CNS involvement.

INTRODUCTION

The purpose of the present investigation is to study the threshold hearing of patients with sickle cell disease, specifically homozygous SS patients. Because of the occurrence of vasoocclusive crises, sickle cell disease may compromise inner ear blood flow and thus cause sensorineural hearing loss. Some studies have reported cases of moderate to severe hearing loss as a consequence of this disease,[1-3] while in other studies only slight to moderate high frequency losses are reported.[4-6] In some of these studies, hearing threshold data were from subjects displaying a variety of hemoglobinopathies.[4,5] In the present study, therefore, we will attempt to clarify the incidence and configuration of sensorineural loss among homozygous SS patients.

Sickle cell anemia is caused by a genetically inherited hemoglobinopathy, in which valine is substituted for glutamic acid in the sixth position of the beta chain of the hemoglobin. When an individual has the heterozygous condition, he inherits the hemoglobin SA pattern. This is considered sickle cell trait. The term sickle cell anemia is used to refer to the symptomatic group of individuals whose hemoglobin contains only hemoglobin SS, the homozygous condition.

The gene for HbS is found predominantly in descendents from sub-Sahara Africa, Mediterranean countries and India. In the United States 8.5% of the black population has the heterozygous genotype (hemoglobin SA) and another 0.3 to 1.3% of the black population has the homozygous genotype (hemoglobin SS).[7]

The initial clinical presentation of sickle cell anemia usually occurs in the first few months of life when the level of normal fetal hemoglobin, HbF, decreases and the HbS concentration increases. Frequently, the first symptom of the disease is dactylitis, or the "hand and foot" syndrome. This syndrome consists of swelling of the hands and feet without erythema and with extreme tenderness. These episodes are self-limited and usually do not appear after the age of three.[8]

The growth and development of these children are abnormal as reflected by a mean weight of approximately two standard deviations below children of the same age. Sexual and skeletal maturity are uniformly delayed. Sickle cell patients have increased susceptibility to infection and this, in combination with painful crises, accounts for the majority of hospitalizations for these patients. The life span and overall prognosis for patients with homozygous sickle cell anemia varies greatly among individuals, and statistics tend to be inconsistent in this area. Lehmann et al note that patients with sickle cell anemia may survive to middle age with good medical care.[8]

Bunn describes the major manifestations of sickle cell disease as follows:[9] 1) chronic hemolytic anemia; 2) systemic manifestations including impairment of growth and development and increased susceptibility to infections; 3) vasoocculsive or painful crises, episodes of pain of varying severity which come on over a few minutes or hours and last a few hours to days. The pain is attributed to the occlusion of small vessels by sickled cells with the release of kinins and, in many instances, microinfarctions. 4) Organ damage is the consequence of multiple microvascular occlusive events and of chronic anemia.

From the Children's Hospital National Medical Center, and the Department of Child Health and Development, George Washington University School of Medicine and Health Sciences, Washington, DC.

Presented at the meeting of the American Otological Society, Inc., Palm Beach, Florida, April 13-14, 1980.

REPRINTS — Gilbert R. Herer, PhD, Children's Hospital National Medical Center, 111 Michigan Avenue, NW, Washington, DC 20010.

The pathophysiology of sickle cell disease has been described by Diggs as an increased viscosity of the blood by crystallization of HbS in the red blood cells.[10] The sickled and rigid red blood cells "log jam" vascular channels and produce stasis, hypoxia, vascular and perivascular lesions.

LITERATURE REVIEW

Morgenstein and Manace report pathologic changes in the temporal bone of a 10-year-old male with chronic sickle cell disease that are quite similar to Diggs' description.[1] The child was known to have a moderate bilateral sensorineural hearing loss. These investigators found absence and abnormality of many inner and outer hair cells, as well as sickle cell engorgement of strial vessels. Venous and capillary channel blockage by clumped sickled cells was found throughout the temporal bone. The organ of Corti showed ischemic changes, and the strial changes were consistent with hypoxia. Middle ear ossicles revealed bone resorption.

Another early report of hearing loss related to sickle cell disease was provided by Urban in 1973.[3] Recovering from coma secondary to sickle cell crisis, a 20-year-old black male displayed a total sensorineural hearing loss. Eleven days following resolution of the crisis, audiograms revealed a significant improvement in hearing. Speech reception thresholds of 27 dB and 50 dB were noted for the left and right ears, respectively. Three months after the first postcrisis hearing test the subject's thresholds improved still further, achieving the 15 dB and 38 dB levels for the left and right ears, respectively.

In a large sample of sickle cell subjects, Todd et al showed a statistically significant percentage of individuals with sensorineural hearing loss.[6] These investigators studied 83 Jamaican sickle cell subjects, ranging in age from 12 to 39 years, along with 83 control subjects in the same age range. Essentially half of each group were males and half were females. Twenty-two percent of the sickle cell group as compared to 4% of the control group displayed hearing loss of at least 25 dB (International Standards Organization, 1964) in one or more frequencies (500-8,000 Hz). Hearing loss in the sickle cell group was predominately in the high frequency region (2,000-8,000 Hz), and occurred as often in right as in left ears. Also, an equal number of males and females displayed hearing loss. Approximately half of the sickle cell group was 12 to 19 years of age, with the other half ranging in age between 20 and 39 years. The incidence of hearing loss among the younger subjects (12-19 years) was 15% of ears, while the rate for the 20 to 39-year-old subjects was 13%, and that for the 30 to 39-year-old group was 27%. The control group in the same oldest age range showed no hearing loss at all. Although the number of ears (26) in the oldest sickle cell subjects was relatively small, these data *may suggest* increased incidence of hearing loss resulting from repeated crises. Todd et al conclude that involvement affecting the auditory system is a two-fold process including severe anemia causing hypoxemia and thrombosis.

Serjeant et al explored the theory that bone marrow engorgement secondary to marrow hyperplasia in sickle cell anemia may similarly affect the petrous bone.[11] Their report examined the possible effect of bone marrow expansion causing narrowing of the internal auditory canal and resultant compression of the eighth nerve. This process could account for a sensorineural hearing loss in sickle cell anemia secondary to pressure necrosis of the auditory nerve. These investigators examined the radiographic measurements of the internal auditory canals of 32 SS subjects with and without abnormal audiograms. They found no correlation between canal size and abnormal audiometric findings and concluded that narrowing of the internal auditory canal is not responsible for hearing loss in sickle cell disease. Serjeant et al speculate that sensorineural loss is due to sickling and impaired blood flow in the cochlear venous system causing anoxia of the hair cells and striae vascularis.

Berry examined the possibility that patients with more sickle cell crises experienced greater sensorineural loss.[4] He reported data on six adults from a veterans hospital who displayed mild to severe high frequency loss and recurrent crises. There were three cases with SA, two with SC and one with SS. Three subjects (1 SA, 2 SC) with more frequent episodes showed 15 to 20 dB greater losses. Due to the small sample size and mixture of hemoglobinopathies, caution must be exercised in generalizing Berry's findings to SS subjects.

In 1977 Orchik and Dunn noted a single case of an 18-year-old male in sickle cell crisis who upon recovery exhibited marked hearing loss.[2] The initial audiograms revealed total bilateral sensorineural deafness, much like the case reported by Urban. Subsequent audiograms revealed no response for the right ear and improvement in the left to the 63 dB level (pure tone average).

Sharp and Orchik report the auditory test findings of nine sickle cell (8 Hb SS and 1 Hb SC) and nine normal subjects.[5] These investigators show that eight of nine sickle cell subjects had normal hearing in each ear from 500 through 8,000 Hz. The remaining subject demonstrated a unilateral high frequency sensorineural hearing loss. From their findings, Sharp and Orchik state that peripheral hearing acuity is not significantly affected by sickle cell anemia. They, therefore, believe their findings differ from those of Todd et al who report 22% of 83 subjects with some hearing loss, primarily in the high frequencies. Although the Sharp and Orchik sample is very small, their data in fact reveal an 11% (1 of 9) hearing loss among their subjects.

The literature, therefore, suggests several configurations of hearing loss in patients with sickle cell disease. A few case studies report profound bilateral losses consequent to severe episodic crisis with partial recovery of hearing over time. Other investigations using larger samples show a significant amount of hearing loss primarily in the high frequency region. Perhaps the former reflect infarctive episodes for some patients, while the latter represents the effects of impaired inner ear circulation resulting from hypoxia. Finally, some reports suggest repeated crises may cause an increased incidence of hearing loss probably due to further compromise of inner ear circulation.

METHODS

The present investigation was undertaken to study the incidence and configuration of hearing loss among homozygous SS patients. The contribution of repeated crises to hearing loss also was explored, although indirectly. Experimental subjects consisted of 43 black children and two adults with sickle cell anemia. Controls included 23 age- and race-matched children with hemoglobin AA.

Since it was difficult to determine accurately the incidence of crises among the SS children of this study, it was assumed that increased age would produce increased crisis episodes. Thus, to explore indirectly the effects of repeated crises upon hearing, the group of experimental children was divided into two age divisions: 7 through 12 years, and 13 through 18 years. The control subjects also were grouped in this manner. In a further attempt to examine the effects of crises on hearing, adult SS subjects were sought for this study. Two such subjects agreed to participate. Obviously the hearing data from these few subjects cannot be considered characteristic of SS adults. However, the findings from them are included for the sake of interest and completeness.

Otological and audiological examinations were conducted with each child in the experimental and control groups. Any cerumen noted during otoscopy was removed. All 43 children in the experimental group were documented as having homozygous SS disease by hemoglobin electrophoresis in cellulase acetate and agar gel, and were followed regularly in the Sickle Cell Clinic of the Children's Hospital National Medical Center, Washington, DC. The control group of 23 children was documented to have normal hemoglobin electrophoreses with AA pattern; no child with sickle cell trait (SA) was included in this latter group. The two adult subjects participating in this study were referred from the Sickle Cell Clinic of the Washington Hospital Center, Washington, DC. This clinic documented that both adults had homozygous SS hemoglobin.

The audiological evaluation of all study subjects consisted of pure tone audiometry, tympanometry and acoustic reflex threshold (AR) measurements. Pure tone audiometers used in this investigation were calibrated to American National Standards Institute, 1969 standards. A Madsen model ZO 73 electroacoustic impedance bridge was used to obtain tympanometric and AR threshold data. Pure tone air conduction thresholds of 0-20 dB hearing level (HL) for test frequencies 250 through 8,000 Hz were considered normal. Any air conduction threshold of 25 dB HL or poorer was considered a hearing loss for the purpose of the present investigation. Jerger's differentiation of tympanograms into types A, B and C was employed to analyze the study data.[12] Also included in this analysis were types A_S and A_D ascribed to Jerger by Northern and Downs.[13] For the purposes of this investigation, contralateral AR thresholds for a subject were considered not normal or "elevated" if the AR threshold was 110 dB or greater (including absent) at two or more frequencies from 500 through 2,000 Hz.

TABLE 1. IDENTIFYING INFORMATION FOR THE SICKLE CELL AND CONTROL GROUPS

Group	Hb Problem	Age Range (yr)	No.	Male/Female Ratio
I	SS	7-12	20	11/9
II	SS	13-18	23	9/14
III	AA	7-12	12	8/4
IV	AA	13-18	11	8/3

RESULTS

As shown in Table 1, 20 of the 43 SS subjects comprised the youngest age group. There were 11 male and 9 female children ranging from 7 years, 2 months to 12 years, 11 months. Twelve of these subjects had normal bilateral pure tone, tympanometry and AR findings. Two subjects displayed a 25 dB loss at 250 Hz in one ear each. One of these subjects had normal tympanometric and AR results. The other had a ventilating tube in the tympanic membrane of the ear with the loss and showed a type C tympanogram in the other ear. Two subjects had air conduction losses at 8,000 Hz in one ear each amounting to 25 dB and 45 dB, respectively, but showed normal bilateral tympanometry and AR results. Four subjects showed normal bilateral hearing thresholds but elevated AR thresholds in one ear each. In every instance with these latter subjects a type A_S or type A_D tympanogram was present suggesting the probability that minor middle ear involvement influenced the AR measurements.

The older age group included 23 SS subjects, 9 males and 14 females ranging in age from 13 years to 18 years, 10 months. Eighteen of these children showed normal bilateral results for pure tones, tympanometry and AR thresholds. Two subjects evidenced high frequency hearing losses in one ear each; a 25 dB loss at 4,000 Hz for one subject and a 25 dB loss at 4,000 Hz and 8,000 Hz for the other subject. Both of these children demonstrated normal tympanometry and AR thresholds (500-2,000 Hz) bilaterally. One 18-year, 9-month-old female subject showed a bilaterally symmetrical high frequency hearing loss for the 3,000 to 8,000 Hz region ranging from 25 to 60 dB HL. Type A tympanograms were noted for each ear. Although air conduction thresholds for each ear of this subject ranged between 0 and 10 dB HL at frequencies 500 through 2,000 Hz, contralateral AR thresholds were 110 dB or greater, and ipsilateral AR thresholds were absent at these test frequencies. Two SS subjects in the older age division displayed normal bilateral hearing but elevated AR thresholds bilaterally. In each instance a type A_D or type C tympanogram was present suggesting the probability of minor middle ear involvement influencing the AR measurements.

The 23 children in the normal control group also

were divided according to age as reported in Table 1. Twelve subjects, eight males and four females, ranged in age from 7 years, 1 month to 12 years, 11 months. All demonstrated normal bilateral air conduction thresholds. Nine in this younger age division revealed type A tympanograms and normal AR thresholds for each ear. The tympanometry-AR threshold results for the remaining three subjects were as follows: one child showed a type A_D tympanogram in one ear and a type A in the other with normal bilateral AR threshold findings. Another subject revealed a type A_S tympanogram in one ear and a type A in the other, also with normal AR results bilaterally. The remaining child evidenced a type C and type A tympanogram in respective ears. Absent AR thresholds were noted when the probe of the impedance bridge was in the ear displaying the type C tympanogram. Normal AR results were observed when the probe was in the ear with the type A configuration.

Eleven of the 23 normal children, eight males and three females, comprised the older age division of the control group. They ranged in age from 13 years to 18 years, 9 months. All of these subjects demonstrated normal bilateral tympanometry and AR threshold results. All but one subject exhibited bilaterally normal air conduction thresholds. The oldest subject in this group, however, did display a 25 dB HL threshold at 250 Hz in one ear, but otherwise normal findings at all other frequencies in each ear.

The two adult SS subjects participating in this investigation were a 39-year-old male and a 43-year-old female. The male subject showed normal air conduction thresholds bilaterally, although a 20 dB HL was noted at 4,000 Hz for one ear. Tympanograms for each ear were type A. However, this subject displayed elevated contralateral AR thresholds for 500 and 1,000 Hz and absent ARs at 2,000 Hz. Ipsilateral reflexes for all test frequencies in each ear also were absent.

The adult female subject exhibited some bilateral high frequency hearing loss. Air conduction thresholds at 6,000 and 8,000 Hz for the left ear were 20 dB and 25 dB HL respectively. Her right ear showed thresholds of 20 dB, 25 dB and 50 dB at 4,000, 6,000 and 8,000 Hz, respectively. Tympanograms for each ear were type A, and both contralateral and ipsilateral AR thresholds across test frequencies were normal.

DISCUSSION

Sickle Cell Subjects. Comparing the air conduction threshold data for each age division of SS children in the present study reveals no trend for an increased incidence of hearing loss with age. If more numerous crises accompanied age in the SS subjects of this study, then these episodes seem not to have caused more hearing loss among the older subjects. It is possible that the sample size might not be large enough to demonstrate such a trend. Or, the present sample of older SS children may not have experienced the expected crisis episodes. Nevertheless, the overall data for each age division are quite similar. Pooling the data from each, therefore, should yield a composite picture of this entire sample of black homozygous SS subjects. The composite for the 43 subjects, 20 males and 23 females, appears as follows.

Thirty-eight subjects, or 88% of the total sample (43), had essentially bilateral hearing within normal limits. Two of these subjects, however, showed a 25 dB loss at 250 Hz in one ear, probably related in at least one instance to middle ear involvement. Among these 38 subjects, 6 displayed elevated acoustic reflex thresholds; but in each instance a type A_S, A_D, or C tympanogram was evident. These tympanometric results suggest the probability that minor middle ear involvement influenced the acoustic reflex measurements. Except as noted, all other subjects in this normal hearing SS group displayed tympanometric and acoustic reflex threshold data within normal limits.

Four subjects, ages 11 through 16 years, showed mild unilateral sensorineural high frequency hearing losses at 4,000 and/or 8,000 Hz ranging from 25 to 45 dB. Three of these subjects had a loss at only one frequency. All four subjects displayed normal type A tympanograms, and normal acoustic reflex thresholds for test frequencies of 500 through 2,000 Hz.

One 18-year, 9-month-old SS subject displayed a bilaterally symmetrical 25 to 60 dB sensorineural hearing loss from 3,000 through 8,000 Hz. Rather interesting AR threshold data were obtained with this subject in the presence of normal tympanometry. Even though air conduction thresholds for each ear ranged between 0-10 dB HL from 500 through 2,000 Hz, contralateral AR thresholds were 110 dB or greater and ipsilateral AR thresholds were absent for these test frequencies. Sharp and Orchik report similar pure tone threshold and AR data for their sickle cell subjects.[5] Perhaps slight middle ear involvement not readily apparent from the other measurements caused these elevated and absent ARs. However, the AR thresholds in this subject could reflect damage to portions of the cochlea not suggested by the subject's air conduction thresholds.

Pollack and Lipscomb summarize current thinking about the pure tone audiogram not illustrating fully the extent of cochlear cell loss.[14] Commenting on studies which compared pure tone audiograms with histopathological findings of human subjects, these investigators conclude "the magnitude of cell damage in the upper half of the cochlea is often not accurately represented by pure-tone audiometry." If this concept holds for the present 18-year-old subject with a high frequency loss, it might give a clue as to why reflex thresholds were elevated or absent in the midfrequency region where air conduction thresholds were normal. Stated differently, perhaps the AR thresholds in this subject express damage to the cochlea not evident by pure tone air conduction thresholds. This speculation seems worthy of further study.

The five subjects of the present investigation with unilateral or bilateral high frequency hearing loss represent a 12% incidence rate of sensorineural loss. In sampling a normal population of children, the incidence of sensorineural loss is expected to be very low. For example, Kessner et al studied the hearing of 1,639 black children, ages 4 through 11 years, from a normal preschool and school population in Washington, DC.[15] The incidence of sensorineural loss reported by these investigators was 0.5%. It would appear, therefore, that the 12% rate of sensorineural loss among the present SS subjects, albeit mostly very mild unilateral high frequency loss, is greater than usual. This finding is similar to that noted by Todd et al.[6]

The presence of any hearing loss in SS patients, albeit extremely mild as seen among the present study subjects, may reflect those patients with more serious complications arising from the disease. A retrospective review of the medical records of the 43 SS subjects was done to document serious complications which might predispose any to hearing abnormality, ie, recurrent otitis media, meningitis, etc. This review showed that six children manifested complications reflecting CNS involvement (cerebral vascular accidents of varying severity). Interestingly, three of these children were among the five who exhibited hearing losses. Chi square analysis revealed a probability of <0.025 that this relation might occur by chance. It would appear, then, that CNS insults significantly increased the risk of hearing loss among the SS subjects in the present study.

The two adult SS subjects revealed essentially normal hearing bilaterally, but one (female) did display some loss in the highest test frequencies (6,000-8,000 Hz) in each ear. Like the 18-year-old sickle cell subject of this study, the adult male demonstrated elevated or absent AR thresholds at frequencies where normal air conduction thresholds were present. Again, perhaps cochlear structures in this subject have been implicated by sickle cell disease which is reflected in the AR findings but not the pure tone thresholds.

Control Subjects. The age distribution of the normal black control group was like that of the SS group. That is, approximately half (12 subjects) was between 7 years and 12 years, 11 months and the other half (11 subjects) was between 13 years and 18 years, 9 months. There was essentially twice the number of male to female subjects for each age division. The male-female distribution in the age divisions of SS subjects, however, was approximately equal.

All 23 control subjects essentially displayed normal hearing bilaterally. No subject evidenced high frequency hearing losses in either ear.

Twenty subjects revealed normal tympanometric and AR threshold findings bilaterally. The three other subjects, all in the younger age division, showed impedance audiometry findings which appear to characterize what is often experienced clinically with younger children in the normal population. That is, the three subjects displayed normal unilateral findings for tympanometry and AR measurements. Two of the three evidenced a unilateral type A_S or A_D tympanogram, coupled with normal AR results. The remaining subject had a type C tympanogram in one ear and absent ARs when that ear became the probe ear. Apparently, the latter subject was experiencing the onset or resolution of middle ear pathology.

CONCLUSIONS

The 23 control subjects displayed hearing, tympanometry and AR threshold data expected of normal children between ages 7 and 18 years. That is, all had normal bilateral air conduction thresholds but some, 3 of 23 (13%), revealed configurations of tympanometric-AR measurements suggesting the probability of past or present middle ear involvement. None of these normal subjects evidenced any sensorineural hearing loss.

Most of the SS subjects (38 of 43) in the 7 to 18-year age range showed findings similar to those of the control group. Bilateral air conduction thresholds were normal, but 6 of these 38 (16%) demonstrated tympanometric-AR results implicating past or present middle ear involvement.

Four of the 43 SS children, 2 in each age division, had very mild (25 to 45 dB) unilateral hearing losses in the 4,000-8,000 Hz range. Since all four subjects showed otherwise normal tympanometric-AR results, these losses are judged to be sensorineural in nature. A fifth subject exhibited a bilateral high frequency loss (25 to 60 dB) in the 3,000-8,000 Hz range. Normal tympanograms (type A) for each ear were noted in this 18-year-old subject confirming the presence of a high frequency sensorineural loss.

Twelve percent of the entire SS group of children (5 of 43 subjects), therefore, revealed some high frequency sensorineural hearing loss. Since the normal non-SS subjects in the same age range did not evidence any such losses, it seems that a mild high frequency sensorineural loss does result from SS disease in some children. Stated another way, a higher than expected amount of mild sensorineural hearing loss seems a concomitance of sickle cell anemia. These findings support those reported by Todd et al and suggest that children with homozygous SS disease should receive periodic hearing evaluations to identify those with auditory complications.

If sickle cell anemia causes sensorineural loss, it might be expected that as SS patients grow older and experience repeated crises, an increased incidence of loss would be found. No such evidence to this effect was observed among the SS children in the present investigation.

Periodic hearing evaluations of SS patients seem particularly appropriate in view of the increased incidence of CNS involvement found among the present investigation's SS subjects with sensorineural losses. Hearing impairment, albeit very mild and unilateral, may be a sensitive indicator of CNS problems. Therefore, if hearing loss is detected in an SS patient, a study should be undertaken to determine if that patient has CNS complications. Such an investigation might require fairly sophisticated examinations such as a careful neurologic evaluation, a CT scan, as well as other tests.[16]

Finally, considering the vasoocclusive nature of sickle cell anemia, it is curious that hearing loss is not more prevalent or severe than found in the present investigation or by Todd et al. Recognizing the sensitivity of the inner ear to ischemia, the crises associated with this disease would be expected to create considerable cochlear damage. Support for this expectation can be found in some histologic evidence of temporal bone damage resulting from sickle cell disease. Perhaps cochlear ischemia produced by sickle cell crises causes damage not reflected by pure tone threshold results. As described earlier, elevated or absent AR thresholds were noted in the midfrequency region of two SS subjects where air conduction thresholds were normal. These data may suggest cochlear involvement resulting from sickle cell disease that is not apparent from pure tone threshold results. Further exploration of this concept seems warranted.

ACKNOWLEDGMENTS — The authors wish to gratefully acknowledge the kind assistance of Camille S. Klein, Claire L. Hermanson and Joan C. Harkin.

REFERENCES

1. Morgenstein K, Manace E. Temporal bone histopathology in sickle cell disease. Laryngoscope 1969; 79:2172-80.

2. Orchik D, Dunn J. Sickle cell anemia and sudden hearing loss. Arch Otolaryngol 1977; 103:369-70.

3. Urban G. Reversible sensorineural hearing loss associated with sickle cell crises. Laryngoscope 1973; 5:633-8.

4. Berry RA. Sickle cell anemia: audiological findings. J Am Audiol Soc 1975; 1:61-3.

5. Sharp M, Orchik D. Auditory function in sickle cell anemia. Arch Otolaryngol 1978; 104:322-4.

6. Todd G, Serjeant G, Larson M. Sensorineural hearing loss in Jamaicans with sickle cell disease. Acta Otolaryngol (Stockh) 1973; 76:268-72.

7. Schwartz HC. Hereditary hemoglobinopathies. In: Cooke R, ed. The biologic basis of pediatric practice. New York: McGraw-Hill, 1968:439.

8. Lehmann H, Huntsman RS, Carey R, Lang A, Lorkin PA, Comings DE. Erythrocyte disorders-anemias related to abnormal globin. In: Williams WJ, ed. Hematology. New York: McGraw-Hill, 1977:495-524.

9. Bunn HF. Hemoglobinopathies. Philadelphia: Saunders, 1977.

10. Diggs LW. The crises in sickle cell anemia. Am J Clin Pathol 1956; 26:1109-18.

11. Serjeant GR, Norman W, Todd GB. The internal auditory canal and sensorineural hearing loss in homozygous sickle cell disease. J Laryngol Otol 1975; 98:453-5.

12. Jerger J. Clinical experience with impedance audiometry. Arch Otolaryngol 1970; 92:311-24.

13. Northern JL, Downs MP. Hearing in children. Baltimore: Williams and Wilkins, 1974:173-91.

14. Pollack MC, Lipscomb DM. Implications of hair cell-pure tone discrepancies for oto-audiological practice. Audiol Hear Ed 1979; 5:16-36.

15. Kessner DM, Snow CK, Singer J. Assessment of medical care for children: contrasts in health status. Vol. 3. Institute of Medicine, National Academy of Sciences, Washington, DC, 1974.

16. Wilmas J, Goff JR, Anderson HR, Langston JW, Thompson E. Efficacy of transfusion therapy for one to two years in patients with sickle cell disease and cerebrovascular accidents. J Pediatr 1980; 96:205-8.

Ann Otol 89:1980

CONGENITAL MALFORMATIONS OF THE EAR
ANALYSIS OF 94 OPERATIONS

ROBERT JAHRSDOERFER, MD
CHARLOTTESVILLE, VIRGINIA

The 94 operations analyzed were performed on 80 ears in 73 patients with congenital malformation of the ear. Operative findings included 13 patients with a congenital absence of the oval window, 5 patients with vascular anomaly of the middle ear, and 6 patients with congenital cholesteatoma. Six of 13 patients with congenital absence of the oval window had a labyrinthotomy performed to create a new opening into the vestibule. The method of surgical repair in atresia was a canalplasty with fascia graft overlay for the substitute tympanic membrane. A Silastic® button was placed over the substitute tympanic membrane to lessen blunting and to anchor the center-hole skin graft in place. A modified face lift procedure was done if necessary to align the external ear with the new ear canal. At present no ear canals are stenosed and no ears are actively discharging. One patient sustained a temporary facial paralysis. The hearing results are discussed.

Congenital ear malformations may be broadly classified into major (M) and minor (m) categories. In the major malformation group there is atresia or stenosis of the external ear canal, the tympanic membrane is rudimentary or absent, and the middle ear architecture is almost always malformed. Microtia is common, but in some cases the auricle may be well formed. In the minor malformations the anomaly is primarily confined to the middle ear. The external ear canal is patent and the tympanic membrane is discernible.

Preoperative evaluation included conventional and impedance audiometry and polytomography of the temporal bones. Early in the series, polytomography was done in an anterior-posterior direction.This was changed to a posterior-anterior direction when it was calculated that this latter position gave only one tenth the amount of irradiation to the lens. Lateral polytomographs were not routinely gotten. Auditory brainstem responses (ABR) and computerized axial tomography of the temporal bones were performed in selected cases.

The patient population included 20 patients with identifiable craniofacial anomalies: osteogenesis imperfecta, 4 patients; hemifacial microsomia, 4 patients; Treacher-Collins syndrome, 3 patients; Crouzon syndrome, 3 patients; Apert's syndrome, 2 patients; Klippel-Feil anomaly, 2 patients; and one patient each had ectodermal dysplasia and Hallermann-Streiff syndrome. Seven other patients had multiple congenital anomalies. Four patients had a congenital facial paralysis.

Ninety-four operations were performed on 80 ears in 73 patients with congenital malformation of the ear. Forty-four operations were performed on 29 patients with a major malformation, and 50 operations were performed on 44 patients with minor malformation. In the major malformation group 19 patients had bilateral atresia or stenosis while 10 patients had unilateral atresia or stenosis. Four patients in this group had surgery on both ears. The minor malformation group was about equally divided into bilateral and unilateral ear involvement.

Operative findings included 13 patients (5M, 8m) with congenital absence of the oval window, 6 patients (2M, 4m) with congenital cholesteatoma, and five patients (1M, 4m) with vascular anomaly of the middle ear. The type of vascular anomaly encountered was a high jugular bulb in two patients, a persistent stapedial artery, an anomalous internal carotid artery, and an ectopic middle ear artery paralleling the facial nerve in a patient with atresia.

There were 9 revision operations in the major malformation group; 4 were for hearing, 2 for postoperative stenosis of the external ear canal, and 3 for infection. At present no external ear canals are stenosed. One patient has a persistent 2 mm perforation in the substitute tympanic membrane and a moist middle ear. No ears are actively discharging. Four revision operations were performed in the minor malformation group; all were for hearing.

One patient with atresia sustained a facial paralysis. In this patient the oval window was recessed beneath the horizontal portion of the facial nerve and could not be visualized. The bony cover of the nerve was purposely removed and the nerve retracted superiorly for exposure of the oval window. Later in the procedure, a modified face lift was performed to align the anteriorly placed auricle with the new ear canal. The patient awoke with a facial paralysis. The cause of the facial paralysis was unclear. It was thought to be either neuropraxia from compression of the facial nerve above the

From the Department of Otolaryngology and Maxillofacial Surgery, University of Virginia School of Medicine, Charlottesville, Virginia.

Presented at the meeting of the American Otological Society, Inc., Palm Beach, Florida, April 13-14, 1980.

REPRINTS — Robert Jahrsdoerfer, Department of Otolaryngology and Maxillofacial Surgery, University of Virginia School of Medicine, Box 430, Charlottesville, VA 22908.

oval window, or transection of the nerve in the face lift procedure. When there was no spontaneous return of function in three weeks, the patient was reoperated. The facial nerve was found to be intact from the geniculate ganglion to its secondary branching in the face. There was a complete return of facial function in three months.

Fenestration was attempted in two cases, both unsuccessful. One patient, a boy with Treacher-Collins syndrome, had the superior semicircular canal fenestrated when a middle ear could not be identified. In another patient with hemifacial microsomia and absent labyrinthine windows, the horizontal semicircular canal could not be located by extensive drilling on the labyrinthine capsule, despite polytomographic evidence of semicircular canals.

Thirteen patients had congenital absence of the oval window. Six of these had a labyrinthotomy to create a new opening into the vestibule. The hearing results were variable, sometimes spectacular, sometimes not. In five patients the air-bone gap was closed to within 10, 12, 12, 20 and 25 dB respectively. In one patient there was no improvement, but in no case was the hearing made worse.

In those ears with an absent oval window, a recognizable round window niche was identified in 4 patients, absent in 5 patients, and not seen in 4 patients. It is not always easy to determine if a round window is present. In many cases severe distortion of the middle ear anatomy concealed the round window. It would be foolhardy to reroute the facial nerve simply to see if it is obscuring the round window. Similarly, it would be adventuresome for the surgeon to drill on the medial wall of the middle ear in search of the round window. Failure to identify the round window should not contraindicate drilling a new oval window. In this series, three of four patients in whom a round window was not seen nonetheless had new oval windows drilled with improvement in hearing.

In the minor malformation group the method of tympanoplasty was determined by the degree of middle ear malformation. Conventional methods of tympanoplasty were used when possible to establish a sound conductive system. When the middle ear architecture was severely malformed innovative techniques were used after carefully weighing the risks against the benefits. A new technique, herein described, was used in those cases in which the oval window was absent, the stapes absent or rudimentary, and the facial nerve displaced inferiorly. Inferior displacement of the facial nerve usually causes it to cross the middle ear in an area where the promontory is normally found. The nerve often runs in a bony trough and may be devoid of a bony covering. Creation of a new oval window by a vestibulotomy depends on both the location and the degree of development of the incus and malleus. These ossicles may be deformed, absent, fused or fixed. The stapes is usually primitive and nonserviceable. The "facial roll" technique involves removing any residual bony cover over the facial nerve, drilling the lip of the bony trough with a diamond burr, and gently rolling the nerve to visualize the floor of the trough. Whether the nerve is rolled inferiorly or superiorly depends on the location of the ossicle to which the prosthesis will be attached. As the nerve is held in a retracted position a new oval window is drilled through the floor of the trough into the vestibule which is usually located directly medially. A wire-piston prosthesis is used with the crook portion of the wire attached to the incus or malleus depending on which ossicle is usable. The facial nerve is then allowed to resume its former position and although it may rest against the prosthesis, facial function is uncompromised and hearing only slightly affected, or affected not at all.

When drilling a new oval window it is preferable to drill down to the endosteal membrane of the vestibule, but not through it. The piston end of the prosthesis may then be placed directly on the membrane. It is not always possible to preserve the endosteal membrane, and if it is torn the piston may still be positioned in the vestibulotomy without need of a tissue graft. It is important to mention that the dense middle layer of bone of the labyrinthine capsule is endochondral bone with poor powers of regeneration. That the vestibulotomy remains open was confirmed in two patients who had revision surgery, one five years after a new oval window had been drilled.

Facial Nerve. In the minor malformation group the course of the facial nerve was aberrant in 12 ears. The most common abnormality was an inferior dislacement of the facial nerve at or below the level of the oval window. The facial nerve was usually uncovered by bone. In one case the nerve was a free hanging strand of soft tissue suspended in air as it crossed the middle ear from the posterior bony annulus to the area of the cochleariform process. No facial nerve injuries were incurred in the minor malformation group in this surgical series. Two patients, however, previously operated on elsewhere, sustained facial nerve paralysis, one temporary, the other partial and permanent. In both cases the facial nerve was mistaken for a fibrous tissue strand on the medial wall of the middle ear and was dissected to improve exposure.

The facial nerve in the atresia/stenosis group often had a short vertical course with an abrupt turn anteriorly to cross the inferior aspect of the middle ear and exit in the area of the temporomandibular joint. On occasion the course of the facial nerve was markedly aberrant. In one atresia patient the nerve was devoid of a vertical segment and was represented by a horizontal knuckle of soft tissue crossing the lower third of the middle ear. In a second patient the facial nerve compartmentalized the middle ear into superior and inferior sections. The inferior compartment housed the eustachian tube, hypotympanum and round window, while the superior compartment contained a fused incus-malleus complex, an underdeveloped stapes, and an oval window.

The appearance of the pinna allowed some prediction as to the degree of development of the middle ear. In general, the more developed the pinna, the more developed were the ossicles and the facial nerve. Patients with Treacher-Collins syndrome were found to have most bizarre anomalies which often defied a rational explanation based on an understanding of contemporary embryology.

Surgical Technique in Atresia and Stenosis. There have been modifications in surgical technique since an earlier presentation two years ago.[1] The fascia graft used for the substitute tympanic membrane is now reflected onto the new bony external ear canal for a short distance only, about 1 or 2 mm. It had become apparent that when the fascia covered a large area of bone, it served as a barrier to vascularization of the overlying split thickness skin graft. Blood vessels, regenerating from the bone, could not pierce the fascia in time to nourish the skin graft and assure a take. On occasion this resulted in partial ischemia and loss of viability of the skin graft.

A second modification is the use of a perforated Silastic button over the substitute tympanic membrane to lessen blunting and to anchor the skin graft in place. It had been found that the medial edge of the skin graft was being pulled away from the new eardrum during the meatoplasty. When the split thickness skin graft was inadvertently displaced laterally in this manner two problems arose: one, squamous epithelium would fail to grow over the substitute tympanic membrane, and two, the mastoid air cell system would be exposed and at risk of becoming infected.

A third modification involved relocating the pinna on the side of the head. In many patients with atresia, in particular those with hemifacial microsomia, the pinna is situated far anterior on the face. Unless the pinna is transposed posteriorly it may be difficult to align the newly drilled ear canal with the new meatus. Various plastic procedures using a rotation flap, pedicle flap, or Z-plasty have been employed to transpose the auricle. I believe a better result can be achieved by a modified face lift procedure. Using the same postauricular incision the pinna and skin of the lateral face are elevated from the underlying soft tissue by blunt and sharp dissection. The facial nerve must be carefully watched for. This technique allows the pinna to be moved posteriorly up to 5 cm. Furthermore, by using the same postauricular incision facial scarring is minimized.

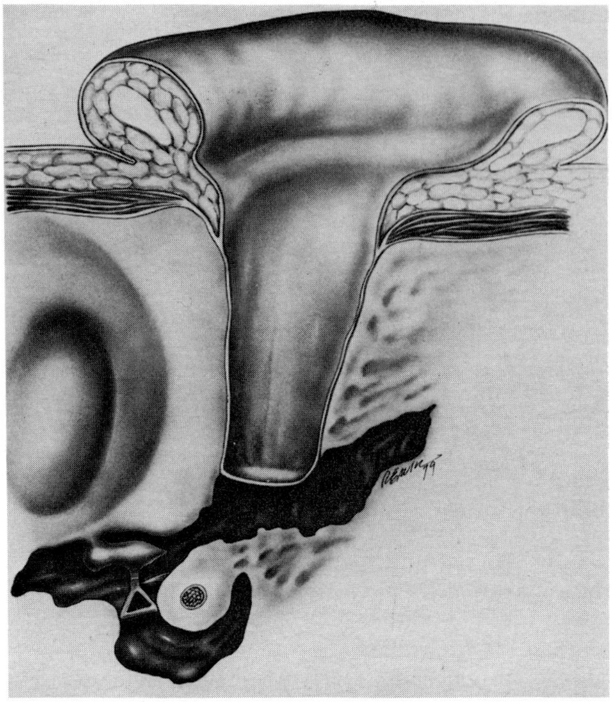

Fig. 1. Pitfalls in atresia repair. A new ear canal had been drilled into the antrum. The surgeon had failed to recognize that the middle ear was located far anteriorly, medial to the temporomandibular joint, and that the malleus was fixed to the atretic plate.

Labyrinthotomy versus Fenestration. Fenestration of the semicircular canal should be avoided in congenital ear malformations. If the labyrinthine windows are absent a labyrinthotomy should be done. Labyrinthotomy offers a better chance of closing the air-bone gap than does fenestration. Moreover, in a severely dysplastic ear the horizontal semicircular canal may not be readily apparent or even accessible. One patient in this series had absent semicircular canals on polytomography and no caloric response to ice water, yet his conductive hearing loss was improved by drilling a new oval window. It is recommended that if a labyrinthotomy has not improved the hearing, a canalplasty should be done and the patient fitted with an ear level hearing aid.

Atretic Plate. Seven atresia patients had been previously operated on elsewhere, with no improvement in hearing. It was apparent that the basic pathology of atresia was either being overlooked or misunderstood. Specifically, when the atretic plate is present, it is always in firm bony union with the malleus. In many cases the previous surgeon apparently had been content to drill an opening into the middle ear or antrum, and then place a graft over the hole. The operation would fail to improve the hearing as the ossicular chain was still fixed to the atretic plate (Fig. 1). In one case a surgeon had opened into the middle ear, found the ossicular

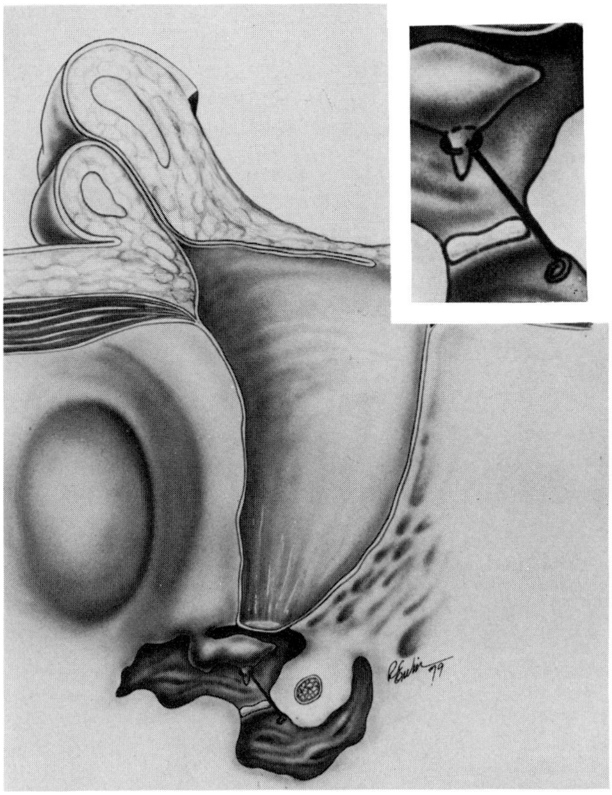

Fig. 2. Pitfalls in atresia repair. An opening had been made into the middle ear, the incus and stapes noted to be fixed, and the stapes suprastructure removed. A wire prosthesis (insert) had been placed onto a mobile footplate and had eroded through the margin to become fixed in the vestibule. The surgeon had overlooked the fact that the malleus was fixed to the atretic plate.

chain to be fixed, and performed a partial stapedectomy with insertion of a wire prosthesis (Figs. 2 and 3).

It is imperative to completely remove the atretic plate. This is done by thinning the dense compact bone of the plate and then dissecting the bone chips from the underlying periosteum. The periosteum should be excised as it prevents adequate exposure of the middle ear and is usually too thick to be used as a substitute tympanic membrane. The new ear canal is then widened at its medial extent to enable the ossicular chain to be situated in the approximate center of the new tympanic membrane. A fascia graft is placed over the ossicles and a center-hole split thickness skin graft, 0.025 cm in thickness, positioned over the fascia. If the problem is stenosis rather than atresia, any remaining skin lining the canal should be preserved. It may then be used in conjunction with a split thickness skin graft.

It is unnecessary to make the new external ear canal two or three times wider than needed in anticipation of a postoperative stenosis. Postoperative stenosis rarely results from new bone growth and soft tissue stenosis can be avoided by covering all raw tissue areas with skin, particularly at the meatus.

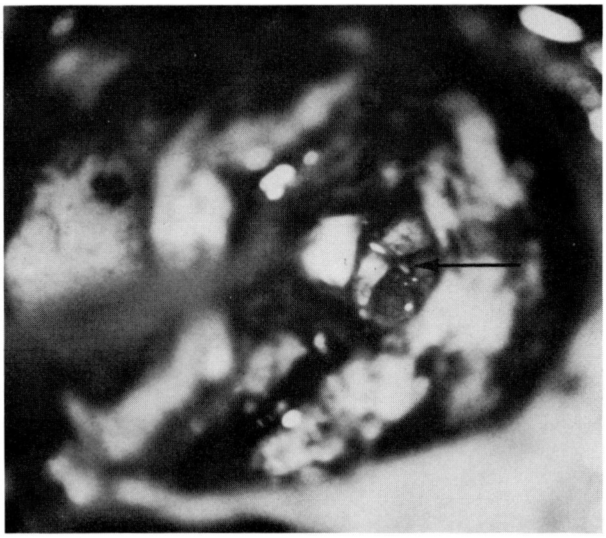

Fig. 3. Photograph of case described in Figure 2. Note wire prosthesis (arrow) on incus.

SURGICAL RESULTS

As a previous presentation dealt with the hearing results in the first 20 cases of atresia repair,[1] and because there have been modifications in surgical technique, only those cases operated on in the past year will be presented. Operations were performed on nine patients with atresia or stenosis of the external ear canal. Eight had surgery for hearing rehabilitation while one had surgery for cholesteatoma. In three of nine ears there was no hearing improvement. Of these three, one patient had absent labyrinthine windows, absent stapes, and a middle ear filled with adipose tissue. Another patient with an absent oval window had an unsuccessful labyrinthotomy. The third patient underwent surgery for cholesteatoma and although the labyrinthine windows were absent the cholesteatoma had created a cochlear fistula on the promontory. A homograft incus was sculptured into the shape of a mushroom and positioned on the fistula membrane.

Six of nine patients achieved a good hearing result (Table 1). The average gain was 38 dB. The air-bone gap was completely closed in one ear and closed to within 8, 10, 10, 11 and 18 dB in the others. In no case was the hearing made worse.

The experience gained in this series enables certain conclusions to be made.

1. Except in carefully selected cases, surgery on a

TABLE 1. HEARING RESULTS IN ATRESIA/STENOSIS IN 1979 (N = 9)

Gain (dB)	*No. Ears*
50 +	1
40-49	1
30-39	4
20-29	0
10-19	0
No change	3

unilateral atretic ear is best postponed until the child reaches young adulthood and can either decide for himself/herself or share in the decision-making process.

2. In bilateral atresia, if a good hearing result has been obtained in one ear, the second ear should be treated in much the same manner as unilateral atresia.

3. Fenestration of the semicircular canals should be avoided. If the labyrinthine windows are absent and labyrinthotomy has not improved the hearing a canalplasty should be done and the patient fitted with an ear level hearing aid.

4. Congenital facial nerve paralysis is not an absolute contraindication to surgery. It may, however, herald severe dysplasia of the middle ear.

REFERENCES

1. Jahrsdoerfer RA. Congenital atresia of the ear. Laryngoscope 1978; 88 Suppl 13:1-48.

≈

OTORHINOLARYNGOLOGY PATIENT OF THE MONTH PROGRAM

ACUTE COCHLEAR DISORDERS: THE COMBINATION OF HEARING LOSS, RECRUITMENT, POOR SPEECH DISCRIMINATION, AND TINNITUS

JUERGEN TONNDORF, MD

NEW YORK, NEW YORK

The combination of hearing loss, recruitment, poor speech discrimination and tinnitus, which is characteristic of acute cochlear disorders, can be accounted for on the basis of a decoupling of hair cells from their drive system, the tectorial membrane. Decoupling may either be caused by a temporary reduction of ciliary stiffness (shown to occur during periods of noise-induced temporary threshold shifts) or by temporary and/or chronic ciliary pathology (demonstrated to exist in cases of antibiotic ototoxicity and in endolymphatic hydrops). Since ciliary coupling is elastic in nature, the decoupling is only partial. The hearing loss and the tinnitus are manifestations of the reduced coupling per se, the magnitude of the loss depending on the degree of decoupling and the number of hair cells involved. Recruitment and poor speech discrimination result from center-clipping of the signal waveform applied to an involved hair cell, the direct corollary of partial, ciliary decoupling.

INTRODUCTION

Acute cochlear disorders are generally characterized by the simultaneous occurrence of sensorineural hearing loss, recruitment, poor speech discrimination and tinnitus. This combination of signs and symptoms is found, for example, during noise-induced temporary threshold shifts (TTS), during attacks of fluctuant hearing loss, and during the early stages of drug-induced ototoxic hearing impairments. The common link between the above disorders is thought to be impairment of hair cell function, suggesting that the four signs and symptoms listed might be traceable to one common cause. The present paper will offer a hypothesis supporting this notion. It grew out of a previous, more tentative publication on the same subject.[1]

During the classical era of light microscopy the functional state of hair cells was simply judged on the basis of their presence or absence in histological follow-up examinations. Absence of hair cells could of course account only for permanent functional losses, but not for temporary ones, such as those taking place in TTS. The first exception to this simple rule came with the observation of opaque, swollen and/or pyknotic hair cell nuclei, following sound exposure.[2,3] These changes were thought to be transient in nature.

STEREOCILIARY CHANGES

Scanning electron microscopy revealed stereociliary changes hitherto unreported. In cases of kanamycin-induced ototoxicity, profound changes were demonstrated:[4] fusion of stereocilia on individual hair cells to a thick stalk or sprouting of giant hairs (Fig. 1). These most certainly were irreversible changes that should eventually lead to the complete degeneration of the involved cells. Occasionally, however, lesser forms of changes were seen that might be reversible: small blebs at or near the tips of individual stereocilia, ie, in places where the cilia are in contact with the tectorial membrane (Fig. 2).

These observations were soon confirmed and extended by others. Kimura,[5] for example, found the

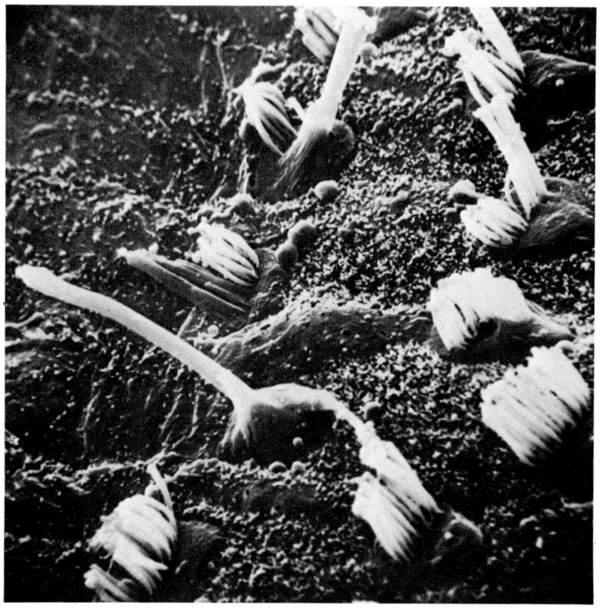

Fig. 1. Scanning electron microscopy of the top surface of the organ of Corti of a cat reveals grave changes of stereocilia caused by kanamycin. (x8,200). (From Bredberg et al.[4] Published with permission.)

From the Department of Otolaryngology, College of Physicians and Surgeons of Columbia University, New York, New York.

Presented at the meeting of the American Otological Society, Inc., Palm Beach, Florida, April 13-14, 1980.

REPRINTS — Juergen Tonndorf, MD, College of Physicians and Surgeons of Columbia University, 630 West 168th Street, New York, NY 10032.

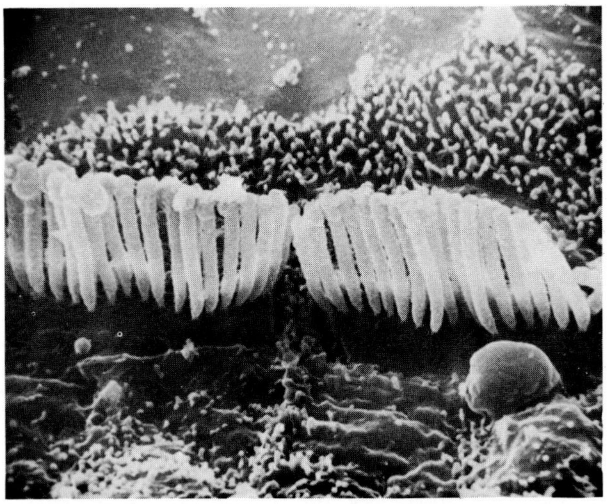

Fig. 2. The ciliary tufts of two inner hair cells showing formation of blebs at the tips of individual hairs (same animal shown in Fig. 1). (x10,600). (From Bredberg et al.[4] Published with permission.)

same changes in postmortem specimens from patients with Menière's disorder of long standing. These findings suggested that the involved hair cells might be *decoupled* to varying degrees from their drive system, the tectorial membrane. This notion became a virtual certainty with another observation.

Stereocilia are known to be very stiff and brittle, breaking on the slightest provocation.[6,7] Hunter-Duvar[8] exposed guinea pigs to 4 kHz tones of sufficient intensity and duration to produce TTS. Immediately after exposure, ie, during the period of TTS, scanning electron microscopy revealed that in the involved cochlear region stereocilia had become quite limp (Fig. 3 A, B). In control animals, sacrificed 24 hours later, ie, at a time when the TTS should have completely recovered, the stereocilia had regained their normal stiffness.

These observations were complemented by the following findings.[9] The core of each stereocilium consists of a bundle of fine filaments, each approximately 5 nm in diameter. These filaments were shown to contain *actin*, a contractile substance, responsible for the stiffness of the entire assembly. Significantly, actin is known to be capable of changing into a paracrystalline state under the effect of certain physiological processes, then rendering the entire assembly of filaments more compliant.

LOSS OF SENSITIVITY

Reduction of ciliary stiffness must *decouple* the involved hair cells to some extent, ie, *partially*, from their drive system, the tectorial membrane; this decoupling should impair signal transmission. (The significance of the term "partial" will become clear presently.) Ciliary pathologies of the kind shown in Figures 1-3 are expected to have essentially the same effect. The resulting loss of auditory sensitivity should vary with the degree of decoupling and with the number of hair cells involved.

TINNITUS

Tinnitus is one of the chief complaints of patients with cochlear disorders. Neurophysiological considerations once prompted Davis[10] to state that tinnitus might be the outcome of a process that renders cochlear nerve fibers "leaky" so that their normal rate of spontaneous discharge is increased. Although intuitively attractive, this was only a descriptive statement, not really an analytical explanation. Tinnitus appears to be a general response of

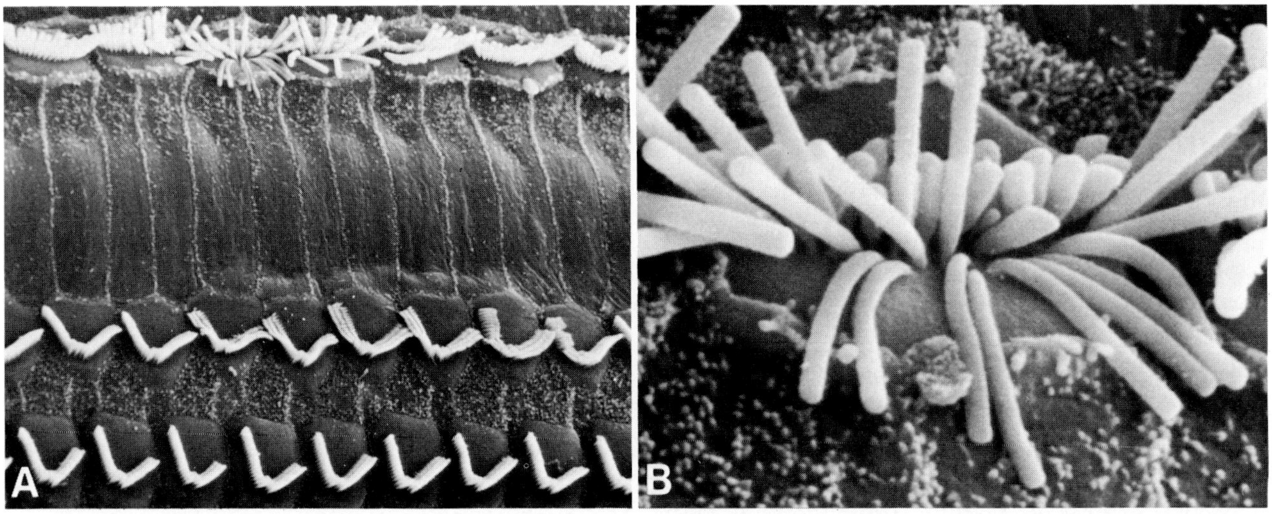

Fig. 3. A) A section of the organ of Corti of a guinea pig in the 4 kHz region. The stereocilia of inner as well as outer hair cells are shown. Note the limpness of stereocilia in a narrow region in the center of the picture. This scanning electron microscopic photograph was obtained immediately after cessation of exposure to a 4 kHz tone. B) Details of A showing the condition of one inner hair cell. During life, stereocilia do not necessarily lean over as extremely as shown in these photomicrographs, since they are pegged to the tectorial membrane, removed here for the sake of preparation. (From Hunter-Duvar IM.[8])

the auditory system to lesions caused by a host of different agents and taking effect at various levels, the cochlea included. The explanation that will be offered here applies only to tinnitus of *cochlear* origin. It will be based on the concept of decoupling of hair cells from the tectorial membrane.

The needed clue was provided by a study of Harris.[11] Harris was interested in determining the noise level at the hair cell input, expecting the hair cell sensitivity, like that of any other receiver, to be limited by the prevailing background noise. On account of the high sensitivity of the ear, he suspected the cochlear noise level to be quite low. In all materials, there exists a low-level noise that is caused by molecular motions of thermal origin, known as *Brownian motion.* Since these motions occur randomly, they constitute a broad-spectrum noise. For constant temperature, their mean velocity is highest in gases, less in fluids, and least in solids. It thus depends on the inverse density of material, or as Harris put it more succintly, on the *coupling* between particles. The tighter the coupling, the lower must be the mean velocity because the mass to be moved becomes effectively larger. Harris therefore decided to calculate the noise level under two extreme conditions, tight coupling between hair cells (large mass) and loose coupling (small mass). With tight coupling, he obtained a noise level approximately 20 dB below the auditory threshold in the most sensitive frequency region. M. Killion* recalculated this value. His result was even closer to threshold. When coupling was loose, however, Harris found the noise level to increase by 55 dB. He concluded that, from the standpoint of his argument, the deduction of tight coupling had been the correct one.

The increase in noise level at the hair cell input when coupling is loose is interesting with respect to the present problem. A large part of the coupling *between* hair cells should be provided by their connection *with* the tectorial membrane. It is suggested that the *increase in noise level caused by a partial decoupling of hair cells from the tectorial membrane is the basis of tinnitus of cochlear origin.* In most patients, the level of tinnitus is surprisingly low, rarely higher than 20 dB above threshold, even though its subjective loudness often appears to be much higher.[12] Thus Harris's result, an increase in noise by as much as 55 dB, appears to be more than ample to account for the tinnitus.

Although it is generated as a broad-band noise, tinnitus may vary from broad-band noises to very narrow-band noises, the latter essentially sounding like pure tones. The apparent filtering is brought about in the following manner. Individual hair cells are very sharply tuned.[13] The center frequency of their respective tuning curves varies with position along the basilar membrane in accordance with the frequency/place principle. When a broad-spectrum noise is applied from the *outside*, it excites a larger number of hair cells distributed over a wide area of the basilar membrane. In response to a narrow band of noise, a lesser number of hair cells is excited and their distribution is limited to a smaller area. The character of a noise generated *within* the cochlea therefore must also depend on the location and on the extent of the region in which the causative lesion, ie, ciliary decoupling, occurred. "Roaring" tinnitus, ie, a low-frequency band of noise, as found in fluctuant hearing loss, indicates a rather broad apical involvement. Significantly, the hearing loss is also of the low-frequency type. A high-pitched, tone-like tinnitus, ie, a very narrow band of high-frequency noise, is typical of TTS. The involvement is limited to quite a narrow area in the basal turn, as was indeed demonstrated by Hunter-Duvar[8] in Figure 3A. The hearing loss as a rule is of the high-frequency notch type. A "hissing" tinnitus, ie, a somewhat broader band of high-frequency noise, is frequently reported in the early stages of drug-induced ototoxic lesions when the hearing loss is still limited to the high-frequency region. In other such cases, when the hearing loss extends well into the speech range, the tinnitus is often described as "wooshing," ie, as a substantially broader band of noise. It is thus seen that there is quite a good correlation between the site of the lesion and its extent, the type of hearing loss occurring, and the character of the noise experienced by the patient.

RECRUITMENT

The decoupling of a given hair cell will rarely be complete, and usually is only partial. On reduction of ciliary stiffness, for example, the tufts of hairs must be deflected for only a certain distance in either direction away from the center position, until they acquire once more an elastic, restoring force sufficient in magnitude to reestablish coupling between the hair cells and the tectorial membrane. There is a "dead play" around the center position similar to that occurring in a worn-out meshed gear, which is alternately moved in opposite directions. In cases of ciliary pathology, decoupling is not necessarily complete either.

When a signal is delivered to a hair cell with ciliary dead play, the loss of amplitude around the center position introduces *center-clipping* of the resultant waveform (Fig. 4 A). The amount of dead play in a given situation is constant. With a rise in signal level, therefore, the *relative* degree of the amplitude reduction must become gradually smaller (compare Fig. 4 A, B), eventually vanishing.

Such changing amplitude relations between input and output signals may be presented quantitatively, in decibels, as so-called *input/output* functions (Fig. 4 C). Curve 1 (Fig. 4 C) represents a function *without* center-clipping. For the sake of il-

*Killion M. Personal communication, 1978.

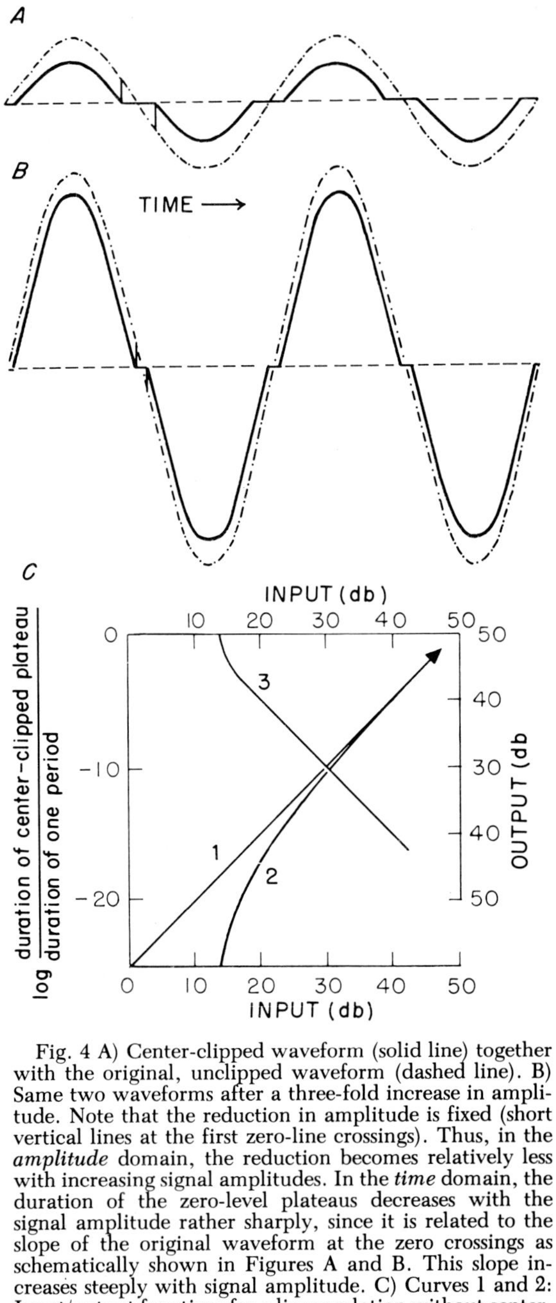

Fig. 4 A) Center-clipped waveform (solid line) together with the original, unclipped waveform (dashed line). B) Same two waveforms after a three-fold increase in amplitude. Note that the reduction in amplitude is fixed (short vertical lines at the first zero-line crossings). Thus, in the *amplitude* domain, the reduction becomes relatively less with increasing signal amplitudes. In the *time* domain, the duration of the zero-level plateaus decreases with the signal amplitude rather sharply, since it is related to the slope of the original waveform at the zero crossings as schematically shown in Figures A and B. This slope increases steeply with signal amplitude. C) Curves 1 and 2: Input/output functions for a linear relation without center-clipping (curve 1) and with center-clipping (curve 2). Curve 3: The fractional duration, in logarithmic values, of the zero-level plateau as function of signal level.

lustration, it is assumed to be perfectly linear. Curve 2 shows a function resulting from center-clipping. It is quite *nonlinear.* There is a threshold shift and, following that, a steeper-than-normal rise in output amplitude. Eventually, but gradually, it joins the corresponding function without center-clipping (curve 1). When the center-clipping is more extensive, the threshold shift simply becomes larger and the entire curve 2 is shifted farther to the right, joining curve 1 at a proportionally higher level.

Curve 2 (Fig. 4 C) is recognized as a typical *recruitment* curve, the equivalent of the laddergram familiar from audiometric charts. This explanation of recruitment, a dead play in the ciliary action, represents *hair cell dysfunction.* As such it is quite compatible with the empirical rule[14] which states that recruitment is invariably associated with *hair cell pathology*, but is never found in retrocochlear lesions.

Partial recruitment is occasionally seen in the presence of space-occupying tumors in the internal auditory meatus. Since it vanishes on removal of the tumor, it is shown to be produced by impairment of the cochlear blood supply, ie, in the last analysis, by a metabolic insufficiency of the hair cells. Hence it is also caused by hair cell dysfunction.[15]

Békésy[16] found evidence for what might be a different kind of recruitment. Using a version of his own audiometer, he recorded the responses of human observers to stimulation of dermal touch receptors. He found that thresholds were sensitive in areas with a high density of touch receptors; in such cases, there were invariably wide-swing tracings. Under either of two other conditions, ie, when an originally sensitive skin area was partially anesthetized, or when an area was chosen with a low density of touch receptors, there were elevated thresholds and narrow-swing tracings. Thus, in contrast to the first set of data, the second and third revealed the presence of recruitment. Békésy then reasoned that the absence of recruitment should require neural integration of responses derived from the action of a large number of peripheral receptors, but that recruitment should result whenever only a small number of receptors contribute to the integrated response.

This reasoning was supported by findings in electronic neuron models,[17,18] in cochlear-microphonic experiments[19] and in cochlear-nerve fiber recordings.[20] Since Békésy registered recruitment only at threshold, it is not readily apparent that this phenomenon should result in an input/output function that would exactly join the corresponding nonrecruiting function and lead to complete recruitment as shown in Figure 4 C. It could conceivably continue to much higher levels. It is therefore suggested that the *relative paucity of available receptors* underlying the findings of Békésy[16] and of the other authors[17-20] might result in *over-recruitment* in the sense of Fowler's classification.[21]

Granted that the above considerations are correct, it appears that underlying all forms of recruitment is hair cell pathology, but that its various forms might have different specific causes. *Complete recruitment* is suggested to be caused by a partial decoupling of a number of hair cells from the tectorial membrane, *over-recruitment* by the complete functional and/or structural loss of hair cells, most likely of *outer* hair cells,[20] and *under-recruitment* by impaired hair cell function due to metabolic insufficiency. It might be added, for the sake of completeness, that "decruitment," in the sense of Fowler's classification,[21] may be brought about by a combination of (hair cell) recruitment and (central) adaptation, as was suggested by Békésy.[22]

POOR SPEECH DISCRIMINATION

Center clipping interferes quite severely with speech perception.[23] That speech discrimination is worse than the pure tone audiogram might indicate, is one of the characteristics of the cochlear disorders under discussion, provided that the hearing loss extends down into the speech frequency range. This is not always the case, for example, in patients with early antibiotic lesions or during TTS.

Although both recruitment and poor speech discrimination are suggested to be causally related to center-clipping, there is an important difference. Recruitment was shown to be merely a manifestation of a fixed loss in the *amplitude* domain. The deterioration of speech perception is suggested to be related to the waveform distortion in the *time* domain, since *peak-clipping*, which also reduces signal amplitude, hardly affects speech discrimination. Even with "infinite" peak-clipping, retaining nothing but the zero-crossings of the input waveform, speech discrimination is surprisingly good.[24]

In the time domain, the duration of the zero-level plateau lessens even more sharply with increasing signal levels than does the relative amplitude reduction (Fig. 4 A, B). Numerically, the fractional duration of the zero-level plateau decreases by approximately one order of magnitude over an input range of a mere 15 dB (curve 3 of Fig. 4 C).

The lessening of center-clipping in the time domain with increasing input levels, however, is of little, if any, help to patients with cochlear disorders for the following reason: running speech signals undergo rapid amplitude fluctuations with time over a range of approximately 30 dB. Many patients with cochlear disorders, when trying to adjust their TV or radio sets to an *acceptable* average level, find this task difficult, if not impossible. The signal is either too loud and uncomfortable on account of the recruitment present, or it is too soft and speech discrimination is severely impaired.

It was stated above that the effects of ciliary pathology on the coupling of hair cells to the tectorial membrane should be essentially similar to those caused by the reduction of ciliary stiffness. No rationale for that statement was given, an omission that shall now be corrected. If the ciliary pathology would merely loosen the connection to the tectorial membrane in the sense of a loss in *frictional coupling*, the output waveform should become *peak-clipped* and that, as just stated, would not affect speech discrimination at all. However, in disorders in which the occurrence of ciliary pathology has been documented, such as endolymphatic hydrops and antibiotic ototoxic lesions, the deterioration of speech perception is very pronounced — provided that the hearing loss involves the speech frequency range. It was therefore concluded a) that the coupling between the stereocilia and the tectorial membrane is *elastic* in nature, and b) that ciliary pathology should therefore affect coupling in the same manner as does the reduction of ciliary stiffness, producing the same type of center-clipping.

CLOSING REMARKS

Admittedly, some portions of the present hypothesis still lack direct experimental proof. Nevertheless, one can derive considerable confidence from its coherence, ie, from the fact that the four characteristic signs and symptoms of acute cochlear disorders (hearing loss, recruitment, poor speech discrimination, and tinnitus) could be explained on the basis of one common phenomenon, ciliary decoupling. I hasten to add, however, that although this may be a very frequent cause of the combined finding, it is not necessarily the exclusive cause of each of the signs and symptoms. Recall the different forms of recruitment and the fact that tinnitus may be generated at various levels of the auditory system.

REFERENCES

1. Tonndorf J. Ein Vorschlag zur gemeinsamen Genese von Hörverlust, Rekruitment und Ohrgeräuschen bei akuten Innenohrveränderungen. Arch Otorhinolaryngol 1977; 217:289-96.

2. Wüstenfeld E, Sprenger FH. Variationsstatistische Untersuchungen an den Sinneszellkernen des Cortischen Organs beim Meerschweinchen. Z Zellforsch Mikrosk Anat 1958; 48:720-34.

3. Beck C, Michler HH. Feinstrukturelle und histochemische Veränderungen an den Strukturen der Cochlea beim Meerschweinchen nach dosierter Reinton Beschallung. Arch Ohrenheilkd 1960; 174:496-567.

4. Bredberg G, Ades HW, Engström H. Scanning electron microscopy of the normal and pathologically altered organ of Corti. Acta Otolaryngol (Stockh) 1972; Suppl 301:3-48.

5. Kimura RS. Experimental pathologenesis of hydrops. Arch Otorhinolaryngol 1976; 212:263-73.

6. Engstrom H, Ades HW, Hawkins JE Jr. Structure and functions of the sensory hairs of the inner ear. J Acoust Soc Am 1962; 34:1356-63.

7. Flock A, Flock B, Murray E. Studies on the sensory hairs of receptor cells in the inner ear. Acta Otolaryngol (Stockh) 1976; 83:85-91.

8. Hunter-Duvar IM. Morphology of the normal and the acoustically damaged cochlea. Scan Electron Microsc 1977; 2:421-7.

9. Flock A, Cheung H. Actin filaments in sensory hairs of the inner ear receptor cells. J Cell Biol 1977; 75:339-43.

10. Davis H. Tinnitus — new aspects on etiology and management: physiological aspects. Trans Am Acad Ophthalmol Otolaryngol 1954; 58:527-8.

11. Harris GG. Brownian motion in the cochlear partition. J Acoust Soc Am 1967; 44:176-86.

12. Vernon JA. The loudness (?) of tinnitus. Hear Speech Action 1976; 44:17-9.

13. Russell IJ, Sellick PM. Tuning properties of cochlear hair cells. Nature 1977; 267:859-69.

14. Dix WR, Hallpike CS, Hood JD. Observation upon the loudness recruitment phenomenon, with especial reference to the differential diagnosis of disorders of the inner ear and VIII nerve. Proc R Soc Med 1948; 41:516-26.

15. Palva T. Finnish speech audiometry. Acta Otolaryngol (Stockh) 1952; Suppl 101.

16. von Békésy G. Neural volleys and the similarity between some sensations produced by tones and by skin vibrations. J Acoust Soc Am 1957; 29:1059-69.

17. Harmon LD. Studies with artificial neurons: I. Properties and functions of an artificial neuron. Kybernetik 1961; 1:7-101.

18. Van Bergeijk WA. Studies with artificial neurons: II. Analog of the external spiral innervation of the cochlea. Kybernetik 1961; 1:102-7.

19. Honrubia V, Ward PA. Cochlear potential recruitment produced by local anesthetics. Surg Forum 1966; 17:471-2.

20. Kiang NYS, Moxon EC, Levine RA. Auditory-nerve activity in cats with normal and abnormal cochleas. In: Wolstenholme GEW, Knight J, eds. Sensorineural hearing loss. London: Churchill, 1970:241-68.

21. Fowler EP. Some attributes of "loudness recruitment" and "loudness decruitment." Trans Am Otol Soc 1965; 53:78-84.

22. von Békésy G. Loudness recruitment. Trans Am Otol Soc 1966; 54:85-93.

23. Licklider JCR. Effects of amplitude distortion upon the intelligibility of speech. J Acoust Soc Am 1946; 18:429-34.

24. Licklider JCR, Pollack I. Effects of differentiation, integration and infinite peak-clipping upon the intelligibility of speech. J Acoust Soc Am 1948; 20:42-57.

≈

REPORT OF THE PANEL ON COMMUNICATIVE DISORDERS

Single copies of the *Report of the Panel on Communicative Disorders to the National Advisory Neurological and Communicative Disorders and Stroke Council* (NIH publication no. 79-1914) may be obtained from: Chief, Office of Scientific and Health Reports, National Institute of Neurological and Communicative Disorders and Stroke, Bldg. 31, Rm 8A08, 9000 Rockville Pike, Bethesda, MD 20205.

IMMUNOPATHOLOGICAL STUDY OF THE LARYNX

IgA DISTRIBUTION AND SECRETORY ACTIVITY

TADASHI NAKASHIMA, MD
SOHTARO KOMIYAMA, MD
KAZUMI MAKISHIMA, MD
KAZUO TAKEDA, MD
IKUICHIRO HIROTO, MD

FUKUOKA, JAPAN

Using immunofluorescent and histopathological techniques, we studied the distribution and secretory activity of the glands of the larynx from 55 humans. The cavity of the larynx was covered with secretory glandular cells with the exception of the true vocal cords, aryepiglottic folds and upper part of the laryngeal surface of the epiglottis. Immunofluorescent study revealed the presence of IgG and other immunoglobulins throughout the connective tissue ground in each laryngeal mucosa. The most striking was seen in the staining pattern of IgA. Diffuse fluorescence for IgA was observed not only in the submucosal or periglandular connective tissue area but also in the intraepithelial or submucosal glands. Secretory component synthesis was found mainly in each serous-type glandular epithelium or acinus. In the submucosal or periglandular area, IgA producing plasma cells were numerous. Our observations suggest that IgA, produced locally, is secreted via the glandular cells as secretory component — SIgA. Secretory activity of SIgA in these glandular tissues indicates that the larynx is possibly an immunologically active organ in the upper respiratory tract.

SC: Secretory component; SIgA: Secretory IgA; FITC: Fluorescein isothiocyanate; PBS: Phosphate-buffered saline; rGG: Rabbit gamma-globulin; Lf: Lactoferrin.

The larynx is situated in the upper respiratory tract and is a significant organ for phonation and respiration. It is well established that the larynx is endowed with a rich supply of glands which are of the exocrine compound tubuloalveolar type.[1] Laryngeal secretions, produced in the glandular tissue, act as lubricants in vocal cord vibration.[2] It has also been suggested that such laryngeal secretions may contribute to the immunological mucosal resistance of the larynx. Most recently Mogi et al reported the biological properties of laryngeal secretions and proposed that such are characterized by exocrine secretion and resembled nasal and tracheobronchial secretions.[3] However, little attention has been given to the immunological role of the larynx regarding the distribution and topography of the laryngeal glands.

The present study was an attempt to demonstrate the distribution of glandular tissue and examine the secretory activity of IgA in the larynx. Since the discovery of IgA in various external secretions, such as parotid saliva, colostrum and nasal secretions, the significance of this immunoglobulin in local immune systems has been reported by various groups.[4,5] In 1965, Tomasi et al demonstrated the presence of 11S IgA, which differs chemically and immunologically from 7S IgA.[6] It is now well established that 11S IgA (so called secretory IgA: SIgA), which is predominant in external secretions, is associated with secretory component (SC) and is synthesized locally in the mucous epithelium or in glandular tissues.[7] It has also been suggested that SC might act as a specific receptor for dimeric IgA and be secreted as SC bound SIgA. Immunohistological analysis concerning the localization of IgA, SC and SIgA in glandular tissue should provide pertinent information on the immunological function of the larynx.

METHODS

Tissue Specimens. Laryngeal tissues were obtained from 55 Japanese patients (35 males, 20 females) and prepared for examination. The age, sex and reasons for excision are summarized in Table 1. Fifteen of 55 larynges were excised from patients who underwent total laryngectomy for cancer lesion. The tissue specimens subjected to immunofluorescent study were determined macroscopically and microscopically to be totally free of cancer. Forty larynges were extracted from autopsied patients who died of other diseases. There were no remarkable changes in these tissues.

After removal, the specimens were placed in 95% ethanol (4 C) for fixation for two to three days, cut into slices of 1 to 2 mm and the fixation was continued for three to five additional days. The fixed tissues were then placed in absolute alcohol (4 C) for dehy-

TABLE 1. TISSUE SPECIMENS (N = 55)

Age	*No. of Patients*	*Sex* *M*	*F*	*Reasons for Excision*	
0-10	3	2	1	Total laryn-	
11-20	1	1	0	gectomy for	
21-30	2	2	0	cancer lesions	15
31-40	3	3	0		
41-50	9	4	5		
51-60	15	9	6		
61-70	15	11	4	Autopsy	40
71-80	7	6	1		

From the Department of Otorhinolaryngology, Faculty of Medicine, Kyushu University, Fukuoka, Japan.

REPRINTS — Tadashi Nakashima, MD, Department of Otorhinolaryngology, Faculty of Medicine, Kyushu University, Fukuoka 812, Japan.

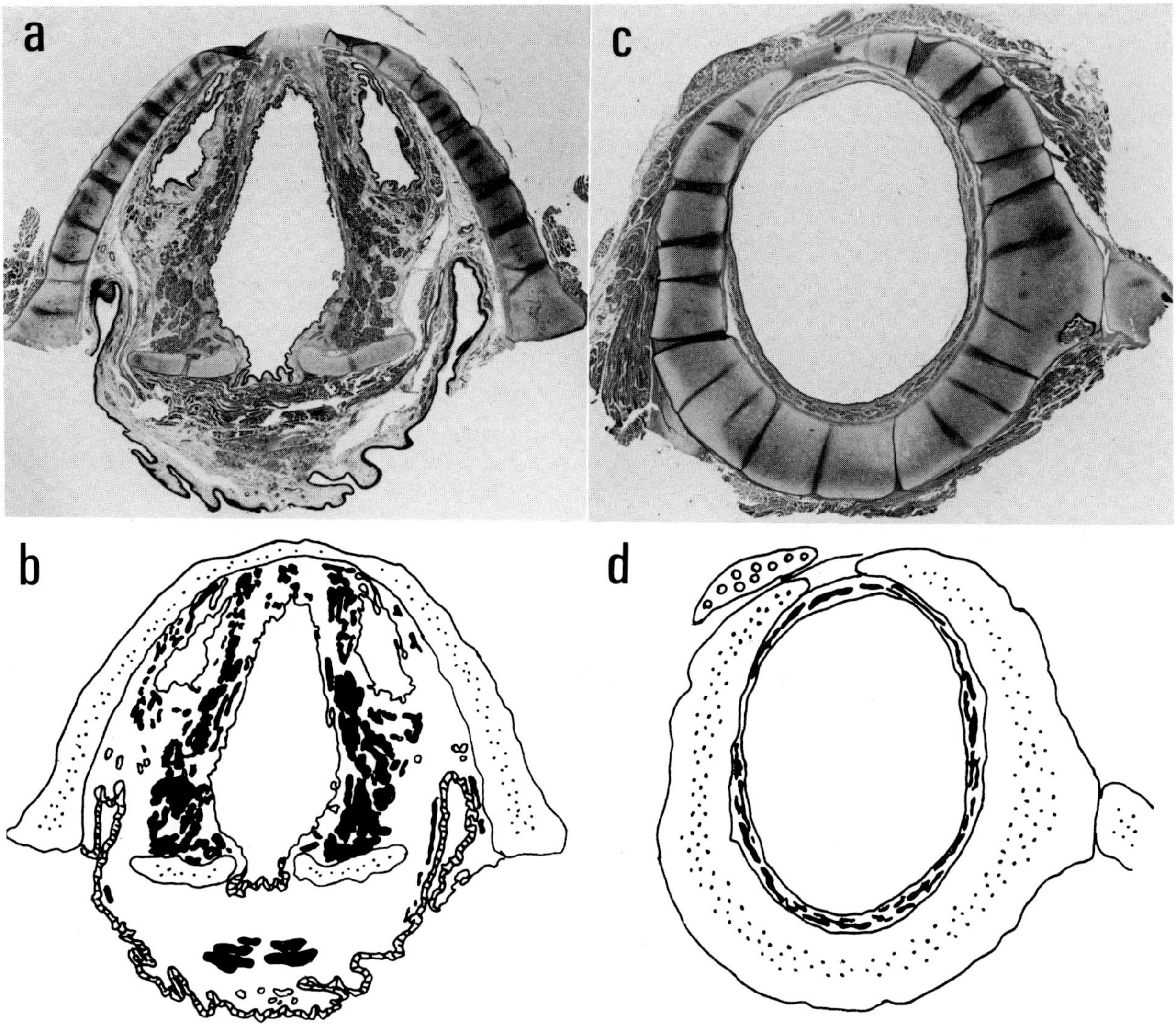

Fig. 1. Horizontal section through ventricle (a,b) and subglottis (c,d). a, c) H & E staining; b, d) Schematic presentation of the glands. (x5). Gland; Bone; Thyroid gland; Squamous epithelium.

dration and were prepared for paraffin sectioning as described elsewhere.[8,9] Embedded sections were cut into serial sections at 4 μ in thickness, deparaffinated and stained using a direct or indirect immunofluorescent technique.[9] The consecutive sections were also stained with H&E or PAS-AB for routine histopathological examination.

Antisera. Antisera to human IgA and IgG were prepared by immunizing rabbits with α-chain or γ-chain component of each immunoglobulin. Rabbit anti-IgM (μ-chain) and anti-IgE (ϵ-chain) were purchased from Boehringer Institute.* Antisera to human SC and lactoferrin (Lf) were gifts.† All these antibodies were adjusted to a protein concentration of 0.2 mg/ml before use. Anti-rabbit gamma-globulin (anti-rGG) goat serum was obtained by immunizing a goat with rGG. Specificities of these antibodies were confirmed by immunodiffusion and immunoelectrophoresis.

Fluorescin-Labeled Antibodies. Antisera to human IgA, IgG and rGG were labeled with fluorescein isothiocyanate (FITC) as described previously.[9,11] Fluorescein-to-protein ratios of labeled anti-IgA, anti-IgG and anti-rGG were 1.2, 0.9 and 1.6.

Immunofluorescent Study. Direct (anti-IgA, anti-IgG) and indirect (anti-IgM, anti-IgE, anti-SC, anti-Lf) immunofluorescent studies were carried out. In the direct immunofluorescent examination, incubation with FITC-labeled antiserum was carried out in a humidified chamber overnight at a room temperature of 20 C and was followed by a wash in four to five changes of cold phosphate-buffered saline (4 C) at pH 7.2 for 15 minutes. The labeled sections were mounted with nonfluorescent glycerin-PBS and observed under a fluorescent microscope.*

For the indirect immunofluorescent techniques, the deparaffinated sections were first incubated with antiserum at 37 C for one hour. After the antiserum was washed out carefully with cold PBS, the sections were reincubated with FITC-labeled anti-rGG overnight followed by washing and mounting as above. In the control studies, unlabeled antiserum was used.

*Hoechst, Japan.

†Goro Mogi, MD, Yamaguchi University School of Medicine, Ube, Japan.

RESULTS

Routine Microscopic Observations. The cavity of the larynx was lined with ciliated or nonciliated respiratory epithelium, with the exception of the true vocal cords and aryepiglottic folds which were covered with stratified squamous epithelium. The

*Nikon Camera Co, Tokyo, Japan.

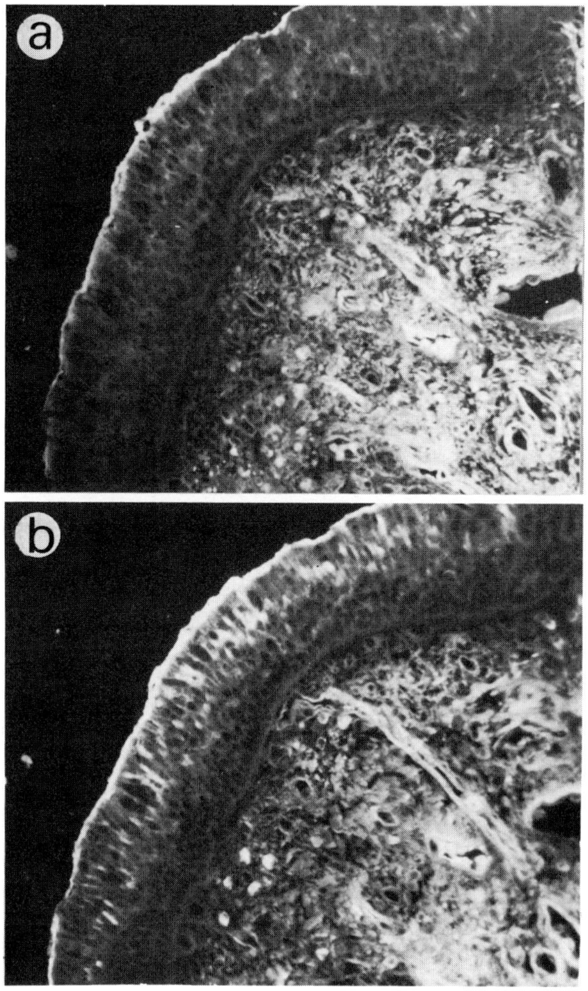

Fig. 2. Immunofluorescent analysis by anti-IgG and anti-IgA in the mucosa of ventricle. Diffuse fluorescence for a) IgG and b) IgA were observed throughout the connective tissue. Plasma cells were also evident. Note the fluorescence for IgA in the secretory epithelium. (x100)

lingual surface of the epiglottis was also covered with squamous epithelium. In the tissues from adults, squamous change was occasionally seen in the mucosa of the upper part of the laryngeal surface of the epiglottis and lip of the false vocal cord, and was most evident in older age groups. The squamocolumnar junction at the lining of the free edge of true vocal cords had shifted to the ventricular or subglottic area in the older age groups. Intraepithelial or submucosal glandular distribution was observed in each laryngeal specimen. Although the pattern and degree of distribution differed more or less from one specimen to the other, the glands were particularly numerous in the false vocal cords, ventricle and subglottis.

In the ventricular area, saccular glands were seen to extend everywhere in the submucosa and further to the submucosa of the false vocal cord. The glands on the ventricular aspects of the false cord were continuous and lateral with those of the saccule. In addition, a few glands were seen to arise from the lateral wall of the ventricle and extend superiorly

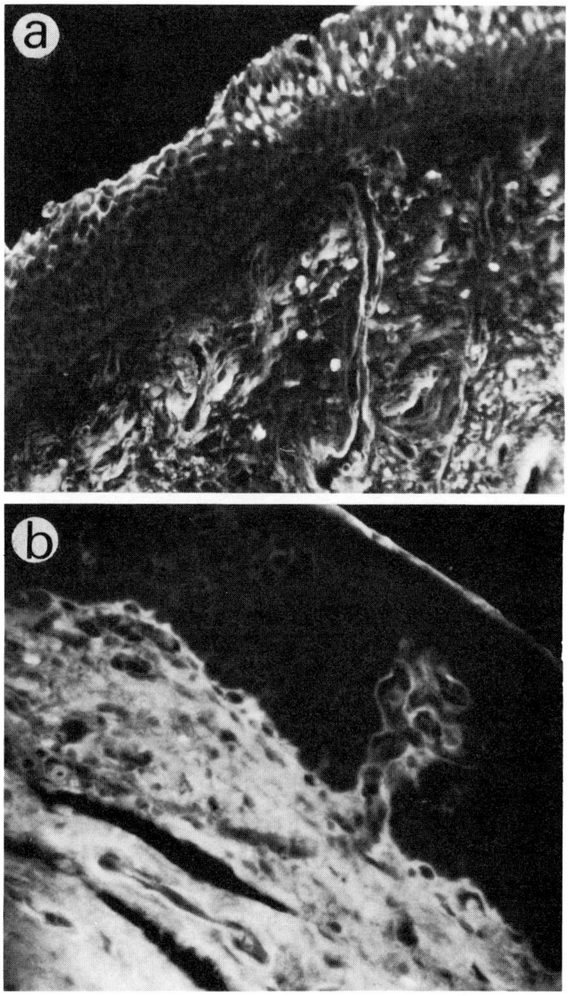

Fig. 3. Staining pattern by anti-IgA conjugate in laryngeal mucosa. a) IgA distribution in the mucosa of false vocal cord. Diffuse fluorescence for IgA distributed in the submucosal stroma. IgA producing plasma cells were also seen. Note the cytoplasmic fluorescence for IgA found in the columnar epithelium. Faint or no fluoresence was found in the squamous epithelium. b) Distribution of IgA in the upper part of the laryngeal surface of epiglottis. Note the clear-cut boundary of the staining pattern at the basement membrane of the epithelium. Fluorescence was also observed in the mucus materials on the mucosa.

and laterally in close proximity to the thyroid cartilage (Fig. 1 a, b). Occasionally, at the level of the vocal process where the ventricle ends, the glands penetrated laterally to the vocal process into the fibers of the vocalis muscles.

A heavy concentration of glands was also found in the subglottic region. As shown in Figure 1 c, d, closely packed glands were found to be distributed in the narrow submucosal connective tissue surrounded by cricoid cartilage. In contrast, glands were rarely found in the submucosa of the true vocal cord or within the underlying vocalis muscle. Only in the ventricular side of the cord did a few ducts proceed downwards. On the epiglottic margin, an extensive tubuloalveolar glandular system extended infraglottically within the deep fibers of the cricothyroid ligament.

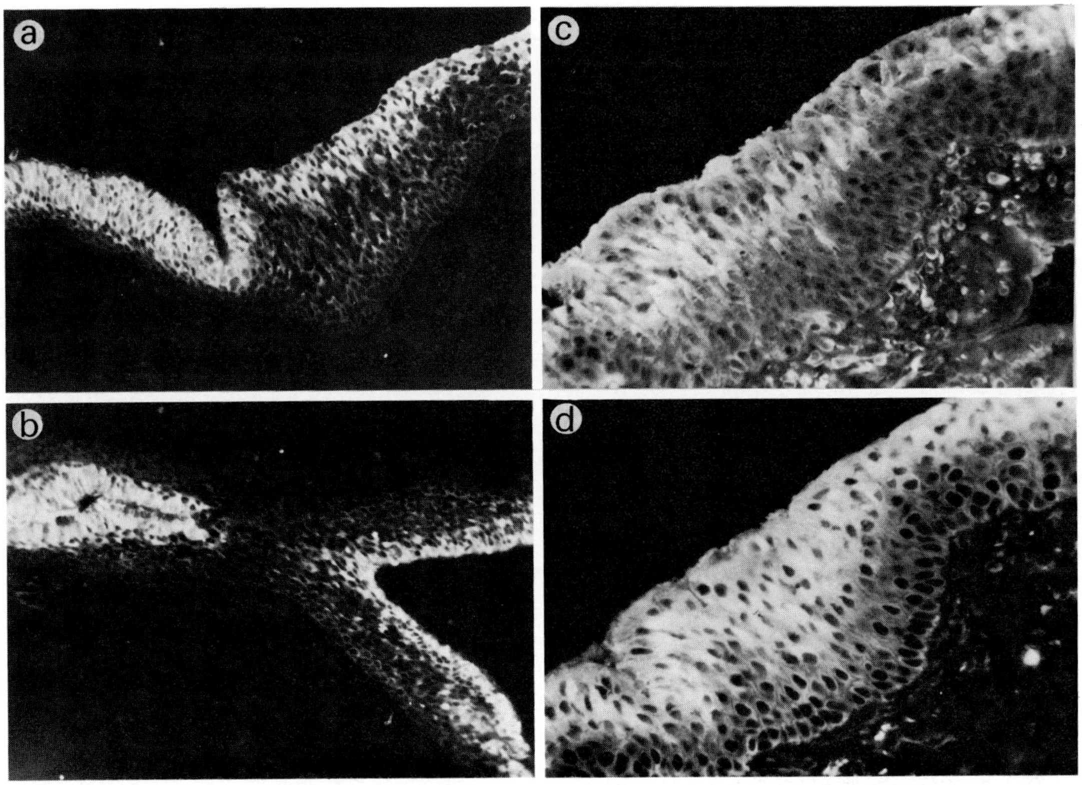

Fig. 4. Immunofluorescent analysis by anti-SC and anti-IgA in the glandular epithelium. a) Glandular epithelium of false vocal cord stained for SC (x200). Bright fluoresence was found in every intraepithelial secretory cell. b) Secretory glands in the ventricle stained for SC (x200). Fluorescence for SC was observed not only in the epithelial glands but also in the glandular ductules. c) Staining pattern by anti-IgA conjugate in the mucosa of the subglottis (x400). Fluorescence for IgA was found in the glandular epithelium and plasma cells just beneath the epithelium. d) Adjacent section to Fig. 4c stained for SC. Note the intense fluorescence found in the cytoplasm of each secretory epithelial cell.

The laryngeal glands were of the mixed seromucinous type. Serous-type glands tended to be predominant in children and young adults. There was no relationship between the distribution of serous- and mucous-type glands in each topographical study. Goblet cells were also found in each specimen. It should be noted that the periglanular adipose tissues increased in number in the older age groups. Round cell infiltration was observed to greater and lesser degrees in each tissue section. In such cells, plasma cells and neutrophils were the most prominent. Plasma cells were present predominantly in the submucosal connective tissue area and around the glandular acini. In some cases, eosinophils were localized in the submucosal connective tissue area.

Immunofluorescent Examination. When tissue sections from laryngeal mucosa were incubated with specific antisera to human IgG, IgA, IgM and IgE, fluorescence for each was observed in almost every case. As demonstrated in Figure 2a, anti-IgG conjugate produced considerable fluorescence not only on the mucoid materials on the mucosa but also in the submucosal connective tissue. IgG producing plasma cells were present in the stroma beneath the epithelium of the false vocal cord, ventricle and subglottis. IgG producing plasma cells were also present around the vessels. Plasma cells producing IgM and IgE also existed in the subepithelial layer of mucosa covering the false vocal cord, ventricle and subglottis. Their numbers, however, were relatively few as compared to findings in the IgG plasma cells. The most intense fluorescence was seen when tissues were incubated with anti-IgA conjugate. Anti-IgA conjugate produced considerable fluorescence in the submucosal connective tissue ground substances not only of the ventricle (Fig. 2) but of the false vocal cord (Fig 3a) and epiglottis (Fig. 3b).

Fluorescence for IgA was also observed in the stroma around the glandular acini or ductules. Fluorescence in mucoid materials on the mucosa also revealed the presence of IgA in the secretion. IgA producing plasma cells were observed in the submucosal connective tissue (Figs. 2b, 3a and 4c), periglandular area (Fig. 5c) and around the vessels. Although the numbers of IgA producing plasma cells varied between different specimens, IgA plasma cells were abundant in specimens taken from the false vocal cord, ventricle and subglottis. In the true vocal cord, the numbers of IgA, IgG, IgM and IgE plasma cells were small despite the presence of such immunoglobulins in the stroma.

The most striking difference between anti-IgA and antisera to other immunoglobulins was in the

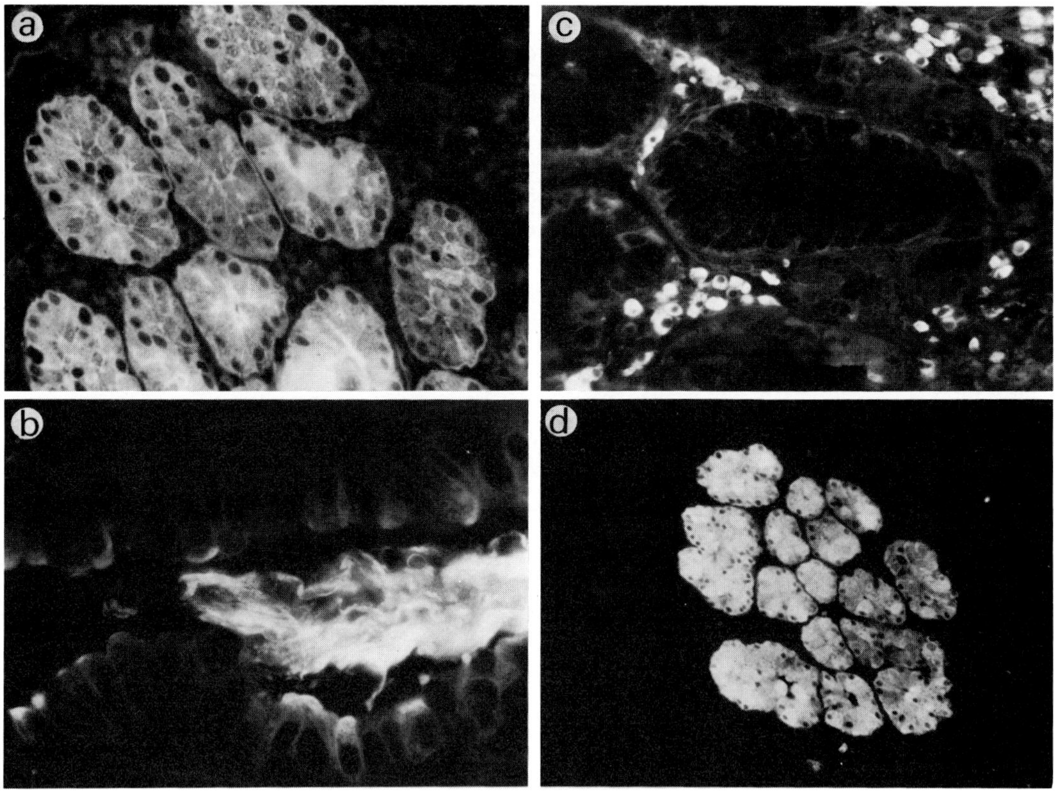

Fig. 5. Secretory glandular acini or ductules in the larynx. a) Closely-packed, tubuloalveolar acini in the ventricular area. Bright fluorescence was found in all the serous-type acinar cells. Intercellular spaces were strongly fluorescent. (Stained for SC, x200). b) Glandular ductules extending to the ventricle. Mucus materials in the lumen were strongly fluorescent. Note the fluorescence in the apical cytoplasm. (Stained for SC, x400). c) Distribution of IgA producing plasma cells around the glandular acini (Stained for IgA, x200). d) Lf synthesis in the closely-packed glandular acini. Fluorescence for Lf was seen in the cytoplasm of serous-type acini. (Stained for Lf, x100).

staining pattern of the laryngeal epithelium. As demonstrated in Figures 2b, 3a and 4c, anti-IgA conjugate revealed a bright fluorescence in the cytoplasm of the intraepithelial secretory glands. Such secretory epithelial cells were commonly seen in the ciliated columnar epithelium of the false vocal cord, ventricle, subglottis and the lower part of the laryngeal surface of the epiglottis. In contrast, IgA secreting glandular cells were not present in the squamous epithelium of the epiglottis (Fig. 3b) and the true vocal cord.

The intense fluorescence for IgA observed on the mucoid materials on the mucosa and the presence of IgA positive cells in the columnar epithelium indicate the significance of this immunoglobulin in the larynx. We, therefore, examined the secretory activity of such glandular tissues by staining with anti-SC and anti-IgA. Bright and regular fluorescence for SC was noted in the glandular epithelial cells of the false vocal cord (Fig. 4a), ventricle (Fig. 4b) and subglottis (Fig. 4d). The fluorescence for SC was most evident in the apical cytoplasm and intercellular spaces of serous-type glandular cells. Mucous-type acinar cells and goblet cells contained very little or no SC.

To assess the secretory process of IgA in glandular epithelium, we observed the staining pattern of IgA and SC in serial sections, as demonstrated in Figure 4c, d. In the glandular epithelial cells of subglottic laryngeal mucosa, SC production was commonly seen in the cytoplasm of secretory cells. When the adjacent section was stained with anti-IgA conjugate, fluorescence was noted not only in the cytoplasm of IgA producing cells but also in the secretory epithelial cells. IgA was also found in the submucosal connective tissue. Mucoid materials on the mucosa also showed positive fluorescence for anti-IgA and anti-SC. It was evident that IgA, produced locally by plasma cells, entered the cytoplasm or intercellular spaces of the secretory cells and was secreted via the secretory epithelium. Mucoid materials, therefore, apparently contained SC bound SIgA.

The secretory process of IgA was most prominent in the submucosal glands. In the closely packed glandular acini, anti-SC revealed the bright staining of cell membrane and also of the cytoplasm, but the most intense staining was from the intercellular spaces of the glands (Fig. 5a). The bright fluorescence for SC was also observed in the glandular ductules (Fig. 5b). Although the fluorescence for SC differed between each glandular cell in such ductules, it was evident that the apical cytoplasm along the ductal lumen fluoresced most intensely. Most of the round cells found around the glandular acini or ductules were IgA producing plasma cells (Fig. 5c). It is considered, therefore, that SIgA production was most prominent in the glands of that area, indicating the presence of SIgA in the laryngeal secretions in the ventricle.

In contrast to the regular and heavy fluorescence for SC obtained from every glandular cell found in laryngeal epithelium, glandular acini and ductules, anti-Lf conjugate produced a brilliant fluorescence only in the submucosal glandular acini (Fig. 5d). Almost no fluorescence for Lf was noted in the secretory cells on the laryngeal mucosa. Lf was usually not detected in the glandular acinar cells positive for PAS-AB staining.

DISCUSSION

The present study demonstrated that most of the mucosa of the laryngeal cavity is lined with ciliated or nonciliated columnar epithelium, showing the predominance of glandular epithelium in the larynx. Stratified epithelium with occasional squamous metaplasia was usually seen in the true vocal cord, epiglottis and also frequently in the lip of the false vocal cord. The fact that the vocal cord is commonly covered with squamous epithelium has been confirmed by others.[1,12,14] Tucker et al, who studied the development of the laryngeal epithelium, reported that the laryngeal surface of the epiglottis is uniformly covered with columnar appearing cells.[13] They also reported that a profile view of such epithelium demonstrated a stratified character. Endo, who examined the laryngeal epithelium histologically, reported that squamous change of the laryngeal surface of the epiglottis increased with aging.[14] Developmental studies of the laryngeal epithelium were also done by Hopp,[12] who demonstrated that the epithelium of the larynx differentiates in a definite pattern throughout embryonic life to achieve its adult appearance, and described it as a result of physiological metaplasia. We found that the stratified squamous epithelium covering the upper part of the laryngeal surface of the epiglottis extended to the ventricular area; such findings revealed evidence of physiological change.

It should be noted, however, that most of the laryngeal cavity is lined with secretory epithelial cells. The presence of intraepithelial or submucosal glandular tissue illustrates the significant role of the secretory system in the larynx. Nassar and Bridger found that the ciliated laryngeal mucosa is generally associated with submucosal glands, and reported that the function is to maintain a lubricated mucosal surface.[1] It was also reported by DeWeese and Saunders that laryngeal secretion acts as a lubricant in vocal cord vibration.[2] The predominance of epithelial or submucosal glands in the ventricular and subglottic areas (Fig. 1) may indicate an active secretion. It should also be considered that the laryngeal mucus may contribute to the immunological mucosal resistance of the larynx.

Mogi et al, who investigated the biological properties of laryngeal secretion, observed that laryngeal secretions have much the same amount of IgG, IgA and other immunoglobulins as those in nasal secretions and tracheobronchial washings.[3] They also emphasized the local immune system by secretory IgA in the laryngeal mucosa. Our immunofluorescent study revealed the presence of IgG (Fig. 2a) and other immunoglobulins in laryngeal mucosa. However, anti-IgA conjugate produced the most intense fluorescence throughout the connective tissue area in each specimen (Figs. 2b and 3). The predominance of IgA producing plasma cells in the submucosal (Figs. 2b, 3a and 4c) or periglandular (Fig. 5c) connective tissue supports the idea of an active local IgA synthesis against antigenic stimuli.[15]

With respect to the local immune system in respiratory passages, numerous studies have been reported.[5,7,10,11] It is now well established that, in such external secretions, SIgA is the predominant immunoglobulin and consists of two antigenically different substances, dimeric IgA and secretory component (SC).[7,16] Recent studies have shown that SC is produced mainly in serous-type glandular acinar cells.[9,10,16] Brandtzaeg reported the presence of dimeric IgA containing plasma cells around the glands.[17] The bright fluorescence for SC localized in the intraepithelial (Fig. 4) or submucosal (Fig. 5a, b) glands and the diffuse distribution of IgA producing plasma cells beneath the mucosa (Fig. 4c) or around the glandular acini (Fig. 5c) provide adequate confirmation. Although the exact mechanism of SIgA transmission is unknown, it is quite probable that interstitial dimeric IgA is secreted via the glandular cells after the binding of SC in the larynx.

Lactoferrin is an antibacterial iron-binding protein in milk and other exocrine secretions.[3,18] Immunofluorescent examination for Lf showed that such is produced only in the closely packed serous-type glandular acini (Fig. 5d), which are negative for PAS-AB staining, whereas glandular cells in the epithelial lining do not react to anti-Lf antibodies. Similar findings were also observed by other workers.[3] Immunohistochemical and cytochemical examinations to determine the differences of Lf synthetic activity between intraepithelial glands and glandular acini are now underway.

ACKNOWLEDGMENTS — We thank Dr. M. Kubomura, Kyushu Chuoh Hospital, for provision of the specimens, and M. Ohara, Kyoto University, for pertinent advice on the manuscript.

REFERENCES

1. Nassar VH, Bridger GP. Topography of the laryngeal mucous glands. Arch Otolaryngol 1971; 94:490-8.

2. DeWeese DD, Saunders WH. Textbook of otolaryngology. St. Louis: CV Mosby, 1960.

3. Mogi G, Watanabe N, Maeda S, et al. Laryngeal secretions. An immunochemical and immunohistological study. Acta Otolaryngol (Stockh) 1979; 87:129-41.

4. Chodirker WB, Tomasi TB Jr. Gamma globulins. Quantitative relationship in human serum and nonvascular fluids. Science 1963; 142:1080-1.

5. Remington JS, Voski KL, Lietze A, et al. Serum proteins and antibody activity in human nasal secretions. J Clin Invest 1964; 43:1613-24.

6. Tomasi TB Jr, Tan EM, Solomon A, et al. Characteristics of an immune system common to certain external secretions. J Exp Med 1965; 121:101-24.

7. Tomasi TB Jr, Bienenstock J. Secretory immunoglobulins. Adv Immunol 1968; 9:1-96.

8. Hamashima Y, Kyogoku M. Immunohistology. Immunofluorescent technique, immuno-electron microscopic technique, radioisotope labeled antibody technique. 3rd ed. Tokyo: Igaku Shoin Ltd, 1974.

9. Nakashima T, Hamashima Y. Loss of secretory activity in the glands of nasal polyps. Ann Otol Rhinol Laryngol 1979; 88:210-6.

10. Mogi G. Secretory immunoglobulin A in oral and respiratory passages in man. Ann Otol Rhinol Laryngol 1975; 84 Suppl 20:3-23.

11. Nakashima T, Hamashima Y. Local immune system of nasal mucosa in inflammation. IgA distribution and secretory activity. Ann Otol Rhinol Laryngol 1980; 89:140-6.

12. Hopp ES. The development of the epithelium of the larynx. Laryngoscope 1955; 65:475-99.

13. Tucker JA, Vidic CB, Tucker GF, Stead J. Survey of the development of laryngeal epithelium. Ann Otol Rhinol Laryngol 1976; 85 Suppl 30:3-16.

14. Endo N. Histological study on the larynx. Its histological change with increasing age. J Jpn Bronchoesophagol Soc 1972; 23:322-44.

15. Heremans JF, Vaerman JP. Biological significance of IgA antibodies in serum and secretions. In: Amos B, ed. Progress in immunology. New York: Academic Press, 1971:875-90.

16. Brandtzaeg P. Mucosal and glandular distribution of immunoglobulin components. Differential localization of free and bound SC in secretory epithelial cells. J Immunol 1974; 112:1553-9.

17. Brandtzaeg P. Two types of IgA immunocytes in man. Nature (New Biol) 1973; 243:142-3.

18. Oram JD, Reiter B. Inhibition of bacteria by lactoferrin and other iron-chelating agents. Biochim Biophys Acta 1968; 170:351-65.

≈

RHINOPLASTY COURSE

The annual course "Rhinoplasty from the Beginning" will be given Sept. 6-10, 1980 in San Francisco. For further information contact: Leslie Bernstein, MD, Otorhinolaryngology, UC Davis Medical Center, 4301 X St., Sacramento, CA 95817. (916) 453-2801.

Ann Otol 89:1980

COMPARATIVE PREOPERATIVE EVALUATION OF EUSTACHIAN TUBE FUNCTION IN PATHOLOGICAL EARS

H. VIRTANEN, MD

T. PALVA, MD

T. JAUHIAINEN, MD

HELSINKI, FINLAND

On 100 pathological ears with tympanic membrane perforation, eustachian tube function was measured by using sonotubometry and the negative pressure equalization test in an attempt to compare these two methods. The pressure equalization test did not appear to be a reliable tool for preoperative clinical determination of tube function because sonotubometry showed tubal opening in 85% (myringoplasty group) and in 49% (radical surgery group) of pathological ears, which were not able to equalize negative middle ear pressure at all during swallowing. The negative pressure equalization test is considered to be unphysiological and may produce a locking phenomenon of the tube. Even a small negative pressure can act like a valve, producing an obstruction that muscle activity of the tube is no longer able to overcome particularly when mucosal changes are present in the tubal orifice. Sonotubometry is a physiological test and as such gives a reliable picture of the opening of the tube during swallowing. Data on tympanic aeration postoperatively will be reported later.

There is general agreement that adequate eustachian tube function is necessary for successful middle ear surgery even if many other factors also influence the results. Opinions have differed on the value of preoperative tubal function tests in chronic otitis media and some investigators have questioned their significance[1,2] because the number of false negative measurements has been too high and their prognostic value in middle ear surgery, poor. Reliable information would, therefore, be welcome in planning the surgical procedures since a well-functioning eustachian tube is an essential prerequisite for postoperative aerated middle ear.

According to many investigators[3-6] the best and most physiological way to examine the tubal function has been the negative pressure equalization method (aspiration method) introduced by Flisberg et al in 1963.[7] The artificially created negative middle ear pressures were equalized with one or two swallowings by normal individuals.[3,4,6,8-11]

The number of ears with the ability to equalize the negative intratympanic pressure completely or partially has varied from 7.5[12] to 70% in different pathological (chronic otitis) materials, the mean being 46%.[13] Good results have been obtained by tympanoplasty even though the negative pressure equalization test has shown the inability of the tube to normalize the altered middle ear pressure.[1,3,8,9,12,14,15] On the basis of this negative correlation some investigators have been of the opinion that the pressure equalization test has very little value in the evaluation of tubal function.

One of the recently worked out methods in the evaluation of physiological auditory tubal opening is sonotubometry, reported by Virtanen.[16,17] In this procedure a pure tone (6, 7, and 8 kHz) delivered into one nostril is recorded from the external ear canal and during swallowing even in 95% of normal ears a sound pressure level change can be registered denoting tubal opening.

Encouraged by these early results which reproduce well, we have started doing the eustachian tube function tests in clinical series in order to compare a simplified negative pressure equalization test and sonotubometry. In the present paper the results of these methods of examination are reported as applied for preoperative assessment of tubal opening in pathological ears scheduled for surgery. Postoperative data will be reported later when sufficient time has elapsed from surgery to evaluate the permanent end result.

METHODS

A total of 100 ears with central or marginal tympanic membrane perforation of 100 patients ranging from 8 to 82 years of age were evaluated. No patient had upper respiratory infection at the time of the test. The patients were divided into two main groups. In the myringoplasty group there were 56 ears which were all dry. The second group consisted of 44 ears with active disease on which radical operations were performed.

Prior to surgery, sonotubometry and the negative middle ear pressure equalization test for eustachian tube function were performed. The main principle in sonotubometry, previously described in detail,[16,17] was to introduce pure tones of 6, 7, or 8 kHz through a nasal oliva tip into the nostril. The test sound passing through the tube during tubal opening was picked up by the microphone embedded in the circumaural ear defender and fitted with a probe of suitable size in the external ear canal. The amplified output of the microphone was fed through the narrow bandpass filter in order to suppress background noise and recorded by a level recorder (Figs. 1 and 2).

The negative middle ear pressure equalization test was performed according to Flisberg et al[7] and Holmquist[18] with some modifications. The eustachian tube function was studied by means of an electroacoustic impedance bridge (Teledyne Model TA-2C), using its manometer section. A negative pressure level of

From the Department of Otolaryngology, University of Helsinki, Helsinki, Finland.

REPRINTS — H. Virtanen, MD, Department of Otolaryngology, University of Helsinki, SF-00290 Helsinki 29, Finland.

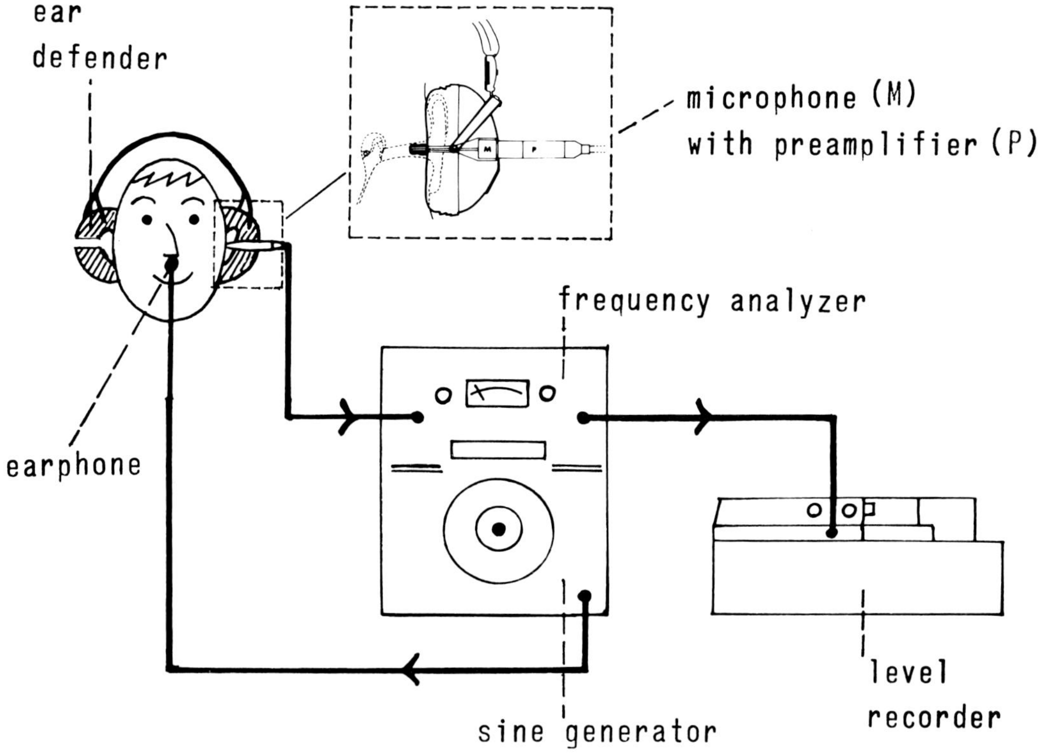

Fig. 1. A block diagram of the equipment.

– 200 mm H_2O was produced by means of the air pressure pump of the impedance meter into the external auditory canal and the middle ear. The patient was then asked to swallow a sip of water repeatedly, as a rule ten times. The associated equilibrating of the artificial negative pressure was registered and this final residual level was recorded.

RESULTS

The results of tubal function by the negative pressure equalization technique were classified into three groups with residual pressure ranges of 0-19, 20-199, and = 200 mm H_2O (Table 1), according to their capacity to normalize negative pressure. In sonotubometry level changes larger than or equal to 5 dB over the base line were accepted and the smaller responses only if these could without doubt be distinquished from the fluctuating base line.

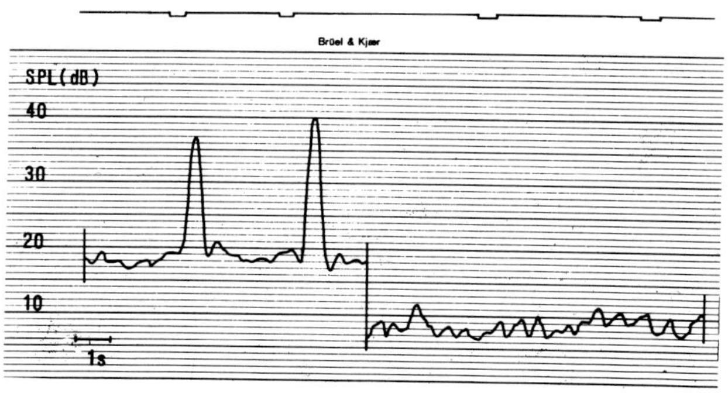

Fig. 2. The general pattern of the tubal opening with 7 kHz tone (left) and without tone (right) introduced into the nose as recorded from the external auditory meatus (SPL re 20 μ Pa). At the top of the chart the markings of the swallowing movements can be seen.

Fifty-six ears underwent myringoplasty with or without tympanoplasty and mastoidectomy. In 44 of the total 100 pathological ears, radical surgery for a chronic ear disease was performed with tympanic membrane, ossicular chain and canal wall reconstruction, combined with mastoid obliteration.[19] In the group of residual negative pressure of 0-19 mm H_2O there was only one ear in the whole series which had entirely "normal" pressure equalization during swallowing preoperatively. The artificially established negative middle ear pressure of 200 mm H_2O was equalized partially (range of 20-199 mm H_2O) in 21 ears in the myr-

TABLE 1. TUBAL FUNCTION OF 100 PATHOLOGICAL EARS DIVIDED ACCORDING TO RESIDUAL NEGATIVE PRESSURE EQUALIZATION TEST AS COMPARED WITH SONOTUBOMETRY

Residual Negative Pressure (mm H_2O)	*No. Ears*	*Sonotubometry*	
		Positive	*Negative*
Myringoplasty			
0-19	1	1	—
20-199	21	20	1
= 200	34	29*	5
Total	56		
Radical surgery			
0-19	—		
20-199	7	7	—
= 200	37	18†	19
Total	44		

*85%
†49%

ingoplasty group and in 7 ears in the radical surgery group. Twenty ears in the former group and seven ears in the latter group had positive sonotubometric results. In the third group, where the negative middle ear pressure was unchanged during swallowing, 29 of 34 myringoplasty ears (85%) and 18 of 37 radical surgery ears (49%), respectively, showed positive tone passage through the tube preoperatively. The detailed results are given in Table 1.

DISCUSSION

Examination of the present data shows a great discrepancy between the sonotubometry and the negative pressure equalization test. This type of result is apparently due to several factors. In cases of a dry ear and normal looking mucosa, the pressure equalization test cannot be considered physiological because the negative air pressure levels applied largely exceed the underpressures which develop normally by gas absorption from the middle ear cavity.[20,21] According to the experiments of Elner[20,21] an underpressure of 30-65 mm H_2O develops in one hour and about 1 ml air is absorbed in 24 hours if the tube does not open, but normally the tube opens once every 1 to 3 minutes.

In the truly pathologically changed middle ears, the mucosal changes often extend to the mucosa of the tube in the form of tissue edema, and sometimes in the form of thick, even polypous or granulating mucosa. In the negative pressure equalization method, the suction power of the negative middle ear pressure on the mucosal surfaces in the tube evidently is capable of further impairing tubal opening during swallowing[8,22] and this locking phenomenon of the tube has also been reported by Holborow.[23] Even a small negative pressure can act just like a valve producing an obstruction that the muscle activity of the tube is no longer able to overcome. Another condition that the equalization technique does not take into account is a perforation which is not connected to the tympanic orifice of the tube and the negative result is directly misleading.

This reasoning accords well with the recent results of Siedentop et al[24] who found no difference between 15 normal and 14 pathological ears with intact tympanic membranes. In their material 60% of normal ears were unable to attain achieved middle ear pressures of -100 mm to -250 mm H_2O when a pressure of -200 mm H_2O was applied to the nasopharynx and the subject asked to swallow. Both the normal and pathological ears required repeated swallows to normalize negative pressures and the repetition was not good.

Our findings indicate clearly that the results of sonotubometry for the identification of tubal dysfunction are not in agreement with those obtained from the pressure equalization method. The sonotubometry was positive in very many cases in which there was no change in the negative pressure equalization test. The preliminary data with sonotubometry results in 18 ears reported by Virtanen[16] showed a much better correlation with surgical results in both the preoperative and postoperative tests.

Enthusiasm for the value of the preoperative eustachian tube function tests has, with the exception of a few workers, greatly declined particularly because the pressure equalization test has not correlated with the surgical results even in the most favorable group, myringoplasty. In dry, normal ears, the surgical results generally testify for a perfect tube function even if the pressure equalization test has been negative. In severely diseased ears surgery around the eustachian tube can greatly modify the end result and it is even logical that the pressure equalization test preoperatively, when negative, is useless. On the other hand, sonotubometry is an entirely physiological test which, when positive, depicts what regularly happens in human ears after each swallow. How well the results will correlate with a successful tympanic aeration will be seen later when this material has had a sufficient follow-up period.

REFERENCES

1. Ekvall L. Eustachian tube function in tympanoplasty. Acta Otolaryngol (Stockh) 1970; Suppl 263:33-42.

2. Smyth GDL, Kerr AG, Goodey RJ. Current thoughts on combined approach tympanoplasty. J Laryngol Otol 1971; 85:205-12.

3. Miller GF Jr. Eustachian tubal function in normal and diseased ears. Arch Otolaryngol 1965; 81:41-8.

4. Holmquist J. Middle ear ventilation. A clinical study. Thesis, University of Göteborg, Göteborg, Sweden, 1969.

5. Elner Å, Ingelstedt S, Ivarsson A. The normal function of the eustachian tube. Acta Otolaryngol (Stockh) 1971; 72:320-8.

6. Kumazawa T, Honjo I, Honda K. Aerodynamic evaluation of eustachian tube function. Preliminary report on normal subjects. Arch Otorhinolaryngol (NY) 1974; 208:147-56.

7. Flisberg K, Ingelstedt S, Örtegren U. Controlled "ear aspiration" of air. Acta Otolaryngol (Stockh) 1963; Suppl 182:35-8.

8. Flisberg K. Ventilatory studies on the eustachian tube. Acta Otolaryngol (Stockh) 1966; Suppl 219.

9. Siedentop KH, Tardy ME, Hamilton LR. Eustachian tube function. Arch Otolaryngol 1968; 88:386-95.

10. Holmquist J. Tympanometry in testing auditory tubal function. Audiology 1972; 11:209-12.

11. Holmquist J. Assessment of eustachian tube function behind an intact tympanic membrane. ORL Digest 1973; 35:21-4.

12. Sharp M. The manometric investigation of tubal function with reference to myringoplasty results. J Laryngol Otol 1970; 84:545-51.

13. Andréasson L, Ivarsson A. On tubal function in the presence of central perforation of drum in chronic otitis media. Acta Otolaryngol (Stockh) 1976; 82:1-10.

14. Holmquist J. The role of the eustachian tube in myringoplasty. Acta Otolaryngol (Stockh) 1968; 66:289-95.

15. Palva A, Kärjä J. Eustachian-tube patency in chronic ears. Pre-operative evaluation correlated to postoperative results. Acta Otolaryngol (Stockh) 1970; Suppl 263:25-8.

16. Virtanen H. Eustachian tube sound conduction. Sonotubometry, an acoustical method for objective measurement of auditory tubal opening. Thesis, University of Helsinki, Helsinki, Finland, 1977.

17. Virtanen H. Sonotubometry. Acta Otolaryngol (Stockh) 1978; 86:93-103.

18. Holmquist J. Eustachian tube function assessed with tympanometry. A new testing procedure in ears with intact tympanic membrane. Acta Otolaryngol (Stockh) 1969; 68:501-8.

19. Palva T. Operative technique in mastoid obliteration. Acta Otolaryngol (Stockh) 1973; 75:289-90.

20. Elner Å. Normal gas exchange in the human middle ear. Ann Otol Rhinol Laryngol 1976; 85 Suppl 25:161-4.

21. Elner Å. Quantitative studies of gas absorption from the normal middle ear. Acta Otolaryngol (Stockh) 1977; 83:25-8.

22. Flisberg K, Ingelstedt S, Örtegren U. The valve "locking" mechanism of the eustachian tube. Acta Otolaryngol (Stockh) 1963; Suppl 182:57-68.

23. Holborow CA. Deafness associated with cleft palate. J Laryngol Otol 1962; 76:762-73.

24. Siedentop KH, Loewy A, Corrigan RA, Osenar SB. Eustachian tube function assessed with tympanometry. Ann Otol Rhinol Laryngol 1978; 87:163-9.

≈

LURIE LIBRARY FUND

Many inquiries have been made about a memorial fund to which friends and colleagues of Dr. Moses Hyman Lurie could contribute. Shortly before his death Dr. Lurie established a modest fund for the purchase of books in Otolaryngology for the Library at the Massachusetts Eye and Ear Infirmary. The Library Committee of the Infirmary has verified that donations can be made in memory of Dr. Lurie to this fund. Contributions may be sent to the "Lurie Library Fund," in care of Mr. Charles Snyder, Librarian, Massachusetts Eye and Ear Infirmary, 243 Charles St., Boston, MA 02114.

Ann Otol 89:1980

VESTIBULAR AND OCULOMOTOR ABNORMALITIES IN VERTEBROBASILAR INSUFFICIENCY

JORGE CORVERA, MD
GUILLERMO LOPEZ-RIOS, MD
LUIS D. BENITEZ, MD
MARIA TERESA RABIELA, MD
MEXICO CITY, MEXICO

The early diagnosis of vertebrobasilar insufficiency in patients with vertigo as their only symptom was attempted using a battery of vestibulo-oculomotor tests. With this testing procedure, we were able to find abnormal vestibulo-oculomotor mechanisms that could account for the vertigo in 41 of 42 patients. These abnormalities, however, did not fall into an easily recognizable pattern that could be considered characteristic of vertebrobasilar insufficiency. The large intersubject variability probably arises from the very different and widespread lesions that occur at the vestibular and neurological levels as a consequence of vertebrobasilar insufficiency.

Of the cerebrovascular diseases, the syndrome of vertebrobasilar insufficiency (VBI) is of particular importance to the neurotologist. It can take two different forms: a) intermittent insufficiency due to transient repetitive occlusion of a major vessel, usually one of the vertebral arteries; and b) steady diminution of the vascular reserve, due to thickening of the walls of small and middle size arteries, with eventual formation of small infarcts. In our experience, the first cause of VBI has been infrequent. By contrast, VBI of the second type is a very common cause of vertigo in patients after the fifth decade of life. In this paper we shall deal only with this form of vascular disease.

It has been established that vertigo is the most common first symptom to appear in VBI[1-4] and that it can exist as an isolated complaint for long periods of time. Vertigo is usually accompanied by unsteadiness more apparent in connection with sudden movements. This cannot be explained by neurological examination and it is only after other major symptoms and physical signs appear, such as diplopia, transient blindness, dysarthria and gait disturbances, that the diagnosis of VBI is established.

The otological examination of these patients has not helped very much in the past. Often, it did not show any abnormality that could explain the vertigo and unsteadiness, and in other cases, the findings could not be interpreted as due to central nervous disease as opposed to labyrinthine origin. The purpose of the present study was to detect abnormalities that could explain the symptoms of vertigo and disequilibrium in patients with VBI, and to explore the possibility of a pattern that could, in turn, help in the early diagnosis of the disease.

METHODS

In the last few years we have studied patients with suspected VBI. These patients can be classified in three groups.

1. Subjects with an established diagnosis of VBI on the basis of neurological studies.

2. Patients with known vascular pathology, like renovascular hypertension, diabetes, etc, who develop vertigo without any other symptom or neurological sign.

3. Vertiginous patients, without vascular or neurological pathology, in whom VBI is suspected based only on the neurotological examination.

In this paper, 42 patients were studied with vertigo as their only symptom, with strong possibility that it could be caused by VBI. This group of patients was followed up, and the diagnosis of VBI was considered confirmed when, in the course of time, the complete neurological picture of VBI or an infarct in the territory of a major cerebral vessel was developed. In five cases, the diagnosis of VBI was confirmed at necropsy; of these, three died of terminal renal insufficiency, one of necrotizing papillitis of diabetic origin and one of hemorrhagic infarct in the territory of the middle cerebral artery.

There were 20 males and 22 females, with a mean age of 63.3 and 64.6 years respectively. The distribution in decades is shown in Figure 1. Ten patients had kidney disease, either pyelonephritis or glomerulonephritis, that caused renovascular hypertension. Eight patients suffered diabetes and 13 arterial hypertension of unknown origin.

It is important to emphasize that, although in many of these patients several nystagmographic tracings had been obtained, only the tracings taken when there were no symptoms other than vertigo and when no neurological abnormalities were detected, were used for the purpose of this paper. For comparison purposes, an age-matched group of 45 normal subjects (with no vertigo or history of ear or neurological disease) was studied.

All patients had complete medical records at the hospital. Otorhinolaryngologic examination included tone and speech audiometry and when needed, Békèsy tracings, SISI and Carhart tests and impedance audiometry. Vestibulo-oculomotor tests included a) standard vestibular tests (spontaneous nystagmus, positional nystagmus and bithermal caloric tests),[5] and b) oculomotor tests with optical stimuli (ocular saccades, pursuit eye movements and optokinetic nystagmus).

From the Department of Otolaryngology, General Hospital and Section of Experimental Neurophysiology, National Medical Center, Instituto Mexicano del Seguro Social, and the Hospital Manuel Gea Gonzalez, Mexico City, Mexico.

REPRINTS — Jorge Corvera, MD, Durango 49-902, Mexico 7, D.F.,Mexico.

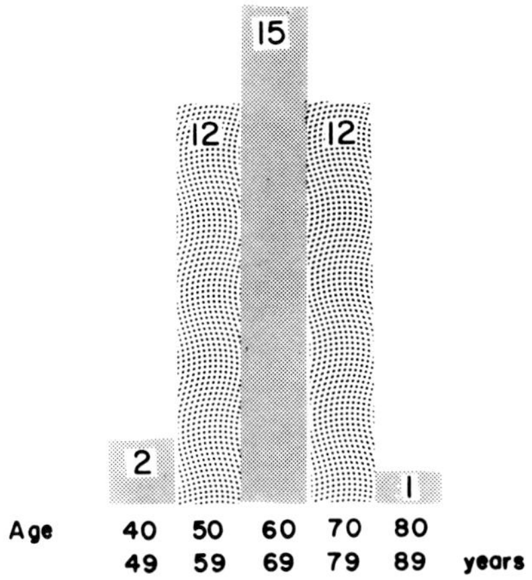

Fig. 1. Age distribution of the 42 patients studied.

The saccadic eye movements were tested by means of two small red lamps separated by an angular distance of 15°. The lights are connected so that when one goes on, the other simultaneously goes off. The pursuit eye movements were studied using the pendular eye tracking tests[6] in which a target swings in front of the patient with a frequency of 0.5 Hz covering an arc of 20-30°. Optokinetic nystagmus was investigated only in the horizontal plane, with the patient looking towards a drum painted with alternate black and white stripes, moving at several speeds, clockwise and counterclockwise.

Optovestibular integration tests were also performed. For this purpose we employed the torsion swing pendulum described by Greiner et al,[7] that oscillates in the vertical axis with a period of 20 seconds. Three tests were performed on each patient.

Vestibular Stimulation. The patient rotates with eyes covered; the eye movements thus produced are due only to vestibular influence. The cumulative nystagmic response is proportional in normals to the angular displacement of the chair and the variation is linear when such displacement is kept between 40 and 280°. The relation of magnitudes, however, varies according to the period; at 0.05 Hz, the total angular displacement of the eyes is equivalent to 40% of the angular displacement of the chair. This value is very constant in normal subjects, the standard variation being equivalent to 17.8% of the mean.[8]

Optovestibular Stimulation. The patient rotates. looking at the stationary surroundings. The vestibular stimulus is thus combined with an optokinetic stimulus, caused by the illusion that the room rotates around the patient. Both vestibular and optokinetic stimuli would produce nystagmus to the same side. The responses to this type of stimulation are known to be very precise; in normals, the cumulative slow phase of the nystagmus corresponds to the amplitude of the stimulatory movement in a one to one relation; that is, the magnitude of the cumulative eye movements equals 100% of the magnitude of the chair displacement.[8]

Vestibular Stimulation with Optical Fixation. The patient rotates, looking at an optical target that moves with the chair. In this test the vestibular nystagmus is inhibited by an optokinetic stimulus that would produce nystagmus to the contralateral side. In normal subjects, no eye movements are produced.[8]

Eye movements were recorded with standard nystagmographic technique, using an 8 channel Grass polygraph. Each eye was tested separately, using both DC coupling and speed derivative. In some cases, an integrator channel was used to facilitate measuring total eye displacement. Vertical leads were used to exclude eye-blinking artifacts. All testing was made with the chair oscillating with a frequency of 0.05 Hz, and responses were measured when the maximum displacement of the chair was in the range of 135 to 180°. The amplitude of oscillation was measured by means of the electrical output of a photocell, recorded in one channel of the polygraph.

The parameter of responses used was the cumulative angular displacement of the eyes due to the slow phase of the nystagmus, measured in degrees. To facilitate analysis of the results, the value of the response was expressed in terms of the percentage of the expected value of normal response. In addition to quantification of the responses, an appreciation of certain qualitative characteristics of the nystagmus was attempted. Montandon[9] described a special configuration of the nystagmus in VBI which he called "petite écriture," a name that can be translated as "micrography." This consists in a decrease of the amplitude of the nystagmic beats with concomitant increase in frequency due to conservation of a normal slow phase speed. To investigate the presence of micrography in our patients, the mean amplitude of the nystagmus was determined by dividing the cumulative displacement of the eyes by the number of nystagmic saccades.

RESULTS

STANDARD VESTIBULAR TESTS

Spontaneous nystagmus was found in 11 patients (26%). In eight it was a "gaze nystagmus" and in three it was "vestibular nystagmus" (VN), according to the classification of Jung and Kornhuber;[10] of these, there was a second degree VN in two cases and first degree VN in one. No spontaneous nystagmus was found in the control group.

Positional nystagmus was found in 12 patients (29%). In nine it was of the "benign paroxysmal" type. In three, a "central" type nystagmus was found. No positional nystagmus was found in the control group, although two patients complained of slight vertigo.

Caloric nystagmus was found abnormal in 14 patients (33%).[11] Six showed bilateral depression, three presented canal paresis and five, directional preponderance. No abnormalities in the caloric test were found in the control group.

OCULOMOTOR TESTS WITH OPTICAL STIMULATION

Saccadic eye movements were abnormal, in 14 patients (33%) classified as follows:

1. "False starts." The eye jumps to the lamp before it is lighted, while the other lamp is still on, so the eye has to go back to the initial point. This is normal when it occurs infrequently, but in seven of the patients in this study, there was a tendency for it to occur almost constantly.

2. Ocular dysmetria. The eyes either stop short of the new target (hypometric dysmetria), or overshoot it, executing a second saccade of opposite direction (hypermetric dysmetria).[12,13] Hypometric dysmetria was observed in five patients, hypermetric dysmetria in one.

3. In one patient, there was continuous tremor and terminal instability of the eyes. No abnormalities of the saccadic eye movement were detected in the control group.

Smooth pursuit movements were abnormal in 28 cases (66%). In 4 patients there was superimposition of fast movements to the smooth sinusoidal

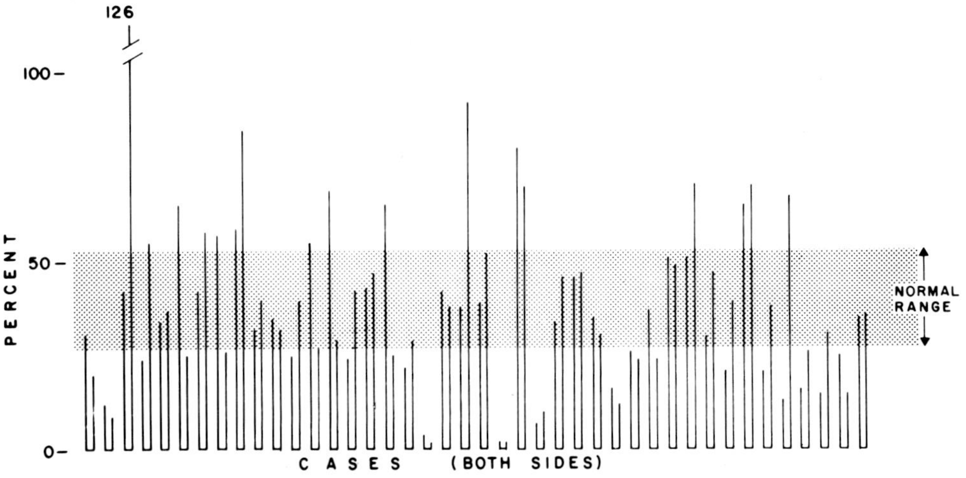

NORMALS 12 (28 %)

ABNORMALS 30 (72 %)

	n	%
DEPRESSION, BILATERAL	8	19
" UNILATERAL	8	19
DEPRESSION + INCREMENT	4	10
INCREMENT, BILATERAL	3	7
" UNILATERAL	7	17

Fig. 2. Magnitude of the integrated eye responses to vestibular stimulation with eyes covered, expressed as percent of the actual rotation of the chair. For each patient the magnitude of the total response to right and left rotation is shown.

curve; in 14, the eye movements were ataxic; eye tracking was abolished in 2 patients; and in 8, there was a fine constant tremor of the eyes. The pursuit eye movements were "ataxic" in three of the patients in the control group.

Optokinetic nystagmus (OKN) was abnormal in 12 patients (29%). The responses were asymetrical in six, symetrically depressed in three, and disorganized in three. Two subjects in the control group had symetrically depressed OKN.

OPTOVESTIBULAR INTEGRATION TESTS

The results, in terms of the percentage of the expected response, are shown in Figures 2 (vestibular stimulation) and 3 (optovestibular stimulation). To be considered abnormal, the responses should devi-

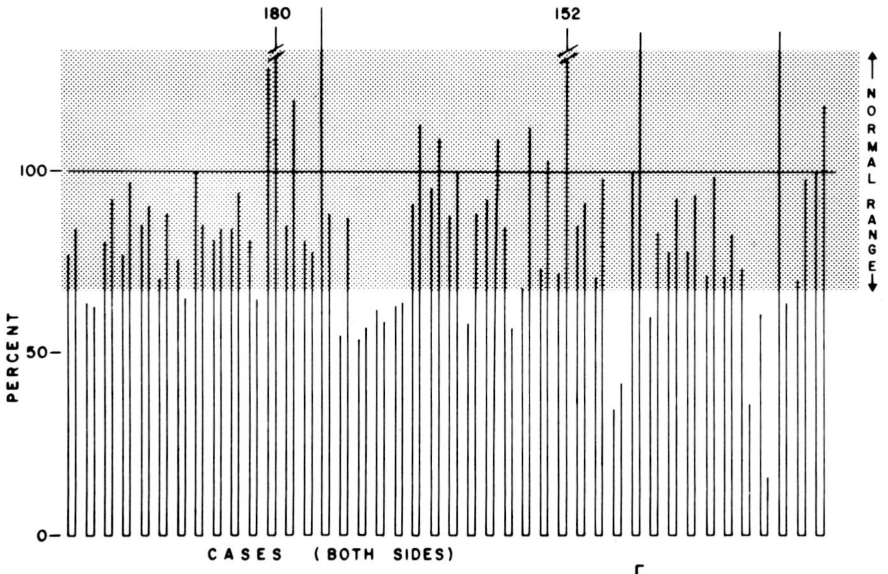

NORMALS 24 (57 %)

ABNORMALS 18 (43 %)

	n	%
DEPRESSION, BILATERAL	6	14
UNILATERAL	7	17
DEPRESSION + INCREMENT	1	2
INCREMENT, BILATERAL	0	0
UNILATERAL	4	10

Fig. 3. Magnitude of the integrated eye responses to optovestibular stimulation (eyes open, illuminated room). Normality (shaded area) falls between 67% to 133% of the chair's angular displacement.

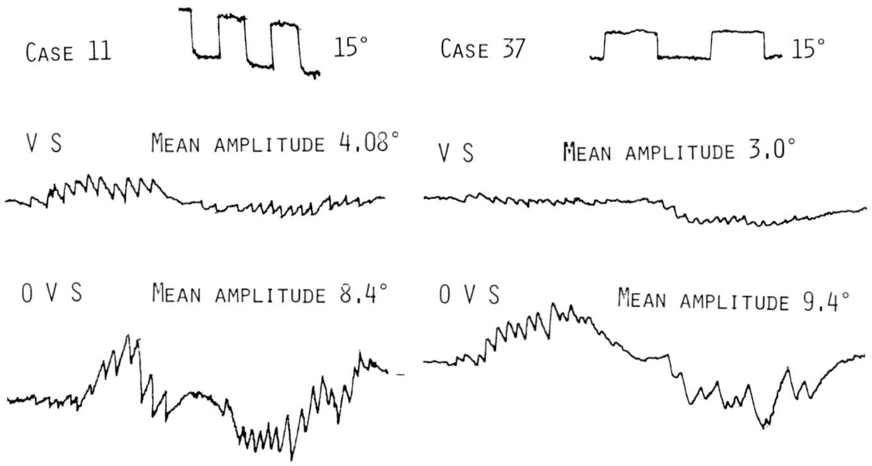

Fig. 4. The two subjects in whom micrography was found. The upper trace corresponds to voluntary saccades of 15° amplitude, the middle shows the eye movements evoked by vestibular stimulation (VS), and the lower by optovestibular stimulation (OVS).

ate more than 33% of the expected value. That means that, in regard to vestibular nystagmus, "depressed" means less than 26% and "increased" more than 53% of the magnitude of the stimulus. In respect to optovestibular stimulation, since the expected normal results are 100%, "depressed" means less than 67% and "increased" more than 133% of the magnitude of the stimulus. In the control group, both the vestibular and optovestibular responses were somewhat depressed. The mean vestibular response was 34.7%, with a standard deviation of 7.2%. The mean optovestibular response was 92.3% with a standard deviation of 19.6%. Individually, three cases showed vestibular depression, with values below the 26% line. No case showed vestibular or optovestibular increase of responses, nor optovestibular depression.

Micrography. The mean amplitude of the nystagmus saccade in normal subjects under the testing conditions was 7.4° for the vestibular and 12.1° for optovestibular stimulation. To be considered abnormal, the mean amplitude of the saccade had to measure 33% less than the normal mean, that is, less than 4.9° in vestibular or 8.1° in optovestibular stimulation. No attempt was made to detect larger than normal saccades. On this criterion, only two vertiginous patients exhibited micrography (Fig. 4); no case showing micrography was found in the control group.

Taking together the results of the different rotatory stimulations only eight patients did not show any abnormality; that is, in more than 80% of patients some alteration could be detected; this compares with the control group, in which only four patients had some abnormality (9%).

DISCUSSION

The frequency of abnormal findings in standard vestibular tests varies among the reports on vertebrobasilar insufficiency. Spontaneous nystagmus appears frequently; its incidence has been reported in 7% to 19% of the patients.[14-16] Positional nystagmus has been reported in 5% to 88% of patients.[16,17] The wide variation of incidence reported is probably due both to the type of patients included in each group, and to the testing technique.

Our series was formed by early cases of VBI, since the patients were selected in such a way that none exhibited neurological signs. Also, the method of examination can be considered gross, since it does not detect the cases where the nystagmus appears only when retinal inhibition is suppressed.

The irrigation of the vestibular nuclei and their nervous pathways is supplied mainly through small paramedian branches of the basilar artery, and thus, is very easily affected by small vessel disease. Postural nystagmus of the "central" type would be indicative of VBI, being caused by a lesion of the cerebellovestibular connections. Postural nystagmus of the "benign paroxysmal" type could be caused by otological disease[5,18,19] or could be due to vascular insufficiency in the internal auditory artery.

The frequency of caloric test abnormalities is more consistent among several reports. Barber[16] found caloric abnormalities in 22% of 100 patients; of those, 11% showed reduced responses and 11% directional preponderance. Thiebaut et al[17] noted bilateral diminution of caloric nystagmus in 66%.

Many authors have pointed out that abnormalities of oculomotor function are early findings in VBI, especially diplopia,[15] transient paresis of conjugate eye movements[14] and internuclear ophthalmoplegia, best noted when testing for OKN.[20] Although we found abnormal saccades in many cases, in half, the alteration consisted in what we have called "false start," in which the significance is obscure.

Alterations of smooth pursuit eye movements was the most common abnormality found in our series.

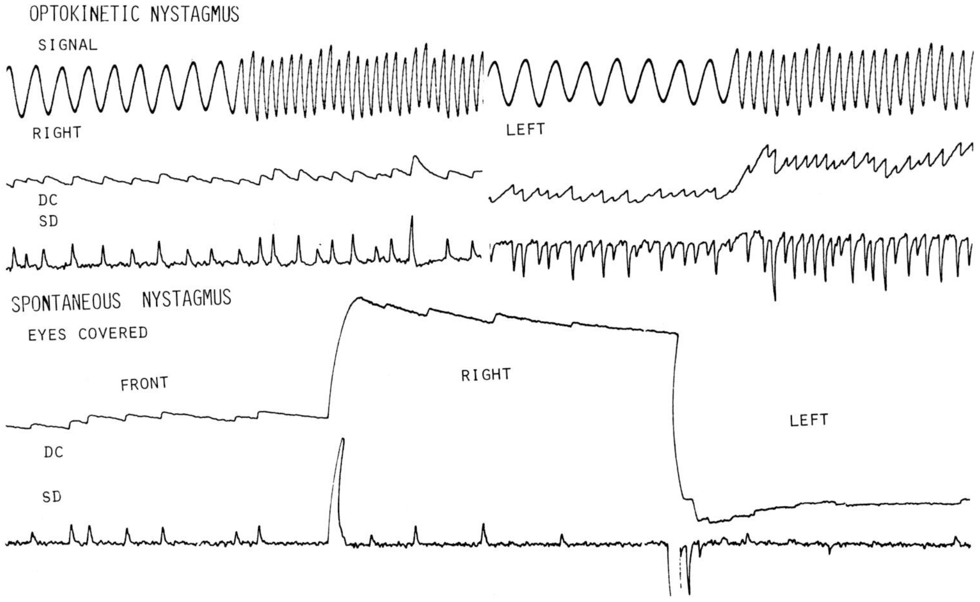

Fig. 5. Patient in whom the vestibular second-degree nystagmus has a direction opposite the preponderance shown by the optokinetic nystagmus. DC - Direct current; SD - Speed derivative.

It has been postulated that substitution of smooth tracking by fast movements is due to damage to cerebellar pathways, while the ataxic disorganization is caused by brainstem disease.[6,21,22] If so, the predominance of ataxia and abolition of pursuit eye movements in comparison with tracking by fast movements in our cases would be in accordance with the pathology of the disease, ischemia being more prominent in the terminal part of the vascular tree. The tremor found in eight patients could be due to involvement of basal ganglia.

Optokinetic nystagmus is not just a succession of pursuit eye movements and compensatory saccades, but a very complex phenomenon in which both optic and vestibular information converge.[23-25] In man, OKN and smooth pursuit eye movements have probably the same physiological basis only at low stimulation speed. Above an apparent angular velocity of the drum of 60° per second, there is evidence that indicates that OKN becomes a triggered phenomenon, with speed, amplitude, and frequency of nystagmus determined, not in relation to the stimuli, but following a preestablished program.[26] This explains the appearance of normal OKN in all kinds of peripheral lesions, as long as the stripes are visible and there is no fusion of images.[27]

Coats[28] has shown that OKN asymmetry due to labyrinthine lesion is accompanied by spontaneous nystagmus with eyes covered, to the side the OKN is more marked. This does not happen when the asymmetry is of central origin. Of our patients with OKN asymmetry, only one had vestibular type nystagmus of second degree, but this nystagmus was of a direction opposite to the OKN preponderance (Fig. 5). On the other hand, two patients with vestibular type nystagmus did not show OKN asymmetry. This points out that the OKN alterations found were probably due to a central lesion.

Although the alternating rotatory chair ("torsion swing" test, "pendular" rotatory test) has been widely used to study VBI,[9,29] no attempt has been made to measure the response and to compare it with the magnitude of the stimulus. This can be done by comparing the instantaneous angular speed of the chair with the angular speed of the eye, but since both vary during the test, it would be necessary to compare two sinusoids. The comparison between total angular displacement of the chair with the cumulative slow phase of the nystagmus during each semiperiod, has been used as a parameter of response in experimental situations, and the values under vestibular, optovestibular and muscular proprioceptor stimulations have been determined for normal humans.[8,30,31] By applying this type of testing to clinical conditions, it has been possible to detect quantitative variations in the responses, comparing responses directly with the magnitude of the stimulus and not, as in other tests, comparing responses only with a statistical value derived from the mean responses of a large population.

Using this testing procedure, the vestibular responses were abnormal in a very high percentage of cases. That this figure is not due to the method of testing is demonstrated by the fact that in a previous study[8] using the same technique in a group of normals, the variability of the results, as measured by the standard deviation of the sample was 17.8 with vestibular stimulation and 10.8 with optovestibular stimulation; expressed in terms of percentage of the means. In no normal case was the variation as great

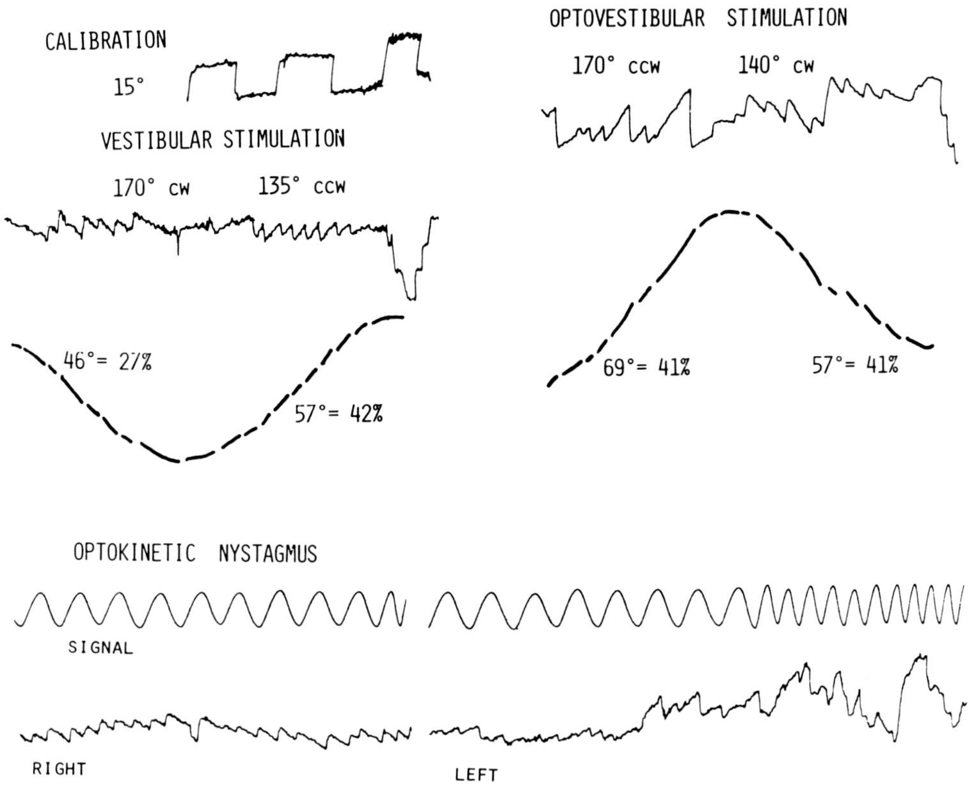

Fig. 6. Tracings showing unilateral depression of the vestibular nystagmus (27%) and bilateral depression of the optovestibular nystagmus (41% and 41%). In this case the optokinetic nystagmus is also depressed.

as 33%, the magnitude chosen in this paper as the threshold of abnormality.

The vestibular abnormalities found in our patients, especially unilateral or bilateral depression, could presumably be demonstrated with caloric testing. This has not happened, however, probably due to a lack of reliable parameters of response, and to problems inherent in the thermic test related to lack of precision in stimulation at the level of vestibular end-organs.

The augmentation of the vestibular responses in our test poses many questions in regard to the physiology of the compensatory eye movements under rotatory stimulation. Probably the 40% figure obtained comparing the magnitude of the vestibular response to the stimulus in normals is not set by the sensibility of the vestibular end-organ, since it is inconceivable that sensibility should increase with disease or old age. It is more likely that this figure would be the result of an interrelation between trigger stimulus from the vestibule apparatus and inhibitory influences from other neurological mechanisms. If so, the increase of the responses could only result from a lesion in the central nervous system that would impair such a mechanism or interrupt its nervous pathways.

The nystagmus obtained when testing with eyes open looking at the room, obviously cannot be due to a simple additon of vestibular plus optokinetic stimuli. Rather, to originate a signal that would be appropriate to make the necessary compensatory eye movements requires computation of the information carried by different sensors. The depression of the response could be due to a defect in the optokinetic mechanisms. However, if such a deficiency exists, it does not show with the classic optokinetical drum test, since of 14 cases with either unilateral or a bilateral depression of optovestibular nystagmus, in only one was the optokinetic test abnormal (Fig. 6). On the other hand, of the 12 patients who showed optokinetic test abnormalities only one had depression of optovestibular nystagmus.

The increase in optovestibular nystagmus responses occurred in few cases, only to one side. Maybe in these cases there was a true summation of optokinetic and vestibular stimuli due to a malfunction of the coordination mechanism.

With the battery of tests performed, most patients showed multiple findings, the most common combination being eye tracking ataxia with vestibular depression. One patient had only postural nystagmus of the "benign paroxysmal" type, and thus the diagnosis could not have been made based on the neurotological examination alone. In one patient, no abnormality was found. We could not confirm the importance of micrography in VBI in this study.

CONCLUSION

With the testing procedure carried out in this group of patients, it was possible to detect abnormalities in the vestibular oculomotor compensatory mechanisms that could explain vertigo in 41 out of 42 patients. We were not able, however, to identify a pattern characteristic of vertebrobasilar insufficiency. The findings were too variable. Perhaps this was to be expected of a disease that causes many different and widespread lesions both at labyrinthine and neurological levels.

REFERENCES

1. Millikan CH, Sickert RG. The syndrome of intermittent insufficiency of the basilar artery system. Proc Staff Meet Mayo Clin 1955; 30:61-8.

2. Williams D, Wilson G. Vertebrobasilar ischemia. Br Med J 1964; 1:84-6.

3. Brandshaw P, McQuaid P. The syndrome of vertebrobasilar insufficiency. Q J Med 1963; 128:279-96.

4. Bosch J. Etude electronystagmographique de l'insuffisance vertebro basilaire. Acta Otorhinolaryngol Belg 1970; 24:418-25.

5. Dix MR, Hallpike CS. The pathology, symptomatology and diagnosis of certain common disorders of the vestibular system. Proc R Soc Med 1952; 45:341-54.

6. Corvera J, Torres-Courtney G, Lopez-Rios G. The neurotological significance of the alterations of pursuit eye movements. Ann Otol Rhinol Laryngol 1973;82:855-67.

7. Greiner GF, Conraux C, Mengus M, et al. La nystagmographie dans l'epreuve rotatoire de type pendulaire. Ann Otolaryngol Chir Cervicofac 1962; 79:129.

8. Romero R, Corvera J. Respuestas oculomotoras reflejas ante estimulos rotatorios alternantes. An Soc Mex Otorrinolaringol 1977; 23:1-12.

9. Montandon A. Vestibulometrie clinique electrnystagmographique. In: Aboulker P, Pialoux M, Neveu M, et al. Syndromes vestibulaires et nystagmographie. Paris, Arnette, 1963; pp 261-80.

10. Jung R, Kornhuber HH. Results of electronystagmography in man. In: Bender MB ed. The oculomotor system. New York, Harper & Row, 1964; pp 428-82.

11. Aschan G, Bergstedt M, Stahle J. The caloric test. Acta Otolaryngol (Stockh) 1956; Suppl 129:157-62.

12. Kornhuber HH. Motor functions of the cerebellum and basal ganglia. Kybernetik 1971; 8:157-62.

13. Haring RD, Simmons FB. Cerebellar defects detectable by ENG calibration. Arch Otolaryngol 1973; 98:14-19.

14. Rosselet E. Vertebral basilar circulatory disorders. Ophthalmologica 1973; 167:288-304.

15. Minor RH, Kearns TP, Millikan CH, et al. Ocular manifestations of occlusive disease of the basilar arterial system. Arch Ophthalmol 1959; 62:112-24.

16. Barber HO, Dionne J. Vestibular findings in vertebrobasilar ischemia. Ann Otol Rhinol Laryngol 1971; 80:805-12.

17. Thiebaut F, Collard M, Conraux C, et al. Les atteintes vestibulaires au cours des syndromes vasculaires du tronc cerebral. Rev Neurol (Paris) 1967; 117:587-8.

18. Lindsay JR. Postural vertigo and positional nystagmus. Ann Otol Rhinol Laryngol 1951; 60:1134-9.

19. Schuknecht HF. Cupulolithiasis. Arch Otolaryngol 1969; 90:765-78.

20. Berkowitz WP, Stroud MH. Early vascular insufficiency and the vestibular syndrome. Laryngoscope 1973; 83:1084-9.

21. Ascoff JC, Cohen B. Changes in saccadic eye movements produced by cerebellar lesions. Exp Neurol 1971; 32:123-33.

22. Baloh RW, Konrad HR, Honrubia V. Vestibulo-ocular function in patients with cerebellar atrophy. Neurology (Minneap) 1975; 25:160-8.

23. Honrubia V, Downey WR, Mitchell DP, et al. Experimental studies in optokinetic nystagmus: II. Normal humans. Acta Otolaryngol (Stockh) 1968; 65:441-8.

24. Honrubia V, Jenkins H, Ward PH. Modifications in the optokinetic nystagmus resulting from monocular stimulation and lateral tilting in normal and pathological cats. Ann Otol Rhinol Laryngol 1971; 80 Suppl 3:34-42.

25. Prince AL. The effect of rotation and unilateral removal of the otic labyrinth in the equilibrium and ocular reactions in kittens. Am J Physiol 1917; 42:308-22.

26. Corvera J, Hernández-Peniche J. Nistagmus optoquinético en el hombre. Rev Hosp Gen 1961; 24:19-29.

27. Corvera J, Torres-Courtney G. Significado clínico de las alteraciones del nistagmus optoquinético. An Soc Mex Oftalmol 1965; 38:105-18.

28. Coats AC. Central and peripheral optokinetic asymmetry. Ann Otol Rhinol Laryngol 1968; 77:938-48.

29. Labaeye P. Insuffisance vertebro basilaire. J Fr Oto-Rhino-Laryngol 1973; 22:215-7.

30. Melvill Jones G. Organization of neural control in the vestibulo-ocular reflex arc. In: Bach-y-Rita, ed. The control of eye movements, New York, Academic Press, 1971; pp 497-518.

31. Meiry JL. Vestibular and proprioceptive stabilization of eye movements. In: Bach-y-Rita, ed. The control of eye movements, New York, Academic Press, 1971, pp 483-96.

CHARACTERISTICS OF CAPILLARY PERMEABILITY IN NASAL MUCOSA

KENSUKE WATANABE, MD
ISAMU WATANABE, MD
YOZO SAITO, MD
VINCI MIZUHIRA, MD

TOKYO, JAPAN

The transendothelial passage of horseradish peroxidase (HRP) and colloidal carbon and diffusion of HRP in pericapillary space, injected intravenously into rats, was studied at the light microscopic and ultrastructural level in the nasal mucosa. In the lamina propria of the mucosa in the middle third of the nasal septum of rats, the capillaries directly beneath the epithelium were mostly with fenestrae, while the capillaries around the nasal gland were without the fenestrae. The permeability of the capillaries in the lamina propria of the nasal mucosa was very high and some of the endothelial cells were wide open, like liver sinusoid, allowing free passage of carbon particles. Marked transendothelial passage was also noted at ten seconds after HRP infusion through the capillaries without fenestrae located around the nasal gland. On the other hand, no extracapillary leakage of HRP was noted even at 150 seconds after its infusion in the capillaries without fenestrae located in the muscles. The permeability of small venules located in the lamina propria of nasal mucosa also was extremely high. The reasons for the greater permeation of HRP through capillaries of nasal mucosa are as follows. First, the endothelial cell junction was loose in the nasal mucosa and in some capillaries endothelium had holes like liver sinusoid. Second, interstitium surrounding the capillary was loose in nasal mucosa.

The blood vessels of the nasal respiratory mucosa play an important role in both thermal regulation and humidification of inhaled air and in the control of the lumen of nasal passages. It is most important to investigate permeability of nasal capillaries, taking nasal function into account.

Regional variations in the permeability of blood capillaries are already known.[1] The permeability increases in the order of capillaries of extremities < intestinal capillaries < liver sinusoids, but studies on the permeability of nasal capillaries are still scanty.

Physiological studies have clarified that the capillary wall of muscles behaved as though it possessed a set each of large[1,2] and small pores.[3] Two components of the capillary endothelium are the candidates for the morphologic counterparts of the pores, the abundant small cytoplasmic vesicles (~500Å) and the junctions among endothelial cells (~90Å).[4-7] Data available for the intestinal capillaries with fenestrae are more limited. The diameter of their small pores is estimated at ~110Å.[1,8]

Electron microscopic studies have shown that the structure of blood capillaries varies from region to region.[9] The morphological characteristics of nasal capillaries consist of the fenestrae of endothelium and the pores of the basement membranes which are apparently responsible for a reduced permeability barrier.[10]

In the present report, horseradish peroxidase (HRP) and colloidal carbon were used as tracers to investigate the permeability of nasal vessels.

METHODS

Under anesthesia with ether, male rats of Wistar strain, each weighing 180-200 gm, were subjected to intravenous injection of HRP (Sigma Type VI, diameter ~50Å) and colloidal carbon (Pelikan ink diameter 230-480Å) via the tail vein in doses of 1 ml saline containing 8 mg of peroxidase or 1.5 ml of colloidal carbon. The tracers were injected over ten seconds. At different times after the tracers were injected (Table 1), the animals were sacrificed by decapitation. Tissue specimens were taken from the middle third of the nasal septum mucosa, intestinal mucosa and femoral muscle.

Experiments with HRP Tracer. The blocks were fixed for one hour at 4C in a formaldehyde-glutaraldehyde fixative.[11] The tissue blocks were then washed for three times in 0.1 M cacodylate buffer with pH 7.3 at 4 C and subsequently sectioned into 40 μ slices with a Sorvall TC-2 tissue sectioner. These slices were incubated for one hour at room temperature in the modified Graham-Karnovsky medium[12] (0.05 M TRIS-HCl buffer, pH 7.6, 10 ml, containing 0.002% H_2O_2 and 8 mg of 3-3′ diaminobenzidine tetrahydrochloride [DAB]), then washed three times in 0.1 M cacodylate buffer, and postfixed for 40 minutes in 2% O_sO_4 and embedded in Epon® 812. Ultrathin cross sections were prepared with a microtome (Poter-Blum MT-2) and stained with uranyl acetate and lead. To compare with endogenous peroxidase, the nasal mucosa of rats not injected with HRP was stained by the DAB method.

Experiments with Colloidal Carbon Tracer. Tissue specimens were fixed for two hours at 4C temperature in 2% glutaraldehyde fixative (0.1 M cacodylate buffer, pH 7.3), washed overnight in 0.1 M cacodylate buffer with pH 7.3, at 4 C, and postfixed for 90 minutes in 2% O_sO_4.

TABLE 1. INTERVALS AND NUMBER OF ANIMALS USED

	Intervals						*Total*
Tracer	*10 sec*	*60 sec*	*90 sec*	*150 sec*	*3 min*	*15 min*	*No. Animals*
HRP	5	2	1	2	2	2	14
Colloidal carbon		1	3		1	2	7

From the Departments of Otolaryngology and Cell Biology of the Medical Research Institute, Tokyo Medical and Dental University, Tokyo, Japan.
REPRINTS — Kensuke Watanabe, MD, Department of Otolaryngology, Tokyo Medical and Dental University, 1-5-45, Yushima Bunkyo-ku, Tokyo, Japan.

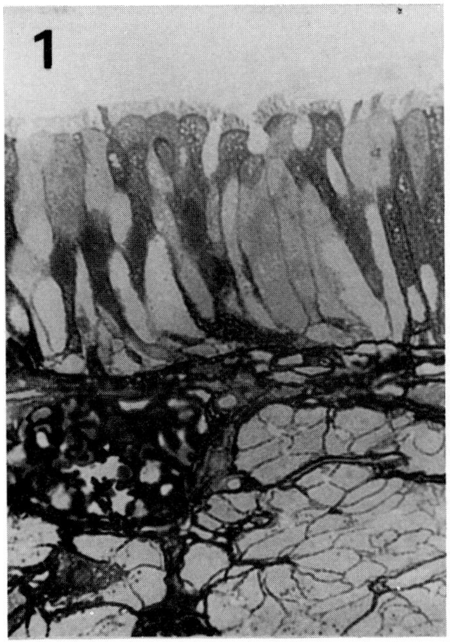

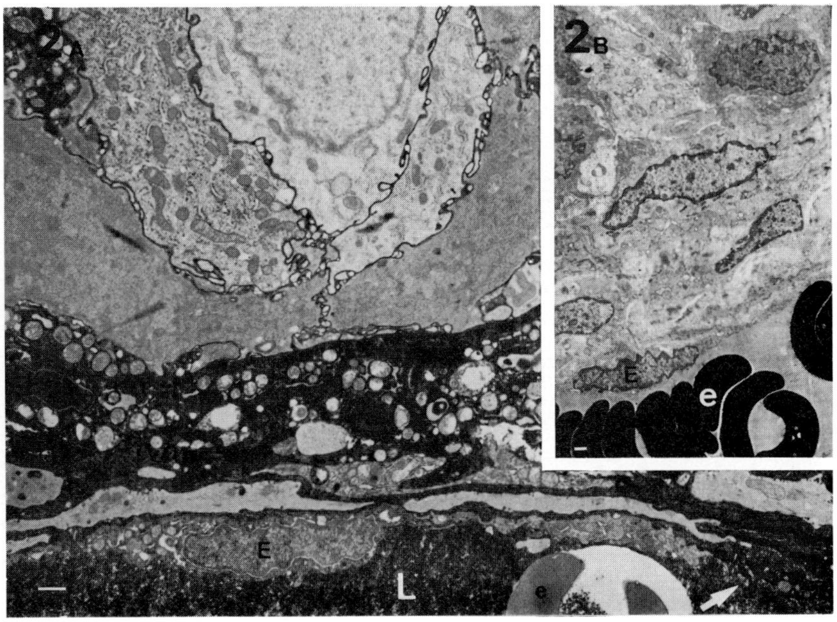

Fig. 1. Light microscopic observation of the mucosa of the nasal septum collected at ten seconds after the start of infusion of HRP indicates that HRP had already passed through the blood vessels and filled the lamina propria of the mucosa. (x800)

Fig. 2. A) Lamina propria of the mucosa around the small venules was filled with HRP at ten seconds after the infusion. HRP could diffusely perfuse through the endothelial cells of the small venule (white arrow). e - Erythrocyte; L - Lumen of the small venule; E - Endothelial cell. (x4000) B) Endogenous peroxidase activity was not found in nasal mucosa except in erythrocytes. The structure of lamina propria of the mucosa of the nasal septum was found to be very loose. (x2000)

RESULTS

The light microscopic inspection of the mucosa of the nasal septum collected at ten seconds after the start of infusion of HRP through the tail vein (Fig. 1) indicated that the HRP tracer had already passed through the blood vessels and filled the lamina propria of the mucosa by the time of the inspection and that it also filled the surroundings of nasal gland and was noted in the intercellular space among the acinar cells.

By the electron microscopic inspection, the permeability of the small venules in the mucosa of nasal septum was so high that, as indicated in Figure 2A, lamina propria of the mucosa around the small venules was filled with HRP as early as ten seconds after the start of infusion. The structure of lamina propria of the mucosa of the nasal septum was found to be very loose, as indicated in Figure 2B, so that HRP which passed through the blood vessels could easily reach the subepithelium. In some regions, HRP could perfuse diffusely through the endothelial cells of the small venule (Fig. 2A, white arrow), while endogenous peroxidase was not detected in the endothelial cells and interstitial tissues except in erythocytes (Fig. 2B). In comparison with that of the small venules in the smooth muscles of intestinal tracts, the permeability of the small venules in the nasal mucosa with diameters of similar size was found to be extremely high. In other words, no extracapillary leakage could be noted in the small venules of the intestinal tracts at ten seconds after the infusion (Fig. 3). The fenestrated capillaries were found directly beneath the nasal epithelium. The passage of HRP from the fenestrae could be readily noted.

Comparison was made between the fenestrated capillaries (Fig. 4) of the intestinal tracts and those of the nasal mucosa. As early as ten seconds after its infusion, HRP could be noted extracapillarily, but the permeability of HRP in the intestinal mucosa was much less than that of the nasal mucosa.

All capillaries existing around the nasal gland were found to be of the type without fenestrae (Figs. 5 and 6). In the capillaries of smooth muscles in the intestinal tracts without fenestrae (Fig. 12) or in the capillaries of femoral muscles (Fig. 13), HRP could not be noted in the extracapillary space at 90 seconds or 150 seconds after its infusion, but in the capillaries around the nasal gland, marked extracapillary passage could be noted at ten seconds after its infusion. The uptake of HRP into the pinocytotic vesicles of endothelial cells was extensive in the capillaries existing around the nasal gland. The electron densities in both the vesicles on the inner side of the capillary wall (Fig. 5, arrow a) and on the outer side of the capillary wall (Fig. 5, arrow c) were high, but the electron density at the middle point (arrow b) was low. Therefore, the HRP shown with the arrow c can be assumed to be based on the intake of HRP from outside the vessels. Consequently, luminal HRP would pass through toward the extracapillary space in the route of arrow A or arrow B in Figure 5 at ten seconds after its infusion. HRP

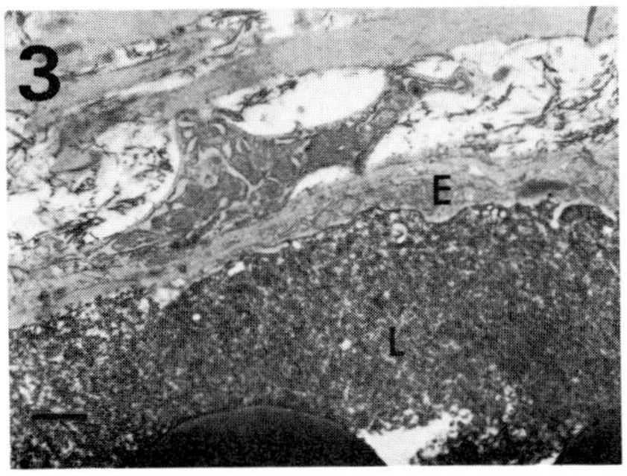

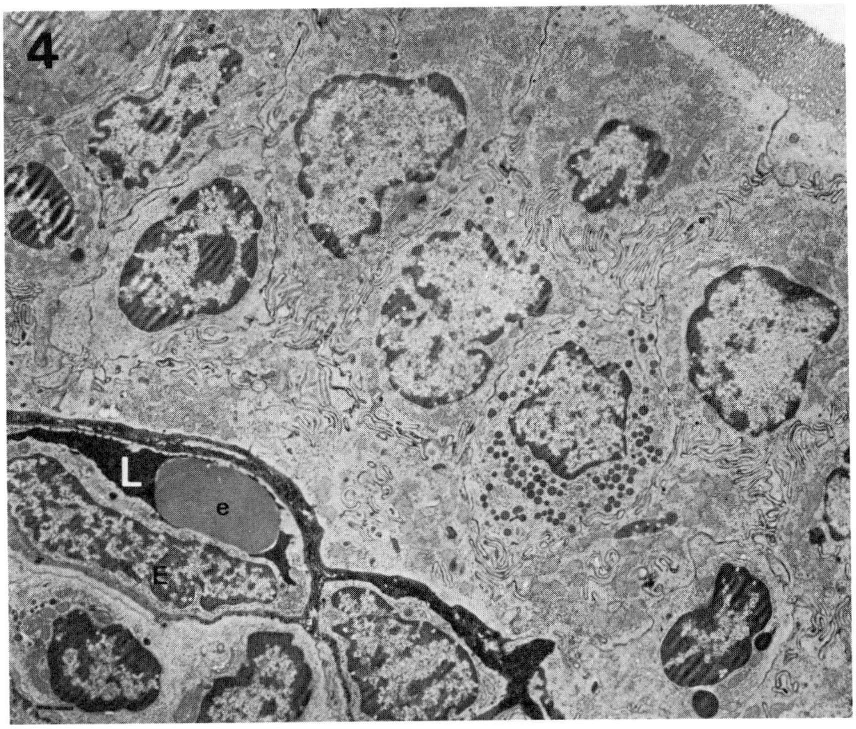

Fig. 3. In the small venule in the smooth muscles of intestinal tracts, no extracapillary leakage could be noted at ten seconds after the infusion. L - Lumen of the small venule; E - Endothelial cell. (x5000)

Fig. 4. At ten seconds after infusion, HRP could be noted extracapillarily in the intestinal mucosa. But the permeability of HRP in the intestinal mucosa was much less than that of the nasal mucosa. L - Lumen of the capillary; e - Erythrocyte; E - Endothelial cell. (x5000)

which perfused through the intercellulary space of acinar cells toward the glandular lumen was not emitted into it due to inhibition by the tight junction (Fig. 6, arrows).

A pattern of greater permeation of venules existing relatively deep in the mucosa and consequent free extracapillary leakage through the intercellular space could be obtained (Fig. 7).

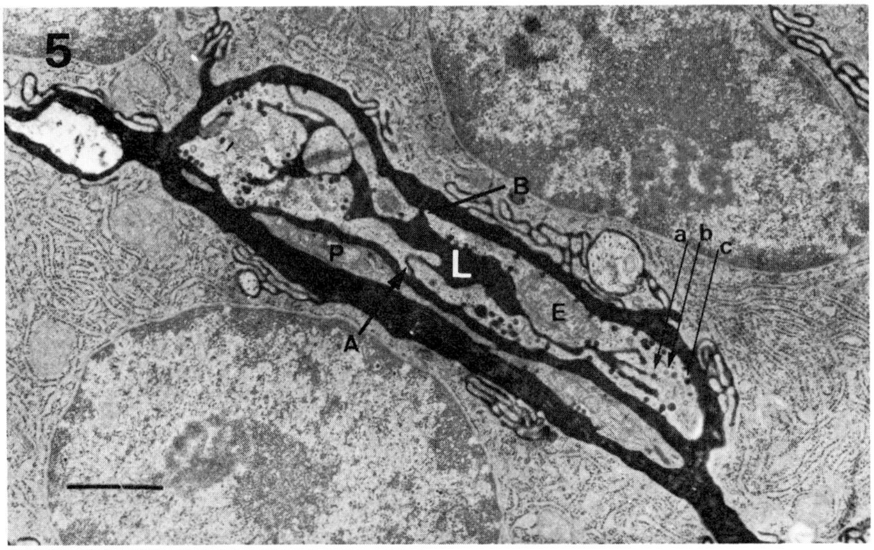

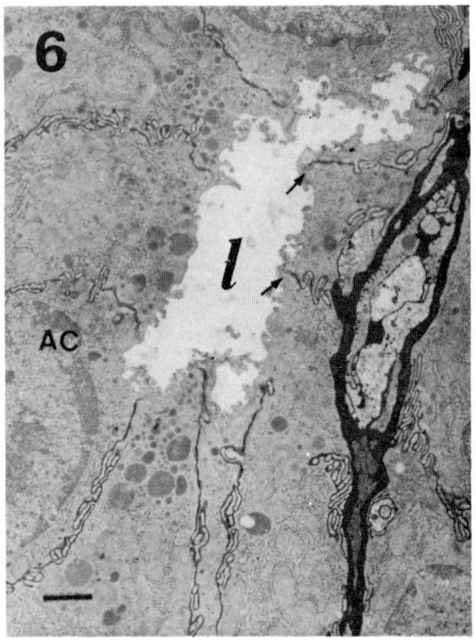

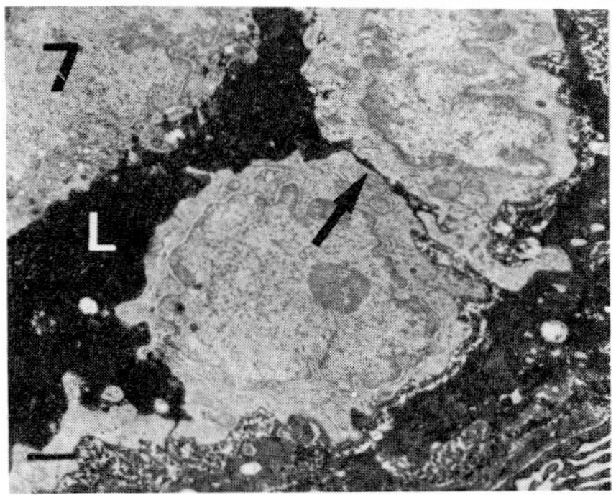

Fig. 5. The capillary existing around the nasal gland was found to be of the type without fenestrae. Marked extracapillary passage could be noted at ten seconds after infusion. The electron densities in both the vesicles on the inner side of the capillary wall (a) and on the outer side of the capillary wall (c) were high, but the electron density at middle point (b) was low. Therefore, it can be assumed likely that HRP could possibly pass through the parts other than the route of a → b → c. The route of extracapillary permeation is deemed to be either A or B. E - Endothelial cell; P - Pericyte; L - Lumen. (x4000)

Fig. 6. HRP which perfused through the intercellulary space of acinar cells (AC) toward the glandular lumen (*l*) was not emitted into it due to inhibition by the tight junction (arrows). (x6000)

Fig. 7. A pattern of high permeation of venule existing relatively deep in the mucosa (arrow) at ten seconds after infusion. L - Lumen of venule. (x5000)

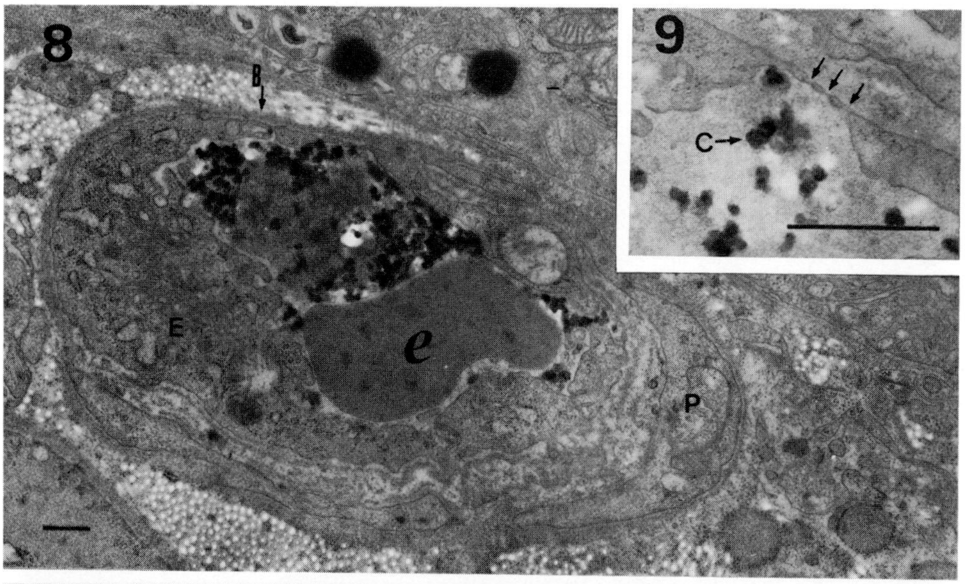

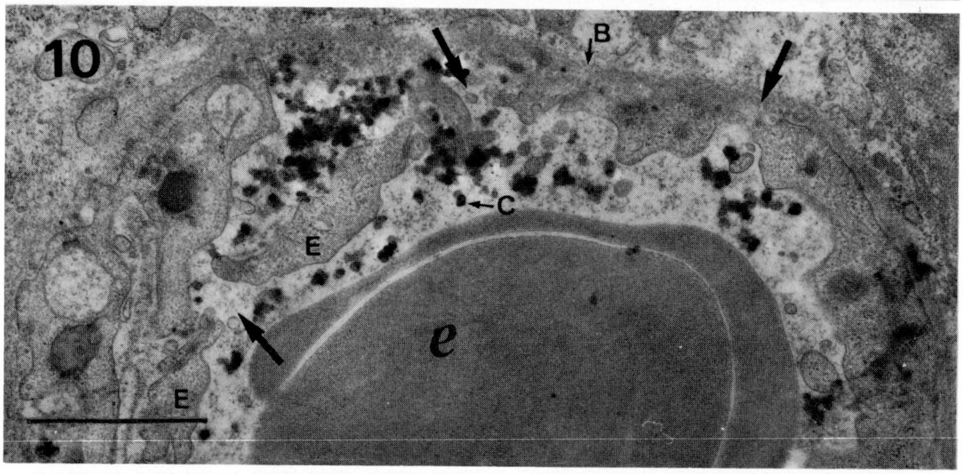

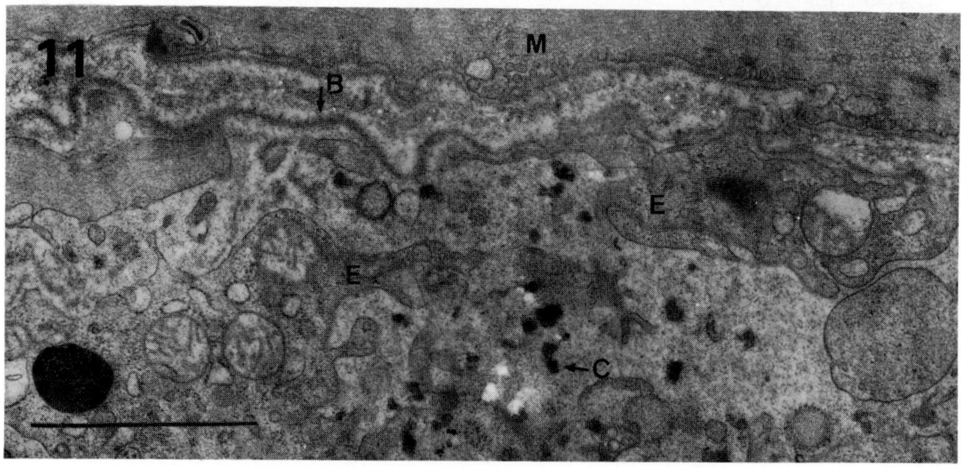

Fig. 8. At 15 minutes after infusion of colloidal carbon. No colloidal carbon passed through the endothelial cells of the capillary. e - Erythrocyte; E - Endothelial cell; P - Pericyte; B - Basement membrane. (x6000)

Fig. 9. At 15 minutes after infusion of colloidal carbon. The carbon particles were larger than the fenestrae (arrows). C - Carbon. (x20,000)

Fig. 10. At 90 seconds after infusion of colloidal carbon. The intercellular space among the endothelial cells (E) was wide open (arrows). e - Erythrocyte; B - Basement membrane; C - Carbon. (x24,000)

Fig. 11. At 90 seconds after infusion of colloidal carbon. The endothelial cells (E) were widely spread in the small venule, and the carbon particles (C) were noted to be able to reach freely the basement membrane (B). M - Smooth muscle. (x30,000)

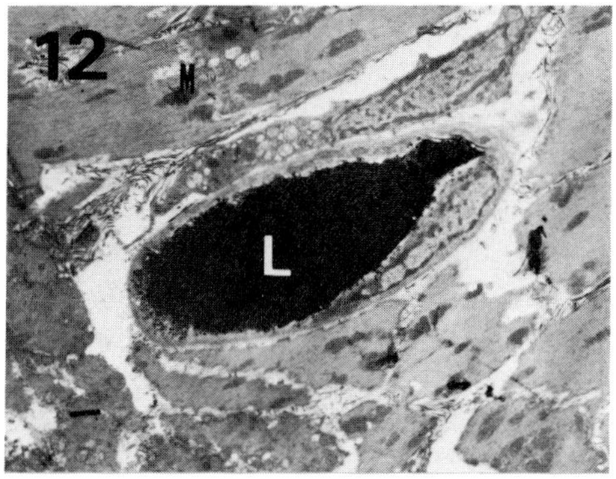

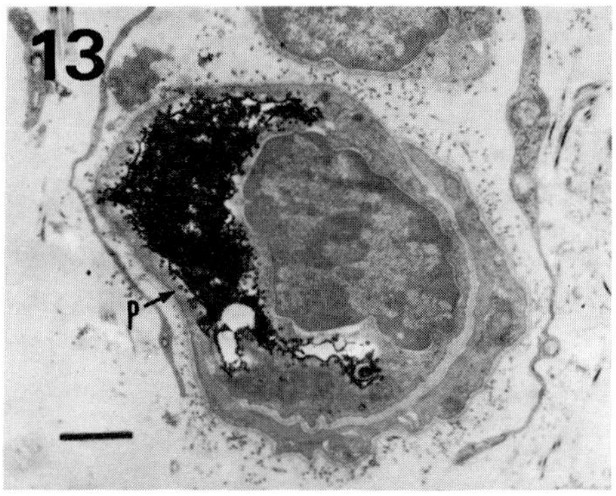

Fig. 12. In the capillary of smooth muscles (M) in the intestinal tracts, HRP could not be noted in the extracapillary space at 90 seconds after infusion. L - Capillary lumen. (x3000)

Fig. 13. In the capillary of femoral muscles, HRP could not be noted in the extracapillary space at 150 seconds after infusion. P - Pinocytotic vesicle. (x7000)

When colloidal carbon was used as the tracer, it did not pass through the basement membrane of the capillary even 15 minutes after its infusion (Fig. 8). The carbon particles were larger than the fenestrae and therefore their passage was deemed unlikely (Fig. 9). Careful observation indicated that the intercellular space among the endothelial cells was wide open (Fig. 10, arrow), like liver sinusoid,[9] and free passage of the carbon particles out of the blood vessels was observed. The carbon particles could not pass through the basement membrane and were pooled in the space between the endothelial cells and the basement membrane. The endothelial cells were also widely spread in the small venules, and the carbon particles were noted to be able to reach the basement membrane freely in some regions (Fig. 11).

DISCUSSION

Variations in the permeability of blood capillaries regionally have been reported by Mayerson et al.[1] Karnovsky[4] also reported that the regional differences were caused by not only the differences in the rates of passage across the endothelium, but also many other factors such as differences in capillary population density per unit volume of tissue, relative proportion of capillaries which are open and perfused, differences in the rates of lymph drainage, etc.

The present investigation concerned the blood capillaries and small venules of the nasal septum mucosa in rats. Much HRP was found to leave the plasma rapidly and to reach the pericapillary spaces in nasal mucosa ten seconds postinjection. Simionescu et al[6] reported that since arrest of the blood flow by the fixative required ~25 seconds, the micrographs of the specimens demonstrated the situation in the endothelium 25 seconds after decapitation; so our findings might have represented the situation 35 seconds postinjection. The fact that even at 35 seconds after infusion of HRP large amounts of reaction products of HRP could be detected in the pericapillary space would mean that the vascular permeability of the mucosa of nasal septum was higher than that of the other organs. In the mucosa of the intestinal tracts having fenestrae, the passage of HRP was much less than in the nasal mucosa, as illustrated in Figure 4. In the capillaries of femoral muscle without fenestrae, the reaction products could not be detected at all in the pericapillary space, even at 150 seconds after the infusion (Fig 13).

The reasons for the greater permeation of HRP through capillaries of nasal mucosa would be identified as the following. First, it was found that the endothelial cell junction was loose in the nasal mucosa and that there were some regions in the nasal mucosa where endothelial cells were wide open like liver sinusoid. Whether the discontinuous portions of the endothelium were the cell junctions or the holes in the endothelial cells could not be firmly concluded, but the carbon particles could freely pass through the wide open parts of the endothelial cells. The carbon particles could not pass through the basement membrane.[8] But it would be considered that a large quantity of HRP would diffuse into the pericapillary tissues from such parts. The endothelial cell junctions located relatively deep in the venules were also loose and the intercellular clefts were also filled with HRP (Fig. 7). Second, it can be considered that the interstitium surrounding the capillaries was loose in the nasal mucosa (Fig. 2B). If the tissues around the capillaries were loose, HRP which passed through capillaries could possibly diffuse into the surrounding tissues within a short period of time. The structure of the interstitium in the mucosa of the intestinal tract was firmer than in the lamina propria of nasal mucosa (Fig. 4), and therefore the diffusion of HRP which passed through the capillaries was inhibited. In the case of glial cells of the central nervous system, where capillary permeability is very low, the processes of glial cells attach themselves closely to the outer surface of the capillary basement membrane.[13,14]

Cotran and Karnovsky[15] found that HRP caused increased vascular permeability in rats and guinea pigs but not in mice. When HRP (Sigma type II) was injected intravenously in a dose of 20 mg/100 gm body weight in rats, the animals developed the typical syndrome of systemic mast cell damage and vascular injury that can be induced by other known histamine liberators. However, Vegge and Haye[16] detected no increase in vascular leakage in guinea pig by using the dosage of HRP which we often used in permeability studies. Cotran and Karnovsky pointed out in their report that there would be no influence of HRP infusion upon vascular permeability unless several minutes elapse after its infusion. However, our experiment indicated passage of a large quantity of HRP through capillaries at as early as ten seconds after HRP infusion. Therefore, the passage of HRP would be deemed to have been prior to the manifestation of the influences of HRP upon the permeability of capillaries. The authors observed that the reaction products of HRP filled the small part of endothelial cytoplasm in small venules and capillaries. It might be considered that the cell membrane of the epithelial cell was damaged by highly concentrated HRP not only in the capillary but also in the pericapillary space where HRP had already permeated out of capillaries. In the capillaries or venules of the other organs, no or negligible leakage was noted at ten seconds after HRP infusion. Taking this into consideration, a higher permeability of capillaries of nasal mucosa than that of the other organs would seem reasonable even though the vascular permeability was elevated by HRP.

Jackson and Burson[17] reported that the nasal mucosa was approximately ten times as permeable to the pertechnetate ion as middle ear mucosa. Nasal mucosa was also permeable to protein, even in the absence of inflammatory mediator, with the physiological technique employed. It was also verified morphologically by our present experiment that the vascular permeability of nasal mucosa is high.

REFERENCES

1. Mayerson HS, Wolfram CG, Shirley HH Jr, Wasserman K. Regional differences in capillary permeability. Am J Physiol 1960; 198:155-60.

2. Grotte G. Passage of dextran molecules across the blood-lymph barrier. Acta Chir Scand 1956; Suppl 211:1-84.

3. Pappenheimer JR. Passage of molecules through capillary walls. Physiol Rev 1953; 33:387-423.

4. Karnovsky MJ. The ultrastructural basis of capillary permeability studied with peroxidase as a tracer. J Cell Biol 1967; 35:213-36.

5. Bruns RR, Palade GE. Studies on blood capillaries: II. Transport of ferritin molecules across the wall of muscle capillaries. J Cell Biol 1968; 37:277-99.

6. Simionescu N, Simionescu M, Palade GE. Permeability of muscle capillaries to small heme-peptides. J Cell Biol 1975; 64:586-607.

7. Williams MC, Wissig SL. The permeability of muscle capillaries to horseradish peroxidase. J Cell Biol 1975; 66:531-55.

8. Clementi F, Palade GE. Intestinal capillaries: I. Permeability to peroxidase and ferritin. J Cell Biol 1969; 41:33-58.

9. Bennett HS, Lift JH, Hampton JC. Morphological classification of vertebrate blood capillaries. Am J Physiol 1959; 196:381-90.

10. Cauna N, Hinderer KH. Fine structure of blood vessels of the human nasal respiratory mucosa. Ann Otol Rhinol Laryngol 1969; 78:865-79.

11. Karnovsky MJ. A formaldehyde-glutaraldehyde fixative of high osmolality for use in electron microscopy. J Cell Biol 1965; 27:137A.

12. Graham RC, Karnovsky MJ. The early stage of absorption of injected horseradish peroxidase in the proximal tubules of mouse kidney. J Histochem Cytochem 1966; 14:291-302.

13. Dempsey EW, Wislocki GB. An electron microscopic study of blood-brain barrier in rat, employing silver nitrate as a vital stain. J Biophys Biochem Cytol 1955; 1:245-56.

14. Luse SA. Electron microscopic observation of the central nervous system. J Biophys Biochem Cytol 1956; 2:531-41.

15. Cotran RS, Karnovsky MJ. Vascular leakage induced by horseradish peroxidase in the rat. Proc Soc Exp Biol Med 1967; 126:557-61.

16. Vegge T, Haye R. Vascular reactions to horseradish peroxidase in the guinea pig. Histochemistry 1977; 53:217-22.

17. Jackson T, Burson J. Effect of inflammatory mediators on nasal mucosa. Arch Otolaryngol 1977; 103:441-4.

GRAND ROUNDS — ALBANY MEDICAL CENTER
DIVISION OF OTOLARYNGOLOGY
JEROME C. GOLDSTEIN, MD, PROFESSOR AND HEAD

SEPTIC OSTEORADIONECROSIS OF THE MANDIBLE

SHARAD S. PARULEKAR, MD, MS, FRCS
DOMINICK F. PAONESSA, MD

Dr. Sharad Parulekar: Septic osteoradionecrosis of the mandible (SORM) is essentially an osteomyelitis of irradiated bone. The term defines an often devastating, and an inexorably progressive, seemingly irreversible complication in the radiotherapeutic management of malignant tumors of the head and neck. Osteoradionecromyelitis of the mandible is suggested as an alternative term.

Irradiation of the bone leads to characteristic dose-related permanent bone changes which have been variously termed radiation osteitis, radiation osteodysplasia, osteonecrosis due to radiation, radiation necrosis of bone and osteoradionecrosis (ORM). Specifically, the osteoclastic and osteoblastic function of the periosteum and marrow spaces are adversely affected and the blood vessels become occluded by thrombosis and proliferating fibrosis. Hence, osteoradioatrophy would perhaps be the more appropriate term with aseptic ORM denoting a more advanced pathology. Infection is characteristically absent in both these conditions. Infection of the bone leads to SORM.

The mandible, because of its superficial location, its compromised blood supply, its intimate relation to the teeth, and dependent sump area of the mouth, and its proximity to both the tumor and the line of resection or mandibulotomy poses special problems. In addition, radiation causes distinct separate deleterious effects on the skin, teeth, mucosa, and salivary glands all of which separately and together contribute to the total outcome.

Howland et al[1] studied radiation changes in the shoulder and radiographically demonstrated atrophic bone changes which were dose-related. There were little or no signs of atrophy with megavoltage or telecobalt radiation with doses up to 4,500 rads given over five weeks. Dosage schedules between 6,000-8,000 rads increased the incidence and severity of atrophic changes. Bedvineck et al[2] found that with radiation of the mandible at dosage levels below 6,000 rads, there was no instance of spontaneous osteonecrosis. The incidence was 1.8% between 6,000-7,000 rads delivered at levels of 1,000 rads weekly. Above 7,000 rads, the incidence rose to 9%. The incidence is higher if the primary tumor is overlying or adjacent to the bone. This is probably because radiation eradication of the tumor results in a more fragile and atrophic mucosa readily susceptible to traumatic breakdown. Guttenberg[3] found that only the introduction of microorganisms in the radioatrophic bone activates the seemingly irreversible course and he proposed the terms SORM and aseptic ORM. He believed that devitalization of the bone is the primary condition, and in an aseptic environment is symptomless. This same condition in a septic situation is manifested by pain and distress. The susceptibility to development of ORM is present anytime from a few weeks after radiotherapy and persists for life.[4]

Several studies done on the health of the teeth reveal an intimate relation to the pathogenesis of SORM. Frank and associates[5] noted that the dental defects occurred whether the teeth were inside or outside the field of radiation and that the common factor in the development of caries was the inclusion of the major salivary glands in the field of radiation. Radiation of the teeth and jaws without inclusion of the salivary glands did not lead to dental pathology. Irradiation of the salivary glands reduces the normal salivary flow and lessens its protection of the teeth by cleansing, lubricating and antibacterial action. The saliva becomes scanty and viscid — an excellent substrate for cariogenic bacterial growth. This bacteria-laden material coats the teeth, thus increasing their susceptibility to caries. The preradiation condition of the teeth, the degree of dietary alteration, the severity of xerostomia, and the ability to maintain oral hygiene are important factors which determine the postradiation integrity of the dentition or possible subsequent SORM.[6] At the M. D. Anderson Hospital, Houston, a policy of elective extraction of teeth in poor condition was followed from 1966 to 1969. Subsequently, the policy was changed to one of vigorous conservation with diligent oral hygiene, restorative dental

From the Division of Otolaryngology, Albany Medical Center, Albany, New York.
REPRINTS — Sharad S. Parulekar, MS, FRCS, Doctors Park, Corbin, KY 40701.

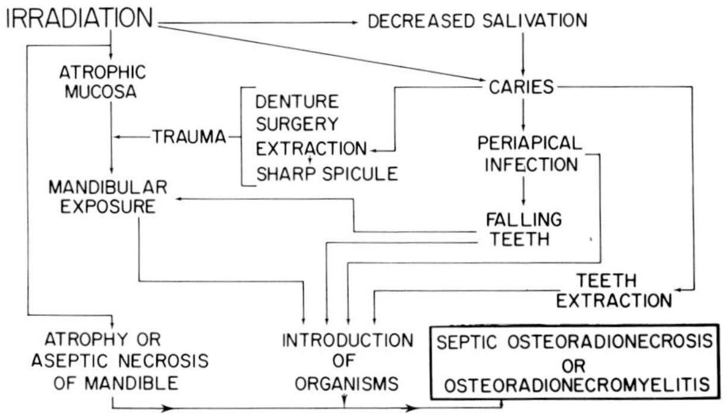

Fig. 1. Diagrammatic representation of the pathogenesis of osteoradionecromyelitis.

procedures and daily fluoride application. The studies indicated a total incidence of osteonecrosis of 14% of 381 patients, the majority occurring within three years of radiation with a peak incidence in the first year. In addition it was found that the incidence of osteonecrosis dropped from 19.7% during the period of elective dental extraction to 7.9% during the period of dental conservation. Bedvineck and associates[2] concluded that preradiation elective extraction did not allow time for complete healing of the extraction site. They further concluded that sharp spicules at the extraction site may later break through the atrophic mucosa and produce bony exposure.

The vitality and resistance to injury of the oral mucosa and gingiva remains impaired. The patient has a mucositis and this discourages adequate oral hygiene predisposing to a worsening of the infection. Pressure from a denture may destroy the integrity of the gingiva and expose the underlying bone. The pathogenesis of SORM is summarized in the diagram (Fig. 1).

A severe deep boring pain in the mandible is usually present for many weeks and leads to facial swelling and increasing trismus. A subcutaneous abscess develops and in its wake there follows a draining sinus which is usually foul-smelling and persistent. The subsequent loss of skin and mucosa results in denudation of the mandible. Sequestration of the mandible is gradual along with the spread of infection to the facial spaces producing a deep cellulitis. If untreated, the symptoms worsen, the patient's condition deteriorates and the prognosis is poor.

It is obvious from the previous discussion that an early evaluation by the dental service is essential in the diagnostic workup of any patient with a suspected cancerous lesion of the head and neck. This becomes even more important with tumors in the vicinity of the mandible and/or when management includes surgery involving the mandible plus radiotherapy. All obviously carious teeth with periodontal infection should be extracted, but vigorous conservation should be practiced with the salvageable teeth. These measures should be started in the pretreatment period and continued during radiotherapy (RT) and indefinitely thereafter.

The occurrence of pain, tenderness, redness and brawny edema or fluctuation over the mandible along with hyperpyrexia, prostration and polymorphonucleocytosis should alert the doctor of the occurrence of a septic complication. Conventional and panorex x-ray views of the mandible should be obtained. If an abscess or draining sinus is formed, Gram stain, aerobic and anaerobic cultures, and blood culture should be obtained. Empiric intravenous high dosage penicillin therapy should be started and this should be either changed to or supplemented with the appropriate antibiotics when the bacteriology reports become available. Meticulous mouth care including irrigation of the sinus tracts and tissues over the exposed mandible is essential. Appropriate remedial measures to correct the patient's anemia or impaired nutritional status should be instituted. Radical surgical procedures such as sequestrectomy may be necessary and may even need repetition, but these lead to disfigurement and dysfunction. A variety of surgical procedures may be required for optimum reconstruction of the surgical defect and each case needs individualization. If either necrosis of skin or fistula formation has occurred, local and distant flaps may be used. Appropriate bone grafts with internal fixation may also become necessary.

In certain centers, hyperbaric oxygen has been used successfully as an adjunct to the combined use of appropriate medical and surgical management.[7-9] It is reported that the symptoms were relieved after 14 days and the sequestra were well demarcated by a bed of vascular granulation tissue. Hyperbaric oxygenation by the inhalation of oxygen under tension multiplies the alveolar oxygen content several fold and with it the tissue oxygen pressure, even if the tissues are compromised by fibrosis, infection or sclerotic bone. This is of particular importance in the mandible which is supplied by end-arteries and lacks the blood supply of the upper jaw. A tissue oxygen pressure of 20-30 mm Hg is optimal to stimulate the fibroblastic and collagen proliferation necessary to promote structural support for the budding and arcading capillaries. Raising the oxygen pressure to 30 mm Hg in hypoxic wounds further increases the leukocyte microbial killing property and simultaneously inhibits the growth of many pathogenic bacteria. The average treatment lasted 45 days. Twenty minutes oxygen was alternated with five minutes of air inhalation to give a daily total of 90 minutes oxygen at 2.4 atmospheric pressure.[7]

I wish to present the following case history: A 70-year-old male, six years earlier, had a $T_2N_1M_0$ moderately differentiated squamous cell carcinoma of the left tonsil for which he underwent a composite resection. In December 1977 he developed a

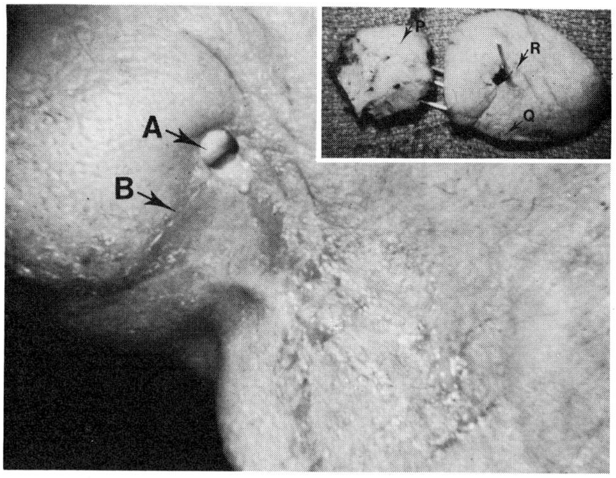

Fig. 2. Orocutaneous fistula with exposed mandible (A) and scarred indurated skin (B). Insert) Excised mandibular sequestrum (P), involved skin (Q) and fistula (R).

recurrence and underwent a full course of RT and received 7,000 rads. Eight months later a dental plate was provided. After wearing the denture for two months he developed pain, odynophagia, swelling, tenderness and hypermia over the left chin region. He subsequently developed intraoral exposure of the mandible over the site of resection and an orocutaneous fistula with constant drainage (Fig. 2). It was in this condition he was admitted to AMCH two months later (December 1978). Since the age of 15 years he smoked two packages of cigarettes per day and was a chronic alcoholic; he appeared to have poor nutrition. His past history was noncontributory. The patient's general clinical condition and his otolaryngologic, laboratory and radiologic examinations were all grossly normal. His oral examination demonstrated ankyloglossia and exposed mandibular sequestrum on the left side in the region of the composite resection. There was a defect in the floor of the mouth and it communicated with the external fistula. There did not appear to be any recurrence of tumor. The external examination demonstrated very hyperemic, indurated, fibrotic and unhealthy skin surrounding the opening of the fistula with foul pus draining from the area. The rest of the neck examination was negative. Conventional, panorex and tomographic x-rays of the mandible were unremarkable. The culture was reported as *Staphylococcus* coagulase negative aerobic, and varieties of *Bacteroides* and fusobacteria on anaerobic cultures. Biopsies of the suspected areas of the mouth and skin followed and were repeated but no cancer recurrence was detected. Aqueous penicillin G intravenous therapy (2.4 million units) q4h and intense hydrogen peroxide and Betadine® irrigations of the mouth and fistula were initiated. The inflammation responded. With the diagnosis of a SORM and a consideration of the potential hazards of operating on a heavily radiated and infected area, the prognosis appeared dismal. The patient was started on very aggressive nutritional therapy. On December 15 a medial based left deltopectoral (DP) flap was raised. After a delay of three weeks, on January 6, 1979, a wide excision of the orocutaneous fistula and sequestrectomy were performed. Immediate repair was accomplished by use of a posterior based tongue flap for lining and the DP flap for cover. The digastric muscle running across the wound was used for approximating and anchoring the tongue and skin flaps (Figs. 2 [insert]-4). The patient generally did very well in the postoperative period with both flaps remaining healthy and covering the mandible. However, a partial separation occurred posteriorly, forming a pocket where food and debris collected, setting up an infection. Antibiotic therapy was changed to intravenous ampicillin 1 gm q6h plus vigorous oral irrigations. On February 17 de-epithelialization and reapproximation of the opposing flaps were performed with good postoperative results. On March 3, 1979 the patient under-

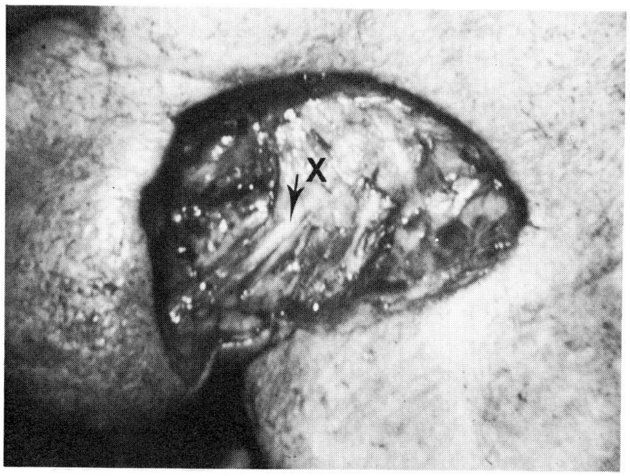

Fig. 3. Defect after excision of the necrotic tissue shown in Fig. 2 insert and showing digastric running across the wound (X).

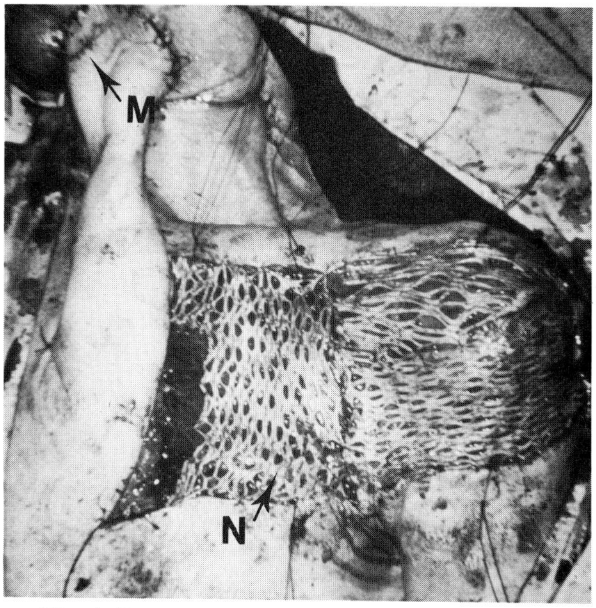

Fig. 4. Reconstruction medial based DP flap (M) and chest cover by meshed split skin (N).

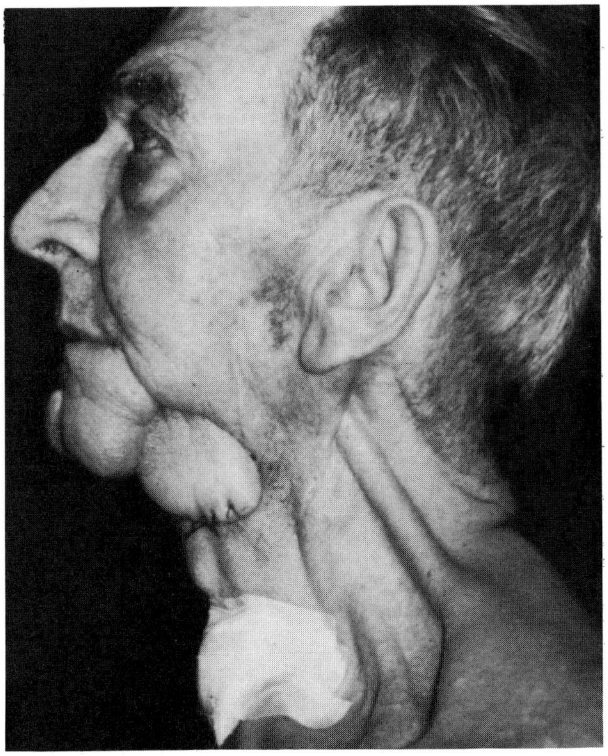

Fig. 5. Final stage of DP flap transfer showing reconstructed and healed defect.

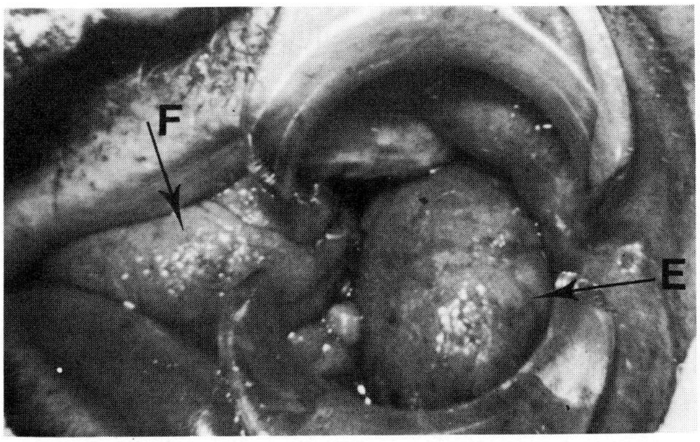

Fig. 6. Picture taken in office in April, three months after use of posterior based lateral tongue flap (E) and also showing mobile tongue (F).

went detachment of the DP flap, the remaining being returned to the chest (Fig. 5), and he was discharged a week later. He was seen after one month and was found to be free of problems (Fig. 6). He had fairly good speech and reported that he will probably never wear a denture again.

Dr. Dominick Paonessa: In their paper on ORM of the mandible, Rankow and Weissman[10] noted a 10-30% possibility of ORM and a 10-20% possibility of death in a patient receiving radiation therapy for his head and neck cancer. The triad of SORM is the history consisting of: 1) radiation therapy to the mandible, 2) trauma to the mandible, and 3) infection. The radiation energy delivered to the mandible as opposed to the surrounding tissue is significantly less today using megavoltage. We do, however, continue to see an uncomfortable incidence of SORM. The radiation effect upon the bone causes an obliterative sclerosis of the nutrient vessels causing impairment of osteogenesis followed by osteoporosis. Trauma to the mandible is usually caused by tooth extraction or dentures. Infection becomes rampant due to the incapacity of the bone with its compromised blood supply to wall off invading organisms. The result is virulent osteomyelitis.

This patient received his dentures about eight months following the termination of 7,000 rads RT. He rapidly developed mucosal breakdown and infection along with fistulization unresponsive to high doses of intravenous penicillin and good oral hygiene with hydrogen peroxide and Betadine. As Dr. Parulekar described, a DP flap was delayed and definitive surgery carried out. Because the entire tissue bed had intense radiation changes and appeared avascular, a posteriorly based lateral tongue flap with its excellent blood supply was chosen. This flap served both as intraoral coverage and to bring additional blood supply to the surrounding tissues. This patient has done well with both speech and deglutition and will continue on ampicillin for several months.

An important question is how long does one wait after the termination of radiation therapy before fitting a patient with dentures. This topic is open for comments and questions.

Dr. Jerome Goldstein: I remember this patient very well. I remarked to Dr. Paonessa about the poor nutritional status and suggested that the raising and delay of the DP flap would allow ample time for aggressive nutritional therapy and for cleansing and hopefully sterilizing the presenting infection. The DP flap would bring in a good unirradiated vascular supply to the debilitated orofacial tissues which had suffered from the effects of radiation and infection. I agree with Dr. Parulekar about the sinister influence of the proximity of the mandibulotomy site in the pathogenesis of ORM. We have at present a patient in the VA Hospital who three years ago had a mandibulotomy for resection of an intraoral lesion and subsequently had RT. He developed a septic ORM complicated by wire sutures. Excision of a fair amount of the mandible was required. One has really to consider several factors before one embarks on combination therapy. Dr. Pressman, what is the dental protocol in the VA Hospital?

Dr. Howard Pressman: The past several years have seen a general decline in the incidence of ORM for the following reasons: 1) Change from orthovoltage to megavoltage and cobalt therapy; 2) greater refinement and sophistication of RT, ie, by shielding of the salivary glands and thereby reduction of xerostomia; 3) advancement by the dental profession in managing head and neck cancer patients by close supervision of oral hygiene and daily topical fluoride application to the dentition and the use of soft tissue conditioners in prosthetic dentistry. The protocol followed by the Dental Service of the Albany Veterans Hospital is as follows: 1) dental extraction of all teeth in the line of RT with thorough alveoplasty of the jaw. The extractions usually involve all the posterior teeth, especially the mandible. A good alveoplasty avoids sharp bony projections or spicules from later piercing the overlaying mucosa. 2) If the remaining dentition (usually anterior teeth) are in poor condition, they are extracted and a thorough alveoplasty performed. 3) If the remaining dentition are in good condition (rarely so), they are retained and the usual meticulous conservative techniques are followed. 4) The patient's oral hygiene, social habits and lifestyle are thoroughly evaluated. If there is any doubt, all teeth are extracted. The key is proper patient selectivity.

The prosthetic dentistry considerations are as follows: 1) If the patient is adequately nourished, has minimal radiation mucositis, is free of recurrence and has healed alveolar ridges, then dentures are considered approximately 6-12 months after completion of RT, only if the patient so desires. 2) The exact length of time without dentures after RT and the need for dentures by the patient is controversial and opinions vary in the different medical centers. In Hines VA Hospital, the patient is not permitted to wear dentures if he has had orthovoltage treatment. If cobalt therapy has been used a minimum waiting period of one year post-RT is required. 3) If the patient wishes to get along without dentures, he is encouraged to do so. 4) Soft tissue conditioners used as denture relining material has greatly reduced complications. 5) If dentures are prepared and used, it is imperative that the dentist or prosthodontist treating and following the patient be aware of and knowledgeable regarding SORM in head and neck cancer patients.

Dr. Ernest Kopp: One often wonders about the need for mandibulotomy to provide access for the resection of intraoral tumors. I personally do a pull-through procedure whenever possible and thereby avoid the risk of SORM.

Dr. Edward Brandow: I feel that a pull-through operation is not always possible, particularly in some posterior oral or oropharyngeal cancers. No one can deny that excellent exposure is obtained by a mandibulotomy or mandibular resection, although it is accompanied by the greater risk of sepsis.

Dr. Nicholas Procino: I would like to emphasize two points. First, I have patients use one-half strength Cēpacol® and one-half strength glycerine as mouth rinses during the period of RT and have found it helpful. Second, during the first year after radiation the dryness of the mouth brings on increased friction and thereby irritation by the dentures. These patients need to be followed very closely. Some of these patients with excessive atrophy of the mandibular ridges may be far better off staying permanently without dentures.

Dr. Sharard Parulekar: I must thank the discussers for their comments which are well appreciated. The patient's management proved very interesting and instructive.

To conclude then:

1. Prevent SORM, if possible.
2. Maintain a high index of suspicion.
3. If prevention is not possible, start antibiotics immediately while obtaining cultures.
4. Start irrigations, mouth washes and debridement.
5. Maintain nutrition and hydration and treat anemia.
6. Use the indicated surgical procedures.
7. Consider referring the patient for hyperbaric oxygenation.

REFERENCES

1. Howland WJ, Loeffler RK, Starchman DE, Johnson RG. Postirradiation atrophic changes of bone and related complications. Radiology 1975; 117:677-85.

2. Bedvinek JM, Shukovsky LJ, Fletcher GH, Daley TE. Osteonecrosis in patients treated with definitive radiotherapy for squamous cell carcinomas of the oral cavity and naso and oropharynx. Radiology 1976; 119:665-7.

3. Guttenberg SA. Osteoradionecrosis of the jaw. Am J Surg 1974; 127:326-32.

4. MacComb WS. Necrosis in treatment of intraoral cancer by radiation. Am J Roentgenol 1962; 87:431-40.

5. Frank RM, Herdley J, Philippe E. Acquired dental defects and salivary gland lesions after irradiation for carcinoma. J Am Dent Assoc 1965; 70:868-83.

6. Karmiol M, Walsh RF. Dental caries after radiotherapy of the oral regions. J Am Dent Assoc 1975; 91:838-45.

7. Davis JC, Dunn JM, Gates GA, Heimbach RD. Hyperbaric oxygen — a new adjunct in the management of radiation necrosis. Arch Otolaryngol 1979; 105:58-61.

8. Goupil MT, Steed DC, Kolodny SC. Hyperbaric oxygen in the adjunctive treatment of chronic osteomyelitis of the mandible: report of case. J Oral Surgery 1978; 36:138-43.

9. Mainous EG, Hart GB. Osteoradionecrosis of the mandible, treatment with hyperbaric oxygen. Arch Otolaryngol 1975; 101:173-7.

10. Rankow RM, Weissman B. Osteoradionecrosis of the mandible. Ann Otol Rhinol Laryngol 1971; 80:603-11.

LETTERS TO THE EDITOR

Dear Editor:

I enjoyed the article by Herzon and Murphy[1] discussing the ultrastructure of cilia in Kartagener's syndrome. I wish, however, to disagree politely with their interpretation of the ultrastructure of the cilia shown in Figure 3.

According to Bloom and Fawcett,[2] two different types of cilia can be characterized, those possessing *isochronal* and those possessing *metachronal* activity (beat). Isochronal activity implies that the cilia all beat together in random fashion. An example of this might be seen in the cilia of the olfactory epithelium. In metachronal activity on the other hand, successive cilia in each row start their beat in sequence so that each is slightly more advanced in the cycle than the preceding one. This sequential activation of cilia results in the formation of waves that sweep slowly over the surface of the epithelium as a whole, regular in periodicity and constant in direction. The effect of this coordinated activity of metachronal beats is to move or propel material (a blanket of mucus) slowly over the epithelium, as opposed to isochronal beats which randomly "stir the pot."

Cilia which possess metachronal activity can be identified by the parallel orientation of the lines drawn between the centers of the two central fibers (tubules).[3] The direction of the effective and recovery beats is in the axis of this line. In cilia beating in isochronal fashion, on the other hand, these lines are randomly oriented. This second situation would seem to be the case in Figure 3 of Herzon and Murphy's article. Obviously, however, additional sections would have to be screened to see if this random, isochronal orientation were a constant finding before a definitive statement could be made. If this were the case, however, then possibly the basic defect in Kartagener's syndrome is an ineffective clearance of the mucus blanket with resultant stasis, suppuration, scar formation and further interference with clearing. Additional work in this area is clearly essential.

REFERENCES

1. Herzon FS, Murphy S. Normal ciliary ultrastructure in children with Kartagener's syndrome. Ann Otol Rhinol Laryngol 1980; 89:81-3.

2. Bloom W, Fawcett DW. Textbook of histology. 10th ed. Philadelphia: WB Saunders, 1975:103.

3. Takasaka T, Sato M, Onodera A. Atypical cilia of the human nasal mucosa. Ann Otol Rhinol Laryngol 1980; 89:37-45.

Sincerely yours,
Bruce W. Jafek, MD, FACS
Mark Lovell, MS
University of Colorado Medical Center
Denver, Colorado

Dear Editor:

I would first like to thank Dr. Jafek and Mr. Lovell for their interest in my article and respond in two ways: first, with an additional microphotograph (Fig. 1) showing a larger cluster of cilia from the patient presented in which all the central tubules except one are oriented in a more parallel fashion.

Second and more importantly, is an examination of their implication that the morphology of cilia, specifically with regard to the orientation of the central tubules, is a prime determiner of chronicity (beat). Dr. Jafek has made the assumption that because there is not a parallel relationship between the central tubules of the cilia presented that they may represent cilia which beat in isochronal fashion. An examination of the available literature would not seem to bear out that conclusion.

One must examine carefully the difference between direction and chronicity (beat). There seems to be clear evidence that the orientation of the central tubules does govern direction. However, the available evidence would seem to indicate that beat is controlled by such things as ATP concentrations, temperature and changes in the number of dynein arms present.[1]

Additionally, a closer look at the significance of the rotation of the central tubules is in order. Although rotation from 5 to 25° is given as the normal variance allowed among central tubules,[2] it would appear that there is some question as to the significance of this rotation and its normal variability. Satir[3] in his examination of the metachronal wave has found central tubules with rotations of up to 90° relevant to one another. Omoto and Kung[4] have shown that the central tubules of paramesium may rotate up to 360°. Depending upon the state in which the tubules are fixed, there would appear to be a greater normal variation of this orientation than previously implied.

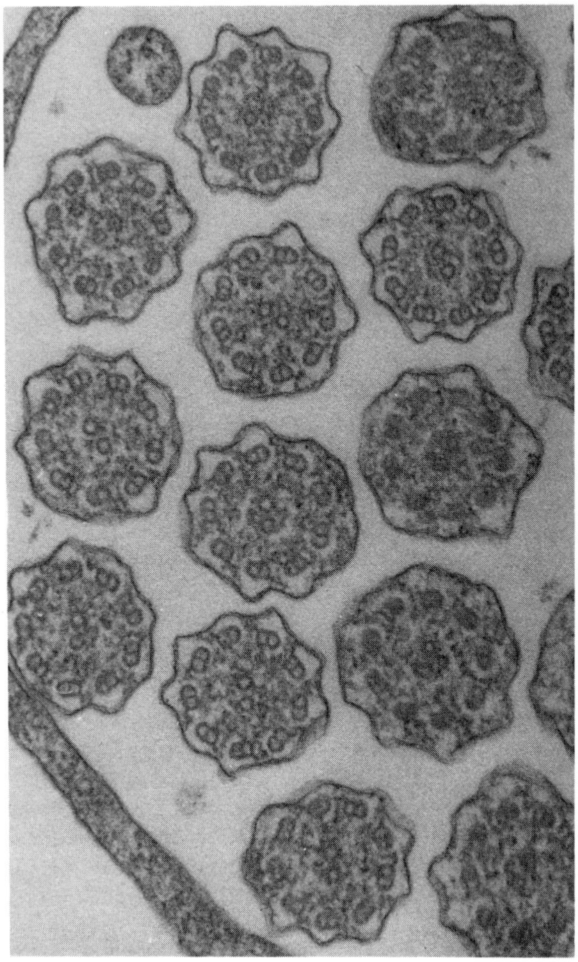

Fig. 1.

So, I will stand by my original statement that the morphologic ultrastructure of the cilia in the presented patient is normal, and would agree with Dr. Jafek and Mr. Lovell that further research in this area is necessary.

REFERENCES

1. Gibbons IR. Structure and function of flagellar microtubules. In: Brinkley RR, Porter KR, eds. International cell biology, 1976-1977. New York: Rockefeller University Press, 1977:348-56.

2. Eliasson R, Mossberg B, Camner P, Afzelius B. The immotile-cilia syndrome, a congenital ciliary abnormality as an etiologic factor in chronic airway infections and male sterility. N Engl J Med 1977; 297:1-6.

3. Satir P. Studies on cilia, the fixation of the metachronal wave. J Cell Biol 1963; 18:345-63.

4. Omoto C, Kung C. The pair of central tubules rotates during ciliary beat in paramecium. Nature 1979; 279:532-4.

Sincerely,
FRED S. HERZON, MD
University of New Mexico
Albuquerque, New Mexico

BOOK REVIEWS

Oculoplastic Surgery

By *Charles E. Iliff*, *W. Jackson Iliff*, and *Nicholas T. Iliff*. Hard cover, black and white illustrations, color illustrations, 348 pp, 1979. W. B. Saunders Company, Philadelphia. Price $110.00.

This volume is not simply a compendium of ophthalmic plastic surgery; rather it represents 30 years of Charles Iliff's creativity and personal experiences. Dr. Iliff has long been recognized as a master surgeon whose comprehension of this subject is so thorough that he has been able to distill the essence of a problem, reduce it to its simplest dimension, and resolve it in the simplest fashion. For many years the Iliff ptosis technique, for example, was widely recognized as a rapid and simple means for correcting ptosis. In this volume, we see the same approach applied to a great variety of oculoplastic problems. Due to his current association with his two sons, the viewpoints of the younger surgeon are added. The drawings by Leon Schlossberg are superb. Many of the photographs, before and after surgery as well at those taken during surgery, are of excellent quality, but unfortunately a number of poorly focused or exposed photos are scattered in with the excellent ones.

Of particular interest to the otolaryngologist will be the chapters dealing with management of thyroid eye disease, including lid retraction and orbital decompression from the lateral (Kronlein) plus inferior approach, mucoceles, tumors of ocular adnexae, and lacrimal tract surgery. The chapter on blepharoplasty may be worth reviewing, although the scope of techniques presented is quite limited.

The first chapter deals with the basics of oculoplastic surgery, particularly the characteristics of lid structures which differ from tissues of other parts of the body.

The ptosis chapter presents a simple, yet very functional anatomical review followed by a discussion of ptosis classification and surgical approaches. Complicated forms of ptosis are described and methods of modifying the appropriate surgery are clearly outlined. The section relating the amount of ptosis to the amount of correction required will be particularly helpful to the novice or to the occasional oculoplastic surgeon. The actual surgical approaches are well illustrated. The frontalis suspension operation is described using a standard technique. The authors present in great detail their favored levator aponeurosis-Mueller's muscle block resection.

The excellent chapter on thyroid disease describes techniques for reducing lid retraction as well as techniques for decompressing the orbit using a lateral orbitotomy together with removal of the orbital floor. It is claimed that this approach is as effective, with less morbidity, than the Ogura antral-ethmoid decompression.

Standard approaches to lacrimal surgery are shown. The section on preoperative diagnosis is sparse, with inadequate attention to the dye tests and other diagnostic entities. The use of a catheter, one of Dr. Iliff's favored techniques for assuring patency of the osteotomy, is nicely shown. Little attention is given to the use of Pyrex® tubes (Jones) or canalicular intubation with silicone tubing for lacerations or obstruction of canaliculi.

The section dealing with tumors of ocular adnexae is highly recommended. The illustrations are superb and very educational. The chapter on congenital defects is good, dealing mainly with the minor problems. It totally omits the approach popularized by Tessier, which is for more radical and serious congenital anomalies. The oculoplastic surgeon should certainly have an understanding of these entities and the most contemporary approach.

In brief, this work is an excellent text if one keeps in mind that it presents the unique Iliff experience. The book is marred by some significant omissions for those looking for a complete textbook. Whether the cost of the book, because of the use of color plates, is warranted, will have to be decided by the purchaser.

BERND SILVER, MD
St. Louis, Mo.

Paediatric Otolaryngology

By *J. F. Birrell*. Hard cover, black and white illustrations, indexed, referenced, 216 pages, 1978. Yearbook Medical Publishers, Chicago.

In this modest volume the author has compiled a rather complete list of the more common and some of the less common head and neck disorders of children encountered in a practice of either otolaryngology or pediatrics. Each section is arranged anatomically and introduced by an appropriate discussion of the embryology of the region. The sections are then subdivided along pathologic considerations such as congenital, infectious, or traumatic. Thus it is easy for someone unfamiliar with otolaryngology to find a general topic. The text is well indexed and specific illnesses are easily found. Illustrations are used effectively.

As the author suggests in his preface, one of the greatest uses of the material in this text may be made by pediatricians. I would add pediatric nurses and perhaps medical students. Because of size limitations, most topics once identified are treated somewhat superficially. This does not mean that some very important concepts are not adequately addressed. For example, the discussion of the indications and expectations of tonsillectomy and adenoidectomy is excellent. The emphasis placed on identifying the hard-of-hearing child early is most important and appropriate. By and large, however, I would hope that any otolaryngologist trained in the United States in the last 15 years would be familiar with the considerations discussed. Also, there are some sections, notably neoplasia, where the author does not seem to be familiar with newer treatment modalities and prognosis.

The greatest failing of this text is its failure to adequately describe modern management of many of the disorders characterized. Undoubtedly there are regional differences which may account for part of this. However, most literature references regarding treatment in this test are at least ten years old and meager at best.

This text provided insight into the nature of a notable otolaryngologic practice of 30 years' duration devoted to children. It certainly represents the great personal experience of the author. As such it provides enjoyable reading. It does not, however, prove to be a source of answers to the management of a difficult pediatric otolaryngologic problem.

RICHARD W. BABIN, MD, FACS
Iowa City, Iowa

Atlas of the Histopathology of Ear Tumors

By *P. G. Gerlings*. Hard cover, black and white illustrations, color illustrations, indexed, 163 pp, 1979. University Park Press, Baltimore. Price $79.50.

In a previous review of this book I have commented on the greatly enhanced interest of otologists and pathologists in the pathology of the ear. Otologists have been masters and pioneers in this field and Dr. Gerlings's *Atlas* bears witness to the profound interest and wide experience of a great otologist.

The *Atlas* has an autobiographical flavor of its own based on the rich material the author has encountered and studied. His papers on paragangliomas of the glomus jugulate were among the first to draw attention to their malignant potential in certain situations. As could be expected this section is particularly rich in interesting material and profusely illustrated (47 of 216 illustrations).

The *Atlas* is recommended to otologists and pathologists as a valuable guide to an important and interesting but still neglected region.

I. FRIEDMANN, MD
Middlesex, England

ABSTRACTS FROM NATIONAL AND INTERNATIONAL JOURNALS

Treatment of Bell's Palsy with Prednisone: A Prospective, Randomized Study

Wolf SM, Wagner JH, Davidson S, et al: Neurology 28:158-161, 1978.

Two hundred thirty-nine patients with idiopathic facial paralysis were randomly distributed into prednisone-treated and control groups to evaluate the benefits of steroids in treatment of Bell's palsy. Electromyographic criteria to evaluate the degree of facial nerve denervation were described. Patients were evaluated monthly until recovery was complete, or for one year. The clinical outcomes were defined as recovery of facial strength and development of motor synkinesis or autonomic synkinesis. Results of the steroid-treated group were superior to the nonsteroid treated group but were statistically significant only for autonomic synkinesis. In the total series, recovery of facial strength was incomplete in 16%. Among patients who recovered completely, the median time to recover was two months for both steroid-treated and control groups. Increased severity of the initial palsy, hyperacusis, and increasing age were all associated with a poor outcome.

J. PORCARO, MD
New York, NY

Ein Beitrag zum operativen Verschluss der Septumperforation (A Contribution to the Closing of Perforations of the Nasal Septum)

Martins M: HNO 26:183-184, 1978.

The problem of closing a perforation of the nasal cartilaginous septum is well-known to otolaryngologists. In this article the author outlines his method which consists of a wide flap of mucoperichondrium based along the inferior margin of the perforation closing the perforation on the one side. On the opposite side, the defect is patched by a composite retroauricular graft, with cartilage carefully shaped to fit the perforation. The flap has a good chance to survive since it is not twisted and the cartilage of the composite graft offers a supportive structure for the mucoperichondrial flap. The author reports good, long-term results. The method is simple and can even be recommended for the less experienced surgeon.

J. INNITZER, MD
Vienna, Austria

Computer Tomography For Small Acoustic Neuromas

Schubiger O, Balabanis A, Menges H: Neuroradiology 15:287-290, 1978.

The authors report on a technique of computer tomography (CT) evaluation for acoustic neuromas measuring 1 cm or less in diameter. The previous limit of resolution with CT scanning had been 1.5-2 cm diameter. Scans were made following injection of contrast (ioxitalamic acid 30%) and using overlapping slices 5 mm thick. The authors state that, using CT machines of the newer generation, small acoustic neuromas 1 cm or less in diameter may be detected. Meatocisternography still remains the only diagnostic method for detecting purely intrameatal tumors or neuromas protruding only a few millimeters into the cerebellopontine angle cistern if CT fails to demonstrate them.

A. JAHN, MD
New York, NY

Computed Tomography of the Larynx

Archer CR, Yeager VL, Friedman WH, Katsantonis GP: J Comput Assisted Tomography 2:404-411, 1978.

The authors demonstrate laryngeal structures and their interrelationships by computed tomography (CT). With improved technology providing faster scanning times and finer resolution, investigation of the larynx by CT is not only feasible but may add a new dimension of diagnostic reliability. Areas including the preepiglottic space, anterior commissure, piriform sinuses, subglottic space, paraglottic soft tissues, and the laryngeal cartilages which are problematic for diagnosis, may be precisely delineated by CT. The transaxial, coronal and sagittal planes have been evaluated and all have diagnostic value. The transaxial plane offers a unique view of laryngeal structures not afforded by any other technique.

T. LAI, MD
New York, NY

Bacteriology of the Chronically Discharging Middle Ear

Karma P, Ojala K, Jokippi AMM: Acta Otolaryngol (Stockh) 86:110-114, 1978.

The authors found anaerobic bacteria in 33% of chronic ears. This contrasts with earlier findings of 1.1% suggesting improved technique, ie, GasPak® system with prereduced anaerobic culture media and bedside inoculations. The anaerobes always grew in mixed cultures. Facultative bacteria are believed to act synergistically in mixed infections: they remove oxygen, produce substances that lower the redoxpotential of the tissues, or provide nutrients of the anaerobic pathogens. Anaerobic bacteria show more frequently in ears with postoperative recurrent infection or with clinical suspicion of cholesteatoma. Treatment with local repeated cleaning is emphasized because anaerobes are resistant to most of the commonly used ototopical antimicrobial medications.

T. LAI, MD
New York, NY

Traumatic Fat Necrosis of the Face in Children

Buswell WA: Br J Plast Surg 32:127, 1979.

This is an interesting article bringing to mind a fact that is fairly well known; namely, that following an injury to a fatty area, resolution and resorption of the fat may take place leaving behind a residual nontender nodule in the subcutaneous tissue. After a period of time spontaneous resolution of the nodule may occur leaving behind a local depression which usually fills in slowly but may leave residual dimpling.

The author brings this series of facts to our attention by stating that this condition is not rare but seems to have been overlooked in the literature. It may cause confusion in diagnosis and management since most cases are seen by practitioners who are not familiar with the problem. He presents an illustrative case and closes with the plea that since the condition is self-limited, no therapy is indicated and simply recognition of its occurrence is sufficient. A single photograph is presented.

M. J. PAYNE, MD
St. Louis, MO

Acoustic Neuroma: Results of Brain Stem Evoked Response Audiometry

Miller GW, Josey AF: South Med J 71:1062-1064, 1978.

The role of brain stem evoked response (BER) audiometry in the assessment of cerebellopontine (CP) angle tumors is assessed. Seventeen patients with CP angle tumors were subjected to BER. In 16 of these patients a tumor was found in the internal auditory canal (15 acoustic neuromas and 1 ependymoma), and the 17th patient had not yet been operated on. In 16 of the 17 cases, wave V on the BER tracing was abnormal: in 12 it was absent, and in 4 the latency was increased. The authors suggest that BER audiometry be included in the battery of tests to evaluate cerebellopontine angle lesions.

A. JAHN, MD
New York, NY

Ann Otol 89:1980

CHEVALIER JACKSON LECTURE

ESOPHAGEAL STENOSIS IN CHILDREN

FLAVIO APRIGLIANO, MD
RIO DE JANEIRO, BRAZIL

Congenital anomalies that can produce esophageal stenosis as well as acquired diseases of the esophagus in children are described. The infant and child who refuse to accept solid foods must be submitted to roentgenologic and endoscopic examination. Dysphagia is sometimes difficult to recognize in infants and children. Endoscopic treatment alone or associated with surgery is successful in many cases if well indicated and precisely done.

This is a never-to-be-forgotten privilege: to have been invited to present before you my best attempt to honor the memory of two world-famous physicians, father and son, whose distinguished name captions the *Chevalier Jackson Lecture.* I know the "Father of Bronchoesophagology" only through the study of his pioneer work; C. L. Jackson I knew well, both as the faithful successor to his father in advancing their work and also as a superb medical ambassador who promoted the friendships that give particular meaning to such a gathering as this. Nor can I forget that my earliest interest in this specialty was generously guided by a man whom the Jacksons trained, the late Dr. Paul Holinger.

Esophageal stenosis in children is a most interesting and extensive chapter of esophageal pathology. I will present our experience and discuss the main aspects of the different types of stenosis. Some of our patients were treated by various methods of dilatation, endoscopic or not, and others had to be operated upon. The cases which underwent surgery were operated upon by Drs. Fernando Paulino and Claudio Souza Leite, in close cooperation with our department. I will mention the surgical pathology including microscopic examination, but will not comment on the surgical technique.

Esophageal stenosis in children is either congenital or acquired. The most common types of congenital anomalies that produce stenosis are 1) congenital webs, 2) congenital stenosis, 3) stenosis due to bronchial remnants, and 4) congenital idiopathic muscular hypertrophy. The congenital anomalies of the esophagus that produce stenosis are not very common. However we must be aware of this diagnostic possibility in every infant or child who presents with difficulty in swallowing and frequent regurgitation.

The clinical history of this group of patients with stenosis is very characteristic. Holinger et al[1] described this in an excellent review of the subject. As a rule, anomalies that reduce the lumen of the esophagus do not do so to the extent that they impede the passage of fluids through the stenotic area. During the first four or five months of life when the infant is on liquid diet there are no symptoms. Thereafter as semisolid foods are added to the diet, feeding problems are apt to manifest themselves. Regurgitation is an important symptom and very often it is mistaken for vomiting by the parents or the physician, and a long series of dietary changes takes place until the child swallows a large piece of food or a solid foreign body that obstructs the esophagus. This interval may last from months to years before diagnosis is made following the removal of the foreign body. The diagnosis of this group of anomalies is made by a roentgenographic study of the esophagus followed by esophagoscopy. Direct examination of the esophagus is of utmost importance, and today we can add to our armamentarium the Storz-Hopkins system of optics which gives a brighter and more detailed image of the mucosa.

Esophageal Web. The congenital esophageal web is a rare condition. We have seen only three cases (ages two years; three years, six months; and six years). The location of the web in the majority of the cases is in the upper esophagus. The x-ray is very characteristic, showing dilatation of the proximal segment, then the zone of the web followed by a normal esophagus. The esophagoscopy is diagnostic and therapeutic because the web is identified through the tube and in advancing the esophagoscope, the membrane is ruptured and the lumen of the esophagus restored (Figs. 1 and 2).

Congenital Esophageal Stenosis. I'm not convinced of the independent existence of so-called congenital stenosis of the esophagus. Some types of

From the Department of Bronchoesophagology, Federal University of Rio de Janeiro, and the Department of Broncho-Esophago-Laryngology, Hospital G. Bonsucesso, INAMPS, Rio de Janeiro, Brazil.

Presented at the meeting of the American Broncho-Esophagological Association, Palm Beach, Florida, April 12-13, 1980.

REPRINTS — Flavio Aprigliano, MD, Rua Terezina, 19, Santa Tereza, 20240 Rio de Janeiro, R.J., Brazil.

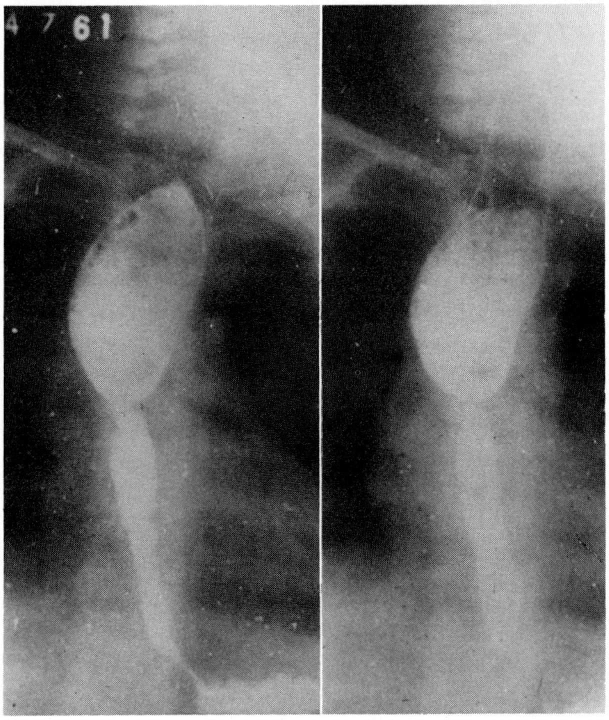

Fig. 1. Esophageal web in an eight-month-old child.

this anomaly have been described in the past, and I myself have made this diagnosis several times. However, in the course of treatment, endoscopically or surgically, other types of pathology, congenital or not, were found and of course we had to change our diagnosis. Now with the advance in pediatric surgery and in the light of our present knowledge there is little pathologic support for so-called true congenital stenosis. In my view, if true congenital stenosis of the esophagus exists at all it is an extremely rare condition, comparable to the congenital short esophagus.

Congenital Stricture due to Tracheobronchial Remnants. This type of congenital stricture is the principal cause of anomaly in our series of six cases (ages eight months to three years). Paulino et al[2,3] described their first cases in 1961 and 1963. Other authors have described various types of bronchial remnants in the esophagus.[4-8]

In five of our cases there was a tight stenosis in

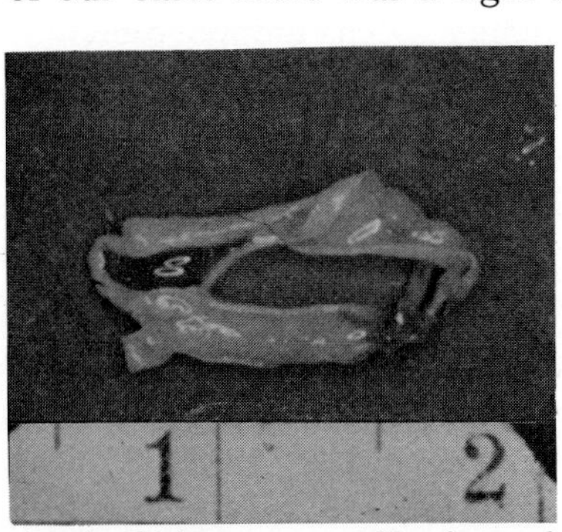

Fig. 2. A web which was ruptured by the esophagoscope and recovered at the tip of the scope.

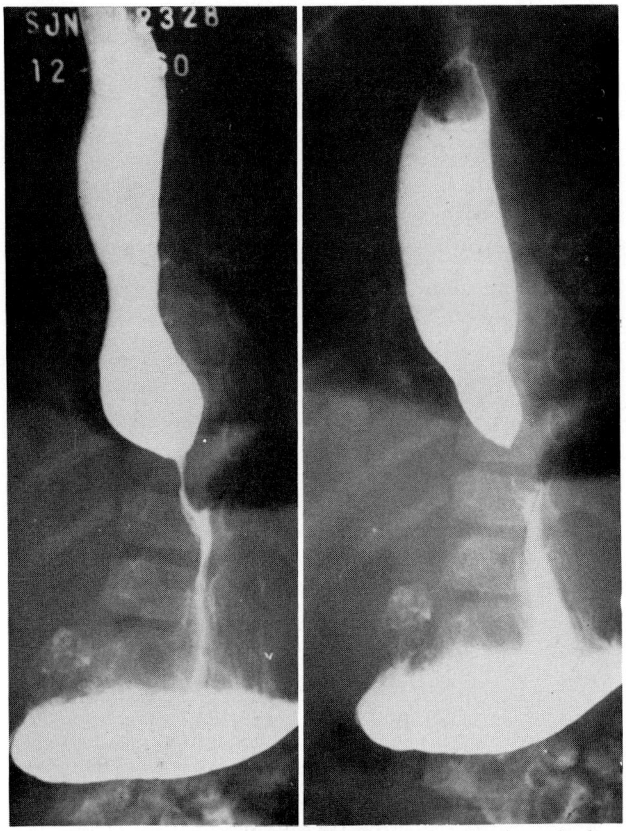

Fig. 3. Congenital stricture due to tracheobronchial remnants. A one-year, eight-month-old child with a cartilaginous ring in the distal esophagus. The x-ray is very suggestive of achalasia of the cardia.

the lower segment of the esophagus, caused by a cartilaginous ring. In each case there was a history of dysphagia since birth and a radiological aspect suggestive of achalasia of the cardia. The differential diagnosis is made through the esophagoscope which shows a rigid stenosis which cannot be dilated with a No. 8 or 10 French Jackson esophageal bougie. The endoscopic finding therefore ruled out achalasia of the cardia (Fig. 3).

The stenosis caused by tracheobronchial remnants does not respond to any type of dilatation and the restoration of the esophageal lumen must be made surgically by sleeve resection and end-to-end anastomosis. All our cases were submitted to surgery and the follow-up for more than three years was satisfactory in that every patient had a normal diet. The histological examination of the resected specimen showed cartilage and tubular arrangements of epithelium typical of respiratory tract origin (Fig. 4). One case, a six-month-old child who had severe dysphagia and was unable to gain weight, showed in the x-ray a lower esophageal stenosis. It was very difficult to dilate through the esophagoscope. She was operated upon and no cartilaginous ring was found (Fig. 5). The histological examination of the surgical specimen did show a fistulous tract with respiratory epithelium. These anomalies result from a failure of separation of the respiratory tract from the primitive esophagus.

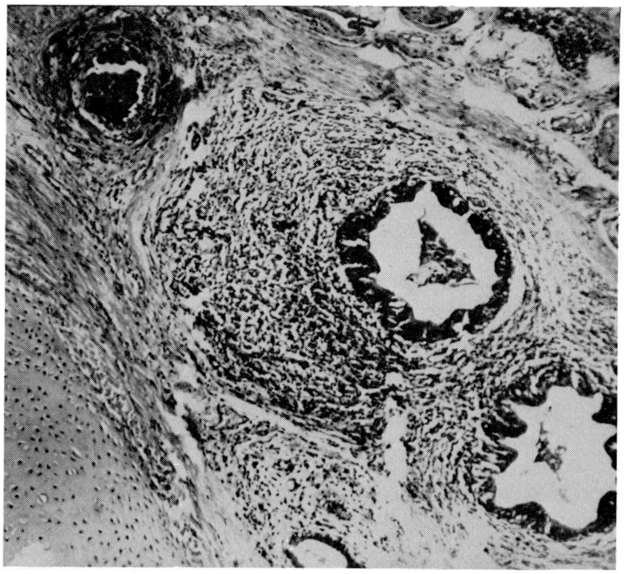

Fig. 4. Histological picture of the resected specimen of a cartilaginous ring stenosis, showing cartilage and respiratory epithelium.

Congenital Idiopathic Muscular Hypertrophy of the Esophagus. This is also a rare entity which was observed in five patients in our clinic. It has been described in adults and children, and some cases published were only diagnosed at autopsy.[5,9-12]

The cause of the thickening of the musculature of the esophagus is not known. Some authors consider it to be analogous to congenital pyloric hypertrophy. In the majority of the cases the hypertrophy was limited to the lower segment of the esophagus, but diffuse hypertrophy of the entire esophagus was also reported[13] (Figs. 6 and 7).

In five cases (ages seven months to three years), the symptoms appeared after birth and worsened when semisolids were added to the diet. The x-ray demonstrated a stenotic area in the lower esophagus without any particular characteristic. At esophagoscopy we found a tight stenosis, difficult to dilate, as well as edema of the mucosa. In two cases the diagnosis was made after the child became obstructed by a foreign body. All patients underwent resection of the stenotic area, and in one case it was necessary to perform an esophagectomy with colon interposition due to muscular hypertrophy of the middle and lower esophagus.

Acquired Stenosis. Acquired stenosis of the esophagus can be divided into these categories: 1) traumatic (after ingestion of lye, or after external trauma, 2) inflammatory, 3) peptic, and 4) after surgery. This is the most common type of esophageal stenosis in children. In my country where lye is still widely used, particularly inland, for home soap making and cleaning purposes, and is sold without any restriction, it is common to see cicatricial stenosis after accidental ingestion of lye in children. We have treated 78 cases of lye stricture in children from five months to six years old. The history is self-explanatory and the x-rays show single or multiple stenotic areas, chiefly in the middle esophagus.

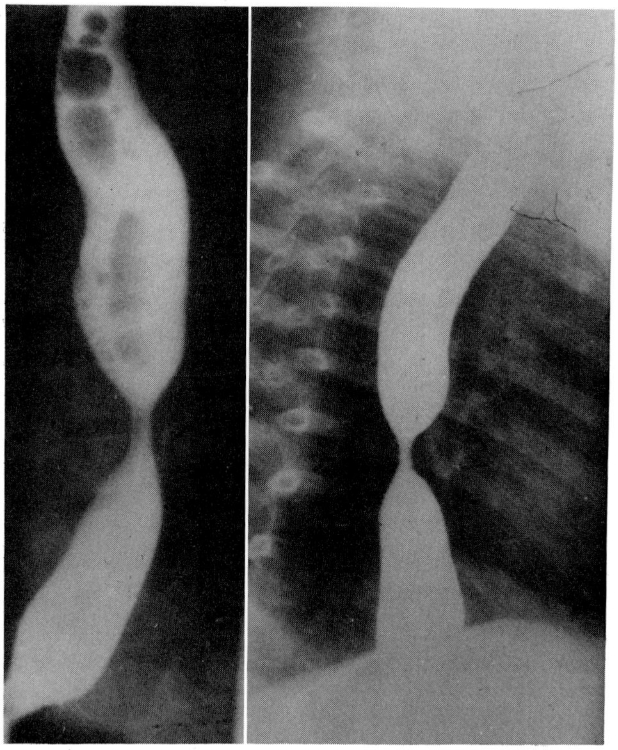

Fig. 5. A six-month-old child with an esophageal stenosis, difficult to dilate, which showed in the histological picture of the resected specimen a fistulous track with respiratory epithelium.

In mild stenosis, dilatation through the esophagoscope guided by a bougie is the best choice, but in severe or multiple strictures, the best approach is to perform a gastrostomy and start a retrograde or prograde dilatation with a string-guided Tucker bougie or the olive-tip metal Plummer bougies. The results are good, but in some cases the dilatation should continue for two or three years, and after that, esophagoscopy should be performed at least every six months. Only in three cases (3.8%) the dilatation did not restore the lumen of the esophagus and the children were sent to surgery.[14,15] When the esophagus is seen by x-ray to be atretic, in almost all cases a lumen can be found with the gentle and patient passage of a urethral catheter through retrograde or per oral esophagoscopy. The catheter is recovered either at the mouth or stomach and a string is tied in the other end for subsequent dilatations.

Inflammatory Stenosis. We have seen only two cases of proven inflammatory stenosis of the esophagus, both due to moniliasis (an infection caused by *Monilia albicans*), and stenosis resulted. One of the patients was dilated successfully through the esophagoscope, but the other had to have a gastrostomy and dilatation with a string-guided bougie.

Peptic Stenosis. Peptic stenosis of the esophagus in children is relatively common. Its etiology is

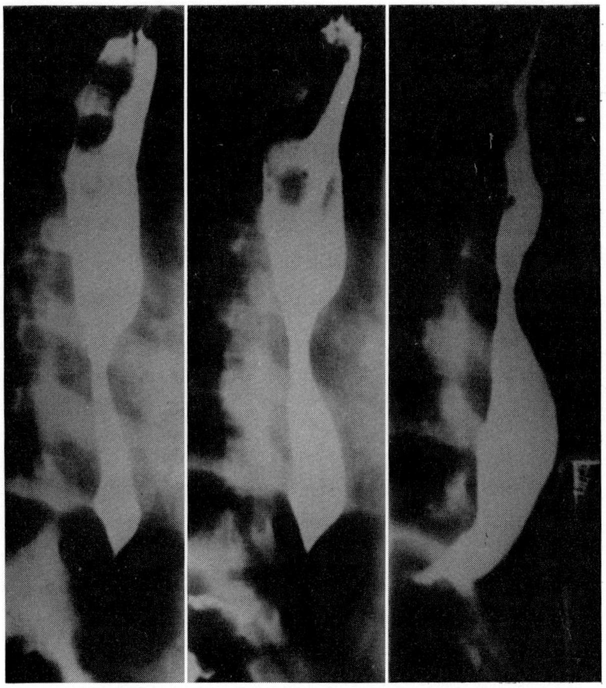

Fig. 6. Esophageal stenosis in a child which by surgery showed a congenital muscular idiopathic hypertrophy of the esophagus.

directly related to incompetence of the gastroesophageal junction. When the mechanism of gastroesophageal competence is disturbed, reflux of gastric contents occurs. This causes severe irritation or ulceration in the esophageal mucosa which is highly sensitive to the action of acid peptic secretion. A common cause of this incompetence is the sliding hiatal hernia. We must stress that reflux and hiatal hernia are different conditions; although they commonly exist together, each can occur independently. The real mechanism of gastroesophageal competence is very complex and it seems that many factors contribute to its normal action. Olsen,[16] and Payne and Olsen[17] made a basic contribution to our understanding of the physiology of this region.

Occasionally the diagnosis of congenital stenosis is posed by the presence of a peptic stricture in a child, because the symptoms of dysphagia, regurgitation, and sometimes bleeding can occur very early in life,[18,19] making this misinterpretation possible. Only a careful roentgenographic study of the esophagus and esophagoscopy with a biopsy can detect the existence of free reflux, severe irritation of the esophageal mucosa, with or without ulcerations and the findings of gastric rugae above the diaphragm when a hiatal hernia exists.

In some cases the x-ray pattern of stricture is not confirmed at esophagoscopy, at which time any mucosal pathology can be detected and the scope is easily advanced into the stomach, proving that it is not, in fact, a real stricture. This is called functional stenosis and is due to motor disturbance (spasm) of

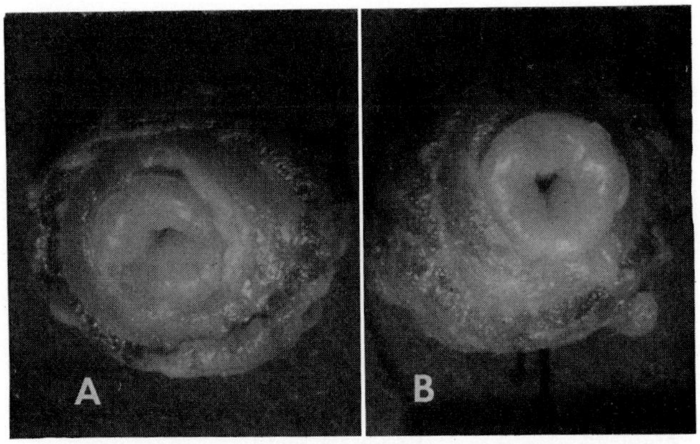

Fig. 7. The surgical specimen of the resected portion of the esophagus, showing a very thick muscular coat.

the muscular coat of the esophagus as a result of constant reflux. We strongly believe that ulcerations of the mucosa and edema of the submucosa are the cause of the stenosis. The true cicatricial stenosis due to reflux is rare and only the histological examination of the resected surgical specimen can prove the transmural fibrosis.

The review of 15 surgical specimens of the esophagus that were resected showed no significant fibrosis in the esophageal wall in five cases. This review was done by one of the surgeons mentioned above, Dr. Fernando Paulino, who, based on his observations, thought that an esophagectomy should be avoided in similar cases, and that recovery from such strictures could be obtained after a good antireflux operation. The proposed surgery was an antrectomy, vagectomy, and a Roux-en-Y anastomosis, as advocated by Holt and Large[20] in 1961, and Payne[21] in 1970.

This procedure is illustrated by the case of a boy who underwent an esophagectomy with an esophagogastric anastomosis to cure a serious peptic stenosis. We know today that this operation is inadequate because the reflux persists and in most cases the stricture recurs. Twelve years after surgery this boy returned with dysphagia, loss of weight, and by x-ray a very tight stenosis that could not be dilated. After a surgical opinion, an antrectomy and a Roux-en-Y anastomosis were performed. Three weeks after the operation a barium swallow showed complete regression of the stricture without any dilatation. The good result persists now seven years after the surgery.[22-24]

A complication that can also occur in children with chronic reflux and esophagitis or stricture is the metaplasia of the stratified squamous epithelium into a columnar type of epithelium which we find high in the esophagus (Barrett syndrome).[18,25-27] In this condition we can detect superficial erosions or deep ulcers similar to peptic ulcers in the stomach (Fig. 8). We must emphasize that esophagoscopy, with the help of an optical system, and multiple biopsies of the esophageal mucosa are mandatory in the diagnosis of this condition.

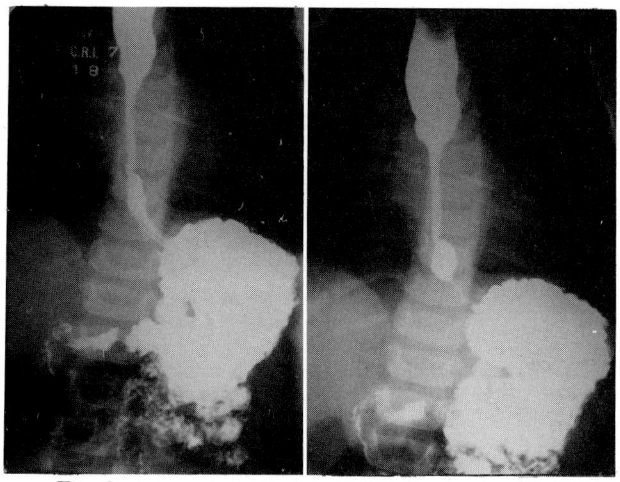

Fig. 8. An esophageal stenosis with hiatus hernia in a child. The terminal esophagus was lined by columnar epithelium (Barrett syndrome).

It is logical that the treatment must be directed to the cause of the disease, that is, the acid-peptic reflux to the esophagus. The form of conducting this treatment is still controversial. Some authors perform primarily a type of antireflux operation, others start with a conservative treatment, based on hygienic-dietetic measures and alkaline drugs. If this does not improve the patient, then surgery is indicated. When dysphagia is severe we can perform a series of dilatations to improve the feeding of the patients, but we did find that in some cases dilatation can be traumatic enough to cause more harm than good, especially when forcing an esophagoscope, guided by a bougie, through the damaged mucosa of the stricture area. We have used more frequently the mercury type of bougie, passed very carefully through the stenosis, associated with antireflux measures already mentioned. We must not forget that the aim of our treatment is the suppression of the gastric esophageal reflux.

Respiratory symptoms can occur in children with esophageal stenosis because of aspiration. These in our experience are more common in cases of the peptic type of stenosis, and they subside when the obstruction and the reflux are improved.

Stricture after Surgery. Esophageal stricture following various types of surgical procedures in the esophagus are not rare. In atresia with tracheoesophageal fistulae, operated by various surgeons in our hospital, 30% of the cases developed a stricture at the site of the anastomosis. Drool saliva is a very early sign. Dilatation should start as soon as the stricture is diagnosed, and it should be made with the Tucker bougie guided by a string, until numbers 28 or 30 are reached, depending on the age and size of the child. At this stage the child is swallowing well and we start to pass a small esophagoscope at different intervals. The results are very good.

Complicating treatment are esophagitis or peptic strictures which develop in patients after dilatation for caustic stricture of the esophagus. After a period without symptoms sour regurgitation and dysphagia recur. This is due to shortening of the esophagus, probably the result of severe burns after ingestion of lye. The treatment is the same as in other peptic pathology.

REFERENCES

1. Holinger PH, Johnston KC, Potts WJ. Congenital anomalies of the esophagus. Ann Otol Rhinol Laryngol 1951; 60:707-28.

2. Paulino F, Roselli A, Aprigliano F, Porto W. Estenose congenita do esofago por anel cartilaginoso. Rev Bras Gastroenterol 1961; 13:117.

3. Paulino F, Roselli A, Aprigliano F. Congenital esophageal stricture due to tracheobronchial remnants. Surgery 1963; 53:547.

4. Bergmann M, Charnas RM. Tracheobronchial rests in the esophagus. J Thoracic Cardiovasc Surg 1958; 35:97.

5. Snyder W Jr. Malformations of the esophagus, small intestine and biliary tract. Surg Clin North Am 1959; 39:1151.

6. Gans SL, Potts WJ. Anomalous lobe of the lung arising from the esophagus. J Thorac Surg 1951; 21:313.

7. Kumar R. A case of congenital oesophageal stricture due to a cartilaginous ring. Br J Surg 1962; 49:533.

8. Fonkalsrud EW. Esophageal stenosis due to tracheobronchial remnants. Am J Surg 1972; 124:101.

9. Sloper JC. Idiopathic diffuse muscular hypertrophy of the lower oesophagus. Thorax 1954; 9:136.

10. Spencer R, Hudson TL. Idiopathic muscular hypertrophy of the gastrointestinal tract in a child. Pediatr Surg 1961; 50:678.

11. Uhrich GI. Idiopathic muscular hypertrophy of the intestinal tract. Am J Surg 1965; 110:973.

12. Vargas LC, Britton RC, Goodman EN. Congenital esophageal stenosis — Report of a case of anular muscle hypertrophy at the esophagogastric junction. N Engl J Med 1956; 422:1224.

13. Blank E, Michael TD. Muscular hypertrophy of esophagus: Report of a case with involvement of the entire esophagus. Pediatrics 1963; 32:595.

14. Barreto PM. Tratamento das lesoes produzidas pelas substancias causticas. J B M 1965; 9:141.

15. Holinger PH. Management of esophageal lesions caused by chemical burns. Ann Otol Rhinol Laryngol 1968; 77:819.

16. Olsen AM. Study of esophageal motility in health and disease. Ann Otol Rhinol Laryngol 1968; 77:892.

17. Payne WS, Olsen AM. The esophagus. Philadelphia: Lea & Febiger, 1974.

18. Atkins JP. Some aspects of benign esophageal diseases in children. Ann Otol Rhinol Laryngol 1968; 77:883.

19. Fearon B. Lower esophageal diseases in infants and children. Ann Otol Rhinol Laryngol 1961; 70:1124.

20. Holt CJ, Large AM. Surgical management of reflux esophagitis. Am Surg 1961; 153:555.

21. Payne WS. Surgical treatment of reflux esophagitis and strictures associated with permanent incompetence of the cardia. Mayo Clin Proc 1970; 45:553.

22. Paulino F. Surgical treatment of peptic strictures and ulcers of the esophagus. XIII Congress of the Pan Pacific Surgical Association, Honolulu, Feb. 1975.

23. Paulino F. Tratamento cirúrgico das estenoses pepticas do

esofago. Anaes do XX Congresso Peruano de Cirurgia. 1975; 28:33.

24. Paulino F, Roselli A. Patologia da esofagite de refluxo. Medicina de Hoje 1977; 3:88.

25. Allison PR, Johnston AS. Oesophagus lined with gastric mucous membrane. Thorax 1953; 8:101.

26. Aprigliano R. Sindrome de Barrett e adenocarcinoma do esofago. Thesis, Faculdade de Medicina da Universida de Federal do Rio de Janeiro, Brasil.

27. Aprigliano R, Cavalcanti A. Epitélio colunar revestindo o esofago, laboratório clínico, 2° Trimestre, 1958.

≈

NINCDS NOTES*

INTERNATIONAL SYMPOSIUM ON TOURETTE SYNDROME: CALL FOR PAPERS

The first international symposium on Gilles de la Tourette syndrome will be held in New York City, May 28-29, 1981.

Sessions will cover the following general topics: pharmacology, biochemistry, clinical aspects of Tourette syndrome, genetics, animal models, and neuropsychology. Each session will feature a state-of-the-art review.

Clinicians and scientists interested in Tourette syndrome and related movement disorders are invited to submit an abstract for consideration by the Program Committee. Deadline for receipt of abstracts is January 31, 1981. Support for expenses will be available to those selected to present a research communication.

Abstract formats and further information about the symposium are available from: Arnold Friedhoff, MD, Director, Millhauser Laboratories, New York University School of Medicine, 550 First Avenue, New York, NY 10016.

NEW PUBLICATIONS

Recent publications from NINCDS include a monograph on language disorders in children, a fact sheet on neurofibromatosis, and special reports prepared at the request of Congress on nine specific areas of the institute's research programs.

The monograph, *The Neurological Bases of Language Disorders in Children: Methods and Directions of Research*, presents proceedings of a two-day symposium sponsored by NINCDS in January 1978. Editors of the 196-page paperback (NINCDS Monograph No. 22) are Christy L. Ludlow, PhD, of NINCDS and Mary Ellen Doran-Quine.

The neurofibromatosis fact sheet answers, in layman's language, some of the questions patients and their families most frequently ask about the disorder.

The special reports to Congress summarize the status of research on amyotrophic lateral sclerosis, epilepsy, Huntington's disease, multiple sclerosis, muscular dystrophy and other neuromuscular disorders, Parkinson's disease, spina bifida and neural tube defects, spinal cord injury and nervous system trauma, and stroke.

Single copies of the monograph and small quantities of the other publications described above are available free from the Office of Scientific and Health Reports, NINCDS, National Institutes of Health, Bldg. 31, Rm. 8A06, Bethesda, MD 20205. (Additional copies of the monograph may be ordered from the Superintendent of Documents, U.S. Government Printing Office, Washington, D.C. 20402; price $6.00.)

OTITIS MEDIA RESEARCH CONFERENCE REPORT AVAILABLE

In May 1979, an international array of basic scientists and clinicians met at Ohio State University College of Medicine for a research conference on recent advances in otitis media with effusion, supported in part by a grant from NINCDS. The purpose of the conference was to reach a consensus on future research directions, to help guide investigators and funding agenices.

A report on the conference has now been published as a supplement to the Annals of Otology, Rhinology & Laryngology (Supplement 69, Vol. 89, May-June, 1980, No. 3, Part 3). Single copies of the supplement are available free to interested members of the scientific community from the Office of Scientific and Health Reports, NINCDS, National Institutes of Health, Bldg. 31, Rm. 8A06, Bethesda, MD 20205.

'CENTERS WITHOUT WALLS' ESTABLISHED

The National Institute of Neurological and Communicative Disorders and Stroke has awarded initial grants of $1,367,000 to establish two "Centers Without Walls" for research on Huntington's disease and related neurological disorders.

Unlike the traditional idea of a specialized disease center consolidated under one roof, Centers Without Walls do not emphasize a central location for research. Instead, a Center Without Walls consists of investigators engaged in basic or clinical research in different departments within a university, or at different universities and medical centers. Patients and their families may be seen in clinical research facilities at any of the institutions comprising the center.

*This information is prepared monthly by the Office of Scientific and Health Reports, National Institute of Neurological and Communicative Disorders and Stroke, National Institutes of Health, Bldg. 31, Rm. 8A06, Bethesda, MD 20205. (301) 496-5751.

ETIOLOGY OF STRIDOR IN THE NEONATE, INFANT AND CHILD

LAUREN D. HOLINGER, MD

CHICAGO, ILLINOIS

Of 219 patients whose primary presenting symptom was stridor, 150 were males, 69 were females. All were under 2½ years of age; more than half were four months of age or younger. Congenital anomalies caused stridor in 191 (87.2%). Congenital laryngeal anomalies accounted for the stridor in 132 (60.3%); there were 35 (16.0%) patients with congenital tracheal anomalies, 11 (5.0%) with congenital bronchial anomalies, 12 (5.5%) with infectious conditions, 12 (5.5%) with internal laryngeal trauma and 15 (6.8%) patients with other conditions. The cause of stridor was undetermined in two patients. Sixteen vascular anomalies were diagnosed and classified according to the part of the tracheobronchial tree which was involved. Twenty-six patients required tracheotomy. Fifty-eight (26.5%) were referred with an erroneous presumptive diagnosis for which they were being treated. The mean length of time from onset of symptoms to determination of the correct diagnosis by endoscopy was four months; it varied from one day to 16 months. The importance of early endoscopy for the diagnosis of conditions causing stridor cannot be overemphasized. The occurrence of more than 1 anomaly in 99 (45.2%) of the 219 patients demonstrates the importance of complete endoscopic examination of all patients with stridor.

Stridor is the audible symptom produced by the rapid, turbulent flow of air through a narrowed segment of the respiratory tract. It is often the most prominent symptom of airway obstruction in the pediatric patient. Proper management is possible only after a precise diagnosis has been established; stridor is a symptom, not a diagnosis, and is not managed on the basis of only a presumptive or inferential diagnosis. This review of the etiology of stridor was undertaken to serve as an aid in determining the correct diagnosis.

METHODS

The data were obtained by a retrospective analysis of 219 patients seen by the author at the Children's Memorial Hospital and Rush-Presbyterian-St. Luke's Medical Center in Chicago, during the four-year period ending June 30, 1979. All patients underwent a thorough evaluation, including complete history and physical examination, posteroanterior and lateral chest x-rays, soft tissue lateral x-ray of the neck, and endoscopic examination. All patients with dysphagia and those patients with moderate or severe stridor had preoperative barium esophagram. Other special studies employed included bronchogram, computed tomography, and radionuclide scan (for gastroesophageal reflux).

Endoscopic examination routinely included initial direct laryngoscopy, without anesthesia, specifically to evaluate vocal cord function; the flexible fiberoptic laryngoscope was occasionally used for this part of the examination. General anesthesia was then used for a more detailed inspection of the larynx and tracheobronchial tree. In cases of immobile vocal cords, the arytenoids were palpated with the patient under deep general anesthesia to rule out vocal cord fixation.[1] Esophagoscopy was done in patients with dysphagia, abnormal esophagram, or gastroesophageal reflux.

Excluded from the study were patients with stridor who were referred for treatment after the diagnosis had been established; thus excluded were typical cases of acute supraglottitis (epiglottitis), laryngotracheobronchitis (croup), most cases of acquired subglottic or laryngeal stenosis secondary to endotracheal intubation, respiratory distress syndrome, most foreign bodies, craniofacial anomalies, tracheoesophageal fistula, bilateral choanal atresia and gross pulmonary abnormalities apparent on chest x-ray.

RESULTS

Of the 219 patients, 150 (68.5%) were males, 69 (31.5%) were females. All 219 patients were less than 2½ years of age; 189 (86.3%) were less than 1 year. More than half (53.4%) were four months of age or younger (Fig. 1).

Congenital anomalies were diagnosed as the cause of stridor in 191 (87.2%) patients; the stridor was due to acquired lesions in 28 (12.8%). Congenital laryngeal anomalies accounted for stridor in 132 (60.3%). The statistics for the most common conditions producing stridor are presented in Table 1. The other causes of stridor included stuffy nose (turbinate hypertrophy) - 2; hypertrophied tonsils and adenoids - 2; bronchial foreign body - 2; base of tongue cyst (thyroglossal duct cyst) - 2; asthma - 2; and 1 each of deviated nasal septum, macroglossia and micrognathia, idiopathic lobar emphysema

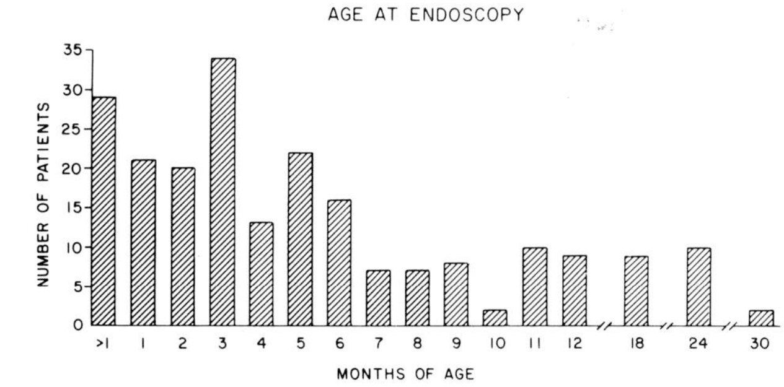

Fig. 1. Age of patients at the time of endoscopic evaluation.

From the Departments of Otolaryngology and Bronchoesophagology, The Children's Memorial Hospital and Rush-Presbyterian-St. Luke's Medical Center, Chicago, Illinois.

Presented at the meeting of the American Broncho-Esophagological Association, Palm Beach, Florida, April 12-13, 1980. Recipient of the Seymour R. Cohen Award for Pediatric Laryngology and Bronchoesophagology.

REPRINTS — Lauren D. Holinger, MD, 700 North Michigan Avenue, Chicago, IL 60611.

TABLE 1. ETIOLOGY

Diagnosis	No. Patients	%
Congenital laryngeal anomalies	132	60.3
Congenital tracheal anomalies	35	16.0
Congenital bronchial anomalies	11	5.0
Infectious conditions	12	5.5
Internal laryngeal trauma	12	5.5
Other	17	7.8
Total	219	100.1*

*Rounding error.

(right upper lobe), agenesis of the right lung, and gastroesophageal reflux. The etiology of stridor remained undetermined in two patients with mild symptoms.

Sixteen vascular anomalies were recognized; they were classified according to the portion of the tracheobronchial tree which was involved. Aberrant innominate artery was diagnosed in 11 patients, vascular sling in 4, and double aortic arch in 1.

Laryngomalacia was the most common condition in the series and the most common congenital laryngeal anomaly (Table 2). In addition to laryngomalacia, subglottic stenosis and neurologic lesions, other congenital laryngeal anomalies included subglottic hemangioma - 2; saccular cyst - 2; and 1 each of laryngocele, cleft larynx, supraglottic, glottic and subglottic laryngeal web.

Of 35 patients with congenital tracheal anomalies (Table 3), 16 (45.7%) had tracheomalacia. Twelve (34.3%) had a compression of the anterior tracheal wall, 11 of which were due to an aberrant innominate artery. Three patients had a vascular sling. Tracheal stenosis was present in two patients. There was one case of a tracheal diverticulum and one case of a double aortic arch.

Congenital bronchial anomalies were present in 11 patients. Six had a narrow left main bronchus, one of which was due to a vascular compression. The right main bronchus was narrow in two; bronchomalacia was present in three.

Stridor due to acquired conditions was of relatively short duration and was due to infectious conditions, endotracheal intubation, foreign body, or tonsil and adenoid hypertrophy. Atypical croup (severe or prolonged laryngotracheobronchitis) produced stridor in 8 of the 12 patients with infectious conditions; exudative laryngotracheitis produced stridor in the other 4 patients. Of these 4, 1 had diphtheria and 1 had *Pseudomonas* tracheitis; more common bacteria were cultured from the other 2 patients. Of the 12 patients whose stridor was related to endotracheal intubation, 9 had acquired subglottic stenosis due to long-term intubation. Three had laryngeal injuries related to the act of intubation; 1 of these had hypertrophy of the right false vocal cord and another had a large granuloma of the right arytenoid. Parents of both patients with bronchial foreign bodies gave no history of an episode of aspiration nor were x-ray findings typical. One was referred with a diagnosis of "atypical asthma"; symptoms had been present for several weeks. The other child had been receiving medical treatment for croup.

TABLE 2. CONGENITAL LARYNGEAL ANOMALIES

Diagnosis	No. Patients	%
Laryngomalacia	79	59.8
Subglottic stenosis	27	20.5
Neurologic	17	12.9
Bilateral vocal cord paralysis 14		
Unilateral vocal cord paralysis 3		
Other	9	6.8
Total	132	100.0

TABLE 3. CONGENITAL TRACHEAL ANOMALIES

Diagnosis	No. Patients	%
Tracheomalacia	16	45.7
Anterior compression	12	34.3
Aberrant innominate artery 11		
Vascular sling	3	8.6
Tracheal stenosis	2	5.7
Tracheal diverticulum	1	2.9
Double aortic arch	1	2.9
Total	35	100.1*

*Rounding error.

Twenty-six (11.9%) of the 219 patients with stridor required tracheotomy, 8 for subglottic stenosis, 7 for atypical croup (severe or prolonged laryngotracheobronchitis), 5 for bilateral vocal cord paralysis, and 1 each for subglottic hemangioma, glottic web, micrognathia and macroglossia, agenesis of the right lung, laryngomalacia (with acquired subglottic stenosis), and supraglottic laryngeal web.

Of the 219 patients, 99 (45.2%) had at least 1 other anomaly. Well over half were anomalies of the respiratory system and may have contributed to the patient's stridor.

Most patients were referred specifically for endoscopic evaluation of stridor, "noisy breathing" or "wheezing"; "congestion" and "hard breathing" were other terms commonly used by the parents. Of the 219 patients, 58 (26.5%) were referred with an erroneous presumptive diagnosis for which they were being treated. In addition to the most common misdiagnoses of asthma, croup, bronchiolitis, laryngomalacia, and bronchitis (Table 4), other diagnoses included URI - 3; allergies - 3; tracheomalacia - 2; hyaline membrane disease - 1; foreign body - 1. The delay from time of onset of symptoms to establishing a diagnosis at endoscopy ranged from one day to 16 months; the mean time was four months.

TABLE 4. ERRONEOUS DIAGNOSES (PRIOR TO ENDOSCOPY)

Diagnosis	*No. Patients*
Asthma	17
Croup	13
Bronchiolitis	9
Laryngomalacia	5
Bronchitis	4
Other	10
Total	58

TABLE 5. SEX DISTRIBUTION

Diagnosis	*No. Patients*	*Male: Female*	*% Male*
Congenital tracheal anomalies	35	27:8	77.1
Congenital subglottic stenosis	27	21:6	77.8
Infectious conditions	12	12:0	100.0
Congenital bronchial anomalies	11	8:3	72.2
Acquired subglottic stenosis	9	8:1	88.9

DISCUSSION

The data accumulated in this study are most representative of chronic stridor: stridor which had been present for more than half of each patient's life. The large majority of cases (87.2%) represents congenital anomalies, although many of these young patients did not have symptoms since birth. Sometimes the stridor appeared shortly thereafter or arose later during infancy or childhood. It often appeared slowly and was not severe except when the infant was stressed with feeding, crying or certain positions. When the onset was slow or presented from birth, the etiology was usually congenital. The patients who presented with symptoms of relatively short duration had acquired lesions: infectious conditions, internal laryngeal trauma, bronchial foreign body, or tonsil and adenoid hypertrophy.

It should not be unexpected that laryngeal anomalies accounted for well over half of all cases of stridor. The dimensions of the triangular aperture of the infant larynx are approximately 7 mm in the anteroposterior direction by 4 mm in width across the posterior commissure. The glottic chink has an area of 14 sq mm; edema of 1 mm of the mucosal surfaces will reduce this area to 5 sq mm, only 35% of the original area.[2] Similarly, 1 mm of edema in the subglottic region of the newborn will reduce the airway to 32% of its former area.[3]

In general, stridor produced by an obstructive lesion above the thoracic inlet is inspiratory. This is due to the dynamic nature of most of these lesions in which the structures collapse inwards with the negative pressure created during inspiration. The exceptions are lesions such as subglottic stenosis which do not change with respiration and therefore produce both inspiratory and expiratory stridor. Lesions of the nasopharynx (eg, adenoid hypertrophy), oropharynx, (eg, micrognathia and macroglossia, tonsil hypertrophy), and hypopharynx (eg, base of tongue mass, retropharyngeal abscess) typically produce a very low-pitched, wet sound similar to snoring; these infants would seem to require suctioning but the audible symptom usually does not clear after suctioning. The inspiratory stridor of laryngomalacia is also low-pitched (and fluttering) but somewhat different in character. In contrast is the high-pitched inspiratory stridor associated with bilateral vocal cord paralysis.

Tracheomalacia and bronchomalacia, like asthma, typically produce stridor during expiration. If the extrathoracic trachea is significantly involved, the stridor may be biphasic; very rarely, when the extrathoracic trachea alone is involved, the patient may have inspiratory stridor due to tracheomalacia. The pitch and phase of the stridor may therefore be extremely helpful in localizing and diagnosing a lesion.

The significance of the male preponderance in this study (a male to female ratio of more than 2:1) is not clear; nor is there an apparent reason for this preponderance. Similar statistics have been reported: of 305 infants with laryngomalacia seen during a seven-year period, 199 (65.2%) were males.[4] An even higher proportion of males occurs in patients with obstructive sleep apnea, an entity which also involves obstruction of the respiratory tract. Guilleminault et al[5] reported 48 (96%) of the 50 patients in their series were male. Gil et al[6] have noted that hypersomnia-sleep apnea (HSA) patients were often difficult to intubate. In addition, they observed that many of these patients had small tracheas with respect to other individuals of comparable size. The preponderance of males in the present series was primarily due to an unusually high percentage of males in the five categories shown in Table 5. In general, males seem to be at greater risk for benign obstructive airway lesions.

One group of patients deserves particular comment. During the late fall and early winter of 1977-78, there were eight patients with croup whose picture was not typical. None had any prior symptoms of airway obstruction; all patients were male and between 3 and 15 months of age. In these atypical patients, either 1) the airway obstruction progressed rapidly to require establishing an airway within hours, or 2) the moderate respiratory distress (with stridor and cough) did not resolve after a period of two weeks of hospital treatment. Endoscopy showed the subglottic larynx to be erythematous and edematous. Purulent tracheobronchitis was present in all but two cases. One of these patients still required a tracheostomy tube 25 months later. During September and October 1979, we observed a repetition of the same pattern, with an epidemic of even more patients who required tracheotomy for atypical croup. The precise etiology remains obscure.

Technique and a high index of suspicion are particularly important in the diagnosis of certain conditions. Less obvious findings of the tracheobronchial tree are more readily observed 1) with the use of a telescopic system, and 2) when the child is breathing quietly and spontaneously under general anesthesia. These factors, as well as an increased awareness of the condition, may account for the relatively frequent finding of aberrant innominate artery. Tracheal compression by the artery produced stridor in 11 patients, none of whom had significant episodes of apnea; innominate arteriopexy was required for obstruction in only 1 case. Most patients who required innominate arteriopexy presented with apnea — not stridor and such patients were not included in this series.

In conclusion, the importance of discovering the etiology of stridor cannot be overemphasized; the fact that 58 (26.5%) of the 219 patients were referred with an erroneous presumptive diagnosis for which they were being treated is indicative of this fact. Jackson[7] stated it this way: "Stridor is of course a symptom and not a disease. In the days when all laryngeal diagnosis in children was inferential, the name stridor was supposed to designate a particular disease. The direct laryngoscope has demonstrated many different pathologic conditions productive of . . . stridor. The name should be retained, however, and applied to a large group of cases that call urgently for accurate differential diagnosis by direct laryngoscopy."

An unexpected finding was the high incidence of associated anomalies: 45.2% of all patients had at least one associated abnormality which usually involved the respiratory tract and may have contributed to the patient's obstructive symptoms. Of the patients with laryngomalacia, 45.6% had associated anomalies. In evaluating stridor, therefore, one does not conclude the procedure with laryngoscopy but rather proceeds with a complete endoscopic examination of the entire tracheobronchial tree.

ACKNOWLEDGMENT — The author thanks Mrs. Rudelia Rosales and Ms. Carla Gaona for their help in preparation of the manuscript.

REFERENCES

1. Cox DJ, Simmons FB. Midline vocal cord fixation in the newborn. Arch Otolaryngol 1974; 100:219.

2. Holinger PH. Pediatric laryngology. American Academy of Ophthalmology and Otolaryngology, Course Instruction Pamphlet, 1952.

3. Holinger PH, Kutnick SL, Schild HA, Holinger LD. Subglottic stenosis in infants and children. Ann Otol Rhinol Laryngol 1976; 85:591-9.

4. Holinger PH, Johnston KC, Schiller F. Congenital anomalies of the larynx. Ann Otol Rhinol Laryngol 1954; 63:581-606.

5. Guilleminault C, van den Hoed J, Mitler MM. Clinical overview of the sleep apnea syndromes. In: Guilleminault C, Dement WC, eds. Sleep apnea syndromes. New York: Allan R. List Inc., 1978:1-12.

6. Gil MW, Simmons FB, Guilleminault C. Tracheostomy and sleep apnea. In: Guilleminault C, Dement WC, eds. Sleep apnea syndromes. New York: Allan R. List Inc., 1978:347-52.

7. Jackson C, Jackson CL. Diseases and injuries of the larynx. New York: MacMillan, 1942:63.

≈

XVII CONGRESS OF PAN AMERICAN ASSOCIATION OF OTOLARYNGOLOGY AND BRONCHOESOPHAGOLOGY

The XVII Congress of the Pan American Association of Otolaryngology and Bronchoesophagology will take place in Santiago, Chile December 7-10, 1980. For further information contact: General Secretary Dr. Jorge Otte, Avenida Vitacura 2653, Santiago, Chile.

Ann Otol 89:1980

INNOMINATE ARTERY COMPRESSION OF THE TRACHEA IN INFANTS WITH REFLEX APNEA

JOSEPH M. ARDITO, MD
GABRIEL F. TUCKER, JR., MD
ROBERT H. OSSOFF, DMD, MD
SERAFIN Y. DELEON, MD

CHICAGO, ILLINOIS

Compression of the trachea by an anomalous innominate artery in association with reflex apnea is a frequent cause of respiratory arrest in infants. Once considered, tracheoscopy is mandatory to rule out this disorder. Surgical correction of this condition by innominate arteriopexy has proven to be a very effective method of management. Seventy-eight patients with tracheal compression by an anomalous innominate artery managed by the authors at The Children's Memorial Hospital in Chicago between January 1977 and December 1979 are presented. In this series, 28 patients had a history of one or more episodes of reflex apnea; all of these patients underwent an innominate arteriopexy. A complete review of this syndrome and methods of its diagnosis are scrutinized. We agree with previous authors that reflex apnea is a definite indication for surgical correction of this vascular anomaly causing tracheal compression, but other indications are delineated.

External tracheal compression, as a result of congenital cardiovascular anomalies, is a rather frequent cause of mechanical upper airway obstruction in children.

Early cases of mechanical tracheal obstruction secondary to congenital cardiovascular anomalies date back as far as the late 18th century. Over the last century and a half several anomalies of the great vessels have been identified and subsequently reported to cause obstructive symptoms in the infant population.

In 1948 Gross and Neuhauser were the first to associate respiratory difficulties with an anomalous innominate artery. Their initial presentation described a four-month-old infant with respiratory distress since birth, describing the anatomic deformity, its related pathophysiology, and the surgical procedure for its correction.[1] In 1955 Gross reviewed four similar cases of anomalous innominate arterial compression of the trachea (AIA) in a major review of 40 cases of congenital cardiovascular anomalies causing respiratory obstruction.[2]

In 1954 Ferguson and Flake discussed the use of tracheography as an aid in diagnosing malformation of the tracheobronchial tree, the aortic arch, and its branches in infants.[3] They concluded that these anomalies were far more common than was generally believed.

Fearon and Shortreed in 1963 reviewed 104 cases of endoscopically documented congenital cardiovascular anomalies causing tracheal compression.[4] The most common cause of tracheal obstruction in this series was anomalous innominate artery (66%). In all cases the diagnosis was definitely made by tracheoscopy. The term reflex apnea was coined by Fearon and his colleagues to describe the episodic apnea sometimes associated with tracheobronchial compression secondary to a double aortic arch or an anomalous innominate artery. It was their opinion that a reflex type respiratory arrest was initiated by irritation of the area of tracheal compression, whether stimulated by a bolus of food or even the tip of a tracheoscope. Interestingly enough, patients who would become apneic during tracheoscopic manipulation under lighter stages of anesthesia, would have no changes in their spontaneous respiratory pattern while under deeper levels of anesthesia. This suggested a reflex mechanism, although there has been no further substantiation from an anatomic or pathophysiologic standpoint as to the features of this reflex.

Six years later Berdon and coworkers reviewed five cases from Babies Hospital of Columbia-Presbyterian Medical Center in New York. Here, the authors emphasized a plain film technique for tracheal evaluation, demonstrating a constant curvilinear anterior tracheal indentation midway between the carina and suprasternal notch on lateral chest x-ray in all five of their cases of AIA.[5]

Later the same year Ericsson and Soderlund[6] presented six similar cases and once again emphasized the value of the plain lateral chest film in diagnosing this anomaly. They felt that its use as a diagnostic tool was such that tracheoscopy, tracheography, and angiography were unnecessary.

Also in 1969, Mustard and his colleagues reviewed 285 patients with the diagnosis of innominate artery

From the Division of Bronchoesophagology-Otolaryngology, The Department of Communicative Disorders, and the Division of Cardiothoracic Surgery, The Children's Memorial Hospital, Chicago, Illinois. Support by the Edward Shedd Wells Fund is gratefully acknowledged.

Presented at the meeting of the American Broncho-Esophagological Association, Palm Beach, Florida, April 12-13, 1980.

REPRINTS — Gabriel F. Tucker, Jr., MD, The Children's Memorial Hospital, Division of Bronchoesophagology, 2300 Children's Plaza, Chicago, IL 60614.

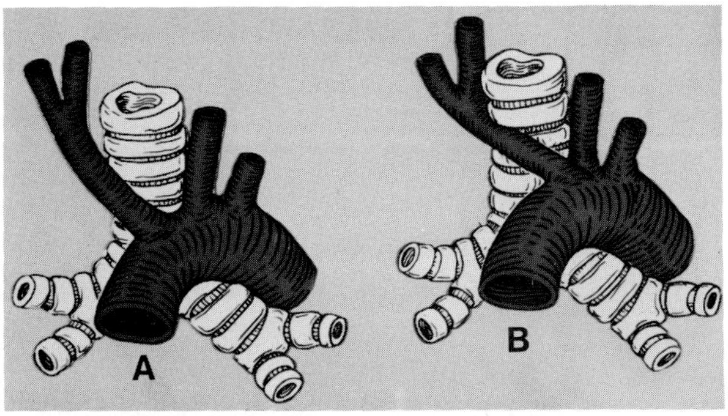

Fig. 1. Gross view of A) normal and B) abnormal relationship between trachea and innominate artery.

compression of the trachea. Of the entire group, only 39 patients were operated on; the remainder being treated medically.[7]

Macdonald and Fearon[8] highlighted the clinical features of this condition in 1971 in their presentation to the American Broncho-Esophagological Association. At the time of their presentation, skepticism still persisted not only as to the clinical significance of this anomaly, but also to its actual existence.

Finally in 1975 Möes and his coworkers reviewed 90 cases of anomalous innominate artery. Two thirds of their patients were treated surgically. They concluded that, aside from reflex apnea being an absolute indication for surgery, patients in respiratory distress with this syndrome who have severe tracheal narrowing, as proven by tracheoscopy, should undergo surgical correction.[9] Since 1971, there have been other scattered case reports of the problem, but in lieu of the historical background of this disease, it is the authors' impression that AIA is an entity whose existence and significance is still not widely appreciated.

This report deals with a series of 78 patients with tracheobronchial compression by an anomalous innominate artery managed by the authors at our hospital between January 1977 and December 1979. The pathologic anatomy and physiology of this congenital cardiovascular anomaly are reviewed. Additionally, the presenting symptoms, accuracy of diagnostic tools, differential diagnosis and indications for surgical correction for this group of patients are discussed.

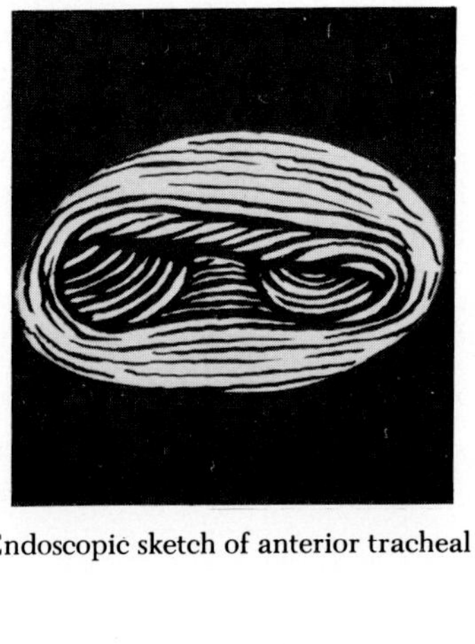

Fig. 2. Endoscopic sketch of anterior tracheal wall compression.

TABLE 1. PRESENTING CONDITIONS SIGNS AND SYMPTOMS

	No. of Patients	*Percent*
Apnea	28	36
Inspiratory stridor	14	18
Biphasic stridor	11	14
Cough	11	14
Recurrent pneumonia	11	14
Others	6	7

PATHOGENESIS

The innominate artery in these cases arises from the aortic arch at a point more distal and posterior than normal. Because it then crosses over the anterior surface of the trachea, usually 1-2 cm above the carina, as it courses superiorly and toward the right apical side of the chest, it forcibly compresses the anterior tracheal wall. This is illustrated in Figure 1. When comparing the normal with the anomalous innominate on the right, it can be readily seen that just the slightest variation in arterial origin causes the artery to behave as a taut sling compressing the trachea anteriorly. The effect this has on the trachea is seen in Figure 2. Note the oblique compression of the anterior tracheal wall, as it extends from left to right.

PRESENTING SYMPTOMS

The average age of onset of symptoms in this series was nine months, ranging from 14 days to eight years of age. However, the vast majority referred to us for endoscopic evaluation were between two and nine months of age. Thirty percent of our patients presented with at least one episode of reflex apnea, clinically described as appearing limp and lifeless following cessation of spontaneous respiration. These episodes usually last less than three minutes. Many of these children will require resuscitation as they enter a formal respiratory arrest while others begin rebreathing spontaneously. They have characteristically assumed a position of opisthotonos to facilitate relief of their airway obstruction.

Other symptoms included recurrent pneumonia in 14% of our patients, unexplained stridor (inspiratory, 18%, and biphasic, 14%), and cough in 14% (Table 1).

Less common symptoms were choking, wheezing, cyanosis, noisy breathing, croup-like symptoms, and respiratory arrest, ranging from 6-10%. Three patients who required tracheotomy, one for a lingual thyroid cyst, and the other two for subglottic stenosis could not be decannulated after their primary problem had been corrected.

TABLE 2. INVESTIGATIVE STUDIES

	Normal	Abnormal	Percent Abnormal
Esophagogram	25	13	34
Chest x-ray	39	20	34
Arteriogram	0	8	100

Innominate artery compression of the trachea may easily be confused with many other common conditions such as asthma, bronchitis, tracheitis, pneumonia, tracheal foreign body and tracheomalacia. In the absence of reflex apnea, the differential diagnosis could also include less common items, such as hiatal hernia, thymic enlargement, pancreatic cystic disease, mediastinal cystic hygroma, mediastinal hemartoma, and thymic capillary hemangioma. However, vascular compression of the trachea must be included in the differential diagnosis when there has been a history of reflex apnea.

FINDINGS

Radiographic. Diagnostic radiography performed on our patients included chest x-ray, esophagogram, and in some cases arteriography. Their studies were reviewed for the most part with the radiologist prior to tracheoscopic evaluation.

Lateral chest x-ray has revealed an indentation of the anterior tracheal wall midway between the thoracic inlet and the carina in 34% of our patients. The remainder of the x-rays revealed no such abnormality, even though they had endoscopically proven tracheal compression. Thirty-four percent of the esophagograms studied were found to be abnormal, but none of this group revealed a specific diagnosis of innominate artery compression. Arteriography was performed on eight patients showing an innominate arterial takeoff arising more distally along the aortic arch than normal. However, arterial compression of the trachea by this anomalous artery cannot be demonstrated by arteriography alone (Table 2).

Endoscopic. Definitive diagnosis of tracheal compression by an anomalous innominate artery can only be made by tracheoscopy. The procedure involves exposure of the endolarynx with a side-slide laryngoscope, and then evaluation of the trachea with a Storz-Hopkins telescope to ensure excellent visualization is carried out. This technique allows diagnostic accuracy without the trauma sometimes encountered by conventional tracheoscopy.

The tracheoscopic appearance is illustrated in Figures 3 and 4. There is a pulsatile compression of the anterior tracheal wall extending from left to right. This compressed segment pulsates synchronously with each cardiac systole and is located 1 to 2 cm above the carina. The right temporal and radial pulses can be diminished or obliterated by bringing the tip of the tracheoscope against the pulsatile compression. The actual percentage of endoscopic compression is recorded in Figure 5.

Also recorded are the corresponding percentages of compression in the operative cases, showing absolutely no relationship between the degree of tracheal compression and clinical need for surgical correction, as suggested by previous authors.[9]

MANAGEMENT

In the absence of reflex apnea, our management consists of conservative medical therapy, including humidified oxygen, and appropriate antibiotics when necessary for the treatment of associated pneumonia or tracheobronchitis. In those patients with reflex apnea, an evaluation by the cardiotho-

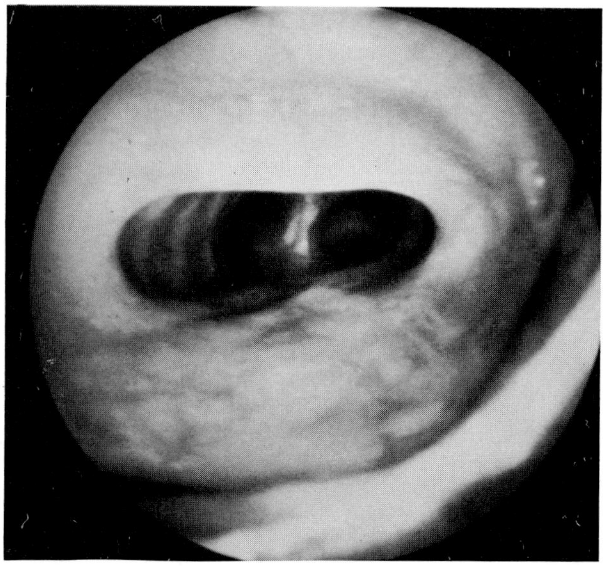

Fig. 3. Tracheoscopic photo of AIA. (Close up - Carina visible.)

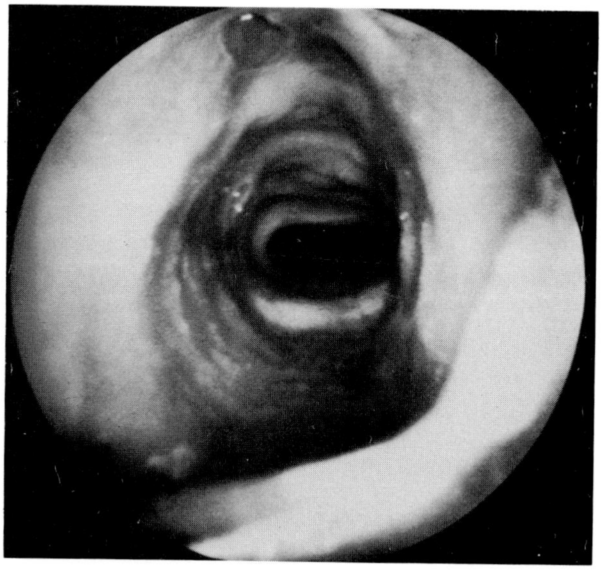

Fig. 4. Tracheoscopic photo of AIA. (Tracheal contour seen through the true cords-inspiration.)

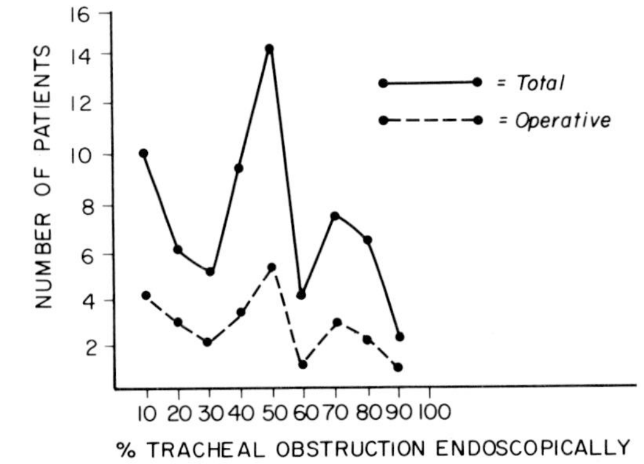

Fig. 5. Percentage of endoscopic compression in operative cases as compared to the total number of cases.

racic surgical service for possible innominate artery suspension or innominate arteriopexy is performed. Reflex apnea remains the one absolute indication for surgery. Recurrent pneumonia in patients with documented AIA, and patients with tracheal obstruction due to AIA, resulting in chronic respiratoy distress on the basis of obstruction, are relative indications for surgery. The effect of the suspension procedure on the tracheal airway is illustrated in Figure 6. Note the familiar anterior tracheal wall compression on the left. Following the suspension procedure, the airway usually opens up significantly as depicted on the right.

DISCUSSION

In 1969 Berdon et al[5] and Ericsson and Soderlund[6] brought forth the concept that the plain lateral chest film shall act as a primary diagnostic tool with reports of positive findings in 70-100%. Ericsson and Soderlund concluded that radiologic evidence of an anterior tracheal wall compression is an adequate tool in making the diagnosis of AIA. Only 34% of our patients had this finding on lateral chest x-ray. A similar percent of esophagograms revealed signs of arterial compression, while 100% of the arteriograms done in this study revealed the anatomic defect. We are able to conclude that chest x-ray may only raise suspicion of the existence of AIA, but is in no way diagnostic of the problem.

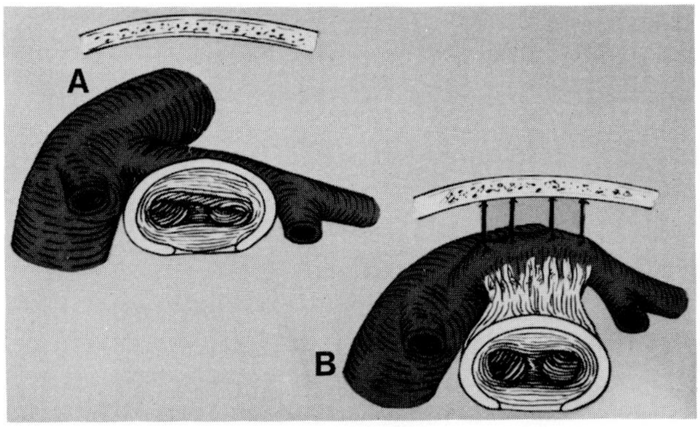

Fig. 6. A) Preoperative and B) postoperative view of trachea.

TABLE 3. OPERATIVE RESULTS

	No. of Cases	Percent
Operative cases	33	—
Operative cases with apnea	28	85
Operative cases with resolution of apnea	22/28	79
Operative cases with resolution of obstructive symptoms	28/33	85
Operative cases with recurrent symptoms	5	15

Esophagograms may also be of some help, but mainly as a method to rule out the presence of other cardiovascular anomalies. Arteriography remains an absolute method of diagnosis, but offers no information about the effects on the trachea.

One hundred percent of our patients were demonstrated to have AIA by tracheoscopy. It should be reemphasized that the diagnosis of this anomaly is readily made by tracheoscopy. However we found that, unlike the opinion of some previous investigators, there is absolutely no relationship between the percentage of tracheal obstruction noted at the time of tracheoscopy and the severity of symptoms. Therefore we conclude that the decision for surgery should not be based on endoscopically proven tracheal compression alone. All the patients with reflex apnea (28 cases) underwent arteriopexy; five others were operated for secondary indications, thus a total of 33 cases were operated (42% of the entire group of 78).

The patients who met the operative criteria and underwent innominate arteriopexy had significant improvement as seen in Table 3. We feel that the five surgical failures (Table 4) are creditable in lieu of their associated upper respiratory problems. The fifth case presented with no known problems other than AIA was felt to have had a technical breakdown of his suspensory repair as seen on repeat tracheoscopy.

It is interesting that such a large percentage of patients with reflex apnea postoperatively resolve this symptom. Unfortunately this alone does not lend any information as to the chemical or electrical nature of this reflex, but most certainly lends support to the efficacy of this surgical procedure.

The potential danger of AIA remains debatable. In 1969 Mustard et al[7] stated "in the case of reflex apnea, death can be sudden and unexpected. Many of our patients with reflex apnea have required mouth to mouth resuscitation by their parents during such an episode." This comment raises the real

TABLE 4. OPERATIVE FAILURES

1. AIA + Acquired subglottic stenosis
2. AIA + Acquired subglottic stenosis
3. AIA + T.E.F + S/P Nisson
4. AIA + S/P Nisson
5. AIA alone

concern that children with reflex apnea are in potential jeopardy. Since almost one third of our series of patients had reflex apnea, we feel that any further skepticism is not only naive, but displays a serious danger to this relatively large group of patients.

It is our practice at the hospital to refer all patients with AIA and associated reflex apnea to the division of cardiothoracic surgery for evaluation for possible innominate arteriopexy. We do not allow the child to be discharged prior to being seen by our cardiothoracic colleagues. Surgery, when indicated, is usually performed during the same hospital admission.

Some previous investigators advocate the endoscopist to be present at the time of arteriopexy, not only to assist, but also to insure accurate repair. We feel this is probably a worthwhile undertaking and should be considered by all.

REFERENCES

1. Gross RE, Neuhauser EBD. Compression of the trachea by an anomalous innomate artery. Am J Dis Child 1948; 75:570-4.

2. Gross RE. Arterial malformations which cause compression of trachea or esophagus. Circulation 1955; 11:124-34.

3. Ferguson CF, Flake CG. Tracheographic and bronchographic studies as aids in the diagnosis of congenital malformations of the tracheobronchial tree and aortic arch in infants and children. Ann Otol Rhinol Laryngol 1954; 63:1056-81.

4. Fearon B, Shortree R. Tracheobronchial compression by congenital cardiovascular anomalies in children: syndrome of apnea. Ann Otol Rhinol Laryngol 1963; 72:949-69.

5. Berdon WE, Baker DH, Bordiuk J, Mellins R. Innominate artery compression of the trachea in infants with stridor and apnea. Radiology 1969; 92:272-8.

6. Ericsson NO, Soderlund S. Compression of the trachea by an anomalous innominate artery. J Pediatr Surg 1969; 4:424-31.

7. Mustard WT, Bayliss CE, Fearon B, Pelton D, Trusler GA. Tracheal compression by an innominate artery in children. Ann Thorac Surg 1969; 8:312-9.

8. Macdonald RE, Fearon B. Innominate artery compression syndrome in children Ann Otol Rhinol Laryngol 1971; 80:535-40.

9. Möes CAF, Toruo I, Trusler GA. Innominate artery compression of the trachea. Arch Otolaryngol 1975; 101:733-8.

≈

CANADIAN OTOLARYNGOLOGICAL SOCIETY

The annual meeting of the Canadian Otolaryngological Society will be held in London, Ontario, June 15-17, 1981. Inquiries may be sent to Dr. William Crysdale, c/o Hospital for Sick Children, 555 University Avenue, Toronto, Ontario.

Ann Otol 89:1980

CONGENITAL TRACHEAL DIVERTICULUM

A CASE REPORT

SAUL FRENKIEL, MD, FRCS(C)

IRENE K. ASSIMES, MD

JOSE K. ROSALES, MD, FRCP(C)

MONTREAL, CANADA

A six-month-old female with a history of recurrent bronchopulmonary infections was admitted to the Montreal Children's Hospital in severe respiratory distress. Cardiac arrest ensued and although ventilation by mask was always possible during the resuscitation procedure, there was a confusing inability to aerate the lungs after successful intubation. A right-sided tracheal diverticulum was identified at autopsy. It was assumed, in retrospect, that the intubating tube entered and abutted against the wall of the diverticulum, thus obstructing its distal lumen. The embryology, morphology and pathophysiology of congenital tracheal diverticuli are discussed. This rare diagnosis should be entertained when successful intubation leads to ineffectual ventilation.

INTRODUCTION

Tracheal diverticuli are relatively rare entities characterized by single or multiple evaginations of the tracheal wall. They usually present in adulthood as the acquired form associated with chronic bronchopulmonary disease. Presenting features include prolonged productive cough, hemoptysis and chest pain. Either bronchography or bronchoscopy can confirm the diagnosis.

The autopsy incidence quoted by MacKinnon is approximately 1%.[1] He discovered eight cases in 867 routine serial necropsies. The diverticuli usually occurred on the right side with the tracheal mucosa protruding through an area of weakness laterally between the cartilaginous rings or posterolaterally through the trachealis muscle. The lining wall consisted of stratified columnar ciliated epithelium with underlying chronic inflammatory reaction and occasional mucous glands communicating with the tracheal lumen via one or more narrow ducts. The walls were characteristically devoid of smooth muscle and cartilage.

The congenital tracheal diverticulum is a completely different entity from the acquired form. Its developmental origin is controversial and difficult to prove. It probably represents vestigial supernumerary lungs[2] or aborted abnormally high divisions of the primary lung bud.[3] When associated with surrounding lung tissue, these evaginations are termed "accessory tracheal bronchi."

The congenital tracheal diverticulum usually occurs in males and emanates from the right side pointing obliquely downward. Their composition is similar to the actual tracheal wall containing both smooth muscle and cartilage.[4] The diverticuli may occur in isolation or in association with other congenital anomalies within the tracheobronchial tree.[5]

Few reports of congenital tracheal diverticuli have appeared in the literature. A recent case, diagnosed at autopsy, is presented to highlight the confusing inability to ventilate the infant while intubated during a cardiopulmonary resuscitation.

CASE REPORT

A six-month-old white female, with normal birth and family history, was first admitted to the Montreal Children's Hospital on August 29, 1978, in moderate respiratory distress. Chest x-ray and barium swallow did not reveal evidence of pneumonia, foreign body or tracheoesophageal fistula. Sweat test and viral cultures were negative. A working diagnosis of bronchiolitis was conferred, although the possibility of laryngotracheomalacia was also considered. Clinically, she improved with conservative treatment consisting of oxygen, humidification, and physiotherapy, and was discharged in satisfactory condition two weeks later.

She returned to hospital on October 8, 1978, with an obvious upper respiratory tract infection and fever of 38.9 C (102 F). On the day of her admission, she became cyanotic momentarily after an episode of vomiting. Physical examination revealed mild inspiratory and expiratory stridor but good air entry in both lung fields. Chest x-ray was within normal limits. She again responded to supportive treatment. No antibiotics were given and she was discharged within 48 hours in satisfactory condition.

One month later, she was admitted for the third time with a mild upper respiratory tract infection and stridor. Her condition improved with humidity and oxygen, and she was discharged two days later. Chest x-ray, bacteriology and virology were negative. The working diagnosis was still bronchiolitis.

From the Departments of Otolaryngology and Anaesthesia, Montreal Children's Hospital, McGill University, Montreal, Canada.

Presented at the meeting of the American Broncho-Esophagological Association, Palm Beach, Florida, April 12-13, 1980.

REPRINTS — S. Frenkiel, MD, Department of Otolaryngology, Montreal Children's Hospital, 2300 Tupper Street, Montreal, Canada H3H 1P3.

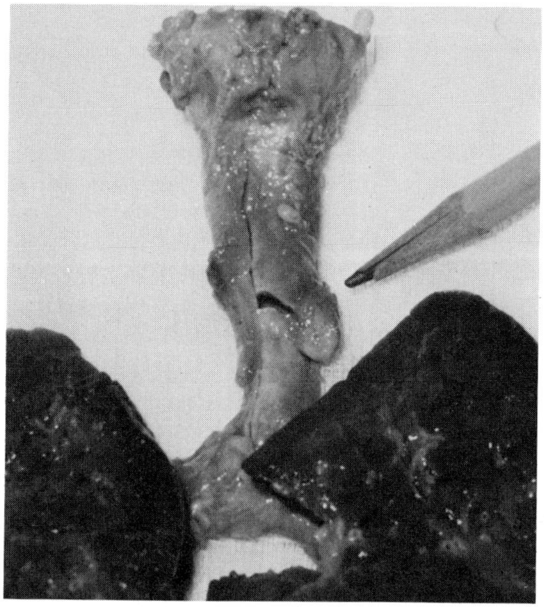

Fig. 1. Posterior view of tracheobronchial specimen indicating the congenital tracheal diverticulum projecting obliquely downward from the right posterolateral wall.

She returned to hospital for the last time on December 12, 1978. One day prior to admission, there was evidence of dyspnea and irritability. She had no fever, feeding difficulty or vomiting. There was no wheezing, cyanosis, or expectoration. Respiratory rate was 54/minute with evidence of intercostal and sternal indrawing. Coarse expiratory rhonchi were heard but air entry was adequate bilaterally.

The infant became more irritable and dyspneic over the next 24 hours. Chest x-ray now showed a rightward mediastinal shift on the basis of an atelectatic right lung. Cardiorespiratory arrest ensued and although successfully intubated alternately with an orotracheal tube and rigid bronchoscope, it was not possible to ventilate the patient. Fulminant bleeding from both lung fields was noted during the bronchoscopy. Ironically, ventilation by mask was extremely adequate during the resuscitative attempts. The child died after the third cardiac arrest when all resuscitative measures failed.

The autopsy indicated an acute bronchopneumonia with superimposed hemorrhage and marked pulmonary edema, presumed to be of viral etiology. A tracheal diverticulum measuring 1 cm in length was found on the right posterolateral wall approximately 2 cm above the carina (Figs. 1 and 2). The surface epithelium showed focal squamous metaplasia and ulceration, with mucus gland hyperplasia and chronic inflammatory infiltrate in the submucosa. The wall of the diverticulum contained smooth muscle and cartilage. Distal to the diverticulum, a stenosis was noted compromising the tracheal lumen to a diameter of 3 mm. No other congenital abnormalities were evident.

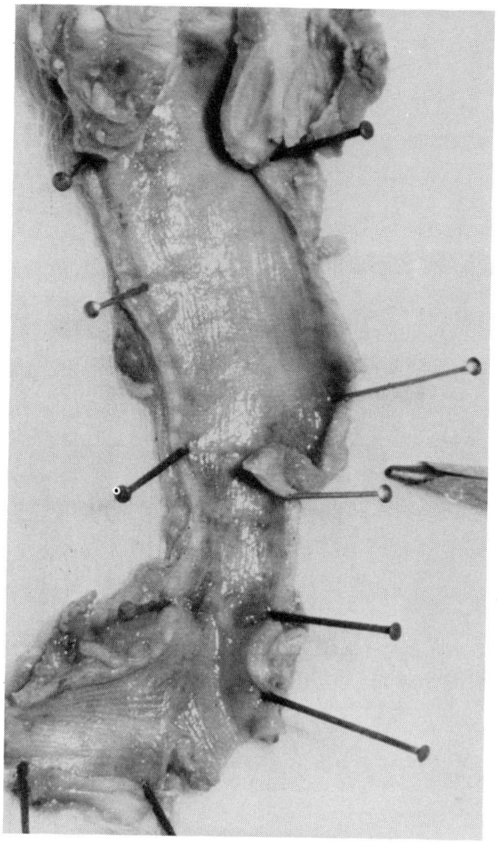

Fig. 2. Posterior view of sectioned tracheal lumen revealing the diverticular evagination with distal stenosis.

DISCUSSION

The classification of congenital malformations of the trachea, bronchi and lung was outlined by Holinger et al in 1952.[6] Recurrent respiratory tract symptomatology in any infant should signal the possibility of a tracheobronchial tree malformation. The preceding case illustrates several important concepts for the pediatric diagnostician and the practicing endoscopist.

The ultimate cause of death in this child was a fulminant bronchopneumonia leading to cardiopulmonary arrest. It is likely that mucus secretions collected within the confines of the tracheal diverticulum, became infected, and periodically spilled over into the lower respiratory tract. Alternatively, stasis of secretions within the diverticulum coagulated into a mucus plug which then proceeded to obstruct the lower airway. Either hypothesis could explain the recurrent episodes of respiratory distress necessitating hospitalization and eventually resulting in the demise of the infant. The stenosis distal to the evagination was a contributing factor.

During the attempted resuscitative procedure, it was possible to adequately ventilate the child at all times by mask. Although per oral intubation was successful, first with a 3.5 mm Portex® endotracheal tube and subsequently with a rigid 3.5 mm bronchoscope, it was not possible to provide ventilation by this route. Retrospectively, it was assumed that the intubation tube distally abutted against the wall of the diverticulum, thus making ventilation ineffectual. Since no difficulty was encountered when the infant was ventilated by mask and because of the immediate urgency of the situation, gradual withdrawal of the artificial airway was not attempted.

CONCLUSIONS

Congenital tracheal diverticuli are rare but potentially fatal lesions. They usually arise from the right lateral trachea and, unlike the acquired variety, contain cartilage within their wall.

A history of repeated respiratory tract infections in infants should signal the possibility of tracheobronchial tree malformation. Contrast bronchography or bronchoscopy is necessary to establish this diagnosis. A tracheal diverticulum should be considered when successful intubation leads to inadequate ventilation.

REFERENCES

1. MacKinnon D. Tracheal diverticula. J Pathol Bacteriol 1953; 65:513-7.

2. Boyden EA. Developmental anomalies of the lungs. Am J Surg 1955; 80:79-89.

3. Peytz F. Congenital tracheal diverticulum. Acta Otolaryngol (Stockh) 1964; 58:81-6.

4. Warkany J. Congenital malformations. Year Book Medical Publishers. 1971; 599-604.

5. Landing BH, Wells TR. Tracheobronchial anomalies in children. Perspect Pediatr Pathol 1973; 1:1-32.

6. Holinger PH, Johnston KC, Parchet VN, Zimmerman AA. Congenital malformations of the trachea, bronchi and lung. Ann Otol Rhinol Laryngol 1952; 61:1159-80.

≈

REPORT OF THE PANEL ON COMMUNICATIVE DISORDERS

Ann Otol 89:1980

INTERNAL LARYNGOCELE AND SACCULAR CYSTS IN CHILDREN

J. OLIVER DONEGAN, MD
JANET L. STRIFE, MD
ROBIN T. COTTON, MD
ALLAN B. SEID, MD
J. SCOTT DUNBAR, MD

CINCINNATI, OHIO

Two children, one with an internal laryngocele and the other with a lateral saccular cyst are described. The anatomy, classification, and history of these unusual lesions are described. The diagnosis and management are discussed. An external approach is suggested for the more persistent cases.

INTRODUCTION

The most common causes of laryngeal stridor in infants and children are laryngotracheal bronchitis and laryngomalacia. Other causes include vascular rings, vocal cord paralysis, foreign bodies, acute epiglottitis and laryngeal webs. To this list may be added congenital laryngeal cysts and laryngoceles, both of which are rare causes of respiratory tract obstruction in children, but when they occur they may present difficulties in diagnosis and management and can be life-threatening.[1] In a review of 200 unselected cases of laryngeal stridor in children Birch had four cases of laryngeal cysts.[2] In Holinger's 30 years experience with laryngeal anomalies he saw 20 cases of congenital cysts and laryngoceles.[3]

ANATOMY

Galen first mentioned the laryngeal ventricle in 300 AD.[4] In 1741 Morgagni described the ventricle in detail,[5] but it was left to Hilton in 1837 to complete the outline of the anatomy of the laryngeal saccule.[6] The saccule arises vertically off the anterior end of the ventricle. This pouch then passes superiorly between the false vocal cord, the base of the epiglottis and the inner surface of the thyroid cartilage.[7] Normally the adult saccule can extend as high as the superior border of the thyroid cartilage.[8] In the fetus approximately 25% of these appendages extend beyond the upper border of the thyroid cartilage and terminate medial to the thyohyoid membrane. The structure is lined by pseudostratified ciliated columnar epithelium and on the surface of its mucous membrane are the openings of 60 to 70 mucous glands.[9] Medial and lateral to the saccule are delicate muscles which compress it to express its secretions upon the vocal cords.[9]

HISTORY OF LARYNGOCELES AND CONGENITAL LARYNGEAL CYSTS

In 1829 Larrey, a surgeon in Napoleon's army, was the first to describe air-containing tumors in the neck.[10] While in Egypt he noted that these lesions were very common among the blind who were employed to chant verses from the Koran from the tops of the minarets every hour of the day and night. Larrey also observed similar air sacs in army drill instructors. Unaware of Larrey's description, Virchow introduced the term "laryngocele" in 1867 to describe an air-filled dilatation of the saccule.[11] Abercrombie introduced the term congenital cyst in 1881 while describing a laryngeal cyst in a newborn.[12]

CLASSIFICATION

DeSanto has clarified the terminology of laryngeal cysts.[13,14] The term saccular cyst has replaced the older term congenital laryngeal cyst. Both the laryngocele and the saccular cyst arise from the saccular appendage. They differ in that the laryngocele communicates freely with the laryngeal lumen and is filled with air, while the saccular cyst has no communication with the laryngeal lumen and is fluid filled. There are two types of saccular cysts. The lateral saccular cyst extends posterosuperiorly into the false vocal cord and aryepiglottic fold from its origin at the nonpatent orifice of the saccule. The anterior saccular cyst extends medially and posteriorly to protrude into the laryngeal lumen from between the true and false vocal cords. Three types of laryngoceles are described. An internal laryngocele is confined to the interior of the larynx and extends posterosuperiorly into the false vocal cord and aryepiglottic fold. An external laryngocele extends superiorly to present laterally in the neck through the opening in the thyrohyoid membrane for the superior laryngeal nerve and vessels. When

From the Department of Otolaryngology and Maxillofacial Surgery, and the Department of Pediatrics, University of Cincinnati Medical Center, Cincinnati, Ohio.

Presented at the meeting of the American Broncho-Esophagological Association, Palm Beach, Florida, April 12-13, 1980.

REPRINTS — J. Oliver Donegan, MD, Department of Otolaryngology and Maxillofacial Surgery, University of Cincinnati Medical Center, 231 Bethesda Ave., Cincinnati, OH 45267.

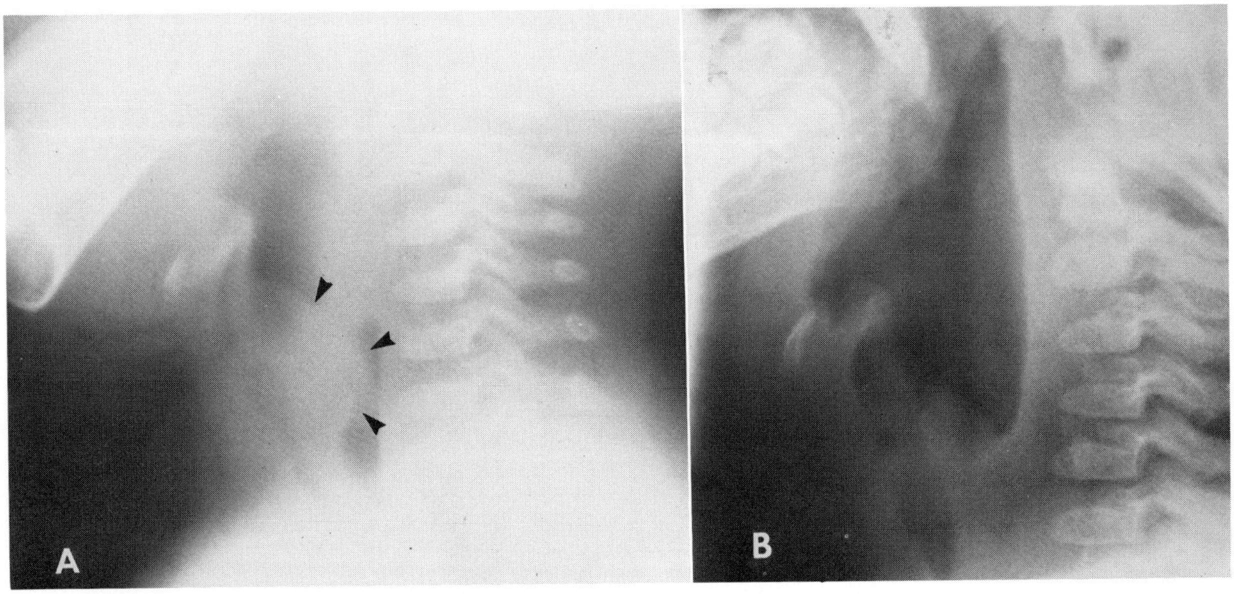

Fig. 1. (Case 1) A) The initial lateral soft tissue film of the neck demonstrates a large supraglottic mass which distorts the pyriform sinus. B) This lateral film was taken 24 hours later and no mass is seen.

the features of both exist simultaneously it is termed a combined laryngocele.

The purpose of this paper is to present two children, one with an internal laryngocele and another with a lateral saccular cyst to highlight the mode of presentation, the diagnostic dilemmas and the management of these unusual lesions.

CASE REPORTS

Case 1. A 12-month-old white female was admitted to Children's Hospital Medical Center on March 17, 1979 on transfer from an outlying hospital. The patient had developed stridor and increasing respiratory difficulty on the day of admission. The mother gave a history of noisy breathing and a hoarse cry which had been intermittent since birth, but these symptoms had gradually increased in severity and frequency. The patient had been admitted to another hospital in August 1978 for wheezing, but no definite diagnosis was made at that time. Physical examination revealed an obese white female infant in moderate respiratory distress with a loud cough. Laboratory data were within normal limits. High kV AP and lateral films of the neck revealed a right supraglottic mass (Fig. 1A). The was seen to vary remarkably in size, at times almost to disappear (Fig. 1B). It was noted to displace the trachea and the larynx anteriorly and to the left. Cine studies of the neck done on admission revealed the mass to be inflatable with crying or straining, and a diagnosis of a laryngocele was made.

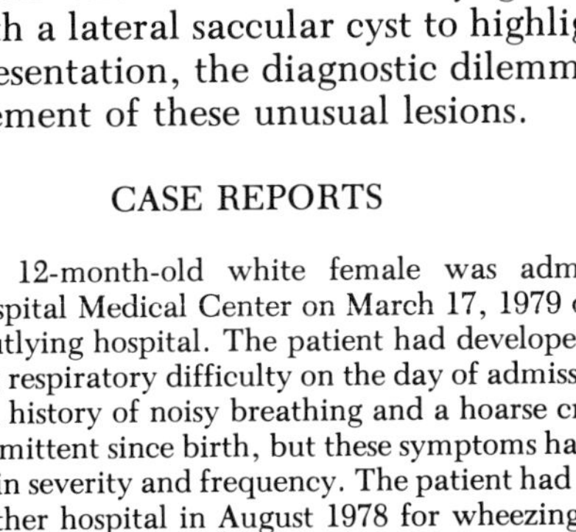

Fig. 2. (Case 1) Right internal laryngocele seen only as a slight fullness of the right false cord and right aryepiglottic fold.

On the afternoon of admission the patient was taken to the operating room and a direct laryngoscopy was performed under general anesthesia. The larynx, hypopharynx, and trachea were noted to be within normal limits. No abnormality was noted on this examination. The patient was observed in the Intensive Care Unit following this examination and it was noted that she did well while sedated, but when agitated and crying the stridor markedly increased. Endoscopy was repeated on March 22, 1979 and again the examination was entirely within normal limits. A laryngogram under general anesthesia was done on March 29, 1979. At that time Dionosil® and air were used as contrast media. During this examination a mass was seen on the right side of the supraglottic larynx, but this was noted to be present only when the patient was breathing and not when apneic. A slight fullness of the right aryepiglottic fold was noted on direct laryngoscopy (Fig. 2). Because of our inability to demonstrate the lesion conclusively on direct laryngoscopy, an external approach was decided upon to excise this mass. Accordingly on April 3, 1979 the patient was returned to the operating room and a tracheostomy was performed. A microlaryngoscopy was then performed and on this examination mucosa was noted to be bulging from the right ventricle. An external approach via a horizontal incision at the level of the thyroid notch was used. The upper half of the right thyroid ala was reflected exposing the paraglottic space (Fig. 3). The sac of the internal laryngocele was identified in this space and was excised without difficulty (Fig. 4). Following surgery the pa-

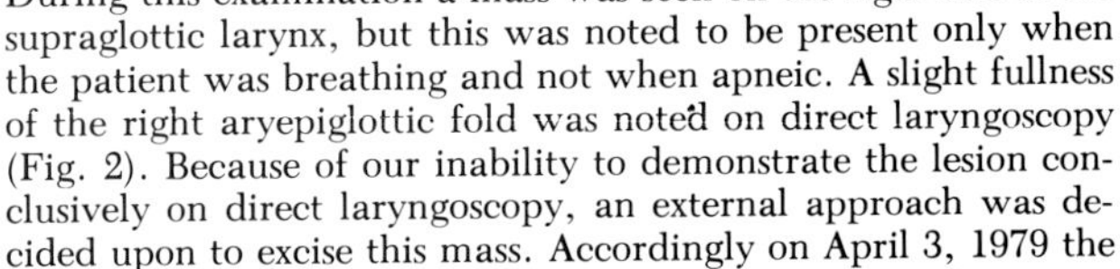

Fig. 3. (Case 1) Incision used to reflect the upper half of the right thyroid ala to expose the paraglottic space.

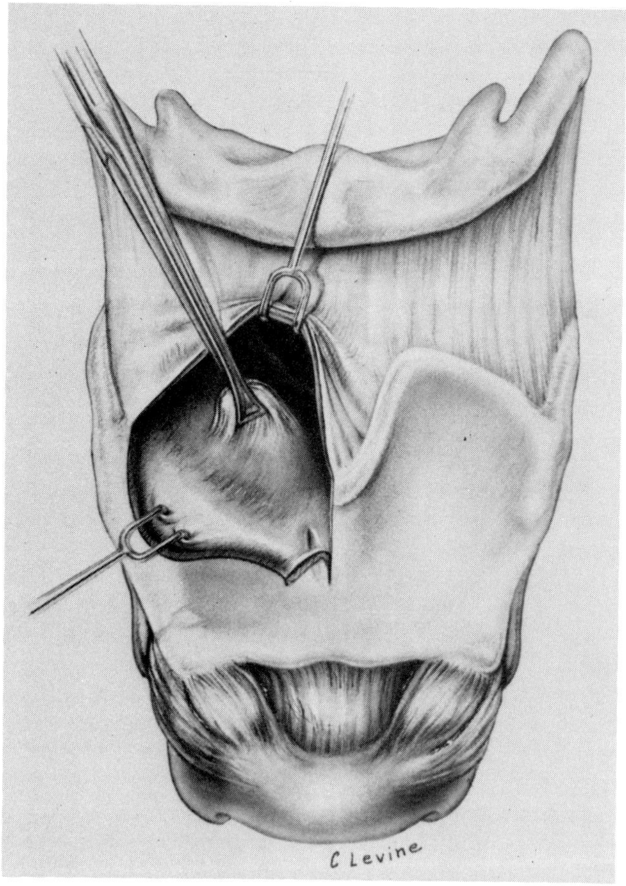

Fig. 4. (Case 1) Right paraglottic space exposed and sac of internal laryngocele identified.

tient did well until the second postoperative day when the tracheostomy tube became dislodged, and as the airway of the infant was obviously adequate the tracheostomy was not replaced. The patient did well following this and has had no further symptoms of respiratory distress.

Case 2. The patient was a white female born on September 1, 1978. At birth the infant had a hoarse cry and gasping respirations and was noted to be dusky. Also, deep suprasternal retractions were noted. A laryngoscopy at this time revealed a $2\frac{1}{2}$ cm mass in the left side of the larynx. An orotracheal tube was passed and the patient was transferred to Children's Hospital Medical Center on the day of birth. On admission a chest x-ray was within normal limits with the endotracheal tube in good position. High kV films of the neck revealed a soft tissue density in the left supraglottic larynx. The mass tended to bow the trachea in an anterior direction. Admission laboratory studies were within normal limits. On September 2, 1978 a microlaryngoscopy was performed under general anesthesia and a large cyst was noted in the left aryepiglottic fold, the left side of the epiglottis and the left pyriform sinus. It was bluish in color and obviously filled with fluid (Fig. 5). A No. 19 spinal needle was used to aspirate the cyst which contained 4-5 cc of a thick mucoid fluid. Following aspiration of this fluid the cyst collapsed. The remainder of the pharynx, endolarynx and the respiratory tract were within normal limits. On September 5, 1978 microlaryngoscopy was repeated and the cyst was again aspirated as the fluid had reaccumulated. On September 6, 1978 microlaryngoscopy was again performed and again the cyst had accumulated more fluid. On this occasion the CO_2 laser was used to uncap the cyst and to drain and marsupialize it. On September 9, 1978 microlaryngoscopy was again repeated and again the cyst had filled with fluid. On this occasion a tracheostomy was performed. Follow-up films of the neck revealed persistence of the large supraglottic mass (Fig. 6). Between September 14, 1978 and October 25, 1978 four further laryngoscopies were performed with aspiration, uncapping, and removal of the cyst wall attempted on each occasion. The examination was repeated on November 9, 1978 and on this occasion no reaccumulation was noted. The patient was discharged shortly afterwards and was readmitted in mid-December 1978 and the larynx was examined and noted to be within normal limits apart from slight thickening of the left aryepiglottic fold. On this admission the patient was successfully decannulated. The larynx was again examined on June 7, 1979 and October 22, 1979 and on both of these occasions it was noted to be within normal limits and the patient had no further evidence of respiratory obstruction.

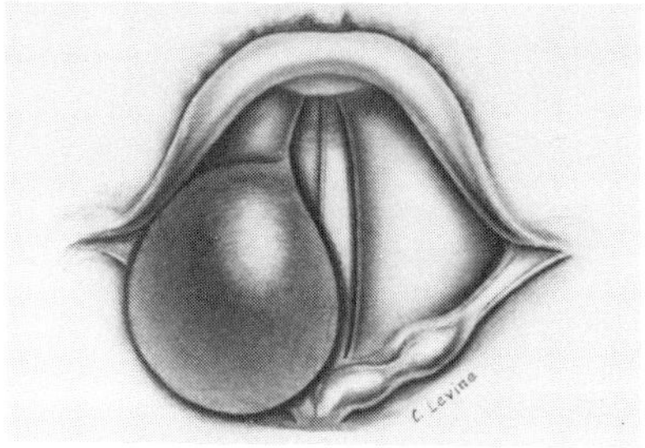

Fig. 5. (Case 2) Left lateral saccular cyst.

DISCUSSION

Internal laryngoceles and lateral saccular cysts may present similar clinical pictures.[1,15-18] They may be present at birth or present at any age. Symptoms may vary, the commonest being respiratory distress, usually with inspiratory stridor.[15,17] There may be a muffled or inaudible cry. Dysphagia may be evident. The symptoms of a saccular cyst are usually persistent while those of an internal laryngocele may be intermittent due to its communication with the laryngeal lumen. A tracheostomy is necessary in most cases.[17,19,20]

The diagnosis of these lesions is based on radiological evaluation and direct laryngoscopy.[18,21] High kV inspiratory and expiratory films in both AP and lateral views will usually demonstrate the ab-

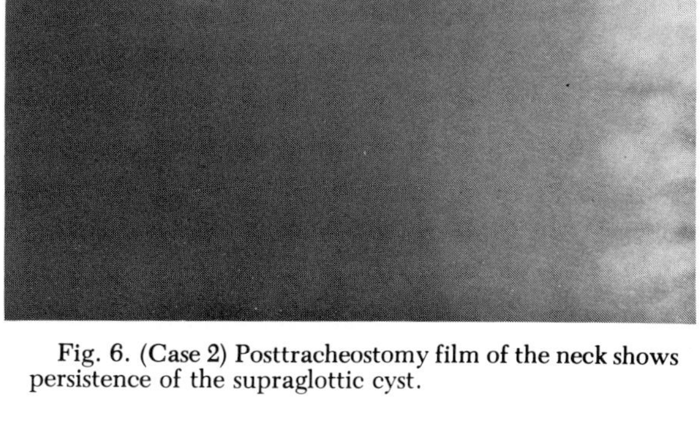

Fig. 6. (Case 2) Posttracheostomy film of the neck shows persistence of the supraglottic cyst.

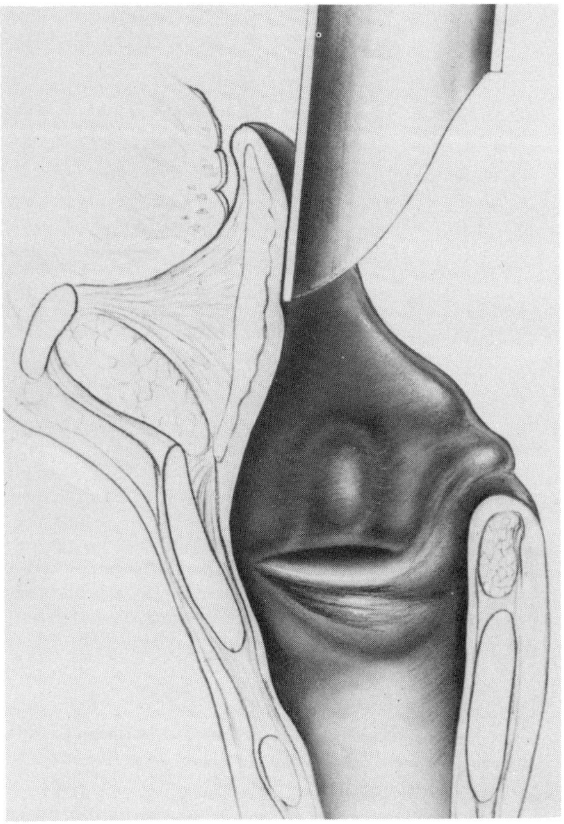

Fig. 7. (Case 1) Laryngoscope in position showing stretching of the right aryepiglottic fold and decompression of the right internal laryngocele.

normality. However, as an internal laryngocele may inflate and deflate several times in a short period, several films may be needed to show the characteristic swelling in the supraglottic area. Both appear as a rounded soft tissue mass involving the false cord, the aryepiglottic fold, the pyriform sinus, the glottis and hypopharynx.[22] Direct laryngoscopy will confirm the diagnosis in most cases but may be inconclusive as pointed out in case 1. These lesions appear as mucosally covered rounded masses expanding the false cord and the aryepiglottic fold, and encroaching on the laryngeal lumen to a significant extent. They may obliterate the pyriform sinus and extend into the hypopharynx. In case 1 we were not able to demonstrate conclusively the laryngocele at direct laryngoscopy which was repeated on three occasions. Presumably this was due to the fact that the air-filled sac collapsed on induction of anesthesia and muscular relaxation, or to the position of the laryngoscope (Fig. 7). Attempts at inflating the lesion with air during one of these examinations were unsuccessful. The diagnosis in this case was made on the history of intermittent airway obstruction and the radiological findings as described.

The treatment of these conditions may be quite troublesome. The saccular cysts can usually be managed by direct laryngoscopy and aspiration.[23] However, the cysts tend to recur again and again, and multiple aspirations may be needed supplemented by unroofing of the cyst with a forceps and attempts to remove all or part of its lining.[24] In Holinger's series a mean of 7.5 laryngoscopies was performed on each infant with one child requiring 14 separate procedures.[20] In our case 2 the child underwent 11 separate procedures before resolution of the problem and successful decannulation. Perhaps in these more persistent cases an external approach and excision of the cyst would be justified.

The treatment of an internal laryngocele may be equally troublesome and frustrating. In Holinger's series two children had laryngoceles, both of which resolved after diagnostic laryngoscopy and no further treatment was tried.[20] There is little in the literature regarding the management of these lesions in infants and children. It is not unreasonable to try a similar approach as that for saccular cysts.[19] Again it is likely that multiple aspirations and attempts at unroofing will be needed. An external approach may also be used to excise the sac. This appeared a more rational approach in our case due to our inability to demonstrate the lesion endoscopically. The external approach allows an extramucosal approach to the enlarged saccules, good exposure and ease of excision with minimal morbidity. Several such approaches are described in the literature.[17,25-28]

REFERENCES

1. Suehs OW, Powell DB. Congenital cyst of the larynx in infants. Laryngoscope 1967; 77:654-61.

2. Birch DA. Laryngeal stridor in infants and children. J Laryngol Otol 1961; 75:833-40.

3. Holinger PH, Brown WT. Congenital webs, cysts, laryngoceles and other anomalies of the larynx. Ann Otol Rhinol Laryngol 1967; 76:744-52.

4. May MT. Galen on the usefulness of the parts of the body. Ithaca: Cornell University Press; 1968:335-84.

5. Canalis RF. Laryngeal ventricle: historical features. Ann Otol Rhinol Laryngol 1980; 89:184-7.

6. Hilton J. Description of the saccules or pouch in the human larynx. Guy's Hosp Rep 1937; 2:519-25.

7. Hast MH. The developmental anatomy of the larynx. Otolaryngol Clin North Am 1970; 3:413-38.

8. Broyles EN. Anatomical observations concerning the laryngeal appendix. Ann Otol Rhinol Laryngol 1959; 68:461-70.

9. Delahunty JE, Cherry J. The laryngeal saccule. J Laryngol Otol 1969; 83:803-14.

10. Larrey DJ. Exercice particularierement dans les camps et les hospitaux militaires depuis 1792 jusqu'en 1892 Paris, Clinique Chircugicale. Paris: Chez Gabon 1829:81-90.

11. Virchow R. Die Krankhafter Geschwulste. Berlin: A Hirschwald, 1867:35-40.

12. Abercrombie J. Congenital cyst in the larynx. Trans Pathol Soc Lond 1881; 32:33-4.

13. DeSanto LW, Devine KD, Weiland LH. Cysts of the larynx — classification. Laryngoscope 1970; 80:145-76.

14. DeSanto LW. Laryngocele, laryngeal mucocele, large saccules and laryngeal saccular cysts: a developmental spectrum. Laryngoscope 1974; 84:1291-6.

15. Cody CC. Laryngocele: diagnosis and management with case report. Eye Ear Nose Throat Mon 1965; 44:68-72.

16. DeRosario JL. Ventricular laryngocele. Int Surg 1966; 46:321-6.

17. English GM, DeBlanc GB. Laryngocele: a case presenting with acute airway obstruction. Laryngoscope 1968; 78:386-95.

18. Holinger PH. Clinical aspects of congenital anomalies of the larynx, trachea, bronchi and esophagus. J Laryngol Otol 1961; 75:1-15.

19. Ferguson GB. Laryngocele. Laryngoscope 1967; 77: 1368-75.

20. Holinger LD, Barnes DR, Smid LJ. Laryngocele and saccular cysts. Ann Otol Rhinol Laryngol 1978; 87:675-85.

21. Holinger PH, Schild JA, Weprin L. Pediatric laryngology. Otolaryngol Clin North Am 1970; 3:625-37.

22. Giovaniello J, Grieco RV, Bartone NF. Laryngocele. Am J Roentgenol Radium Ther Nucl Med 1970; 108:825-9.

23. Shackelford GD, McAllister WH. Congenital laryngeal cyst. Am J Roentgenol Radium Ther Nucl Med 1972; 114:289-92.

24. Van DeWater FW. Laryngeal cysts — their surgical management. Laryngoscope 1973; 83:1185-91.

25. Putney FJ. Laryngocele. Trans Pac Coast Oto-Ophthalmol Soc 1968; 49:749-55.

26. Walpita PR. Laryngocele in an infant. J Pediatr Surg 1975; 10:843-4.

27. Yarington CT, Frazer JP. An approach to the internal laryngocele and other submucosal lesions of the larynx. Ann Otol Rhinol Laryngol 1966; 75:956-60.

28. Montgomery WW. Surgery of the larynx. In: Montgomery WW, ed. Surgery of the upper respiratory system. Philadelphia: Lea and Febiger, 1973:445-514.

≈

ASSOCIATION FOR RESEARCH IN OTOLARYNGOLOGY

The 4th Mid Winter Research Meeting of the Association for Research in Otolaryngology will be held at the Happy Dolphin Inn, St. Petersburg Beach, Florida, January 19-21, 1981. In addition to the contributed paper sessions, a colloquium honoring Dr. Catherine A. Smith will be held entitled "Some Unresolved Problems in the Auditory System."

Ann Otol 89:1980

PEDIATRIC FLEXIBLE BRONCHOSCOPY

ROBERT E. WOOD, PhD, MD JAMES M. SHERMAN, MD

CLEVELAND, OHIO

We have utilized a prototype pediatric flexible bronchoscope to perform diagnostic and therapeutic procedures on pediatric patients ranging from 840 gm to 14 years of age. Flexible bronchoscopy, with appropriate instrumentation and careful attention to physiological requirements of the patient, is safe and effective in pediatric patients. The availability of new instrumentation promises to have as great an impact on pediatric pulmonology as the standard flexible bronchoscopes did on adult pulmonology. With this instrument, the indications for bronchoscopy may be considerably expanded.

The introduction of the flexible bronchoscope in the early 1970s led to a veritable explosion in the applications of pulmonary endoscopy.[1] Unfortunately, however, applications in the pediatric population have been severely limited because of the lack of adequate suction capability in available small instruments and the small size of the airways in relation to the size of standard instruments. Most authorities suggest that flexible bronchoscopy cannot (or should not) be performed on children younger than about ten years.

We previously reported[2] the use of a modified 3.5 mm flexible bronchoscope (Olympus BF3C2, which has no suction channel but does have controlled flexion at the tip) in infants as young as 18 months. This instrument was modified by attaching an external suction channel (polyethylene or Teflon® tubing 1.5-1.8 mm in diameter). Although this was useful for many applications, it had limitations, and could not be used in smaller infants.

In late 1978, the Olympus Corporation developed an experimental prototype of a pediatric bronchoscope (BF3C4), which we have used since that date. This instrument has an outside diameter of 3.5 mm, and a 1.2 mm suction channel. In every other respect it is very similar to the standard Olympus bronchoscopes. We have utilized this instrument for 211 procedures in patients aged 14 years or less, and here report a summary of our experience.

TABLE 1. INDICATIONS FOR ENDOSCOPIC PROCEDURES

Atelectasis	58
Stridor	53
Suspected foreign body	12
Recurrent pneumonia	9
Persistent pneumonia	12
Bronchial toilet	9
Intubation	5
Hemoptysis	7
Miscellaneous	24
Wheezing	7
Cough	8

METHODS

Inpatients (as well as selected outpatients) at Rainbow Babies & Childrens Hospital underwent diagnostic or therapeutic procedures (bronchoscopy or transnasal direct laryngoscopy) for a variety of clinical indications (Table 1). Of these procedures 175 were bronchoscopies; 36 were transnasal laryngoscopies only. Two thirds of the patients were under one year of age: the age distribution is shown in Table 2.

Procedures were performed either in the Pediatric Endoscopy Laboratory or in one of the several intensive care units in the hospital. Patients were fasted for at least six hours (four hours in small infants) prior to the procedure, and in infants under two years of age the stomach was routinely aspirated prior to the procedure. The nose, posterior pharynx and larynx were anesthetized with 2% lidocaine in all cases. Infants younger than 3-4 months were not sedated unless necessary, while older infants and children were sedated with a "cocktail" of meperidine, promethazine, and chlorpromazine or with meperidine alone. Occasionally this was supplemented with intravenous diazepam. Patients 12-14 years or older were given the opportunity to undergo the procedure with topical anesthesia only (if appropriate) supplemented with hypnoanalgesia; many of them were quite interested to view the interior of their lungs through the teaching head of the bronchoscope and desired to remain awake. An occasional older child needed or requested sedation after initially declining; intravenous diazepam was then used.

All procedures were performed by a transnasal approach unless there was an artificial airway in place large enough to pass the bronchoscope (at least 4.5 mm ID). In several infants with a tracheostomy the instrument was passed transnasally, and then behind the tracheostomy tube while mechanical ventilation was continued. In one infant with severe subglottic stenosis the bronchoscope was passed through the tracheostomy stoma after replacing the tracheostomy tube with a 3.0 mm (ID) endotracheal tube passed through the stoma.

TABLE 2. AGE OF PATIENTS

Age	*Bronchoscopy*	*Laryngoscopy only*
0-3 months	53	13
4-12 months	54	13
1 year	25	5
2-6 years	20	5
7-14 years	23	0

From the Rainbow Babies & Childrens Hospital, Case Western Reserve University, Cleveland, Ohio. This study was supported by grants from the National Institutes of Health (HL 17776, HL 07415, and AM 08305) and the Parker B. Francis Foundation.

Presented at the meeting of the American Broncho-Esophagological Association, Palm Beach, Florida, April 12-13, 1980.

REPRINTS — Robert E. Wood, PhD, MD, Rainbow Babies & Childrens Hospital, Case Western Reserve University, 2101 Adelbert Road, Cleveland, OH 44106.

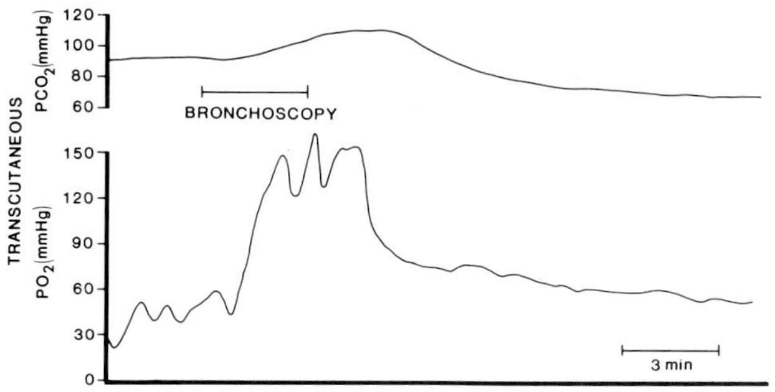

Fig. 1. Recording of transcutaneous oxygen and carbon dioxide tension in an 1,100 gm infant with massive atelectasis during therapeutic bronchoscopy. The patient was receiving 50% oxygen by CPAP prior to the procedure; the same concentration was given afterwards. Note the increase in both oxygen and carbon dioxide tension during the procedure (oxygen was insufflated through the suction channel of the bronchoscope while it was below the cords). Removal of a large mucus plug resulted in improvement in clinical condition and in oxygenation. The direct reading of the CO_2 electrode is approximately 20% too high (compared to arterial) and its response is delayed for 1½ to 2 minutes.

Specimen Collection. Direct aspiration of secretions into a suction trap was performed in the same fashion as with larger flexible bronchoscopes. Small-volume saline lavages (5-20 cc) for diagnostic purposes (culture and cytological examination) were also performed as with larger instruments. Biopsies are not obtainable with this instrument at present.

Monitoring of Patients. Procedures are performed with complete monitoring and resuscitative equipment at hand and with at least two physicians and one nurse in attendance. The second physician has the responsibility to monitor the patient for breath sounds, heart rate, color, respiratory distress, or any other signs of problems. EKG monitoring is done in small infants or in patients with hypoxemia or who are considered to be at risk. When appropriate, monitoring of oxygenation is done by ear oximetry (oxygen saturation) or a transcutaneous oxygen electrode. Supplemental oxygen is given by face mask as necessary; in very small infants ($<$ 2,000 gm) oxygen is insufflated down the suction channel at a rate of 1 liter/minute when the tip of the bronchoscope is above the larynx. This is done by attaching an oxygen line to the suction adapter of the bronchoscope and occluding the outlet of the adapter with the fingertip in the same way as suction would normally be applied. When the tip of the instrument is below the larynx, the outlet of the suction adapter is occluded intermittently for one-half to one second, in phase with the patient's inspiratory efforts, thus delivering 10-20 cc of oxygen down the suction channel. When suctioning is needed, the oxygen line is removed and a suction line attached.

RESULTS AND DISCUSSION

Flexible bronchoscopy is well tolerated by infants and children as long as due care is taken to provide for adequate topical anesthesia, sedation, and monitoring for airway patency. Newborn (full-term) infants are able to breathe spontaneously around the instrument, with minimal to no evidence of airway obstruction. Smaller infants cannot ventilate around the instrument, and special care must be taken to avoid hypoxia. By flushing oxygen down the suction channel intermittently (as described above) we have been able to maintain adequate oxygenation in infants as small as 840 gm. However, despite adequacy of oxygenation, this procedure may lead to transient hypercapnea (Fig. 1) in these very small infants. In older infants there has seldom been evidence (clinically or by ear oximetry) of significant hypoxia except in patients with preexisting hypoxia and extensive secretions. Supplemental oxygen delivered to the face has been sufficient in these cases.

TABLE 3. DIAGNOSES (LOWER AIRWAY)

Mucus plug	46
Bronchial stenosis or compression	25
Tracheomalacia	15
Inflammation (only)	13
Foreign body	7
Tracheal stenosis	6
Granulation tissue	5
Miscellaneous	14
No anatomic diagnosis	33

The most frequent indication for bronchoscopy (Table 1) in our series has been atelectasis (55 patients), particularly in infants under three months of age. Many of the 53 bronchoscopies in infants under three months were in premature infants or newborns with postextubation atelectasis. Our indication for bronchoscopy in these patients is failure to respond to conventional therapy (suctioning, chest physiotherapy) for at least 48 hours; often the patients had been reintubated for suctioning without success. In infants who were in distress with massive atelectasis, bronchoscopic intervention was undertaken earlier. In 25 of 29 infants less than 3,800 gm with atelectasis there was radiographic resolution within one hour; three infants resolved within 12-24 hours, and one did not resolve. These patients are the subject of a separate report. Several of the smallest infants (840-1,200 gm) required more than one procedure because of recurrence of massive atelectasis; each responded well on each occasion to removal of thick mucus plugs.

The diagnoses established at bronchoscopy are shown in Table 3. As might be anticipated from the indications (Table 1), the most common finding was mucus plugs, closely followed by anatomical obstruction of the airways. Compression of a bronchus (most often the left main stem) was a common finding in infants with congenital heart disease and cardiomegaly or enlargement of the great vessels. In some of these patients atelectasis was relieved by lavage and suctioning despite the anatomic abnormality.

The small (1.2 mm) suction channel in the bronchoscope might be presumed an impediment to effective suctioning. However, this has not been the case. In many infants (especially the premature infants) thick mucus plugs were removed by sucking a portion of the plug up into the suction channel and then slowly removing the bronchoscope from the airway, pulling the mucus plug along with the bronchoscope, which was then cleared and reinserted. The ability to direct the tip and to assess the results of suctioning visually make this an extremely

TABLE 4. DIAGNOSES (UPPER AIRWAY)

Laryngomalacia	31
Subglottic stenosis or edema	19
Cord paralysis	3
Miscellaneous (cysts, hemangiomas)	4

effective method for airway toilet, even in the smallest infants.

Children known to have aspirated a foreign body were referred directly for open tube bronchoscopy. In several patients however, foreign body was not suspected clinically. In others, the diagnosis was equivocal on clinical grounds. All but one foreign body was found in the left main stem bronchus or in the left lower lobe. These patients were subsequently treated by open tube bronchoscopy, but in several cases flexible bronchoscopy was later necessary to remove mucus plugs. Those children who had had extensive granulation tissue at the site of foreign body were examined with the flexible instrument several weeks later; one had to be referred back for removal of additional foreign material. The superior optics of the flexible instrument (in comparison to a standard open tube bronchoscope) and the relative ease and safety with which the procedure can be performed may make the flexible procedure the method of choice for initial evaluation of questionable foreign bodies and for follow-up examinations.

In 33 patients no anatomical diagnosis was made at bronchoscopy. Ten of these patients had radiographic evidence of atelectasis; washings of the affected lobes revealed evidence of infection in six, two had numerous eosinophils in the washings, and two had normal cytology and negative culture.

The small bronchoscope makes an excellent laryngoscope, and was often used in the investigation of stridor (53 patients). The diagnoses established at transnasal direct laryngoscopy are shown in Table 4. In a number of infants with stridor we noted that direct laryngoscopy in the conventional fashion revealed no abnormalities, while a transnasal layngoscopy revealed a very floppy epiglottis. Other infants with short aryepiglottic folds or with prolapse of the arytenoids into the glottis were also seen. In several infants being investigated for possible obstructive apnea the laryngeal examination was initially completely normal, but when the patient was sedated, stridor developed. In these cases we noted collapse of the lateral pharyngeal walls, softening of the epiglottis, and prolapse of the aryepiglottic folds or arytenoids into the glottis, apparently resulting from a loss of muscle tone during sleep.

TABLE 5. RESULTS (N = 211)

Resolution of atelectasis	44/58
Establishment of diagnosis:	
Anatomical	121/163
Bacteriological (only)	16/163
No useful information	12/211

Stridor was the most common indication for transnasal laryngoscopy, and variations on the theme of laryngomalacia (floppy epiglottis, short aryepiglottic folds, redundant arytenoids/aryepiglottic folds) were the most common findings. Other findings included subglottic stenosis, laryngeal edema, laryngeal cysts, laryngeal webs, papillomatosis, and subglottic hemangioma.

The pediatric bronchoscope is a very useful tool for nasotracheal intubation[3] in infants large enough to take a 4.5 mm (ID) endotracheal tube. The average time required for nasotracheal intubation with this method has been about 30 seconds. Tubes larger than 6.5 mm, however, are too stiff to use easily with this small instrument.

The overall outcome of the patients in this series is summarized in Table 5. It is noteworthy that useful information or therapeutic result was obtained in 94% of the patients. We estimate that approximately 25 of these patients would have been considered candidates for bronchoscopy if only open tube instruments had been available.

Few complications occurred in our series of patients. There was one episode of transient laryngospasm associated with intrabronchial instillation of N-acetyl cysteine in an eight-year-old girl with a persistent mucus plug. A three-month-old infant with severe stenosis of the left main stem bronchus developed a pneumothorax during an attempt to dilate the stenosis with the tip of the bronchoscope. Neither patient had lasting effects from these complications. One infant (2,200 gm) had a seizure one hour after bronchoscopy; in retrospect this might have been related to the topical anesthetic (lidocaine) used, although this was not documented. This infant was critically ill, with complex cyanotic heart disease (single ventricle) and massive atelectasis. She required immediate reintubation after the procedure and mechanical ventilation; the atelectasis resolved by the following morning. No neurologic sequelae could be identified, and it is not known whether the seizure was causally related to the procedure. However, this patient does emphasize the point that one must be careful with drug dosages in children, and even more so with very small infants.

ACKNOWLEDGMENTS — The authors thank Mr. Richard Gerstin of the Olympus Corporation for providing the prototype bronchoscope, and Mark Pultusker and Dr. Richard Martin for assistance with the transcutaneous oxygen and carbon dioxide measurements.

REFERENCES

1. Sackner MA. State of the art: bronchofiberoscopy. Am Rev Respir Dis 1975; 111:62.

2. Wood RE, Fink RJ. Applications of flexible fiberoptic bronchoscopes in infants and children. Chest 1978; 73:737.

3. Rucker RW, Silva WJ, Worcester CC. Fiberoptic bronchoscopic nasotracheal intubation in children. Chest 1979; 76:56.

ACUTE UPPER AIRWAY OBSTRUCTION IN INFANTS AND CHILDREN

EVALUATION BY THE FIBEROPTIC BRONCHOSCOPE

PIERRE A. VAUTHY, MD RAMALINGA REDDY, MD

TOLEDO, OHIO

All infants and children seen by the pediatric pulmonary service who display symptoms of upper airway obstruction undergo transnasal fiberoptic evaluation with the 3.2 mm flexible instrument. The procedure enables the observer to immediately visualize the nasopharynx, supraglottic, glottic and subglottic structures. Instrumentation is done in the sitting upright position and takes the skilled observer about 20 seconds to perform. The differentiation of epiglottitis from subglottic croup, foreign body aspiration and other less common causes of airway obstruction is easily performed and well tolerated. The fiberoptic instrument is often utilized both as a diagnostic and therapeutic tool. It can be utilized to intubate cases of epiglottitis and to evaluate the epiglottis to determine the appropriate time for extubation. This procedure is superior to oral airway examination because it does not distort airway anatomy, can be performed in the upright position, and does not further exacerbate airway obstruction.

The use of fiberoptic bronchoscopes in infants and children to evaluate both the upper airway and the tracheobronchial tree has received little attention in the medical literature. During the past four years, fiberoptic instruments have been utilized at The Pediatric Pulmonary Center of The Toledo Hospital and The Medical College of Ohio at Toledo in over 800 procedures. The patients range in age from premature infants to adolescents. Indications for instrumentation include history of apnea or aspiration, nasal obstruction, stridor, dysphagia, dysphonia, localized wheezing, localized airway turbulence, persistent atelectasis, lobar hyperaeration and suspected foreign body aspiration.

TECHNIQUE

The 3.2 mm and 5.3 mm Olympus fiberoptic bronchoscopes are utilized in the evaluation of patients, however the smaller instrument is the preferred diagnostic tool. This bronchoscope does not have a suction or instrument channel, but has good mobility and optics which provide the observer with an excellent view of the airway. Its small size makes it ideally suited for infants, children and adults.

Patients do not routinely receive premedication. Two percent Xylocaine® jelly is inserted into the nasal alae which provides both lubrication and topical anesthesia. Topical Cetacaine® spray is at times administered to the oropharynx if bronchoscopy is contemplated. Infants are restrained by a blanket wrapped circumferentially around the body. Children under five years of age are usually restrained by a papoose board and are studied with the head elevated at 40-45°. Older children rarely need restraints. All patients presenting with acute airway obstruction are studied in the upright position.

Upper airway evaluation is performed by inserting the fiberoptic instrument transnasally. This provides excellent visualization of the nasal passage, posterior pharynx, tonsils, epiglottis, arytenoids, vocal cords, and subglottic space. If the upper airway evaluation is nondiagnostic then the instrument is inserted through the glottis into the tracheobronchial tree. The patient is monitored by a nurse during the entire procedure. Electrocardiac monitoring is utilized on acutely ill patients and those undergoing bronchoscopy. Oxygen, suction and resuscitation equipment is always present in the procedure room. All procedures excluding those performed in the Emergency Department are videotaped by the Circon color video system. This allows for immediate playback and documentation of the procedure.

AIRWAY OBSTRUCTION IN INFANTS

The diagnosis of upper airway obstruction in infants is most easily made when the upper airway structures can be evaluated without distorting their anatomy or normal physiology. Direct laryngoscopy or straight bronchoscopy does not permit such an evaluation. The fiberoptic instrument can be inserted via the nasal route in infants as small as 1 kg permitting visualization of the upper airway during normal breathing. The infant can be studied in both the prone and supine positions which is not possible with conventional techniques.

Clinical conditions which produce airway obstruction in infants differs from those of older children. Table 1 lists the diagnoses made over the past four years at the Pulmonary Center. The most common diagnosis is that of laryngomalacia. The effects of changes in body position on the floppy epiglottis and arytenoids can be well documented with the fiberoptic instrument. Differentiation of obstructive from central apnea is performed by leaving the instrument in the posterior pharynx of a sleeping infant. Continuous monitoring of the patient's airway is recorded by the video system. The findings are correlated with cardiac and respiratory tracings

TABLE 1. AIRWAY OBSTRUCTION IN INFANTS

Laryngomalacia	Vocal cord trauma
Aryepiglottic cysts	Subglottic polyps
Vocal cord paralysis	Subglottic stenosis
Vocal cord web	Obstructive apnea
Vocal cord polyps	Congenital anomalies
Nasal polyps	Iatrogenic

From the Toledo Hospital Pediatric Pulmonary Center and the Department of Pediatrics, the Medical College of Ohio at Toledo, Toledo, Ohio.
Presented at the meeting of the American Broncho-Esophagological Association, Palm Beach, Florida, April 12-13, 1980.
REPRINTS — Pierre A. Vauthy, MD, The Toledo Hospital, 2142 North Cove Boulevard, Toledo, OH 43606.

TABLE 2. ACUTE AIRWAY OBSTRUCTION IN CHILDREN

Epiglottitis	Tonsillar edema
Croup	Bacterial
Supraglottic	Viral
Subglottic	Foreign body
Membranous tracheitis	Trauma

which are obtained simultaneously. Evaluation of swallowing and aspiration is also performed with this type of monitoring.

AIRWAY OBSTRUCTION IN OLDER CHILDREN

Airway obstruction postinfancy is usually more acute and life threatening and demands rapid diagnosis. Tables 2 and 3 list the causes of acute and chronic airway obstruction diagnosed at the Center. Patients with acute onset of stridor with significant respiratory difficulty undergo an upper airway evaluation within minutes of reaching the Center. All patients are evaluated in the sitting position in an attempt to prevent acute airway obstruction. The most common diagnoses that have been made include epiglottitis, supraglottic and subglottic croup, membranous tracheitis, and foreign body aspiration. Patients with epiglottitis are immediately intubated while awake by passing a nasotracheal tube over the bronchoscope which has been placed into the patient's trachea. The optimal time for extubation is also determined by direct visualization of the supraglottic structures of the intubated patient. Patients with croup and obstructive tracheitis can also be intubated in this manner, if the airway diameter permits. Foreign bodies are removed by conventional straight bronchoscopy under general anesthesia once the diagnosis is made. Patients with a history of airway obstruction with changes in body position are evaluated in the prone, supine, and upright positions. This is especially important in evaluating airway obstruction in children with large tonsils or facial anomalies. Sleep apnea studies are performed with little sleep disturbance as described in infants.

TABLE 3. CHRONIC AIRWAY OBSTRUCTION IN CHILDREN

Enlarged tonsils and adenoids	Foreign body
Congenital subglottic stenosis	Facial anomalies
Acquired subglottic stenosis	Obstructive sleep apnea
Vocal cord	Tracheomalacia
Trauma	Tracheal compression, extrinsic
Paralysis	Iatrogenic
Polyps	
Granuloma	

DISCUSSION

Fiberoptic bronchoscopy in this center has become a routine procedure for the evaluation of airway problems in the pediatric age group. Transnasal fiberoptic study appears to be superior to conventional evaluation of the airway in that it does not significantly distort the anatomy or physiology of normal breathing. It is tolerated much better than laryngoscopy or straight bronchoscopy and does not necessitate the use of heavy sedation or the risks of general anesthesia. In addition, patients can be studied in various anatomical positions and long-term visualization and video recordings can be performed. Most importantly, in acute airway obstruction, the procedure can be performed rapidly, usually in less than one minute. This provides the physician with a quick diagnosis, and in some cases, such as epiglottitis, the instrument can also be used as a therapeutic tool to intubate the patient. Our present experience demonstrates its efficacy in infants and children. They tolerate both upper airway and lower airway examinations without significant complication. Short-term complications include mild epistaxis and transient hoarseness. Two complications secondary to Cetacaine topical anesthesia have been recorded. Methemoglobinemia in a three-year-old child and laryngospasm in an adult occurred immediately after application of the spray. No major problems have been noted secondary to the actual fiberoptic procedure.

Ann Otol 89:1980

HEMOPTYSIS IN CHILDREN

LAWRENCE W. C. TOM, MD
ROBERT A. WEISMAN, MD
STEVEN D. HANDLER, MD
PHILADELPHIA, PENNSYLVANIA

Hemoptysis is uncommon in the pediatric age group. There is little mentioned regarding this problem in either the pediatric or the otolaryngologic literature. A review of the past ten years' experience at the Children's Hospital of Philadelphia identified 40 patients whose presenting symptoms included hemoptysis. Causes of the hemoptysis included tumor, infection, trauma, and foreign bodies, as well as a variety of other conditions. Based on these findings, a systematic approach to the diagnostic evaluation of the pediatric patient with hemoptysis has been developed. A thorough endoscopic examination of the upper aerodigestive tract is essential in most cases, and can have both diagnostic and therapeutic value. Particular attention is directed toward airway management in patients with massive hemorrhage. Close cooperation among the bronchoesophagologist, pediatrician, and anesthesiologist is mandatory for optimal care of the child with hemoptysis.

Hemoptysis is defined as the expectoration of blood or blood-tinged sputum. It is a startling symptom which often brings the patient to the physician and which may be anxiety-provoking to both. The source of blood may be anywhere in the respiratory tract from the nose to the lungs.

Although the ancient Greeks noted many causes for hemoptysis as early as 2,000 years ago, for subsequent centuries hemoptysis was regarded as pathognomonic of tuberculosis.[1] With the development of modern diagnostic techniques, the numerous causes of this potentially life-threatening symptom have been established, and in the majority of cases, the physician is able to determine the etiology of the hemoptysis.

While hemoptysis is a relatively common symptom in adults, it occurs rarely in the pediatric group. Although the list of possible etiologies is considerably smaller in children than adults, the diagnosis of hemoptysis is more difficult in the pediatric age group. Children are poor historians, more difficult to examine, and rarely expectorate sputum, even with extensive coaching. Therefore, the diagnostic evaluation differs in adults and children.

The physician must first determine if the patient is experiencing hemoptysis. Hematemesis, the vomiting of blood, may be confused with hemoptysis, particularly in children. Once hemoptysis is established, the physician must attempt to establish the etiology. In many cases this will require an extensive diagnostic evaluation. The otolaryngologist is ideally suited for evaluating hemoptysis, since he can evaluate the respiratory and upper digestive tracts in the search for a site of hemorrhage.

The literature concerning hemoptysis in children has dealt with this symptom as it relates to specific diseases.[2,3] To our knowledge, there have been no previous papers which address the problem of hemoptysis in children. A review of ten years' experience at the Children's Hospital of Philadelphia identified 40 patients whose presenting symptoms included hemoptysis. Based on this review, a systematic approach to the diagnosis and management of the pediatric patient with hemoptysis has been developed. Particular attention is directed toward airway management in patients with massive hemoptysis. In addition, three cases are presented which illustrate unique problems in children with hemoptysis.

METHODS

A thorough analysis was performed on the inpatient records of those patients who were admitted to the Children's Hospital of Philadelphia from January 1970 through December 1979 whose presenting symptoms included hemoptysis. Children with post-adenotonsillectomy hemorrhage were specifically excluded. Forty patients were identified and comprise the material for this study. All of the charts were carefully reviewed for the following variables: age, sex, quantity of blood, associated symptoms, chest radiograph findings, bacteriology of sputum specimens, endoscopic evaluation, special diagnostic studies, and etiology of hemoptysis.

RESULTS

Age. The ages of the patients ranged from 6 weeks to 20 years with a mean of 6.6 years (Fig. 1).

Sex. There was no sex predominance with 20 females and 20 males.

Quantity of Blood. In many of the records, the amount of blood was not quantitated. In the great majority of patients, the amount of blood was

From the Departments of Otorhinolaryngology and Human Communication, Children's Hospital of Philadelphia, and the University of Pennsylvania, Philadelphia, Pennsylvania.

Presented at the meeting of the American Broncho-Esophagological Association, Palm Beach, Florida, April 12-13, 1980.

REPRINTS — Steven D. Handler, MD, Department of Otorhinolaryngology, Children's Hospital of Philadelphia, 34th and Civic Center Blvd., Philadelphia, PA 19104.

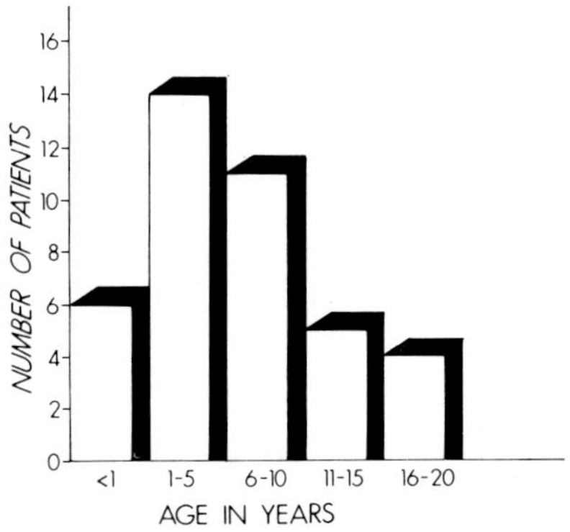

Fig. 1. Bar graph depicting the age distribution of the 40 patients with hemoptysis.

small. Only two patients experienced a blood loss in excess of 200 ml.

Associated Symptoms. Hemoptysis was the sole presenting symptom in seven patients (18%). In the remaining 33 patients, hemoptysis was most often associated with the symptoms of a respiratory tract infection. Coughing was noted in 18 patients while 121 presented with fever.

Chest Radiograph Findings. Chest radiographs were performed on all patients. In 13 patients (32%) these films were normal. In 6 of these 13 patients a pulmonary cause for hemoptysis was ultimately discovered. Atelectasis, parenchymal infiltrates, and interstial infiltrates were the most common abnormal chest x-ray findings. A variety of other findings were noted, including air trapping, cardiomegaly, pulmonary nodules, pleural effusion, pneumothorax and foreign bodies.

Bacteriology and Sputum Specimens. Sputum specimens were obtained for culture and sensitivity in 17 patients (42%). No growth was demonstrated in the specimens from eight patients. There was a wide variety of organisms identified in the positive cultures, with the most common organism being streptococci. Acid fast bacilli were not identified in any specimen.

Endoscopy. Bronchoscopy was performed on 34 patients (85%). In nine patients, bronchoscopy revealed a normal tracheobronchial tree. The next most common finding was a foreign body which was noted in five patients. Other common findings included inflammation of the tracheobronchial tree and purulent secretions. Bronchoscopy was not performed on six patients. Three of these patients were known to have preexisting pulmonary disease which was assumed to be the cause of the hemoptysis. In two patients, the amount of bleeding was not considered significant enough to warrant the procedure. The parents of one patient refused to permit the surgery. Esophagoscopy was performed on three patients, and no bleeding sites were found. Nasopharyngoscopy was performed on two patients, and a nasopharyngeal bleeding site was identified in one of these children.

TABLE 1. CAUSES OF HEMOPTYSIS

Pneumonia	8
Foreign body	6
Tracheobronchitis	6
Unknown	6
Cystic fibrosis	3
Trauma	2
Neoplasm	2
A-V malformation	2
Cardiac disease	1
Hemosiderosis	1
Laryngitis	1
Nasopharyngeal bleeding	1
Tuberculosis	1
Total	40

Special Studies. Eight patients (20%) underwent additional diagnostic procedures which included upper gastrointestinal series, cardiac catheterization, and pulmonary angiography. In only one patient, a child with congenital heart disease, did these studies establish a diagnosis.

Etiology. There were a variety of causes for hemoptysis (Table 1). In this series, the most frequent causes were pneumonia, bronchitis, and foreign bodies. No cause was found in seven patients.

CASE HISTORIES

The following case histories are presented to illustrate some of the unique features of hemoptysis in pediatric patients.

Case 1. A three-year-old male was first admitted at 21 months of age for treatment of pneumonia. Chest x-ray revealed hyperlucency of the left lung with a mediastinal shift to the right. Bronchoscopy demonstrated narrowing of the left main bronchus. After resolution of the pneumonia, he was discharged but experienced intermittent episodes of nonproductive coughing. Sixteen months later, he was admitted for evaluation of hemoptysis described as a "handful" of blood mixed with sputum. There was no recent history of fever, upper respiratory tract infection, or choking.

Physical examination revealed a healthy male child. There was dullness to percussion and rhonchi were heard in the left lower lobe. Blood count, coagulation studies, and electrolytes were normal. Intermediate strength PPD was negative. Chest x-ray demonstrated a left lower lobe interstial infiltrate.

On the day of admission, bronchoscopy demonstrated purulent secretions originating from the left main bronchus. Cultures were taken. Irrigation of this area revealed inflammation of the left lower lobe orifice. A small sunflower seed was noted at this orifice and was removed. The patient's postoperative course was unremarkable.

COMMENT. In a child with hemoptysis and persistent or recurrent pneumonia, the possibility of foreign body aspiration should be considered.

Case 2. An 18-year-old female with cystic fibrosis was admitted for evaluation and treatment of hemoptysis of 225 to 300 ml of bright red blood. Three days prior to admission she had an upper respiratory tract infection with pharyngitis and coughing. She did have one previous admission for treatment of pneumonia.

She presented as an adolescent female in no distress. There was an increase in the A-P diameter of her chest, but her physical examination was otherwise normal. Complete blood count, coagulation studies, and electrolytes were normal. Chest x-ray revealed increased hilar markings in the right lung and diffuse peribronchial thickening.

While in the hospital, she continued to cough blood-tinged sputum. Sputum was obtained for cultures, and intravenous carbenicillin and gentamycin were begun. Two strains of *Pseudomonas* were identified from the cultures. She was treated with gentle chest percussion, postural drainage, mucolytic agents and intravenous antibiotics. No hemoptysis occurred after the second day of hospitalization.

COMMENT. Bleeding in cystic fibrosis tends to occur in adolescence, may be massive, and is often associated with *Pseudomonas* bronchitis. Endoscopy is generally not performed unless the hemorrhage causes respiratory distress.

Case 3. A four-year-old female was well until two days before admission when she coughed several milliliters of blood. Over the next 24-36 hours, she lost 60-70 ml of blood during six episodes of hemoptysis. She was transferred from another hospital to Children's Hospital for evaluation.

She presented in moderate distress with hemoptysis consisting of bright red blood and blood-streaked sputum. No blood was noted in her nose or oral cavity. Her chest examination revealed diffuse rhonchi in the right lung. Her hematocrit was 35.1% and WBC was 12,200. Coagulation studies and chest x-ray were normal. Shortly after admission, another episode of hemoptysis amounting to 250 ml took place.

Because of persistent hemoptysis, it was decided to perform bronchoscopy. Blood was typed and cross-matched for possible transfusion, and a thoracic surgeon was notified that a child with significant hemoptysis was undergoing bronchoscopy.

Bronchoscopy revealed inflammation of the right main bronchus and bronchus intermedius. Blood was noted in the right middle lobe orifice. The bronchoscope was brought back to the carina. On reinspection of the orifices of the right lobes, bleeding was noted from all these orifices, with the most blood from the middle lobe. Attempts to tamponade the bleeding with the bronchoscope were unsuccessful. The bronchoscope became obstructed with blood and was replaced with an endotracheal tube. The patient was suctioned through this tube, and bleeding ceased. An exploratory thoractomy was performed immediately. A diffuse vascular lesion involving the right lung was identified and a right pneumonectomy was performed.

Histologic examination of the excised lung revealed an extensive arteriovenous malformation. Postoperative course was uneventful.

COMMENT. In a young child with massive airway hemorrhage, neoplasm or arteriovenous malformation should be considered. Cooperation between endoscopist and anesthesiologist is mandatory for proper management of these patients. Emergency thoracotomy may be necessary for control of hemorrhage.

DISCUSSION

In the pediatric age group, hemoptysis is an infrequent but potentially life-threatening symptom. Fortunately, for the great majority of pediatric patients, hemoptysis is not massive. This permits the physician to proceed with an orderly and systematic evaluation of this symptom. Practically any disease or trauma affecting the respiratory tract may cause hemoptysis.

In a child the more common causes include: infections, foreign bodies, trauma, cystic fibrosis, neoplasm, pulmonary hemosiderosis, cardiac disease, and congenital pulmonary vascular abnormalities.

In this study, infections were the most frequent cause of hemoptysis with 16 patients (40%) having an infection which was believed to be the cause of their hemoptysis. There are several ways in which infections may produce hemoptysis. In acute tracheobronchitis, the mucosa of the respiratory tract is friable and bleeds easily. Pneumonia, especially the necrotizing variety, may cause destruction of the lung parenchyma and erosion of blood vessels resulting in hemoptysis. Infections may also predispose the patient to bronchiectasis, a well-recognized cause of hemoptysis. Studying 137 cases of bronchiectasis unrelated to cystic fibrosis, Glauser et al noted that hemoptysis occurred in 15% of these patients.[4] Tuberculosis, which was once regarded as a major cause of hemoptysis in children, was believed to be responsible for only one of our cases of hemoptysis.[5] The most likely explanation for the decline in importance of tuberculosis as a cause for hemoptysis is the decreasing incidence of this disease.

An aspirated foreign body is a well-known cause of hemoptysis especially in children (in whom 70% of foreign bodies of the aerodigestive tract occur).[6] With foreign bodies, hemoptysis may result from mechanical trauma, inflammatory reaction in the respiratory tract, or infection distal to the site of obstruction. An aspirated foreign body should be suspected as a reason for hemoptysis in most children with pronounced coughing or persistent wheezing even with a negative history and a normal chest radiograph.

Hemoptysis may occur secondary to trauma of the face, neck, or chest. In these cases the etiology is readily apparent. Trauma to the nasal cavity, nasopharynx, or oral cavity may not be as obvious, and it is important to examine these areas carefully for a source of hemorrhage.

With the improved life expectancy in patients with cystic fibrosis, there has been an increasing frequency of bronchiectasis and hemoptysis secondary to this disease. Cystic fibrosis is now a major cause of hemoptysis in adolescents and young adults, and often the bleeding is profuse.[3,7,8] Stern et al noted a 5% incidence of massive hemoptysis in 728 children with cystic fibrosis.[8] In cystic fibrosis there is proliferation of blood vessels in the areas of bronchiectasis, and an increase in the size and tortousity of the bronchial arteries. Erosion of peribronchial abscesses into these vessels is believed to be the cause of the massive hemoptysis.

Neoplasms of the upper aerodigestive tract, while uncommon in the pediatric age group, should be considered in the differential diagnosis of hemoptysis. Both primary and metastatic tumors may present with hemoptysis. Two of the patients in our series presented with hemoptysis from pulmonary metastases.

Pulmonary hemosiderosis is an uncomon disease which occurs primarily in children and young adults and is associated with diffuse, recurrent or persistent intra-alveolar hemorrhage. This disease is characterized by hemoptysis usually consisting of pink frothy sputum, diffuse parenchymal infiltrates on chest x-ray, and iron deficiency anemia. Pulmonary hemosiderosis may be classified into three categories: idiopathic pulmonary hemosiderosis; primary pulmonary hemosiderosis with cow's milk hypersensitivity, glomerulonephritis, or myocarditis; and secondary pulmonary hemosiderosis associated with collagen vascular disease or hemorrhagic diseases.[9]

Congenital heart disease is a well-recognized cause of hemoptysis. Hemoptysis is most frequently found in conditions leading to pulmonary vascular hypertension in which the bleeding is believed to originate from dilated arterioles. Hemoptysis has also been noted in patients with increased bronchial circulation and with pulmonary venous congestion.[2] These patients usually have a mild or moderate degree of hemoptysis with occurrence at irregular intervals.

Hemoptysis may be a presenting symptom in patients with congenital pulmonary venous abnormalities, especially arteriovenous fistulas.[2,10] Since most of these fistulas are a manifestation of hereditary telangectasia, any patient with hemoptysis and cutaneous telangectases should be suspected of having a pulmonary arteriovenous fistula.

Management. In approaching the pediatric patient with hemoptysis, a thorough history is mandatory. In children, certain points need emphasis. The physician must attempt to distinguish among hemoptysis, hematemesis, and spitting of blood. To a child or worried parent, these three may appear to be the same. One should seek a history of recent trauma or surgery of the upper aerodigestive tract. Questions should also be asked about the possibility of foreign body aspiration. Choking, wheezing, or "asthma" which has not responded to medical therapy are highly suggestive of an aspirated foreign body. Reviewing a series of patients with unsuspected foreign bodies of the aerodigestive tract, Banks and Potsic reported that four patients with foreign bodies in their tracheobronchial trees experienced hemoptysis.[11,12]

A complete physical examination is always performed with particular attention to evaluation of the head, neck, and chest. Examination of the oral cavity and nose is usually performed without difficulty in most children. The nasopharynx, pharynx, and larynx should also be inspected although this part of the examination may be limited by the child's ability to cooperate. Auscultation of the chest may reveal wheezing, rales, and signs of consolidation which will not only help to localize the disease but may suggest the pathology.

Laboratory evaluation is often useful in evaluating patients with hemoptysis. Complete blood count, platelet count, and coagulation studies are performed in every case.

The chest radiograph is often invaluable in arriving at a diagnosis. It may demonstrate both the nature and site of the pathology. However, in several reported series, 25-50% of adults with hemoptysis have normal chest x-rays.[13-16] Our experience correlates well with these results, with 32% of children with hemoptysis having normal chest x-rays. If a patient with a normal chest x-ray has significant or persistent hemoptysis, further evaluation is still necessary.

Since children may be unable to expectorate sputum, specimens for stains and culture are not always obtained. If the physician suspects that a respiratory tract infection is the cause for hemoptysis, it is recommended that sputum specimens be obtained for bacterial studies. If a child is unable to produce sputum, specimens may be obtained by nasotracheal suctioning or bronchoscopy.

If the diagnosis has not been discovered with the above maneuvers, endoscopy is recommended. In most patients, bronchoscopy will be indicated, and in some cases, nasopharyngoscopy, laryngoscopy, and esophagoscopy will be necessary. In one case in our series, nasopharyngoscopy located the site of hemoptysis.

In adults, the flexible fiberoptic bronchoscope is usually used because it permits a detailed examination of the distal bronchial tree.[17-19] Although a pediatric flexible fiberoptic bronchoscope is now available,[20] the open ventilating bronchoscope should be used in children since most flexible bronchoscopes are too large to allow simultaneous ventilation and inspection of the pediatric airway. Flexible scopes are also impractical for removal of most foreign bodies. In addition, in patients with substantial hemoptysis, visualization in the flexible instrument may be obstructed by relatively small amounts of blood. This is less likely to occur with an open bronchoscope, which is ideally suited for suctioning and clearing the airway. Its relatively large lumen provides an excellent route for ventilation. Fiberoptic telescopic attachments are available which permit superb visualization of the tracheobronchial tree through the open bronchoscope.

In both adults and children with hemoptysis, the timing of bronchoscopy remains controversial. It must be emphasized that bronchoscopy is not recommended for all patients with hemoptysis. Patients in whom the diagnosis has already been made or who have one episode of blood-tinged sputum do not always require bronchoscopy. We do recommend bronchoscopy in children with hemoptysis where no cause is immediately apparent, and bleeding is recurrent or substantial. In these cases bronchoscopy can be both diagnostic and therapeutic.

Experience in adults supports the idea that bronchoscopy should be done during active bleeding. Pursel and Lindskog[1] and Smiddy and Elliott[19] believe that one is more likely to identify the bleeding site if bronchoscopy is performed during active bleeding. Our data support bronchoscopy for active bleeding only if the bleeding is persistent or profuse. If the diagnosis is not made by endoscopy, additional studies, including bronchography, upper gastrointestinal series, pulmonary angiography, and cardiac catheterization may be needed.

Despite a thorough evaluation, the cause of hemoptysis may not be discovered. In our study 18% of the patients fell into this category, and this is comparable to the results of studies in adults.[1,16,21] The prognosis for this group is excellent.[22] It is suggested that all of these patients be followed for a year, and if hemoptysis recurs, the evaluation should be repeated.[18,22]

Most acute episodes of hemoptysis last less than 24 hours and gradually subside. Patients with mild or moderate hemoptysis should have a history, physical examination and laboratory studies. These may be done as outpatient procedures depending upon the frequency and severity of the bleeding and associated symptoms.

Occasionally, a child is bleeding profusely when first examined. The immediate objectives are to protect the airway, stop the hemorrhage and to prevent shock. Since these patients are at risk for developing life-threatening hemorrhage, equipment for suctioning, intubation and tracheostomy should be near the patient's bedside. An anesthesiologist, pediatrician, and thoracic surgeon should be available to participate in the care of the patient should an emergency arise. Fortunately, in most of the patients, hemoptysis will usually stop spontaneously.

Massive hemoptysis is an uncommon life-threatening condition and is best defined as respiratory tract bleeding which causes respiratory distress. Rather than exsanguination, the patient's greatest danger is asphyxiation from the aspirated blood. In adults, tuberculosis is recognized as the most frequent cause of massive hemoptysis[23-25] while in the pediatric age group cystic fibrosis is probably the most common cause.[3,7,8]

The role of the bronchoesophagologist is to protect the airway, locate and stop the hemorrhage. The open ventilating bronchoscope with a telescopic lens system is the instrument we prefer. It may be used to protect the airway and to tamponade the bleeding site. If bleeding is so profuse that the bleeding site cannot be identified, the bronchoscope is left in place to clear blood and maintain the airway. If the bronchoscope becomes occluded, we recommend that it be replaced by a large endotracheal tube to facilitate endotracheal suctioning.

The treatments for massive hemoptysis include endoscopic tamponade, angiographic embolization, or surgical resection.[23-28] Thus, it is mandatory that a thoracic surgeon participate in the care of any patient with significant hemoptysis.

CONCLUSION

Hemoptysis is an uncommon symptom in the pediatric age group. A review of 40 children with hemoptysis indicates that in most cases the amount of bleeding is small. The most frequent cause of hemoptysis in this series was respiratory tract infection.

All children with hemoptysis must be thoroughly evaluated. The initial diagnostic evaluation consists of a complete history, physical examination and chest radiograph. If there is evidence of a respiratory tract infection, sputum specimens for stains and cultures should be obtained. If no diagnosis has been established or hemoptysis continues, endoscopy, most often bronchoscopy, is indicated. Other diagnostic procedures may be necessary if no etiology is identified. Despite complete evaluations, 18% of the patients in our study had no demonstrable cause for hemoptysis.

In the initial operative management of massive hemoptysis, the open ventilating bronchoscope with fiberoptic telescopic lens system is preferred. With its proper use, the bronchoesophagologist is capable of protecting the airway, localizing the bleeding site, and controlling the hemorrhage. Definitive control of bleeding in some of these patients may require thoracotomy. Close cooperation between the endoscopist, thoracic surgeon, and anesthesiologist, is mandatory if these children are to be managed successfully.

ACKNOWLEDGMENT — The authors would like to acknowledge Drs. Sylvan Stool and William Potsic for their management of many of the patients in this series.

REFERENCES

1. Pursel SE, Lindskog GE. Hemoptysis. Am Rev Respir Dis 1961; 84:329-36.

2. Haroutunian LM, Neill CA. Pulmonary complications of congenital heart disease: hemoptysis. Am Heart J 1972; 84:540-59.

3. Holsclaw DS, Grand RJ, Shwachman H. Massive hemoptysis in cystic fibrosis. J Pediatr Surg 1970; 76:829-38.

4. Glauser EM, Cook CD, Harris GBC. Bronchiectasis: a review of 187 cases in children with follow-up pulmonary function studies in 58. Acta Pediatr Scand 1966; Suppl 165.

5. Andosca JB, Foley JA. Nontuberculous hemoptysis. Int Clin 1942; 1:153-8.

6. Holinger PH. Foreign bodies in the air passages. In: Gellis SS, Kagen BM. Current pediatric therapy 7. Philadelphia: WB Saunders, 1976.

7. Schuster SR, Fellows KE. Management of major hemoptysis in patients with cystic fibrosis. J Pediatr Surg 1977; 12:889-96.

8. Stern RC, Wood RE, Boat TF, Matthews LW, Tucker AS, Doershuk CF. Treatment and prognosis of massive hemoptysis in cystic fibrosis. Am Rev Respir Dis 1978; 117:825-8.

9. Bluestone CD. Pulmonary hemosiderosis. In: Vaughn VC, McKay RJ, Behrmann RE, eds. Nelson's textbook of pediatrics. Philadelphia: WB Saunders, 1979:1222-4.

10. Parsons GH, Lillingtor GA. Hemoptysis. J Fam Pract 1978; 7:353-9.

11. Banks W, Potsic WP. Unsuspected foreign bodies of the aerodigestive tract. Ann Otol Rhinol Laryngol 1978; 87:515-8.

12. Potsic WP, Banks W. Unsuspected foreign bodies of the aerodigestive tract. Trans Pa Acad Ophthalmol Otolaryngol 1978; 31:84-9.

13. Jackson CL, Diamond S. Hemorrhage from trachea, bronchi, and lungs of nontuberculous origin. Am Rev Tuberc 1942; 46:126-38.

14. Johnston RN, Lockhart W, Ritchie RT, Smith DH. Haemoptysis. Br Med J 1960; 1:592-5.

15. Poole G, Stradling P. Routine radiography for hemoptysis. Br Med J 1964; 1:341-2.

16. Souders CR, Smith AT. The clinical significance of hemoptysis. N Engl J Med 1952; 247:790-8.

17. Kovnet DM, Roth GS, Anderson WM. Maximal extent of visualization of bronchial tree by fiberoptic bronchoscopy. Am Rev Respir Dis 1974; 110:88-90.

18. Selecky PA. Evaluation of hemoptysis through the bronchoscope. Chest 1978; 73:741-5.

19. Smiddy JF, Elliott RC. The evaluation of hemoptysis with fiberoptic bronchoscopy. Chest 1973; 64:158-62.

20. Tucker JA, Silberman HD. Flexible fiberoptic pediatric bronchoscope: a new instrument. Ann Otol Rhinol Laryngol 1978; 87:558-9.

21. Moersch HJ. Clinical significance of hemoptysis. JAMA 1952; 148:1461-5.

22. Barrett RJ, Tuttle WM. A study of essential hemoptysis. J Thorac Cardiovasc Surg 1960; 40:468-74.

23. Crocco JA, Rooney JJ, Fankushen DS, Di Benedetto RJ, Lyons HA. Massive hemoptysis. Arch Int Med 1968; 121:494-8.

24. Gourin A, Garzon AA. Operative treatment of massive hemoptysis. Ann Thorac Surg 1974; 18:52-60.

25. McCollum WB, Mattox RL, Guinn CA, Beall AC. Immediate operative treatment for massive hemoptysis. Chest 1975; 67:152-4.

26. Hiebert CA. Balloon catheter control of life-threatening hemoptysis. Chest 1974; 66:308-9.

27. Remy J, Arnaud A, Fardou H, Giraud R, Voisin C. Treatment of hemoptysis by embolization of bronchial arteries. Radiology 1977; 122:33-7.

28. Garzon AA, Gourin A. Surgical management of massive hemoptysis. Ann Surg 1978; 187:267-71.

Ann Otol 89:1980

CARCINOID AND MUCOEPIDERMOID CARCINOMA OF BRONCHUS IN CHILDREN

J. C. McDougall MD
K. Unni, MD
A. Gorenstein, DDS, MD
E. J. O'Connell, MD

Rochester, Minnesota

Four patients with bronchial carcinoid and two patients with mucoepidermoid carcinoma of the bronchus are presented. Presenting symptoms of these rare childhood tumors are chronic cough, hemoptysis, repeated bouts of pulmonary infection, and chest pain. Bronchoscopic examination should be considered in patients with these symptoms and is highly reliable in diagnosing these tumors. Surgical resection is the treatment of choice. Bronchial carcinoid and mucoepidermoid carcinoma have an excellent prognosis following conservative surgical resection.

INTRODUCTION

Carcinoid and mucoepidermoid carcinoma of the bronchus are rarely found in children. Chronic cough, repeated respiratory infections, and hemoptysis are the most common presenting features. These slowly growing malignancies were previously described as bronchial adenomas. This is a misnomer because their true malignant nature is now well recognized. We report our series of six pediatric patients with carcinoid and mucoepidermoid carcinoma of the bronchus.

METHODS

Medical records of all pediatric patients seen at Mayo Clinic between 1941 and 1976 were screened and the charts of all pediatric patients with bronchogenic tumors were reviewed. Histologic sections were available on all cases and were reviewed by one of us (KKU). Patients beyond the age of 15 years were excluded from this series.

CLINICAL FINDINGS

Six pediatric patients with histologically proven malignant bronchial tumors were seen at Mayo Clinic from 1941 to 1976 (Table 1). The median age was 10 years with the range of 6 to 15 years. There was no sexual predominance. A history of repeated pulmonary infections was obtained in each case and all had a history of cough which had been present from 2 to 20 months prior to diagnosis. Three of six patients had had hemoptysis. Fever had occurred in all patients. Physical examination revealed localized wheezing in two patients. The average duration of symptoms prior to diagnosis was 11 months. No patient had symptoms or laboratory findings suggestive of carcinoid syndrome. Chest x-rays revealed persistent or recurrent lobar infiltrates in all six patients. No patient underwent bronchography.

Bronchoscopy was performed in each case and in five of the six patients, a polypoid tumor mass could be seen partially or totally obstructing a bronchus. In one patient only bronchial narrowing with mucoid secretions in the affected area were seen. Four of the lesions were on the right side and two were on the left.

PATHOLOGY

Microscopic Appearance. Of the six tumors four

TABLE 1. PEDIATRIC PATIENTS WITH PROVEN MALIGNANT BRONCHIAL TUMORS (1941-1976)

Patient No.	*Age (yr)*	*Sex*	*Tumor Type*	*Tumor Location*	*Cough*	*Hemoptysis*	*Localized Wheeze*
1	6	F	ME	Left lower lobe	+	–	–
2	10	F	ME	Right main & upper lobe	+	–	+
3	10	M	C	Right lower lobe	+	–	+
4	11	F	C	Bronchus intermedius	+	+	–
5	14	M	C	Right upper lobe	+	+	–
6	15	M	C	Left lower lobe	+	+	–

ME - Mucoepidermoid; C - Carcinoid; + - Present; – - Absent

From the Department of Internal Medicine, Mayo Graduate School of Medicine, Rochester, Minnesota.
Presented at the meeting of the American Broncho-Esophagological Association, Palm Beach, Florida, April 12-13, 1980.
REPRINTS — J. C. McDougall, MD, ℅ Section of Publications, Mayo Clinic, 200 First Street SW, Rochester, MN 55901.

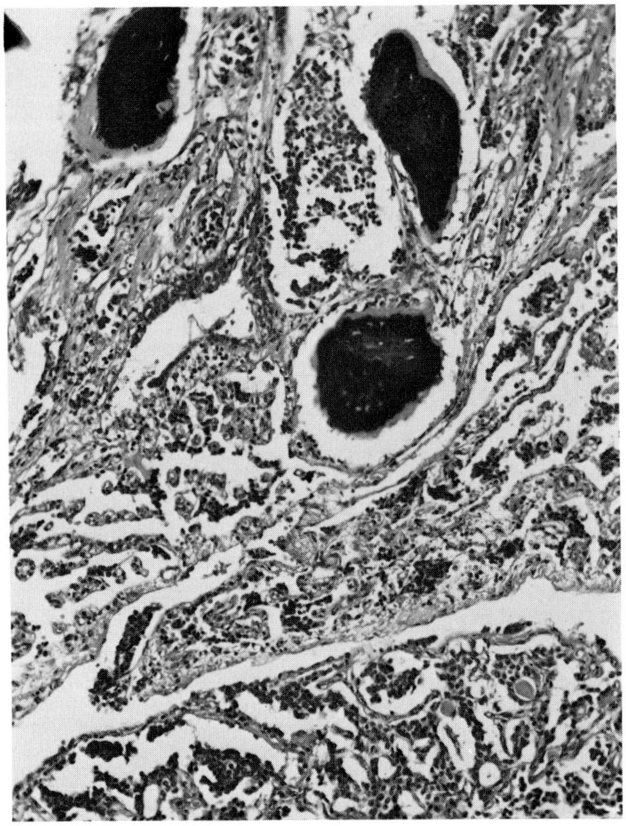

Fig. 1. Carcinoid tumor of bronchus. Small round cells with irregular nuclei are arranged in clusters. There is bone formation in the tumor. (H & E, x160)

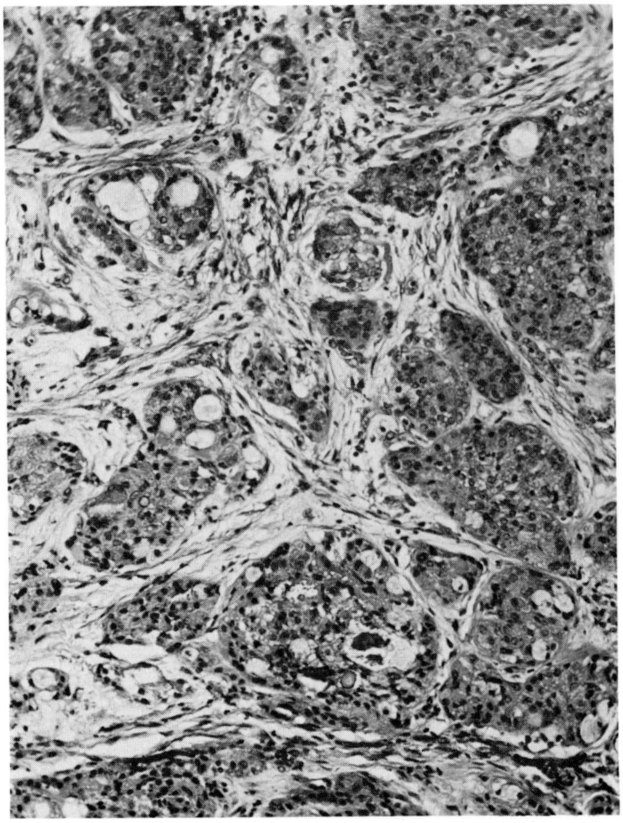

Fig. 2. Mucoepidermoid carcinoma of bronchus. Polygonal cells with slightly granular cytoplasm are arranged in clusters which contain pools of mucus. (H & E, x160)

were carcinoid and two were low-grade mucoepidural carcinoma. The four carcinoid tumors were histologically typical (Fig. 1). All the tumors were invasive penetrating through the bronchial cartilage but none invaded pulmonary parenchyma. The cells were small with round to oval nuclei and were arranged in a microglandular or trabecular pattern. The nuclei lacked pleomorphism. Areas of necrosis and mitotic activity were not seen. One tumor showed foci of squamous metaplasia and another, focal osteoid production.

The other two tumors were distinctly different. They were well circumscribed and lacked invasive growth pattern. The cells were polygonal, arranged in sheets with few glandular spaces. Some of the cells contained clear cytoplasm and some of the glandular lumina contained mucus. Although clear-cut squamous differentiation was not seen, some of the cells were elongated suggestive of the transitional cells seen in mucoepidermoid tumors of salivary glands. These two tumors were classified as low-grade (grade 1) mucoepidermoid carcinoma (Fig. 2).

TREATMENT

All six patients had resection of the tumor. Four patients had lobectomy, one patient had resection of two lobes, and one patient had a pneumonectomy. There was no evidence of nodal metastasis in any case as judged by chest x-ray and surgical exploration. The patient who had two lobes resected had an accumulation of pleural fluid postoperatively which prolonged the recovery. No patient received radiotherapy or chemotherapy and none required a second surgical procedure for recurrent disease. All patients are alive and well with no evidence of recurrence of their tumor at 2, 13, 14, 18, 20, and 24 years following treatment.

COMMENT

In 1882, Mueller[1] reported a case of bronchial adenoma, the term by which carcinoid, mucoepidermoid and adenoid cystic carcinoma of the bronchus were originally known. Further cases were described by Jackson and Konzelmann.[2] Hamperl[3] in 1937 classified adenomas of the bronchus as being of the carcinoid or the cylindroid type. Liebow[4] in 1952 described a third type, a mucoepidermoid tumor occurring in the bronchus and histologically similar to that found in the salivary glands. The term bronchial adenoma implies that they are benign tumors and is no longer acceptable in referring to this group of tumors. Their malignant potential is well recognized and reports of metastasis to mediastinal lymph nodes and extrathoracic structures are found in the literature.[5,6]

A careful search of the literature reveals reports of 66 pediatric patients with low-grade malignant bronchogenic tumors.[2,5-22] Twenty of these cases can only be identified as bronchial adenomas without further characterization. Thirty-five carcinoid tumors, six mucoepidermoid carcinomas, and five adenoid cystic carcinomas of the bronchus have previously been reported in children.

Bronchogenic neoplasm must be conisdered in a child who presents with persistent cough, hemoptysis, chest pain, repeated bouts of pulmonary infection and atelectasis. Aspirated foreign body, cystic fibrosis, bronchiectasis, tuberculosis, and intrabronchial hamartomas more commonly cause these findings. The presenting symptoms of bronchogenic neoplasm depend upon the location in the bronchial tree, rate of growth, vascularity, and the malignant potential. Hemoptysis, repeated pulmonary infection in the same lobe or segment of the lung, persistent chest pain, or localized wheezing are indications for bronchoscopy. In nearly every case, bronchogenic tumors can be identified at the time of bronchoscopy. Caution should be used in biopsying these tumors and the bronchoscopist should be prepared to manage bleeding following biopsy. Carcinoid tumors are highly vascular and mortality due to hemorrhage following biopsy of this tumor has been reported.

Bronchoscopic removal is not recommended as treatment of bronchogenic neoplasms. Local recurrences and stricture formation are sequela of this method of management. The treatment of choice is surgical resection. Lobectomy is recommended for lesions located in the lobar bronchus or more peripherally. Bilobectomy or sleeve resection is recommended for a neoplasm in the intermediate bronchus. Pneumonectomy may be necessary for lesions in the main stem bronchus but every attempt for conservative resection should be made in view of the low degree of malignancy of these tumors and the rare occurrence of spread to regional lymph nodes.

REFERENCES

1. Muller H. Zur Entstehungsgeschichle der Bronchiolerweiterunger. Ermsleben: Busch, 1882.

2. Jackson CL, Konzelman FW. Bronchoscopic aspects of bronchial tumors: with special reference to so-called bronchial adenoma (reports of 12 cases). J Thorac Surg 1937; 6:312-29.

3. Hamperl H. Über gutartige Bronchialtumoren (Cylindrome und Carcinoide). Virchows Arch Pathol Anat 1937; 300:46-88.

4. Liebow AA. Tumors of the lower respiratory tract. In: Atlas of tumor pathology, Section 5, Fascicle 17. Washington: Armed Forces Institute of Pathology, 1960:26-53.

5. Cathala J, Galey AP, Saada B, Bertrand N. Tumeur carcinöde de bronche avec metastase ganglionnaire chez une fille de 10 ans. Arch Pediatr 1960; 17:816-21.

6. Fu Y-S, McWilliams NB, Stratford TP, Kay S. Bronchial carcinoid with choroidal metastasis in an adolescent: case report and ultrastructural study. Cancer 1974; 33:707-15.

7. Weisel W, Lepley D. Tracheal and bronchial adenomas in childhood. Pediatrics 1961; 28:394-8.

8. Condon VR, Phillips EW. Bronchial adenoma in children: a review of the literature and report of three cases. Am J Roentgenol 1962; 88:543-54.

9. Wilkins EW Jr, Darling RC, Soutter L, Sniffen RC. A continuing clinical survey of adenomas of the trachea and bronchus in a general hospital. J Thorac Cardiovasc Surg 1963; 46:279-89.

10. Nunez VA, Spjut HJ, Rosenberg HS. Bronchial adenomas in children. Tex State J Med 1965; 61:683-6.

11. Verska JJ, Connolly JE. Bronchial adenomas in children. J Thorac Cardiovasc Surg 1968; 55:411-7.

12. de Paredes CG, Pierce WS, Groff DB, Waldhausen JA. Bronchogenic tumors in children. Arch Surg 1970; 100:574-6.

13. Logan WD Jr, Sehdeva J, Hatcher CR Jr, Abbott OA. Tracheobronchial adenomas. Am Surg 1970; 36:359-64.

14. DeBuse PJ, Lewis MJ, Shepherd JJ. Muco-epidermoid tumour of the bronchus in a child. Br J Dis Chest 1971; 65:130-3.

15. Koikkalainen K, Keskitalo E, Luosto R, Taskinen E. Carcinoid tumours and cylindromas of the tracheobronchial tree. Ann Chir Gynaecol Fenn 1974; 63:332-41.

16. Miller RE, Hopeman AR. Bronchial adenoma. Ann Thorac Surg 1975; 19:378-85.

17. Lawson RM, Ramanathan L, Hurley G, Hinson KW, Lennox SC. Bronchial adenoma: review of an 18-year experience at the Brompton Hospital. Thorax 1976; 31:245-53.

18. Bean DM, Haldenby DA. Endobronchial adenomata in children. J Otolaryngol 1976; 5:519-22.

19. Buschi AJ, Smith TH. Bronchial carcinoid. V Med Mon 1975; 102:1027-31.

20. Madani MA. Mucoepidermoid bronchial adenoma: with unusual pattern of growth. NY State J Med 1977; 77:1283-5.

21. Marks C, Marks M. Bronchial adenoma: a clinicopathologic study. Chest 1977; 71:376-80.

22. Andrassy RJ, Feldtman RW, Stanford W. Bronchial carcinoid tumors in children and adolescents. J Pediatr Surg 1977; 12:513-7.

Ann Otol 89:1980

EPIDERMOLYSIS BULLOSA DYSTROPHICA OF THE LARYNX AND TRACHEA

ACUTE AIRWAY OBSTRUCTION

JEROME W. THOMPSON, MD

A. RAZZAQUE AHMED, MD JAMES P. DUDLEY, MD

LOS ANGELES, CALIFORNIA

Epidermolysis bullosa dystrophica (EBD) is a rare inherited skin disease generally presenting in newborns. It is characterized by noninflammatory bullous lesions which can involve the mucous membranes of the oral cavity and oropharynx. If death occurs, it is usually the result of septicemia or fluid and electrolyte imbalance. Although mucous membrane involvement may be extensive and despite the reported evidence of tracheal and indirect evidence of laryngeal involvement, airway obstruction has not been implicated as a possible contributor to mortality in these patients. Since the presence of EBD in the larynx of a newborn might be expected to produce upper airway obstruction, however, and because of the absence of reports of laryngeal EBD, a case is presented of EBD-induced airway obstruction accompanied by photographic evidence of laryngeal and tracheal involvement with EBD. A three-week-old boy with biopsy-proven EBD present at birth was admitted to UCLA Medical Center with increasing stridor. The patient's extremities, diaper area, and numerous pressure-bearing sites on the back and elbows demonstrated erythematous denuded skin with occasional bullae up to 2 cm in size. The mucous membranes of the mouth and oropharynx showed similar denuded lesions. A tracheotomy was performed followed by a direct microlaryngoscopy and bronchoscopy revealing EBD on the supraglottic structures, vocal cords, and trachea. Otolaryngologists who are involved in the care of newborns should be aware of the possible, nearly fatal laryngeal involvement that can accompany this disease.

Epidermolysis bullosa dystrophica is a rare hereditary skin disease of infancy that can involve the mucous membranes of the oral cavity[1] and the esophagus.[2] A separation of the epidermis from the underlying dermis leads to the formation of bullae, and the erosions that occur due to the rupture of the bullae may lead to scarring on the skin and mucous membranes. Esophageal involvement resulting in stenosis brings the otolaryngologist into the management of the larynx in patients with epidermolysis bullosa.[3] The reports of laryngeal involvement have been few. Ramadass and Thangavelu noted the presence of laryngeal stenosis in a child with the disease.[4] Cohen reported progressive laryngeal obstruction in a six-month-old infant with epidermolysis bullosa necessitating a tracheotomy.[5] These two reports indicated that chronic disease could produce airway obstruction. It is because there have been no reports of the laryngeal complications of acute disease that this case is presented.

CASE REPORT

A three-week-old infant was admitted to the UCLA Medical Center with ulcerations involving the skin of the buttocks, inguinal areas, hands, elbows, and feet. The lesions were noted at birth. A skin biopsy examined by routine histology and by electron microscopy showed the characteristic features of epidermolysis bullosa.[6] The child is the second of parents who are first cousins. On admission he showed no signs of dehydration or feeding problems. His cry was normal, and no retractions or any other signs of respiratory distress were present. Although no bullae were seen, there were erythematous, moist, denuded areas which involved the skin of the diaper area, feet, elbows and hands affecting 30% of his total body surface. Patchy ulcerations but no bullae were noted on the mucous membranes of the oral cavity. Although cultures of the skin ulcerations revealed *Staphylococcus aureus*, *Proteus vulgaris*, *Escherichia coli*, and *Corynebacterium* species, therapy at various times with gentamicin, ampicillin, oxacillin, and dicloxacillin was successful in preventing bacteremia. The day after admission, inspiratory stridor and retractions began to develop. Because of increasing respiratory distress on the following day, a tracheotomy was performed. A direct microlaryngoscopy done at the time revealed a glottis narrowed by epithelial debris with areas of denuded epithelium and an interarytenoid vesicle (Fig. 1). Inspection of the tracheobronchial tree using 3.0 mm Hopkins telescopic bronchoscope demonstrated ruptured vesicles and ulcerations of the tracheal wall, and a single unruptured vesicle on the posterior tracheal wall was noted (Fig. 2). Reinspection of the larynx after removal of the bronchoscope from the larynx demonstrated the friability of the laryngeal mucosa. When the larynx was reexamined eight days after the initial inspection, however, it was found to be covered with normal mucosa. The tracheotomy tube was removed at that time, and the area of surgical incision healed quickly. Although the skin

From the Division of Head and Neck Surgery, Department of Surgery, and Division of Dermatology, Department of Medicine, UCLA School of Medicine, Los Angeles, California.

Presented at the meeting of the American Broncho-Esophagological Association, Palm Beach, Florida, April 12-13, 1980.

REPRINTS — James P. Dudley, MD, Division of Head and Neck Surgery, Room 62-158 CHS, UCLA Medical Center, Los Angeles, CA 90024.

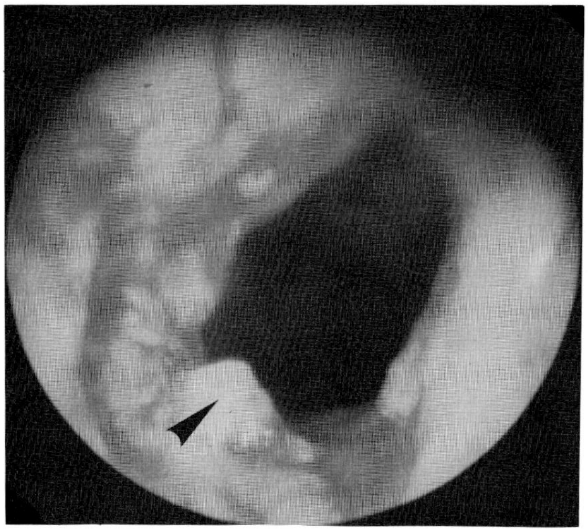

Fig. 1. Epidermolysis bullosa dystrophica of the larynx. Interarytenoid vesicle (arrow) whose presence was noted after suction removal of epithelial debris.

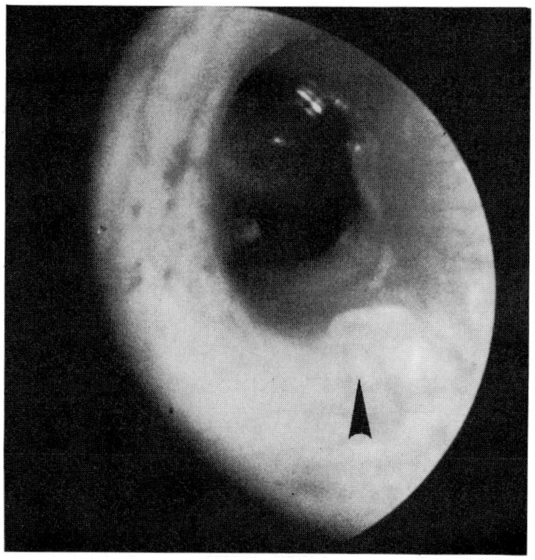

Fig. 2. Epidermolysis bullosa dystrophica of the trachea. A single unruptured vesicle (arrow) on the posterior tracheal wall.

lesions had not disappeared at the time of his discharge, no further laryngeal problem was noted during the remainder of his 18-day hospitalization.

DISCUSSION

Although the involvement of the larynx during the acute stage of this infant's disease should not be unexpected in a pathologial process which can be as diffuse and widespread as epidermolysis bullosa dystrophica, the sudden onset of respiratory distress is previously unreported. The changes in the larynx which precipitated this infant's respiratory distress were morphologically similar to those on the skin or other mucous membranes, but a rapid disappearance of these laryngeal lesions was observed while the skin lesions were considerably slower to resolve. Despite the normal appearance of the laryngeal mucosa at the time of discharge, there always remains the possibility of long-term laryngeal stenosis even though the acute disease resolved.

Three clinically distinct forms of this disease have been described: 1) simplex, 2) hereditaria letalis, and 3) dystrophica.[7] Epidermolysis bullosa simplex is autosomal dominant, and the mildest form of the disease. The bullae develop at sites of trauma to skin and resolve in a short period of time leaving only a transient hyperpigmentation. Mucosal involvement is rare. Epidermolysis bullosa hereditaria letalis is characterized by the large bullae on sites of trauma, and it is autosomal recessive. The bullae occur shortly after birth and rupture easily, leaving large denuded areas. Death usually occurs within days to months from sepsis or electrolyte imbalance. In those few patients who survive, residual scarring is rarely seen. Epidermolysis bullosa dystrophica may be either inherited or acquired. The clinical presentation is similar to the two previous forms. The formation of bullae at birth usually occurs on areas of trauma. The infant may die within a few days, but survivors suffer mutilating deformities with webbing of the digits, contractures, and occasionally esophageal stenosis.

The case presented in this report had laryngeal and tracheal involvement during infancy which required a tracheotomy. After an 18-day hospitalization, a complete clinical resolution of the laryngeal and tracheal disease was noted. Though rare, this potentially fatal disease should be recognized early and treated promptly to avoid complications or death.

REFERENCES

1. Pearson RW. The mechanobullous diseases. In: Fitzpatrick TB, Arndt KA, Clark WH, eds. Dermatology in general medicine. New York: McGraw Hill, 1971:621-43.

2. Orlando RC, Bozymski EM, Briggaman RA, Bream CA. Epidermolysis bullosa: gastrointestinal manifestations. Ann Intern Med 1974; 81:203-6.

3. Schild JA, Vander Aarde SB, Hollinger P. Esophageal stricture associated with epidermolysis dystrophica. Laryngoscope 1972; 82:510-4.

4. Ramadass T, Thangavelu TA. Epidermolysis and its ENT manifestations. Two case reports. J Laryngol Otol 1978; 92:441-6.

5. Cohen SR, Landing BH, Isaacs H. Epidermolysis bullosa associated with laryngeal stenosis. Ann Otol Rhinol Laryngol 1978; 87 Suppl 52:25-8.

6. Lever WF, Gudula-Lever G. Histopatholgy of skin. 5th ed. Philadelphia: JB Lippincott, 1975:69-70.

7. Pearson RW, Potter B, Strauss F. Epidermolysis bullosa hereditaria letalis. Arch Dermatol 1974; 109:349-55.

Ann Otol 89:1980

UPPER AIRWAY OBSTRUCTION IN INFECTIOUS MONONUCLEOSIS

JUDITH A. WOLFE, MD
PHILADELPHIA, PENNSYLVANIA

LEE D. ROWE, MD
SAN FRANCISCO, CALIFORNIA

Life-threatening upper respiratory obstruction is an unusual complication of infectious mononucleosis. Although the majority of fatalities result from progressive bulbar paralysis or the Guillain-Barré syndrome, airway impairment primarily occurs as a result of pharyngeal lymphoid hyperplasia and associated faucial arch edema. Recent experience in a young child with infectious mononucleosis who exhibited progressive hypersomnolence, sleep apnea, and stridor during sleep is presented. In addition, a retrospective analysis of 72 cases of respiratory complications of infectious mononucleosis provides guidelines for specific airway management. Mild upper respiratory obstruction with persistent fever, severe odynophagia, and malaise is treated with parenteral corticosteroids. Immediate tonsillectomy using a halothane and oxygen induction technique is recommended for severe airway occlusion. Tracheotomy is currently reserved for those patients with progressive alveolar hypoventilation, hypercarbia, atelectasis, and bulbar paralysis. In general, tonsillectomy is well-tolerated, eliminating airway obstruction, improving swallowing function, and rapidly resolving pharyngeal discomfort.

INTRODUCTION

Upper airway obstruction in children and young adults is an unusual but potentially fatal complication of infectious mononucleosis. More commonly, the disease is a benign, self-limited disorder of the lymphopoietic system manifested by fever, pharyngitis, generalized lymphadenopathy, and splenomegaly.[1] Because the development of acute, life-threatening respiratory difficulty is uncommon, its successful treatment remains uncertain, as evidenced by the recent death of a 15-year-old male with serologically proven pharyngeal (anginose) mononucleosis.[2]

Our experience with severe upper airway obstruction in a young child secondary to infectious mononucleosis prompted an investigation into its proper management. A retrospective analysis of reported airway complications of infectious mononucleosis during the preceding 90 years is presented, reviewing current methods of airway control with attention to the role of corticosteroids, tonsillectomy, and tracheotomy.

CASE REPORT

A seven-year-old black female was admitted to San Francisco General Hospital with a four-day history of odynophagia, dysphagia, fever, and progressive upper airway obstruction characterized by hypersomnolence, sleep apnea, and stridor during sleep. Two days prior to admission a diagnosis of exudative pharyngotonsillitis was made and she received phenoxymethyl penicillin (250 mg orally, four times per day). A pharyngeal culture for group A beta-hemolytic streptococci was negative.

However, because of bizarre behavior including eight to ten episodes of disorientation and auditory hallucinations, the mother returned the child to the hospital. In addition, she had fallen asleep at inappropriate times, exhibiting episodes of obstructive apnea. The past medical history was negative for the pickwickian syndrome, adenoidal or tonsillar hyperplasia, or obstructive sleep apnea. There was no history of known allergies and diphtheria-pertussis-tetanus immunizations were complete.

Physical examination disclosed a lethargic, thin, black female with denasal voice, sonorous oral respirations, and a temperature of 38.33 C (101 F). While falling asleep in her mother's arms, she developed coarse inspiratory stridor, substernal retractions, and episodes of obstructive apnea lasting 10-20 seconds. In addition to an exudative erythematous pharyngotonsillitis, massive symmetrical tonsillar hypertrophy was observed with nearly complete oropharyngeal occlusion. Bilateral, tender anterior and posterior cervical lymphadenopathy was present; however, generalized lymphadenopathy and hepatosplenomegaly were not detected.

Because of severe upper airway obstruction, an emergency adenotonsillectomy was performed with immediate relief of stridor, rapid resolution of fever within 24 hours, and improvement in swallowing. Subsequent laboratory data revealed an absolute lymphocytosis, many atypical lymphocytes, and a positive Monospot® test. The child was discharged on the third hospital day on oral penicillin without fever, stridor, oropharyngeal hemorrhage or odynophagia. Microscopic sections of lymphoid tonsillar tissue demonstrated an increased number of polymorphonuclear leukocytes, lymphocytes, and plasma cells which in some necrotic areas coalesced to form microabscesses.

LITERATURE REVIEW

Including the most recent case reported in 1978, there have been a total of 33 documented fatalities related to respiratory complications of infectious mononucleosis.[2-15] The majority (28) are attributed to bulbar paralysis or Guillain-Barré syndrome with associated alveolar hypoventilation, poor tussive ability, aspiration, and pneumonia.[3-14]

Four fatalities are recorded as a result of upper airway obstruction from massive edema of Waldeyer's ring and the surrounding pharynx.[2,7,13,15] Only one fatal case of pharyngeal hemorrhage following severe mucosal ulceration was found in an extensive review of the world's literature.[7] In 79% of patients a complete autopsy was performed. Autopsy findings common to those patients with respiratory obstruction included marked mem-

From the Department of Otorhinolaryngology and Human Communication, University of Pennsylvania, School of Medicine, Philadelphia, Pennsylvania, and the Department of Otolaryngology, University of California, San Francisco, California.

Presented at the meeting of the American Broncho-Esophagological Association, Palm Beach, Florida, April 12-13, 1980.

REPRINTS — Lee D. Rowe, MD, 400 Parnassus Avenue, Suite A-717, San Francisco, CA 94143.

branous tonsillitis, pharyngotonsillar and faucial arch edema, and focal and diffuse mononuclear infiltration of the mucosa and submucosa.[2,7,13,15]

Following World War II, until the early 1960s, the vast majority of patients with pharyngeal obstruction secondary to infectious mononucleosis were treated with tracheotomy.[15-28] Although the age range was from 11 months to 22 years, the clinical pattern is strikingly similar: a membranous exudate, variable amounts of faucial arch edema, and prominent posterior cervical lymphadenopathy. Signs varied from dysphagia, muffled voice, drooling, and dyspnea to inspiratory stridor exacerbated by the recumbent position. The mean length of illness prior to tracheotomy was six days, requiring an average of eight days before successful decannulation.

Although tonsillectomy for severe upper airway obstruction complicating infectious mononucleosis was reported as early as 1956,[29] only two case reports have appeared in the English literature in the intervening years.[29-33] Indeed, marked clinical improvement was observed in all cases including rapid resolution of fever, improved swallowing, and relief of upper airway obstruction.

DISCUSSION

Following Filatof's and Pfeiffer's clinical descriptions of glandular fever or *Drüsenfieber* in 1885 and 1889, respectively, little additional information regarding the pathogenesis of this disease was provided until 1920.[34,35] In that year Sprunt and Evans reported the presence of an absolute lymphocytosis and atypical mononuclear cells in the blood of patients with this illness, which the authors referred to an infectious mononucleosis.[1] Twelve years later, Paul and Bunnell discovered in the serum the characteristic heterophile antibody which is capable of agglutinating sheep erythrocytes.[36] Most recently, in 1968, Henle and coworkers established the important relationships between infectious mononucleosis and Epstein-Barr virus, a herpes group virus.[37] Although Koch's postulates have not been fulfilled, the ability of infectious mononucleosis cells to undergo lymphoblastoid transformation, the appearance of at least 10% atypical cells, and the development of persistent antibody to Epstein-Barr virus raises the possibility of an associative relationship with the virus.[38,39]

The incubation period ranges from a few days to several weeks, and the disease is heralded by malaise, chills, headache, and intermittent fever (38.33-39.44 C {101-103 F}).[1] Currently, infectious mononucleosis is confirmed by the presence of a positive Monospot test, rising heterophile agglutination titers, and absolute lymphocytosis with atypical lymphocytes: large cells exhibiting oval, horseshoe-shaped or indented nuclei and a basophilic, vacuolated foamy cytoplasm.[40] Characteristically, the diagnosis is made by the fourth to fifth day of the disease, which commonly persists for two to eight weeks.

Complications of infectious mononucleosis primarily include hepatic dysfunction with elevated liver function tests and neurologic disorders including peripheral neuritis, cranial neuropathy, meningoencephalitis, and the Guillain-Barré syndrome.[41] Thrombocytopenic purpura, pericarditis and splenic rupture are uncommon. Even more unusual are respiratory complications which now total 73 reported cases.

Although the Guillain-Barré syndrome accounts for the majority of fatalities, massive Waldeyer's ring lymphoid hyperplasia and faucial arch edema are primarily responsible for upper airway obstruction.[29-33] In addition, edema of the epiglottis, aryepiglottic folds and arytenoids, massive enlargement of mediastinal lymph nodes, and formation of a pseudomembrane similar to diphtheria, are implicated in the pathogenesis of airway obstruction.[5,16,42,43]

The appearance of a pseudomembrane in the presence of progressive upper respiratory tract obstruction mimics diphtheria, and many patients who were previously unsuccessfully treated with antidiphtheria serum probably had infectious mononucleosis.[27]

The absence of an absolute lymphocytosis, generalized lymphadenopathy or hepatosplenomegaly, and findings of a panleukocytosis and Klebs-Löffler bacilli confirm the diagnosis of diphtheria.[44] Although the diphtheritic pseudomembrane is similar to that observed in infectious mononucleosis, it persists for a shorter period of time and separates readily from the pharynx with associated hemorrhage when the fever falls.[44]

Early management of infectious mononucleosis is primarily symptomatic, employing saline gargles, salicylates, and bed rest. Quarantine is totally unnecessary. If severe pharyngotonsillitis complicated by beta-hemolytic streptococci supervenes, antibiotics are warranted. Penicillin is the recommended drug, while ampicillin is contraindicated because of a frequent associated severe papular rash similar to the Jarisch-Herxheimer reaction.[45]

With progressive systemic toxicity manifested by persistent fever, severe odynophagia, and mild upper respiratory obstruction, parenteral steroids are recommended. This degree of airway obstruction is characterized by *intermittent* nasal alar flaring, suprasternal retractions, and inspiratory stridor induced by the supine position. A dramatic reduction in odynophagia, Waldeyer's ring and faucial arch edema, cervical adenopathy, and respiratory distress is observed within 6-24 hours.[46-49] Also the duration of malaise, asthenia, and fever is significantly shortened, in addition to a measurable decrease in the leukocyte count.[47,50]

The rapid defervescence of lymphoid hypertrophy, faucial arch edema, and subsequent airway improvement is attributed to steroid-induced lysis of the lymphocytic perivascular infiltration.[51] Currently, adolescents and young adults receive 60-80 mg of prednisone intravenously the first day, reducing the dosage 5 mg daily over a seven to ten-day period.[27,45]

The majority of patients with mild respiratory obstruction can be successfully managed with corticosteroids. When signs and symptoms progress to moderate or severe airway obstruction close attention to this development is necessary. Moderate airway obstruction includes nasal alar flaring, suprasternal retractions and stridor which is exacerbated by the supine position. Airway obstruction may progress to the severe stage manifested by tachycardia, tachypnea, hypercarbia, and hypoxia. Clinical findings may be more subtle, however, as evidenced by development of hypersomnolence and obstructive sleep apnea in this child.

Severe airway obstruction requires operative intervention. Using halothane and oxygen anesthesia and avoiding muscle relaxants, the patient is perorally intubated in the operating room with the otolaryngologist prepared to perform bronchoscopy and/or tracheotomy. Because the primary etiology of acute upper respiratory tract obstruction is massive lymphoid hyperplasia, we recommend immediate tonsillectomy rather than prolonged intubation or tracheotomy.

Prior to tonsillectomy, direct laryngoscopy is performed to evaluate the extent of edema. Tonsillectomy appears to be well tolerated in infectious mononucleosis; upper respiratory tract obstruction is rapidly relieved, swallowing is improved, and there are no reported complications.[29-33] Many of the objections to tonsillectomy are similar to those raised for quinsy tonsillectomy: 1) the danger posed by a general anesthetic; 2) the increased risk of systemic bacteremia and sepsis; and 3) intraoperative or postoperative tonsillar hemorrhage.[52] Most deaths associated with tonsillectomy are caused by hemorrhage in which blood is not replaced. In acute bacterial tonsillitis, the objections to tonsillectomy are theoretical. No increased immediate or delayed postoperative hemorrhage has been observed, and there is no data to support the contention of an increased incidence of septicemia or risk of general anesthesia.[53-55]

In general, tonsillar hypertrophy obstructing the airway or deglutition is an absolute indication for tonsillectomy.[55,56] After reviewing the respiratory complications of infectious mononucleosis, we recommend immediate tonsillectomy for moderate or severe airway obstruction or unremitting tonsillar hemorrhage. Tracheotomy is reserved for those patients with the Guillain-Barré syndrome who develop alveolar hypoventilation, atelectasis, hypercarbia, and hypoxia.[57]

REFERENCES

1. Sprunt TP, Evans FA. Mononuclear leukocytosis in reaction to acute infections (infectious mononucleosis). Johns Hopkins Hosp Bull 1920; 31:410-7.

2. Regan WA. Mononucleosis patient dies of asphyxiation. Hosp Prog 1978; 59:80-2.

3. Gooding SEF. On glandular fever or infective mononucleosis. Practitioner 1931; 127:468.

4. Thomsen S, Vimtrup B. 6 Lethale tilfaelde af mononucleosis infectiosa. Nord Med 1939; 4:3295.

5. Jersild T. Mononucleosis infectiosa med letald forlob. Nord Med 1942; 14:1705.

6. Ricker W, Blumberg A, Peters CH, Widerman A. The association of the Guillain-Barré syndrome with infectious mononucleosis: report of two fatal cases. Blood 1947; 2:217-26.

7. Custer RP, Smith EB. The pathology of infectious mononucleosis. Blood 1948; 3:831-57.

8. Haymaker W, Kernohan J. The Landry-Guillain-Barre syndrome: clinical pathologic report of 50 fatal cases and critique of the literature. Medicine 1949; 28:59-141.

9. Silversides JD, Richardson JP. Neurologic complications of infectious mononucleosis. Can Med Assoc J 1950; 63:138-43.

10. Dolgopol VB, Husson GS. Infectious mononucleosis with neurological complications — report of a fatal case. Arch Intern Med 1949; 83:179-96.

11. Bernstein TC, Wolff HG. Involvement of the nervous system in infectious mononucleosis. Ann Intern Med 1950; 33:1120-38.

12. Shinton NK, Hawkins CF. A fatal case of glandular fever. Lancet 1956; 2:708-9.

13. Erwin W, Weber RW, Manning RT. Complications of infectious mononucleosis. Am J Med Sci 1959; 238:699-712.

14. Rahal J Jr, Henle G. Infectious mononucleosis and Reye's syndrome: a fatal case with studies for Epstein-Barr virus. Pediatrics 190; 46:776-80.

15. Lemierre A, Morin M, Alison M. The serious occurrence of suffocation in two cases in infectious mononucleosis. Bull Mem Soc Med Hosp Paris 1948; 64:51-4.

16. Chen KC, Teng CT. Infectious mononucleosis in a Chinese simulating laryngeal diphtheria with laryngeal obstruction. Chin Med J (Engl) 1941; 59:116-30.

17. Story GBT, MacCabe AF. A case of infectious mononucleosis requiring tracheotomy. Br Med J 1946; 2:652.

18. Jones GP, Jones E. Anginose type of glandular fever requiring tracheotomy. Br Med J 1949; 2:1212.

19. Bower AG, Affeldt JE, West H. Treatment of the angina type of infectious mononucleosis with gamma globulin. J Pediatr 1949; 35:58-62.

20. Librach IM. Anginose type of glandular fever requiring tracheotomy. Lancet 1951; 1:1105.

21. Delaney AJ, Nelson BA. Anginose type of infectious mononucleosis requiring tracheotomy. Ann Otol Rhinol Laryngol 1953; 62:213-6.

22. Specter S, Bautista A. Respiratory obstruction caused by acute tonsillitis and acute adenoiditis. NY J Med 1956; 56:2118-9.

23. Parsons HN, Dodds EJA. A case of glandular fever causing acute respiratory obstruction. J Laryngol Otol 1958; 72:910-1.

24. Dodds EJA. A case of glandular fever causing respiratory obstruction. Practitioner 1959; 182:595-7.

25. Grier J. The tonsils and adenoids causing respiratory obstruction. J Laryngol Otol 1962; 76:978-80.

26. Marfatia PT. Anginose type of infectious mononucleosis requiring tracheostomy. J Laryngol Otol 1968; 82:831-2.

27. Lee MD. Respiratory obstruction in glandular fever. J Laryngol Otol 1969; 83:617-22.

28. Gutgesell HP Jr. Acute airway obstruction in infectious mononucleosis. Pediatrics 1971; 47:141-3.

29. Ranta LJ, Grahne B. Tonsillectomy during infectious mononucleosis. Pract Oto-Rhino-Laryngol 1956; 18:65-71.

30. Yeager HP. Airway obstruction in infectious mononucleosis. Arch Otolaryngol 1964; 80:583-6.

31. Feroli EJ, Mella GW, Pedreira FA, Storch RT. Indications for tonsillectomy in infectious mononucleosis. Pediatrics 1971; 48:338.

32. Nessel VE. Die operative Behandlung der Komplizierten monosytenangina. Tracheotomie oder Tonsillektomie? Z Laryngol Rhinol Otol Ihre Grenzgeb 1962; 41:182-6.

33. Sinios A, Rossberg G, Lennartz H. Tonsillektomie im okuten Stadium der infektiosen Monokleose. Monatsschr Kinderheilkd 1977; 125:535.

34. Filatof NF. Vorlesungen uber acute infectious Krankheiten im Kindesalter. 1, Moscow: A. Lang, 1885; 1:229-59.

35. Pfeiffer E. Drusenfieber. Jahrbuch für Kinderheilkunde. Basel: S Karger 1889; 29:257.

36. Paul JR, Bunnell WW. The presence of heterophile antibodies in infectious mononucleosis. Am J Med Sci 1932; 183:90-104.

37. Henle G, Henle W, Diehl V. Relation of Burkitt's tumor-associated herpes-type virus to infectious mononucleosis. Proc Natl Acad Sci USA 1968; 59:94-101.

38. Niederman JC. Infectious mononucleosis. In: Wintrobe MM, ed. Harrison's principles of internal medicine. New York: McGraw-Hill Inc, 1974:1063-8.

39. Paublini H, Meech RJ, Lambert HP. The glandular fever syndrome revisited. Practitioner 1977; 219:713-7.

40. Strauss M. Burkitt's lymphoma, nasopharyngeal carcinoma, infectious mononucleosis and the Epstein-Barr virus. Laryngoscope 1972; 82:2049-58.

41. Smith EB, Custer RP. Rupture of the spleen in infectious mononucleosis. Blood 1946; 1:317-33.

42. Ravenna P, Snyder J. The occurrence of edema of the pharynx and larynx in infectious mononucleosis. Ann Intern Med 1948; 28:861-6.

43. Weinstein L, Brown RB. Otolaryngologic manifestations of extrinsic infectious diseases. Otolaryngol Clin North Am 1976; 9:645-53.

44. Tidy HL. Glandular fever and infectious mononucleosis. Lancet 1934; 2:180-6, 236-40.

45. Lai PT. Infectious mononucleosis: recognition and management. Hosp Pract 1977; 8:47-52.

46. Mandel W, Marilley RJ Jr, Gaines LM Jr. Corticotropin in severe anginose infectious mononucleosis. JAMA 1955; 158:1021-2.

47. Creditor MC, McCurdy HW. Severe infectious mononucleosis treated with prednisolone. Ann Intern Med 1959; 50:218-22.

48. Nye FJ. Problems in the diagnosis and treatment of infectious mononucleosis. Practitioner 1977; 218:367-70.

49. Relkin R. The use of steroids in infectious mononucleosis. NY State J Med 1960; 60:3876-9.

50. Mollica V, Grasso E. Manifestazioni otorinolaringologiche della mononucleosi infettiva e suo trattamento con ormoni steroidi corticali. Minerva Otorinolaryngol 1962; 12:243-75.

51. Doran JK, Weisberger AS. The used of ACTH in infectious mononucleosis. Ann Intern Med 1958; 38:1058-62.

52. Yung AK, Cantrell RW. Quinsy tonsillectomy. Laryngoscope 1976; 86:1714-7.

53. Sumner E. Quinsy tonsillectomy: a safe procedure. Anaesthesia 1973; 28:558-61.

54. Ritter FN. Tonsillectomy and adenoidectomy: indications and complications. Postgrad Med 1967; 41:342-7.

55. Kornblut A, Kornblut AD. Tonsillectomy and adenoidectomy. In: Paparella MM, Shumrick DA, eds. Otolaryngology. Vol 3. Philadelphia: WB Saunders 1973:296-316.

56. Reid JM. Donaldson JA. The indications for tonsillectomy and adenoidectomy. Otolaryngol Clin North Am 1970; 3:339-44.

57. Eaton OM, Stevens H, Silver HM. Respiratory failure in polyradiculoneuritis associated with infectious mononucleosis. JAMA 1965; 194:609-11.

Ann Otol 89:1980

FOREIGN BODIES IN THE LARYNX AND TRACHEOBRONCHIAL TREE IN CHILDREN

A REVIEW OF 225 CASES

BRUCE F. ROTHMANN, MD CLIFFORD R. BOECKMAN, MD

AKRON, OHIO

In a study of 225 patients with foreign bodies in the larynx, trachea and bronchi, 77% were 36 months of age or less. The male-female ratio was 2:1. Food or food derivatives were the causative agent in 70% of the cases, with 38% due to a portion of nut. The foreign body involved the right and left bronchus with equal frequency. A choking episode followed by an audible wheeze (55%) was the most common presenting complaint. Obstructive emphysema was demonstrated in 60% and was best demonstrated by inspiration-expiration chest roentgenograms or fluoroscopy. A radio-opaque object was seen in 13%. Two hundred ten foreign objects (93%) were removed by endoscopy. Four patients required pulmonary resection for bronchiectasis and in three patients bronchotomy was performed. Five patients expelled the foreign body spontaneously, two patients were transferred to another hospital, and one foreign body was not recovered. There was no mortality.

The sudden aspiration of a foreign object into the larynx, trachea or bronchus of a child is usually accompanied by respiratory distress. The event is most commonly referred to as a choking episode. A wheeze and persistent cough often follows. Diagnosis of the presence of a foreign body and the rapidity with which it is established is dependent on many factors. Two hundred twenty-five patients with confirmed diagnosis have been treated at the Children's Hospital Medical Center of Akron, Ohio, during the 25-year period May 1954 to December 1979. Analysis of these patients forms the basis of this report.

One hundred forty-two patients were male and 83 were female. This almost 2:1 incidence in males has been noted by others,[1] but no plausible reason has been proposed for this observation.

One hundred two objects were situated in the right bronchial tree and 100 in the left. The almost equal incidence[2] is quite different from the adult experience where the right side predominates. This might be explained by the fact that the left main stem bronchus has a more acute angle from the trachea in children. Eighteen objects (8%) were in the trachea and only 5 (2%) in the larynx.

TABLE 1. AGE OF PATIENTS

Years	*No.*
1	39
2	93
3	42
4	12
5	11
6	5
7	6
8	3
9	3
10 & Over	11

One hundred seventy-four incidents (77%) occurred in the first three years of life (Table 1). The youngest was five months of age. The exploring child in this age group is often partially edentulous and has a tendency to place any object in the mouth. A solid object entering the pharynx elicits a startle response permitting the foreign body to enter the open larynx during forced inspiration.

Food or food products accounted for 157 instances (70%) (Table 2). A portion of nut, particu-

TABLE 2. TYPE OF FOREIGN BODY

	No.
Portion of Nut	86
Food	32
Carrot	18
Popcorn	8
Fruit (Stem, Seed)	5
Bone	8
Plastic	27
Metal	19
Tooth	4
Stone	4
Timothy Hay	4
Miscellaneous	
Bead	2
Mucus	2
Balloon	1
Crayon	1
Wood	1
Paper	1
Acorn	1
Pine Needle	1

From the Surgical Service of the Children's Hospital Medical Center of Akron, Akron, Ohio.

Presented at the meeting of the American Broncho-Esophagological Association, Palm Beach, Florida, April 12-13, 1980.

REPRINTS — Bruce F. Rothmann, MD, Surgical Service, Children's Hospital Medical Center of Akron, Akron, OH 44308.

TABLE 3. PRESENTING HISTORY AND SIGNS

History of Aspiration	191
Wheeze	123
Fever	60
Recurrent Pneumonia	17
Respiratory Distress	14

larly peanut, is most frequently found and is the causative agent in 38% of all cases. It is obvious that these foods should neither be offered nor made accessible to small children. It is of importance that plastic objects are seen more frequently than metal in recent years. This may delay diagnosis as plastic is rarely radio-opaque. Timothy grass, while present in only four patients, is particularly treacherous, as discussed by Jewett and Butsch.[3] In two patients a timothy grass head was extracted from the posterior basal segment because it was suspected. It could not be visualized with the bronchoscope.

One hundred ninety-one patients (85%) had a history of a definite event, either of aspiration or choking, most often accompanied by paroxysms of coughing (Table 3). This may be followed by a relatively asymptomatic interval. The actual event was often recalled only after the diagnosis had been established. It is significant, however, that in 40 patients (18%) the diagnosis was established more than one week after the event and in 19 (8%) more than one month later. In 123 (55%), a wheeze was present. Auscultation often revealed this to be present only on the side involved. The sudden appearance of a wheeze in a child who has not previously manifested asthma should arouse a strong suspicion of the presence of a foreign body.

Fever was present in 60 cases (27%) and usually subsided promptly once the foreign body was removed.

Recurrent pneumonia was the prominent finding in 17 patients (7.5%). This was most commonly segmental in type and did not respond to antibiotic therapy. A history of repeated or persistent lobar or segmental pneumonia demands investigation for foreign body.

Only 14 (6%) presented with acute respiratory distress. This was most frequently seen in patients with laryngeal or tracheal obstruction. Two patients manifested transient evidence of cerebral hypoxia.

Obstructive emphysema was found in 135 (60%) patients on the chest roentgenogram (Table 4). The "expansile check valve" action[4] of the foreign body, allowing the air to enter but not exit, is most easily demonstrated on the inspiration-expiration views. The expiration film shows the involved lung to be overdistended and the mediastinal structures displaced to the opposite side.

TABLE 4. X-RAY FINDINGS

Obstructive Emphysema	135
Foreign Body Visualized	31
Atelectasis	27
Pneumonia	18
Normal	17
Mediastinal Emphysema	4

Fluoroscopy was done if the films were not conclusive. In occasional patients, air-trapping and mediastinal swing can be demonstrated only by fluoroscopy during vigorous ventilation.[1] This was added to the diagnostic work-up if a suggestive history was present and the diagnosis was not established on the inspiration-expiration views.

Complete obstruction to the flow of air will produce atelectasis (12%) and/or pneumonia (8%).

No change is seen in the minimally obstructed airway and the chest roentgenogram was interpreted as normal in 17 cases (7.5%).

The foreign body was visualized in 31 instances (13%).

Four patients manifested mediastinal emphysema indicating disruption of the bronchial wall.

The foreign body was removed by bronchoscopy or laryngoscopy in 208 (93%) of the patients (Table 5). All procedures were performed under general anesthesia. Two objects were removed by direct laryngoscopy in the emergency room. Thirteen required more than one bronchoscopic procedure with removal of the foreign body in eight. The rigid, distally lighted bronchoscope (Jackson) was used in most instances. The Hopkins rod-lens bronchoscope (Storz)[5] with self-contained grasping forceps, recently introduced, has been a valuable addition to the instrumentation. Removal of a small round foreign body may be facilitated by performing bronchoscopy in a head down position. In this position, the foreign object is less likely to be advanced to a segmental bronchus, and gravity may permit it to pass readily through the bronchoscope. The foreign body usually is impinged against the bronchoscope with the forceps and both instruments withdrawn together. The bronchoscope is then reinserted and careful examination is done to assure that no foreign body remains.

Lobectomy or segmental resection was performed

TABLE 5. TREATMENT

Bronchoscopy with Removal	205
Laryngoscopy with Removal	5
Spontaneous Expulsion	5
Lobectomy	4
Thoracotomy with Removal	3
Unsuccessful Treatment	3
Tracheostomy	6

in four patients. Bronchiectasis was present in all specimens. The foreign body involved (peanuts - 2, timothy grass - 1, plastic - 1) was not suspected in three of the four patients. The foreign body was identified in the specimen. It is of interest that no pulmonary resection has been done in the last 145 cases.

Three patients required thoracotomy for removal of a distal foreign body. A tooth was present in two patients and metal in the other. In each instance, the foreign object was removed by bronchotomy without sacrifice of significant lung tissue.

Tube thoracostomy with water seal drainage was required for pneumothorax following bronchoscopy in two patients.

Tracheostomy was performed on six patients. Three were performed prior to removal of the foreign body and three were done after endoscopic removal of the foreign body.

Five patients (2%) spontaneously expelled an identifiable foreign body. Postural drainage as suggested by Burrington and Cotton[6] and Cotton et al[7] has not been utilized. The danger of dislodging a foreign body to the opposite side[8] seems to be greater with this method than in endoscopy which is expertly done and performed under excellent pediatric anesthesia. Close cooperation between the anesthesiologist and endoscopist is of paramount importance. The well-ventilated, relaxed patient affords the best situation for successful removal of the foreign body.

REFERENCES

1. Brown BSTJ, Ma H, Dunbar JS, MacEwan DW. Foreign bodies in the tracheobronchial tree in childhood. J Assoc Can Radiol 1963; 14:158-71.

2. Keith FM, Charrette EJP, Lynn RB, Salerno TA. Inhalation of foreign bodies by children: a continuing challenge in management. Can Med Assoc J 1980; 122:52-7.

3. Jewett TC, Butsch WL. Trials with treacherous timothy grass. J Thorac Cardiovasc Surg 1965; 50:124-6.

4. Jackson C. Bronchial obstruction. Dis Chest 1950; 17:125-50.

5. Gans S, Berci G. Advances in endoscopy of infants and children. J Pediatr Surg 1971; 6:199.

6. Burrington JD, Cotton EK. Removal of foreign bodies from the tracheobronchial tree. J Pediatr Surg 1972; 7:119-22.

7. Cotton EK, Abrams G, VanHoutte J, Burrington J. Removal of aspirated foreign bodies by inhalation and postural drainage. Clin Pediatr 1973; 12:271-6.

8. Law D, Kosloske AM. Management of tracheobronchial foreign bodies in children: a reevaluation of postural drainage and bronchoscopy. Pediatrics 1976; 58:362.

≈

ADVANCED COURSE IN PEDIATRIC OTOLARYNGOLOGY

A one-week course in Pediatric Otolaryngology will be held at the Institute of Child Health, University of London, November 17-21, 1980, in association with the Hospital for Sick Children. Applications are available from: Dean's secretary, Institute of Child Health, 30 Guilford St., London WC1N 1EH. (Tel: 01 242 9789.)

Ann Otol 89:1980

FOREIGN BODIES IN THE AIRWAY

FIVE-YEAR RETROSPECTIVE STUDY WITH SPECIAL REFERENCE TO MANAGEMENT

SEYMOUR R. COHEN, MD
GEORGE B. LEWIS, JR., MD
WAYNE I. HERBERT, MD
KENNETH A. GELLER, MD
LOS ANGELES, CALIFORNIA

The charts of 143 patients with foreign bodies in the larynx and tracheobronchial tree who were admitted to the Childrens Hospital of Los Angeles during the period 1973 to 1978 were reviewed. Of these children 84 were male and 59 were female. One hundred were private patients and forty-three were clinic patients. Of these foreign bodies 60 were nut meat which is by far the most common foreign body of the tracheobronchial tree. All foreign bodies were successfully removed. One hundred twenty-six were discharged within the first 24 hours after admission and treatment. Fifty-one or 36% of these patients were discharged on the same day after the foreign body was removed. Sixty-two of the foreign bodies were in the left bronchial tree, while 55 were in the right bronchial tree. One hundred thirty-eight were endoscoped under general anesthesia using the apneic technique and five patients were treated with oxygen standby only because of severe respiratory obstruction. A detailed description of the use of apneic technique with profound muscle relaxation, the avoidance of preoperative medication and the team approach to ventilating the patients are all described. The advantage of general anesthesia, and the potential intraoperative and postoperative problems are reviewed. Of the total number of cases 13% were between 4 and 11 months of age, 44% were between 12 and 23 months of age and 57% were over 23 months of age.

INTRODUCTION

During the era of the Jacksons and many of their disciples (Clerf, Tucker, Van Loon, Atkins and Holinger, to name a few), removal of foreign bodies from the larynx and tracheobronchial tree was performed without anesthesia. For many years the use of anesthesia was considered dangerous and contraindicated for the pediatric endoscopic procedure. However, with the development of newer methods, drugs and techniques and the advances of anesthesiology as a specialty, general anesthesia has been used increasingly for endoscopic procedures in children. General anesthesia remains contraindicated in cases where there are severe obstructive diseases from whatever cause or where the airway cannot be controlled.

General anesthesia facilitates both the endoscopic procedure and the removal of the foreign body. It reduces trauma to the anatomic structures invaded by the endoscope, eliminates discomfort and trauma to the psyche, and gives complete compliance on the part of the patient without restraints. The ease of endoscopy and more effective and delicate application of a forceps under general anesthesia makes for less trauma and fewer complications. It is not, however, a substitute for the skill and competence of the endoscopist.

In the removal of foreign bodies in children there is no substitute for the open rigid endoscope. All techniques which are used for aiding the obstructed patient in an emergency, such as pounding the back, postural drainage, bronchodilators, finger probing of the throat and Heimlich procedures, are dangerous and should be discouraged unless there is no choice because of obstruction of the airway which is unrelieved by the patient's own reflexes. These techniques may result in further impaction and the possibility of total obstruction not present prior to these attempts. These efforts may also delay transfer of a child to a proper facility for medical care.

Foreign bodies produce varying degrees of airway obstruction. In children who at first examination have little or no obstruction, attempts at extraction or improper use of a general anesthetic may increase obstruction. Thus there may be an unnecessary toll in increased morbidity and mortality unless intense attention to details is observed.

The purpose of this paper is to outline some of the statistics of the foreign bodies in the airway which were treated over a five-year period at the Childrens Hospital of Los Angeles and to detail the methods of anesthesia used in the management of these cases.

LITERATURE REVIEW

Choking on foods has been the cause of between 2,500 to 3,900 deaths per year in this country.[1] It is the sixth most common cause of accidental deaths. Fifty-five percent of aspirated foreign bodies involve the respiratory tract in children six months to four years of age.[2] It is estimated that in over one third of these children the accident is neither observed nor suspected, a fact which has contributed to many complications and a high incidence of un-

From the Department of Surgery, Divisions of Otolaryngology and Anesthesiology, Childrens Hospital of Los Angeles and University of Southern California Medical School, Los Angeles, California.

Presented at the meeting of the American Broncho-Esophagological Association, Palm Beach, Florida, April 12-13, 1980.

REPRINTS — Seymour R. Cohen, MD, 1300 North Vermont Avenue, Los Angeles, CA 90027.

TABLE 1. STATISTICAL ANALYSIS OF CASES (N = 143)

1973-1978

Sex		Age	
Male	- 84	4-11 mos	- 19
Female	- 59	12-23 mos	- 63
		2 yrs	- 23
		3 yrs	- 9
		4 yrs	- 3
		5 yrs	- 4
Financial Status		6 yrs	- 8
Private patients	- 100	7-12 yrs	- 12
Clinical patients	- 43	Over 12 yrs	- 2

necessary morbidity. The severity of the potential dangers during foreign body extractions under general anesthesia are well documented by Ward and Benumof.[3] For many years the mere suggestion of the use of general anesthesia for endoscopy in the pediatric age group generated considerable heat. Tucker in his Chevalier Jackson lecture noted the advances and increasing acceptance of general anesthesia for endoscopy.[4] Leigh and Belton[5] described the use of a profound muscle relaxant in combination with Fluothane® and succinylcholine given intravenously in multiple doses or by intravenous drip. This technique had been used at Childrens Hospital of Los Angeles for at least three or four years prior to the publication of their book. In 1966 the discussion following Morse and Hartman's paper[6] presented before The American Broncho-Esophagological Association reflected the diversity of opinion of that day regarding general anesthesia and the use of apneic technique specifically.

In a symposium before The American Broncho-Esophagological Association Fearon[7] opens his discussion of anesthesia in pediatric peroral endoscopy with the statement that it is like the title of a popular song, "All or Nothing at All." He reinforces an attitude gained from many years of experience that halfway measures, a little of this and a little of that, are unsuitable for endoscopy in the pediatric age group.

STATISTICAL ANALYSIS OF PATIENTS

The charts of 143 cases of foreign bodies in the larynx and tracheobronchial tree treated over a five-year period were reviewed. Eighty-four (59%) were male and 59 (41%) were female; 19 of these children (13%) were under one year of age, 63 were 12 to 23 months of age, and 23 were under three years of age (Table 1).

Nut meat was by far the most common type of foreign body, occurring in 78 (55%) of the cases.

TABLE 2. TYPES OF FOREIGN BODY

Peanuts	49	Rocks	5
Food particles	29	Watermelon seeds	4
Metal	24	Foil and paper	2
Other nuts	11	Glass	1
Sunflower seeds	10	Miscellaneous	2
Plastic	6		

TABLE 3. SITE OF ENLODGEMENT

Left bronchus	- 62
Right bronchus	- 55
Trachea	- 13
Larynx	- 6
Trachea and bronchus	- 3
Bilateral bronchus	- 3
Bilateral bronchus & trachea	- 1

Food particles were aspirated in 29 cases (20%) and metallic objects were next most common, seen in 24 cases (16.7%) (Table 2). Of great interest is the occurrence of more foreign bodies in the left bronchial tree (62 cases, or 43%), a fact which is contrary to common belief based on anatomic details. Fifty-five (38%) were found in the right bronchial tree. Only six (4%) of the cases were in the larynx, and the remaining 19% were in the trachea or were multiple, in the trachea and one or both bronchi (Table 3).

Foreign bodies were lodged for a varying length of time. Fifty-nine (41%) were recognized and treated within the first 24 hours after aspiration. The remainder of the cases were scattered between five days to one year with the longest impaction of a foreign body being present for over one year (Table 4).

General anesthesia was used in 138 cases (96.5%) and oxygen standby without any anesthesia was used in five of the cases (3.5%) (Table 5). A general anesthetic was not used in children in whom there was severe airway obstruction and in those children in whom the airway could not be controlled. Of these five patients, three had impacted laryngeal foreign bodies and two had sunflower seeds severely obstructing the tracheal lumen.

The postoperative discharge of patients following the endoscopic procedure was as follows. One hundred twenty-five (88%) were discharged within the first 24 hours after the endoscopic procedure. Of these 51 (36%) were discharged soon after recovery from the general anesthetic. Seventy-five (52%) of the patients were discharged by the following day making a total of 125 (88%) being discharged within 24 hours of the endoscopic procedure. Fifteen cases (10%) were discharged within 48 hours and two cases remained hospitalized for 72 hours because of postoperative laryngitis or social problems (Table 6).

The postoperative problems were chiefly those related to the foreign body reactions and occasionally due to the endoscopic procedure. The most common was subglottic laryngeal edema in 22 chil-

TABLE 4. DURATION OF ENLODGEMENT

2-8 hrs	- 24
8-24 hrs	- 35
1-5 days	- 14
5-10 days	- 14
10-30 days	- 19
1-6 mos	- 9
6 mos - 1 yr	- 2
Longer	- 1

TABLE 5. ANESTHESIA

General	- 138
Standby O_2	- 5

dren; in most of these only humidified air and an extra dose or two of dexamethasone were required. A number of these children had been referred after having had an endoscopic procedure performed elsewhere (15 patients). Bronchitis occurred in six children more often due to the foreign body reaction and three had edema and fever due to the manipulation of the foreign body in an already infected area. Pneumonia occurred in two, the result of impaction and longstanding foreign bodies in the airway. Laryngotracheobronchitis (LTB) occurred in two patients (Table 7).

Twenty-six children required a second procedure because of the presence, at the time of the removal of the foreign body, of a granulomatous reaction, bronchial stenosis, persistent pneumonia or suppurative process. The procedure was performed in order to insure complete resolution and to prevent chronic stenotic lesions in the bronchi. A second procedure was performed on one patient who was referred from another hospital after an unsuccessful attempt to remove a metallic foreign body with a fiberoptic bronchoscope. The foreign body was distal to the visibility afforded by the bronchoscope and this patient required removal with a second procedure which was successful, using the image intensifier.

ANESTHESIA MANAGEMENT

The technique described requires an experienced, skillful endoscopist in concert with a compatible, experienced anesthesiologist. A team approach is of utmost importance. A competent operating room technician or nurse in a well equipped surgical amphitheater and available consultation with a pediatrician, radiologist and thoracic surgeon all are essential. A thoracic surgeon is rarely required except in cases in which the foreign body has wandered to the periphery of the lung and cannot be removed with the image intensifier. Thoracotomy then may be necessary but is rarely justified and was not required in any of the patients reported in this series.

The airway is shared by both endoscopist and anesthesiologist and therefore the maintenance of adequate ventilation, which is of the highest priority, is totally dependent on these two members of the team. Each must concentrate on maintaining the airway with adequate ventilation at all times.

TABLE 6. POSTOPERATIVE DISCHARGE

Same day	- 51
Next day	- 75
Two days	- 15
Over three days*	- 2

*Either croup or parental-social problem.

TABLE 7. POSTOPERATIVE COMPLICATIONS

Croup	- 22
Bronchitis	- 6
Edema	- 3
Fever	- 3
Pneumonia	- 2
LTB	- 2

There can be no compromising of this need for even a single moment.

The skilled operating room technician is aware of the endoscopist's needs and wastes no time in ensuring adequate lighting, change in instrumentation and adequate suctioning and maintenance of the equipment.

The pediatrician is most important in the early recognition of the disease and should seek immediate consultation with the endoscopist. He will aid in the treatment of pneumonia, bronchiectasis or bronchial suppuration which may persist after removal of the foreign bodies of long sojourn. The earlier the diagnosis, the fewer will be the laryngeal, bronchial and pulmonary complications and the easier will be the extraction of the foreign body.

PREOPERATIVE EVALUATION

The presentation and complications of foreign bodies affect the duration of the procedure, make removal difficult and may require modification of the type of anesthesia. These are bronchial suppuration, bronchial ulceration and granulation tissue formation, bronchial stenosis, peribronchial and peritracheal lymphadenopathy with compression of the bronchi, pneumonitis, atelectasis, obstructive emphysema, pneumomediastinum, pneumothorax, hemoptysis and variable degrees of airway obstruction. These will be determined by the history of the foreign body presence, physical examination and roentgen studies.

A. Look for signs of airway obstruction, quantitate the respiratory distress, note the respiratory rate, characteristics of breathing (such as stridor, retractions, presence or absence of cyanosis, anxiety) and finally evaluate the child's sensorium.

B. If possible determine whether the foreign body is in the larynx, trachea or bronchus. This is very important in determining the general approach and deciding whether a general anesthetic can be used. It is helpful to know the type of foreign body which was aspirated. This will permit determination as to whether it can be removed through the larynx. Encapsulated dry vegetable substances such as beans can swell in the presence of moisture and create difficulties in delivering the foreign body in one piece. This type of foreign body must be broken into smaller pieces to avoid total obstruction of the trachea when attempts are made to remove it intact from the bronchus. Close observation is necessary when breaking up the foreign body to prevent some of the pieces from occluding the originally unobstructed bronchus. It is important to determine by examination whether the larynx is obstructed by or edematous from the foreign body or whether there has been laryneal edema due to previous instrumentation. Voice change and a barking croupy cough will indicate this possibility. Where the foreign body is in the larynx or within the trachea, obstruction can be more severe. It is in these two areas that obstruction is most likely to create severe airway problems under general anesthesia. If multiple removals are necessary, preparation for reintroduction of the bronchoscope should be made soon after the first removal.

C. There is a higher incidence of laryngeal edema in children who have been previously endoscoped elsewhere. This complication may require postponement of the endoscopic procedure unless airway obstruction is major. The child may then be treated during this waiting period with antibiotics, humidified air and multiple sequential doses of steroids.

POTENTIAL INTRAOPERATIVE PROBLEMS

The greatest hazards of the entire procedure most frequently occur during the operative period. These arise from defective equipment, inability to ventilate the patient due to mechanical obstruction, hypoventilation (usually due to poor teamwork between anesthesiologist and endoscopist) leading to hypercarbia with respiratory acidosis, or hypoxia followed by arrhythmias which may lead to cardiac arrest. The longer the period of instrumentation and the larger the bronchoscope, the more likely laryngeal edema will occur. The endoscopist's skill and the use of proper-sized instruments will reduce further edema. The preference should be for the smallest bronchoscope to permit removal of the foreign body. Trauma is also reduced by adequate immobilization of the child's larynx with the appropriate anesthetic.

The loss of the intravenous cannula can result in a serious problem since the sudden need for a relaxant may not be instantly satisfied. During this very light period, the patient splints and ventilation can be difficult or impossible. This splinting has been interpreted as being due to bronchospasm, and calls for immediate relaxation and not bronchodilators. A plastic intravenous cannula is preferable since it is more dependable and secure.

To adequately ventilate the patient, the bronchoscope must be in direct alignment with the airway. Precautions against hyperextension of the head, especially in the very young infant, is mandatory. Hyperextension causes the bronchoscope to be directed anteriorly and makes ventilation difficult to impossible. The endoscopist must be aware of the difficulties in ventilating a patient when the bronchoscope is inserted deeply into the obstructed bronchus so that the normal lung cannot be ventilated. By judicious manipulation of the endoscope to a more proximal level this hazard can be prevented.

Cardiac arrhythmias, succinylcholine bradycardia and asystole have effectively been controlled or prevented by proper atropinization before the relaxant drug is administered. One milligram doses of atropine are sufficient and may be repeated as necessary.

Faulty equipment such as a loose anesthetic tube or a disconnection from the gas machine or bronchoscope should be immediately recognized by the endoscopist who with experience can detect any change in the color of the mucous membrane long before any change in the cardiac status is evident to the anesthesiologist with his monitors.

Another serious intraoperative problem is the removal of a large obstructive foreign body from the bronchus into the trachea or by stripping the foreign body off at the laryngeal level. This would impair ventilation and immediate steps should be taken to remove the object from the larynx or upper trachea. If this is not possible, the foreign object should be pushed into one of the bronchi so that ventilation can proceed with the unobstructed lung. Should none of these alternatives be possible, the foreign body will require fragmentation to allow ventilation. It can then be removed when the patient's condition has been stabilized by proper ventilation.

POTENTIAL POSTOPERATIVE PROBLEMS

For the immediate postoperative care of the patient a competent recovery room staff is essential. Postbronchoscopic laryngospasm is rare in our experience. Spraying of the larynx with local anesthetics has been advised to prevent such an occurrence. It was not used, however, in this series of patients. Laryngospasm becomes a problem and occurs when the anesthetized patient is not deep enough or light enough to have permitted all of his reflexes to have returned. It will never occur when the patient is adequately relaxed. To prevent laryngospasm, the bronchoscope should never be removed unless the patient is either wide awake with all reflexes having been recovered, or is still under the influence of succinylcholine. It will not occur if the patient has not been given preoperative medication or if the larynx or pharynx has not been sprayed with local anesthesia, thus allowing for rapid recovery of the protective reflexes. Laryngeal edema is prevented by the use of a proper-sized bronchoscope and with minimal manipulation of the bronchoscope so that the larynx is not the fulcrum of the force of those manipulations. The use of Decadron® (dexamethasone) preoperatively and at times postoperatively when necessary effectively reduces airway obstruction from laryngeal edema. Intravenous fluids and high humidification with a solosphere in the recovery room will usually suffice to correct any minor laryngeal involvement. Racemic epinephrine has rarely if ever been necessary.

AWAKE TECHNIQUE

The child is mummified with a large cotton blanket and a reliable intravenous route is established in an ankle or foot vein. After preoxygenation with the patient being monitored by the anesthesiologist, the foreign body is extracted through the laryngoscope while a high flow of oxygen is insufflated into the mouth by means of a catheter. Basal and preoperative local anesthesia were never used because they create hypoventilation or will interfere with the protective reflexes of the respiratory tract in the immediate postoperative period. If bronchoscopy is required with the patient breathing spontaneously the oxygen adapter can be applied to the side arm of the bronchoscope and the patient can be aided in his ventilation.

ANESTHESIA METHODS

Preanesthetic Medication. Narcotics and sedative drugs including scopolamine are contraindicated because they may depress respirations and contribute to further respiratory embarrassment with resultant hypoventilation. These drugs also delay emergence from anesthesia and prolong recovery, thus interfering with the protective cough and gag reflex.

Preinduction. Before the anesthetic is started the patient is placed on a circulatory water mattress and the body temperature is monitored continuously from a Thermister probe inserted deeply into the axilla. The cardiovascular system is monitored by means of a precordial stethoscope, blood pressure cuff and electrocardiograph.

Intraoperative Management. A choice of whether to use oxygen standby only or a general anesthetic will be determined by the anesthetist and endoscopist in consultation. During the past five years, general anesthesia was employed in 96.5% of the patients in this series. The remaining patients were treated on an emergency basis and general anesthesia was not employed because of the presence of severe respiratory obstruction. Usually, obstruction resulted from the foreign body being within the larynx or in the upper trachea lumen almost occluding the airway. In a rare instance where marked cardiopulmonary distress was associated with extensive air-trapping or mediastinal shift, pneumomediastinum or pneumothorax caused by ball valve action of the foreign body, general anesthesia was not used. However it is not contraindicated in those patients with these complications if the airway is secure and ventilation is adequate.

Induction. Anesthesia is induced with a mixture of nitrous oxide, halothane and oxygen. As soon as the patient is unconscious, the respirations are assisted by manual compression of the breathing bag, and the character of each breath is carefully evaluated for adequacy. The tidal air can usually be evaluated and must be adequate and assured before paralyzing the patient. If inadequate ventilation occurs not expected from preoperative evaluation, the child should be awakened and the awake technique should be used.

Maintenance of Anesthesia. Once the decision has been made to continue with the anesthesia, the anesthetic route is one which permits intermittent ease of ventilating the lungs and allows sufficient time for the atraumatic manipulations of the bronchoscope. These needs can be fulfilled with the apneic relaxant technique, which consists of a light plane of general anesthesia accompanied by a muscle relaxant. Safety of the anesthesia is enhanced by the administration of 95 to 100% oxygen just prior to and during the induced apnea. This procedure establishes a high pulmonary reservoir of oxygen as well as complete saturation of the arterial blood and delays the onset of hypoxia. Inasmuch as carbon dioxide will accumulate during the periods of apnea, it is essential to ventilate the lungs at frequent intervals to prevent hypercarbia and respiratory acidosis. This requires a very close interplay between endoscopist and anesthesiologist.

The anesthetic procedure is as follows. Just prior to the endoscopic procedure, the nitrous oxide is discontinued. The halothane concentration is reduced to 0.5% or less and the lungs are hyperventilated with a high concentration of oxygen for one to two minutes. Ideal conditions are obtained by profound muscular relaxation which is achieved by the use of a short-acting depolarizing muscle relaxant, succinylcholine, given intravenously in one or more boluses as required. Succinylcholine may be given as a continuous drip of a dilute concentration of 0.2% when this is occasionally required for prolonged procedures. When given as a bolus, the dose is 2 mg per kg body weight, and it must be initially preceded by atropine 0.1 mg given intravenously in order to prevent nodal bradycardia or cardiac asystole, which are often associated with the cholinergic properties of succinylcholine. If multiple doses are required the atropine dose may be repeated as necessary. Long-acting muscle relaxants such as curare and Pavulon® are avoided because muscle relaxation with these drugs is inadequate except with very high doses. Large amounts of these drugs may be difficult to reverse with Prostigmin® thus making it necessary to ventilate the patient for a considerable length of time after the procedure has been completed.

Ventilation of the lungs via the mask technique continues as the patient becomes fully paralyzed. As soon as the bronchoscope is placed into the trachea, the side arm of the bronchoscope is attached to the circle absorption system by means of a short, flexible rubber tube, and the lungs are ventilated again with a high concentration of oxygen. At frequent intervals throughout the procedure, the respirations are intermittently controlled by simultaneous occlusion of the open end of the bronchoscope with the endoscopist's thumb while the anesthesiologist manually compresses the breathing bag. This aspect of the procedure is facilitated by having the patient completely relaxed, but requires a high degree of cooperation between the surgeon and the anesthesiologist.

In patients with multiple foreign bodies or where the foreign body requires fragmentation, it is necessary to repeatedly remove and introduce the bronchoscope. The respirations may be controlled by face mask technique after the bronchoscope is removed. However, where the endoscopist is skillful, the interval between removing the fragment and reintroducing the bronchoscope may be no more than five to ten seconds and mask anesthesia may not be necessary. It is extremely important to maintain profound muscular relaxation with succinylcholine until the total extraction of the foreign body objects is completed, in order to facilitate instrumentation and ventilation of the lungs. In older children, and during prolonged procedures, halothane anesthesia becomes inadequate and it is necessary to administer very small increments of thiopental intravenously to maintain unconsciousness.

Emergence from Anesthesia. After extraction of the foreign body and completion of the procedure, there is a general tendency for the entire team to become elated and thus attention may be diverted from the care of the patient. The anesthesiologist and the endoscopist must not join in this celebration but must instantly carry out an organized plan of ventilating the patient without distractions of any kind.

In those children with food in the stomach and where the procedure is urgent and cannot be postponed because of severe obstruction to the airway, postbronchoscopic intubation of the patient with an endotracheal tube of a smaller size than usual for this age should be performed. The tube should be left in place while the patient is ventilated until fully awake. In children where the stomach is empty, face mask ventilation after removing the bronchoscope will suffice to give assisted or controlled respirations until the residual succinylcholine is metabolized and the patient is awake, crying and breathing adequately. Laryngospasm or so-called bronchospasm is rarely seen during the emergence when the bronchoscope is removed at the proper depth of anesthesia.

Because of instrumentation and frequent inflammatory problems from the foreign body, dexamethasone phosphate is given in intravenous doses, 4 mg to infants and 8 mg to older children, prior to the endoscopic procedure. This will reduce and minimize subglottic edema. Because preanesthetic medication has not been used and intravenous depressants are minimal during the procedure, the patients are expected to awaken and cry or talk before they leave the operating room. Complications have been minimal with the described technique above. One patient had a prolonged apnea from succinylcholine as a result of a pseudocholinesterase deficiency. This patient required ventilation for approximately three hours after the endoscopic procedure had been completed.

CONCLUSIONS

General anesthesia using a controlled apneic technique with light halothane anesthesia associated with profound relaxation using a short-acting muscle relaxant, succcinylcholine, has given ideal conditions for the successful removal of foreign bodies. This technique has been used for well over 30 years at The Childrens Hospital of Los Angeles. Of the 143 cases of laryngeal and tracheobronchial foreign bodies, 138 were treated with the techniques described within this paper. The avoidance of preoperative basal anesthesia and spraying of the throat with local anesthesia make possible rapid emergence from the anesthesia with rapid return of normal protective reflexes. These features make for ideal, atraumatic operating room endoscopic experiences. There were no serious complications and no deaths in this series of patients.

REFERENCES

1. Eller WC, Haugen RK. Food asphyxiation. N Engl J Med 1973; 289:81.

2. Anderson DL. Death from improper mastication. Int Dent J 1977; 27:349-54.

3. Ward CF, Benumof JL. Anesthesia for airway foreign body extraction in children. Anesthesiol Rev 1977; Dec:13-5.

4. Tucker GF Jr. Pediatric laryngobronchoesophagology. Ann Otol Rhinol Laryngol 1979; 88:784-93.

5. Leigh MD, Belton MK. Pediatric anesthesiology. 2nd ed. New York: MacMillan, 1960.

6. Morse HR, Hartman MM. General anesthesia for peroral endoscopy: apneic technique. Ann Otol Rhinol Laryngol 1966; 75:1040-8.

7. Fearon B. Anesthesia in pediatric peroral endoscopy. Ann Otol Rhinol Laryngol 1969; 78:469-75.

Ann Otol 89:1980

ENDOSCOPY AND BIOPSY IN GASTROESOPHAGEAL REFLUX IN INFANTS AND CHILDREN

BRUCE BENJAMIN, FRACS

DAVID POHL, MB, BS

PATRICIA M. BALE, FRCPA

SYDNEY, AUSTRALIA

The clinical features of abnormal gastroesophageal reflux in infants and children extend beyond repeated vomiting and include dysphagia, pain, bleeding, failure to thrive, esophageal stricture, and recurrent respiratory symptoms including aspiration pneumonitis and cyanotic attacks. The unreliability of the traditional barium swallow examination as a diagnostic test is well known. This study reports the results of endoscopic assessment and esophageal biopsy in 100 infants and children and relates them to the clinical findings and the changes in the contrast esophagogram. The results show that further valuable diagnostic information can be gained from endoscopic examination of the esophageal mucosa, especially when there is esophagitis with ulceration, bleeding, or stricture. Endoscopic biopsies are useful to confirm the presence of esophagitis but biopsies alone do not give absolute diagnostic information.

Gastroesophageal reflux is a common problem which occurs when the lower esophageal sphincter is incompetent and characteristically commences in the neonatal period with vomiting occurring at any time during or between feedings. The clinical features of gastroesophageal reflux are known to extend beyond repeated vomiting. They include failure to thrive, dysphagia, pain, bleeding, anemia, esophageal stricture and recurrent respiratory symptoms including aspiration pneumonitis and cyanotic attacks due to aspiration.[1] There is still confusion as to the etiology and the nature of abnormal gastroesophageal reflux and the mechanism of action of the distal esophageal sphincter.[2]

Besides the clinical features and the fact that gastroesphageal reflux may be demonstrated by contrast esophagogram, any test that gives objective supplemental evidence is useful. The tests available include esophagoscopy and endoscopic assessment, esophageal biopsy,[3,4] manometric studies and 24-hour pH monitoring of the distal esophagus.[5,6] We are reporting our experience with esophagoscopy and esophageal biopsy in 100 infants and children.

METHODS

All children were in-patients at the Royal Alexandra Hospital for Children, Sydney, Australia, between 1970 and 1979. The records of 100 infants and children who had esophageal biopsy were reviewed. Ninety-four patients in the group studied had clinical features suggesting gastroesophageal reflux sufficient to warrant study in hospital. Six patients with purely respiratory symptoms had esophagoscopy as part of a diagnostic endoscopic examination and biopsies were taken as controls. The group studied represented not only patients with straightforward gastroesophageal reflux but also those in whom it was associated with repaired tracheoesophageal fistula, cerebral palsy, or other congenital anomalies. Also in the group were patients who presented a diagnostic problem where the clinical features and the contrast esophagogram did not clearly indicate the diagnosis. Others again were of a severe nature, unresponsive to medical treatment and were being considered for antireflux surgery.

All examinations were performed under general anesthetic. A rigid Negus esophagoscope was used and the mucosa of the esophageal wall was assessed first with the naked eye and then with the Hopkins telescope in all cases.

The biopsies were taken using sharp, double-action cup biopsy forceps 3 mm in diameter. Multiple biopsies were usually taken from the posterior esophageal wall, the first biopsy 2 or 3 cm above the gastroesophageal mucosal junction and a further biopsy or biopsies at measured intervals above this. There were no complications. The biopsies were examined histologically for elongation of the papillae greater than two thirds, thickening of the basal cell layer to more than three or four cells, ulceration, severe inflammation and fibrosis. The result of the endoscopic assessment and the esophageal biopsy was related to the clinical features and the changes in the contrast esophagogram.

RESULTS

The age range of the children was from 3 days to 15 years. The average age was 35 months. Of the 94 patients with gastroesophageal reflux 59 were male and 35 were female, showing a marked male preponderance, almost 2 to 1.

The clinical features are shown in Table 1. Although vomiting was by far the commonest symptom, many patients had multiple symptoms.

The barium swallow was positive in 65% according to the technique used in our radiology department. Screening examination with spot films is performed, using thin barium with the patient lying supine and slightly turned to the right.

The endoscopic findings were positive in 81% as judged by the presence of localized or generalized changes including granularity, bleeding to touch, slough, ulceration, exudate or stricture. Erythema alone was not considered a diagnostic abnormality.

From the Royal Alexandra Hospital for Children, Sydney, Australia.

Presented at the meeting of the American Broncho-Esophagological Association, Palm Beach, Florida, April 12-13, 1980.

REPRINTS — Bruce Benjamin, FRACS, 229 Macquarie Street, Sydney NSW 2000, Australia.

TABLE 1. CLINICAL FEATURES

Clinical Features	*(%)*
Vomiting	59
Hematemesis	14
Feeding difficulty	10
Cyanotic attacks	10
Pain	8
Cough	7
Dysphagia	4

Histologically, the criteria used for "reflux change" were elongation of papillae to two thirds of the mucosal thickness, in addition to basal hyperplasia to at least three to four layers thick. There were 66 positive biopsies (70%). These included 28 with reflux change only, 18 with ulceration or severe inflammation, 16 with reflux change combined with ulceration, severe inflammation or columnar epithelium and 3 with fibrosis. There were 34 negative biopsies (17 normal, 8 minor nondiagnostic change and 9 columnar epithelium only which could have come from the stomach).

When microscopic findings included 1) ulceration or fibrosis; or 2) reflux change combined with columnar epithelium, ulcer, or inflammation, the correlation with positive endoscopic and radiological findings was very high. However, when microscopy revealed reflux change alone, the correlation was poor, 7 of 28 having normal barium swallow and endoscopic appearance. Similarly 9 of 17 histologically normal mucosae had reflux on barium swallow and redness on endoscopy.

DISCUSSION

It is highly probable that all infants have some degree of gastroesophageal reflux at some time and the distinction from vomiting, regurgitation and possetting may be impossible. It is often difficult to make a reliable diagnosis on the clinical features alone. Although the barium swallow has traditionally been regarded as a diagnostic radiological investigation, the unreliability of a single barium swallow examination even when performed by an experienced pediatric radiologist is well known. We found the barium swallow positive in 66% of cases and it is obvious that further diagnostic information would be valuable.

The endoscopic assessment of esophageal mucosa is reliable when there is ulceration, bleeding, or stricture and our study showed positive endoscopic findings in 81%. The significance of the findings is less reliable when there is merely redness, granularity, or the appearance reported as "erythematous."

The biopsy specimen with the Storz double action cup forceps is more satisfactory than that reported by others in adults where the biopsies were taken with small cup forceps through a flexible fiberoptic endoscope. In our opinion it seems reasonable that multiple biopsies of larger diameter are more satisfactory than a single small biopsy and reflect the changes through the length of the esophageal wall more adequately. Our study showed positive changes in 70%.

Ismail-Beigi et al[3] in 1970 reexamined the currently accepted histological features of esophagitis. They stated that the histological changes in the esophagus in the presence of gastroesophageal reflux in man included thickness of the basal zone more than 15% of the normal thickness of the epithelium and extension of the papillae more than two thirds of the distance to the epithelial surface. The presence of round cells such as lymphocytes and plasma cells in the lamina propria was designated as normal.

Behar and Sheahan[4] in 1975 found that the coexistence in at least two biopsy specimens of lamina propria papillae height greater than 50% of mucosal thickness, and basal cell proliferation that was greater than 15% of mucosal thickness, occurred in 95% of patients with reflux esophagitis and in none of the asymptomatic patients. They stressed that both changes could be present in a patient with clinical evidence of mild esophagitis but with an esophagus which appeared endoscopically normal. They also confirmed that lymphocyte, histiocyte, eosinophil or plasma cell infiltrates of the lamina propria do not correlate with the symptoms or objective findings in patients with reflux esophagitis. Intraepithelial and lamina propria neutrophil infiltrates were considered to have a low sensitivity as a criterion of esophagitis.

So far as we know there have been no previous studies relating endoscopy and biopsy in the pediatric age group. The diagnosis of gastroesophageal reflux is notoriously difficult to make with certainty and may remain inconclusive. Consequently we feel that it is reasonable to assume that patients with positive barium study, endoscopic findings, and biopsy findings have true gastroseophageal reflux. In our study only 45 of 94 (48%) met these triple criteria. It is interesting to note that the biopsy findings increased the diagnosis by only 2 cases, as 47 had positive barium and endoscopic findings.

Obviously in many patients only one of these three investigations showed a positive result. If we regard these as the false positive rates for the individual procedures, there were 4 false positives for barium swallow, 3 for endoscopy and 11 for biopsy of the total of 94 cases. It seems to us that such a high false positive rate for biopsy precludes its usefulness as an absolute diagnostic procedure, but it is useful to confirm the presence of esophagitis which has already been seen at endoscopy. This study in infants and children is in contrast to those in adults[3,4] which report a high correlation with biopsy.

Gastroesophageal reflux in infants and children is

a challenging diagnostic problem. The clinical features are of foremost importance and the barium swallow may not be diagnostic. The presence of esophagitis and ulceration is best determined by esophagoscopy with confirmatory biopsy. Endoscopic examination gives valuable information in guiding the clinician in management, especially in cases which are complicated or are diagnostic problems, eg, in repaired tracheoesophageal fistula, where there is aspiration pneumonitis or where asthma is thought to be on the basis of inhalation or in patients who have cyanotic or apneic attacks. The added information that esophagitis from reflux is present is also valuable in patients being considered for antireflux surgery.

We now favor placement of a pH probe and 24-hour pH monitoring following the endoscopic assessment. We have not sufficient experience with pH study to correlate it with our endoscopic findings but we believe it may be another important test in defining the presence or absence of significant gastroesophageal reflux.

REFERENCES

1. Christie DL, O'Grady LR, Mack DV. Incompetent lower esophageal sphincter and gastroesophageal reflux in current acute pulmonary disease of infancy and childhood. J Pediatr 1978; 93:23-7.

2. Moroz SP, Espinoza J, Cumming WA, Diamant NE. Lower esophageal sphincter function in children with and without gastroesophageal reflux. Gastroenterology 1976; 71:236-46.

3. Ismail-Beigi F, Horton PH, Pope CE. Histological consequences of gastroesophageal reflux in man. Gastroenterology 1970; 58:163-74.

4. Behar J, Sheehan DC. Histologic abnormalities in reflux esophagitis. Arch Pathol 1975; 99:387-91.

5. Hill JL, Pelligrini CA, Burrington JD, Reyes HM, DeMeester TR. Technique and experience with 24-hour esophageal pH monitoring in children. J Pediatr Surg 1977; 12:877-87.

6. Johnson LF, DeMeester TR. Twenty-four-hour pH monitoring of the distal esophagus. Am J Gastroenterol 1974; 62:325-32.

≈

LURIE LIBRARY FUND

Many inquiries have been made about a memorial fund to which friends and colleagues of Dr. Moses Hyman Lurie could contribute. Shortly before his death Dr. Lurie established a modest fund for the purchase of books in Otolaryngology for the Library at the Massachusetts Eye and Ear Infirmary. The Library Committee of the Infirmary has verified that donations can be made in memory of Dr. Lurie to this fund. Contributions may be sent to the "Lurie Library Fund," in care of Mr. Charles Snyder, Librarian, Massachusetts Eye and Ear Infirmary, 243 Charles St., Boston, MA 02114.

Ann Otol 89:1980

THE CRICOPHARYNGEUS IN THE NEONATE

TIMOTHY J. REICHERT, MD   KENNETH D. FAW, MD

ST. LOUIS, MISSOURI

The cricopharyngeus muscle in neonates and infants has not been well established. It is found, like other laryngopharyngeal structures in infants, to be relatively much larger than its counterpart in the adult but not large enough to correlate with the total length of reported sphincter function. It also varies significantly in size, and therefore probably does not contribute completely to the function of the upper esophageal sphincter. Its relationship to airway protection, regurgitation and respiration needs to be more thoroughly studied.

In 1717, Valsalva[1] first described the cricopharyngeus muscle and distinguished it from the inferior pharyngeal constrictor. Killian[2] in 1908 later subdivided the cricopharyngeus muscle into its two portions: the pars obliquus and the lower pars fundiformis. He felt the pars fundiformis was a constrictor and the muscle which formed the lip of the esophagus and acted to close the mouth of the esophagus. He also found in his dissections no definite anatomic division between the pharynx and the esophagus, but was able to separate distinctly the pars obliquus from the pars fundiformis.

More recent studies have concentrated on the neuromuscular dysfunctions of the upper esophageal sphincter. Cohen's observations[3] regarding neuromuscular dysfunction in swallowing and Kirchner's studies[4] on the cricopharyngeus in dogs have been major examples.

Review of the literature, however, reveals a paucity of information regarding the anatomy of the cricopharyngeus muscle in infants and children. Other parts of the laryngopharynx, the larynx, position, and anatomy have been noted to be significantly different in infants than in adults. An adequately functioning sphincter system of the upper esophagus would seem extremely important in neonates since their diet is liquid and their predominantly supine position would make regurgitation a significant possibility and increase the risk of tracheobronchial tree aspiration. This report, therefore, focuses on an anatomic study of the cricopharyngeus muscle. Results of this pilot study are presented, their significance related to reported esophageal motility studies, and differences from adult studies regarding the site of the sphincter are discussed.

METHODS

Six laryngopharynges from neonates were obtained for study. The specimens were obtained by transecting the cervical esophagus and trachea at the level of the fourth tracheal ring and dissecting it from the vertebral fascia superiorly to the level of the hyoid bone. The pharynx was then transected above the level of the hyoid bone and placed in formalin. Gross dissections were performed utilizing a dissecting microscope as demonstrated in Figure 1. The pharynx was inspected first posteriorly to identify the inferior border of the median raphe. The cricopharyngeus muscle was then identified at its origin at the cricoid and followed posteriorly to the median raphe. Its superior and inferior borders were defined from this dissection. Vertical dimensions in the posterior midline measured under the microscope, gross relations to the cricothyroid muscle, the superior thyropharyngeus and inferior circular esophageal fibers were noted.

Vertical muscle segments were then taken from the specimen from the upper esophagus to the superior border of the cricopharyngeus for histologic studies as seen in Figures 2 and 3. Measurements were made of the specimens prior to embedding in order to identify the level of the cricopharyngeus on the slides. The specimens were stained with hematoxylin and eosin and inspected for myenteric plexuses.

RESULTS

Gross Anatomic Directions. The superior to inferior height of the cricopharyngeus muscle was noted to vary from 1.9 to 4.5 mm as summarized in Table 1. It was found to have a horizontal direction in two cases and an oblique direction from posterosuperior to anteroinferior in four cases. The muscles blended continuously with the circular esophageal fibers below and the thyropharyngeus muscle above. The median raphe of the thyropharyngeus muscle above was easily identified in all specimens. No obvious oblique fibers of the cricopharynx that inserted into the median raphe were noted. The cricopharyngeus muscle was not overlapped by the thyropharyngeus nor did it overlap the circular esophageal fibers. The Killian-Jamerson area was noted to be prominent in only one specimen and the Lamier area below the cricopharyngeus on the posterior wall was easily identified in each specimen.

Histologic Studies. Specimens were inspected for myenteric plexuses. Myenteric plexuses were noted only in the area of the superior esophagus and none was seen in the area of the cricopharyngeus. Numerical counts were not performed of myenteric plexuses but rather their existence or absence was noted.

From the Division of Pediatric Otolaryngology, St. Louis Children's Hospital, St. Louis, Missouri.

Presented at the meeting of the American Broncho-Esophagological Association, Palm Beach, Florida, April 12-13, 1980.

REPRINTS — Timothy J. Reichert, MD, 777 South New Ballas Rd., St. Louis, MO 63141.

TABLE 1. SUMMARY OF GROSS ANATOMIC FINDINGS OF THE CRICOPHARYNGEUS IN THE NEONATE

Age According to Estimated Gestational Age (wk)	*Maximum Vertical Dimension of Muscle (mm)*	*Direction of Muscle Fibers*
21	4.5	Oblique
23	2.0	Transverse
25	1.9	Transverse
27	2.2	Oblique
30	4.5	Oblique
31	4.4	Oblique

DISCUSSION

Function of the Cricopharyngeus Muscle. Most studies in infants and indeed in adults regarding the cricopharyngeus muscle are related to the physiology and pathophysiology of the laryngopharynx in deglutition. Killian[2] in his description was impressed on hypopharyngeal examination that, upon drawing the larynx forward, a portion of the pharynx immediately posterior to the larynx was also drawn forward. Even by grasping the cricoid cartilage with a hook through a tracheotomy and exerting intense traction, the entrance to the esophagus could not be made to gap. On gross dissections he found circularly arranged fibers in the muscle arising from the cricoid and looping around the entrance to the esophagus which he felt "guarded the entrance to the esophagus." Later, Jackson and Jackson[5] termed this guardian to the esophagus, *Bab el Mandeb* (gate of tears), because of the danger of perforating the esophagus at this point during esophagoscopy. He also noted the effectiveness of the cricopharyngeus in its ability to force foreign bodies from the pharynx into the esophagus, resulting in the high incidence of retained foreign bodies immediately below the cricopharyngeus muscle.

The cricopharyngeus muscle has primarily been studied as a sphincter related to deglutition. It must open at the proper time to allow a bolus to pass from the pharynx into the esophagus and then close to prevent regurgitation while the bolus is moved by peristalsis through the esophagus toward the stomach. Indeed, it is so effective in this role that regurgitation will not occur in man even while swallowing with one's head down.

However, the cricopharyngeus or the upper esophageal sphincter in addition has a second and perhaps equally important role in protecting the airway from regurgitation. Euler et al[6] reported that some 17 of 30 children with recurrent pulmonary disease were found to have evidence of gastroesophageal reflux. In evaluating these patients with radiographic, manometric and endoscopic studies the efficiency of the lower esophageal sphincter was found to be defective in 17 patients and a diagnosis of gastroesophageal reflux made. Other reports and studies have also implicated tracheobronchial aspiration from regurgitation in cases of recurrent pulmonary disease, wheezing, and cough in children as well as adults. In addition in a recent study, injection of milk into the tracheas of piglets produced respiratory arrest, while injections of saline in control animals have produced no changes in respiration. Such information raises the possibility of tracheobronchial tree aspiration contributing to the syndrome of sudden death in infants under six months of age.[7]

Site of the Upper Esophageal Sphincter. Recent authors had disputed the question of the actual site of the upper esophageal sphincter. Batson[8] in an interesting study of cadavera noted a prominent bar protruding into the pharynx in adults. The bar was formed by the cricopharyngeus muscle. He noted in

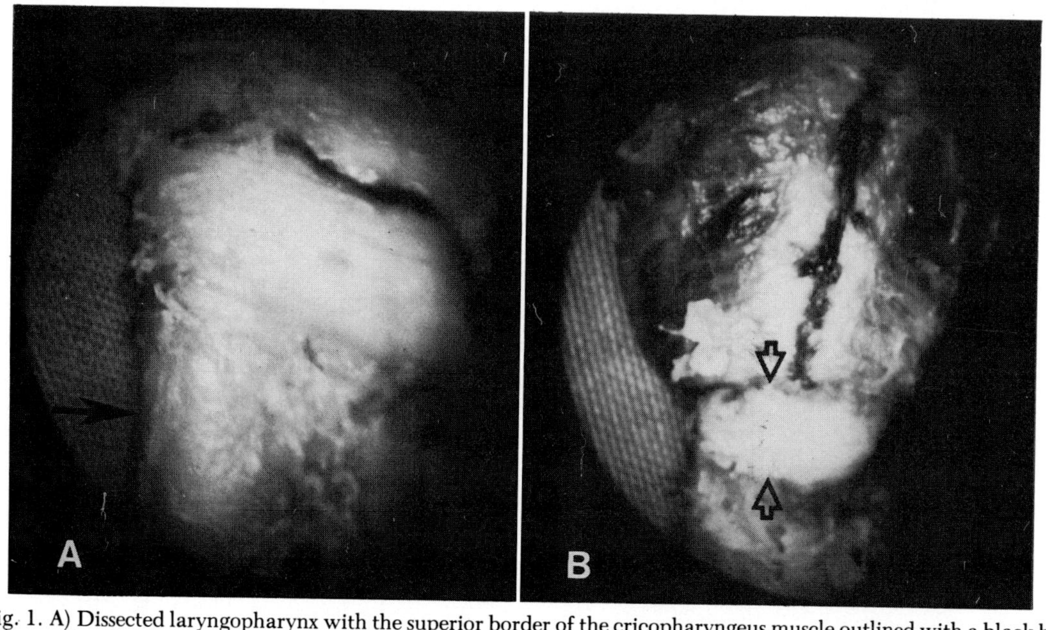

Fig. 1. A) Dissected laryngopharynx with the superior border of the cricopharyngeus muscle outlined with a black band. The oblique direction is easily noted from the posterosuperior on the left to anteroinferior on the right. B) Posterior view of the pharynx. The median raphe is marked by a black band and the cricopharyngeus is noted between two arrows.

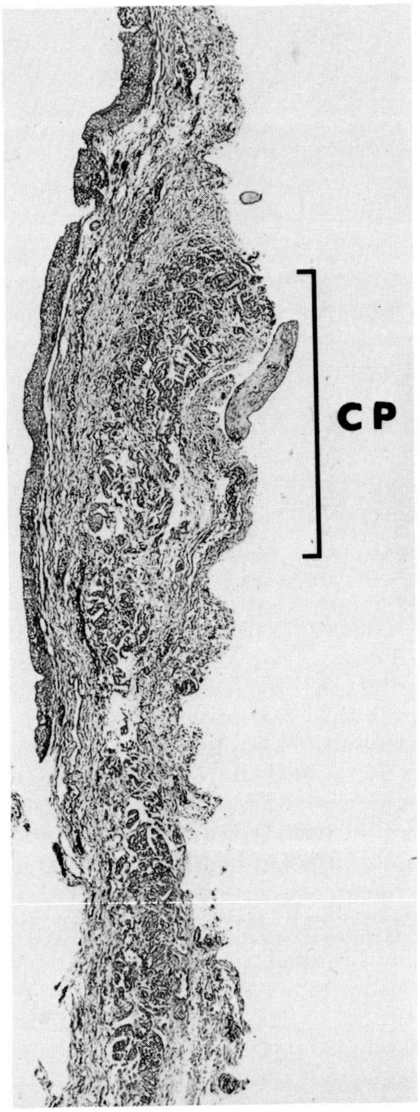

Fig. 2. Low power of a histologic section. The thicker cricopharyngeus (CP) is seen at the top while the thinner superior esophagus is seen at the bottom. (x40)

a study of dogs in the laboratory, that the cricopharyngeus became markedly more prominent after formalin was injected intravenously. In one picture provided by Batson the muscle actually measured 8 mm high by 12 mm in thickness.

Other authors have noted a hypopharyngeal bar on endoscopic and radiologic contrast studies. The significance of this hypopharyngeal bar has been widely disputed, however. As many as 72% of patients with no symptoms have been noted to have this hypopharyngeal bar on contrast studies.[9] Others[10] have noted the indentation to be present in as few as 5% and felt that the finding was definitely pathological.

Zaino et al[11] felt the sphincter zone was below the level of the cricopharyngeus and demonstrated the difference on anatomic studies as well as radiographic studies. They noted and demonstrated a hy-

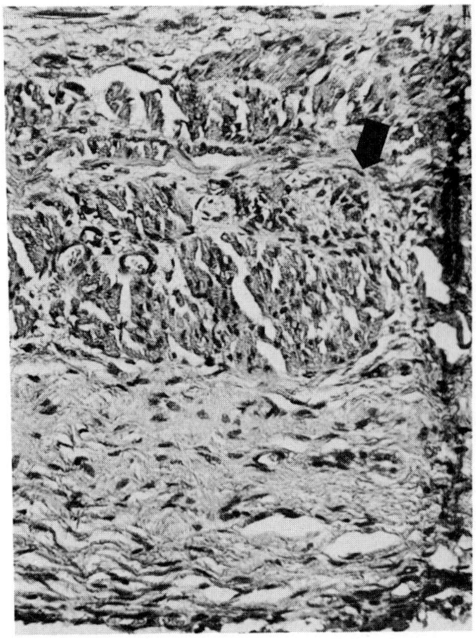

Fig. 3. High power section of Figure 2. The ganglion cells marked by the arrow are seen between the circular and longitudinal muscle bundles. (x350)

popharyngeal bar with a contracted sphincter zone below. They felt the zone of elevated pressure was below the cricopharyngeus muscle. Gates[12] in 1979 also presented evidence to argue for contribution of the upper esophageal muscle fibers to what he termed the pharyngoesophageal sphincter. He felt the zone of high pressure extended beyond the isolated cricopharyngeus muscle. Leavitt et al[13] noted the high pressure zone of the esophageal sphincter measured approximately 2-4 cm in distance but felt this did not correlate with the actual anatomic sphincter length of 1-2 cm (the length of the cricopharyngeus muscle in the adult) because of the artifact created by catheters necessary for the motility studies. Furthermore, he felt the laryngeal motion altered and increased the length of the sphincter zone. Cohen and Wolf[14] in an excellent study combining pressure and cineradiographic recordings in the esophagus identified a high pressure zone at the site of the cricopharyngeus and correlated this with contrast studies. However, they did not discuss the length of the segment or relationship of the length of this contracted segment with the width of the cricopharyngeus muscle.

Gryboski[15] noted in studies of neonates as well as premature infants that the upper esophageal sphincter zone varied in length from 0.5 to 1 cm, an area much longer than that comprised by the cricopharyngeus muscle. She did note the constancy of results in motility studies which not only included measurements of the upper esophageal sphincter but esophageal motility in lower esophageal sphincter function as well. She also noted an increase in tone of the lower esophageal sphincter in neonates 60 to 72 hours after birth. Interestingly, there was no related increase in tone of the upper esophageal sphincter either in the study group as a whole or those who seemed to have poor lower sphincter function.

The use of formalin in this study may also have affected the measurements of cricopharyngeus size. As noted previously, Batson[8] viewed a change in the size of the hypopharyngeal bar while freshly sacrificed dogs were perfused with formalin. Formalin, however, does allow dissection of small structures because it fixes the tissue. Zaino et al[11] found they could not utilize fresh infant pharynges for gross anatomic studies; initial dissections with fresh specimens of the present study confirmed this finding.

The present anatomic study then correlates well with previous physiologic and other anatomic observations made by those studying adults. Though the cricopharyngeus muscle seemed to have a great variation in width even at its maximum, it does not seem to be large enough to contribute to the total upper esophageal sphincter function found in infants. It does have a large enough variation in its dimensions to raise questions about its consistent effectiveness as a sphincter if considered alone. However, not enough information is available to speculate further on this issue.

The significance of the myenteric plexus related to the pharynx and esophagus has not been well delineated. The present study confirms the findings of Zaino et al[11] whose histologic studies were almost exclusively related to infants. They found a lack of myenteric plexuses in the pharynx and cricopharyngeus muscle. Since other sphincters in the gastrointestinal tract are noted to have markedly increased numbers of ganglion cells, Zaino et al used this information to confirm their feeling that the upper esophageal sphincter was located in the upper esophagus and not at the cricopharyngeus.

The presence or absence of myenteric plexuses, however, may be of questionable significance. The myenteric ganglion plexuses of Auerbach which occur within the muscles are noted to be primarily associated with the smooth musculature. Smooth muscle does appear in the cervical esophagus to a minimal degree and is either between the muscularis mucosa and the circular fibers or between the circular fibers and transverse fibers. It would seem that the amount of smooth muscle and the numbers of ganglion plexuses would have to be correlated in order to associate properly the ganglionated plexuses with the site of an upper esophageal sphincter.

In addition this area has embryological contributions from the fifth and sixth branchial arches and it would seem logical that a major portion of the efferent nerve supply would be controlled by the nucleus ambiguus. Indeed, studies have demonstrated the effect of the nucleus ambiguus and vagus nerve on this area. Since in other animals and in other studies the sphincter function has been related to respiration as well as vagus nerve section, the pharyngoesophageal sphincter most probably has a cranial nerve supply.

REFERENCES

1. Valsalva AM. De aure humano trachtatus quibus interponta es museulorum uvula stgue pharyngea. Utrecht, 1717.
2. Killian G. Uber den Mund der Spreiserohre Zestracchea. Z Ohrenheilkd 1908; 55:1-41.
3. Cohen SR. Congenital dysphagia: neurogenic considerations. Laryngoscope 1955; 65:515-43.
4. Kirchner JA. The motor activity of the cricopharyngeus muscle. Laryngoscope 1958; 68:1119-59.
5. Jackson C, Jackson CL. Bronchoesophagology. Philadelphia: WB Saunders, 1950.
6. Euler AR, Byrne WJ, Ament ME, et al. Recurrent pulmonary disease in children: a complication of gastroesophageal reflux. Pediatrics 1979; 63:47-51.
7. Downing SE, Lee JC. Laryngeal chemosensitivity: a possible mechanism for sudden infant death. Pediatrics 1975; 55:640-9.
8. Batson OV. The cricopharyngeus muscle. Ann Otol Rhinol Laryngol 1955; 64:47-54.
9. Siebert TL, Stein J, Poppel MH. Variations in the roentgen appearance of the "esophageal lips." Am J Roentgenol 1959; 81:570-5.
10. Seaman WB. Cineroentgenographic observations of the cricopharyngeus. Am J Roentgenol 1966; 96:922-31.
11. Zaino C, Jacobsen HG, Lepon M, et al. Pharyngoesophageal sphincter. Springfield: Charles C Thomas, 1970.
12. Gates GA. Upper esophageal sphincter: pre and post laryngectomy — a normative study. Laryngoscope 1980; 90: 454-64.
13. Leavitt NM, Dedo HH, Ogura JH. The cricopharyngeus muscle: an electromyographic study in the dog. Laryngoscope 1965; 75:122-36.
14. Cohen BR, Wolf BS. Handbook of physiology. Washington: American Physiologic Society, 1968.
15. Gryboski JD. The swallowing mechanism of the neonate: esophageal and gastric motility. Pediatrics 1965; 35:445-52.

HIGH INCIDENCE OF PULMONARY SYMPTOMS IN INFANTS EVALUATED FOR ESOPHAGEAL DISEASE

FRED C. ROTHSTEIN, MD THOMAS C. HALPIN, MD

CLEVELAND, OHIO

Of 62 children (1-24 months of age) evaluated for esophageal disease, 22 were found to have pulmonary symptoms of apnea, pneumonia, wheezing, cyanosis, cough and stridor. Upper gastrointestinal series showed free gastroesophageal reflux in 10 of 22 infants; 3 were thought to have stricture. Acid-reflux test was positive in 13 of 15 and correlated with the presence of esophagitis in 12. In addition to esophagitis, endoscopic examination found two foreign bodies and an esophageal stricture unrecognized during fluoroscopy. Endoscopic grasp biopsy was inadequate in most infants for the histologic evaluation of esophagitis. However, suction biopsy correlated well with endoscopically diagnosed esophagitis. In infants where medical therapy failed and symptoms were life-threatening, a Nissen fundoplication resulted in excellent resolution of symptoms. In children who present with prolonged and often life-threatening symptoms, esophageal dysfunction should be evaluated by rigorous testing.

INTRODUCTION

With the increasing awareness of gastroesophageal reflux (GER), more infants are being referred for the evaluation of esophageal dysfunction. The complications of this can be severe and include failure to thrive, iron deficiency anemia, esophagitis, esophageal stricture, developmental delay and Sandifer's syndrome.[1-4] Recently, reports in children and adults have linked esophageal dysfunction with pulmonary disease, especially asthma, recurrent bronchitis and chronic pulmonary infections.[5-8] Case reports have attempted to associate GER with the sudden infant death syndrome (SIDS).[9,10] In the pediatric literature, there are relatively few reports of infants with esophageal disease which present mainly with pulmonary complaints.[5,6,11] The study reported here reflects our experience.

METHODS

Sixty-two infants (age 1-24 months) were referred to the Pediatric Gastroenterology Service at Rainbow Babies and Childrens Hospital from September 1977 to August 1979 for evaluation of esophageal disease. Symptoms referrable to esophageal dysfunction included vomiting (33), hematemesis (11), dysphagia (15), odynophagia (6) and abnormal deglutition (2). Of these 62 infants, 22 also had pulmonary complaints and are the subject of this study.

Evaluation included barium swallow and upper gastrointestinal series in all patients. Presence or absence of pharyngeal dysfunction was noted during deglutition. In addition to observing the presence or absence of spontaneous reflux of barium, the patients were studied in both the upright and supine positions and during maneuvers to increase abdominal pressure.

Acid-reflux tests were performed in 15 of these patients according to the method of Euler as modified for children.[12] Gastroesophageal reflux was considered present if esophageal pH dropped below four on two occasions. In addition, all symptoms occurring during episodes of reflux were recorded and the ability of the infant to clear acid was assessed with glucose water-feeding.

Esophagoscopy was performed with an Olympus GIF-P_2 fiberoptic endoscope. Preparation for the procedure included sedation with intravenous meperidine, 1-2 mg/kg and 0.5-1.0 mg/kg of diazepam.[13] All patients had had nothing by mouth for at least four hours prior to esophagoscopy. A specially trained pediatric nurse was present during the procedure. Esophagitis was diagnosed endoscopically if erythema and friability or frank ulceration and exudation were present. Ten biopsy specimens were taken by grasp forceps (Olympus FB14K) during the procedure. Four biopsies were taken under direct endoscopic vision using the Rubin multipurpose biopsy with a 1.6 mm port. Specimens were mounted on a monofilament nylon mesh and fixed in Bouin's solution.[14] Microscopically, esophagitis was defined by the presence of polymorphonuclear leukocytes and/or lymphocytes in the lamina propria, basal cell hyperplasia of the squamous epithelium and changes in the height of the dermal papillae.[15]

RESULTS

Thirty-five percent of infants referred for evaluation had pulmonary symptoms, many of which were life-threatening (Table 1). Table 2 gives the age, sex and results of the esophageal evaluation of these infants.

Gastroesophageal reflux during barium fluoroscopy was demonstrated in 10 of 22 infants. No patient had any evidence of antral, pyloric, duodenal or small bowel obstruction. No documentation of symptoms associated with reflux was made at the time of fluoroscopy. A possible stricture of the midesophagus was seen on fluoroscopy in one infant and was confirmed by endoscopy. Hiatal hernia was noted radiographically in one infant. One child was noted to have an irregular mucosal pattern of

TABLE 1. PULMONARY SIGNS AND SYMPTOMS IN INFANTS (N = 62)

Apnea	9	Cough	2
Pneumonia	9	Stridor	1
Wheezing	6	Tachypnea	1
Cyanosis	6		

From the Department of Pediatrics, Case Western Reserve University and Rainbow Babies and Childrens Hospital, Cleveland, Ohio.

Presented at the meeting of the American Broncho-Esophagological Association, Palm Beach, Florida, April 12-13, 1980.

REPRINTS — Thomas C. Halpin, MD, Rainbow Babies and Childrens Hospital, Department of Pediatrics, 2101 Adelbert Road, Cleveland, OH 44106.

TABLE 2. RESULTS OF ESOPHAGEAL EVALUATION IN INFANTS WITH PULMONARY SYMPTOMS

Case	*Age (Mo)*	*Sex*	*Esophagogram*	*Tuttle*	*Endoscopy*	*Dx*
1	2	F	Reflux	Pos	LES/Inf	Inf
2	3	F	Normal	Pos	LES/Inf	NPD
3	1	M	Reflux	Pos	LES/Inf	NPD
4	7	M	Reflux	Pos	LES/Inf	NPD
5	8	F	Reflux	Pos	Patulous LES	ND
6	24	M	Hiatal hernia without reflux	Pos	Inf/Hiatal hernia	Inf
7	18	F	Irreg. esophagus	ND	FB with ulcer	ND
8	5	M	Normal	Neg	LES/Inf	ND
9	1	F	Reflux	Pos	Milk-coated esophagus	NPD
10	7	M	Normal	Pos	LES/Inf	Inf
11	6	F	Normal	Pos	LES/Inf	ND
12	6	M	Reflux	ND	LES/Inf	NPD
13	12	M	Reflux	ND	LES/Inf	ND
14	3	M	Reflux	Pos	LES/Inf	NPD
15	12	F	Esophageal stricture	Pos	Stricture	NPD
16	2	F	Reflux	ND	Inf	ND
17	2	M	Normal	Pos	Inf	NPD
18	18	M	Soft-tissue swelling	ND	FB	ND
19	12	M	Normal	Neg	Inf	Inf
20	8	F	Normal	Pos	Inf	NPD
21	7	M	Reflux	Pos	Patulous LES	ND
22	4	M	Normal	ND	Blood in esophagus	NPD

ND - Not done; NPD - No pathologic diagnosis; FB - Foreign body; LES - Lower esophageal sphincter; Inf - Inflammation.

his esophagus just below the thoracic inlet with an area of increased opacification. Endoscopic examination identified a foreign body which was removed with a basket forceps. An additional child was noted to have an irregular mucosal pattern with a narrowed esophagus, but no foreign body was visualized radiographically. Additionally, there was soft-tissue swelling with compression of the membranous portion of the trachea. An embedded plastic foreign body was found at endoscopy.

Thirteen of 15 infants tested had positive acid-reflux tests. Informal observation of symptoms at time of reflux was dramatic in many infants. Apnea with low pulse rate, opisthotnic posturing, extreme irritability and tachycardia and flushing were seen variously in eight children. These observations often correlated with the presenting clinical complaints.

Esophagogastroduodenoscopy revealed the following abnormalities: clinical esophagitis (15), foreign body (2), patulous lower esophageal sphincter with bile reflux (2), esophageal stricture (1) and hiatal hernia (1). The last child had blood on the esophageal walls without evidence of a bleeding lesion. Later at bronchoscopy he was found to have a bleeding pulmonary hemangioma.

Twelve of 14 children with endoscopically diagnosed esophagitis had biopsies performed. Seven of eight biopsies performed using the FB14K grasp forceps were poorly suited for morphologic interpretation because of crush artifact and small tissue samples. One did show acute inflammation. Esophageal suction biopsies were performed in four patients. Histologically, three showed changes of acute and/or chronic inflammation. Suction biopsies were uniformly superior for morphologic evaluation of esophageal histology.

Management of Symptoms (Table 3). Most infants were given a trial of medical management for GER which included upright posturing and thickened feeds. If esophagitis was present, antacids were used with a modified Fordtran regimen for a minimun of six weeks.[16] Caloric support was provided by parenteral nutrition in patients with failure to thrive and intractable GER. Eight of 22 infants improved with medical management. These tended to be infants who were less ill on presentation and who responded promptly to medical therapy. No infants in this group had apnea after therapy was initiated. At follow-up, none have had pulmonary complaints. Nissen fundoplication was performed if GER was unresponsive to medical management. Ten infants required surgical intervention. These were infants most at risk for SIDS — those with apnea and/or recurrent pulmonary consolidation. Two infants with foreign bodies were treated with endoscopic removal and prompt resolution of symptoms. Two infants who had a Nissen fundoplication died more than six months after the operation, one from carbon monoxide poisoning and the second with intractable seizures and a cardiopulmonary arrest. At follow-up, the remaining patients are asymptomatic and thriving. One patient on medical therapy left the hospital against medical advice and follow-up was not available.

DISCUSSION

It is important that physicians be aware that

TABLE 3. MANAGEMENT OF PULMONARY SYMPTOMS AND ESOPHAGEAL DISEASE IN INFANTS

Case	*Major Pulmonary Symptoms*	*Duration of Symptoms*	*Management*
1	Apnea, cyanosis, acute pneumonia	2-3 weeks	Med
2	Apnea, chronic pneumonia	3 months	Med
3	Apnea, cyanosis	Days	AMA
4	Apnea, wheezing, chronic pneumonia	5 months	Nissen
5	Apnea, cyanosis	2 weeks	Nissen
6	Chronic pneumonia	18 months	Nissen
7	Stridor	6 months	FBR
8	Acute pneumonia	2 months	Med
9	Apnea	Days	Med
10	Wheezing, acute pneumonia	5 months	Med
11	Wheezing	5 months	Med
12	Wheezing	4 months	Nissen
13	Cough	12 months	Med
14	Apnea, cyanosis	3 months	Nissen
15	Cough	1 month	Nissen
16	Apnea, cyanosis, acute pneumonia	Days	Nissen
17	Apnea, cyanosis, tachypnea	2 months	Nissen
18	Wheezing, dysphagia	5 months	FBR
19	Chronic pneumonia	3 months	Med
20	Wheezing	4 months	Missen
21	Chronic pneumonia	7 months	Nissen
22	Wheezing	1 month	Med

Med - Medical management; AMA - Discharged against medical advice; Nissen - Nissen fundoplication; FBR - Foreign body removed.

esophageal disease can cause a variety of respiratory symptoms. In our experience, the most common respiratory complaints were apnea, pneumonia and wheezing. The most common clinical presentation in those infants less than six months of age was apnea and pneumonia; and in those greater than six months wheezing and vomiting.

In the present study, 86% of infants with pulmonary symptoms tested had positive acid-reflux tests. All had an abnormality at the time of endoscopy. These findings support the hypothesis that reflux of gastric contents can play a significant role in the development of respiratory symptoms and even respiratory arrest. Several mechanisms have been postulated. Downey and Lee have demonstrated the chemosensitivity of the larynx in newborn piglets by instilling H_2O or milk which produced a reflux central apnea.[17] A similar reflex has been reproduced in newborn lambs.[18] However, central apnea could not be reproduced in older piglets.[17] Of interest, older infants in this series did not present with apnea, but rather were more likely to present with wheezing, cough or recurrent pneumonia.

Another life-threatening mechanism that has been identified is secondary to reflux of gastric contents into the posterior pharynx, resulting in laryngospasm. Pathologic specimens from children dying with SIDS supports the view that gastric contents need not be aspirated to cause death.[19] Our observations during the acid-reflux tests demonstrated apnea, opisthotnic posturing, tachycardia and rapid fall in pulse rate when esophageal pH dropped to less than four. The above findings are reinforced by the epidemiologic data that note the peak age of SIDS is less than six months, that it frequently occurs in infants who have been recently fed and 25-45% of these patients had respiratory symptoms which may have been unrecognized sequelae of GER.[11,20,21] Two of our patients with apnea had siblings who died of SIDS.

The association of GER with recurrent pulmonary disease has been made previously in adults and children.[6,11,22,23] Gastric contents may be aspirated and cause obstruction to air flow, leading to respiratory compromise, pneumonia and possible cardiac arrest. Reflux with aspiration has been demonstrated in newborns with chronic pulmonary disease.[22] The large number of children with pneumonia and positive acid-reflux tests lends additional support to that hypothesis.

Two of our cases also point out that esophageal foreign body must be considered in infants who present with respiratory symptoms. Esophageal foreign body can cause a variety of respiratory symptoms and is most commonly reported in children less than three years of age. The most frequent site of foreign body impaction is the cervical esophagus just below the cricopharygeus constrictor at the thoracic inlet.[24] This lesion is *not* always appreciated with radiographic studies. Newman has noted that respiratory symptoms may be caused by: 1) compression of the soft membranous portion of the posterior trachea; 2) aspiration of contents secondary to esophageal obstruction; 3) direct extension of the inflammatory process from esophagus to trachea, causing compression; or 4) erosion of foreign body into trachea, causing tracheoesophageal fistula formation and obstruction of the trachea.[25]

Esophagoscopy, when performed in association with the acid-reflux test in this study, added another dimension to the evaluation of the esophageal-related disease. Ten of 13 infants with positive acid-reflux tests had clinical esophagitis. However, this finding was not confirmed with esophageal grasp biopsy. Limited by the 2 mm size of the grasp forceps, only superficial specimens could be taken and morphologic evaluation was very difficult. The poor correlation between biopsy findings and the endoscopic presence of esophagitis was corrected with the use of suction-type biopsies.

In conclusion, we have found that 1) respiratory disease associated with esophageal dysfunction is common in a large pediatric center; 2) infants with esophageal disease often present with pulmonary symptoms; 3) infants younger than six months are more likely to present with apnea and pneumonia, while those older than six months present with wheezing and vomiting; 4) GER should be suspected as a cause of SIDS, especially when acid-reflux test is positive and esophagitis is present; 5) foreign body should be considered in any child who presents with prolonged respiratory symptoms; and 6) grasp biopsy appears to be an inadequate technique for evaluation of infant esophageal mucosa because of crush artifact, poor orientation and the limited depth of the biopsy.

REFERENCES

1. Darling DB, Fisher JH, Gellis SS. Hiatal hernia and gastroesophageal reflux in infants and children: analysis of the incidence in North American children. Pediatrics 1974; 54:450-4.

2. Rohatigi M, Shandling B, Stephins CA. Hiatal hernia in infants and children: results of surgical treatment. Surgery 1971; 69:456-61.

3. Randolph HG, Lilly JR, Anderson KD. Surgical treatment of gastroesophageal reflux in infants. Ann Surg 1974; 180:479-84.

4. Carre IJ. A historical review of the clinical consequences of hiatal hernia (partial thoracic stomach) and gastroesophageal reflux. In: report of the seventy-fifth Ross conference on pediatric research. Columbus: Ross Laboratories, 1979:1-8.

5. Euler AR, Byrne WB, Ament ME, et al. Recurrent pulmonary disease in children: a complication of gastroesophageal reflux. Pediatrics 1979; 63:47-51.

6. Christie DL, O'Grady LR, Mack DV. Incompetent lower esophageal sphincter and gastroesophageal reflux in recurrent acute pulmonary disease of infancy and childhood. J Pediatr 1978; 93:23-7.

7. Davis VM. Relationship between pulmonary disease, hiatal hernia and gastroesophageal reflux. NY State J Med 1972; 72:935-40.

8. Dees SC. The role of gastroesophageal reflux in nocturnal asthma in children. NC Med J 1974; 35:230-3.

9. Leape LL, Holder TM, Franklin JD, Amoury RA, Ashcraft KW. Respiratory arrest in infants secondary to gastroesophageal reflux. Pediatrics 1977; 60:924-6.

10. Herbst JJ, Book LS, Bray PF. Gastroesophageal reflux in the "near miss" sudden infant death syndrome. J Pediatr 1978; 92:73-5.

11. Danus O, Casar C, Lorrain A, Pope CE. Esophageal reflux — an unrecognized cause of recurrent obstructive bronchitis in children. J Pediatr 1976; 89:220-4.

12. Euler AR, Ament ME. Detection of gastroesophageal reflux by Tuttle test. Pediatrics 1977; 60:65-8.

13. Ament ME, Christie DL. Upper gastrointestinal fiberoptic endoscopy in pediatric patients. Gastroenterology 1977; 72:1244-6.

14. Perera DR, Weinstein W, Rubin CE. Small intestinal biopsy. Hum Pathol 1975; 6:157-217.

15. Ismail-Beige F, Horton PF, Pope CE. Histologic consequences of gastroesophageal reflux in man. Gastroenterology 1970; 58:163.

16. Peterson WL, Sturdevant RAL, Frankl HD, et al. Healing of duodenal ulcer with an antacid regimen. N Engl J Med 1977; 297:341-5.

17. Downing SE, Lee JC. Laryngeal chemosensitivity: a possible mechanism for sudden infant death. Pediatrics 1975; 55:640-9.

18. Kovar I, Selstam U, Catterton WZ, Stahlman MT, Sundell HW. Laryngeal chemoreflex in newborn lambs: respiratory and swallowing response to salts, acids and sugars. Pediatr Res 1979; 13:1144-9.

19. Beckwith JB. The sudden infant death syndrome. Curr Probl Pediatr 1973; 3:1-29.

20. Beckwith JB. Pathology discussion. In: Bergman AB, Beckwith JB, Ray CG, eds. Sudden infant death syndrome. Seattle: University of Washington Press, 1970:122-38.

21. Froggatt P. Sudden death in babies: epidemiology. Am J Cardiol 1968; 22:457-61.

22. Herbst JJ, Minton SD, Book LS. Gastroesophageal reflux causing respiratory distress and apnea in newborn infants. J Pediatr 1979; 95:763-8.

23. Darling DB, McCauley RG, Leonidas JC, Schwartz AM. Gastroesophageal reflux in infants and children: correlation of radiological severity and pulmonary pathology. Radiology 1978; 127:735-40.

24. Jackson C, Jackson CL. Bronchoesophagoscopy. Philadelphia: WB Saunders, 1950:13-7.

25. Newman DE. The radiolucent esophageal foreign body: an often forgotten cause of respiratory problems. J Pediatr 1978; 92:60-3.

Ann Otol 89:1980

LARYNGEAL STENOSIS FROM ENDOTRACHEAL INTUBATION

A REVIEW OF 58 CASES

DONALD B. HAWKINS, MD WILLIAM M. LUXFORD, MD

LOS ANGELES, CALIFORNIA

During the decade of the 1970s, the Department of Otolaryngology at the Los Angeles County - University of Southern California Medical Center encountered 58 patients who required tracheotomy for laryngeal stenosis secondary to endotracheal intubation. This included 19 children and 39 adults. We treated 50 of these patients, of whom 35 (70%) were decannulated after endoscopic management alone. One other patient could have been decannulated but needed the tracheotomy for medical reasons. Two others will probably be decannulated in the near future. Eight patients underwent open reconstructive procedures.

Laryngeal stenosis as a complication of endotracheal intubation develops in only a small percentage of intubated patients. When it does occur, however, it presents difficult and frustrating problems for both the patient and the physician. During the decade of the 1970s, we saw a large number of patients at the Los Angeles County - University of Southern California Medical Center who had sustained trauma to the larynx from intubation. Many of these could be managed without tracheotomy, but 58 patients did require tracheotomy. In this paper we are reporting our experiences, good and bad, with these 58 patients.

AGE AND SEX DISTRIBUTION

Seventeen patients were five years of age or younger. Fifteen of these were under one year and ten were under one month. Two patients were nine years old. Twenty-seven were between 16 and 40 years, and 12 were over 40 years of age. In the remainder of this paper, those patients under 15 years of age will be referred to as children and those over 15 as adults.

There were 38 females and 20 males. Among the children, the distribution was almost even, 9 females and 10 males, but adult females outnumbered adult males almost three to one, with 29 females to 10 males.

CONDITIONS REQUIRING INTUBATION

The most common condition overall for which intubation was required was a medical illness, accounting for 22 patients. The second most common condition was drug overdose in 19 patients. Twelve patients were intubated for various types of trauma, while five were intubated for postsurgical complications. Fourteen of the 22 with medical illnesses were children. Ten of the 14 were neonates with respiratory distress syndrome. Five of these ten were intubated with Cole tubes. As reported in an earlier publication,[1] Cole tubes resulted in a high incidence of laryngeal stenosis on the newborn service at our institution until their use was discontinued in April 1971. Of the other 5 children, 3 were intubated for trauma, 1 for drug overdose, and 1 for postsurgical complications.

Among adults, the most common condition was drug overdose in 18 patients, compared to 9 with trauma, 8 with medical illness, and 4 with postsurgical complications. The high incidence of drug overdose accounts for the three to one ratio of females to males in our adult patients, because all but one of our drug overdose patients were females. The smaller female larynx, sometimes cited as a reason for a larger proportion of females with postintubation stenosis,[2,3] may or may not have been a factor in our series.

FACTORS IN INTUBATION STENOSIS

In the adults, duration of intubation varied from less than 1 day to 20 days, with an average of 6.5 days. The average duration for the 19 children was 15 days. Among the 10 neonates, 1 who developed central nervous system problems was intubated for 90 days; the other 9 averaged 17 days. The nine children older than one month averaged only five days of intubation.

A number of our patients, especially those with longer periods of intubation, had several extubations and reintubations. Some also had histories of difficult and probably traumatic intubations. Other factors which we were unable to determine in many patients were the size and type of endotracheal tube used. Although these are not as easy to measure as duration of intubation, all are important causative factors in stenosis of the larynx.

From the Department of Otolaryngology, University of Southern California School of Medicine, Los Angeles, California.
Presented at the meeting of the American Broncho-Esophagological Association, Palm Beach, Florida, April 12-13, 1980.
REPRINTS — Donald B. Hawkins, MD, 1200 North State Street, Box 296, Los Angeles, CA 90033.

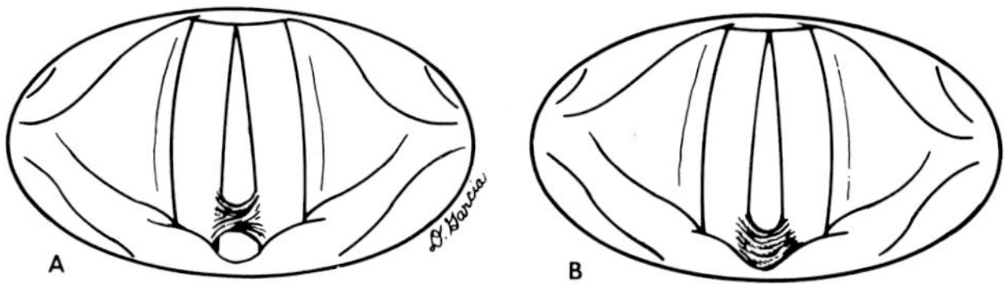

Fig. 1. A) Glottic stenosis: a fibrous band extending between the vocal processes of the arytenoid cartilages preventing abduction of the vocal cords. B) Glottic stenosis: submucosal accumulation of scar tissue in the interarytenoid space preventing abduction of the vocal cords. This is more subtle than the fibrous band and more difficult to identify. (Reprinted with permission.[4])

TYPES OF STENOSIS

In 16 patients, scarring at the glottic level prevented sufficient abduction of the vocal cords to maintain an airway. Stenosis at this level alone was found in one child and 15 adults. Subglottic stenosis was found in 18 patients, 8 children and 10 adults. Seventeen patients, nine children and eight adults, had combined glottic and subglottic stenosis in which the obstruction at either level would have been sufficient to have required tracheotomy. Of the 9 children with combined stenosis, 6 had been intubated with Cole tubes, the 5 neonates mentioned earlier and 1 intubated for postsurgical complications. A seventh had been intubated with a rubber endotracheal tube. Only two children developed this more severe type of stenosis from polyvinylchloride uniform-diameter tubes that have been used almost exclusively in pediatrics for the past several years. Both were burn victims with apparent heat damage to their larynges.

In three adults, large granulations or granulomas in the subglottic area produced airway obstruction. These arose principally from the arytenoid vocal processes, and the posterior and lateral portions of the cricoid cartilage. In addition to these three in whom granulations were the obstructing element, some of the patients with glottic and subglottic stenosis also had granulations which were not obstructive. Acute chondritis involving the cricoid cartilage and vocal processes of the arytenoids with tissue swelling, exudate, and granulations constituted the obstruction in one child and three adults.

Considering glottic stenosis, isolated scar tissue bands between the vocal cords (Fig. 1A) were found in six adults and one child as the only obstructing element. Isolated bands were also the glottic component of combined stenosis in two children.

A more subtle type of submucosal scarring (Fig. 1B) may develop in an interarytenoid area ulcerated by an endotracheal tube. Submucosal interarytenoid scarring was the cause of pure glottic stenosis in 9 adults and as the glottic component of combined stenosis in 8 adults and 7 children.

MANAGEMENT

Eight patients, seven children and one adult, were not treated by us for correction of their laryngeal stenosis. The 7 children, 2 with subglottic stenosis and 5 with combined stenosis, were all under one year of age. Three died of complications of their underlying disease; four moved or were transferred elsewhere. Of these 4, we have learned that 1 was decannulated at 18 months of age, 1 died of tracheotomy tube obstruction, and 2 still have tracheotomies at eight years of age. The one adult had combined stenosis. She was 77 years old and in poor medical condition, so we elected not to try to correct her stenosis. Of the 50 remaining patients whom we treated, 16 had glottic stenosis, 16 had subglottic stenosis, 11 had combined stenosis, 3 had granulations, and 4 had acute chondritis.

Our method of managing patients with laryngeal stenosis has been described in a previous publication.[4] We examine each patient closely for glottic scarring as well as for subglottic and tracheal involvement. We attempt to correct the stenosis by endoscopic management. This involves dividing glottic scar tissue with a knife, and dilating the glottic and subglottic areas with Jackson laryngeal dilators followed by bronchoscopes. Granulations and necrotic debris are removed. All dilatations in these tracheotomized patients are performed under general anesthesia with complete succinylcholine-induced muscle relaxation.

The shorter the interval between dilatations, the better the results are in most cases. Dilatations every one to two weeks is our preferred schedule, but for various reasons we often have to settle for longer intervals. In the acute cases steroids and antibiotics are given for approximately two weeks. Perioperative steroids are given for almost all of the endoscopic procedures. Methylprednisolone (Depo Medrol®, Upjohn Co.) was injected into the stenosis in several patients. Although it may have helped in one or two patients, it did not appear to be beneficial in most.

RESULTS

Thirty-five of the 50 patients were able to have their tracheotomies removed after endoscopic management alone. All four of the patients with acute chondritis and all three with obstruction due to granulations were decannulated in an average of four weeks after beginning therapy. Those with acute chondritis might have recovered as well with antibiotic and steroid treatment alone, as others have who did not require tracheotomies. However, since they had tracheotomies which provided a safe airway for anesthesia, we performed one or two endoscopies in each of the four to remove necrotic tissue, gently dilate, and to drain an arytenoid abscess in one.

Thirteen of the 16 patients with glottic stenosis were decannulated in an average of five weeks. All seven of those with isolated glottic bands were decannulated in an average of two weeks after beginning therapy. Of the nine patients with submucosal glottic scarring, six were decannulated after an average of eight weeks and four procedures.

Of the 16 patients with subglottic stenosis, 10 had their tracheotomies removed after an average of 18 weeks. This included four of six children and six of ten adults.

Five of the 11 patients with combined stenosis were decannulated after an average of 19 weeks. Included were two of four children and three of seven adults.

Of the 15 patients not decannulated with endoscopic management, 8 underwent open reconstructive procedures to correct their stenosis. The courses of the other seven are as follows: One infant with subglottic stenosis from intubation as a neonate is still being dilated at seven months of age. Her prognosis is good for decannulation before one year of age. Another child with subglottic stenosis has an adequate airway after six months of dilatations, but decannulation has been delayed because of tracheomalacia at the tracheotomy site, as described by Crysdale.[5] One child with severe combined stenosis from intubation trauma superimposed on heat injury to the larynx died suddenly at home, apparently from tracheotomy obstruction. He had been undergoing dilatations approximately every five weeks for three years; this was maintaining an airway for speech. He was to have an open procedure eventually, but his larynx was so severely damaged that even this probably would not have been successful. Another child with severe combined stenosis from neonatal intubation with a Cole tube was decannulated at age three years after multiple dilatations. The tracheotomy had to be replaced one month later. She was then referred to Childrens Hospital of Los Angeles where she has undergone multiple dilatations and recently laser treatments, so far without success.

One adult has a good laryngeal airway after two procedures to correct glottic submucosal stenosis. She could be decannulated, but she needs the tracheotomy for medical reasons. A second adult with combined stenosis had dilatations for one year, then declined a recommended open procedure. She keeps her tracheotomy plugged most of the time, but her glottic airway is not sufficient for its removal. A third adult, one of the earlier patients in this series, underwent stenting for two years without success. She moved to another city with her tracheotomy still in place.

Open or external reconstructive procedures were performed on eight patients; all eight were adults. Two had glottic stenosis, four had subglottic stenosis, and two had combined stenosis.

One patient with glottic submucosal stenosis underwent external arytenoidectomy in 1972. This was unsuccessful because the interarytenoid scar tissue still prevented the cords from separating enough to provide an adequate airway. The patient declined further surgery. In 1975, another patient underwent a successful arytenoidectomy with submucosal excision of interarytenoid scar tissue by a thyrotomy approach.

For subglottic stenosis, our first external procedure in 1973 was interposition of a portion of thyroid cartilage to the anterior cricoid ring after submucosal excision of subglottic scar tissue. This patient was ultimately successful in removing her tracheotomy. However, decannulation was delayed because of posterior glottic scarring, apparently the result of over one year of unsuccessful stenting earlier in her course.

The hyoid bone muscle-pedicle interposition, popularized by Ward et al[6] and others,[7] has been performed for subglottic stenosis on three patients in the past two years. In all three, the stenosis involved the cricoid and upper trachea. In all three we excised submucosal scar while attempting to preserve mucosa. The first was successful, but only after three endoscopic procedures to remove granulations and dilate a relative stenosis that developed at the point of scar tissue excision. In the second patient the subglottic lumen remained open, but the upper tracheal stenosis re-formed. We planned to reoperate, but the patient died three months after surgery when her tracheotomy tube was removed at a party. The third procedure was done only a few weeks ago. In this one, we applied a split thickness skin graft over a soft stent, as advocated by Olson,[8] after excising subglottic and upper tracheal scar tissue. It is too early to be certain of a good result, and we have not yet removed the tracheotomy, but the subglottic and tracheal lumen appears to be adequate.

In two patients with combined stenosis we performed hyoid interposition, as for subglottic stenosis, combining it with a posterior cricoid section through a thyrotomy approach. This technique was described by Reithi[9] and modified by Grahne.[10] It has also been used by Crysdale and Platt,[11] Fearon et al,[12] and Cotton.[13] In this procedure, the posterior cricoid lamina is incised and separated vertically in the midline, widening the interarytenoid space. In each of our patients, stents were left in place for two months. Both were successful with good glottic airways, but required several endoscopic procedures to remove granulations from the undersurface of the interposed hyoid before the subglottic airways were adequate. One patient was decannulated four months after removal of the stents. The other patient kept her tracheotomy plugged 99% of the time and could have removed it, but wanted to keep it as a crutch when she felt nervous. She died of drug overdose five months after surgery.

DISCUSSION

The sequence of events leading to stenosis involves ulceration of mucosa and cartilage, inflammatory reaction with granulation and fibrous tissue formation, and contraction of fibrous scar. The degree of stenosis depends upon the severity of injury and the amount of local tissue reaction. The stenosis becomes firmer with the passage of time. Once a dense fibrous stenosis has formed, it is difficult to correct by endoscopic measures. On the other hand, endoscopic dilatations started before the stenosis becomes firm and refractory, and repeated frequently and persistently will often be successful. This was the case in our series in which 35 of 50, or 70% were decannulated by endoscopic measures alone.

For maximum effectiveness, dilatations should be done under general anesthesia with total relaxation. If too gentle the dilatations will be useless; they must be firm to be effective. If too forceful, however, they may aggravate the stenosis. We agree with Fearon et al[12] that the greater the vertical extent of the stenosis, the greater will be the problem with treatment. The 11 patients with combined glottic and subglottic stenosis were the only group with less than 50% success by endoscopic measures. Those most difficult to manage also had stenosis involving the upper trachea.

Of the glottic stenoses, the isolated posterior band forms most often in patients who had elective tracheotomies at the time the endotracheal tubes were removed. This was the case with seven of nine patients who developed glottic bands, as pure glottic stenosis or as part of combined stenosis. In patients with tracheotomies, the larynx is bypassed in breathing and the cords remain in relatively close approximation. Mucous and fibrinous connections between ulcerated vocal processes become adhesions that organize into scar tissue bands. On the other hand, two patients were extubated without tracheotomy, but required tracheotomy three and six weeks later for airway obstruction from glottic bands. In both, limited activity and limited vocal cord abduction apparently allowed mucous connections to persist and become fibrous bands.

In managing isolated glottic bands, often only one endoscopic division of the band is necessary. The tracheotomy is plugged the next day to insure laryngeal breathing with vocal cord abduction. It is left in for 7 to 14 days, however, because a second procedure is occasionally necessary. Glottic submucosal scarring, which seems to have no relationship to tracheotomy at the time of extubation, is more difficult to correct than glottic bands because it is less obvious. This type responds much better to dilatations if it is divided with a knife before dilating.

Regarding the use of stents or lumen-keepers, there is considerable difference of opinion.[8] Stents were used in two of the early patients in this series for over one year. Their subglottic stenoses were not improved, and we thought the stents had created or aggravated glottic scarring. Since then, we have used stents only after open reconstructive procedures. Although indwelling stents are likely to aggravate glottic scarring, Goode and Shinn,[14] and Kotton[15] reported some success with stents in subglottic stenosis. Their average duration of stenting was 6 to 12 months. Subtracting our two patients with unsuccessful stenting, 10 of 14 with subglottic stenosis were decannulated after an average of 4½ months by dilatations without stents.

If after an adequate trial of dilatations, approximately four or five procedures, no improvement is noted, an open reconstructive procedure should be considered. From our relatively limited experience with open procedures in eight patients, we prefer the hyoid muscle-pedicle interposition for subglottic stenosis, the Rethi-Grahne posterior cricoid section for glottic stenosis, and a combination of the two for combined stenoses.

REFERENCES

1. Hawkins DB. Hyaline membrane disease of the neonate. Prolonged intubation in management: effects on the larynx. Laryngoscope 1978; 88:201-24.

2. Harrison GA, Tonkin JP. Prolonged (therapeutic) endotracheal intubation. Br J Anaesth 1968; 40:241-8.

3. Dixon TC, Sando MJW, Bolton JM, Gilligan JE. A report of 342 cases of prolonged endotracheal intubation. Med J Aust 1968; 2:529-33.

4. Hawkins DB. Glottic and subglottic stenosis from endotracheal intubation. Laryngoscope 1977; 87:339-46.

5. Crysdale WS. Nasotracheal intubation in management of delayed decannulation. Ann Otol Rhinol Laryngol 1974; 83:802-9.

6. Ward PH, Canalis R, Fee W, Smith G. Composite hyoid sternohyoid muscle grafts in humans. Arch Otolaryngol 1977; 103:531-4.

7. Wong ML, Finnegan DA, Kashima HK, Jafek BW. Vascularized hyoid interposition for subglottic and upper tracheal stenosis. Ann Otol Rhinol Laryngol 1978; 87:491-7.

8. Olson NR. Wound healing by primary intention in the larynx. Otolaryngol Clin North Am 1979; 12:735-40.

9. Rethi A. An operation for cicatricial stenosis of the larynx. J Laryngol Otol 1956; 70:283-93.

10. Grahne B. Operative treatment of severe chronic traumatic laryngeal stenosis in infants up to three years old. Acta Otolaryngol (Stockh) 1971; 72:134-7.

11. Crysdale WS, Platt LJ. Division of posterior cricoid plate in young children with subglottic stenosis. Laryngoscope 1976; 86:1451-8.

12. Fearon B, Crysdale WS, Bird R. Subglottic stenosis of the larynx in the infant and child. Ann Otol Rhinol Laryngol 1978; 87:645-8.

13. Cotton R. Management of subglottic stenosis in infancy and childhood. Ann Otol Rhinol Laryngol 1978; 87:649-56.

14. Goode RL, Shinn JB. Long-term stenting in the treatment of subglottic stenosis. Ann Otol Rhinol Laryngol 1977; 86:795-8.

15. Kotton B. The treatment of subglottic stenosis in children by prolonged dilatation. Laryngoscope 1979; 89:1983-90.

ADDENDUM

Three patients who were under active treatment at the time this paper was presented have had changes in the status of their airways. The infant whose subglottic stenosis was still being dilated at seven months of age was successfully decannulated at ten months of age. The child whose decannulation was delayed because of tracheomalacia at the tracheotomy site underwent open resection of a necrotic depressed fragment of anterior tracheal wall immediately above the tracheal opening. The tracheotomy cannula was replaced by a nasotracheal tube at surgery. The nasotracheal tube was removed 24 hours later. Except for mild stridor with crying during the first week the patient had no further airway difficulty. The adult patient who had a split thickness skin graft and hyoid interposition, and whose airway appeared adequate at the time the paper was presented, developed another stenosis. The lower portion of the hyoid graft sloughed into the lumen creating an anterior stenosis. The skin graft took in some areas but not enough to prevent restenosis at the site of scar excision. He recently underwent a revision procedure in which we opened, but did not excise, the stenosis. The hyoid graft was replaced by a graft of costal cartilage over a polyvinylchloride stent. We plan to leave the stent in place for several months.

≈

SECOND INTERNATIONAL CONFERENCE ON CHOLESTEATOMA AND MASTOID SURGERY

The Second International Conference on Cholesteatoma and Mastoid Surgery will be held March 22-27, 1981 in Tel-Aviv, Israel under the auspices of Tel-Aviv University and Weizmann Institute of Science. For further information contact: Professor J. Sade, P. O. Box 16271, Tel-Aviv, Israel. Telex: 342272 (Kenes) Tel-Aviv.

PROLONGED OROTRACHEAL INTUBATION IN THE NEWBORN

GEORGE H. CONNER, MD

MICHAEL J. BUSHEY, MD

M. JEFFREY MAISELS, MD, BCh

HERSHEY, PENNSYLVANIA

One hundred seventy-four consecutive cases of newborn infants who required orotracheal intubation for longer than three days were studied retrospectively. The duration of intubation varied from 3 to 211 days with an overall mortality rate of 22.9%. There was one complication directly related to orotracheal intubation. One tracheotomy was performed. Orotracheal intubation is felt to be superior to nasal tracheal intubation and tracheotomy in managing infants in this age group who require prolonged assisted ventilation.

INTRODUCTION

Prolonged or repeated endotracheal intubation in the newborn has been felt to produce irreversible laryngeal and tracheal damage.[1-5] For this reason Pickard and Oropeza have recommended tracheotomies for infants with respiratory insufficiency for more than 24 hours,[2] while Gibson and Byrne recommended waiting 72 hours.[6] Heroy et al recommended tracheotomies for those infants requiring ventilatory assistance for longer than seven days.[5]

In a previous study, two of the authors (GHC and MJM) presented data suggesting that orotracheal intubation in the newborn was apparently well tolerated for extended periods of time in the adequately equipped and staffed newborn intensive care unit. That study dealt with 100 consecutive newborn intubations of six hours or greater duration. A significant number were intubated less than 72 hours.[7] In this presentation we will be dealing only with newborn infants who have been intubated 72 hours or longer.

It is the purpose of this presentation to show that prolonged or repeated orotracheal intubation properly managed in the premature or term infant does not appear to produce significant damage to the larynx and trachea and should not be a factor in determining whether or not a tracheotomy is to be done. Furthermore, it is our opinion that tracheotomy is seldom, if ever, necessary in this age group and is indicated only in relation to the underlying disease process.

METHODS

One hundred and seventy-four consecutive neonates who were intubated three days (72+ hours) or longer in the newborn intensive care unit (NICU) of The Milton S. Hershey Medical Center were studied retrospectively. The duration of intubation ranged from 3 to 211 days. The majority of cases were admitted for prematurity which was usually associated with hyaline membrane disease (84%). Congenital and other disorders requiring ventilatory assistance accounted for the remainder. Follow-up for this group ranged from three months to five years and covered the period between January 1974 and December 1978.

In order to assess the possible deleterious effects of duration of intubation, the 174 infants were separated into four groups according to the length of time intubated (Table 1).

RESULTS

There were no deaths attributable to orotracheal intubation.

No tracheotomies were performed because of duration of intubation or frequency of reintubation.

One tracheotomy was performed on an infant who had been intubated and ventilated for 72 days. She had a generalized neuromuscular defect with gradual improvement. She was found to have a partial bilateral cord paralysis which did not improve. The tracheotomy was performed so that she could feed orally. Bronchoscopic examination of this child three years later showed no evidence of damage to the larynx or trachea as a result of her prolonged intubation.

Two infants intubated 211 and 72 days had 29 and 23 reintubations, respectively, without clinical evidence of untoward effects on the larynx or trachea.

Complications related to prolonged orotracheal intubation included:

TABLE 1. DURATION OF INTUBATION

Group	*Duration Intubation (days)*	*No. Patients*
I	3- 7	107
II	7-14	37
III	14-30	18
IV	30+	12

From the Division of Otorhinolaryngology, Department of Surgery, and the Division of Newborn Medicine, Department of Pediatrics, The Milton S. Hershey Medical Center, The Pennsylvania State University, Hershey, Pennsylvania.

Presented at the meeting of the American Broncho-Esophagological Association, Palm Beach, Florida, April 12-13, 1980.

REPRINTS — George H. Conner, MD, Division of Otorhinolaryngology, Department of Surgery, The Milton S. Hershey Medical Center, The Pennsylvania State University, Hershey, PA 17033.

TABLE 2. RELATIONSHIP OF BIRTH WEIGHT AND MORTALITY

Birth Weight (gm)	*No. Patients*	*Mortality (%)*
< 1250	31	54
1250-2000	75	22
> 2000	68	18

1. Accidental dislodgment of the tube requiring reintubation — 22 cases.

2. Suspected obstruction of the tube by secretions requiring reintubation — 36 cases.

3. Tracheal ulceration and necrosis — 1 case.

Sepsis as a complication of intubation is difficult to assess. Sepsis is a common problem in these infants and it is often impossible to determine an exact etiology. They are extremely ill, have numerous arterial and other catheters, and are highly susceptible to infection. Tracheal aspirates are submitted weekly for culture, but it has not always been possible to show a direct correlation between a positive culture and clinical sepsis.

The overall mortality of the 174 infants was 22.9% and was directly related to the underlying disease process, especially prematurity and low birth weight (Table 2).

Follow-up on the 134 survivors was carried out largely through the outpatient pediatric clinic by one of the authors (MJM) at three to six-month intervals. The follow-up period ranged from three months to five years. There were seven lost to follow-up. Pulmonary ventilatory studies[8] were not done.

Postmortem examination was performed on 36 infants. The larynx and trachea were grossly examined in all postmortem examinations but routine microscopic examination of this tissue was not performed. A study is now in progress to evaluate more precisely what microscopic damage does occur with prolonged orotracheal intubation and whether or not there is a correlation between the degree of microscopic damage and the duration of intubation.

DISCUSSION

Proper orotracheal intubation technique, especially in relation to the selection of the correct tube size, was felt to be essential to avoid airway damage with these infants. All intubations were carried out by the pediatric staff and residents using Portex® * disposable orotracheal tubes.

Prior to attempting orotracheal intubation the following general principles are recommended:

1. Endotracheal intubation in this group is usually not an emergency. It should be done when there is adequate personnel and equipment.

2. Never intubate an hypoxic infant. Always oxygenate well with a bag before attempting to expose the larynx and pass the tube.

3. Have someone timing the efforts. If the tube is not in place within 30 seconds, withdraw the laryngoscope and reventilate.

4. Monitor the heart rate at all times. If for any reason bradycardia occurs, withdraw the laryngoscope and reventilate.

By following these principles, cardiac arrest can largely be avoided.

Intubation is accomplished with the infant laryngoscope inserted into the vallecula and the tongue elevated. Gentle counterpressure on the external surface of the larynx can be accomplished with the little finger against the thyroid cartilage or by an assistant. The epiglottis is visualized and the orotracheal tube passed easily through the glottis. The infant is ventilated and both lung fields listened to in order to help determine the position of the tube. The tip of the tube should be at about the sternal notch which corresponds to the midportion of the infant trachea.

Following insertion of the tube, it is essential that auscultation at the mouth with a stethoscope is done to confirm that there is a leak of air around the tube when a positive pressure of 25-30 cm of water is applied. If no leak can be heard, the tube is removed and the next smaller size is inserted. A straight Portex tube is used, the size varying from 2.5 ± 3.5 mm. The Cole tube with a narrow diameter at the tip is not used because of the possibility of causing pressure necrosis of the vocal cords.

Adequate securing of the orotracheal tube is extremely important. The tape and suture technique as described by Gregory[9] has been quite effective and has allowed for very few accidental tube dislodgments all of which were easily corrected. The position of the orotracheal tube at the midportion of the trachea is always confirmed by x-ray examination of the chest. The tube is left in place indefinitely and is removed only when extubation or reintubation is deemed appropriate.

The management of the orotracheal tube is also of critical importance. Only warm and humidified gas is used. The tube is suctioned every hour by instilling 0.25 ml saline into the tube and gently suctioning it out. After each pass with the suction catheter, the baby is ventilated with deep "sighing" positive pressure ventilation for one to two minutes. Sterile technique is always used.

Extubation is carried out when the infant can breathe spontaneously without assistance and is able to maintain satisfactory blood gas levels. After

*General Medical Co., Div. of Smith Industries, Wilmington, Mass.

extubation the infant is watched continuously and blood gases monitored. No steroids are given. If satisfactory blood gases cannot be maintained, the baby is reintubated.

Nasal tracheal intubation is not done at our institution because of possible damage to the nasal structures. In addition, compression of the nasal structures can cause secondary nasal and sinus blockage resulting in local infection.[9-11] Since nasotracheal tubes require changing every 48 to 72 hours, contamination can be carried into the trachea. Finally, the technique of nasal tracheal intubation is significantly more difficult than that of orotracheal intubation.

CONCLUSIONS

It is our thesis that orotracheal intubation is the superior method of providing a safe and effective airway for newborn infants who require prolonged ventilatory assistance. Tracheotomy does not appear to be indicated on the basis of duration or repeated reintubation and should be performed only if the underlying disease state would warrant it. The fact that only one tracheotomy was done for this large group of neonates justifies this conclusion. We feel that orotracheal intubation largely avoids the serious complications of tracheotomy caused by accidental dislodgment of the tracheotomy tube, the obvious direct trauma to the trachea, and the problem of decannulation of the tracheotomized infant.[3,6,12-16] Orotracheal intubation is felt to be preferable to nasal tracheal intubation because of its greater technical ease and avoidance of local nasal tissue damage.

REFERENCES

1. Fearon B, McDonald R, Smith C, Mitchell D. Airway problems in children following prolonged endotracheal intubation. Ann Otol Rhinol Laryngol 1966; 75:975-86.

2. Pickard RE, Oropeza G. Tracheotomy in premature infants. Laryngoscope 1971; 81:418-22.

3. Joshi VV, Mandavia SG, Stearn L, Wigglesworth FW. Acute lesions induced by endotracheal intubation. Am J Dis Child 1972; 124:646-9.

4. Hengerer AS, Strome M, Jaffe BF. Injuries to the neonatal larynx from long-term endotracheal tube intubation and suggestive tube modification for prevention. Ann Otol Rhinol Laryngol 1975; 84:764-70.

5. Heroy JH, MacDonald JG, Plazzi E, Risemberg HM. Airway management in the premature infant. Ann Otol Rhinol Laryngol 1978; 87:53-9.

6. Gibson R, Bryne JET. Tracheotomy in neonates. Laryngoscope 1972; 82:643-50.

7. Conner GH, Maisels MJ. Orotracheal intubation in the newborn. Laryngoscope 1977; 87:87-91.

8. Schuller DE, Birck HG. The safety of intubation in croup epiglottitis: an 8-year follow-up. Laryngoscope 1975; 85:33-46.

9. Gregory GA. Respiratory care of newborn infants. Ped Clin North Am 1972; 5:311-24.

10. McDonald IH, Stocks JG. Prolonged nasotracheal intubation. Br J Anaesth 1965; 37:161-73.

11. Striker WT, Stool S, Downes JJ. Prolonged nasotracheal intubation in infants and children. Arch Otolaryngol 1967; 85:210-3.

12. Ardan GM, Caust LJ. Delayed decannulation after tracheostomy in infants. J Laryngol Otol 1963; 77:555-66.

13. Oliver P, Richardson JR, Clubb RW, Flake CG. Tracheotomy in children. N Engl J Med 1962; 267:631-7.

14. Putney FJ. Complications and postoperative care after tracheostomy. Arch Otolaryngol 1955; 62:272-6.

15. McClelland RMA. Complications of tracheotomy. Br Med J 1965; 2:267-9.

16. Mattila MAK, Suutarinen T, Sulamaa M. Prolonged endotracheal intubation or tracheostomy in infants and children. J Pediatr Surg 1969; 4:674-82.

Ann Otol 89:1980

LARYNGEAL REGULATION OF AIRWAY RESISTANCE
II. PULMONARY RECEPTOR REFLEXES

THOMAS V. MCCAFFREY, MD EUGENE B. KERN, MD

ROCHESTER, MINNESOTA

The response of laryngeal airway resistance to pulmonary receptor stimulation was studied in 20 mongrel dogs anesthetized with α-chloralose (80 mg/kg). Stimulation of pulmonary stretch receptors by lung inflation inhibited the phasic variation of laryngeal resistance during respiration and produced a sustained reduction of laryngeal resistance, which was related to lung inflation pressure. Stimulation of pulmonary J-receptors with capsaicin produced apnea and a large increase in laryngeal resistance. Capsaicin produced this reflex when injected into the pulmonary circulation but not when injected into the systemic circulation. Irritant receptor stimulation with histamine hydrochloride produced tachypnea and a reduction in inspiratory laryngeal resistance. Pulmonary receptor reflexes were abolished by dividing the vagus nerves distal to the origin of the recurrent laryngeal nerves. Laryngeal reflexes may be important in the regulation of respiration and the production of physiologic and pathologic alterations in pulmonary function.

INTRODUCTION

The respiratory functions of the larynx include protection of lower airway and regulation of airway resistance. Resistance properties of the larynx have been largely neglected because of the difficulty in measuring the laryngeal airway resistance in isolation from the resistance of the tracheobronchial airway. The unique property of the laryngeal airway is its ability to undergo rapid adjustments corresponding to the phase of respiration and the physiologic status of the lower airway. This integration results in part from reflexes initiated by receptors in the lower airway and lung parenchyma.

There are three types of pulmonary receptors: stretch, irritant, and unmyelinated (J-receptors).[1] Although there are some species variations, the general characteristics of these receptors are similar for man and for the most widely studied laboratory animal species (cat, rabbit, and dog). Each receptor type evokes a specific reflex pattern that is associated with characteristic changes in the rate and depth of respiration, heart rate, and blood pressure (Table 1).

The purpose of the present study is to describe and quantitate the effect of pulmonary receptor stimulation on laryngeal airway resistance in the dog. This study examines the laryngeal airway resistance in response to stretch receptor, irritant receptor, and J-receptor stimulation.

METHODS

Twenty mongrel dogs weighing from 15 to 25 kg were used in the study. The dogs were anesthetized with ketamine hydrochloride (8 mg/kg intramuscularly) and α-chloralose (80 mg/kg intravenously). Further doses of α-chloralose (5 to 10 mg/kg intravenously) were given at appropriate intervals to maintain a constant level of anesthesia. The left femoral vein was catheterized, and the catheter was advanced into the right atrium for the administration of drugs into the pulmonary circulation. The left femoral artery was catheterized, and the catheter was advanced into the left ventricle for administration of drugs into the systemic circulation.

The trachea was cannulated in the neck after the recurrent laryngeal nerves were identified and preserved. Without assistance, the dogs breathed 100% O_2 from a nine-liter spirometer (Collins, Braintree, MA) containing a CO_2 absorber. Tidal volume (V_T), respiratory frequency (f), and minute ventilation ($\dot{V}_E$) were determined from the spirometer recording. Airway pressure (P_{ao}) was measured using a pressure transducer (Statham PM131) attached to the side arm of the tracheal cannula.

Laryngeal resistance was determined by passing a continuous flow of humidified air through the upper airway at the rate of 1 liter/sec. Airflow was measured continuously by means of a pneumotachograph and a gas pressure transducer (Hewlett-

TABLE 1. CHARACTERISTICS OF PULMONARY RECEPTORS IN THE DOG

Pulmonary Receptor	*Location*	*Fiber Conduction Velocity (m/sec)*	*Respiratory Effects*	*Stimulus*
Stretch	Associated with smooth muscle of large bronchi[2]	32.3±11.8[3]	Inhibits inspiration[1] and (?) bronchodilation	Lung inflation[1] and veratrum alkaloids
Irritant	Epithelium of medium and small-size bronchi[4]	23.3± 7.1[5]	Tachypnea[1]; decrease in tidal volume; bronchoconstriction	Smoke[1]; mechanical irritation; histamine; lung hyperinflation; lung deflation
"J"	(?) Near pulmonary capillaries (juxta-alveolar capillaries[6])	1.4±0.13[7]	Apnea[1,8] and (?) bronchoconstriction	(?) Pulmonary edema;[9-11] (?) increased pulmonary artery pressure; capsaicin

From the Department of Otorhinolaryngology, Mayo Clinic, Rochester, Minnesota. This study was supported in part by the St. Jude Fund for Otolaryngology Education and Research.

Presented at the meeting of the American Broncho-Esophagological Association, Palm Beach, Florida, April 12-13, 1980.

REPRINTS — T. V. McCaffrey, MD, Mayo Clinic, 200 First Street SW, Rochester, MN 55901.

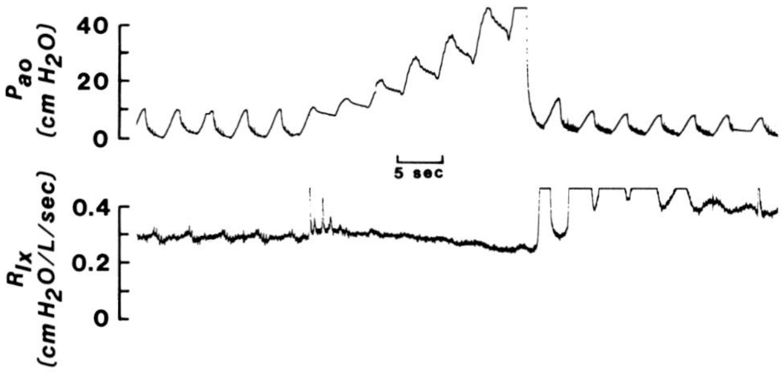

Fig. 1. Lung inflation — vagi intact. Response of laryngeal airway resistance (R_{lx}) to stepwise lung inflations as measured by airway pressure (P_{ao}).

Packard model 270). Transglottic pressure difference was recorded using another pressure transducer (model 270). Laryngeal airway resistance was calculated as the transglottic pressure divided by the airflow through the larynx. This technique permitted measurement of the laryngeal resistance with the larynx functionally isolated from the lower airway, except for its innervation. A complete description of the method of measuring laryngeal resistance has been given.[12]

Tidal volume (V_T), airway pressure (P_{ao}), laryngeal airflow, and transglottic pressure were simultaneously recorded on a chart recorder (Hewlett-Packard).

At intervals throughout the procedure, PaO_2 and $PaCO_2$ were measured. PaO_2 was maintained greater than 180 mm Hg, and $PaCO_2$ was maintained between 35 and 45 mm Hg to minimize chemoreceptor reflexes. Pulmonary receptor stimulation was done before and after the afferent pulmonary nerves were divided. The afferent innervation of the lungs is carried in the vagus nerves. To interrupt the afferent vagal fibers without destroying the efferent motor fibers to the larynx, the vagus nerves were divided in the chest below the origins of the recurrent laryngeal nerves.[13,14]

Stretch Receptor Stimulation. Pulmonary stretch receptor reflexes were stimulated in eight dogs by controlled lung inflation. The chest of each dog was opened widely through a bilateral thoracotomy. Ventilation was maintained by a pump respirator (Harvard Apparatus) using 100% O_2. Airway pressure was measured using a pressure transducer (Statham PM131) attached to the side arm of the tracheal cannula. For the prevention of atelectasis, a positive pressure of 3 cm of water was maintained in the airway by placing the expiratory line under water.

While laryngeal resistance and airway pressure were recorded, lung inflations were performed by closing the expiratory line of the respirator. With each respirator pump stroke, the lungs were inflated by an increment of one tidal volume (350 ml). Inflations were done to an airway pressure of 30 cm of water.

Lung inflations were repeated after the vagus nerves were divided bilaterally below the recurrent laryngeal nerves.

J-Receptor Stimulation. J-receptor reflexes were stimulated in ten spontaneously breathing dogs by the injection of capsaicin. The capsaicin was injected in solution prepared as described by Coleridge et al.[11] Capsaicin (10 μg/kg) was injected into either the right atrium or the left ventricle while laryngeal resistance and tidal volume were recorded.

J-receptors were denervated in three dogs by dividing the vagus nerves bilaterally below the recurrent laryngeal nerves. Capsaicin injections were then repeated while laryngeal resistance was recorded.

Irritant Receptor Stimulation. Irritant receptor reflexes were stimulated in 14 spontaneously breathing dogs with histamine hydrochloride. Histamine hydrochloride (10 μg/kg) was injected intravenously while laryngeal resistance and tidal volume were recorded.

The irritant receptors were denervated in four dogs by sectioning the vagus nerves bilaterally below the recurrent laryngeal nerves. Histamine injections were repeated while laryngeal resistance was recorded.

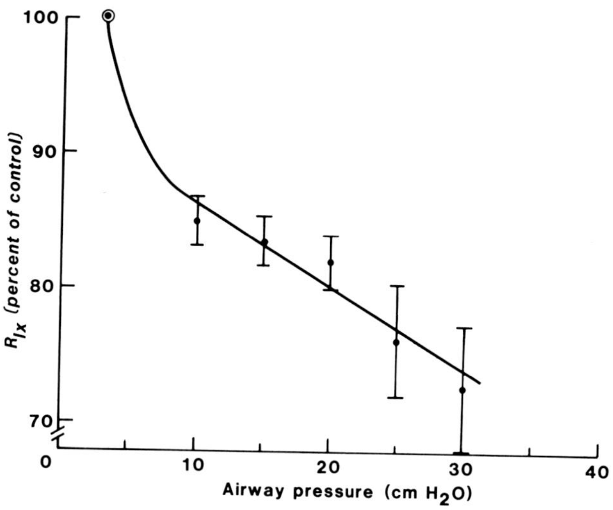

Fig. 2. Effect of lung inflation of laryngeal resistance in five dogs. Vertical bars indicate standard error of mean.

RESULTS

Stretch Receptors. Stretch receptor stimulation by progressive lung inflation in the open-chest dog produced two responses in laryngeal resistance: 1) lung inflation inhibited the phasic inspiratory activity of the laryngeal abductors when this was present, and 2) progressive lung inflation decreased laryngeal resistance which was related to the degree of lung inflation (Fig. 1). The first effect is a counterpart of the Hering-Breuer inhibito-inspiratory reflex, which inhibits inspiratory phased respiratory muscles, whereas the second reflex does not affect the phasic muscle activity but produces a continuous decrease in laryngeal resistance. Progressive lung inflation significantly decreased ($P<0.05$) laryngeal resistance (Fig. 2 and Table 2).

At the termination of lung inflation, the rapid deflation of the lung produced a large increase in laryngeal resistance (Fig. 1). This response may be due to the rapid inhibition of stretch receptor activity or to the stimulation of irritant receptors by rapid lung deflation.

After the vagus nerves were divided below the

TABLE 2. RELATIONSHIP OF AIRWAY PRESSURE TO LARYNGEAL AIRWAY RESISTANCE IN THE DOG

P_{ao} (cm H_2O)	N	R_{lx} ($M \pm SE$), % Control
3	8	100
10	8	85.1±1.80*
15	8	83.5±1.84*
20	8	82.1±2.00*
25	8	76.3±4.20*
30	8	72.8±4.80*

*Significantly decreased from control value (Wilcoxon's signed-rank test, $P<0.05$).

P_{ao} - Airway pressure; R_{lx} - Laryngeal airway resistance.

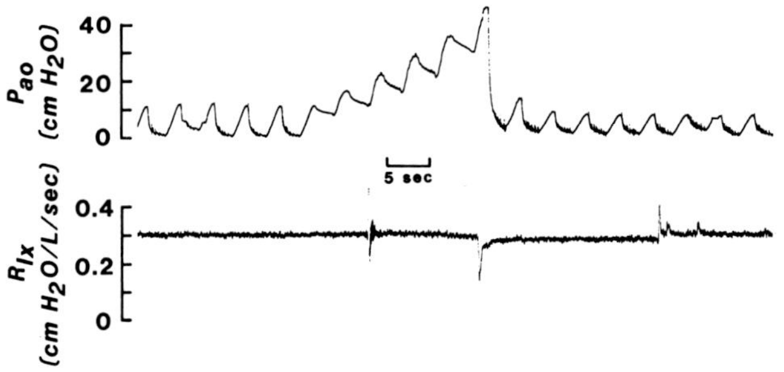

Fig. 3. Response of laryngeal airway resistance (R_{lx}) to stepwise lung inflations after sectioning the vagus nerves below the origin of recurrent laryngeal nerves.

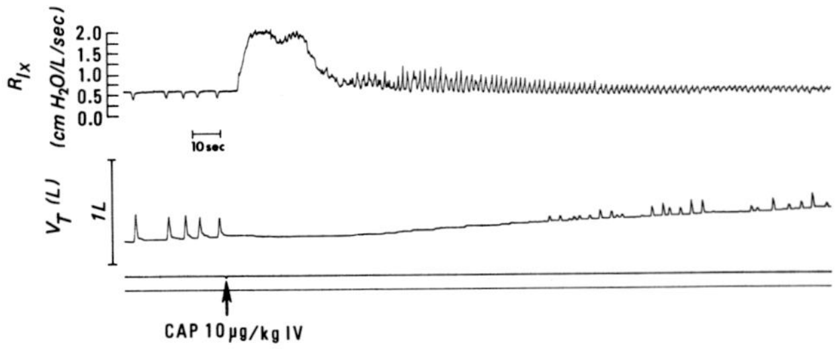

Fig. 4. Effect of intravenous injection of capsaicin (CAP, 10 µg/kg) into right atrium on laryngeal airway resistance (R_{lx}) and tidal volume (V_T).

origin of the recurrent laryngeal nerves, the effect of lung inflation on laryngeal resistance was abolished (Fig. 3).

J-Receptors. The injection of capsaicin (10 µg/kg) into the right atrium produced apnea and a significant increase ($P<0.05$) in laryngeal resistance after a latency of 4.8±0.33 seconds (Fig. 4 and Table 3). The short latency suggests that the effect is produced by stimulation of receptors in the pulmonary circulation. This is confirmed by the absence of a response to capsaicin when injected into the left ventricle (Fig. 5 and Table 3).

The response of laryngeal resistance to capsaicin is mediated by afferent vagal fibers arising from the lung, since dividing the vagus nerves below the origin of the recurrent laryngeal nerves abolishes the response to capsaicin injected into the right atrium (Table 3).

Irritant Receptors. Stimulation of pulmonary irritant receptors by intravenously administered histamine (10 µg/kg) produced tachypnea with a decreased tidal volume and a decrease in both inspiratory and expiratory laryngeal airway resistances (Fig. 6). However, only the decrease in inspiratory resistance was statistically significant ($P<0.05$). Histamine injections into the left ventricle failed to produce a response (Table 4). Sectioning the vagus nerves below the origin of the recurrent laryngeal nerves abolished the response to intravenous histamine injection (Table 4). These observations indicate that the response to histamine injection is mediated by pulmonary receptors with vagal afferent fibers.

DISCUSSION

Stretch Receptors. Pulmonary stretch receptors have been the most widely investigated of the pulmonary receptor types.[1-3,15-18] Lung inflation stimulates stretch receptors by the tension produced in the walls of the larger bronchi where the receptors are concentrated. The effect of stretch receptor stimulation is an inhibition of the inspiratory muscles of respiration — the classic Hering-Breuer reflex.

The effect of stretch receptor stimulation on the larynx is consistent with the action on other respiratory muscles. Lung inflation inhibits the inspiratory muscles of the larynx (the posterior cricoarytenoid muscles).[19] This has the effect of inhibiting the phasic reduction of laryngeal resistance during inspiration. Moreover, sustained lung inflation produces a tonic decrease in the laryngeal airway resistance. The decrease in laryngeal resistance is related to the inflation pressure of the lungs. This reflex arises from intrapulmonary receptors and is not merely a mechanical effect of lung inflation since it is effectively abolished by section of the afferent vagal fibers. It cannot be determined from the present study whether lung inflation inhibits vocal fold adductors or stimulates vocal fold abductors. Studies by Green and Neil[20] have shown inhibition of inspiratory phased vagal fibers and stimulation of expiratory phased vagal fibers with lung inflation. This corresponds with the observed inhibition of the phasic activity of the laryngeal resistance observed in the present study. Moreover, studies on human subjects[21] have shown that laryngeal resistance is lower at large lung volumes than at small lung volumes. This is consistent with the second observation that lung inflation produces a tonic decrease in laryngeal resistance related to the transpulmonary pressure.

The effect of a decrease in laryngeal resistance with lung inflation would tend to stabilize functional residual capacity during ventilation. With

TABLE 3. EFFECT OF CAPSAICIN* ON LARYNGEAL AIRWAY RESISTANCE IN THE DOG

Route of Administration	*Afferent Vagus*	*N*	*Latency (M±SE), sec*	R_{lx} *(M±SE), % Control*
Right atrium	Intact	10	4.8±0.33	150±30†
Left ventricle	Intact	5	—	104± 3
Right atrium	Sectioned	3	—	93±14

*Dose of 10 µg/kg.

†Significantly increased from control value (Wilcoxon's signed-rank test, $P<0.05$).

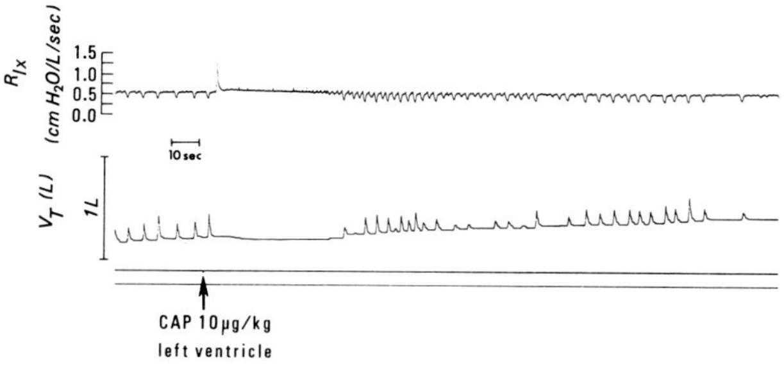

Fig. 5. Effect of injection of capsaicin (CAP, 10 μg/kg) into left ventricle on laryngeal airway resistance (R_{lx}) and tidal volume (V_T).

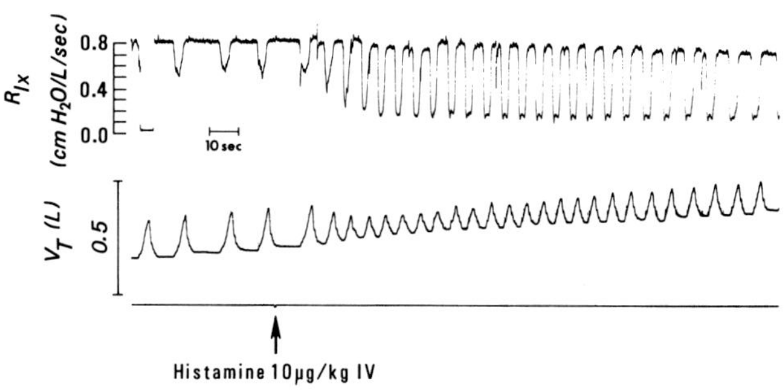

Fig. 6. Effect of intravenous injection of histamine hydrochloride (10 μg/kg) on laryngeal resistance (R_{lx}) and tidal volume (V_T).

large lung inflation, laryngeal resistance would decrease, thus facilitating lung emptying. With small inflation, laryngeal resistance would be higher, slowing lung deflation. In these cases, the lung would tend to reach a constant functional residual capacity during expiration for both large and small inflations.

J-Receptors. The unmyelinated J-receptors have been examined in several species: the dog, cat, and rabbit. The reflex produced by J-receptor stimulation is generally the same in these species; there is a decrease in blood pressure and apnea, followed by tachypnea and bradycardia.[1] However, there is peculiar variability in the chemical stimuli producing these reflexes. In the cat and rabbit, phenyldiguanide produces the J-receptor reflex.[1] However, this agent is ineffective in producing this reflex in the dog and in man.[22-24] In the dog, capsaicin produces a typical J-receptor reflex.[6] The reasons for the difference in sensitivity of J-receptors to these agents is not known. The physiologic stimulus for the J-receptor is not known with certainty, although pulmonary edema and pulmonary vascular congestion have been suggested as effective stimuli.[1]

The effect of J-receptor stimulation on the larynx is a striking increase in laryngeal resistance during the apnea induced by the stimulation. This effect of J-receptor stimulation has been observed in the cat during stimulation of J-receptors by phenyldiguanide.[17,18]

The J-receptors are physiologically located in the region of the lung supplied by the pulmonary circulation. This is consistent with the anatomic localization in the juxta-alveolar capillaries (hence the name J-receptor).[1]

The physiologic role of these receptors is not known, and the powerful laryngospasm produced by their stimulation is equally unexplained. Reflex laryngospasm probably is not a protective reflex because J-receptors cannot be stimulated until the irritant agent reaches the alveoli. However, if pulmonary edema is the effective physiologic stimulus for J-receptors, laryngospasm may have a beneficial effect by producing elevated airway pressure during expiratory apnea, thus forcing edema fluid into the pulmonary blood vessels and lymphatic vessels. This reflex must remain speculative, however, until more is known about the physiologic stimulus of J-receptors.

Irritant Receptors. Pulmonary irritant receptors produce a tachypnea with a decrease in tidal volume in response to airway irritations, histamine, and lung deflation. Although histamine may produce some nonvagal actions, the main action of histamine on breathing is by stimulation of lung irritant receptors. Some reports indicate that histamine can stimulate pulmonary J-receptors, but the difference between the action of capsaicin (a powerful J-receptor stimulant) and of histamine in the dog suggests that histamine does not produce significant reflex action through J-receptor stimulation in this species.

That the observed decrease in laryngeal resistance after histamine injection is secondary to pulmonary receptor stimulation is established by the absence of a response after the afferent vagal fibers are sectioned.

The physiologic role of laryngeal resistance changes during irritant receptor stimulation is uncertain, although a decrease in laryngeal resistance and tachypnea would tend to expel irritant substances from the airway.

TABLE 4. EFFECT OF HISTAMINE HYDROCHLORIDE* ON LARYNGEAL AIRWAY RESISTANCE IN THE DOG

Route of Administration	*Afferent Vagus*	*N*	*Latency (M ± SE), sec*	R_{lx} *(M ± SE), % Control* *Inspiration*	*Expiration*
Right atrium	Intact	14	10.8 ± 1.1	59 ± 10†	96 ± 3
Left ventricle	Intact	3	9.3 ± 0.33	109 ± 8	106 ± 7
Right atrium	Sectioned	4	—	94 ± 4	95 ± 3

*Dose 10 μg/kg.

†Significantly decreased from control value (Wilcoxon's signed-rank test, $P < 0.05$).

CONCLUSIONS

The larynx is a rapidly adjustable resistance in series with the bronchopulmonary airway. Breath-to-breath variations in laryngeal airway resistance provide a means of adjusting expiratory airflow and thereby lung volume. This function of the larynx is regulated by a reflex originating with lung stretch receptors within the intrathoracic airways. In addition to stretch receptors, pulmonary irritant receptors and pulmonary J-receptors can modify laryngeal resistance. However, the physiologic role of these pulmonary receptor reflexes is unclear at the present time. The laryngeal airway is closely integrated with the function of the lower airways by a network of reflex arcs which uniquely provides for rapid and reversible modification of airway resistance.

REFERENCES

1. Paintal AS. Vagal sensory receptors and their reflex effects. Physiol Rev 1973; 53:159-227.

2. Miserocchi G, Sant'Ambrogio G. Distribution of pulmonary stretch receptors in the intrapulmonary airways of the dog. Respir Physiol 1974; 21:71-5.

3. Miserocchi G, Sant'Ambrogio G. Responses of pulmonary stretch receptors to static pressure inflations. Respir Physiol 1974; 21:77-85.

4. Mortola J. Sant'Ambrogio G, Clement MG. Localization of irritant receptors in the airways of the dog. Respir Physiol 1975; 24:107-14.

5. Sampson SR, Vidruk EH. Properties of 'irritant' receptors in canine lung. Respir Physiol 1975; 25:9-22.

6. Coleridge HM, Coleridge JCG. Impulse activity in afferent vagal C-fibres with endings in the intrapulmonary airways of dogs. Respir Physiol 1977; 29:125-42.

7. Coleridge HM, Coleridge JCG, Luck JC. Pulmonary afferent fibres of small diameter stimulated by capsaicin and by hyperinflation of the lungs. J Physiol (Lond) 1965; 179: 248-62.

8. Pórszász J, György L, Pórszász-Gibiszer K. Cardiovascular and respiratory effects of capsaicin. Acta Physiol Acad Sci Hung 1955; 8:61-76.

9. Paintal AS. Mechanism of stimulation of type J pulmonary receptors. J Physiol (Lond) 1969; 203:511-32.

10. Paintal AS. The influence of certain chemical substances on the initiation of sensory discharges in pulmonary and gastric stretch receptors and atrial receptors. J Physiol (Lond) 1957; 135:486-510.

11. Coleridge HM, Coleridge JCG, Kidd C. Role of the pulmonary arterial baroreceptors in the effects produced by capsaicin in the dog. J Physiol (Lond) 1964; 170:272-85.

12. McCaffrey TV, Kern EB. Laryngeal regulation of airway resistance. I. Chemoreceptor reflexes. Ann Otol Rhinol Laryngol 1980; 89:209-14.

13. Hilsabeck JR, Hill FC. Anatomy of the thoracic vagus in the dog and a technic for its interruption. Proc Soc Exp Biol Med 1950; 73:633-7.

14. Mizeres NJ. The anatomy of the autonomic nervous system in the dog. Am J Anat 1955; 96:285-318.

15. Lazarus S, Gross P, Buxton R, et al. Mechanisms of changes in airflow resistance with changing transpulmonary pressure. Abstract. Clin Res 1968; 16:133.

16. Campbell CJ, Murtagh JA, Raber CF. Laryngeal resistance to airflow. Ann Otol Rhinol Laryngol 1963; 72:5-30.

17. Dixon M, Szereda-Przestaszewska M, Widdicombe JG, et al. Studies on laryngeal calibre during stimulation of peripheral and central chemoreceptors, pneumothorax and increased respiratory loads. J Physiol (Lond) 1974; 239:347-63.

18. Stransky A, Szereda-Przestaszewska M, Widdicombe JG. The effects of lung reflexes on laryngeal resistance and motoneurone discharge. J Physiol (Lond) 1973; 231:417-38.

19. Fukuda H. Sasaki CT, Kirchner JA. Vagal afferent influences on the phasic activity of the posterior cricoarytenoid muscle. Acta Otolaryngol (Stockh) 1973; 75:112-8.

20. Green JH, Neil E. The respiratory function of the laryngeal muscles. J Physiol (Lond) 1955; 129:134-41.

21. Spann RW, Hyatt RE. Factors affecting upper airway resistance in conscious man. J Appl Physiol 1971; 31:708-12.

22. Dawes GS, Mott JC. Circulatory and respiratory reflexes caused by aromatic guanidines. Br J Pharmacol 1950; 5:65-76.

23. Dawes GS, Mott JC, Widdicombe JG. Chemoreceptor reflexes in the dog and the action of phenyl diguanide. Arch Int Pharmacodyn Ther 1952; 90:203-22.

24. Jain SK, Subramanian S, Julka DB, et al. Search for evidence of lung chemoreflexes in man: study of respiratory and circulatory effects of phenyldiguanide and lobeline. Clin Sci 1972; 42:163-77.

RELATIONSHIP BETWEEN CONDYLOMATA AND LARYNGEAL PAPILLOMATA

CLINICAL AND MOLECULAR VIROLOGICAL EVIDENCE

CEDRIC A. QUICK, MD
PETERSBURG, VIRGINIA

SUSAN L. WATTS, PhD
MINNEAPOLIS, MINNESOTA

R. A. KRZYZEK, PhD
MINNEAPOLIS, MINNESOTA

A. J. FARAS, PhD
MINNEAPOLIS, MINNESOTA

In a survey of 49 papilloma patients accurate maternal condyloma history was obtained in 31 instances and of these, 21 were positive for the presence of condyloma during pregnancy or parturition. Molecular virological studies indicate that positive hybridization could be demonstrated to human papilloma virus 2 in both laryngeal papilloma and condyloma by the Southern blot technique. Immunoperoxidase staining illustrated the presence of virus-related particles only near the surface of the mucous membrane papilloma, which is in contrast to the definite staining of the stratum granulosum and stratum corneum of verrucae. Collectively this provides convincing evidence for an etiological relationship between condyloma acuminata and some laryngeal papillomata. The highly contagious nature of human papilloma virus infection is discussed and the possibility of cesarian section in the presence of active condyloma must be considered.

INTRODUCTION

A viral etiology for all warty growth has been suspected for a long time. This opinion was based upon the common histological pattern of the growths, and on the typical clinical course of the lesions which tend to recur and spread despite seemingly adequate ablation of the tumors, but eventually spontaneously regress. Early light histological studies demonstrated inclusion bodies in the stratum spinosum and granulosum of keratinizing varieties of papillomas. Electron microscopy studies later confirmed the presence of virus crystals in these situations. However, only a few isolated reports suggest the presence of virus particles in mucous membrane papillomata such as laryngeal papilloma or papilloma of the vagina and uterine cervix.[1,2] Other workers have failed to find virus material in laryngeal papillomas even after exhaustive searches.[3] This apparent discrepancy may now be explained in light of recent evidence to be presented later.

Further evidence for a viral etiology was strongly indicated by the experiments of Ullman.[4] Excised laryngeal papilloma tissue was self-inoculated into the forearm. After 90 days typical flat warts were visible. Suspecting a virus Ullman then inoculated cell-free extracts of laryngeal tissue into his own arm and that of an assistant. Warty growths occurred after a similar latent period. This work was substantiated by Ishikawa in 1936.[5] These findings led to the hypothesis that warts or papillomas from all locations were caused by the same viral agent. Although in the literature papilloma, condyloma, wart and verruca are often used synonymously, in this paper the term wart or verruca will be used to describe the papillary tumors of cutaneous surfaces and the term papilloma will be used only to describe mucous membrane lesions. Condyloma acuminata are lesions that occur in the genital area of males or females and will be designated cutaneous or mucous membrane condyloma according to the histological presence or absence of a stratum corneum and distinct stratum granulosum.

The coincidental presence of skin warts in patients with laryngeal papillomas was cited as additional evidence for a virus etiology and for the possibility of self-inoculation. Majoros et al reviewed the incidence of laryngeal papillomas and found that the greatest incidence of onset occurred before five years of age.[6] Zur Hausen et al in an epidemiological survey showed that there was a bimodal distribution of laryngeal papillomas that did not correspond to the distribution of verruca vulgaris.[7] An etiological relationship between laryngeal papilloma in children and condyloma acuminata of the mother has also been suspected and sporadic case reports have appeared describing this phenomenon.[8-10]

Cook and coworkers performed an analysis of 13 patients with laryngeal papillomas and found that the mothers of five of nine children had condyloma at the time of delivery.[11]

As yet no whole virus has been isolated from laryngeal papillomas but recent virological techniques have clearly shown the presence of free human papilloma virus (HPV) DNA.[12] To date no reproducible in vitro model has been established

From the Department of Otolaryngology, West Virginia University Medical Center, Morgantown, West Virginia, and the Department of Microbiology, University of Minnesota, Minneapolis, Minnesota. This study was supported by NIH grant from NCI 7 R01 CA 25124-01.

Presented at the meeting of the American Broncho-Esophagological Association, Palm Beach, Florida, April 12-13, 1980.

REPRINTS — Cedric A. Quick, MD, 700 S. Sycamore Street, Petersburg, VA 23803.

TABLE 1. SUMMARY OF CLINICAL CONDYLOMA HISTORY IN MOTHERS OF CHILDREN WITH LARYNGEAL PAPILLOMA

Institution	*No. of Patients*	*Condyloma Positive*	*Condyloma Negative*	*Unable to Determine*	*Lost to Follow-Up*
1	14	7	4	1	2
2	35	8	7	15	5
		(14)	(6)	(10)	(5)
Total	49	21	10	11	7

Positive incidence maternal condyloma — definitive group - 67%; overall group - 42%.

Parentheses indicate the change from initial history by the more detailed gynecological investigation.

that permits the growth and replication of HPV. However, using techniques of DNA reassociation, hybridization and restriction endonuclease mapping several distinct strains of HPV have been isolated.[13]

The purpose of this paper is to present clinical evidence of the association of condyloma and laryngeal papilloma which is supported by molecular virological and immunohistochemical studies.

CLINICAL EVALUATION

Personal observation, reviews of obstetric and gynecologic charts, direct questioning of patients' mothers and their physicians, as well as pelvic examinations by these physicians were used in extracting the following data. The patients were drawn from the otolaryngologic practice at two teaching institutions. A total of 49 patients were collected (Table 1). Seven patients were lost to follow-up and in 11 patients we were unable to determine if condylomata had been present. In the remaining 31 patients, 21 had a positive maternal history of condyloma and 10 had a definite negative history. The majority of those patients with a negative history had a late (adult) onset of papillomata. The mother of one female patient whose papilloma appeared at 16 years of age following intubation for tonsillectomy did have a confirmed history of condyloma at delivery. Frequently the presence of condyloma was initially denied by the mother but on further investigation the information was found to be forgotten or the individual had been unaware of the presence of these lesions which had disappeared after local treatment (Table 1). In some instances the vulva and vagina were free of clinical condyloma but small flattened lesions were reported on the cervix.

The age of onset of laryngeal symptoms ranged from the neonatal period to 64 years of age, with the majority occurring within the first 5 years of life. The histological pattern of atypia correlated with the frequency of recurrence as has been described previously.[14]

MOLECULAR VIROLOGICAL STUDIES

The virus isolation scheme employed has been documented in a previous publication.[12] (Fig. 1). We have been unable to isolate whole HPV particles banding after cesium chloride density gradient centrifugation from extracts of laryngeal papillomas, even though virus particles could be isolated easily by this procedure from equivalent amounts of skin warts. We have also failed to identify form 1 HPV DNA by cesium chloride-propidium diiodide centrifugation and electron microscopy of the Hirt supernatant fraction[15] of laryngeal papillomas.[12] Separation of cellular DNA species by agarose gel electrophoresis followed by ethidium bromide staining allows visualization by ultraviolet light of as little as 10 ng of DNA migrating in a single band.[16] In 20 μg of electrophoretically separated cellular DNA, bands corresponding to viral DNA forms 1, 2, or 3 could be discerned in many samples fron anogenital warts but none from laryngeal papillomas.

Laryngeal papillomas were also assayed for HPV

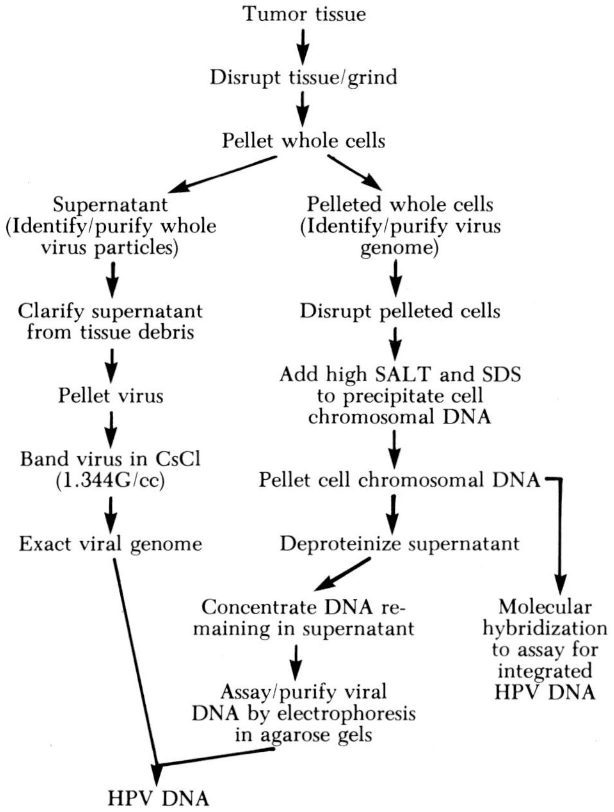

Fig. 1. Scheme of human papilloma virus genome purification and identification (Reprinted with permission of Quick et al.[12])

DNA by nucleic acid hybridization procedures. Hybridization analyses by DNA-DNA reassociation using purified HPV DNA probes labeled by nick translation[17] were designed to detect approximately 0.2 genome equivalents of viral DNA per diploid cell genome. Results of such hybridization analyses with laryngeal DNA and HPV 1 probe were negative.[12,18] Using our HPV-2 probe low levels of hybridization were found.*

Since there are apparently such small quantities of free viral DNA in laryngeal papillomas we have resorted to the more sensitive Southern's technique of blot hybridization.[19]

Cellular or viral DNA is separated by molecular weight in a 1% (w/v) agarose gel by electrophoresis. For Southern blotting, the DNA contained in the gel is denatured in situ by treatment with sodium hydroxide (NaOH) and then transferred to a piece of nitrocellulose paper by placing the gel on the paper, dripping high salt buffer on top of the gel, and pulling the buffer through the gel and the paper by vacuum filtration. The gradient of salt through the gel transfers the DNA onto the nitrocellulose paper. The paper is then baked to bind the DNA irreversibly to the paper. Transfer of the DNA from the gel to the paper may be confirmed by restaining the gel after transfer.

For hybridization, the nitrocellulose paper is sealed in a plastic bag containing a reaction mixture with unlabeled RNA and DNA and incubated to reduce background hybridization. Viral DNA labeled in vitro with ^{32}P by nick translation is added to the reaction mixture and the bag is further incubated. After completion of hybridization incubation, the nitrocellulose filter is washed exhaustively to remove unhybridized ^{32}P-DNA. The paper is then autoradiographed to detect hybridizing viral DNA. As little as 1 pg of viral DNA in a single band may be detected by this procedure.

Furthermore, the use of hybridization reaction mixtures containing different strengths of formamide allows us to vary the stringency of hybrid formation. Under less stringent hybridization conditions, additional viral DNA hybrids may be detected which are incompletely homologous to the viral DNA probe. Under stringent hybridization conditions (50% formamide, 42 C) only HPV DNA will be detected that is completely homologous to the viral DNA probe, that is, an HPV 2 DNA probe will only detect HPV 2 DNA. Under less stringent hybridization conditions (20% formamide, 37 C), a given HPV probe will detect any type of HPV DNA, ie, an HPV 2 or HPV 5 probe will detect HPV 1, HPV 2, HPV 3, HPV 4, or HPV 5 DNA in the sample.

Laryngeal papillomata assayed for HPV sequences by Southern blot hybridization was not cleaved with restriction endonuclease prior to agarose gel electrophoresis. Therefore, free, unintegrated viral DNA could be detected as forms 1, 2 or 3. Positive hybridization results indicating the presence of viral DNA forms were obtained under two types of hybridization conditions (Table 2). Under stringent conditions positive hybridization was seen both in a sample of laryngeal papilloma and condyloma acuminata, strongly indicating that the same virus (HPV 2) was responsible for both lesions. Under less stringent conditions positive hybridization was obtained in 5 (of 9) laryngeal papilloma samples, 2 condyloma samples from females and 1 condyloma sample from a male. These results indicate that an HPV was responsible for these lesions, but not necessarily the same HPV strain in each instance. One sample of inverted papilloma of the nose used as a control showed no hybridization.

*Watts S, Krzyzek R, Faras A, Quick CA. Identification of papilloma virus DNA in laryngeal papillomas. Submitted for publication 1980.

TABLE 2. STRINGENT AND LESS STRINGENT HYBRIDIZATION TO HPV 2 (SOUTHERN TECHNIQUE)

DNA Source	*Stringent*	*Less Stringent*
Larng. pap.	+	+
Condyl. acum. (vulva)	+	+
Condyl. acum. (vagina)	–	+
Condyl. acum. (penis)	–	+
Laryng. pap.	–	+
Laryng. pap.	+	+
Inverted pap. (nose)	–	–

+ - Positive hybridization in papilloma tissue. Laryng. pap. - Laryngeal papilloma; Condyl. acum. - Condyloma accuminata.

IMMUNOHISTOCHEMISTRY

An indirect immunoperoxidase stain* was used on formalin-fixed histological sections of laryngeal papillomata and condyloma acuminata to ascertain if viral staining could be detected and if so, to determine the site of virus particle production.

Immunoperoxidase staining utilizes an enzymatically generated histochemical reaction to mark the site of antigen-antibody reaction where 3,3-diaminobenzidine in the presence of hydrogen peroxide and peroxidase is oxidized to form an insoluble brown polymer.[20] The antiviral antibody used was produced in rabbits. Human papilloma virus was isolated from pooled plantar warts and internally disrupted by the detergent sodium dodocyl sulphate to reveal the common antigenicity to all known HPVs.[21] Our controls included the use of normal tissue, heat inactivated antivirus serum and omission of antivirus serum.

Positive staining was achieved in sections of laryngeal papilloma and sections of mucous membrane condyloma acuminata. The type of staining in mucous membrane papilloma was markedly dif-

*Jensen B. Personal communication, 1979.

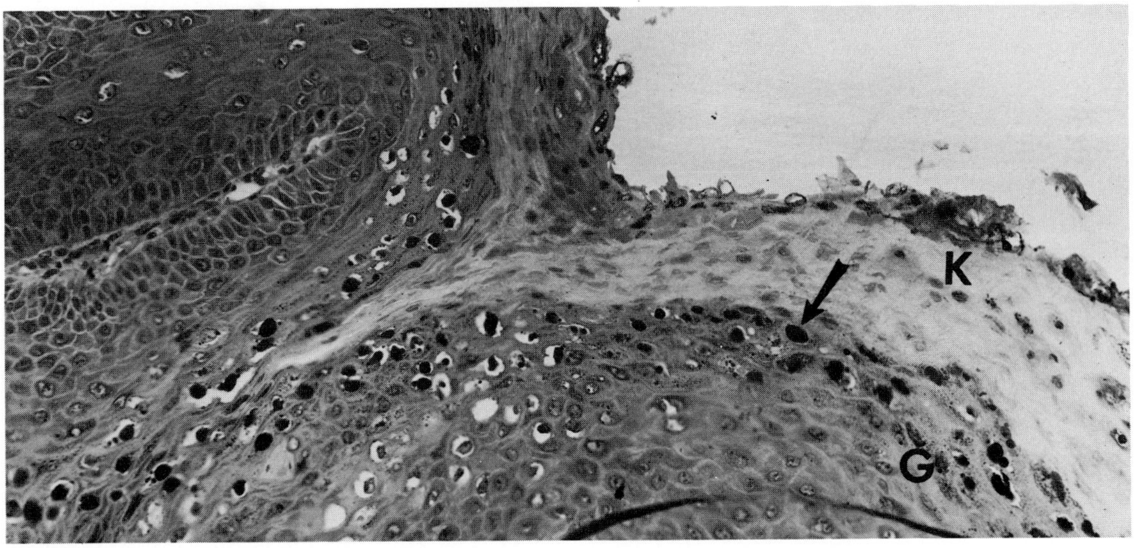

Fig. 2. Immunoperoxidase stain of verruca of lower lip. Discrete areas of positive staining (arrowed) is seen in the stratum granulosum (G) and scattered staining is seen in the stratum corneum (K). (Approx. x250)

ferent from that of cutaneous warts such as a verucca of the lip.* In the cutaneous variety the red-brown precipitate was clearly seen as spherical masses within the cells of the stratum granulosum and scattered staining was present throughout the stratum corneum (Fig. 2). Staining of the mucous membrane varieties were seen as a sparsely distributed precipitate occurring in the most superficial single cell layer (Fig. 3A,B). Frequently it was evident that this positively staining layer could be lost in vivo, or during handling, or in processing the tissue.

*Quick CA, Gnepp D, Bouquot G. Papilloma of the head and neck. In preparation.

Occasionally in a tangential cut of the superficial prickle cell layer, intracellular diffuse staining was seen which was concentrated in the vicinity of the cell nucleus.

DISCUSSION

In our small series of patients about 60% of the definitive group or 40% of the overall group of children were born of mothers who had condyloma either during pregnancy or at parturition. This is in agreement with other authors. The peak incidence for laryngeal papillomas is within the first five years of life and frequently there is a history that from the

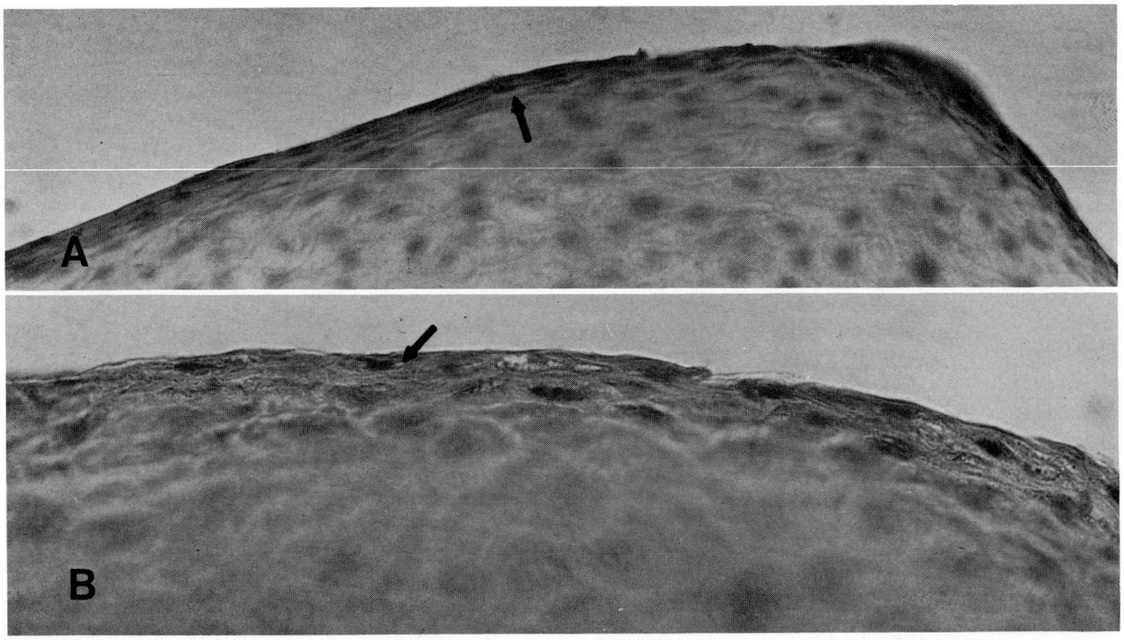

Fig. 3. A) Immunoperoxidase stain of papilloma of uterine cervix showing staining (arrow) confined to the superficial layer (approx. x350). B) Immunoperoxidase staining of laryngeal papilloma showing positive staining (arrow) of the superficial layer only (approx. x500).

earliest days of life the child had a "poor cry." Perinatally acquired viral infections are well recognized,[22] therefore, the acquisition of human papilloma virus during passage through the contaminated birth canal seems a plausible explanation for the above phenomenon. Perhaps the minor trauma of suctioning the meconium from the pharynx may help to implant the virus. Furthermore, it is recognized that HPV virus can remain dormant for long periods and that minor trauma and the presence of moisture can produce overt disease. The ease of transmission of condyloma by sexual contact[23] and spread of laryngeal lesions by "papilloma fluid" during surgical excision or instrumentation[24] are readily appreciated in the light of the immunohistochemical evidence of viral particles on the superficial layers of the tumor where they are easily dislodged.

Our virological studies are highly indicative of a role for HPV in laryngeal papillomatosis where it exists rarely as whole virus but usually as minute quantities of free DNA and more probably as integrated DNA in the host cell chromosome. Although we have only confirmed the presence of type 2 HPV DNA in laryngeal papilloma, less stringent Southern blot results suggest that other HPV are present which have not yet been identified with respect to type. Furthermore, the presence of HPV 2 in both condyloma acuminata and laryngeal papilloma provides good evidence of a direct etiologic link between these lesions. Our new evidence also indicates that several distinct types of HPVs may be associated with a single type of papilloma and different types of lesions may be caused by a single type of HPV. This latter aspect is partial vindication of the view of early workers who believed that all papillomas were caused by the same virus. The mucous membrane papillomas have usually been regarded as nonpermissive for whole virus replication but our immunoperoxidase experiments suggest that only the most superficial layer or two will demonstrate any viral activity. Although the exact nature of the viral protein antibody produced by the detergent-disrupted virus is yet to be determined, the product is highly specific for papilloma virus. Without the keratin layer of cutaneous warts to "trap" the maturing virions it is not surprising that electron microscopic identification of virus in laryngeal papilloma has been at best, serendipitous.

In view of the highly infectious nature of HPV, of fundamental importance is whether overt condyloma in a pregnant female is sufficient indication for cesarian section. Unfortunately there is no way to predict which infants will develop laryngeal papilloma since it is unlikely that all infants born in the presence of condyloma will acquire this disease. At this stage the decision for an alternative method of delivery must be left to the clinical judgment of the informed obstetrician in consultation with the patient.

ACKNOWLEDGMENTS — The authors are indebted to Dr. F. Pass for the supply of his antiviral serum and to Dr. Bennett Jensen for his cooperation in establishing the immunoperoxidase technique.

REFERENCES

1. Boyle WF, McCoy EG, Fogarty WA. Electron microscopic identification of virus like particles in laryngeal papilloma. Ann Otol Rhinol Laryngol 1971; 80:693-8.

2. Oriel JD, Almeida JD. Demonstration of virus particles in human genital warts. Br J Vener Dis 1971; 47:1-13.

3. Svoboda DJ, Kirchner FR, Proud GO. Electron microscopic study of human laryngeal papillomatosis. Cancer Res 1963; 23:1084-9.

4. Ullman EV. On the etiology of the laryngeal papilloma. Acta Otolaryngol (Stockh) 1923; 5:317-25.

5. Ishikawa K. Experimentalle Studien uer die Transplantation des Papilloma. Fukuoka Otol 1936; 8:68-76.

6. Majoros M, Parkhill E, Devine KD. Papilloma of the larynx in children. Am J Surg 1964; 108:470-5.

7. zur Hausen H, Gessman L, Steiner W, Dippold W, Dreger J. Human papilloma viruses and cancer. Bibl Haematol 1975; 43:569-71.

8. Hajek E. Contributions to the etiology of laryngeal papilloma in children. J Laryngol Otol 1956; 70:166-8.

9. Kaufman RS, Balogh K. Verrucas and juvenile laryngeal papillomas. Arch Otolaryngol 1969; 89:748-9.

10. Duff TB. Laryngeal papillomatosis. J Laryngol Otol 1971; 85:947-56.

11. Cook T, Cohn A, Brunschwig JP, Goepfert H, Butel J, Rawls W. Laryngeal papilloma: etioloic and therapeutic considerations. Ann Otol Rhinol Laryngol 1973; 82:649-55.

12. Quick CA, Faras A, Krzyzek R. The etiology of laryngeal papillomatosis. Laryngoscope 1978; 88:1789-95.

13. Coggin JR. Workshop on papillomaviruses and cancer. Cancer Res 1979; 39:545-6.

14. Quick CA, Foucar E, Dehner LP. Frequency and significance of epithelial atypia in laryngeal papillomatosis. Laryngoscope 1979; 89:550-60.

15. Hirt B. Selective extraction of polyoma DNA from infected mouse cell cultures. J Mol Biol 1967; 26:365-9.

16. Gissmann L, Pfister H, zur Hausen H. Human papilloma viruses (HPV): characterization of 4 different isolates. Virology 1977; 76:569-80.

17. Maniatis T, Jeffrey A, Kleid D. Nucleotide sequence of the rightward operator of phage lombda. Proc Natl Acad Sci USA 1975; 72:1184-8.

18. Pfister H, zur Hausen H. Seroepidemiological studies of human papilloma virus (HPV-1) infections. Int J Cancer 1978; 21:161-5.

19. Southern EM. Detection of specific sequences among DNA fragments separated by gel electrophoresis. J Mol Biol 1975; 98:503-17.

20. Pearse AGE. Histochemistry: theoretical and applied. Boston: Little Brown Co, 1961:517-20.

21. Pass F, Maizel JV. Wart-associated antigen: II. Human immunity to viral structural proteins. J Invest Dermatol 1973; 60:307-11.

22. Plotkin SA. Perinataly acquired viral infections. Curr Top Microbiol Immunol 1977; 78:111-20.

23. Oriel J. Natural history of genital warts. Br J Vener Dis 1971; 47:1-13.

24. Kirchner J. Papilloma of the larynx with extensive lung involvement. Laryngoscope 1951; 61:1022-9.

Ann Otol 89:1980

TOPICAL CHEMOTHERAPY OF RECURRENT RESPIRATORY PAPILLOMATOSIS

A PRELIMINARY REPORT

HOWARD G. SMITH, MD
CHARLES W. VAUGHAN, MD
GERALD B. HEALY, MD
M. STUART STRONG, MD

BOSTON, MASSACHUSETTS

Topical chemotherapy with the antimetabolite 5-fluorouracil (5-FU) has been used as an adjunct to surgical laser excision of squamous papillomas arising in the larynx and in the tracheobronchial tree. The drug has been administered intensively to eight patients with tracheotomies and disease in both anatomic regions. These patients received repeated instillations of 5-FU at concentrations from 0.5 to 5% into the larynx and tracheobronchial tree while in the hospital and at home. More than 4,500 doses of the drug have been administered during our phase 1 study. There has been no significant toxicity associated with repeated 5-FU instillation into the airway. Several patients developed blood-tinged tracheal secretions after the repeated use of high concentrations of the agent. Other complications included coughing, bronchospasm, and peristomal irritation. These symptoms all disappeared after temporary discontinuation of the drug. No patient has developed a systemic hypersensitivity response to the drug either detectable clinically or by repeated skin testing. There were no adverse effects on the hematologic or hepatic systems. Use of 5-FU was associated with inhibition of papilloma regrowth in six of eight patients. The major limitation to drug effectiveness is the requirement for its frequent administration.

INTRODUCTION

Squamous papillomas arising in the larynx and other portions of the upper respiratory tract have been described for over 300 years. First differentiated from other laryngeal masses by MacKenzie[1] in the late 19th century, papillomas are the most common benign neoplasm of the larynx in the pediatric age group.

The mechanical and physical treatment regimens for respiratory papillomatosis are varied.[2-4] These include complete mechanical surgical excision,[3] cryosurgery,[5] electrofulguration,[3] ultrasound,[6] and laser excision.[2] Each technique can eradicate clinically evident lesions to temporarily control the disease; none has been demonstrated to either eliminate or reduce the rate of recurrences.

For this reason, topical or locally injected agents have been utilized as adjuncts to surgical excision. These include the steroid hormone diethylstilbestrol,[7] podophyllum,[8] tetracycline,[9] and idoxuridine, an antiviral agent.[10] Each of these agents has produced promising initial results, but no long-term advantage over surgery alone has been demonstrated.

The antimetabolite 5-fluorouracil (5-FU) is an antineoplastic agent usually administered systemically for treatment of a variety of malignant neoplasms. This drug was first tested extensively as a topical agent by Dr. Edmund Klein of the Roswell Park Memorial Institute. Repetitive application of 5-FU effectively inhibited the growth of a variety of cutaneous neoplasms and preneoplastic lesions.[11-13]

This agent has several modes of action. It is a competitive inhibitor of thymidine synthetase and thereby blocks the methylation of deoxyuridylic acid to thymidylic acid. This effect directly interferes with the synthesis of deoxyribonucleic acids (DNA) and indirectly inhibits the synthesis of DNA-dependent ribonucleic acids (RNA).[14] The drug can also directly inhibit RNA synthesis by acting as a "false"-base.[15]

Repeated topical application of 5-FU in varying concentrations can eradicate or inhibit the growth of cutaneous squamous cell carcinomas, bell carcinomas, dysplastic keratoses, and intraoral leukoplakia.[16,17] If utilized over extended periods of time, 5-FU produced resolution of existing cutaneous lesions and prevented the outgrowth of predicted new lesions.

Topical 5-FU has been previously utilized to treat papillomatous and verrucoid lesions of the skin and mucous membranes. Hursthouse,[18] in a controlled study, demonstrated that 5% 5-FU ointment produced an absolute cure rate of 60% compared with a rate of 7% for a placebo ointment. Dretler and Klein[19] showed that intraurethral applications of 5% 5-FU aqueous cream could eradicate genital condylomata in each of 20 patients treated.

Singer et al* initiated the use of topical and local-

*Singer H, Tingwald F, Harris H. Personal communication, Nov. 1977.

From the Departments of Otolaryngology, The Children's Hospital Medical Center and the University Hospital, Boston, Massachusetts. This work was supported by No. 1 K07 NS00405-01 from the National Institute of Neurological Disorders and Stroke.

Presented at the meeting of the American Broncho-Esophagological Association, Palm Beach, Florida, April 12-13, 1980.

REPRINTS — Howard G. Smith, MD, Department of Otolaryngology, The Children's Hospital Medical Center, 300 Longwood Avenue, Boston, MA 02115.

TABLE 1. PATIENT PROFILE

Pt.	Sex	Age at Onset (yr)	Parental Genital Pap.	No. Prior Procedures	Age at Rx Onset (yr)	Pap.	Notes
1	M	2	M-F	57	13.3	LTBP	Auto-vaccine levamisole, MTX
2	M	0.5	M	50	12.0	LTB	Cryo, MTX
3	F	4	F	11	7.4	LTB	Asthma
4	M	2	UK	19	8.5	LT	
5	F	2	M	18	6.5	LTB	
6	M	1.1	N	17	3.5	LT	
7	M	3	N	50	12.9	LT	
8	F	1	M	17	3.0	LT	

L - Laryngeal; B - Bronchial; T - Tracheal; P - Pulmonary; MTX - Systemic methotrexate; M - Maternal disease; F - Paternal disease; UK - Unknown information; Pap. - Papillomata; Cryo - Cryotherapy.

ly injected 5-FU as adjuvant treatment for respiratory papillomatosis at the Cleveland Clinic, beginning in 1969. These investigators noted a decreased incidence of recurrent disease as well as regression of some otherwise untreated lesions. They noted no significant side effects or airway problems.

The present study was instituted as a phase 1 investigation of the safety and efficacy of topical 5-FU preparations as adjuvants to laser excision of rapidly recurrent papillomatosis of the larynx and tracheobronchial tree.

METHODS

Patient Population. The eight patients chosen for entry into this study protocol were drawn from more than 95 children and adolescents with recurrent respiratory papillomatosis followed since 1972 by the investigators at the Children's Hospital Medical Center and at the University Hospital, Boston, Massachusetts. Each subject had extensive respiratory papillomatosis involving the larynx and the tracheobronchial tree; all were undergoing frequent laser excisions of their disease in order to maintain an adequate airway.

A patient profile is shown in Table 1. There were five males and three females ranging in age from 3 to 13 years at the time of therapy initiation. All patients had clinical onset of disease at a young age (median two years). Five of seven children were born to parents known to have had genital papillomata in the perinatal period.

An indwelling tracheotomy tube was a requirement for study entry in order to provide ready access to the tracheobronchial tree for both medication administration and airway management in the event of an untoward reaction to the drug.

Each child had undergone multiple microlaryngoscopic and bronchoscopic procedures at our institutions and elsewhere prior to entry into the study. All patients had active papillomatosis in the larynx and trachea. Four of eight also had active disease in one or both mainstem bronchi. One patient had pulmonary papillomatosis; he had previously been treated unsuccessfully with autogenous vaccine and levamisole. Two patients with severe bronchial papillomatosis had received low dose systemic methotrexate with limited success. Our experience with this treatment modality will be reported elsewhere.*

Treatment Protocol. The nature of the therapy, its risks and possible benefits were discussed in detail with the parents/guardians and, where possible, with the patients themselves. A standard informed consent instrument was formally executed before onset of therapy.

Prior to each endoscopy, a patch test of 5% 5-FU aqueous cream on an adhesive bandage was placed on the patient's volar forearm to monitor for the development of an immediate or delayed cutaneous hypersensitivity response. Hematologic tests (complete blood count, differential, and platelet count), and a battery of liver function tests (SGOT, LDH, alkaline phosphatase, total/direct bilirubin) were obtained.

At the time of endoscopy, the patch test was examined for local erythema and induration. During the direct microlaryngoscopy and bronchoscopy, the investigators produced drawings and notations of the anatomic extent of disease. After laser excision of visible papillomatous disease, 5% 5-FU aqueous cream (0.5 cc = 25 mg) was applied to all involved mucosal surfaces. A second aliquot of cream was also applied to the tracheotomy tube prior to its reinsertion. Early in the study, some children received 5% 5-FU solution for injection into the bases of laryngeal lesions.

During the postoperative period, each parent or guardian was instructed about the home care to be administered after the patient left the hospital. An instruction sheet and treatment diary were provided to maintain treatment compliance. Each patient began therapy with 0.25 mg/kg of 5-FU topical solution instilled into the tracheotomy tube twice daily for four consecutive days each week. The tracheotomy tube was to be partially or completely removed, coated with approximately 0.5 cc (25 mg) of the 5-FU aqueous cream, and reinserted. Patients were instructed to inhale and then subsequently cough after intratracheal instillation.

In later treatment cycles, the protocol was expanded to administer 5-FU into the larynx and hypopharynx. A volume of 0.2 cc of a 2.5% 5-FU solution (5 mg) was administered twice a day on four consecutive days per week. Patients were instructed to inhale deeply during instillation in order to distribute the medication as far as possible into the glottic and subglottic areas.

Parents/guardians were instructed to discontinue medication and to immediately contact the investigators if tracheal bleeding, wheezing, coughing, or dyspnea occurred or persisted.

Medication. Fluorouracil was provided as a 5% aqueous cream, a 5% sterile injectable solution, and a 5% topical solution by Roche Laboratories. The agent has been granted an investigational drug status for use in this protocol by the Food and Drug Administration, Department of Health, Education, and Welfare.

The topical 5-FU for intratracheal instillation was diluted to a total volume of 1 cc and instilled into the tracheotomy tube with a tuberculin syringe and a modified No. 22 gauge needle.

The 2.5% 5-FU solution was administered using a DeVilbiss No. 15 sprayer. The 5% 5-FU cream was applied to the tracheotomy tube with a sterile cotton applicator stick.

Analysis of Treatment Results. The efficacy of topical 5-FU treatment was assessed by determination of the prevalence of papillomatous disease before and after therapy. The mucosal surfaces of the larynx, the trachea, and the proximal bronchial tree were divided into 42 distinct anatomic sites (18 supraglottic, 6 glottic, 4 subglottic, 12 tracheal, and 2 bronchial areas) (Fig. 1). Using our intraoperative drawings and operative notes, each site was scored for the presence or absence of clinically detectable papillomatous disease. If any portion of the anatomic site con-

*Smith HG, Frantz C, Healy GB. Treatment of severe respiratory papillomatosis with systemic methotrexate. In preparation.

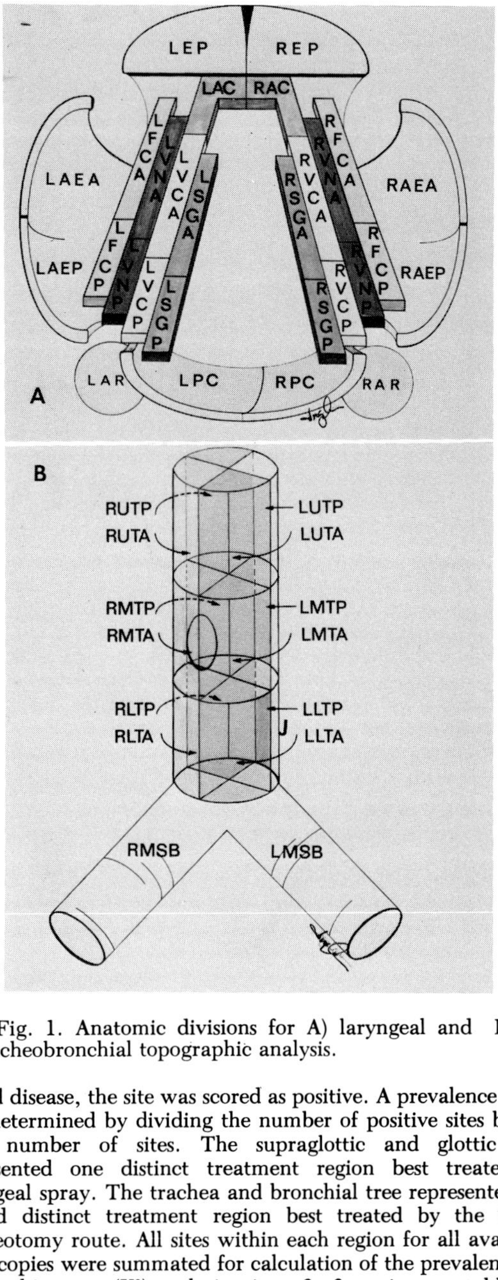

Fig. 1. Anatomic divisions for A) laryngeal and B) tracheobronchial topographic analysis.

tained disease, the site was scored as positive. A prevalence index was determined by dividing the number of positive sites by the total number of sites. The supraglottic and glottic sites represented one distinct treatment region best treated by laryngeal spray. The trachea and bronchial tree represented the second distinct treatment region best treated by the trans-tracheotomy route. All sites within each region for all available endoscopies were summated for calculation of the prevalence index. A chi-square (X^2) analysis using a 2 x 2 contingency table was used to evaluate the statistical significance of differences in disease present at the pretreatment and the treatment endoscopies.

RESULTS

Patient Compliance. We were working very closely with a small group of parents and guardians; their compliance to the regimen was excellent. Parents/guardians informed us promptly whenever a complication occurred, and were genuinely interested in working together with us to arrive at an individualized regimen well tolerated by the child.

In each case, a primary working relationship was established with only one responsible adult, comfortable with manipulating the tracheotomy tube. Four of eight parents/guardians were regularly changing their child's tracheotomy tube prior to entry into the study. The remaining four parents were given instruction and practical experience by our nursing staff. However, two parents continued to be uneasy about completely removing their child's tube; therefore they were encouraged to withdraw the tube as far as possible for coating with aqueous cream.

Table 2 is a summary of the medication administered. At the time of writing, the children had been on protocol from between 17 to 74 weeks with a median of 42.5 weeks. A total of 1,955 doses of topical solution, 1,684 doses of cream, and 1,009 doses of peroral spray have now been administered. The doses administered represent over two thirds of the prescribed doses. The difference between the two values represents doses omitted due to the onset of complications. These will be discussed below. Six of eight patients received more than 80% of their prescribed doses.

The majority of patients tolerated the medication well. At each endoscopy, the dose of topical solution instilled into the trachea was increased by 50%. The maximum dose reached without complication was 20 mg twice daily. Two patients whose dosages escalated above this level to 25 mg and 30 mg, respectively, developed profuse bleeding. The dosage of aqueous cream was increased by adding additional days of administration. The maximal number of doses administered was ten per week. At the present time, the intralaryngeal spray is being administered to seven patients on a regular basis. Six are utilizing the spray at the initial dosage. One patient is receiving the spray on a daily basis.

Complications. Table 3 reviews the complications which occurred during the trial for each patient and for the group as a whole. Whenever one of

TABLE 2. SUMMARY OF TOPICAL 5-FLUOROURACIL ADMINISTRATION

		Doses Administered/Prescribed (%)		
Pt.	*Wks on Rx*	*Solution*	*Cream*	*Spray*
1	74	600/790 (75.9)	503/658 (76.4)	378/462 (80.0)
2	55	360/440 (81.8)	360/440 (81.8)	16/120 (13.3)
3	52	36/416 (8.7)	19/416 (4.6)	77/224 (34.3)
4	43	322/344 (93.6)	322/344 (93.6)	163/176 (92.6)
5	42	164/344 (47.7)	15/168 (8.9)	88/176 (50.0)
6	29	226/232 (97.4)	218/226 (96.4)	202/226 (89.3)
7	18	144/144 (100.0)	144/144 (100.0)	96/96 (100.0)
8	17	103/106 (97.2)	103/106 (97.2)	39/40 (97.5)
	Totals	1955/2816 (69.4)	1684/2502 (67.3)	1009/1520 (66.4)

TABLE 3. COMPLICATIONS DURING TOPICAL 5-FLUOROURACIL ADMINISTRATION

	Significant Episodes of				
Pt.	*Tracheal Bleeding*	*Peristomal Inflammation*	*Bronchospasm*	*Prolonged Coughing*	*Other Illness*
1	10	7	—	5	2
2	—	—	—	2	3
3	3	—	—	—	—
4	8	—	—	—	—
5	12	—	6	2	1
6	—	—	—	—	—
7	—	—	—	1	—
8	1	2	1	3	—
Totals	34	9	7	13	7
(%)	(48.6)	(12.9)	(10.0)	(18.5)	(10.0)

these symptoms occurred and persisted, the medication was discontinued for the remainder of the week during which it occurred. If the symptom did not immediately stop upon cessation of medication, the drug was also omitted during the subsequent week. After that time, the medication was resumed but the dosage was adjusted downward by 50%.

At no time did any patient experience airway compromise. No patient required hospitalization for any symptoms related to the 5-FU administration. None of the patients demonstrated any changes in their hematologic status or in liver function during therapy. The administration of 5-FU did not appear to interfere with healing of the larynx or the tracheobronchial tree after laser surgery.

The most frequently encountered complication was tracheal bleeding. This symptom was associated with the administration of both intratracheal 5-FU medications. Although every patient treated had occasional pink tracheal secretions, there were 34 significant episodes of more marked tracheal bleeding in five patients. In no case was the bleeding uncontrollable nor were there any associated episodes of airway compromise. Three patients had no significant bleeding episodes.

The bleeding would usually occur 10 to 14 days after initiation of the treatment regimen. It would begin first as a blood tinged aspirate. In cases where the medication was continued, frank but self-limited bleeding would occasionally occur with coughing or suctioning. Four of five patients had cessation of bleeding after temporary discontinuation of the 5-FU cream. One patient required discontinuation of both the cream and the topical solution.

Two of the patients (3 and 5) experienced sufficient tracheal bleeding to seriously curtail administration of the intratracheal medications. Because of this reaction, these patients received between 4 and 48% of their prescribed doses of topical solution and cream. Dosages of both medications have now been adjusted downward to levels which, to date, have been well tolerated.

Prolonged coughing after medication administration was the second most common complication. Thirteen episodes accounted for 19% of all significant complications reported. In all cases, the symptom recurred immediately after 5-FU administration and ceased several hours after the time of administration. This problem usually stopped after reduction of medication dosage.

One patient (2) developed violent coughing approximately one hour after the administration of the 5-FU spray. The coughing lasted uninterrupted for several hours. For this reason, the spray was discontinued after only 13% of the prescribed doses were administered. The cream and topical solution, instilled into the trachea, produced no such complication. No other patient had an undesirable reaction to the spray.

Two patients had significant problems with inflammation developing around their tracheotomy incisions after prolonged administration of 5-FU cream. In each case, the peristomal rash resolved after discontinuation of the 5-FU cream. No other topical or systemic treatment was necessary.

Wheezing occurred in two patients. This complication along with tracheal bleeding severely limited the administration of 5-FU to patient 5. In addition to wheezing, this patient also noted the onset of a sensation of throat swelling and dysphagia. She experienced only a slight change in her voice. She had no difficulties with dyspnea or cough.

There were four episodes of intercurrent illness during which 5-FU administration was halted. There were two episodes of pneumonia and five episodes of upper respiratory infection. There was no increase in the incidence of upper respiratory illness in any patient on the protocol.

Therapeutic Results. We emphasize that the present study was a phase 1 investigation. As such, there was no matched control group for comparison with the treated group. However, each of the eight patients participating had undergone multiple endoscopic procedures prior to initiation of 5-FU therapy. A careful review of these procedures yielded data which defined an expected prevalence

TABLE 4. EXTENT OF RESPIRATORY PAPILLOMATOSIS BEFORE AND AFTER TOPICAL 5-FLUOROURACIL ADMINISTRATION

Pt.	Analysis Period	Prevailing Region of Disease: Laryngeal	Prevailing Region of Disease: Tracheobronchial	Total
1	Pre-Rx-8	71/224 (.31)	47/112 (.42)	118/336 (.35)
	Rx-2	PT 4/56 (.07)*	T 4/28 (.14)x	8/84 (.09)*
	Rx-2′	PT 11/56 (.19)	T 9/28 (.32)	20/84 (.24)
	Rx-4	T 37/112 (.33)	T20/56 (.35)	57/168 (.33)
	Rx-Total	52/224 (.23)	33/112 (.29)	85/336 (.25)†
2	Pre-Rx-8	16/224 (.07)	53/112 (.47)	69/336 (.21)
	Rx-2	PT 4/56 (.07)	T 4/28 (.14)‡	8/84 (.09)x
3	Pre-Rx-8	82/224 (.37)	14/112 (.13)‡	96/336 (.28)
	Rx-2	NT 24/56 (.42)	T11/28 (.39)	35/84 (.41)
4	Pre-Rx-11	179/308 (.88)	22/154 (.14)	201/462 (.43)
	Rx-1	NT 21/28 (.75)	T 1/14 (.07)	22/42 (.52)
5	Pre-Rx-7	126/196 (.64)	65/98 (.66)	191/294 (.65)
	Rx-1	NT 18/28 (.64)	T 1/14 (.07)	19/42 (.45)
6	Pre-Rx-4	51/112 (.46)	23/56 (.41)	74/168 (.44)
	Rx-1	NT 22/28 (.79)	T 5/14 (.35)	27/42 (.64)
	Rx-1′	T 1/28 (.04)*	T 2/14 (.14)	3/42 (.07)*
7	Pre-Rx-2	28/56 (.50)	18/28 (.64)	46/84 (.58)
	Rx-3	T 7/84 (.08)*	T 3/42 (.07)*	10/126 (.08)*
8	Pre-Rx-6	18/28 (.64)	6/14 (.43)	24/42 (.57)
	Rx-3	NT 12/84 (.14)*	T 2/42 (.05)†	14/126 (.11)*

Prob. Pre-Rx = Rx by x^2; * - $P<.0005$; ‡ - $P<.001$; † - $P<.01$; x - $P<.025$.

T - Area treated; NT - Area not treated; PT - Area partially treated; Rx-No. - No. of endoscopic Rx's summed; Rx-No.′ - Subsequent group of Rx's.

of papillomatous disease at each anatomic site. These "expected" values were compared with the "observed" frequencies of disease prevalence found at endoscopic procedures carried out during the conduct of 5-FU therapy.

Six of eight patients had a statistically significant decrease in the prevalence of papillomatous disease at treated sites (Table 4). Of the two nonresponders, one (3) received relatively few doses of medication. The other (4) did not begin treatment with 5-FU spray to his larynx, the major site of papilloma involvement, until several months ago. A follow-up endoscopy has not yet taken place.

One patient (1) has undergone an adequate number of endoscopic procedures after initiation of 5-FU therapy. Initially, the prevalence of disease decreased in the directly treated tracheobronchial tree and in the indirectly treated endolarynx. The larynx, treated at the time of endoscopy, was treated as part of the home treatment regimen by repetitively coughing and expelling the medication from the trachea into the larynx. Subsequently, however, the prevalence of disease became insignificantly different from that noted prior to therapy. Despite the widespread involvement, the growth of papillary lesions was not as luxuriant as seen in the pretherapy period.

It is important to emphasize the preliminary nature of these therapeutic results. The majority of patients have undergone only one to three endoscopies since treatment onset; four of eight patients have not had a complete evaluation since beginning therapy with the 5-FU spray to the larynx.

The two patients who have demonstrated the most dramatic response to the 5-FU treatment (7 and 8) both had extensive disease in the larynx and the upper portion of the trachea. Both tolerated the medication well and received a very high proportion of prescribed doses. When examined at endoscopy, both patients had a marked erythematous reaction in the mucosae of the trachea and bronchi. Neither patient has had a significant complication of the therapy to date.

Another indicator of therapeutic effectiveness was an increase in the time intervals between recommended endoscopies. For three patients (1, 2, and 8) this interval at least doubled; in each case the difference in time interval was statistically significant as assessed by the Student *t*-test. Two other cases had a decrease in recommended interval but insufficient data were available for statistical analysis.

Six of eight parents/guardians reported that their child showed improvement in eating habits, voice, and/or general well-being while on the 5-FU therapy. Two children (8 and 6) communicated for the first time with laryngeal speech while on the drug. This type of information, while subjective and anecdotal, is nonetheless gratifying.

DISCUSSION

Recurrect respiratory papillomatosis is a disease affecting large geographic fields of mucosa in the upper airway of children and adults.[2-4] The lesions tend to recur at sites of previous involvement and spread to new sites lower in the airway, particularly after creation of a tracheotomy.[2]

Despite the precise and complete eradication of visible disease using instruments such as the CO_2 surgical laser, the papillomatosis can recur and progress. An adjuvant treatment is needed which can effectively eradicate microscopic deposits of papillomatosis and preneoplastic lesions. Such an agent must be readily administered, safe, and uniformly effective. Since the agent must be applied to large areas of mucosa, it should have a minimal effect on the growth and healing of normal tissue.

The properties of 5-FU reported in the literature suggested that this drug may be a useful adjuvant. Our study confirms the observations of others[17,19,22] that topical 5-FU can be applied repeatedly to mucosal surfaces without severe complications or interference with normal healing functions. This phenomenon is explained by the studies of Eaglstein et al[15] which demonstrate that topically applied 5-FU selectively penetrates neoplastic and dysplastic tissue. In contrast, intradermally injected 5-FU effected DNA synthesis in both normal and neoplastic tissue.

As in Klein's studies[17] on cutaneous and intraoral lesions, the success of 5-FU treatment in this study was dependent upon the repeated application of the drug and the accessibility of the lesions to be treated. It was disappointing to us that the patient on the protocol for the longest period of time (1) seemed to have developed disease at least partially resistant to therapy. Klein also found that certain, very aggressive tumors previously and unsuccessfully treated with other modalities, tended to become resistant to 5-FU therapy.

In order to investigate this phenomenon, we have begun to collect tissue specimens of the residual fragment 3 of papillomatous disease. The preliminary data from three of our patients indicates that residual papillomas are more hyperplastic and, in some fields, more dysplastic than the papilloma tissue biopsied prior to therapy. More tissue specimens must be studied in order to draw any definite conclusions.

It is likely that the 5-FU therapy is selecting out more aggressive papilloma cells rather than creating dysplastic changes in the tissue. Studies of long-term administration of 5-FU for treatment of preneoplastic lesions indicates that the drug eliminates such lesions and prevents rather than fosters the outgrowth of cutaneous malignant neoplasms.[14]

It is interesting that none of our patients developed cutaneous hypersensitivity to the 5-FU. Mansell et al[20] found that 11 of 15 patients undergoing topical 5-FU therapy for cutaneous neoplasms developed a positive skin test to the drug. In that series, the success of therapy correlated positively with the development of this systemic hypersensitivity. Several of our patients did develop mucosal erythma, but it is likely that this phenomenon is due to a direct effect of the 5-FU on the mucosa. Strong et al[2] has previously reported the results of a preliminary study which suggested that patients with severe papillomatosis may have partial or complete suppression of their cell-mediated immune functions. Such a phenomenon may render our patients incapable of producing a cutaneous reaction to 5-FU and may inhibit the development of any immune reaction to the drug.

This study represents a beginning. To prove that topical 5-FU is a valuable adjuvant to surgical excision of respiratory papillomas will require a large controlled, randomized study. Since the majority of patients with respiratory papillomatosis fortunately do not require a tracheotomy, drug administration must be carried out via a peroral route. We are currently conducting such a study in older adolescents and adults with papillomatosis.

ACKNOWLEDGMENTS — The authors wish to thank Drs. Edmund Klein and Edward Miller for their help in initiating this study.

REFERENCES

1. MacKenzie M. Essays of growths in the larynx with reports and an analysis of 100 consecutive cases treated by the author. Philadelphia: Lindsay & Blakiston, 1871.

2. Strong MS, Vaughan CW, Healy GB, Cooperband SR, Clemente MACP. Recurrent respiratory papillomatosis: management with the CO_2 surgical laser. Ann Otol Rhinol Laryngol 1976; 85:508-16.

3. Holinger PH, Schild JA, Mauriz DG. Laryngeal papilloma: a review of etiology and therapy. Laryngoscope 1968; 78:1462-74.

4. Bone RC, Fearon AP, Nahum AM, Winkelhake BG. Laryngeal papillomatosis: immunologic and viral basis for therapy. Laryngoscope 1976; 86:341-7.

5. Singleton GT, Adkins WY. Cryosurgical therapy of juvenile laryngeal papillomatosis. An 8 year experience. Ann Otol Rhinol Laryngol 1972; 81:784-90.

6. Birck HG, Mankart HE. Ultrasound for juvenile laryngeal papillomas. Arch Otolaryngol 1963; 77:603-8.

7. Szpunar J. Laryngeal papillomatosis. Acta Otolaryngol (Stockh) 1967; 63:74-86.

8. Hollingsworth J, Kohlmoss H, McNaught R. Treatment of juvenile papillomas with podophyllum. Arch Otolaryngol 1950; 52:82-5.

9. Holinger PH, Johnson KC, Anison GC. Papilloma of the larynx. A review of 109 cases with a preliminary report of aureomycin therapy. Ann Otol Rhinol Laryngol 1950; 59:547-64.

10. Cook TA, Cohn AM, Brunschwig JP, Goepfert H, Butel JS, Rawls WE. Laryngeal papilloma: etiologic and therapeutic considerations. Ann Otol Rhinol Laryngol 1973; 82:649-54.

11. Klein E, Milgrom H, Helm F, Ambrus J, Traenkle HL, Stoll HL. Tumors of the skin II: keratoacanthoma-local effect of 5-fluorouracil. Skin 1962; 1:153-6.

12. Klein E. Tumors of the skin VIII. Local chemotherapy of metastatic neoplasms in the skin. NY State Med J 1968; 68:877-84.

13. Klein E, Stoll HL, Milgrom H, Traenkle HL, Graham S, Helm F. Tumors of the skin. VI. Study of the effects of local administration of 5-fluorouracil in basal cell carcinoma. J Invest Dermatol 1966; 47:22-9.

14. Miller E. The metabolism and pharmacology of 5-fluorouracil. J Surg Oncol 1971; 3:309-15.

15. Eaglstein WH, Weinstein GD, Frost P. Fluorouracil:

mechanism of action in human skin and actinic keratosis. I. Effect on DNA synthesis *in vivo*. Arch Dermatol 1970; 101:132-9.

16. Klein E, Stoll HL, Milgrom H, et al. Tumors of the skin V. Local administration of anti-tumor agents to multiple superficial basal cell carcinomas. J Invest Dermatol 1965; 45:489-95.

17. Klein E. Tumors of the skin X. Immunotherapy for cutaneous and mucosal neoplasms. NY State Med J 1968; 68:900-11.

18. Hursthouse MW. A controlled trial in the use of topical 5-fluorouracil on viral warts. Br J Dermatol 1975; 92:93-6.

19. Dretler S, Klein LA. The eradication of intraurethral condyloma accuminata with 5% 5-fluorouracil cream. J Urol 1975; 113:195-8.

20. Mansell PWA, Litwin MS, Ichinose H, Krementz ET. Delayed hypersensitivity to 5-fluorouracil following topical therapy of cutaneous cancers. Cancer Res 1975; 35:1288-94.

≈

GUIDELINES FOR GRANTS
TRUSTEES OF THE RESEARCH FUND OF THE AMERICAN OTOLOGICAL SOCIETY, INC.

The members of the Board of Trustees of the Research Fund of the American Otological Society have determined guidelines for making grants from the Fund. The following is the formulation of policy.

Grants will be given in the area of otosclerosis: its diagnosis and management, the possible causes and underlying conditions, and an understanding of the disorder that may lead eventually to its prevention or cure.

The present lack of understanding of the disorder and the absence of similar conditions in other animals makes research in this field difficult. A direct approach to the disease may or may not be feasible; therefore, a sound strategy would be to use other approaches, such as the investigation of bone development, growth and repair under various conditions, and the study of other diseases that may be similar to otosclerosis. It is possible that investigations which may seem initially remote from otosclerosis may provide information which will eventually lead to a substantive further understanding of the disease process which underlies otosclerosis. The applicant should describe correlations between proposed research with the clinical pathological entity of otosclerosis.

The policy is to aid and encourage research in the immediate field of otosclerosis and also in adjoining fields, if, in the opinion of the Board, there is a substantial promise that results obtained will be of assistance in the ways indicated, and may lead to the attainment of the objective of the further understanding of otosclerosis.

Applications for a research grant from the Research Fund of the American Otological Society may be obtained from the Office of the Secretary-Treasurer of the Research Fund of the American Otological Society. Write to Robert J. Ruben, M.D., Secretary-Treasurer, Department of Otolaryngology, Albert Einstein College of Medicine, 1300 Morris Park Avenue, Bronx, New York 10461; (212) 430-3036.

All grant requests must be submitted by January 31, 1981.

EXPERIMENTAL OTITIS MEDIA FOLLOWING MIDDLE EAR INOCULATION OF NONVIABLE *STREPTOCOCCUS PNEUMONIAE*

SETH H. LOWELL, MD, PhD
ORMOND BEACH, FLORIDA

S. K. JUHN, MD
MINNEAPOLIS, MINNESOTA

G. SCOTT GIEBINK, MD
MINNEAPOLIS, MINNESOTA

The pathogenesis of otitis media is poorly understood, and the events leading to bacterial invasion of the middle ear cleft and resulting inflammation are a matter of conjecture. While *Streptococcus pneumoniae* is the most frequent microbe cultured from acute, purulent middle ear effusions, it is infrequently cultured from nonsuppurative serous and mucoid effusion. To explore the possibility that nonviable pneumococci persisting in the middle ear cleft might produce mucosal inflammation, a solution of heat-killed pneumococci was placed in the middle ear cavity of experimental animals. Mucoperiosteal pathology which followed inoculation included an active, early subepithelial inflammatory response, metaplasia of the lining epithelium and later new bone formation. Thus, nonviable pneumococci are capable of producing middle ear inflammation, and it is possible that persistence of whole nonviable organisms or subcellular components in either middle ear effusion or mucoperiosteum may lead to continued middle ear inflammation or nonsuppurative otitis media.

INTRODUCTION

Otitis media is a common disease and a significant world health problem. Although otitis media is well recognized at a clinical level, its pathophysiology is poorly understood. In experimental acute pneumococcal otitis media, an acute inflammatory response is established soon after the introduction of pneumococci into the middle ear cavity.[1] An acute infiltration of polymorphonuclear leukocytes in the subepithelial layer, often with disruption of the overlying epithelium, leads to purulent middle ear effusion.[1-6] Infection with *Streptococcus pneumoniae* in humans is associated with rapid multiplication of bacteria which may be possible because this organism possesses a capsule which resists phagocytosis.[7] The mechanism of host injury, however, is not known. In recent years, bacterial surface structures and many by-products of bacterial growth have been biochemically and immunologically characterized. These antigenic and enzymatic components are capable of inducing host reactions ranging from immediate anaphylaxis to delayed hypersensitivity. It is reasonable that similar mechanisms play a role in the development of purulent otitis media, and

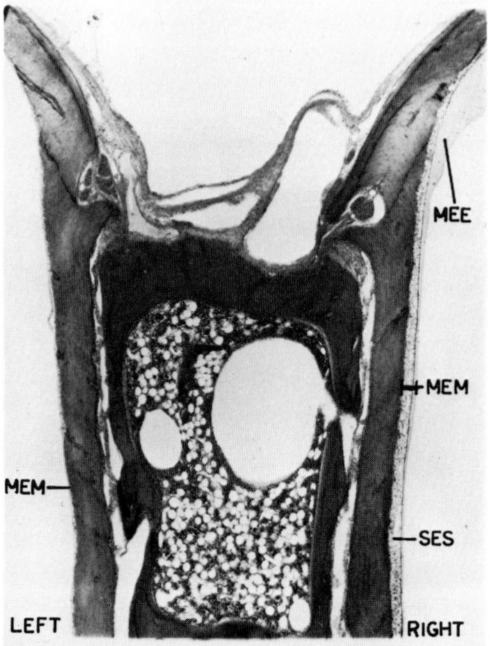

Fig. 1. A comparison of the middle ear mucosa (MEM) in the right and left middle ear cavities. The MEM on the right is thickened, with a widened subepithelial space (SES) three days after a heat-killed pneumococci solution was introduced. The middle ear effusion (MEE) is evident superiorly on the right side. (x40)

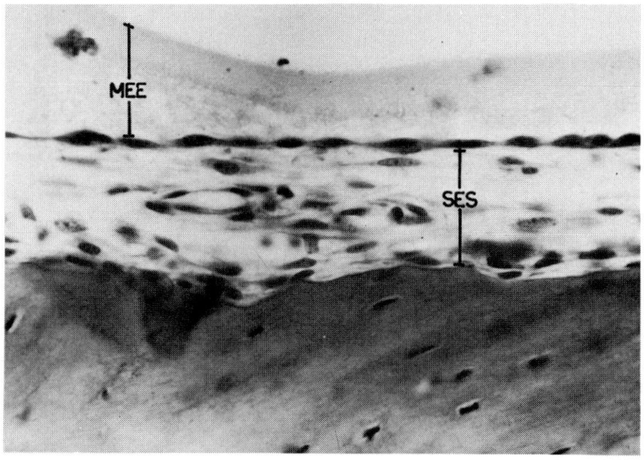

Fig. 2. A high magnification view of the MEM in right middle ear cavity, seen in Figure 1. The SES is widened, with increased intercellular spaces and dilated vessels. Occasional WBCs are present and the MEE is visible overlying the epithelium. (x500)

From the Department of Otolaryngology and Department of Pediatrics, University of Minnesota School of Medicine, Minneapolis, Minnesota. This research was supported by USPHS grant No. NS14538.

REPRINTS — Seth H. Lowell, MD, 565 Memorial Circle, Suite B, Ormond Beach, FL 32074.

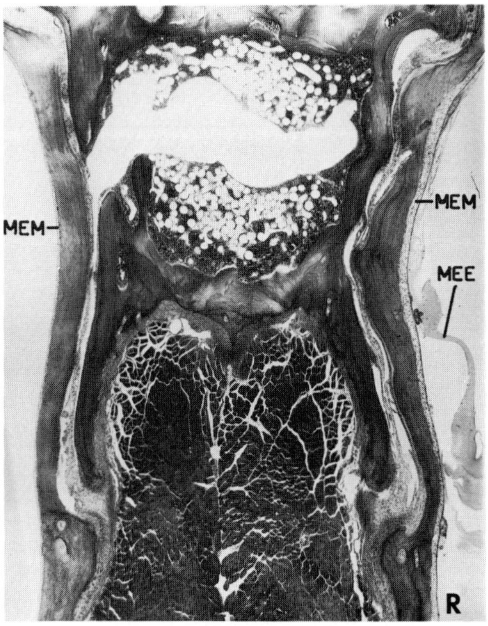

Fig. 3. A comparison of the MEM in the right and left middle ear cavities seven days after the HKB solution was introduced on the right side. A MEE is present on the right side and the MEM is thickened. (x40)

possibly of nonsuppurative middle ear effusions. As pneumococci are cultured most frequently from acute purulent effusions in man,[8,9] this study was designed to examine the possibility that nonviable pneumococci persisting after the acute phase of infection might lead to nonsuppurative effusion with mucoperiosteal pathology.

METHODS

Streptococcus pneumoniae type 23B (type 65 by American nomenclature) was used.[1] The organism was passed through mice each month, to maintain encapsulation and virulence. Pneumococci were subcultured for use in each experiment in beef heart infusion broth with neopeptone. Stationary phase pneumococci were washed and suspended in phosphate buffered saline (PBS) to 10^8 colony forming units (cfu) per milliliter. Intact, nonviable heat-killed pneumococci (HKB) were obtained by

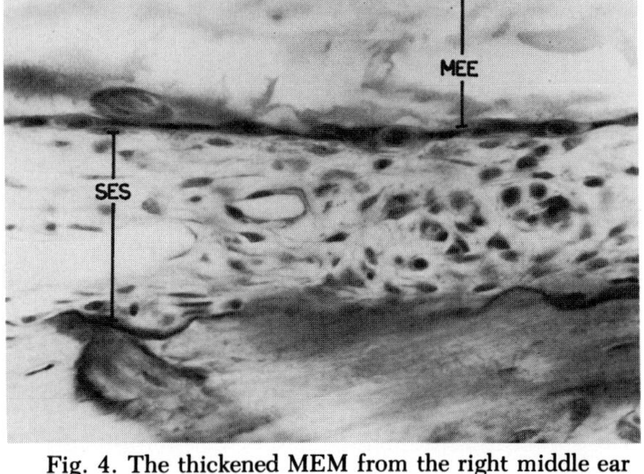

Fig. 4. The thickened MEM from the right middle ear cavity in Figure 3 is seen in high magnification. Dilated vessels are present as are a number of mononuclear leukocytes in the widened SES. A MEE is present in the middle ear cavity. (x500)

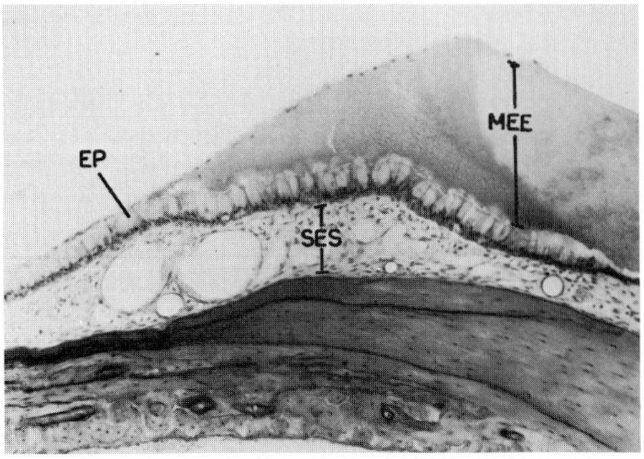

Fig. 5. Field shows metaplastic epithelium overlying the apex of the cochlea in the right middle ear cavity from Figure 3. A secretory epithelium has replaced the normally simple squamous one. EP - Epithelium. (x350)

heat-killing the bacterial suspension in a water bath at 18.3 C (65F) for 45 minutes.[7,10] Culture of HKB consistently showed sterility. Quellung reaction using type 23 antiserum (Statens Serums-institut, Copenhagen, Denmark) showed capsular swelling in all HKB suspensions.

Healthy adult chinchillas served as the experimental animal in this study. An experimental model of acute otitis media due to S *pneumoniae* has been previously described using this animal, and results of this study may be compared with the previous data.[1,11] For the experiments, 0.1 cc of the HKB solution or sterile PBS was inoculated into the right middle ear cavity via a transbulla approach under ether anesthesia, and animals were sacrificed 3, 7, 14 and 21 days later for histologic evaluation. The left ear of each animal served as a normal control for histologic comparison. Standard techniques were used for the preparation of temporal bone specimens.[1] After sacrifice, the animal was perfused with Heidenhain-Susa solution. Specimens were washed, decalcified, dehydrated and embedded in celloidin. Horizontal cuts through the temporal bones were stained with hematoxylin and eosin for subsequent histological evaluation.

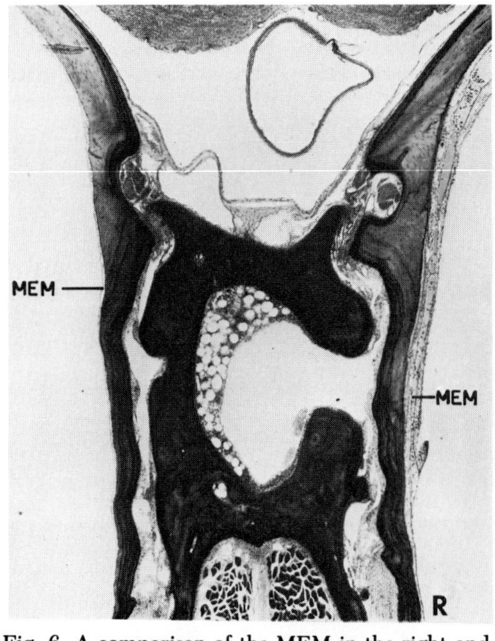

Fig. 6. A comparison of the MEM in the right and left middle ear cavities 14 days after the HKB solution was introduced on the right side. The right side continues to have dilated vessels in a widened SES. (x40)

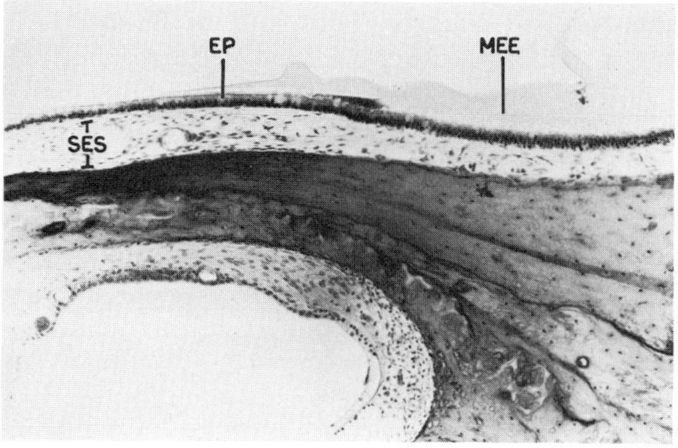

Fig. 7. The MEM over the apex of the cochlea shows secretory metaplasia in a higher magnification view of the right middle ear cavity of Figure 6. A small amount of MEE and some chronic inflammatory cells are also present. (x120)

RESULTS

In a preliminary study, 1.5 cc of the sterile PBS solution was injected into both ears of five animals. No evidence of middle ear effusion or other pathological change was present after three or seven days in any animal, and cultures of the middle ear cavities at sacrifice of these animals were sterile.

Three and seven days following unilateral inoculation of HKB serous effusions were present in the middle ear cavities of all experimental animals (Fig. 1). Histologic changes of the middle ear mucoperiosteum at day three included mucosal thickening with an edematous subepithelial space containing occasional polymorphonuclear leukocytes (PMNs) (Fig. 2). These same changes were visible at day seven (Figs. 3 and 4), but mononuclear leukocytes replaced the PMNs. Subepithelial space thickening persisted through day 14 (Fig. 6). Epithelial metaplasia developed by day seven with replacement of squamous epithelium by secretory epithelial cells (Figs. 5 and 7). Evidence of new bone formation was present in the subepithelial space at days 14

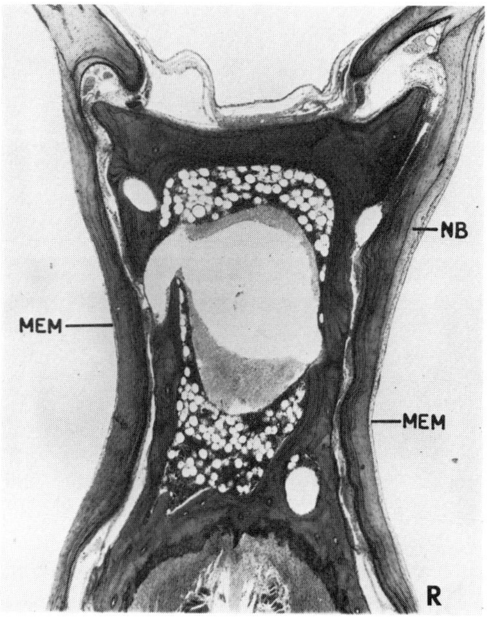

Fig. 9. This is a comparison of the MEM in the right and left middle ear 21 days after an HKB solution was introduced into the right side. The MEM is thickened, with widening of the SES and evidence of new bone formation. (x40)

and 21 (Figs. 8, 9 and 11). The mononuclear cell infiltrate persisted in the subepithelial space through day 21 (Fig. 10). Cultures from the middle ear cavity taken at sacrifice from all animals were sterile. No histologic changes were seen at any time in the contralateral control ear, and inner ear histology was normal bilaterally in all animals.

DISCUSSION

The pattern of injury in the middle ear of experimental animals following the inoculation of nonviable HKB consisted of edema of the subepithelial space accompanied by a mild inflammatory response and epithelial metaplasia. Within three weeks, new bone formation was seen in the subepithelial space. These changes appear to be non-

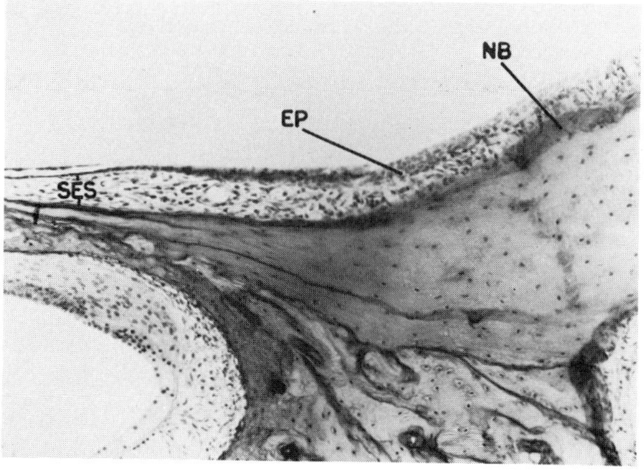

Fig. 8. Focal areas of new bone formation are visible in other areas of the SES of the MEM in the right middle ear cavity of Figure 6. Mild squamous metaplasia of the epithelial layer is also present. NB - New bone. (x120)

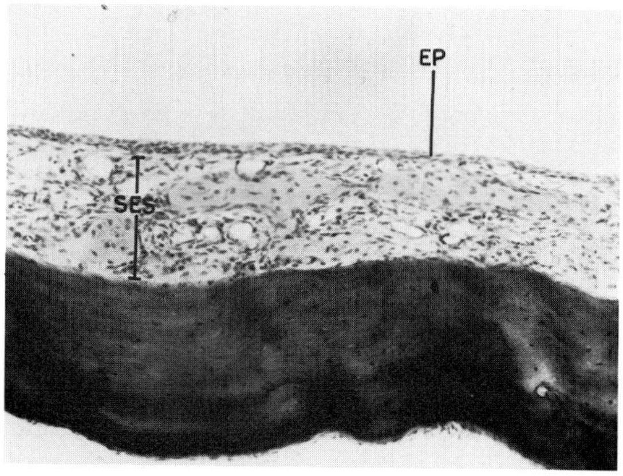

Fig. 10. The epithelial layer of the MEM in the right middle ear cavity shows mild squamous metaplasia, in a higher magnification of Figure 9. Frequent mononuclear WBCs are present in the SES. (x120)

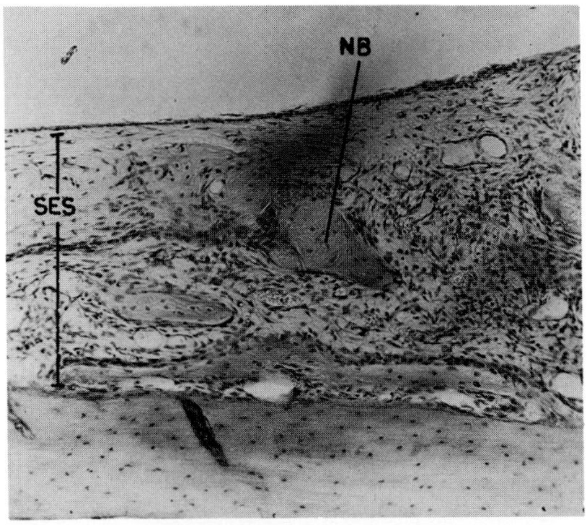

Fig. 11. Areas of new bone formation in the SES and numerous mononuclear leukocytes are present in other areas of the SES in the right middle ear at 21 days. (x120)

specific reactions to injury and common sequelae of the inflammatory response,[12,13] as the subepithelial space appears to play a key role in the recognition of foreign materials as well as mounting portions of the immune response.[4,14] Similar nonspecific changes can be found in serous and mucoid otitis media in humans.

Pneumococci produce a number of intracellular enzymes and are surrounded by a complex peptidoglycan-teichoic acid cell wall and type-specific capsular polysaccharides. Thus, the mechanism of injury from HKB may be related to these subcellular products or surface antigenic components. Some aspects of the role of the bacterial enzymes in damaging the middle ear have recently been discussed,[15] and it appears that the pneumococci possesses enzymes which are capable of causing epithelial disruption and a brisk inflammatory response. The exact nature and role of these components remains to be clarified.

The results of this investigation may apply to some types of otitis media in humans. Bacteria may play a role in the pathogenesis of serous and mucoid otitis media since culture of these effusions yields aerobic pathogens in approximately 30% of cases.[16-19] The presence of immunoglobulins, lysozyme and other host-produced bacteriostatic substances provides further indirect evidence that bacteria contribute to the development or persistence of these nonsuppurative types of otitis media. This study suggests that the presence of nonviable pneumococci in the middle ear cleft causes histopathological changes in the mucoperiosteum and sterile serous effusion for a prolonged period. This observation lends further support to antimicrobial and immunologic prophylaxis which might prevent initial colonization of the middle ear left by pneumococci.

REFERENCES

1. Giebink GS, Payne EE, Mills EL, Juhn SK, Quie PG. Experimental otitis media due to *Streptococcus pneumoniae:* immunopathogenic response in the chinchilla. J Infect Dis 1976; 134:595-604.

2. Dickson DR. Anatomy of normal and cleft palate eustachian tube. Ann Otol Rhinol Laryngol 1976; 85 Suppl 25:25-9.

3. Hentzer E. Ultrastructure of middle ear mucosa. Ann Otol Rhinol Laryngol 1976; 85 Suppl 25:30-5.

4. Lim DJ. Functional morphology of the mucosa of the middle ear and eustachian tube. Ann Otol Rhinol Laryngol 1976; 85 Suppl 25:36-43.

5. Vuori M. Middle ear fluid in acute otitis media. Acta Otolaryngol (Stockh) 1959; Suppl 153:1-64.

6. Hersh EM, Bodey GP. Leukocytic mechanisms in inflammation. Ann Rev Med 1970; 21:105-32.

7. White B. Biology of the Pneumococcus. London: Oxford Press, 1938:65-102, 214-37.

8. Sprinkle PM, Veltri RW. Microbiology of the middle ear and nasopharynx. Ann Otol Rhinol Laryngol 1971; 80:354-64.

9. Howie VM, Ploussard JH, Lester RL. Otitis media: clinical and bacteriological correlation. Pediatrics 1970; 45:29-35.

10. Rahn O. Sterilization of micro-organisms. Bacteriol Rev 1945; 9:24-35.

11. Juhn SK, Giebink GS, Hanson DG, Paparella MM. Experimentally induced acute otitis media — an experimental model. Arch Otorhinolaryngol (NY) 1977; 215:95-6.

12. Arnold W. The reactions of the human middle ear mucous membrane. Arch Otorhinolaryngol (NY) 1977; 216:369-473.

13. Robbins SL. Pathologic basis of disease. Philadelphia: WB Saunders, 1974:357.

14. Kastenbauer ER. The immunological function of the middle ear mucosa membrane during inflammation. Presented at the Symposium of Physiology and Pathophysiology of the Eustachian Tube, Frieberg, Germany, September, 1977.

15. Lowell SH, Juhn SK. The role of bacterial enzymes in inducing inflammation in the middle ear cavity. Otolaryngol Head Neck Surg 1979; 87:859-70.

16. Senturia BH, Gessert CF, Carr CD, Baumann ES. Studies concerned with tubotympanitis. Ann Otol Rhinol Laryngol 1958; 67:440-67.

17. Healy GB, Teele DW. The microbiology of chronic middle ear effusions in children. Laryngoscope 1977; 87:1472-8.

18. Liu YS, Lim DJ, Lang RW, Birck HG. Chronic middle ear effusions: immunological and bacteriological investigations. Arch Otolaryngol 1975; 101:278-86.

19. Giebink GS, Mills EL, Huff JS, et al. The microbiology of serous and mucoid otitis media. Pediatrics 1979; 63:915-9.

Ann Otol 89:1980

X-RAY OF THE MONTH

PITUITARY ADENOMA PRESENTING AS A SPHENOID SINUS LESION

JAMES M. DAVIS, MD   ALFRED L. WEBER, MD

BOSTON, MASSACHUSETTS

PATIENT

This 24-year-old female presented to an ophthalmologist with a three-month history of blurred vision. On physical examination, an upper bitemporal hemianopsia was noted. No other neurological abnormalities were present. Because of the radiographic findings (discussed below) an endocrinological consult was obtained. No hormonal abnormalities were discovered. However, on physical examination, bilateral galactorrhea was noted. There was no history of amenorrhea.

RADIOGRAPHS

Radiographic evaluation included skull films and pluridirectional tomography of the sella. These showed a sella normal in size, but with erosion of the postero-inferior floor. There was diffuse increased density within the sphenoid sinus (Fig. 1). A contrast-enhanced computerized tomographic scan (CT) was obtained. This revealed a large, contrast-enhancing mass within the sphenoid sinus and sella, which extended into the suprasellar region (Fig. 2). A metrizamide cisternogram (6 cc metrizamide, 170 mg I_2/cc) was performed to further delineate the suprasellar extent. A transphenoidal operation was then performed. A large pituitary adenoma was removed.

DISCUSSION

This case illustrates the evaluation of a mass which occupies the sphenoid sinus, sella turcica, and suprasellar region. There are several excellent articles which discuss the differential diagnosis of lesions in each of these areas.[1-3] The differential diagnosis is extensive and it is beyond the scope of this report to discuss each diagnosis in detail. The main diagnoses in this case include pituitary adenoma and sphenoid sinus mucocele.

Pituitary adenomas comprise 8-10% of intracranial tumors. Routine views and tomography of the sella may reveal sellar enlargement, erosion of the lamina dura of the sella, and/or calcification (1-6%). Involvement of the sphenoid sinus, to the extent of our case, is unusual. Computed tomography with intravenous or intrathecal contrast material is superior to pluridirectional tomography in demonstrating the extent of the tumor in important contiguous areas (infratemporal fossa, nasopharynx, orbit, suprasellar and/or parasellar).[4] Pituitary adenomas frequently demonstrate moderate or marked contrast enhancement with intravenous contrast material, particularly the suprasellar and extrasellar extensions. Confusion with an internal carotid artery aneurysm may exist and angiography is indicated. The use of metrizamide, a water-soluble nonionic contrast agent, is helpful in further defining the outlines of the tumor in the suprasellar region, as the tumor may destroy the adjacent suprasellar cistern.

Mucoceles of the sphenoid sinus are evaluated with plain films of the sinuses and pluridirectional tomography. Findings include expansion of the sinus, with or without thinning and interruption or sclerosis of the sinus walls. When bone destruction is advanced, the diagnosis is particularly difficult, and differentiation from large rapidly growing pituitary neoplasms and primary or metastatic neoplasms may be impossible. However, CT with intravenous contrast enhancement shows no increase in density. If in the rare event there is an intracranial extension, the mucus and/or purulent contents are of lower density than the surrounding cerebral tissues. In both pituitary adenomas and sphenoid sinus mucoceles, coronal as well as axial CT images are preferable.[5-9]

In summary, the distinction between these two entities may be confusing clinically as well as radiographically. If there is extension of a mucocele superiorly into the sella and suprasellar region, or if there is spread of a pituitary adenoma inferiorly into the sphenoid sinus, the plain film and tomographic findings may be identical. However, differentiation may be made by CT with utilization of contrast-enhancement since sphenoid mucoceles rarely enhance whereas pituitary tumors frequently do so.

From the Department of Radiology, Massachusetts Eye and Ear Infirmary, Boston, Massachusetts.

REPRINTS — Alfred L. Weber, MD, Department of Radiology, Massachusetts Eye and Ear Infirmary, 243 Charles Street, Boston, MA 02114.

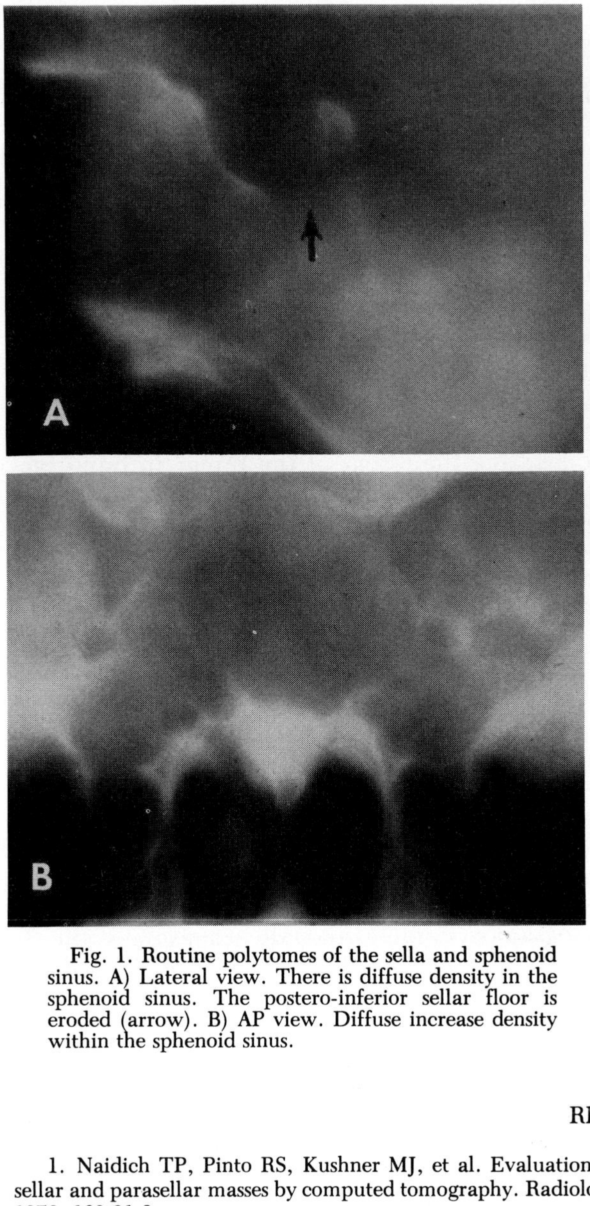

Fig. 1. Routine polytomes of the sella and sphenoid sinus. A) Lateral view. There is diffuse density in the sphenoid sinus. The postero-inferior sellar floor is eroded (arrow). B) AP view. Diffuse increase density within the sphenoid sinus.

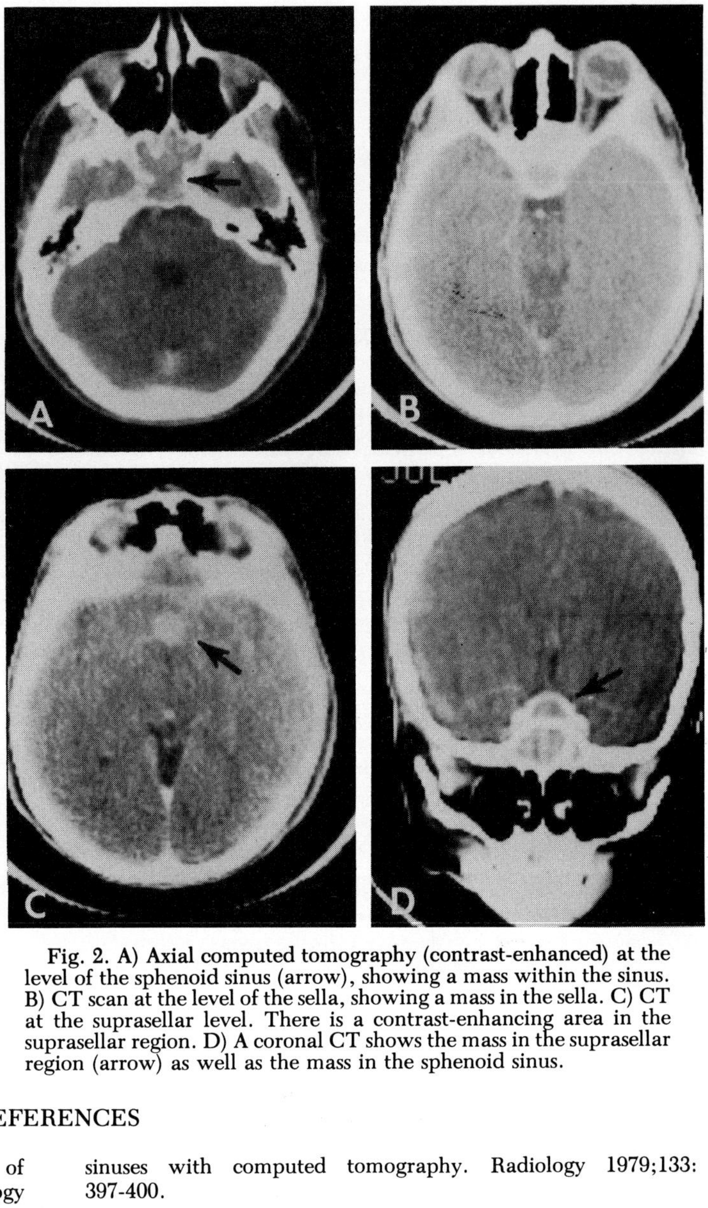

Fig. 2. A) Axial computed tomography (contrast-enhanced) at the level of the sphenoid sinus (arrow), showing a mass within the sinus. B) CT scan at the level of the sella, showing a mass in the sella. C) CT at the suprasellar level. There is a contrast-enhancing area in the suprasellar region. D) A coronal CT shows the mass in the suprasellar region (arrow) as well as the mass in the sphenoid sinus.

REFERENCES

1. Naidich TP, Pinto RS, Kushner MJ, et al. Evaluation of sellar and parasellar masses by computed tomography. Radiology 1976; 120:91-9.

2. Gyldensted C, Karle A. Computed tomography of intra and juxtasellar lesions. Neuroradiology 1977; 14:5-13.

3. New PFJ, Davis KR. Intrasellar and perisellar lesions. In: Wolpert SM, ed. Multiple imaging procedures. Vol 2. New York: Grune and Stratton, 1979:57-81.

4. Drayer B, Rosenbaum A, Kennerdell J, Robinson A, Bank W, Deeb Z. Computed tomographic diagnosis of suprasellar masses by intrathecal enhancement. Radiology 1977; 123:339-44.

5. Hesselink JR, Weber AL, New PFJ, Davis KR, Roberson GH, Taveras JM. Evaluation of mucoceles of the paranasal sinuses with computed tomography. Radiology 1979;133: 397-400.

6. Osborne AG, Johnson L, Roberts TS. Sphenoidal mucoceles with intracranial extension. J Comput Assist Tomogr 1979; 3:335-8.

7. Takahashi M, Jingu K, Nakayama T. Roentgenologic appearances of sphenoethmoidal mucocele. Neuroradiology 1973; 6:45-9.

8. Diaz F, Latchaw R, Duvall AJ, Quick CA, Erickson DL. Mucoceles with intracranial and extracranial extensions. J Neurosurg 1978; 48:284-8.

9. Dubois PJ, Schultz JC, Perrin RL, Dastur KJ. Tomography in expansile lesions of the nasal and paranasal sinuses. Radiology 1977; 125:149-58.

BOOK REVIEWS

Diseases of the External Ear: An Otologic-Dermatologic Manual

By *Ben H. Senturia*, *Morris D. Marcus*, and *Frank E. Lucente*. Second edition. Hard cover, black and white and color illustrations, indexed, 194 pages, 1980. Grune & Stratton, New York. Price: $30.00

It was a pleasure to have the opportunity to review the second edition of *Diseases of the External Ear*. The authors set forth their objectives for this book in their preface in a very lucid way and then adhere to these objectives in the text. A marked evolution in both content and style has occurred when compared and contrasted with the first edition.

This book is appropriate for otolaryngologists at every level and all physicians who treat patients with diseases of the head and neck. It is also well referenced and makes a good source book. It has been written with great attention to including only the most important features that a practitioner should need. The section on anatomy is much better illustrated than it was in the first edition and presents not only the anatomy, but also the very important subject of production and the contents of cerumen, and its importance in the external auditory meatus. It also presents the important microbiology in summary form rather than going into great detail.

Techniques of examination were not included in the first text, but are in the second. This section is very well illustrated and emphasizes the practical points of examination in detail. This is an extremely important section and makes excellent reading for beginning residents in otolaryngology and family practitioners.

The principles of therapy and prophylaxis for infections in the external ear are discussed thoroughly. These principles are dermatologic in nature, consequently the therapy for skin disorders is outlined. This important information can be applied by head and neck physicians not only in treatment of diseases of the external ear but in diseases of skin elsewhere in the head and neck region.

The section on diseases due to infection is excellent, and has incorporated in a much more readable and lucid manner the aspects which made up separate chapters in the first edition. This section has been updated and the out-of-date remedies have been omitted and the etiology, diagnosis, management and prophylaxis are discussed stepwise and details are provided for the interested reader.

The remaining sections on treatment of various other diseases have been expanded, brought up-to-date, and much improved. Of particular interest are the chapters on malformations and tumors, which were only hinted at previously. These are well described and nicely illustrated.

The book is profusely illustrated with color plates. The quality of the reproduction of color is not as good as one would have desired, but in most cases, the points are made in a dramatic way.

In summary, this is a very useful and very readable book which provides the details necessary for good understanding and diagnosis of management of diseases of the external ear.

EUGENE N. MYERS, MD, FACS
Pittsburgh, Pennsylvania

Diseases of the Oral Mucosa

By *Philip L. McCarthy* and *Gerald Shklar*. Hard cover, black and white illustrations, indexed, 559 pp, 1980. Lea & Febiger, Philadelphia. Price $47.50.

This outstanding book was written by Dr. McCarthy, a Diplomate of the American Board of Dermatology and Dr. Shklar, a Diplomate of the American Board of Oral Pathology and of the American Board of Periodontology. The authors have continued to be active in teaching, practice and in research at Tufts University School of Dental Medicine and Harvard School of Dental Medicine. The unusually broad coverage of the book is clearly a result of the excellent background and training of the authors.

It has been some 15 years since the first edition of the book which has been unavailable for the past several years. The authors are interested in introducing in the revised book the many advancements of ultrastructural and experimental studies and describe the significant advances particularly with regard to new diagnostic procedures, therapy, and management. The text has been expanded to include chapters on immunopathology and genetic disease, experimental pathology and vestibulobullous diseases. The book contains a large number of black and white illustrations, some good ultrastructural illustrations and black and white drawings. Illustrations are evident throughout the book dealing with oral manifestations of systemic diseases. The total absence of color illustrations is a striking deficiency.

One is impressed by the extensive experimental studies performed by Dr. Shklar especially in experimental pathology of oral mucous membrane diseases. There are outstanding chapters oriented towards the histochemistry and histopathology of dermatologic lesions which involve the oral cavity. There is a well-written and well-illustrated chapter dealing with benign tumors and tumor-like lesions. This book will be of particular interest to the otolaryngologist, who observes all forms and varieties of lesions of the oral cavity in his routine, everyday practice and needs some authoritative text to identify the nature and seriousness of these findings. It will also be of interest to the dermatologist, dentist, pediatrician, and general practitioner.

BEN H. SENTURIA, MD
St. Louis, Missouri

Hals-Nasen-Ohren-Heilkunde in Praxis und Klinik, Band 5, Ohr (The Ear)

Edited by *J. Berendes*, *R. Link*, and *F. Zollner*. Hard cover, 982 color and black and white illustrations, 56 tables, indexed, 1240 pages, 1979. Georg Thieme Verlag, Stuttgart. Price: DM 648.

The new edition of this volume has 26 chapters written by 37 authors of international renown.

Embryology, anatomy and histology of the ear are extensively covered, including a chapter on the ultrastructure of the labyrinth. In seven different chapters the physiology and pathophysiology of middle and inner ear are thoroughly and masterfully presented. Audiometry in all its different and most modern aspects is described in three chapters. One chapter deals with the current x-ray examination of the temporal bone, another chapter very thoroughly covers the latest on eustachian tube function testing. Inflammatory diseases of the ear and their manifestations take up four special chapters. Temporal bone neoplasms, facial paralysis, otosclerosis, traumatic injuries of the ear and traumatic injuries of the temporal bone each have a special chapter. Two chapters deal with vestibular function testing and vestibular physiology. The science of otology and its up-to-date achievements are thoroughly and scholarly presented in depth.

Most illustrations are clear and convincing. Bibliography is extensive and complete.

This well-written volume is recommended for medical schools, university clinics and teaching insitutions, as well as researchers in the field. Since it appears in the German language, it does not serve the needs of the practicing otolaryngologist in the English-speaking countries.

KARL H. SIEDENTOP, MD
Chicago, Illinois

Sensory Systems and Communication in the Elderly, Volume 10, Aging

Edited by *J. Mark Ordy* and *Ken R. Brizzee*. Hard cover, black and white illustrations, indexed, referenced, 322 pages, 1979. Raven Press, New York. Price: $25.00

Presbycusis is one of the largest categories of hearing impairment. However, it has defied good understanding or clarification because of 1) the difficulty of separating peripheral from central contributions, 2) the multiplicity of probable causes for both peripheral and central dysfunctions with age, and 3) the difficulty of excluding other factors, eg, prolonged noise exposure, as the cause of hearing impairment in old persons. Understanding of the basis for or treatment of presbycusis will not be easy to derive from this book for two reasons. First, about half of the book is about vision with several other chapters given to chemical, vestibular and somesthetic sense, autonomic mechanisms, motor control systems and psychologic coping. Second, the two chapters devoted specifically to audition and verbal communication are of limited value. "Age differences in the functional and structural organization of the auditory system in man" by the editors and their colleagues is a sketchy literature review without much sophistication. "Aging and speech understanding" by Pickett, Bergman and Levitt was adapted from a CHABA report. Its main value is its identification of the issues relative to speech understanding as a function of age, its review of contemporary studies, and its call for the partialing out of the variables in central processing as well as the variables of peripheral pathology in any study of speech discrimination.

The chapters on vision, particularly those reporting the results of specific behavioral and electrophysiologic studies, do give some insight into both peripheral and central changes with age which may be generalized to the ear and auditory function. In particular, the chapter by Bartus (Effects of Aging On Visual Memory, Sensory Processing and Discrimination Learning in a Nonhuman Primate) and by Elias (A Life-Span Perspective on Cerebral Asymmetry and Information Processing with an Emphasis on the Aging Adult) provide some insightful overviews. An extended quotation from the former illustrates this point.

". . . many of the age-related impairments in learning ability do not necessarily reflect a deficit in associative mechanisms, per se, but rather are manifested because of deficiencies in motivation, attention, color discrimination and visual acuity, . . . and increases in behavioral rigidity or perseverative tendencies . . . It is clear that when the task is arranged so that the aged subject (a) is properly motivated, (b) is familiar with the task situation, (c) can easily attend to, process, and discriminate the relevant information, (d) can easily execute choice responses, and (e) does not have to contend with competing response predispositions, the simple formation of new associations may not be consistently or seriously impaired. Whether this should be considered evidence of a lack of genuine learning disabilities in the aged is not the central issue here. Rather what is important is that if this analysis is accurate and the ability to form new associations does not necessarily decline with old age, it should be possible (through careful planning) to arrange many situations so that the learning of new tasks or the formation of new habits is not seriously impaired in the aged population."

ROBERT GOLDSTEIN, PhD
JUDITH E. HIRSCH, PhD
Madison, Wisconsin

Evaluating Research in Speech Pathology and Audiology

By *Ira M. Ventry* and *Nicholas Schiavetti*, with a chapter by *Teri A. Denson*. Hard cover, black and white illustrations, indexed, referenced, 356 pp, 1980. Addison-Wesley Publishing Co., Reading, Massachusetts.

This is intended to be a textbook for a course designed to teach graduate students in speech pathology and audiology how to understand and critically evaluate research. Few such textbooks exist and, as the authors note, related books from the fields of psychology and education are only peripherally related. The need for such a textbook is evident.

The vast majority of practicing professionals in speech pathology and audiology have only limited training in evaluating research. In fact, the elimination of master degree theses requirements from training programs in recent years has reduced the emphasis on research evaluation. Yet licensure requirements and competent clinical practice necessitate that professionals be able to critically evaluate research articles. This textbook then should also be of some benefit to many practicing clinicians.

The book is organized into three major sections, each containing a number of separate chapters. The first section categorizes the types of research found in speech pathology and audiology journals and describes some of the general considerations related to research design. It ends with a chapter covering the organization, manipulation and presentation of research data. The second section separately defines and explains the major divisions of typical research articles. It describes the introduction, method, results, discussion, and conclusion portions of research articles. The final section employs a pragmatic summary of the previous two sections. Published articles existing in the literature, one in language and one in audiology, are reprinted in their entirety and critically evaluated with respect to the concepts presented in the first two sections.

This well-written textbook achieves its purpose. Although many different organizational schemes could have been used, the existing organization is particularly appropriate. It is logical, consistent, and relevant to the needs of the student. The exercises at the end of each chapter are directly related to the current literature in speech pathology and audiology and are generally quite thorough. The individual concepts presented in a chapter should be well understood if the exercises are completed.

The text has some inadequacies, however. First, some important concepts were treated superficially. For example, concepts related to differences between descriptive and inferential statistics, operational definitions, and relevant differences vs statistically significant differences, are mentioned but should be covered in greater depth. The issues related to data presentation are covered too briefly. Second, some minor errors exist. The authors' own presentation of data shows an inadequate, or lack, of labeling on certain axes of some graphs. Some nominal data which should be presented with bar graphs were connected with straight lines. Some important terms (such as asymptote) were used incorrectly.

These criticisms are not serious however. In fact, since most of the major points are covered and errors are minor, the text can serve as a springboard for excellent class discussions. I see this text becoming widely used in speech pathology and audiology training programs for seminar courses, independent study courses, and journal clubs. It should also become a reference for practicing clinicians.

GERALD R. POPELKA, PhD
St. Louis, Missouri

Microlaryngoscopy and Endolaryngeal Microscopy

By *Professor Dr. med. O. Kleinsasser*. Translated by P. M. Stell. Hard cover, black and white and color illustrations, 167 pages, 1979. University Park Press, Baltimore. Price:$64.50

Kleinsasser's primary work in endolaryngeal microsurgery was well documented in the first (1968) edition of this work. The second German edition (1976) and its English translation (1979) are even more beautifully illustrated. Not only has the number of illustrations increased by about one third but many of the original illustrations have been replaced. The result is most pleasing; the photographs have a three-dimensional realism perhaps unequaled in any other such work. The text has been updated (to 1976) and increased in length by 40% reflecting the author's experience with over 3000 cases.

Professor Kleinsasser has given us not only a handsome atlas but a text which is a testament to the place which microsurgery holds in the practice of modern laryngology.

GABRIEL F. TUCKER, JR., MD
Chicago, Illinois

BOOKS RECEIVED

New Directions in Public Health Care. A Prescription for the 1980s

Edited by Cotton M. Lindsay, MD. Index, black and white illustrations, soft cover, 300 pages, 3rd edition, revised, Institute for Contemporary Studies, San Francisco. $6.95.

Rocca Pneumatica e Vacuum Petrosum

By Prof. Alessandro Fioretti. Index, black and white illustrations, hard cover, summary in English, French, German, Italian and Spanish, 138 pages, Piccin Editore S.A.S., Italy.

Terminology of Communication Disorders

By Lucille Nicolosi, MA, Elizabeth Harryman, MA, and Janet Kresheck, PhD. Black and white illustrations, soft cover, 273 pages, Book Review Audit, The Williams & Wilkins Company, Baltimore. $14.50.

Thalamocortical Organization of the Auditory System in the Cat Studied by Retrograde Axonal Transport of Horseradish Peroxidase

By Prof. Dr. Kahee Niimi and Hiroaki Matsuoka. Index, black and white illustrations, soft cover, 51 pages, Springer-Verlag New York, Inc. $19.25.

Environmental Noise Control

Selected reprints edited by Thomas D. Rossing, PhD. Black and white illustrations, soft cover, 196 pages, Publications Department of American Association of Physics Teachers, Stony Brook, New York. $6.00.

Mammalian Vestibular Physiology

By Victor J. Wilson and Geoffrey M. Jones. Index, black and white illustrations, hard cover, 366 pages, Plenum Publishing Co., New York. $32.50.

Tumors of the Head and Neck

By John G. Batsakis, MD. Second edition, black and white illustrations, hard cover, 561 pages, The Williams & Wilkins Company, Baltimore. $46.00.

Acoustic Tumors — Volume I: Diagnosis: Volume II: Management

Edited by William F. House, MD, and Charles M. Luetje, MD. Index, black and white illustrations, hard cover, 297 pages, $29.50 for Volume I, and 280 pages, $19.50 for Volume II. University Park Press, Baltimore.

Recent Advances in Otolaryngology, No. 5

Edited by T.R. Bull, FRCS, Joselen Ransome, FRCS, and Harold B. Holden, FRCS. Index, black and white illustrations, hard cover, 242 pages, Churchill Livingston/Medical Division of Longman Inc., New York. $32.50.

Neurological Surgery of the Ear, Volume II

By Herbert Silverstein, MD, and Horace Norrell, MD. Black and white illustrations, index, hard cover, 396 pages, Aesculapius Publishing Co., Birmingham. $60.

Respiratory Tract Mucus

By the Ciba Foundation Symposium 54. Black and white illustrations, index, hard cover, 325 pages, Elsevier/Excerpta Medica/North Holland, Amsterdam.

External Ear Malformations: Epidemiology, Genetics, and Natural History

By Michael Melnick, DDS, PhD, and Nitnos C. Myrianthopoulos, PhD. Index, black and white illustrations, hard cover, 128 pages, Alan R. Liss, Inc., New York. $18.

ABSTRACTS

Sternocleidomastoid Regional Flaps: A New Look at an Old Concept

Jabaley ME, Heckler FR, Wallace WH, Knott LH: Br J Plast Surg 32:106, 1979.

The authors present a very thorough resume of the use of the sternocleidomastoid (SCM) regional flap. They studied the SCM flap in three ways: by cadaver dissections; by dissections in the living such as neck node excisions and rhytidectomy; and by fluorescein injections after raising SCM flaps.

The blood supply of the skin overlying the SCM muscle has a tripartite blood supply from the perforating branches of the occipital and posterior auricular arteries superiorly; branches of the transverse cervical branch of the thyrocervical trunk inferiorly; and a myocutaneous supply from the SCM muscle itself. The clinical applications of the use of the flap are in a number of areas about the neck, cheek and jaw, and oral cavity and it has been used also to release burn contractures when the flap donor site has been lightly burned. Although it has uses in the cheek, these authors have not used it there before because of the limitation of the cases presented. Whereas other authors have reported necrosis of a part or all of the flap, these authors state that this is generally due to the fact that there has been either previous irradiation in the area, or interruption of the vessel at its superior pedicle has taken place. In addition, the flap may be unavailable or at least, in part, may be a poorer choice because of its proximity to the area of potential use. They do not advocate the use of the flap in irradiated necks and point out the criticisms other authors make regarding the use of the flap.

The authors present a good schematic diagram of three figures outlining the use of the flap and a total of 12 photographs illustrating its use. There are 15 references presented.

M. Payne, MD
St. Louis, Mo

Evaluation of Speech after Correction of Rhinophonia with Pushback Palatoplasty Combined with Pharyngeal Flap

Dixon VL, Bzoch KR, Habal MB: Plast Reconstr Surg 64:77, 1979

The authors present a total of 35 patients who have been operated on by the technique they describe as a balanced technique of anatomical repair based on a functional restoration of balanced speech. They have complete speech evaluations in 15 of these patients; these were selected because they had had preoperative evaluation tests and were available for postoperative tests.

Tables are given listing the sex, age, classification of the causative factor for the speech problem, age at the time of surgery, precipitating medical condition producing the speech derangement, and the time for evaluation postoperatively. The methods for evaluation consist of 1) the Bzoch Error Pattern Screening Articulation Test; 2) the phonation test consisting of having each patient prolong three vowels "A," "E" and "O"; 3) a nasal emission index was recorded; 4) the hypernasality "cul-de-sac" test; and 5) the hyponasality "cul-de-sac" test.

The statistical analysis of these findings are described in elaborate detail, possibly more than the average reader would be interested in; however, it is an excellent statistical review and the findings that are listed as their conclusions include the following: 1) The palatal pushback with pharyngeal flap surgery appears to be as effective for males as for females. 2) This surgical technique can be used for patients with a cleft palate as well as for patients with congenital velopharyngeal insufficiency. 3) The same results can be obtained whether the patient has had previous palatal surgery or not. 4) The amount of time elapsing from surgery to postoperative evaluation is not an important factor affecting the speech and voice results.

Eighty-six percent of the patients examined showed no abnormal nasal emission and no evidence of significant hypernasality during word production. Other items were recorded such as the presence or absence of snoring and the presence or absence of mouth breathing preoperatively and postoperatively.

There are five tables presented, one figure showing the outline of the defect in the velopharyngeal mechanism, and a total of 19 references.

M. Payne, MD
St. Louis, Mo

The Significance of Secretory IgA in Middle-Ear Fluid

Jones EA Jr, Thomas LR, Davis NC: J Allergy Clin Immunol 42:236-240, 1979.

Middle ear fluid was obtained from 23 patients at therapeutic myringotomy and immunoglobulin levels were analyzed using immunodiffusion and antiserum precipitation technique. In acute otitis media, middle ear fluid immunoglobulin levels were commensurate with serum levels. In chronic otitis media, middle ear fluid immunoglobulins were nearly always higher than serum levels, and middle ear fluid IgA levels were proportionately higher than other immunoglobulin values from middle ear fluid as compared to serum. The authors speculate that the higher levels of IgA suggest the presence of a secretory epithelium lining the middle ear, ie, that a proportion of middle ear fluid IgA is secretory in nature. They suggest that in the course of development of serous otitis media the mucoperiostial lining of the middle ear is converted to a secretory membrane which may continue to pour secretion into the tympanic cavity even after the initial inciting factor has been eliminated. The presence of secretory IgA in middle ear fluid suggests that the inflammatory process has continued long enough for a secretory epithelium to evolve. Removal of the serous middle ear fluid and ventilation using transtympanic membrane ventilation tubes is felt to hasten reestablishment of a normal mucoperiostium.

A. Jahn, MD
New York, NY

Orbital Floor Fractures — Should They Be Explored Early?

Sacks AC, Friedland JA: Plast Reconstr Surg 64:190, 1979

One hundred consecutive cases of orbital floor fractures were retrospectively reviewed. These cases were evaluated to compare preoperative findings with postoperative surgical results and to attempt to clarify the relationship between signs and symptoms on admission as compared with the late results. Early findings of diplopia, infraorbital rim step-off, and hypesthesia became an indication for exploration of the orbital floor and placement of silicone sheeting. It was noted that when this was done, minimal complications resulted.

A total of five figures are presented, including an interesting bar graph arrangement of the postoperative results as compared with preoperative findings and the operative treatment; and a figure to demonstrate the area of involvement in orbital floor fractures. Fourteen references are provided.

M. Payne, MD
St. Louis, Mo

Ann Otol 89:1980

SIXTH DANIEL C. BAKER, JR. MEMORIAL LECTURE

INDUCTION OF CANCER BY DNA VIRUSES

JAMES D. WATSON, PhD

COLD SPRING HARBOR, NEW YORK

The life cycles of the tumor virus SV40 and polyoma are discussed with particular emphasis on the role of the viral coded proteins which mediate the transformation of normal cells into their cancerous equivalents. One or more of these proteins possibly act by stimulating directly the synthesis of cellular DNA, while others may mimic the action of polypeptide mitogens that act at the cell surface.

How tumor viruses induce cancer has long been a classical puzzle for biologists. Until we knew what viruses were and began to understand the molecular tricks by which they replicated, there was no way to even superficially attack this problem. We have had to wait until most of the basic facts of molecular virology were worked out before we could even make intelligent guesses as to what was happening when infection by a tumor virus changed (transformed) a normal cell into the cancerous equivalent.

Though at first we hoped for a unitary answer, the discovery that both DNA viruses (eg, wart viruses) and RNA viruses (eg, Rous sarcoma virus) could transform cells made us suspect that there might be many different ways by which viral-induced cell transformation occurred. Now as firm facts have begun to appear over the past decade, we see this to be the case, with the generalization emerging that the transforming activity of the DNA tumor resides in the properties of viral genes needed for their own replication. In contrast, the transforming potential of the RNA tumor viruses results from their having accidentally picked up normal cellular genes that play no role in viral replication, but which when expressed at high levels change the cells in which they reside into cancer cells.

The first tumor virus that looked suitable for the molecular biologist was the Shope papilloma virus. The warts which it produces on wild cottontail rabbits are rich sources of infectious virus particles, and already by the late 1940s, through the work of Joseph Beard,[1] we knew the molecular weight of the virus to be about 50 million and, from its DNA content, its chromosome was estimated to have a molecular weight of about 5 million. This suggested that papilloma DNA might be smaller than any other DNA molecule. So encouraged, John Littlefield and I[2] did some preliminary work at Massachusetts General Hospital in 1959 measuring its sedimentation constant and observing its reversible melting as a function of temperature. We did not use the EM to look at our molecules, however, and missed the crucial fact that they were circular. Moreover, the inability to work with the Shope virus in cell culture meant that most experiments of the type that intrigues the molecular biologist were out of our reach, and I retreated back to work on bacterial viruses, soon focusing on the very small RNA phages whose chromosomes at most could contain only several genes.

Since then papilloma viruses have been implicated as the causative agents for warts in a variety of animals as well as humans (Table 1), and they clearly should receive much more attention than they now get. Nonetheless, the great holdup remains of our inability to effectively either grow them in cell culture or routinely use them as transforming agents. With, however, the recent major advances achieved by Howard Green's MIT lab[3] in the growing of normal epithelial cells in culture, we may soon witness the development of good in vitro systems for work on the papilloma viruses. But for the time being, virtually all our hard data on tumor viruses comes from work on those viruses that animal virologists have been able to domesticate for routine work in cultured cells.

In this lecture therefore I shall focus on the small monkey DNA virus SV40 (Fig. 1), whose tumorogenous potential was discovered almost 20 years ago and on which we began intensive work at Cold Spring Harbor some 10 years ago. SV40 both replicates in and transforms cells that grow well in culture, and with its close relative, the mouse virus polyoma, are the best understood viruses at the molecular level.

The key factor that intially led the molecular biologists to devote so much attention to SV40 and polyoma was their small size. They are among the smallest of DNA viruses with their chromosomes being circular DNA molecules (Fig. 2) made up only

From the Cold Spring Harbor Laboratory, Cold Spring Harbor, New York.

Presented at the meeting of the American Laryngological Association, Palm Beach, Florida, April 14-15, 1980.

REPRINTS — James D. Watson, PhD, Cold Spring Harbor Laboratory, Cold Spring Harbor, NY 11724.

TABLE 1. HUMAN AND BOVINE PAPILLOMAS AND ASSOCIATED VIRUSES

Papilloma	Observed Malignant Conversion	Virus
Human		
Common wart (verruca vulgaris)	–	3 Distinct types and 2 subtypes of the most prevalent type (HPV-1); the 2 additional types are designated HPV-2 and HPV-4
Flat wart (verruca plana)	–	1 Distinct type HPV-3
Epidermodysplasia verruciformis	+ + +	2 Distinct types HPV-3 and HPV-5
Genital warts (condyloma acuminatum)	+	Virus-specific DNA has been tentatively identified; at least 1 serotype revealed by indirect immunofluorescence
"Juvenile" type of laryngeal papilloma	+	?
Bovine		
Fibroepithelioma	?	2 Distinct types, BPV-1 and BPV-2
Epithelial warts	?	1 Type (BPV-3) distinct from BPV-1 and BPV-2

HPV - Human papilloma virus; BPV - Bovine papilloma virus.

of 5,200 base pairs. This fact led us to suspect they might contain only 3-7 genes. Even so, the possibility of knowing their exact molecular sequences seemed a most remote idea, conceivably two to three decades away. Thanks, however, to the discovery of 1) enzymes that cut DNA molecules at specific points (the restriction enzymes, Table 2), 2) the development of electrophoretic methods for separating the resulting fragments, and 3) the development of powerful, quick ways for nucleotide sequence determination, the exact nucleotide sequence of both the SV40 and polyoma chromosomes are now known. They provide a wealth of key molecular detail that not even the most optimistic of molecular virologists would have dreamed attainable a decade ago.

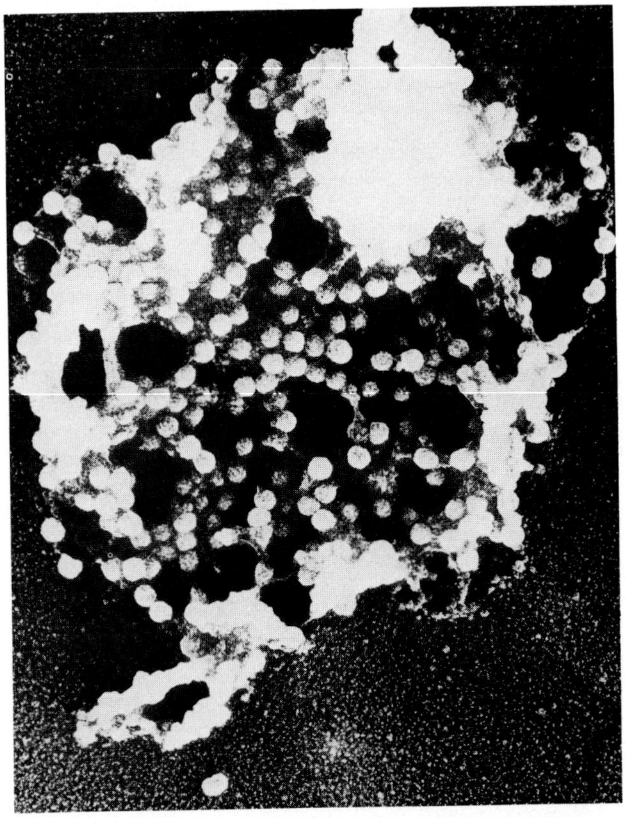

Fig. 1. SV40 particles seen on the surface of a nuclear membrane fragment of an SV40-infected CV-1 (monkey) cell. (From Tooze J, ed. DNA tumor viruses. Part 2, Molecular biology of tumor viruses. Cold Spring Harbor: Cold Spring Harbor Laboratory, 1980. Reprinted with permission.)

With SV40 and polyoma, like all other DNA tumor viruses, no trace of infectious virus particles are seen within the cells they transform. This is not surprising, since when DNA viruses multiply in cells, they invariably kill them. So DNA tumor viruses only transform "nonpermissive" cells in which they cannot carry out a complete infectious cycle (Table 3). For example, in studying transformation by SV40, we infect, say, mouse or hamster cells, while when we wish to study the normal replication cycle of SV40, we employ a "permissive" monkey cell line like CV-1. In contrast to lytic multiplication which can occur in virtually all permissive cells, transformation (Fig. 3) is a much rarer event, and we generally do not study the transformation event itself. Instead we focus attention on the properties of the transformed cell lines, hoping from their properties (Table 4) to work backward to the molecular events which initiate them.

From the very start of molecular tumor virology

TABLE 2. SOME EXAMPLES OF CLEAVAGE OF POLYOMA VIRUS DNA AND SV40 DNA BY RESTRICTION ENDONUCLEASES

Microorganism	Abbrev.	Sequence (5′→3′ / 3′→5′)	No. of Sites Polyoma	SV40
B albidum	*Bal*I	CGG↓CCG GCC↑GGC	0	0
H parainfluenzae	*Hpa*I	GTT↓AAC CAA↑TTG	0	4
B amyloliquefaciens H	*Bam*I	G↓GATCC CCTAG↑G	1	1
E coli RY13	*Eco*RI	G↓AATTC CTTAA↑G	1	1
H aegyptius	*Hae*II	RGCGC↓Y Y↑CGCGR	2	1
H influenzae R_d	*Hind*II	GTY↓RAC CAR↑YTG	2	7
H influenzae R_d	*Hind*III	A↓AGCTT TTCGA↑A	2	6
H haemolyticus	*Hha*I	GCG↓C C↑GCG	4	2
H parainfluenzae	*Hpa*II	C↓CGG GGC↑C	8	1
H aegyptius	*Hae*III	GG↓CC CC↑GG	24	19

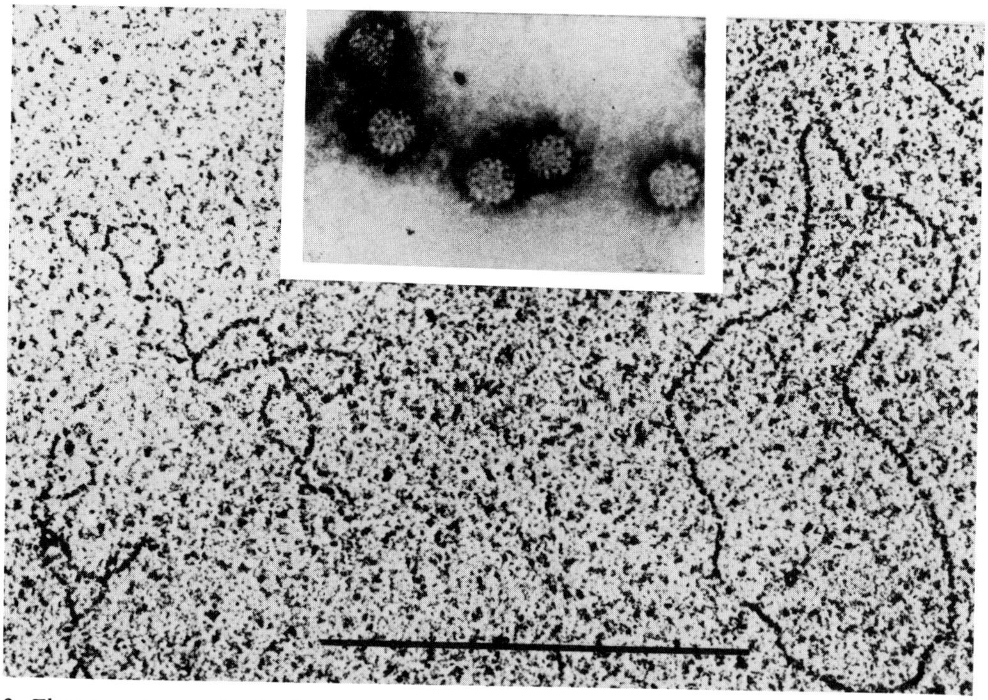

Fig. 2. Electron micrograph of polyoma virus particles and DNA (inset). Polyoma virus particles: left) polyoma superhelical (form I) DNA; right) polyoma circular (form II) DNA. A single nick in the DNA converts form I to form II. In this micrograph, the same scale was used for viral particles and DNAs. Bar represents 5000 Å. (From Tooze J, ed. DNA tumor viruses. Part 2, Molecular biology of tumor viruses. Cold Spring Harbor: Cold Spring Harbor Laboratory, 1980. Reprinted with permission.)

in the early 1960s, our way of thinking was strongly influenced by earlier research on the bacterial viruses (bacteriophages). In the first place, we knew that certain phage chromosomes not only contained genes which specified their structural proteins, but also genes which functioned to ensure the replication of their own nucleic acids. Conceivably the DNA animal viruses were similarly constructed, carrying genes that would not only speed up the replication of their own chromosomes but also that of their host cell's chromosomes. In the second place we had learned that phage chromosomes could become inserted into bacterial chromosomes under conditions where some of phage genes could function. If tumor viruses' chromosomes could similarly become part of their host cell's chromosomes, some of these integration events might yield transformed

TABLE 3. RESPONSE OF CELLS OF DIFFERENT SPECIES TO INFECTION BY SV40 AND POLYOMA VIRUS

Species	*Infection by SV40*	*Infection by Polyoma Virus*
Human	Semipermissive	Nonpermissive
Mouse	Nonpermissive	Permissive
African green monkey	Permissive	Nonpermissive
Rat	Nonpermissive or semipermissive	Semipermissive
Guinea pig	Nonpermissive or semipermissive	NT
Rabbit	Nonpermissive or semipermissive	NT
Cow	Nonpermissive or semipermissive	NT
Hamster	Semipermissive	Semipermissive
Lizzard	Semipermissive	NT

NT - Not tested.

cells because of the subsequent expression of the viral genes coding for DNA replication.

The first strong hint that SV40 transformed cells, in fact, contained viral specific genes, came from observations of SV40 specific antigen found in transformed cells. Called the T(tumor) antigen, it

TABLE 4. PROPERTIES OF CELLS TRANSFORMED BY SV40 OR POLYOMA VIRUS*

Growth
- High or indefinite saturation density†
- Different, usually reduced, serum requirement†
- Growth in agar or methocel suspension — anchorage independence†
- Tumor formation upon injection into susceptible animals
- Not susceptible to contact inhibition of movement
- Growth in a less-oriented manner†
- Growth on monolayers of normal cells†

Surface
- Increased agglutinability of plant lectins†
- Changes in composition of glycoproteins and glycolipids
- Tight junctions missing
- Fetal antigens revealed
- Virus-specific transplantation antigen
- Different staining properties
- Increased rate of transport of nutrients
- Increased secretion of proteases or activators†

Intracellular
- Disruption of the cytoskeleton
- Changed amounts of cyclic nucleotides

Evidence of virus
- Virus-specific antigenic proteins detectable
- Viral DNA sequences detected
- Viral mRNA present
- Virus can be rescued in some cases

*Transformed cells show many, if not all, of these properties, which are not shared by untransformed parental cells.

†Several of these properties have formed the basis of selection procedures for isolating transformants.

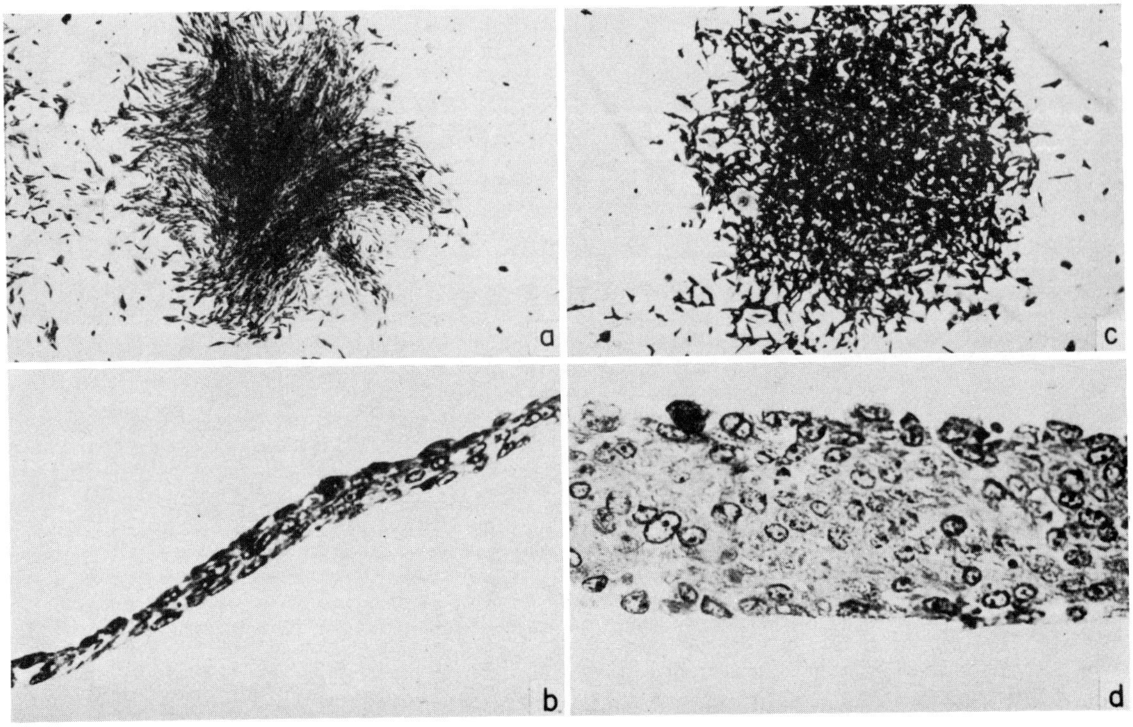

Fig. 3. Transformation of BHK-21 cells by polyoma virus. a) Colony illustrating the regular parallel arrangement of the elongated fibroblastic cells. b) Section of the colony shown in 3a stained with hematoxylin and eosin. c) BHL-21 cells transformed by polyoma virus, illustrating the random orientation of more rounded cells. d) Section of the colony shown in c stained with hematoxylin and eosin. (From Tooze J, ed. DNA tumor viruses. Part 2, Molecular biology of tumor viruses. Cold Spring Harbor: Cold Spring Harbor Laboratory, 1980. Reprinted with permission.)

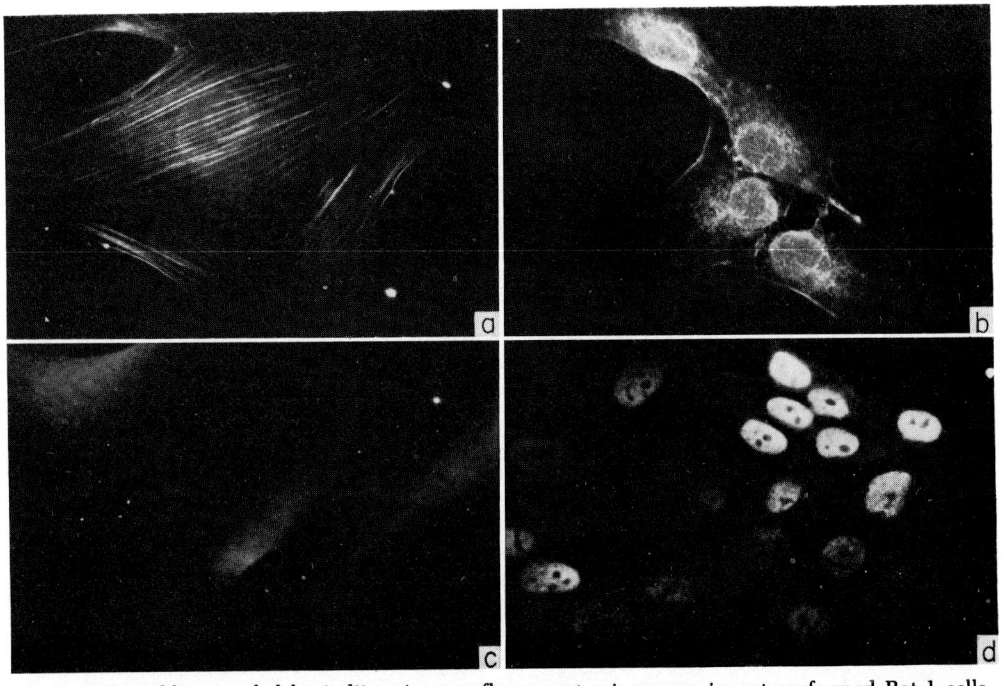

Fig. 4. a) Actin cables revealed by indirect immunofluorescent microscopy in untransformed Rat-1 cells. b) Actin distribution in an SV40-transformed cell line (14B) derived from Rat-1 cells. c) Untransformed Rat-1 cells stained with hamster anti-SV40-tumor serum. d) SV40-transformed Rat-1 cells (14B line) stained with the same serum and revealing the nuclear localization of SV40 large T antigen. All the micrographs were taken at the same magnification. (From Tooze J, ed. DNA tumor viruses. Part 2, Molecular biology of tumor viruses. Cold Spring Harbor: Cold Spring Harbor Laboratory, 1980. Reprinted with permission.)

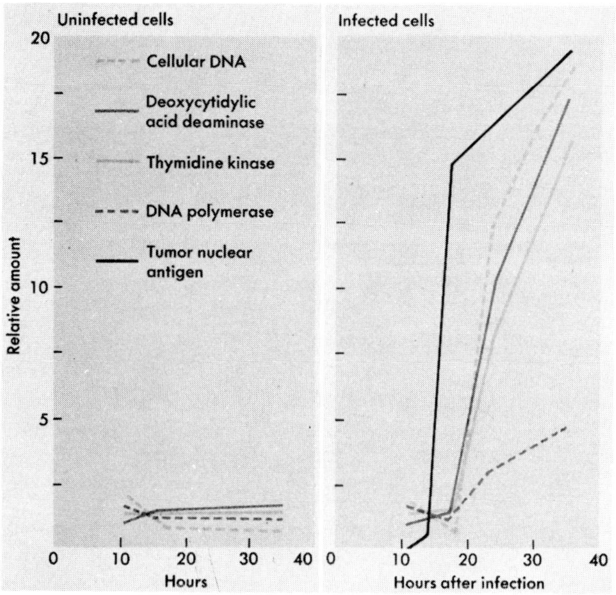

Fig. 5. Induction of enzymes involved with DNA synthesis following infection of permissive monkey cells by SV40 virus. Before these cellular-coded enzymes appear, synthesis of the viral-specific protein, the "T" nuclear antigen, has begun. (From Watson JD. Molecular biology of the gene. 3rd ed. Menlo Park: WA Benjamin, 1976. Reprinted with permission.)

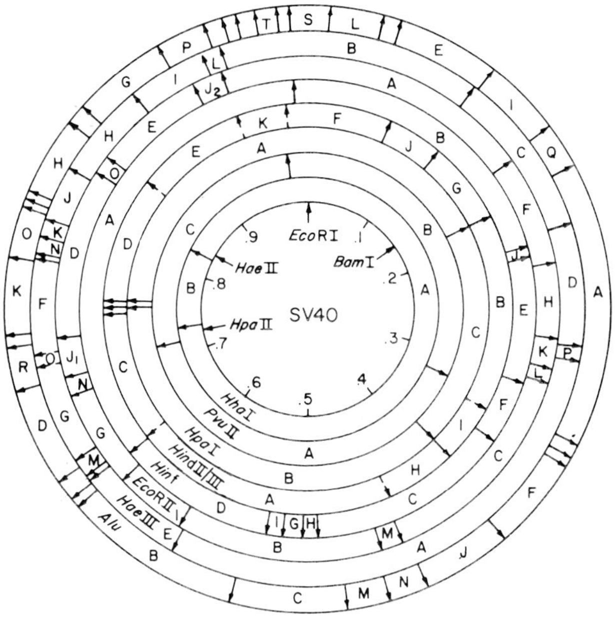

Fig. 6. Cleavage map of SV40 DNA. Enzyme-producing single scissions of SV40 DNA are noted inside the circle; the *Eco*RI site is defined as the zero coordinate. Each concentric ring shows sites of cleavage by individual enzymes.

was observed not only in transformed cells (Fig. 4) but also was present in the monkey cells during SV40 replication. Most importantly, the T antigen bore no relation to any protein used to make up the viral capsid and so was not a structural protein. It might then be an enzyme involved, needed in DNA replication, a hypothesis strengthened by the fact that appeared only in the viral life cycle before viral DNA replication started (Fig. 5). Moreover, it was located almost exclusively in the nucleus, the site of all viral DNA synthesis as well as of normal chromosomal DNA synthesis. Likewise, in SV40 transformed cells the T antigen was exclusively located in the nucleus.

If this way of thinking is correct, we should expect to find direct evidence for the presence of SV40 DNA sequences within SV40 transformed cells. This first came from work in Dulbecco's Salk Institute lab[4] that showed the presence of not only SV40 specific messenger RNA, but also of SV40 DNA integrated into large pieces of host chromosomal DNA. Cell transformation thus appeared to be due to the insertion of viral specific genes into host chromosomes, and their subsequent functioning to produce viral specific proteins like the T antigen.

To go further in this analysis required the working out of the fundamental events in the lytic cycle through which SV40 DNA was replicated and the synthesis of the viral specific protein was insured. Here we were effectively stymied until the restriction enzymes became available to cut DNA at specific sites. We could then produce and isolate small chromosomal fragments whose arrangement within the circular SV40 chromosome could be precisely defined (Fig. 6). Given these fragments it was

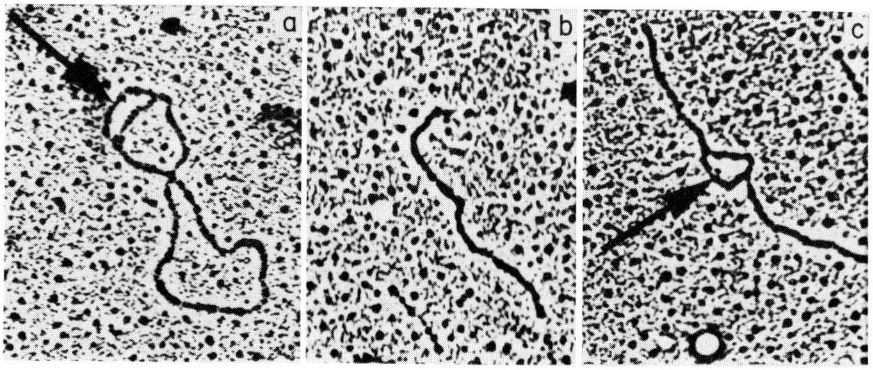

Fig. 7. Electron micrographs of replicating polyoma virus DNA. Arrow indicates replicating bubble. a) Polyoma virus DNA replicating molecule less than 50% replicated. b,c) Replicating molecule cleaved with *Hin*dIII, which cleaves polyoma virus DNA into two fragments of unequal sizes. The larger of the two fragments, c, has the replicating bubble, which is located 25±3% from one end and 30±3% from the other. (x26,100)

possible to localize a single site at which DNA replication commenced (the origin) (Fig. 7) as well as to show that the SV40 messenger RNA molecules were divided into two classes, one (the early mRNA) which apparently coded for only the T antigen, the other (the late mRNA) which coded for the viral capsid proteins used in the construction of the viral particles (Fig. 8). The early mRNA was synthesized counterclockwise from the origin, while the late mRNA was synthesized in the clockwise direction. The early and late mRNAs thus came from mutually exclusive RNA regions, each occupying approximately one half the genome.

When similar experiments were done on transformed cells, only the early T antigen coding mRNA was found. In contrast, no late mRNA was found in agreement with the fact that no structural (late) proteins are found in transformed cells. Conceivably the only protein mediating cell transformation was the T antigen since its size as revealed by its movement on SDS gels (Fig. 9) was in the neighborhood of 100,000 molecular weight (MW) corresponding to virtually all the coding capacity contained within the early DNA region.

Clearly the T antigen had to be studied as a pure protein, but this was not initially easy since it is present in only very small amounts either during lytic infection or in transformed cells. Only when certain hybrid SV40 adenovirus particles were found here at Cold Spring Harbor to produce much larger amounts of T antigen could it be properly studied as a molecular entity. Then Bob Tjian[5] could definitively show that the T antigen bound specifically to several specific sites around the origin

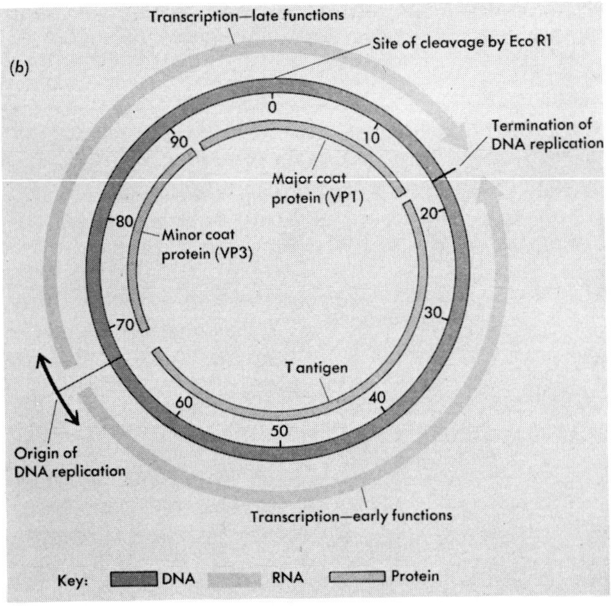

Fig. 8. The circular chromosome of SV40 (polyoma) showing its three genes, the initiation points for DNA replication, and the transcription pattern of its early and late genes. (From Watson JD. Molecular biology of the gene. 3rd ed. Menlo Park: WA Benjamin, 1976. Reprinted with permission.)

Fig. 9. Immunoprecipitations from monkey (CV-1) cells lytically infected with SV40. Cells were starved from methionine one hour prior to labelling with 250 uCi^{35}S-methionine. After incubation with radioactive label for one hour, the cells were disrupted and their proteins precipitated either with a rabbit immune serum directed against the SV40 large T-related protein purified from Ad2^{++}D2 or with hamster anti-SV40-tumor serum. The anti-D2 serum recognizes only the large T protein, while the anti-tumor serum recognizes both large T and small t (data of W. Topp, Cold Spring Harbor Laboratory).

of DNA replication. This was a most pleasing result, since Tjian, with Fey and Graessman, furthermore could show using microinjection experiments that the presence of T leads to the initiation of cellular DNA synthesis as well as of SV40 DNA. The nucleotide sequences at which cellular DNA synthesis is initiated thus must closely resemble those at the SV40 origin.

At the molecular level, how T antigen stimulates the initiation of DNA synthesis is still unknown. Our only clue is the presence of ATPase activity in highly purified T antigen. A similar activity is found on certain proteins involved in the replication of phage DNA, and hopefully through the use of in vitro systems derived from mammalian cells the exact step where T antigen acts can be elucidated in the not too distant future.

It was thus almost possible to believe that the entire role of SV40 in transformation lay through its ability to initiate DNA synthesis, thereby giving to a cell blocked before DNA synthesis the capacity of double its DNA and to go through a complete cell cycle to yield two daughter cells. But a bad snag to this idea arose in late 1976, when SV40 mutants were found that were unable to transform well but which multiplied normally in monkey cells and induced normal complements of T antigen. This suggested that a still undiscovered protein might be the key to the transformed phenotype, a most bothersome idea, since the T antigen seemed to require all the "early region" to code for all its some 900 amino acids.

The resolution of this paradox came in the spring of 1977 from the discovery of RNA splicing. Through this process a given primary RNA transcript can be so modified to give rise to several different smaller mRNA molecules, each coding for a different protein. Within a month after the discovery of adenovirus splicing this phenomenon was extended to SV40 where it was shown that the early as well as the late transcripts have several splicing pathways, each generating one specific protein product (Fig. 10). Through splicing, the early SV40 region gives rise not only to T (large) MW 100,000 but to t (small) MW 17,000. It is t which is functionally absent in cells infected with the replicating nontransforming mutants, and so t must play a vital role in transformation. Mere stimulation of the initiation of DNA synthesis is thus not by itself sufficient to make cells cancerous.

In contrast to T, t is not located in the nucleus, but at a cytoplasmic site yet to be determined. Up until now t has not been sufficiently purified to let the protein chemist study it, but this should happen soon. Our main clue so far is that in absence of t, but in the presence of T, the recipient cells resemble normal cells and do not take up the less adhesive, rounded character of the truly transformed cancer cell (Fig. 4). This "roundness" reflects the absence

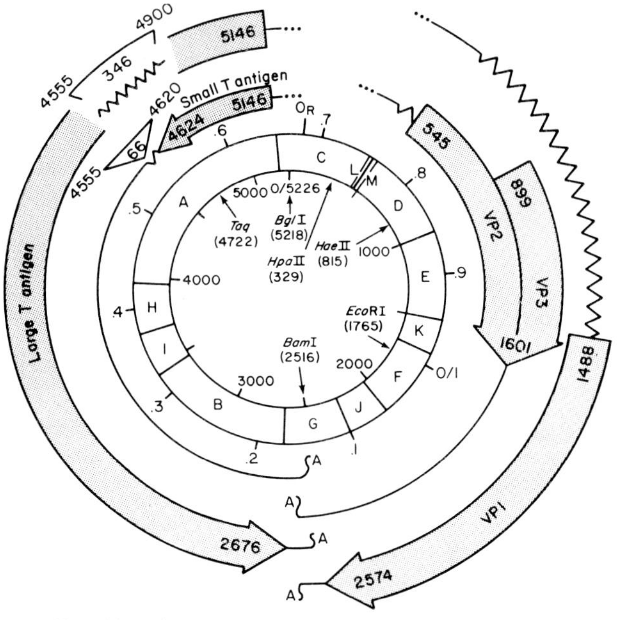

Fig. 10. Schematic representation of SV40 genome indicating locations of some principal features. The genome is represented as a circle with the origin of replication at the top. (From Tooze J, ed. DNA tumor viruses. Part 2, Molecular biology of tumor viruses. Cold Spring Harbor: Cold Spring Harbor Laboratory, 1980. Reprinted with permission.)

of the large actin-myosin-containing stress fibers that are so characteristic of the flattened adhesive normal cells. We can thus hypothesize that "t" by somehow interfering with a normal cytoskeletal component mimics a normal mitogenic stimuli that lets a cell move from G_1 into the S (DNA synthesis) phase of the cell cycle.

Here we should note the parallel with recent results on the Rous sarcoma virus whose integrated presence also leads to rounded cells. Its "sarc" gene codes for a 55,000 MW protein that acts within the cytoplasm most likely after combining with (inserting into) the cytoplasmic surface of the exterior plasma membrane.

We must also ask whether, in fact, T is at all necessary for cell transformation, as distinct from its unambiguous necessity for viral DNA replication. Here the answer for SV40 is most probably yes, since in order for fragments of SV40 DNA to transform DNA, they must contain all the DNA sequences needed to encode T. But for its close relative polyoma it now seems totally clear that T plays no essential role in transformation. A decisive experiment here uses recombinant DNA procedures to create hybrid DNA molecules lacking sufficient DNA sequences to code for polyoma T, but containing all the bases needed to make polyoma t. Cells infected with such DNAs can be transformed to yield stable clones capable of growing in agar (a key diagnostic feature of the transformed cell), and which lack significant numbers of the actin-myosin-containing stress fibers. The situation is here complicated by the fact that polyoma codes for still another protein from the early region that is called middle T. What middle T does is totally obscure except for the tendency to associate with the outer plasma membrane. There it somehow is able to generate a cell-mediated immunological response that can prevent tumors forming in mice containing polyoma transformed cells. Somehow SV40 T also leads to a protective cell-mediated immunological response that may explain why SV40 infection so seldom leads to cancers within the animals it infects. This suggests that the SV40 T must also associate sometimes with the plasma membrane, but of this we yet have no evidence.

Clearly we also have to learn much more about t, asking among other things why it is always coded in native SV40 DNA even though it is not necessary for viral replication in cells in culture. One possible answer is that in nature SV40 often infects nondividing cells which are blocked in from further DNA synthesis. Such cells may only be unleashed to make any DNA by the receipt of a mitogenic signal. Conceivably even with T present, the many other enzymes needed to carry out DNA synthesis are not present unless a t-like molecule has acted. We might ask here whether t mimics a normal cellular gene product that works only at specific times in the cell cycle, say in G_1. If that is the case, then t is likely to be evolutionarily derived from such a protein.

In so suggesting that a viral gene has an ancestral origin in a cellular gene, we are much influenced by a very recent result obtained by David Lane at Cold Spring Harbor.[6] In order to better define chemically T, he has generated a number of different hybridomas, each yielding a monoclonal antibody specific for T. Most of these, as expected, showed no cross reactivity for any normal cell component. One, however, to our initial surprise, yielded antibodies which bind also to a "normal" cell protein of MW 80,000 that is found in the nucleus and whose amount increases in cells transformed by a variety of carcinogenic agents. This cross reaction could possibly be accidental. We prefer to believe that all normal cells contain a T-like molecule which functions to initiate DNA synthesis in normal cells. If this is the correct hypothesis, then it seems simplest to assume that the T represents a modified cellular protein whose gene has been positioned within the viral chromosome in a way that optimizes its appearance during the early phase of the lytic cycle.

The exquisitely powerful tools now available to the molecular biologist also let us ask whether by integrating into human chromosomes a given DNA tumor virus is a significant cause of cancer. Here the evidence for SV40, as well as the closely related human viruses BK and JV, looks largely negative. While several positive claims have been made over the past five years, one in particular for meningiomas, they have not been repeatable. These negative results are not the result of the lack of suitable human infections, since virtually all adults have been infected with and are carriers of BK and JV viruses. Since it could be most surprising if some human cells were not transformed by either BK or JV, we suspect they fail to generate such tumors because the presence of T invariably leads to an immunological response. Given the increasingly sophisticated experiments made possible by recombinant DNA techniques, we are now in a position to answer this question. Hopefully, within several years our effective immunity to transformed cells generated by SV40-like viruses will be explained.

To conclude, we thus see that by studying tumor viruses at the molecular level, we may be also coming to grips with many of the key events involved in the transversal of a cell through the cell cycle. Hopefully, we shall soon isolate key cell-cycle proteins whose very existence we might have remained ignorant of had we not so heavily focused on tumor virology. Thus, even if SV40-like viruses turn out not to be the cause of much human disease, they may remain increasingly indispensable for the serious study of the cancerous state.

REFERENCES

1. Taylor AR, Beard D, Sharp DG, Beard JW. Nucleic acid of rabbit papilloma virus protein. J Infect Dis 1942; 71:110-4.

2. Watson JD, Littlefield JW. Some properties of DNA from Shope papilloma virus, letter to the editor. J Mol Biol 1962; 2:161-5.

3. Green H, Thomas J. Pattern formation by cultured human epidermal cells: development of curved ridges resembling dermatoglyphs. Science 1978; 200:1385-8.

4. Dulbecco R. From the molecular biology of oncogenic DNA viruses to cancer. Science 1976; 192:437-40.

5. Tjian R, Fey G, Graessmann A. Biological activity of purified simian virus 40T antigen proteins. Proc Natl Acad Sci USA 1978; 75:1279-83.

6. Lane DP, Hoeffler KK. SV 40 large T shares an antigenic determinant with a 68,000 mwt cellular protein. Nature (in press).

Ann Otol 89:1980

PAPILLOMA OF THE LARYNX AND TRACHEOBRONCHIAL TREE IN CHILDREN

A RETROSPECTIVE STUDY

SEYMOUR R. COHEN, MD
SHARON SELTZER, MD
KENNETH A. GELLER, MD
JEROME W. THOMPSON, MD
LOS ANGELES, CALIFORNIA

One hundred and forty cases of papilloma of the larynx and tracheobronchial tree are documented in the records of the Childrens Hospital of Los Angeles. The records of 90 patients were available and were reviewed intensively. The method of direct laryngoscopy with general anesthesia using apneic technique in most patients and intubation in some was an adequate method of treating patients with laryngeal papillomata. A general anesthetic was never used where obstruction was severe and the airway could not be controlled. The low incidence of papilloma of the tracheobronchial tree and an absence of parenchymal lung seeding in this series is attributed to the avoidance of a tracheotomy and fewer intubation anesthetics thus avoiding trauma to the trachea and bronchi. The immediate removal of the tracheotomy tube seems an alternative if the surgical procedure had been performed. In the patients in this series decannulation was accomplished in a very short period of time. The establishment of an airway seems to be a priority in the treatment of this disease and this can be accomplished by repeated endoscopic procedures rather than tracheotomy. Statistics are given, and prognosis based on the type of lesion and histopathology is documented.

INTRODUCTION

Ubiquitous but not a common laryngeal lesion in children, treacherous in its potential, defying all forms of treatment, eluding successful research into its cause, papilloma of the larynx remains a serious challenge to the clinical laryngologist. The most common benign tumor of the child's larynx, papilloma causes serious compromise of the important functions of the larynx and is a potential threat to the life of the child it invades. Papilloma of the larynx and tracheobronchial tree is responsible for a very high degree of morbidity and economic cost in this country as well as in other countries worldwide.

This retrospective study reviews the charts of patients with papilloma of the larynx and tracheobronchial tree, treated at the Childrens Hospital of Los Angeles (CHLA) in the prelaser days. All of the patients in this study were treated with cup or Patterson forceps removal of the tumor by direct laryngoscopy under general anesthesia either using apneic technique or less often intubation. A general anesthetic was not used when severe airway obstruction was encountered.

In a chapter on papilloma of the larynx in *The Practice of Medicine*,[1] published in 1897, the proposed treatment for papilloma of the larynx was the use of "causticum, sanguinaria, thuja, belladonna, calcarea phosp, conium silicea and when all else failed surgery." The authorities of that day felt surgery should be used only when the tumor threatened the airway but reminded the reader that surgery caused these tumors to recur more rapidly.

A review of the more recent literature indicates very little has changed in regard to the many and varied forms of medical, physical and surgical forms of therapy which have been suggested in dealing with this most frustrating disease. That treatment is no closer to a cure is disappointing in the light of remarkable advancements which have been made in basic immunological research and medical technology. Surgical extirpation remains the essence of therapy and will remain so until a cure is found.

As documented almost 100 years ago[1] and still remaining a mystery, it is unknown why papilloma will suddenly disappear or regress in some patients regardless of the form of therapy which was instituted.

REVIEW OF LITERATURE

Etiology. The most likely cause of laryngeal papilloma is viral.[2] It is thought to be produced by a double-stranded tumor-producing DNA-containing virus belonging to the papovavirus group. Zur Hansen[3] distinguishes between juvenile and adult papilloma as follows: 1) that virus particles are sometimes demonstrable in the juvenile form but not in the adult, 2) that transmissibility by experiment has been possible in the juvenile and not in the adult type, 3) that malignant transformation is common in the adult but rare in the juvenile form except after irradiation, and 4) that the type of

From the Department of Surgery, Division of Otolaryngology, Childrens Hospital of Los Angeles and University of Southern California Medical School, Los Angeles, California.

Presented at the meeting of the American Laryngological Association, Palm Beach, Florida, April 14-15, 1980.

REPRINTS — Seymour R. Cohen, MD, 1300 N. Vermont Ave., Los Angeles, CA 90027.

human papovavirus 1, 2, 3, 4 has not been determined while virus-like particles have been described repeatedly in juvenile forms of papilloma. "Most of these findings do not withstand a severe scrutiny and are not sufficiently distinguished from other nuclear inclusions such as perichromatin granula which are thought to be inactive chromatin found in most nuclei in varying amounts."[3]

Spoendlin and Kistler[4] point out that in rapidly growing papilloma, the virus is less likely to be found than in slow-growing lesions such as skin warts in which the virus is frequently demonstrated and a high tendency to cure rate is known. Critically minded authors have been unable to demonstrate the virus in juvenile laryngeal papilloma either in extracts or in electron microscopy sections. They conclude that the papovavirus in laryngeal papilloma exists most of the time as invisible genomes in the nuclear chromatin and that the mature virus particles are only found under certain, thus far not well-defined conditions. They conclude that the viral theory remains the etiology of papilloma of the larynx in theory only.[4]

Ullman[5] and Ishikawa,[6] were able to transfer children's laryngeal papilloma to laboratory animals and to the human skin using a filtrate of papilloma tissue. Holinger et al[7] gave some evidence of the viral theory by serological tests, animal inoculations and tissue cultures.

Boyle et al[8] produced strong evidence to support the viral theory showing the presence of virus-like particles similar in configuration to the papovavirus in lesions removed from patients.

Ahmed[2] reviews the literature regarding nuclear bodies in laryngeal papilloma and states there is a suggestion that there is a relationship between the presence of nuclear bodies and viruses. He, however, points out that while his studies provide further support for a viral theory, "present observations do not permit any conclusion to be drawn concerning the exact relationship of nuclear bodies to papilloma virus other than that it may be associated with some stage of virus formation." He suggests further studies such as tissue culture, morphological and histochemical, be carried out to establish whether there is indeed a relationship between nuclear bodies and papilloma virus and how these nuclear bodies are formed and what their fate may be.

Many other etiological agents such as endocrine factors, allergy, infection, chronic irritation, racial, sexual, geographic, abnormalities of calcium, magnesium or zinc metabolism, are all factors which have never been consistently proven in any large series of patients.

Therapeutics. The literature has been rampant with offers of potentially hopeful curative measures. The most common form of therapy has been surgical, at times conservative and at other times very radical. The most common surgery is endoscopic removal with forceps with other forms such as microlaryngeal cautery, laser surgery, laryngofissure and tracheotomy. The latter surgery once was suggested in order to place the larynx at complete rest but at this time most laryngologists will do this procedure only to protect the airway rather than for any effect it may have on the intralaryngeal disease.

Tetracycline, advised by Holinger et al,[9] has not proven beneficial as at first had been hoped. Corticosteroids[10] have been discarded. Estrogen[11] and podophyllin[12] applied locally and magnesium and calcium given systemically[13] have been disappointing. Immunological measures such as local injection of smallpox vaccine[14] and bovine vaccination[15] have given poor results and have been proven harmful.

Of the physical methods, electrocautery[7] has been used but may result in permanent damage unless used extremely carefully. Ultrasound[16] has some enthusiastic supporters but has not been universally accepted.

Cryosurgery[17] has been used with varying degrees of success. Miller[18] cautions that cryotherapy in children without a prior tracheotomy should be avoided. The CO_2 laser is now preferred by many in the field of laryngology and is probably the most accurate for removing small lesions in crucial areas of the larynx.[19] It, however, like all other methods may produce serious damage if used injudiciously and has not reduced the recurrence rate significantly.

METHODS

Although the records at CHLA show there were 140 patients who were admitted with the diagnosis of papilloma in the larynx and tracheobronchial tree, only 90 charts were available for review. Because as in all retrospective studies certain data were desired but not documented, the statistical analysis of the group of patients in this study was not complete in a number of aspects of this study. Therefore it was not possible to document the birth history of the patient nor whether the mother had condylomata. Also, because of the number of years which have passed since many of these patients were treated, the follow-up was not always possible.

The following items could be completely studied in the group of patients: the age at onset of symptoms, sex and race, birthplace, symptoms which led to the diagnosis, other sites of involvement by papilloma, patients with tracheotomy, the presence of lesions in the tracheobronchial tree, the site and type of papilloma, preoperative diagnosis, the histological presence of atypia and its effect on the prognosis, complications, the number of procedures, the time of resolution, method of treatment and anesthesia, and the mortality.

STATISTICAL ANALYSIS

Of the total of 90 patients whose charts were available and were reviewed, 47 were male and 43 were female. Unfortunately the birth history, type of delivery, and absence or presence of venereal

TABLE 1. INCIDENCE OF LARYNGEAL PAPILLOMA ACCORDING TO SEX AND RACE

Sex	*No.*	*Race*	*No.*
Male	47	White	75
Female	43	Black	14
		Mixed	1

warts in the mother were not documented. Only one child whose mother had vaginal condylomata was noted to have been born by vaginal route and had perineal warts and papilloma of the larynx with onset of symptoms at birth.

Of the 90 children, 75 were white, 14 were black and 1 was mixed. There were no Orientals in this study. While the birthplace of most of the patients was California, patients in the study and referred for therapy came from many other states in the north, south, east and midwest areas. No geographic significance could be elicited (Table 1).

SYMPTOMS

The most common symptom was voice change, occurring in 81 (90%) of the patients. It was usually moderately severe and progressive and in some children aphonia was present. Airway obstruction was documented in 40 (44%) of the children, but varied from moderate to very severe, some children requiring immediate attention. Stridor was documented in 35 (39%) of the patients and in many of these children the treatment prior to the accurate diagnosis was misdirected to croup, allergy or asthma (Table 2).

TABLE 2. LARYNGEAL PAPILLOMA: SYMPTOMS (N = 90)

	No.	*%*
Voice change	81	90
Airway obstruction	40	44
Stridor	35	39

SITES OF PAPILLOMA OTHER THAN LARYNX

In addition to their laryngeal papilloma, ten children had palatal lesions, two had lesions in the tonsil area, three had tracheobronchial lesions, one on the skin of the hand and one had papilloma covering her perineum. These lesions responded to treatment much more rapidly than the laryngeal papilloma. It is noteworthy that no parenchymal lung lesions were seen in this series of patients (Table 3).

TRACHEOBRONCHIAL PAPILLOMA

Only three patients were found to have tracheal and bronchial papilloma, an exceedingly low incidence in a large series of patients. A breakdown of these patients is of interest. Tracheobronchial papilloma are rare in patients without laryngeal lesions and uncommon where a tracheotomy has not been performed.

TABLE 3. LARYNGEAL PAPILLOMA: OTHER SITES

Palate	10	Tracheobronchial	3
Tonsil	2	Skin	1
Pharynx	1	Perineum	1

TABLE 4. LARYNGEAL PAPILLOMA: TRACHEOBRONCHIAL LESIONS*

Primary without laryngeal lesion	1
Laryngeal without tracheotomy	1
Laryngeal with tracheotomy†	1

*No pulmonary lesions.

†One bronchogenic CA.

One child, an $8^1/_2$-year-old female had a perfectly normal larynx, no other papilloma in the body, and had severe stridor for many years diagnosed as emphysema. At bronchoscopy she had almost total obstruction of her trachea by a large papillomatous mass which was cored out and with two endoscopic procedures was apparently cured. One year later another bronchoscopy was performed and the trachea and bronchi were found to be normal. One of the patients who had many procedures performed elsewhere for the removal of laryngeal papilloma, who had been intubated repeatedly for the laryngeal surgery, developed wheezing and airway obstruction and was found to have a large number of papilloma in the trachea and right bronchus. He responded to three procedures with complete resolution and is now free of disease for over two years. The third patient with tracheobronchial papilloma following a tracheotomy, and who had never been irradiated, developed transformation to a bronchogenic carcinoma and succumbed from metastatic disease at age 20 years.[20] His laryngeal lesions had been controlled for many years (Table 4).

AGE AT ONSET OF SYMPTOMS

The age at the onset of the papilloma could be correlated with the age at the onset of symptoms. The symptoms such as voice change, stridor and/or airway obstruction were most prominent. Twenty-one patients developed symptoms between birth and six months of age. Fourteen patients developed symptoms between one to two years of age and 12 patients developed symptoms between three to four years of age. Sixty-one (68%) of the children had symptoms of papilloma prior to four years of age. Decreasing frequency of the disease, as evidenced by the development of symptoms, occurred as the child became older than six years. Only one child had his onset of symptoms between ages 10 and 11 (Table 5).

TRACHEOTOMY

Of the patients who received all of their treat-

TABLE 5. AGE AT ONSET OF SYMPTOMS

Birth-6 Mo	21	5- 6 Yr	3
7-12 Mo	8	6- 7 Yr	2
1- 2 Yr	14	7- 8 Yr	2
2- 3 Yr	6	8- 9 Yr	2
3- 4 Yr	12	9-10 Yr	2
4- 5 Yr	3	10-11 Yr	1

TABLE 6. LARYNGEAL PAPILLOMA: TRACHEOTOMY*

CHLA	4 (4%)
Elsewhere	9 (10%)

*All decannulated except 1 who was treated a short period of time and moved.

ment at CHLA only four were tracheotomized. One child was tracheotomized on the ward soon after admission because of coma and asphyxia. Soon after the diagnosis of papilloma was confirmed by direct laryngoscopy and treatment was instituted, he was decannulated and he made an uneventful recovery. One child was admitted for airway obstruction misdiagnosed as croup, and was tracheotomized only to find that he had papilloma. He was decannulated when his condition stabilized and after surgical management of the papilloma underwent resolution. Another patient, the third in this series, was tracheotomized for a rhabdomyolysis after anesthesia and succumbed to his disease. He had no papilloma at the time of his death. The fourth patient required a tracheotomy for the treatment of tracheal obstruction due to an associated tuberculous compressive and invasive tracheal lesion. He was lost to follow-up after being transferred to a tuberculosis sanitorium.

Eight of the nine patients who were referred for treatment with a tracheotomy in place performed elsewhere, were decannulated within one to two months after surgical therapy for their laryngeal papilloma. The ninth patient with a tracheotomy and tracheal papilloma was lost to follow-up and is being treated in a midwestern children's hospital.* For the past ten years a tracheotomy has not been performed for the treatment of this disease at CHLA (Table 6).

ERRORS OF DIAGNOSIS

Less than one third of the patients had a correct diagnosis made prior to direct laryngoscopy. The usual erroneous diagnoses were vocal nodules, vocal paralysis, bronchitis, asthma, allergy, croup, tracheoesophageal fistula, obstructive tonsils and adenoids, and laryngomalacia. Two children had tonsillectomies and adenoidectomies performed for airway obstruction. In both of these children the airway obstruction was in actuality due to laryngeal papillomatosis. In older children indirect laryngoscopy with a positive diagnosis was occasionally possible. It was quite clear in this study however that direct laryngoscopy was the only method of making a correct diagnosis (Table 7).

TABLE 7. LARYNGEAL PAPILLOMA: INITIAL DIAGNOSIS

Nodules	TEF
Vocal paralysis	Obstructive T&A
Bronchitis	Laryngomalacia
Asthma	Emphysema
Allergy	Croup

TEF - Tracheoesophageal fistula.

*Belenky W. Personal communication.

TABLE 8. LARYNGEAL PAPILLOMA: TYPE OF LESION

	SL	*ML*	*MD*
Total no.	13.0	6.0	60.0
Mean no. procedures	3.8	12.8	15.9
Mean age onset (yr)	2.8	3.0	3.2
Mean duration of symptoms (yr)	3.2	11.9	5.34

SL - Solitary local; ML - Multiple local; MD - Multiple diffuse.

TYPE OF LESION AND COURSE OF DISEASE

The lesions in the larynx were divided into solitary local, multiple local, and multiple diffuse. Thirteen patients with solitary localized lesions had an average number of procedures of 3.8. The mean age at onset of symptoms in this group was 2.8 years and the mean duration of symptoms was 3.2 years.

There were six patients in the multiple localized laryngeal lesions. This group had an average of 12.8 procedures with a mean age at onset of symptoms of three years and a mean duration of symptoms of 11.9 years.

Sixty patients with multiple diffuse lesions were in the majority and had an average of 15.9 procedures. The mean age of onset was 3.2 years and the mean duration of symptoms was 5.34 years. While these figures may not be statistically valid, it would appear that the solitary localized lesion occurred in the younger child and these patients may undergo resolution at an earlier age and would require fewer procedures. The least common, those with multiple localized papilloma, carried the poorest prognosis with symptoms lasting the longest of the three groups. Fortunately this was the least common of the three types.

The most common form, the multiple diffuse lesions, occurred in most of the patients, required the largest number of procedures, but resolved at a much earlier age (Table 8).

HISTOLOGICAL CONSIDERATIONS

Since there was good documentation of the pathology by the Surgical Pathology Division, the results were reviewed. In almost all cases biopsies were taken at each procedure. The usual pathology was "papillary formation composed of stratified squamous epithelium on a fibrovascular core." If nuclear atypia was present, this was so stated in the report of the pathologist. Seventy-six of the 90 patients had reports which could be analyzed. Forty percent (36) showed atypia in their biopsies quite frequently. Fifty-one (56%) showed no atypical nuclei. The patients with atypia had a total of 896 procedures with an average of 25. The patients without nuclear atypia had 406 procedures or an

TABLE 9. LARYNGEAL PAPILLOMA: HISTOLOGY

	Atypia	*No Atypia*
Patients	36 (40%)	51 (56%)
Procedures	896	406
Mean	25	8

TABLE 10. LARYNGEAL PAPILLOMA: COMPLICATIONS OF FORCEPS REMOVAL

Webs	9	(10%)
Hoarseness	10	(11%)
Laryngeal stenosis	4	(4.5%)
Keel surgery	2	

average of 8 per patient. Thus, atypia was associated with three times more procedures than the patients in the nonatypia group (Table 9).

COMPLICATIONS OF FORCEPS REMOVAL

Forceps removal of papilloma, while commonplace and effective, produces complications. Many of the patients in this group had been referred after having had initial or multiple procedures performed elsewhere. As in all forms of therapy, the potential scarring, usually from excesses of the method, is hazardous to the larynx, resulting in voice change or obstruction of varying degrees.

In nine of the patients, webs formed in the anterior commissure usually from injudicious use of forceps and denuding of both vocal cords at the same time. Of the 10% of these patients only two required keel surgery. These were some of the earliest patients treated in this series. Ten patients (11%) had hoarseness of varying degrees, one quite severe and still under treatment. Laryngeal stenosis occurred in four patients (4.5%) but was never severe enough to require tracheotomy or intralaryngeal treatment. Obstruction was never severe enough to produce functional disability (Table 10).

NUMBER OF PROCEDURES

The number of procedures varied with the age of onset, type of laryngeal papilloma and the degree of obstruction. The smallest number required for resolution was two procedures in one infant while 110 procedures were required in one female child. Another patient (male) had 109 procedures and succumbed from metastases secondary to transformation to bronchogenic carcinoma. The total number of procedures among the 90 patients was 1,047, an average of 11.8 procedures per patient. However, this figure is meaningless since eliminating those that had the largest number of procedures would bring this number down to a mean of nine. Also, many of the procedures were for follow-up care and no treatment in many of the children was necessary when they were found to be free of disease (Table 11).

RESOLUTION OR CURE

As previously stated and well known among laryngologists, the disease can recur after years of being quiescent. One of the patients, a black female, was free of disease for two years and returned with massive papilloma. The recurrences were eradicated with three procedures and she is now still being followed. Thirty-three patients, or approximately 30%, were followed for a sufficient length of time to be able to say that they had undergone resolution. This group was followed for at least two years and is known to have been free of disease. Many of the patients had no papilloma when they were last seen but their follow-up was of insufficient length of time to regard them as having undergone resolution.

TABLE 11. LARYNGEAL PAPILLOMA: NUMBER OF PROCEDURES

Total no. 90 patients	1047	
Smallest no.	2	
Largest no.	110	(1 F)
	109*	(1 M)

*Developed bronchogenic CA — No irradiation.

SURGERY AND ANESTHESIA

The methods of anesthesia varied among the three principle operators who followed these patients. Seven hundred and sixteen of the procedures were performed with the apneic technique. Two hundred and ninety-eight procedures were performed with intubation anesthesia and 21 procedures were performed with the anesthetic being given through the tracheotomy tube. When severe obstruction of the airway was present the bulk of the tumor was removed without anesthesia and when the airway was secure the general anesthetic was given. Only 10 procedures of the total 1,047 were performed with suspension laryngoscopy and intubation. All the other procedures were performed with hand-held laryngoscopic technique. Two patients were treated without general anesthesia having had local anesthetic sprayed to the larynx (Table 12).

MORTALITY

There were three deaths in this series of patients. One developed rhabdomyolysis after anesthesia and was found to be free of disease at autopsy. Another patient died of accidental extrusion of the tracheotomy after revision surgery for severe tracheal stenosis. He had no laryngeal papilloma when he was referred for therapy and had no laryngeal papilloma at death. The third patient died of metastatic disease from transformation of his papilloma to bronchogenic carcinoma. He had been tracheotomized and had had no laryngeal papilloma for many years prior to his death.

SUMMARY AND CONCLUSIONS

Of the total of 140 patients seen and treated with

TABLE 12. LARYNGEAL PAPILLOMA: METHOD AND ANESTHESIA

Apneic tech	716
Intubation D.L.	298
Trach	21
Intubation — Susp	10
Local spray	2

D.L. - Direct laryngoscopy.

papilloma of the larynx at CHLA, the charts of 90 patients were available and were reviewed. The literature on etiology and therapy was also reviewed. Of the 90 patients all were children under 11 years of age at the onset of their therapy. Forty-seven of the children were male and 43 were female. Seventy-five of this group of children with laryngeal papilloma were white and fourteen were black. One patient was of mixed racial heritage and none were of the Oriental race. Ninety percent of the patients had moderately severe and progressive voice change, and this was the most common symptom of the disease. Forty-four percent of the children had varying degrees of airway obstruction from moderate to very severe. Stridor was found in 39% of the children, a symptom frequently misinterpreted as being due to another cause. The most common extralaryngeal site of the lesion was on the palate and the least common was on the skin.

Notable in this series is the extremely few cases of tracheobronchial lesions. This low incidence is ascribed to the avoidance of a tracheotomy or, when it had been performed, to make all efforts to remove it as soon as possible. The method of endoscopy and anesthesia may also be a factor in that with the use of apneic technique, trauma to the trachea and bronchi was avoided.

In this series of patients 21 developed symptoms between birth and six months, 14 patients between one to two years of age and 12 patients between three to four years of age. Sixty-one of the 90 patients developed their symptoms prior to four years of age.

Of the types of laryngeal papilloma the localized solitary form required the fewest number of procedures before resolution. The majority of patients had multiple diffuse lesions and required an average of 15.9 procedures. The best prognosis, with resolution and a mean duration of symptoms of 3.2 years, was found in the localized solitary lesion.

Of the 90 patients only 76 had sufficient histological studies to allow critical evaluation of the pathological report. Of these 76, 60 (40%) showed atypia in their biopsies. This group of patients required 896 procedures, an average of 25 procedures per patient as compared with those without atypia who required 406 procedures or an average of 8 procedures per patient. Atypia was therefore associated with three times more procedures than the group without nuclear atypia. The complication rate was acceptable in the study since no patient had severe enough laryngeal stenosis to require surgical intervention. Only two patients with severe webs causing hoarseness required keel surgery.

The chief method of anesthesia was the performance of the direct laryngoscopy by the apneic technique in 716 of the total procedures. Two hundred and ninety-eight were performed with intubation anesthesia and only ten procedures were performed with suspension laryngoscopy and intubation.

Of the three patients with a fatal outcome, one died of bronchogenic carcinoma with embolic metastases, one of rhabdomyloysis after anesthesia, and another from accidental extrusion of the tracheotomy tube after revision of the tracheotomy site.

Over the almost 25 years of this study, only four patients had a tracheotomy performed at CHLA. On two of those occasions it was performed for the wrong diagnosis. Eight of the nine patients in the series who were tracheotomized elsewhere were decannulated within a one- to two-month period and one was lost to follow-up. A tracheotomy has not been performed for the treatment of papilloma of the larynx at CHLA.

Direct laryngoscopy with apneic technique has been a successful method of treatment of papilloma of the larynx in children. A tracheotomy is rarely required or necessary or justified for the treatment of this disease. Radical surgery is also not recommended. It is hoped that with interferon the ultimate cure may be obtained.

REFERENCES

1. Goodno WC. Practice of medicine. Vol II. Philadelphia: Hahnemann Press, 1897:207-9.

2. Ahmed MM. Nuclear bodies in laryngeal papilloma. Acta Otolaryngol (Stockh) 1977; 84:429-33.

3. Zur Hansen H. Human papilloma virus and their possible role in squamous cell carcinomas. Curr Top Microbiol Immunol 1977; 78:1-30.

4. Spoendlin H, Kistler G. Papova virus in human laryngeal papillomas. Arch Otorhinolaryngol (NY) 1978; 218:289-92.

5. Ullman EV. On the aetiology of laryngeal papilloma. Acta Otolaryngol (Stockh) 1923; 5:317-25.

6. Ishikawa K. Klinische und experimentalle Untersuchungen uber die Entstchungsurachen der Papillome. Acta Med (Fukuoka) 1936; 29:87-8.

7. Holinger PH, Schild JA, Mauriz DG. Laryngeal papilloma, review of etiology and therapy. Laryngoscope 1968; 78:1462-74.

8. Boyle WF, Riggs JL, Oshiro LS, Lennette EH. Electron microscopic identification of papova virus in laryngeal papilloma. Laryngoscope 1973; 83:1102-8.

9. Holinger PH, Johnson KC, Anison GC. Papilloma of the larynx. A review of 109 cases with a preliminary report of aureomycin therapy. Ann Otol Rhinol Laryngol 1950; 59:547-64.

10. Broyles EN. Treatment of laryngeal papilloma in children. South Med J 1941; 34:239-42.

11. Spunar J. Laryngeal papillomatosis. Acta Otolaryngol (Stockh) 1967; 63:74-86.

12. Hollinsworth J, Kohlmoss H, McNaught R. Treatment of juvenile papilloma with resin of podophylline. Arch Otolaryngol 1950; 52:82-5.

13. Shilovtseva AS. The complex treatment of patients affected with papillomatosis of the larynx and trachea. Est Otol 1967; 29:74-9.

14. McGee AR. Apparent antagonism of vaccines and wart viruses. Cancer 1967; 20:1643-53.

15. Moffit O. Treatment of laryngeal papillomatosis with bovine wart vaccine. Laryngoscope 1959; 59:1421-6.

16. Buck HG, Manhart HE. Ultrasound for juvenile laryngeal papillomatosis. Arch Otolaryngol 1968; 77:603-8.

17. Singleton GT, Adkins WY. Cryosurgical treatment of juvenile laryngeal papillomatosis. Ann Otol Rhinol Laryngol 1972; 81:784-90.

18. Miller D. Does cryosurgery have a place in the treatment of papillomata or carcinoma of the larynx? Ann Otol Rhinol Laryngol 1973; 82:656-60.

19. Strong MS, Vaughn CW, Healy GB, Cooperband SR, Clemente MACP. Recurrent respiratory papillomatosis: management with the CO_2 laser. Ann Otol Rhinol Laryngol 1976; 85:508-16.

20. Siegel SE, Cohen SR, Isaacs H Jr, Stanley P. Malignant transformation of tracheobronchial juvenile papillomatosis without prior radiotherapy. Ann Otol Rhinol Laryngol 1979; 88:192-7.

≈

REPORT OF THE PANEL ON COMMUNICATIVE DISORDERS

Single copies of the *Report of the Panel on Communicative Disorders to the National Advisory Neurological and Communicative Disorders and Stroke Council* (NIH publication no. 79-1914) may be obtained from: Chief, Office of Scientific and Health Reports, National Institute of Neurological and Communicative Disorders and Stroke, Bldg. 31, Rm 8A08, 9000 Rockville Pike, Bethesda, MD 20205.

Ann Otol 89:1980

DOUBLE-BARRELED (DIVERSIONARY)TRACHEOSTOMY IN THE MANAGEMENT OF JUVENILE LARYNGEAL PAPILLOMATOSIS

HARVEY M. TUCKER, MD

CLEVELAND, OHIO

A two-year-old female presented to the author with a 1½ year history of multiple recurrences of juvenile laryngeal papillomatosis which when first seen had progressed to and below the tracheotomy site. The entire supraglottic larynx, glottis, and subglottic area were completely filled with exuberant papillomata. There was active growth of papilloma at and below the tracheotomy site and the tube had to be inserted through papilloma in order to reach a clear area in the trachea. In hopes of preventing further spread of papilloma below the area already involved and in order to control the airway and provide access to the subglottic area for laser removal, a double-barreled tracheostomy was performed. Laser treatment and/or spontaneous resolution ultimately resulted in complete clearing of all papillomata from the upper and lower tracheal segments. Four years and nine months after the initial procedure it was felt safe to attempt reconstruction. Her postoperative course was uneventful and she was successfully extubated three months later. Both vocal cords are normally mobile and her voice is quite clear although slightly hoarse as a result probably of slight changes in the edges of the cords because of the repeated surgical interventions. There has been no recurrence of papilloma now, over one year since reconstruction of the trachea. This somewhat radical approach to a life-threatening growth of endotracheal papilloma was successful in preventing further spread below the level of tracheostomy and ultimately permitted total reconstruction of an intact tracheal bronchial tree in the case reported.

The carbon dioxide surgical laser has revolutionized the management of juvenile laryngeal papillomatosis. Several recent reports[1,2] confirm that this lesion can be managed with a high degree of success and with maximal preservation of a normal-functioning larynx by the use of the laser. Because this instrument instantaneously vaporizes lesions in an almost bloodless field and further permits very meticulous removal with minimal damage to adjacent soft tissues, papillomatosis can be managed with greater facility, and the need for tracheostomy to maintain an adequate airway should be diminished even in very small children. Such improved management is due at least in part to the minimal laryngeal edema which results from use of the laser as compared to other techniques available.

Most authors agree that juvenile papillomatosis spreads by viral transmission, possibly the same one that causes condyloma acuminata, coupled with as yet poorly understood immunologic factors. Fortunately, spread into the tracheobronchial tree below the larynx is a relatively uncommon occurrence, especially in the absence of direct tracheal trauma such as might result when tracheotomy is required. For this reason, even before the laser was available, every effort was made to avoid the need for tracheotomy because of the significant risk that papillomatous involvement of the tracheotomy site would result.

This report is prompted by the author's experience with a single case of virulent and rapidly progressive papillomatosis of the tracheobronchial tree in a small child. Because of the imminent risk of spread of papilloma beyond the level at which a tracheotomy could bypass it, a life-saving and somewhat radical procedure was undertaken for the first time with success.

CASE REPORT

A two-year-old female presented to the author with a 1½ year history of multiple recurrences of biopsy proven juvenile laryngeal papillomatosis, which when first seen had progressed to and below the tracheotomy site. The child had undergone seven separate endoscopic procedures for control of her airway and, following the sixth procedure it had become necessary to perform a tracheotomy. At the seventh endoscopic procedure, the attending surgeon became aware that there was exuberant spread of papilloma below the vocal cords to the point where it was approaching the level of the tracheotomy itself. The child was referred for further evaluation and management. Upon admission she presented as an attractive two-year-old with a tracheotomy tube in place and in no acute distress. She was essentially aphonic. Growth and development were otherwise normal and there was no other significant medical history, except for the fact that the mother had been known to have condyloma acuminata at the time that the child was delivered. After suitable preoperative evaluation, endoscopy was undertaken. This showed that the entire supraglottic larynx and glottic chink were completely occluded by massive, frondular papillomata. The tracheotomy tube was removed and the subglottic area and upper trachea were inspected. A large prolongation of papilloma was present on the posterior wall of the trachea and had reached and even passed slightly beyond the level of the tracheotomy tube (Fig. 1). The circumference of the tracheotomy wound itself and the anterior wall of the trachea seemed to be uninvolved. The subglottic portion of the vocal cords was involved bilaterally. Bronchoscopy beyond the site of the tracheotomy tube showed no evidence of distal spread of the papilloma. Since this represented a rapid progression of disease even in the ten days between the last observation by the referring surgeon and the current observation by the author, it was felt that there was imminent danger of rapid spread of the lesions to the

From the Department of Otolaryngology and Communicative Disorders, The Cleveland Clinic Foundation, Cleveland.

Presented at the meeting of the American Laryngological Association, Palm Beach, Florida, April 14-15, 1980.

REPRINTS — Harvey M. Tucker, MD, Department of Otolaryngology and Communicative Disorders, The Cleveland Clinic Foundation, 9500 Euclid Ave., Cleveland OH 44106.

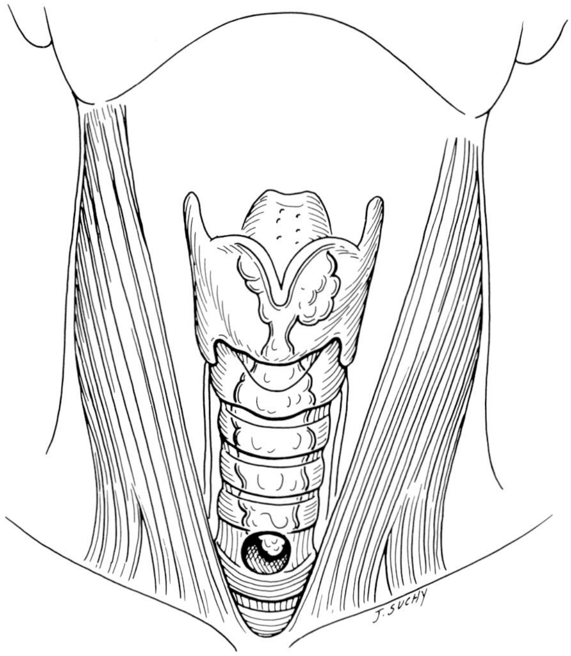

Fig. 1. Complete occlusion of the larynx and subglottic trachea by persistent papilloma. The leading edge of the tumor mass extends to the level of the tracheotomy.

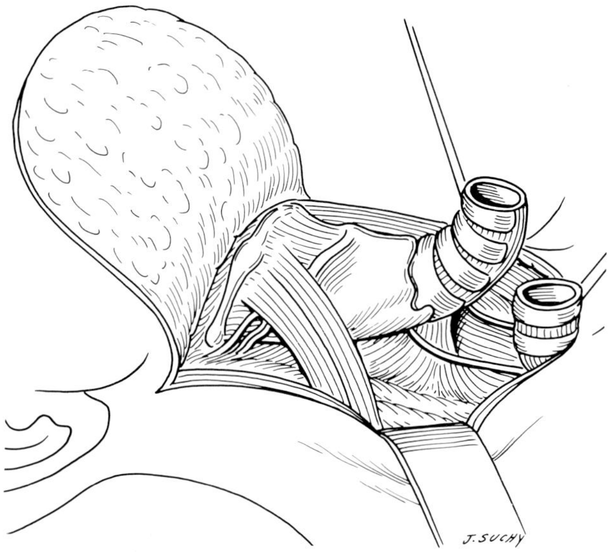

Fig. 2. Transection of the trachea with mobilization of proximal and distal segments. Note that the recurrent laryngeal nerves are preserved.

point where a tracheotomy tube would no longer be adequate to maintain an airway. It seemed apparent, therefore, that some intervention was indicated in hopes of preventing further spread. Consultation was obtained with two recognized experts in the field and the plans of the author were agreed to. The parents were carefully appraised of the experimental nature of the procedure and the potential risks. They agreed to the procedure.

SURGICAL TECHNIQUE

The patient was prepared and draped for sterile surgery with a cuffed endotracheal tube in place. A slightly curved transverse incision was made crossing the midline just below the existing tracheotomy site, the skin of which was excised in the process. Superior and inferior skin flaps were elevated in the subplatysmal plane. The great vessels and sternocleidomastoid muscles were mobilized and retracted bilaterally and the tracheal-laryngeal complex was isolated in the midline. The strap muscles were separated and retracted, thus exposing the trachea and the existing tracheotomy site. Both recurrent laryngeal nerves were carefully identified at the point of entry into the larynx at the cricothyroid joint and then traced inferiorly to a point below the intended site of transection. The space between the trachea and esophagus was mobilized so that the esophagus could be protected. The trachea was then transected one ring below the existing tracheotomy site (at approximately the junction between the third and fourth tracheal rings). The distal trachea was inspected and was noted to be free of papilloma. This was brought out in the midline as a standard laryngostoma (Fig. 2). The proximal tracheal segment was inspected from below and was noted to be involved with papilloma in its posterior 50%. The lesion reached almost to the level of the tracheotomy site although it appeared to have extended further because of a leading edge of tumor mass which was not actually growing from the posterior wall. No attempt was made at this time to excise any of the lesion. The right sternocleidomastoid muscle was mobilized and the fibers separated at roughly the midpoint, at a level appropriate to the distal end of the proximal tracheal segment. The cartilage of the lowermost tracheal ring of the proximal segment was carefully removed leaving the mucosa and inner perichondrium intact (Fig. 3). The distal end of the proximal trachea was then lead between the two portions of the right sternocleidomastoid muscle and the cartilage tacked to the muscle with nonabsorbable sutures. A stab wound was made at an appropriate level in the skin

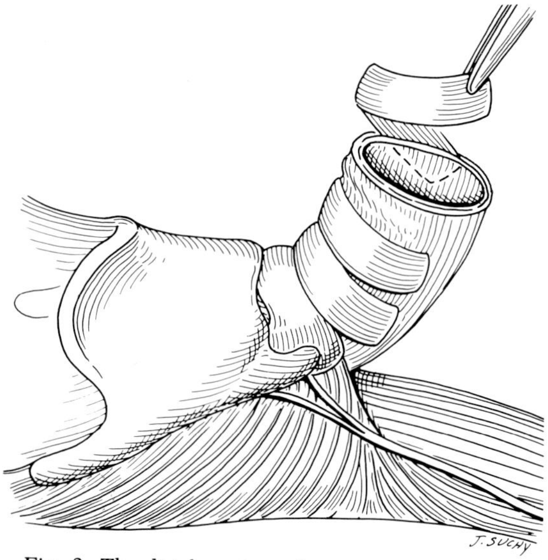

Fig. 3. The distal most cartilage ring of the proximal segment is removed leaving the underlying soft tissue of the trachea intact.

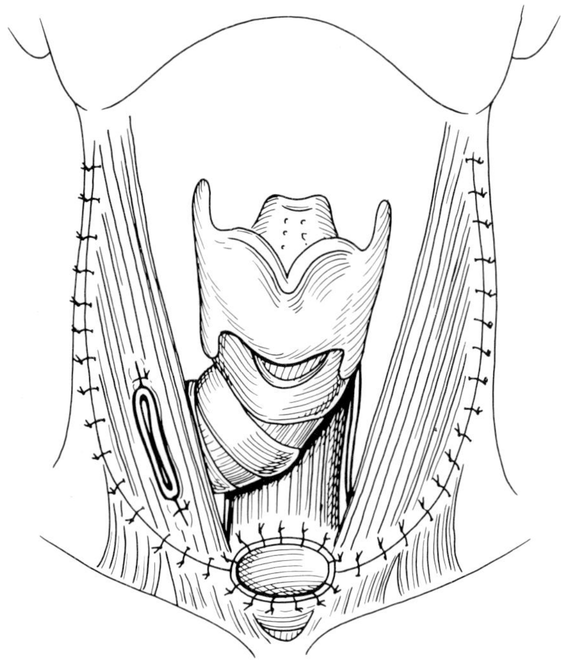

Fig. 4. Distal trachea brought out as a laryngostoma. Proximal trachea brought between heads of the sternocleidomastoid muscle as a mucous fistula.

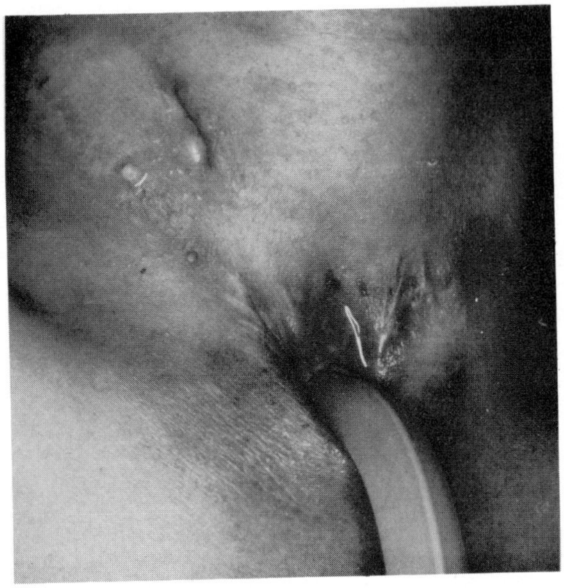

Fig. 5. Status of neck five years later following successful treatment of papillomata by laser surgery.

of the right side of the neck to allow the mucoperichondrium of the distal portion of the proximal trachea to be brought out through it and sutured mucosa-to-skin to produce a mucous fistula (Fig. 4). The neck incision was closed after placing a small hemovac drain. A small Foley® catheter was placed in the proximal mucous fistula and the balloon inflated to allow suction drainage of any secretions that might collect in this segment initially. A standard pediatric tracheotomy tube was modified to fit the tracheal stoma. The postoperative course was uneventful. The child healed promptly and was discharged from the hospital seven days after the surgical procedure. At this time there was little or no leakage from the proximal mucous fistula, possibly because of the obstruction due to the papillomata.

FURTHER MANAGEMENT

The child was referred to Dr. Stuart Strong and his associates in Boston for direct management of the papillomata by laser surgery, inasmuch as his was one of the few institutions in the country which had one at that time. After multiple laserings, most of which were directed at disease in the distal trachea, all residual papillomata disappeared. When a period of six months had elapsed since the last lasering with no evidence of recurrent disease, the child was referred back to the author for consideration of reconstruction of the trachea. During this period of time she was aphonic, although she did manage to communicate verbally using forced air expulsion from the oral cavity not unlike the type of speech used in certain African dialects ("click" speech). Her progress in school, although limited by her ability to communicate, was excellent and she was clearly of above average intelligence. With the exception of her airway problems, her health was excellent.

When seen again by the author the child had a well-healed functioning midline laryngectomy stoma and a very small mucous fistula on the right side of the neck (Fig. 5). There was little or no drainage from it even during swallowing. When endoscopic evaluation again confirmed no recurrence of papilloma one year from the last lasering, it was decided that an attempt could be made to repair the trachea. Under general anesthesia, the original skin incision was opened and was carried somewhat more superiorly on the right side to encompass the mucous fistula, which was excised. Skin flaps were elevated and the ends of the tracheal segments were freshened. The proximal trachea was remobilized so that it could be returned to the midline and an end-to-end anastomosis was accomplished between the two ends of the trachea (Fig. 6A, B). A Silastic® T-tube was placed and she wore this for a period of three months following the anastomosis. When re-endoscoped for removal of the T-tube, a well-healed anastomotic segment was noted above the new tracheotomy site. Therefore, a standard tracheotomy tube was inserted and another three months were allowed to elapse to be sure that there would be no secondary stenosis. During this time the tracheotomy tube was kept corked continually and she was able to talk. At first she was troubled by a tendency to persist in her oral speech mechanism, but with suitable speech therapy and practice she quickly overcame this habit and began to phonate in a more normal fashion. Although her voice is somewhat hoarse and rather deep for a child her age, it is really surprisingly good. Both vocal cords are normally mobile.

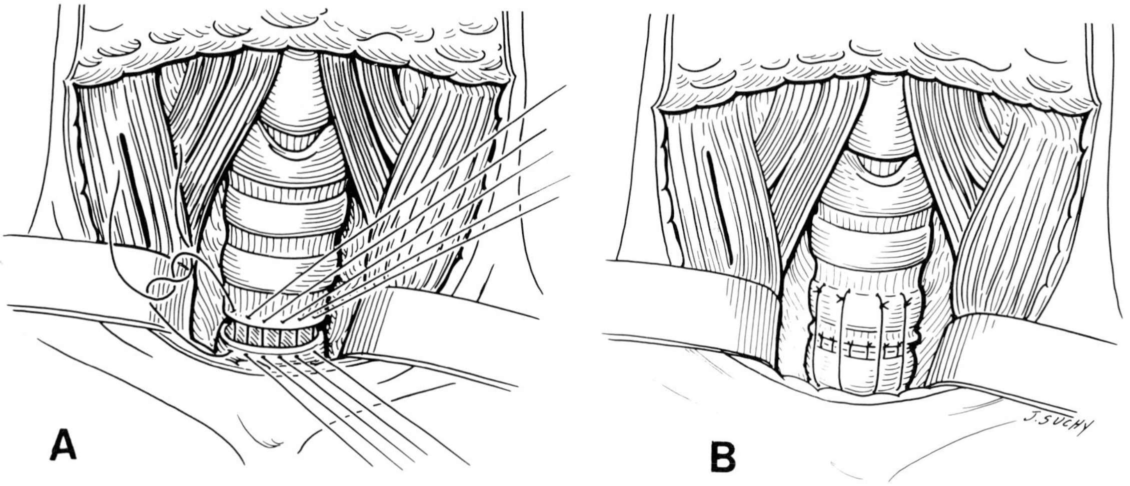

Fig. 6. End-to-end anastomosis of proximal and distal tracheal segments.

At the time of this writing an additional year has elapsed since the final removal of her tracheotomy tube and the surgical closure of the stoma. There is no evidence of either recurrence of papilloma or of any deterioration in either voice or airway since that time.

DISCUSSION

Possible spread of papilloma to a traumatized area in the trachea, particularly after tracheotomy, is to be avoided at all costs. For this reason, the first priority in the management of juvenile papillomatosis is maintenance of as satisfactory a glottic airway as possible. The laser has been a great improvement in this effort. Nevertheless, even with the laser it is not always possible to maintain an adequate airway and tracheotomy is sometimes necessary. Fortunately not all patients with juvenile papillomatosis who require tracheotomy also exhibit such exuberant growth as was manifested in this case, but on occasion a truly life-threatening situation will occur. Because there seems to be evidence that spread of papilloma virus may be to adjacent cells and/or because of "drop" metastases to traumatized areas, it was felt in this case that separating the uninvolved distal trachea from the traumatized proximal trachea might prevent further spread of the disease into the trachea and also might offer better access for the laser to the existing disease.

The concept of "double-barreled" (diversionary) tracheotomy is not a new one. It has been recommended in the management of uncontrollable aspiration where total laryngectomy is not appropriate.[3,4] The technique most widely recommended is to divert the distal end of the proximal trachea into the esophagus and to bring the proximal end of the distal trachea out as a stoma. This would not have been suitable in the case described since there might have been progression of growth down into the esophagus. Furthermore, access to the subglottic area from below would not have been possible.

This procedure was a radical one undertaken in what was felt to be a life-threatening situation. It was successful in managing this case although it did not prevent spread of papilloma into the distal trachea. Certainly there is insufficient clinical experience to warrant recommending it as a routine procedure. Moreover, with the availability of the laser and other better means of managing papillomatosis, perhaps on an immunologic basis, uncontrolled growth down the trachea should be even more uncommon.

CONCLUSION

Life-threatening growth of papilloma into the distal trachea following tracheotomy in a small child was managed in one case by transection of the trachea with double-barreled (diversionary) tracheotomy. Such an approach not only can maintain a safe airway but may allow access to the subglottic area and upper trachea through the mucous fistula for laser treatment.

REFERENCES

1. Strong MS, Vaughan CW, Healy GB, Cooperband SR, Clemente M. Recurrent respiratory papillomatosis: management with the CO_2 laser. Ann Otol Rhinol Laryngol 1976; 85:508-16.

2. Jako GJ. Microsurgery of the larynx with the CO_2 laser. In: Otolaryngology, vol. 3. Hagerstown: Harper & Row, 1979, chap 49.

3. Lindeman RC. Diverting the paralyzed larynx: a reversible procedure for intractable aspiration. Laryngoscope 1975; 85:157-80.

4. Lindeman RC, Yarington CT, Sutton D. Clinical experience with the tracheoesophageal anastomosis for intractable aspiration. Ann Otol Rhinol Laryngol 1976; 88:609-12.

Ann Otol 89:1980

MANAGEMENT OF THE EXTUBATION PROBLEM IN THE PREMATURE CHILD

ANTERIOR CRICOID SPLIT AS AN ALTERNATIVE TO TRACHEOTOMY

ROBIN T. COTTON, MD

ALLAN B. SEID, MD

CINCINNATI, OHIO

Long-term endotracheal intubation is a widely established means of giving ventilatory support in the newborn period. Though such long-term intubation is well tolerated by the premature infant, laryngeal complications do occur and extubation may be impossible even though the initial disease process for which the intubation was performed has resolved. In such a situation, careful endoscopic evaluation of the upper respiratory tract is advocated to identify the site of the problem. If subglottic edema or mucosal ulceration in the subglottic area is the site of the damage and if, during endoscopic evaluation immediately following removal of the endotracheal tube, the subglottic area starts to narrow because of edema formation or edema fluid filling up compressed granulation tissue, then a split of the cricoid in the midline anteriorly, leaving the endotracheal tube in as a stent, appears to be a preferable alternative to performing a tracheotomy. Of 12 consecutive patients, 9 have been successfully extubated.

INTRODUCTION

Long-term endotracheal intubation as a means of prolonged respiratory support was reintroduced by McDonald and Stocks in 1965.[1] Since that time this method of support has been widely practiced in many countries throughout the world. A common clinical situation in which long-term endotracheal intubation is used is in the care of the premature infant with respiratory distress syndrome or other cardiopulmonary problems. Approximately 45% of admissions to a premature nursery in the United States will require endotracheal intubation for longer than seven days.[2]

There is no adequately documented prospective study of the incidence of subglottic stenosis following this method of ventilatory support. Various retrospective studies, however, suggest that the complication rate is in the region of 2.5%.[2] Certainly the incidence of complications is relatively low and otolaryngologists as a group must commend our pediatric and anesthetic colleagues for a job well done in the care of the indwelling endotracheal tube in the premature.

It is an established fact that the premature infant can withstand endotracheal intubation better than the full-term neonate or the older child.[3] This is all the more remarkable when considering the fact that it is often impossible to place an endotracheal tube with a leak around it as should be standard practice with the placement of an endotracheal tube in a larger child. The reason for this is merely the initial small size of the larynx in the neonate and even a 3.0 mm tube fits snugly into the larynx.

Complications, however, do occasionally occur (Table 1).[4-6] In the larynx we have not seen supraglottic disease as a sequela of intubation in the premature child. In the glottis, however, lesions that may prevent successful extubation include edema, anterior web, granuloma formation, posterior glottic stenosis, vocal cord lacerations and vocal cord paralysis.

Subglottic complications are more common than glottic problems[3] and when they occur are usually more serious in nature.

A third site for significant problems is in the carina area or in the region of the take-off of the right upper lobe bronchus, secondary to erosion of the mucosa in the region of the tip of the endotracheal tube. Finally, any combination of the above lesions may be seen.

Avoidance of complications is of paramount importance. To do so the factors contributing to the complications must be adequately documented; however, there is no such study and all factors mentioned must therefore be anecdotal. The pathological sequence of events in the subglottis, however, is well established.[3] Initially edema and mucosal hemorrhage is seen. After some days mucosal ulceration, particularly posteriorly in the cricoid area, is the striking feature, followed by cartilaginous exposure. Subglottic ulcerations beneath the arytenoids were seen in 15 of 16 neonatal larynges intubated six days or longer.[3] In the process of repair, granulation tissue forms in the ulcers, maturing to form collagen tissue, which in some cases is later covered with epithelium. Secondary

From the Department of Otolaryngology and Maxillofacial Surgery, University of Cincinnati Medical Center, Cincinnati, Ohio.

Presented at the meeting of the American Laryngological Association, Palm Beach, Florida, April 14-15, 1980.

REPRINTS — Robin T. Cotton, MD, Department of Otolaryngology and Maxillofacial Surgery, Children's Hospital Medical Center, Cincinnati, OH 45229.

TABLE 1. COMPLICATIONS OF ENDOTRACHEAL INTUBATION IN NEONATES

Supraglottis	
	No complications in our series
Glottis	
	Edema
	Anterior web
	Granuloma formation
	Posterior glottic stenosis
	Vocal cord lacerations
	Vocal cord paralysis
Subglottis	
	Edema
	Mucosal ulceration
	Granulation tissue
	Perichondritis
Carina	
	Granulation tissue
Right upper lobe orifice	
	Granulation tissue

perichondritis may occur, producing both submucosal fibrosis and cartilaginous thickening.

The cricoid in the premature infant is the most likely site of damage for two reasons: it is the smallest part of the upper airway in this age group, and it is the only complete cartilaginous ring. Certainly two important factors in the avoidance of complications include the skill of the initial intubation and any subsequent tube changes, and the size of the endotracheal tube that is placed.

With regard to subglottic damage, the typical history is that of a premature infant who developed respiratory distress syndrome soon after birth, requiring intubation. From days to weeks later, the pulmonary pathology has healed to the point where extubation may be attempted. Following extubation, the infant does well for several minutes to hours and then respiratory distress, slowly advancing in nature, recurs and reintubation is necessary. Often this sequence of events has occurred several times prior to an otolaryngological consultation.

At this point, endoscopy should be performed, using a laryngoscope in the vallecula and the 2.8 mm 0° Storz Hopkins rod telescope. Adequate preoxygenation and spontaneous ventilation allow for a leisurely examination. The various pathologies mentioned above are specifically looked for during the evaluation. If the subglottis is healthy, then complete endoscopy with the 2.5 mm sheath is performed.

The most common site of the lesion is in the subglottic area. It is important to realize, however, that the endotracheal tube acts as a stent and it is often necessary to observe the subglottic area for several minutes following the removal of the endotracheal tube, looking for subglottic swelling secondary to edema formation or granulation tissue that has been compressed by the endotracheal tube. It is the reappearance of this swelling that causes the recurrence of symptoms of respiratory distress and a reintubation to be performed.

Previously, in the management of this type of case, a tracheotomy has been reluctantly considered with the strong possibility that with the removal of the endotracheal tube and the loss of its stent-like action, subglottic stenosis will develop. These stenoses have been among the most severe that we have had to manage and have necessitated dilation in the early phases to keep the airway patent, followed in some cases by external laryngotracheoplasty techniques to remove the scar tissue. Certainly many of these children have a tracheotomy in place for several months or years. For thc past three years in such cases, we have performed an alternate procedure to the tracheotomy. This has been termed the "anterior cricoid split."

METHODS

Under local anesthesia and with the endotracheal tube in place, a horizontal skin incision is made over the cricoid to expose the cricoid and upper two tracheal rings. A single vertical incision is made through the anterior cartilaginous ring of the cricoid and through the mucosa, to expose the endotracheal tube. This incision is extended inferiorly to divide the upper two tracheal rings in the midline. When the incision is made through the cricoid, the cricoid springs open and the endotracheal tube is readily visible in the lumen, and an air leak is heard. The skin is loosely approximated around an elastic band drain. The endotracheal tube is left in place for two to three weeks, at which time extubation is attempted. Endoscopy is not performed at this time.

The rationale behind this procedure is to decompress the area of the cricoid, the only complete circumferential cartilaginous ring, thus decreasing the pressure of the tube on the mucosa. Secondly, leaving the endotracheal tube in place for approximately two weeks allows it to act as a stent and prevent the subglottic lumen from becoming obliterated with edema secondary to the mucosal damage already established. Our concept is that after the cricoid is decompressed the pressure factors contributing to the mucosal damage are lessened, allowing a decrease in mucosal inflammation. When two weeks have elapsed there has been sufficient resolution of the edema that extubation may be accomplished.

RESULTS

We have results to date in 12 patients treated in this manner, 9 of whom have been successfully extubated. In three, extubation was unsuccessful and a tracheotomy was performed. Two of the three failures deserve some explanation. Encouraged by the initial success of the procedure for cases of isolated subglottic problems, the authors extended the indications for the procedure to include cases with visible glottic complications combined with subglottic pathology (cases 4 and 5, Table 2). In these cases, an incision in the lower third of the thyroid cartilage, immediately inferior to the anterior commissure, was also made in addition to the incision through the cricoid and the upper two tracheal rings. Both these cases could not be extubated and required a subsequent tracheotomy. With this in mind, we have decided not to perform

TABLE 2. DATA SUMMARY OF PATIENTS

Case	Age at Birth (wk)	Intubations	Weight at Surgery (kg)	Extubation
1	30	8	1.4	+
2	28	5	1.5	+
3	30	3	2.0	+
4	27	3	1.0	−
5	28	2	1.2	−
6	30	5	1.6	+
7	27	4	2.0	+
8	28	3	1.2	+
9	30	3	1.7	−
10	27	4	2.1	+
11	30	2	1.6	+
12	28	5	2.0	+

this procedure on any child in whom there is significant glottic involvement. The third failure (case 9, Table 2) was in a child with an isolated subglottic complication; at the time of initial assessment there was extensive mucosal ulceration and granulation tissue formation with cartilage exposure and active perichondritis which subsequently formed a dense subglottic stenosis. One significant complication has occurred and that was in a child who developed an infection of the neck wound with a persistent air leak that took approximately three weeks to close spontaneously. The endotracheal tube was successfully removed at three weeks in this case.

None of the nine children successfully extubated have developed any subsequent airway problems.

Two deaths occurred unrelated to surgery. One child developed septicemia four months after leaving the hospital and a second child died six weeks after the procedure, secondary to severe congenital cardiac disease. Both children, however, had been successfully extubated.

The gross larynx of the first child was obtained and the cricoid examined by microscopic transverse

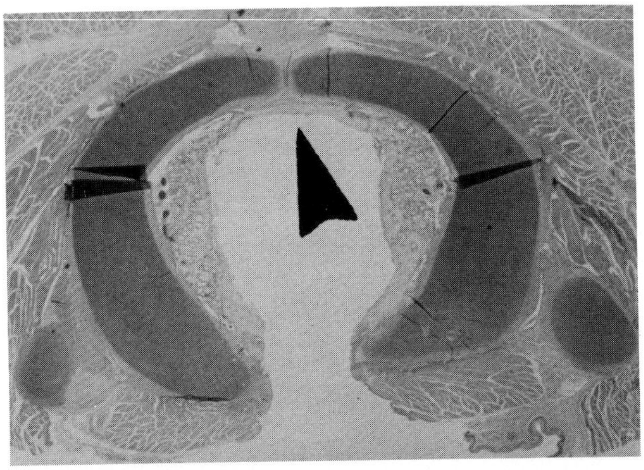

Fig. 1. Cross section of cricoid, four months after anterior cricoid split showing some degree of submucosal thickening, and the site of the anterior cricoid split (arrow). (The larger posterior opening is secondary to a posterior incision performed by the pathologist at time of autopsy.)

TABLE 3. CRITERIA FOR ANTERIOR CRICOID SPLIT

- Neonate
- Appropriate extubation status
- Minimal glottic pathology
- Subglottic pathology
  - Edema
  - Mucosal ulceration
  - Granulation tissue
- The alternative would be a tracheotomy

section. Figure 1 illustrates a representative transverse section of the cricoid showing some element of submucosal thickening and also the site of the healing where the cricoid split was performed four months earlier. There is no evidence of cartilaginous irregularity or cricoid collapse.

DISCUSSION

It is important to stress that this operation should be considered only in those neonates in whom extubation is not possible because of subglottic pathology secondary to endotracheal tube damage. Formerly, in this group a tracheotomy would be performed. The incidence of performing the operation should be low. In three years we have performed the operation on nine patients from our neonatology service which has 1,500 admissions per year. Three patients have been referred from other regional nurseries.

It may be argued that these patients could have been extubated without performing the anterior cricoid split. Review of our cases, however, indicates that since the introduction of the anterior cricoid split our incidence of tracheotomy and subsequent subglottic stenosis in the neonatal group has markedly decreased. Thus, our incidence of tracheotomy for neonatal extubation problems secondary to subglottic pathology in 1974-1977 was reviewed. In this three-year period, 11 tracheotomies were performed of which 8 subsequently developed severe subglottic stenosis. Since the introduction of the anterior cricoid split only four tracheotomies have been performed, three of which were the failures of the anterior cricoid split operation (cases 4, 5, 9; Table 2). The fourth case was an infant with severe glottic pathology in whom the split was not attempted. Evaluation of these figures strongly suggest that the anterior cricoid split has indeed lowered our incidence of tracheotomy for 11 in three years to 4 in three years. More significantly the incidence of neonatal subglottic stenosis has reduced from eight in three years to three in three years. Based on this data it is strongly our opinion that the anterior cricoid split has prevented a significant percentage of neonates from developing subglottic stenosis secondary to endotracheal tube damage.

Our criteria for performing the procedure are outlined in Table 3. At this point we have only performed the procedure on the premature neonate.

The largest child weighed 2.1 kg. The neonate should in all other respects be ready for extubation. Extensive glottic pathology is a contraindication to the procedure. Two of our three failures had extensive glottic scarring at the time of initial endoscopy. With regard to the subglottis, the procedure has been successful in cases where there is evidence of mucosal ulceration and granulation tissue. In one case where there was extensive active perichondritis the procedure was unsuccessful. Finally, we performed the procedure only in those infants in whom further prolonged intubation seemed contraindicated and in whom the alternative would have been a tracheotomy.

REFERENCES

1. McDonald IH, Stocks J. Prolonged nasotracheal intubation. Br J Anaesth 1965; 37:161-7.

2. Parkin JL, Stevens MH, Jung AL. Acquired and congenital subglottic stenosis in the infant. Ann Otol Rhinol Laryngol 1976; 85:573-81.

3. Hawkins DB. Hyaline membrane disease of the neonate, prolonged intubation in the management: effects on the larynx. Laryngoscope 1978; 88:201-24.

4. Joshi VV, Mandavia SG, Stern L, Wiglesworth FW. Acute lesions induced by endotracheal intubation. Am J Dis Child 1972; 124:646-9.

5. Hengerer AS, Strome M, Jaffe BF. Injuries to the neonatal larynx from long-term endotracheal tube intubation and suggested tube modification for prevention. Ann Otol Rhinol Laryngol 1975; 84:764-70.

6. Lindholm CD. Prolonged endotracheal intubation. Acta Anaesthesiol Scand 1969; Suppl 33.

≈

ASSOCIATION FOR RESEARCH IN OTOLARYNGOLOGY

The 4th Mid Winter Research Meeting of the Association for Research in Otolaryngology will be held at the Happy Dolphin Inn, St. Petersburg Beach, Florida, January 19-21, 1981. In addition to the contributed paper sessions, a colloquium honoring Dr. Catherine A. Smith will be held entitled "Some Unresolved Problems in the Auditory System."

ACQUIRED STENOSIS OF THE UPPER AIRWAY IN NEONATES
AN INCREASING PROBLEM

MICHAEL J. PAPSIDERO, MD NIGEL R. T. PASHLEY, MB, FRCS(C)
ANN ARBOR, MICHIGAN

Thirty neonates with acquired airway stenosis were treated between 1975 and 1979 at the C. S. Mott Children's Hospital of the University of Michigan. Neonates surviving a period of ventilation are at risk of developing subglottic stenosis (8.3%). The stenosis is often severe. Children with respiratory distress syndrome and/or neurologic disorders were particularly prone to developing a stenosis (37%). Following treatment, 43% were successfully decannulated and decannulation occurred in a biphasic pattern. Thirty-seven percent were still tracheostomy-dependent but had a voice and were developing normal speech patterns. The mean decannulation time was 92.5 weeks, confirming that acquired subglottic stenosis in the neonate is a serious problem with long-term disability.

INTRODUCTION

Advances in neonatology have resulted in an increased survival of critically ill newborn infants. Many children who previously did not survive are now living after a period of endotracheal intubation and mechanical ventilation. In this particularly susceptible group of infants the apparent incidence of upper airway damage, and later stenosis, might be expected to increase with prolonged survivals.[1-6]

The purpose of this study is to report the incidence of acquired stenosis of the airway in the neonatal age group and to examine the treatment outcome. An attempt is made to characterize those "at risk" infants and to study those factors which may be used as predictors of outcome.

METHODS

In the five-year period 1975 to 1979, 75 infants were treated at the C. S. Mott Children's Hospital, University of Michigan, with airway stenosis; of these 74 required a tracheostomy. Children in whom the stenosis could be related to congenital cricoid hypoplasia, eg, congenital subglottic stenosis, were not included in this study. Thirty neonates were identified as having survived a period of endotracheal intubation (and often assisted ventilation). All these babies had developed an airway stenosis following a period of intubation. The study group contained 20 males and 10 females, of whom 26 were white, 3 black, and 1 Oriental. The birthweights ranged from 910 to 3,200 gm and the gestational ages from 26 to 40 weeks (Fig. 1).

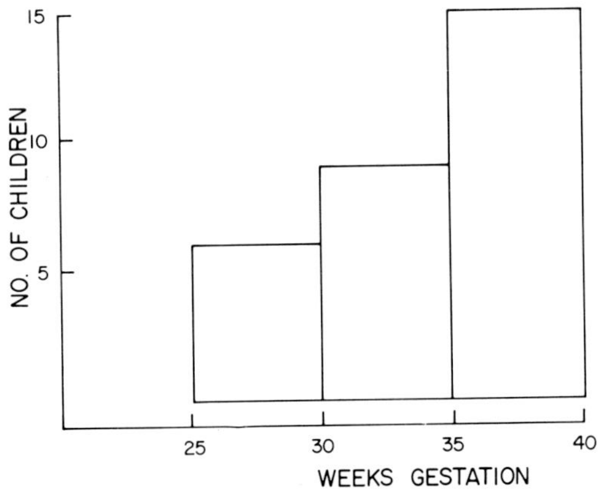

Fig. 1. Histogram showing the gestational age of children who acquired subglottic stenosis following a period of intubation and ventilatory support.

During the years 1975 to 1979 there were 1,827 admissions to the Neonatal Intensive Care Unit. Five hundred sixty-two children required intubation and ventilatory support and 199 (35.4%) died. Three hundred sixty-three neonates (64.6%) survived a period of assisted ventilation, of whom 30 (8.26%) developed significant airway stenosis precluding prompt extubation.

Twenty-nine infants (96.6%) required a tracheostomy and in all those the degree of airway damage was seen to be severe at the time of endoscopy. The extent of stenosis varied. However, in no patient was a thin, easily dilated, short scar or web encountered. All stenoses were seen to involve at least two cartilaginous rings (the cricoid cartilage was involved in all cases). In many the stenosis extended from the cricoid cartilage to the tracheostomy site and constituted a complete stenosis along its length. The anatomic site of stenosis is shown in Table 1.

In an attempt to characterize those infants developing stenosis maternal antenatal and infant-related problems were identified (Tables 2 and 3).

The length of time intubated and/or ventilated was studied (Fig. 2). The range of time intubated was 1 to 110 days (mean 35 days). The range of time ventilated was 2 to 110 days (mean 36 days).

Multiple intubations were common with a prolonged intubation both for toilet purposes and during the period of attempted extubation. The number of intubations performed is shown in Figure 3.

In 16.6% of infants (5/30) the intubation was precipitated by a respiratory arrest at birth, implying less than optimal endoscopic conditions. The tube was inserted by a neonatologist in 76% of our study group.

TABLE 1. ANATOMIC SITE OF STENOSIS (N = 30)

	Percentage
Tracheal stenosis	3
Subglottic stenosis	100
Glottic stenosis	6

From the Department of Otolaryngology, University of Michigan, Ann Arbor.
Presented at the meeting of the American Laryngological Association, Palm Beach, Florida, April 14-15, 1980.
REPRINTS — Nigel R. T. Pashley, MB, BS, FRCS(C), Department of Otolaryngology, University of Michigan, Ann Arbor, MI 48109.

TABLE 2. PROBLEMS OCCURRING IN THE MOTHERS OF NEONATES WITH ACQUIRED STENOSIS (N = 30)

	Percentage
Polyhydramnios	6.6
Premature membrane rupture/labor	3.3
Mid-trimester hemorrhage	3.3

Once damage precluding extubation was present a tracheostomy was performed. All stenoses were assessed endoscopically and managed according to the degree of structural loss in the area (Table 4). Dilation was used as both a primary treatment, and as a surgical adjunct following resection of the stenosis and reconstruction.

An open surgical resection of scar with free buccal mucosal grafts attached to a stent was used. Usually the stent was attached to a tracheostomy tube allowing synchronous motion of the larynx, stent, and tracheostomy tube to occur during swallowing. Posterior cricoidotomy and pedicled hyoid interpositioning were sometimes used.

TABLE 3. ASSOCIATED PROBLEMS OCCURRING IN THE NEONATE WITH ACQUIRED STENOSIS (N = 30)

	Percentage
Respiratory distress syndrome	36.6
CNS disorders	36.6
Congenital heart disease	20.0
Congenital/hereditary disorders	20.0
Severe jaundice	13.3
Septicemia	6.6

There were three deaths in the study group. One child with multiple congenital anomalies died of recurrent pneumonia unrelated to the stenosis or treatment. One death was tracheostomy-related. An overly long Silastic® tube for the 910 gm child eroded the carina. There was one death which occurred six days following surgery. An autopsy revealed no abnormal findings other than bronchopulmonary dysplasia.

In our study group the follow-up period was three months to five years. Forty-three percent of our infants (13/30) were successfully decannulated and had a voice. Thirty-seven percent (11/30) infants were still tracheostomy-dependent but a voice was present and they were developing normal speech patterns. Twenty percent (6/30) of the infants had an obligatory tracheostomy and were aphonic. The time relationships of decannulation and tracheostomy were examined (Fig. 4).

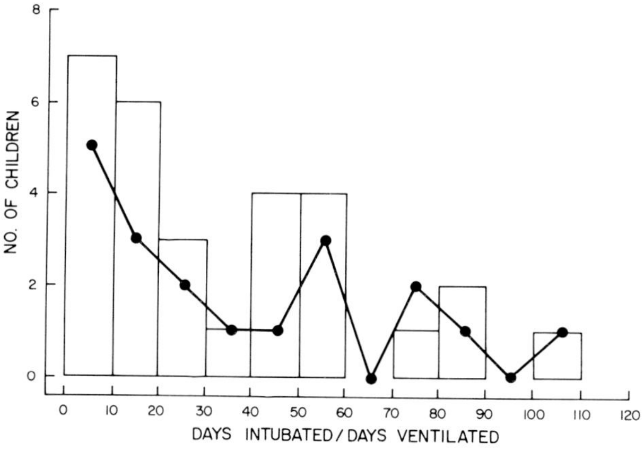

Fig. 2. Graph showing the number of days intubated (histogram) and the number of days of assisted ventilation (line graph) in children with acquired stenosis of upper airway.

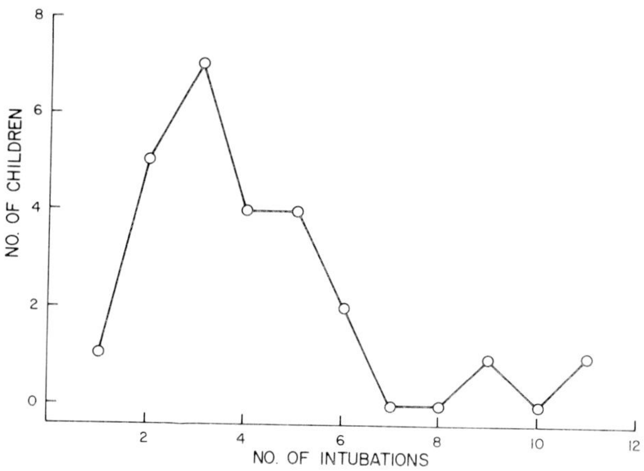

Fig. 3. Graph showing the number of intubations experienced by children with acquired stenosis of upper airway.

DISCUSSION

Neonates who survive a period of intensive care with intubation and/or mechanical ventilation carry a risk of 8.3% of developing an airway stenosis which is located in the laryngeal subglottis. There is a conspicuous absence of stenosis in the tracheal or glottic regions in our study.

Prenatal maternal problems do not seem to be contributory. Children with respiratory distress syndrome and/or a neurologic disorder (including spinal dysrhaphism) seem to be predisposed to airway stenosis (37% in each case).

TABLE 4. TREATMENT OF ACQUIRED AIRWAY STENOSIS

	N	*Deaths*
Tracheostomy	29/30	3.3%
Dilation	15/30	0.0%
Surgical reconstruction	7/30	3.3%

The therapeutic aim was a child with no tracheostomy, a normal voice, and subsequently normal laryngeal development. A relative therapeutic success rate of 80% was achieved (43% of infants

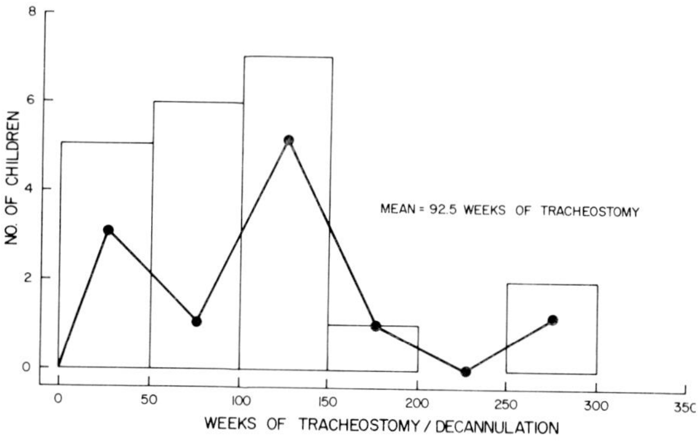

Fig. 4. Graph showing the number of weeks of tracheostomy required in children with acquired stenosis of upper airway (histogram) and the time of decannulation (line graph).

were decannulated and had a voice: 37% had a voice but were still reliant upon a tracheostomy).

A spectrum of results was seen over the follow-up period of from three months to five years. As this is a continuing series, some of the recently treated infants may be expected to change their category.

There is a low mortality for both tracheostomy and surgical intervention in these delicate patients (3.3% in each case).

Decannulation occurs in a biphasic pattern. Early decannulation (0 to 50 weeks after tracheostomy) was possible in three patients (23% of those decannulated). Later decannulation peaked between 100 to 150 weeks after tracheostomy (38.5% of those decannulated). This does not reflect differences in degrees of stenosis as almost all our patients had severe stenosis. We postulate that growth may contribute significantly to this second peak of the biphasic decannulation pattern.

It is of interest that the mean decannulation time was 92.5 weeks, confirming that acquired subglottic stenosis in the neonate is a serious problem with significant long-term disability.

REFERENCES

1. Holinger P, Kutnick SL, Schild J, Holinger LD. Subglottic stenosis in infants and children. Ann Otol Rhinol Laryngol 1976; 85:591-9.

2. Parkin J, Stevens M, Jung A. Acquired and congenital subglottic stenosis in the infant. Ann Otol Rhinol Laryngol 1976; 85:573-81.

3. Hawkins D. Glottic and subglottic stenosis from endotracheal intubation. Laryngoscope 1977; 85:349-56.

4. Fearon B, MacDonald R, Smith C, Mitchell D. Airway problems in children following prolonged endotracheal intubation. Ann Otol Rhinol Laryngol 1966; 75:975-86.

5. Fearon B, Cotton R. Surgical correction of subglottic stenosis of the larynx in infants and children. Ann Otol Rhinol Laryngol 1974; 83:428-38.

6. Markus N, Schild J, Holinger P. Tracheostomy in the first year of life. Trans Am Acad Ophthalmol Otolaryngol 1976; 82:466-77.

≈

CANADIAN OTOLARYNGOLOGICAL SOCIETY

The annual meeting of the Canadian Otolaryngological Society will be held in London, Ontario, June 15-17, 1981. Inquiries may be sent to Dr. William Crysdale, c/o Hospital for Sick Children, 555 University Avenue, Toronto, Ontario.

Ann Otol 89:1980

LONG-TERM STENTING FOR LARYNGOTRACHEAL STENOSIS

DAVID E. SCHULLER, MD
COLUMBUS, OHIO

The use of an inert stent as an adjunct to surgical procedures to correct laryngotracheal stenoses remains somewhat controversial. It is the purpose of this report to describe the use of long-term stents in seven patients with either acute or chronic laryngotracheal stenoses. The conclusion from this series is that stenting for prolonged periods of time represents a valuable adjunctive technique in the correction of the more severe airway reconstruction problems.

INTRODUCTION

The management of acute injuries and chronic stenoses of the larynx and trachea continues to be a difficult problem. A number of therapeutic approaches have been recommended over the years. No one surgical procedure has received uniform acceptance to the total exclusion of other techniques. The primary problem can be defined as the need to maintain adequate patency of a hollow organ that has been traumatized and, therefore, becomes vulnerable to progressive narrowing of the lumen as a result of the normal dynamics of healing, namely, wound contraction. The advisability of stenting the surgical repairs of these injuries has been actively debated among otolaryngologists. Earlier reports in the literature seem to generally favor the use of some type of a stent, whereas newer techniques have minimized the use of such a mechanism to maintain lumen patency. The purpose of this report is to describe the results of long-term adjunctive stenting in seven patients who had either severe acute laryngeal injuries or tracheal stenosis problems and to illustrate the value of this treatment in selected clinical situations.

LITERATURE REVIEW

The otolaryngological literature continues to contain an abundance of reports describing surgical techniques being advocated for the correction of acute and chronic endotracheal injuries. In many cases, the technique chosen is a function of the anatomical area which is damaged. Techniques differ for the repair of a supraglottic,[1] a glottic,[2,3] or a subglottic[4] stenosis. The management of tracheal stenosis has evolved to the point where resection with end-to-end anastomosis is considered the treatment of choice. When the stenotic length is substantial, some type of release mechanism, either in the form of a superior suprahyoid laryngeal release or inferior mobilization of the trachea through a thoracotomy approach is necessary.[5] However, as these stenosis problems increase in severity, more elaborate procedures have been advocated.

Alonso et al[6,7] have recently reported on the use of a free hyoid arch autograft interposed between thyroid cartilage and even cricoid cartilage for the management of laryngeal and even upper tracheal stenosis. Krizek and Kirchner[8] in 1972, and more recently Toohill,[9] have reported on the use of autogenous mucoperichondrial grafts from the nasal septum in the repair of selected cases of laryngeal and upper tracheal stenoses.

The special problem of subglottic stenosis in children has been intensively studied by Fearon and Cotton.[10,11] Cotton[12] has reported his successful management of subglottic stenosis in 18 children accomplished with a composite graft of the perichondrium and costal cartilage used as an elliptical wedge placed through a midline incision. The incision includes the cricoid and upper tracheal rings to increase the diameter of the airway lumen.

The successful management of extended combined laryngeal and tracheal stenosis has been described by Friedman et al.[13] Their procedure involves first developing a trough, then inserting Marlex® adjacent to the trough, and subsequently closing the defect with a local flap including the Marlex for rigid anterior tracheal wall support. An in-depth discussion of the problems and techniques employed in reconstruction of the larynx and trachea was recently published.[14]

The literature contains many descriptions of the role of inert stents to maintain patency after reconstruction of laryngotracheal stenoses. Most reports agree that stenting should be used;[15,16] however, Olson[17] has advocated not using stents. Not only is there a lack of agreement about whether a stent should be used, there is also no uniformly accepted optimal time duration for stent placement. Most authors recommend keeping a stent in place for a period of six to eight weeks. However others' recom-

From the Department of Otolaryngology, Ohio State University and Children's Hospital, Columbus. This study was supported in part by grant 1 K07 NS00417-01 from the National Institute of Neurological and Communicative Disorders and Stroke (Teacher-Investigator Award).

Presented at the meeting of the American Laryngological Association, Palm Beach, Florida, April 14-15, 1980.

REPRINTS — David E. Schuller, MD, Department of Otolaryngology, The Ohio State University, 456 Clinic Drive, Columbus, OH 43210.

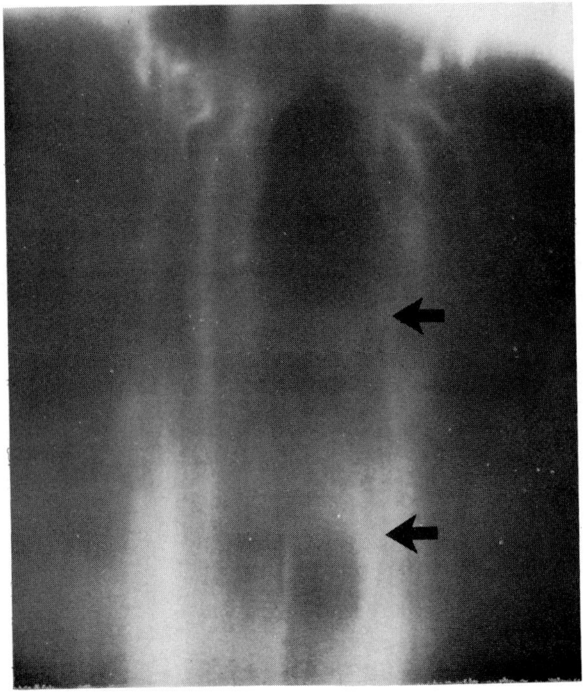

Fig. 1. (Case 2) Polytome radiograph demonstrating complete stenosis (arrows) of trachea following a previous tracheal resection.

mendations can vary from as short as two or three weeks to as long as three or four months.[18] Harris and co-workers[19,20] advocated earlier removal of any stent in the management of acute laryngeal injuries and reported excellent results in a large series of patients. In 1977, Goode and Shinn[21] reported their favorable results using long-term (3-12 months) silicone rubber stenting in the successful management of 12 of 14 cases of severe subglottic stenosis. Such long-term stenting evolved after the authors experienced failures following placements of stents for the usually recommended shorter time period.

CASE REPORTS

This report is based on the experience gained from treating seven patients with long-term stenting for various acute laryngeal or chronic laryngotracheal stenoses seen by the author at the Ohio State University Department of Otolaryngology and Columbus Children's Hospital in the last 30 months. It will be necessary to individually describe each of these patients to further define unique features of their health problems that played a role in the

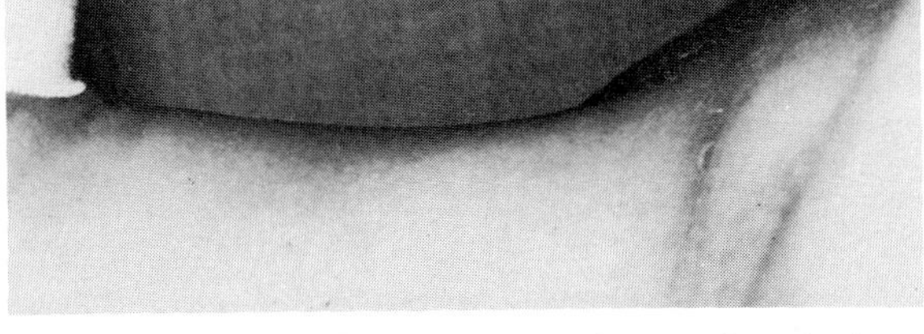

Fig. 2. (Case 3) The loss of any laryngeal projection when viewing the patient's neck is a physical finding consistent with a laryngeal fracture which has decreased the anterior-posterior length of the larynx.

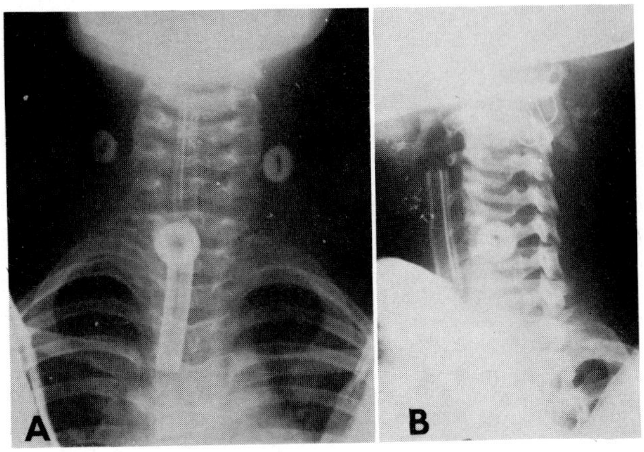

Fig. 3. (Case 3) A) Postoperative radiograph documents proper position for modified Portex endotracheal tube laryngeal stent being held by external neck skin buttons. B) Lateral radiograph demonstrates laryngeal stent position and wires placed to stabilize C1-2 cervical spine dislocation.

use of long-term stenting for the correction of their airway problems.

Case 1. An eight-year-old male sustained blunt trauma over the larynx resulting in a laryngeal fracture requiring lifesaving tracheotomy. This was followed by open reduction and repair of soft tissue and cartilaginous injuries and subsequent insertion of a modified Portex® endotracheal tube laryngeal stent as described by Birck.[22] The stent was removed after six weeks and the boy subsequently developed stenosis within two weeks. Laryngeal dilatations and steroid injections were unsuccessfully used on five different occasions to correct this stenosis problem. He ultimately underwent laryngofissure and excision of a glottic supraglottic stenosis with insertion of another identical laryngeal stent. The stent was kept in place for ten months and he has been decannulated for the last ten months. He is now back to normal activities, including acting as a mascot for the local minor league baseball

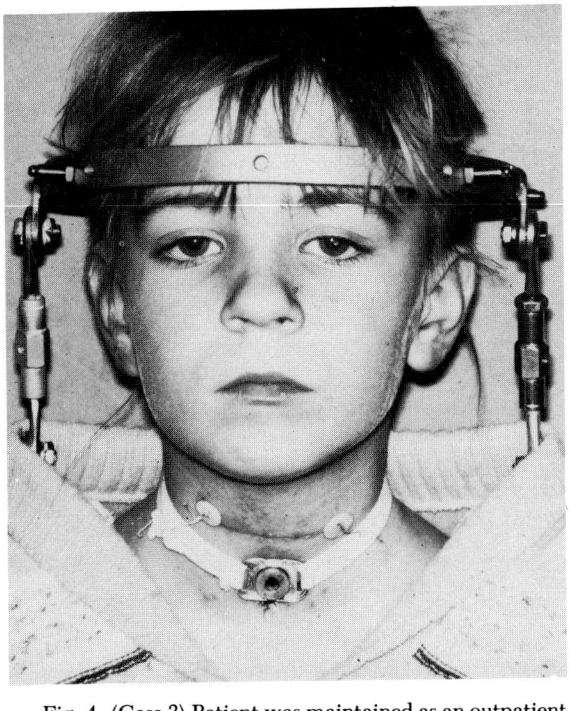

Fig. 4. (Case 3) Patient was maintained as an outpatient in an external cervical fixation apparatus concomitant with laryngeal stent and tracheotomy.

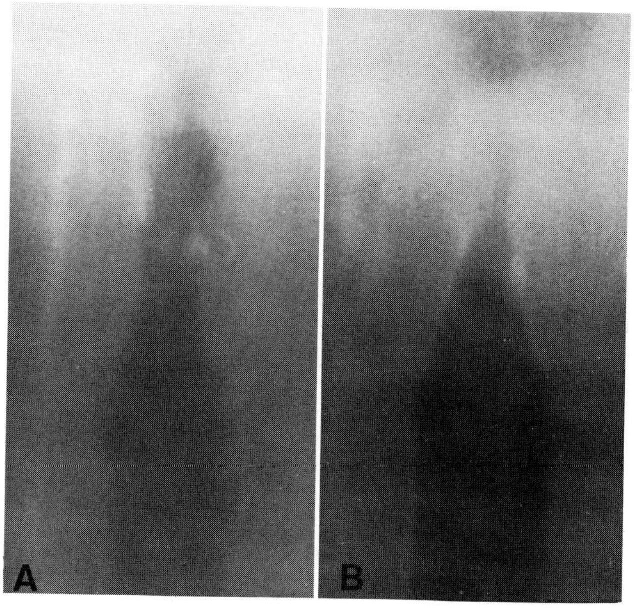

Fig. 5. (Case 3) A) Poststent-removal polytomographic evidence of an adequate laryngeal airway during inspiration, and B) showing some glottic and supraglottic closing during phonation.

team. The patient speaks in a readily intelligible voice, but with decreased intensity.

Case 2. A 53-year-old female developed a tracheal stenosis following a prolonged endotracheal intubation for pneumonia. This was treated by another physician with multiple surgical procedures, the last being a tracheal resection. She was then referred to Ohio State University with a total tracheal stenosis measuring 4 cm long (Fig. 1). This patient underwent a tracheal resection encompassing 5 cm of the trachea which necessitated a suprahyoid laryngeal and transthoracic tracheal release. Because of the tension on the reanastomosis secondary to the extraordinary length of the stenosis coupled with a previous tracheal resection, a Montgomery tracheal T-tube[23] was placed and removed three months postoperatively. The patient began to experience some audible respiratory activity two weeks after removal of the stent, and underwent a second procedure to have the T-tube reinserted. This was then left in place for a period of 13 months. The patient has now been decannulated for the last 16 months and is back to normal activity with bilateral vocal cord mobility.

Case 3. Another eight-year-old female sustained blunt trauma to the larynx with severe laryngeal injury involving the soft tissue and multiple comminuted thyroid cartilage fractures (Fig. 2). The diagnosis of this injury required flexible fiberoptic laryngoscopy because of a concomitant C 1,2 cervical spine dislocation with no neurologic injury. She underwent open reduction and laryngeal stenting at the same time that she had stabilization of the cervical spine dislocation (Fig. 3 A,B). Cervical immobilization was maintained with an external fixation apparatus concomitant with tracheotomy and laryngeal stenting (Fig. 4). The patient has been decannulated for the last nine months and is back to normal activity which includes active participation in a local amateur dance troupe. Postoperative polytome radiographs reveal bilateral vocal cord mobility (Fig. 5 A,B) and the patient speaks in a readily intelligible voice, but with decreased intensity.

Case 4. This patient sustained a shotgun injury to the neck treated with tracheotomy approximately ten years prior to referral. The injury involved destruction of the lower half of the larynx and cervical trachea (Fig. 6). He had been totally aphonic since the injury. Evaluation revealed a total stenosis at the level of the glottis except for a pinpoint opening in the posterior commissure. However, there seemed to be some slight arytenoid movement when he was asked to phonate. Below the level of the true vocal cords, there was total destruction of the subglottic region and the

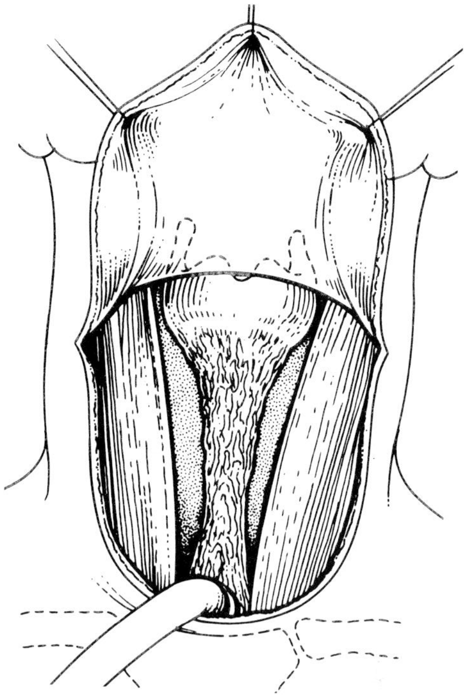

Fig. 6. (Case 4) Diagram of severe laryngeal and upper tracheal destruction following a gunshot wound ten years ago.

upper 5 cm of trachea with only a string-like opening from the level of the glottis down to the tracheotomy site. The rest of the subglottic and upper tracheal area were replaced by scar tissue. The patient underwent a laryngotracheal reconstruction by excising the glottic stenosis and then resecting all of the scar tissue in the subglottic and upper tracheal area. There was no remaining subglottic or tracheal mucosa and no usable cricoid cartilage or tracheal rings. The patient had one buccal mucosal graft sutured around the upper end of the modified Portex endotracheal tube stent. Then another larger buccal graft was sutured around a tracheal T-tube to hopefully provide mucosal lining for the posterior and lateral walls of the upper trachea (Fig. 7). The buccal muco-

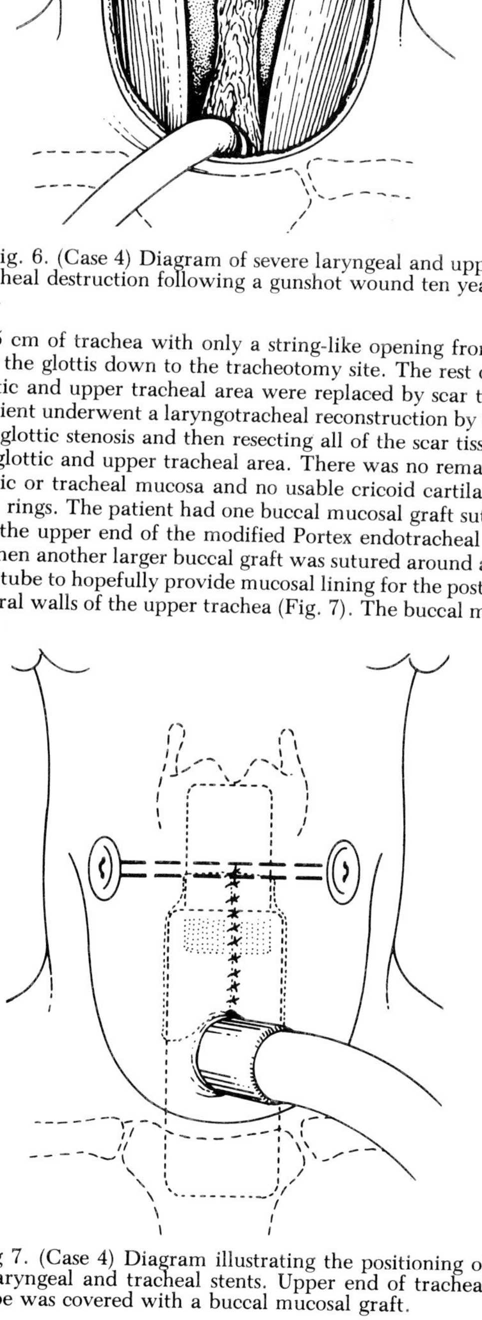

Fig 7. (Case 4) Diagram illustrating the positioning of the laryngeal and tracheal stents. Upper end of tracheal T-tube was covered with a buccal mucosal graft.

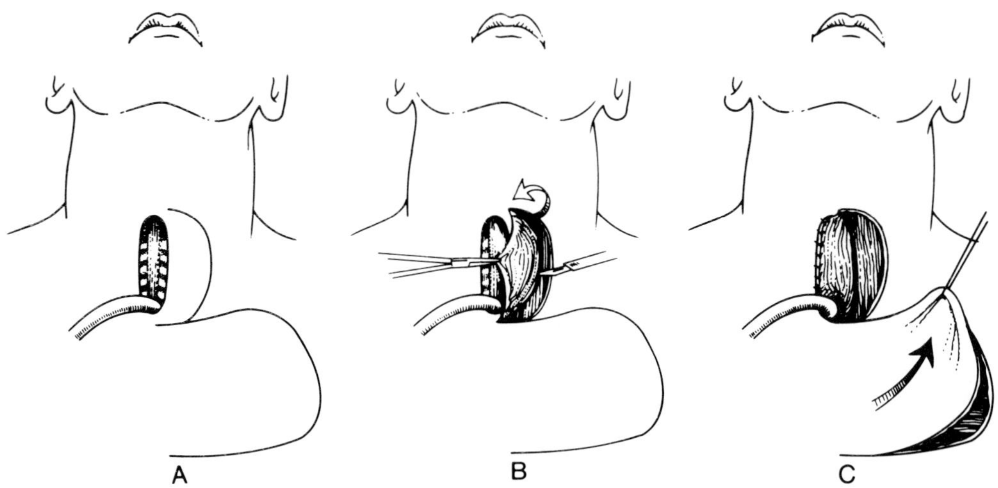

Fig. 8. (Case 4) The second operation involved reconstructing the anterior tracheal wall with A) a local "turnover" and a regional rotation flap with B) "turnover" flap providing inner epithelial coverage, and C) tracheal T-tube maintaining patency with a rotation chest flap used for neck skin resurfacing.

sal graft for the tracheal reconstruction was supplemented with rotation flaps developed from the posterior tracheal wall at the level of the tracheotomy tube. These two stents were left in place for four months. When they were removed, the patient had mucosal continuity of the reconstructed larynx and posterior and lateral walls of the upper trachea with the normal distal trachea. A second stage operation involved reconstruction of the anterior wall using a local "turnover" flap for the inner tracheal epithelium and a regional upper chest rotation flap for neck skin coverage (Fig. 8 A-C). No rigid implants were placed, but rather a tracheal T-tube was inserted to permit fibrous accumulation in the subepithelial tissues of these flaps around the T-tube to provide the rigidity needed to maintain lumen patency. This T-tube was kept in position for six months and the man has now been decannulated for the last four months with only a small tracheocutaneous fistula. He now has laryngeal speech for the first time in ten years and his level of activity has returned to a normal status.

Case 5. The patient, following a total laryngectomy, developed a tracheal stenosis that extended from his stoma down to 2 cm proximal to the carina. Because of the extensive length of this stenosis, surgical resection with reconstruction was not feasible. Therefore, the patient had the stenosis dilated followed immediately by insertion of a specially designed and manufactured Silastic® tracheal tube (Fig. 9). This total tracheal stent has now been in place for 14 months and shows no radiographic evidence of adversely affecting the trachea. Whereas prior to insertion of this stent the patient was at bedrest with partial airway obstruction, he is now back to normal activity and has resumed communication with esophageal speech which he could not successfully perform when he was obstructed. The plan is to leave this tracheal tube in place for an indeterminate period of time.

Case 6. A quadraplegic male developed a tracheal stenosis at the level of the endotracheal tube cuff following a prolonged intubation for treatment of pneumonia. Because the patient's cord

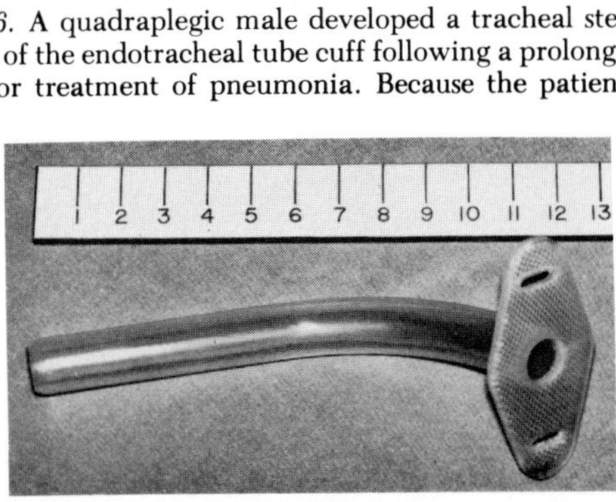

Fig. 9. (Case 5) Specially designed and manufactured tracheal tube used to maintain patency.

level was such that he had restricted thoracic cage movement, a tracheal resection with primary reanastomosis was felt to represent an excessive risk for him. Therefore, he underwent transtracheal excision of the granulation tissue and insertion of a T-tube. This tube has now been placed for six months and will be kept in place for an indefinite period. The patient's ability to communicate and his activities are not at all restricted with the T-tube.

Case 7. A mentally retarded male developed a tracheal stenosis at the site of an endotracheal tube cuff following prolonged endotracheal intubation used during treatment of a mediastinal hematoma. The patient underwent tracheal resection and primary reanastomosis with insertion of a T-tube as an airway safeguard for this individual whose mental capabilities limit his ability to manage any insidious airway restriction which could develop without the use of the T-tube. The tube was kept in place for six months and then removed. However, the patient developed some audible respirations two weeks after removal. He had no airway distress, but because of his mental retardation,it was felt prudent to assure his airway with reinsertion of the T-tube. It has now been in place for a total of ten months and the patient's level of activity is back to normal, as is his ability to communicate, which is important for this particular individual. Plans are to keep this tube in place for an extended period.

DISCUSSION

The successful correction of acute and chronic laryngotracheal injuries has been and continues to be one of the toughest problems facing otolaryngologists. Its complexity rivals the multiple variables associated with treatment decisions for head and neck cancers. The ultimate goal is to reconstruct an adequate airway for breathing without the need for permanent tracheotomy and also to maintain a voice quality adequate for communication. It is not possible to speak in terms of only one technique which is suitable for correction because the problems differ according to what portion(s) of the larynx and/or trachea are involved. Even when the anatomical area of the injury has been defined, there are still a multitude of techniques that have been advocated for the successful correction of a particular problem. The extensive variety of surgical procedures probably attests to the fact that not one procedure gives consistent results in all cases. This report has tried to illustrate the positive contribution of long-term stenting in the management of some of these difficult airway reconstructive problems.

Recent reports in the literature suggest that stenting may be deleterious. Thomas and Stevens[24] conducted an animal study to compare the use of three stenting materials with no stent at all following intentional acute laryngeal injuries to dogs. Their study showed that those animals who had no stents had the most complete and uncomplicated healing. It was their conclusion that stenting must be selected carefully depending on the severity of the clinical complication because of its potential adverse effect on wound healing. The results of this animal study are counterbalanced by the favorable results reported in 1977 by Goode and Shinn.[21] Their report followed an earlier report[25] describing the successful management of a posttraumatic tracheal stenosis with long-term stenting for nine months in one patient.

It is important to emphasize that long-term stenting is not being advocated for every laryngotracheal injury encountered by the physician. A review of this series of patients indicates that their problems were complex for a variety of reasons. The two children with acute laryngeal injuries had not only cartilaginous fractures, but also severe laryngeal soft tissue injuries. There are certain features of laryngeal soft tissue which provide a significant challenge for uneventful healing to occur. The laryngeal mucosa is loose and oftentimes there is no or minimal submucosa. Even with microsurgical techniques, which were used to reapproximate the tissues in these two children (cases 1 and 3), it is still difficult to place sutures which can be expected to maintain epithelial continuity in this less than ideal tissue whose healing capabilities have been stressed even more by the edema and cell destruction associated with such an injury.

Another patient (case 2) had previously undergone a tracheal resection and needed an additional 5 cm removal of this already shortened trachea. Even when the maximal surgical release techniques were used both superiorly and inferiorly, there was no way to achieve primary closure without considerable tension at the anastomosis site. Some reports[26,27] in the literature state that the amount of tension involved with a tracheal resection of more than 4 cm is excessive and significantly decreases the chances of success

No remaining mucosa or cartilage was present in the subglottis or trachea in this patient. He not only needed epithelium but also rigid support. The next patient (case 5) really had no options for treatment except long-term stenting. Temporary stenting for a distal tracheal stenosis with a long tracheotomy tube has been previously reported.[28] In view of the fact that this man most probably will require a lifelong stent, an inert, specially made tracheal tube was designed and manufactured specifically for this patient to minimize tissue trauma. The other two patients (cases 6 and 7) have concomitant health problems which favored a more conservative therapeutic approach to their tracheal stenoses. It becomes apparent that long-term stenting seems to be especially useful in the cases that are more complicated either by magnitude of the severity of the laryngotracheal injury or by concomitant health problems.

When the dynamics of wound healing are considered specifically in the context of the repair of laryngotracheal injuries, there seems to be a rationale for the use of stents. It is obvious that the ultimate goal is to restore epithelial continuity to minimize development of granulation tissue and subsequent collagen deposition which undergoes contraction. As previously mentioned, there are certain features of laryngeal soft tissue which increase the difficulty in maintaining epithelial contact. Yet, the need to restore epithelial continuity is of paramount importance to decrease this inherent tendency for wound contraction. It is important to realize that there is still the problem of wound contraction even with restoration of epithelial coverage, especially with epithelial grafts. Both skin and mucosal grafts undergo contraction. Contraction which narrows the diameter of the airway by as little as 1 mm can result in partial airway obstruction. There is no safe margin of tolerance. The amount of contraction which occurs is less with skin flaps. However, the use of skin flaps has limited applicability due to the size of the areas being reconstructed in the laryngotracheal complex. The contraction seen with an epithelial graft is most probably a function of the collagen deposition in the subepithelial tissues. This is not necessarily an adverse factor. In fact, one patient (case 4) had total subglottic and upper tracheal reconstruction based on the hypothesis that the amount of inelastic firm tissue deposited in the subepithelial tissues around a skin graft being maintained by a long-term stent would provide adequate rigidity, and indeed this was the case. The intent of such long-term stenting is to permit the dynamics of wound healing to occur about a relatively inert object which resists the contraction process. When it is felt that wound healing has stabilized, the stent can safely be removed.

Another variable which some authors fail to mention when discussing the inadvisability of stenting is that the phenomenon of wound healing is being specifically challenged within the reconstructed laryngotrachea by an increased predilection for infection. This adds additional stress which is not a part of wound healing when it occurs in other parts of the body that are not subjected to the prevalence of airway microflora.

There are disadvantages to long-term stenting. In three of the patients, it resulted in persistent tracheocutaneous fistulae which then had to be closed in a secondary procedure. The maintenance of the laryngeal stents with external neck skin buttons has increased the chance of infection with granulation tissue formation on the neck skin. This can be a moderate problem. But the major problem is determining the appropriate time for stent removal. In those four patients who have been successfully decannulated, the duration of stenting ranged from 7-13 months with the average being 10 months. There does not appear to be any danger in leaving the stents in too long as attested to by the fact that one patient has had a stent in place for 14 months with no radiographic evidence of any irritation of the tracheal mucosa. Rather the problem seems to be at the other end of the spectrum, namely removing the stent too soon. There seems to be no means of assessing the best time except for removing the tube and observing the patient for airway problems after tube removal. One patient (case 7) had the tube removed after six months of intubation and then developed audible respirations three weeks afterwards, in spite of the absence of any granulation tissue at the tube site. The timing of the stent period should be based on the individual circumstances relative to the patient's laryngotracheal problem and other health considerations.

CONCLUSION

The surgeon attempting to successfully treat acute or chronic laryngotracheal injuries needs a variety of surgical approaches in his armamentarium. The approach decided upon is a function of the location and extent of the injury. Buccal grafts, local flaps, regional flaps and tracheal resections with primary reanastomosis are just some of the commonly used approaches. The favorable experience reported in this series of seven patients with severe laryngotracheal injuries supports Goode and Shinn's report[21] that the critical feature of any treatment program is the maintenance of lumen patency with a stent which is inert enough to permit long-term placement. It is emphasized that this technique is not advocated for all clinical situations. It seems especially valuable in the more severe injuries.

ACKNOWLEDGMENTS — The author appreciates the contributions of Gerard Kakos, MD, Division of Thoracic Surgery, who performed the transthoracic inferior tracheal release in case 2 and of Edward Kosnik, MD, Division of Neurologic Surgery, and John Kean, MD, Division of Orthopedics, who performed the C1-2 stabilization in case 3. Nancy Sally, illustrator, created the diagrams for case 4.

REFERENCES

1. Ogura JH. Management of traumatic injuries of the larynx and trachea including stenosis. J Laryngol Otol 1971; 85:1259-61.

2. McNaught RD. Surgical correction of anterior web of larynx. Laryngoscope 1950; 60:264-72.

3. Negus VE. Treatment of chronic stenosis of the larynx with special reference to skin grafting. Trans Am Laryngol Assoc 1938; 60:82-92.

4. Holinger PH, Brown WT. Congenital webs, cysts, laryngoceles, and other anomalies of the larynx. Ann Otol Rhinol Laryngol 1967; 76:744-52.

5. Dedo AH, Fishman NH. Laryngeal release and sleeve resection for tracheostenosis. Ann Otol Rhinol Laryngol 1969; 78:285-6.

6. Alonso WA, Druck NS, Griffiths CM, Summer HW, Ogura JH. Cricoid arch replacement in dogs. Arch Otolaryngol 1975; 101:42-5.

7. Alonso WA, Druck NS, Ogura JH. Clinical experiences in hyoid arch transposition. Laryngoscope 1976; 86:617-24.

8. Krizek TJ, Kirchner JA. Tracheal reconstruction with an autogenous mucochondrial graft. Plast Reconstr Surg 1972; 50:123-30.

9. Toohill RJ. Autogenous graft reconstruction of the larynx and upper trachea. Otolaryngol Clin North Am 1979; 12:909-17.

10. Fearon B, Cotton R. Subglottic stenosis in infants and children: the clinical problem and experimental surgical correction. Can J Otolaryngol 1972; 9:281-9.

11. Fearon B, Cotton R. Surgical correction of subglottic stenosis of the larynx in infants and children: progress report. Ann Otol Rhinol Laryngol 1974; 83:428-31.

12. Cotton R. Management of subglottic stenosis in infancy and childhood. Ann Otol Rhinol Laryngol 1978; 87:649-57.

13. Friedman WH, Biller HF, Som ML. Repair of extended laryngotracheal stenosis. Arch Otolaryngol 1975; 101:151-6.

14. Lehman RH, Toohill RJ, Schmitz GL. Reconstruction of the larynx and trachea. Otolaryngol Clin North Am 1979; 12:733-932.

15. Maran AGD, Geissler PR. A new material for laryngeal prosthesis. J Laryngol Otol 1970; 84:1147-51.

16. Miller LH. Laryngotracheal trauma in combat casualities. Ann Otol Rhinol Laryngol 1970; 79:1088-90.

17. Olson NR. Wound healing by primary tension in the larynx. Symposium on Reconstruction of the Larynx and Trachea, Milwaukee, April 1-2, 1977. Otolaryngol Clin North Am 1979; 12:735-40.

18. Curtin JW, Holinger PH, Greeley PW. Blunt trauma to the larynx and upper trachea. J Trauma 1966; 6:493-502.

19. Harris HA, Ainsworth JZ. Immediate management of laryngeal and tracheal injuries. Laryngoscope 1965; 75:1105-15.

20. Harris HA, Tobin HA. Acute injuries of the larynx and trachea in 49 patients. Laryngoscope 1970; 80:1376-84.

21. Goode RL, Shinn JB. Long-term stenting in the treatment of subglottic stenosis. Ann Otol Rhinol Laryngol 1977; 86:295-8.

22. Birck HG. Endoscopic repair of laryngeal stenosis. Trans Am Acad Ophthalmol Otolaryngol 1970; 74:140-3.

23. Montgomery WW. T-tube tracheal stent. Arch Otolaryngol 1965; 82:320-1.

24. Thomas GK, Stevens MH. Stenting in experimental laryngeal injuries. Arch Otolaryngol 1975; 101:217-21.

25. Fredrickson JM, Strahan RW, Goode RL. Reinforced t-tube tracheal stent. Arch Otolaryngol 1969; 90:120-3.

26. Cantrell JR, Folse JR. The repair of circumferential defects of the trachea by direct anastomosis: experimental evaluation. J Thorac Cardiovasc Surg 1961; 42:589-98.

27. Mathey J, Binet JP, Galey JJ, Evrard C, Lemoine G, Denis B. Tracheal and tracheobronchial resections: techniques and results in 20 cases. J Thorac Cardiovasc Surg 1966; 51:1-13.

28. Levine PA, Sasaki CT, Kirchner JA. The long tracheostomy tube. Arch Otolaryngol 1978; 104:108-10.

Ann Otol 89:1980

SILICONE TRACHEAL CANNULA

WILLIAM W. MONTGOMERY, MD
BOSTON, MASSACHUSETTS

This presentation is to introduce a silicone tracheal cannula which has been designed for use in selected cases instead of a tracheotomy tube. The design of the cannula was developed in the laboratory and has now been used clinically over a period of four years in 26 cases. Special features of the cannula include a one-size diameter which is suitable for all adults. An inner flange is shaped so as to conform with the inner aspect of the anterior wall of the trachea and to prevent rotation and anterior displacement of the cannula. The inner flange is angulated to allow for proper direction of the long axis of the cannula. An outer flange fits into one of a number of grooves and prevents posterior displacement of the cannula. Thus far the silicone tracheal cannula has been used in cases of sleep apnea, bilateral vocal cord paralysis in the position of adduction, intermittent glottic insufficiency, laryngeal carcinoma, chronic lung disease, and short-term necessity for a tracheotomy. Special equipment has been designed for ease of the surgical procedure required for insertion of the cannula. A one-way valve has been designed which is easily applied to the cannula. A variation of the silicone tracheal cannula has been designed for long-term use.

DESCRIPTION

The silicone tracheal cannula (Fig. 1 A) has been designed to be used in place of a tracheotomy tube. The *main advantage* is that there is no foreign body projecting into the trachea as the silicone tracheal cannula extends only to the inner surface of the anterior tracheal wall. The silicone tracheal cannula is constructed from vulcanized silicone material to which there is no tissue reaction. It is flexible and nonirritating. The cannula has an inside diameter of 8 mm which is an adequate airway for both male and female adults of all ages. The *component parts* of the silicone tracheal cannula include an inner flange which is thin and shaped so as to fit against the contour of the inner anterior tracheal wall. This inner flange is designed so that the vertical dimension is greater than the horizontal dimension. This allows for *ease of insertion* into the opening of the anterior tracheal wall and also *prevents rotation* of the cannula once it is in place. The inner flange is fashioned at a 27° angle (Fig. 1 B) to the long axis of the tracheal cannula so that the cannula will project straight forward or in a slightly superior direction when inserted. The 27° angle was the end result of studying the angular relationship between the trachea and plane of the anterior cervical skin using soft tissue x-rays of 100 larynges and cervical tracheas. There are ten circumferential ridges on the shaft of the tracheal cannula. The three inner ridges are in the shape of circumferential barbs. This design allows the tracheal cannula to be easily inserted but prevents it from being anteriorly displaced once it is fixed in place. The outer ridges are rounded. The grooves between these ridges serve to secure the face plate in the desired position according to the thickness of the wall between the trachea and the anterior cervical skin. There is a groove along the inferior surface of the shaft of the cannula. This serves to allow for the drainage of serum and products of inflammation which may occur during the immediate postoperative period and also to identify the inferior aspect of the tube, thus being a point of reference to indicate if the inner flange has been accidentally rotated out of its proper position.

The silicone tracheal cannula set also includes a wing-shaped face plate, a plug, and a ring washer. The wing-shaped face plate serves to secure the cannula in place at the time of surgery. It is sutured to the skin with 3-0 polyethylene suture material. The plug is used to obstruct the cannula when the cannula airway is not needed (Fig. 1 B). It is fixed in place simply by inserting and twisting it in a clockwise direction. The plug has a head so that it cannot be introduced too far into the tracheal cannula. This also facilitates its insertion and removal. After the silicone tracheal cannula has been in place for a week, the wing-shaped face plate can be replaced by the ring washer (Fig. 1 C). The washer is less bulky and prevents irritation of the skin surrounding the silicone tracheal cannula. The cannula has now been used over a period of four years in 26 very carefully selected cases (Table 1).

METHODS

Either a vertical or a horizontal skin incision can be made to insert the silicone tracheal cannula (Boston Medical Products). I prefer the vertical incision made with an electrical knife (Fig. 2 a). The median raphe between the sternohyoid and sternothyroid muscles is identified and incised. The thyroid isthmus is divided and suture ligated (Fig. 2 b). The anterior wall of the trachea is exposed so that the fenestration can be made at the proper level (Fig. 2 c).

The fenestration of the anterior tracheal wall is made with the *tracheal trephine fenestrator* (Figs. 2 d and 3 A). This tracheal fenestrator consists of an outer trephine knife which fits over an inner cannula. The trephine knife is 6 cm in length. The diameter of the trephine knife is 8 mm, which is 2 mm less than the outside diameter of the silicone tracheal cannula. Once the trephine

From the Department of Otolaryngology, Harvard Medical School and Massachusetts Eye and Ear Infirmary, Boston.
Presented at the meeting of the American Laryngological Association, Palm Beach, Florida, April 14-15, 1980.
REPRINTS — William W. Montgomery, MD, Massachusetts Eye and Ear Infirmary, 243 Charles Street, Boston, MA 02114.

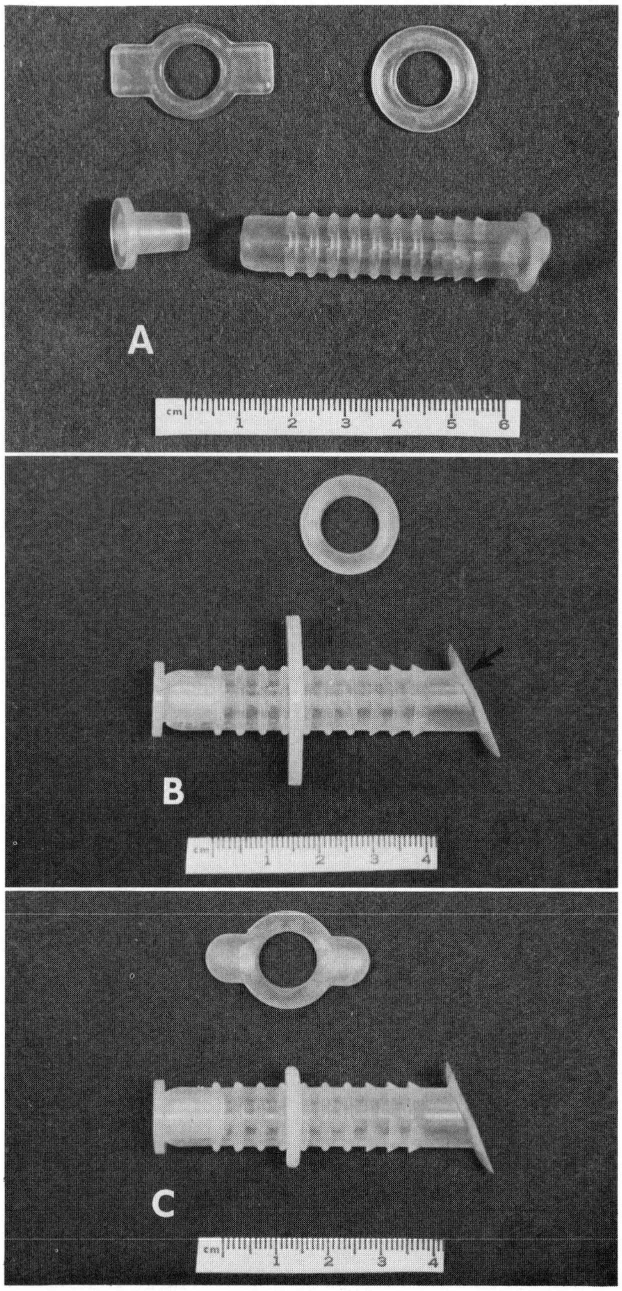

Fig. 1. A) The silicone tracheal cannula is shown along with the wing-shaped face plate, plug and ring washer. The outside diameter of the cannula is 10 mm, the inside diameter is 8 mm, and its length is 6 cm. The cannula is viewed from the bottom where there is a groove along its long axis. This groove serves both for drainage and also as a reference point to identify the inferior aspect of the cannula. The first three rings adjacent to the flange are roughly triangular in shape (circumferential barbs). This design assists in fixing the cannula in place and making it much more difficult to displace anteriorly. The remaining rings and grooves serve to secure the silicone face plate in place. The plug has a head so that it cannot be introduced too far into the lumen of the cannula. B) The silicone tracheal cannula is viewed from the side. The flange (arrow), the only portion of the cannula to remain intraluminal, is placed at a 27° angle to the long axis of the cannula. The vertical dimension of this flange is much longer than its width. This shape permits it to fit snuggly against the concave contour of the anterior intraluminal tracheal wall. The silicone plug has been inserted and the face plate is placed in the fourth groove of the cannula. C) The face plate has been removed from the cannula and is replaced by the ring washer in the fourth groove.

TABLE 1. INDICATIONS FOR USE

Sleep apnea		— tube plugged except when sleeping
Bilateral vocal cord paralysis (position of adduction)		
	Temporary	— after trauma to larynx
		— following thyroid or thoracic surgery
	Permanent	— when a corrective procedure such as an arytenoidectomy is contraindicated
Intermittent laryngeal (glottic) insufficiency		
	Neurological disorders	— head trauma
		— myasthenia gravis
		— amyotrophic lateral sclerosis
	Laryngeal arthritis (cricoarytenoid)	
	Intermittent laryngeal stridor	— chronic laryngitis
		— laryngeal edema postradiation therapy
Laryngeal carcinoma with glottic insufficiency		(used while receiving radiation therapy)
Chronic lung disease		
Short-term tracheotomy		(when cuffed tracheotomy tube not required)
Following T-tube removal		(until certain that airway is adequate)

opening is made with this 8-mm trephine knife, it stretches so that it will easily allow the 10-mm diameter tracheal cannula. The cutting edge of the trephine knife is designed so that it can both cut and saw. The cutting effect is for the soft tissues of the anterior tracheal wall and the teeth are placed in order to cut through cartilage which has become ossified.

The second portion of the tracheal trephine fenestrator is an inner cannula which fits snuggly inside the trephine fenestrator. This is $8\frac{1}{2}$ mm in length. The serrated end fits into the suction tubing.

To use the tracheal trephine fenestrator, the inner cannula is first attached to suction tubing (Fig. 3 B). The fenestrator is placed over the inner cannula so that the inner cannula projects beyond the cutting edge of the fenestrator (Fig. 2 d). The projecting edge of the inner cannula is then placed against the anterior tracheal wall to which it immediately adheres due to the negative pressure inside (Fig. 2 d). The outer, or trephine, portion of the tracheal fenestrator is advanced to the anterior tracheal wall and rotated in a clockwise direction to incise a core of anterior tracheal wall (Fig. 4 a). The core of trachea thus removed either remains adherent to the end of the inner cannula or is aspirated into the suction tubing.

The *advantages* of this instrument over the previous methods for making a tracheotomy fenestration are that it is simpler, less traumatic to the trachea, and a perfectly round fenestration can be made in the anterior tracheal wall (Fig. 4 b).

To insert the end of the silicone tracheal cannula into the trachea, its end is compressed using a curved hemostat. In so doing, this end forms a point (Fig. 4 c) which can easily be inserted into the lumen of the trachea (Fig. 4 d). The tracheal cannula is then pulled anteriorly until the inner flange fits snuggly against the intraluminal anterior tracheal wall (Fig. 5 a, b).

The wound is closed in layers above and below the silicone tracheal cannula (Fig. 5 c). The face plate is applied over the tracheal cannula and is then advanced until it fits fairly closely but not too tightly against the skin (Fig. 5 c). One 3-0 polyethylene suture is placed in each wing of the face plate to secure it to the skin (Fig. 5 d). Anesthesia or oxygen can be administered by way of the tracheal cannula as the patient recovers from general anesthesia. If there is a significant loss of air superiorly into the upper respiratory system, or if anesthesia is to be continued, then a Fogarty® catheter* is inserted and inflated superior to the level of the silicone tracheal cannula.

*American Hospital Supply Corp, Irvine, Calif.

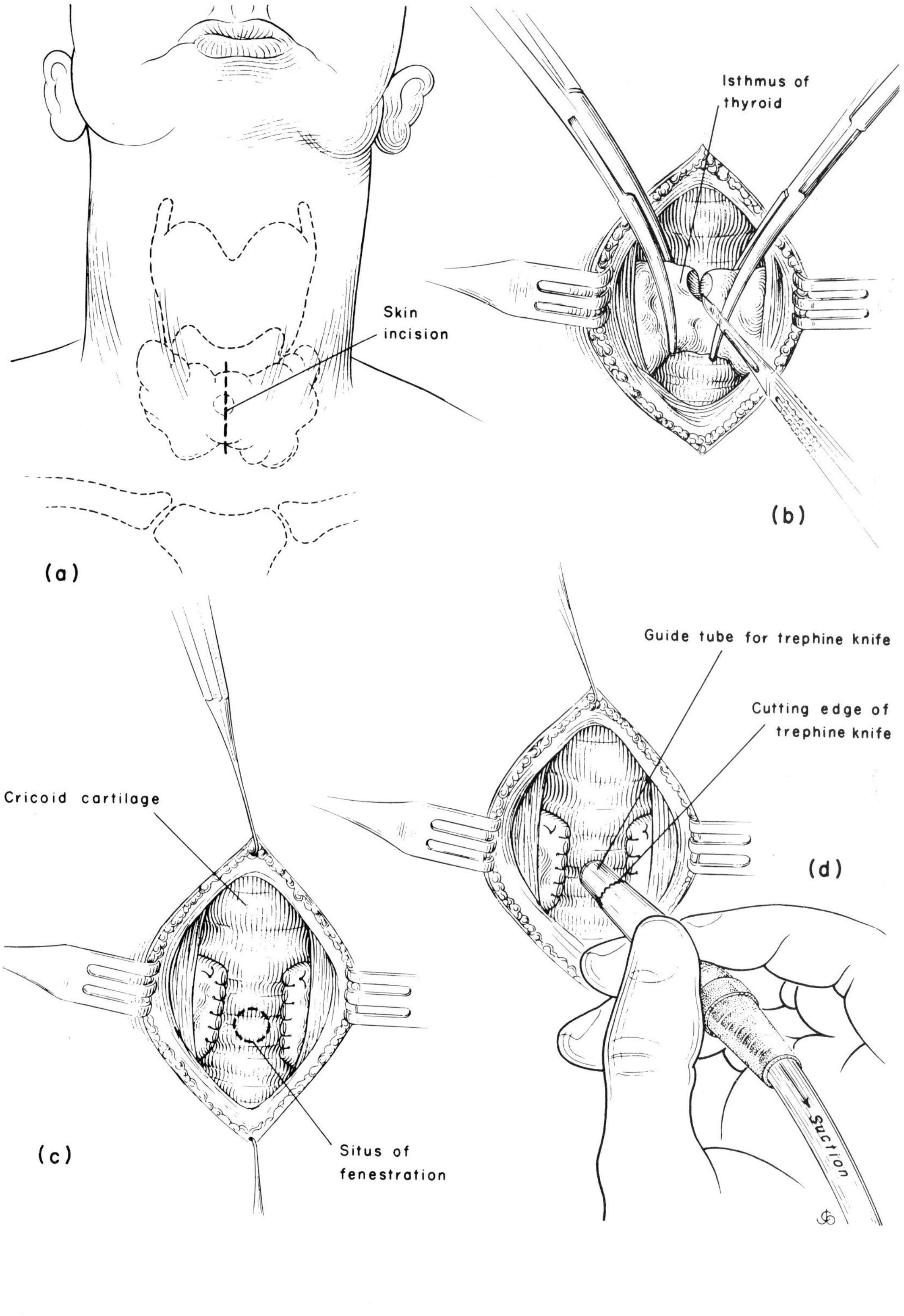

Fig. 2. a) A vertical skin incision is made to expose the thyroid isthmus, and b) it is divided and suture ligated. c) The divided segments have been dissected away from the anterior tracheal wall. The site for the fenestration is indicated. d) The tracheal trephine fenestrator has been placed over its inner cannula which in turn is connected to suction tubing and placed against the anterior tracheal wall.

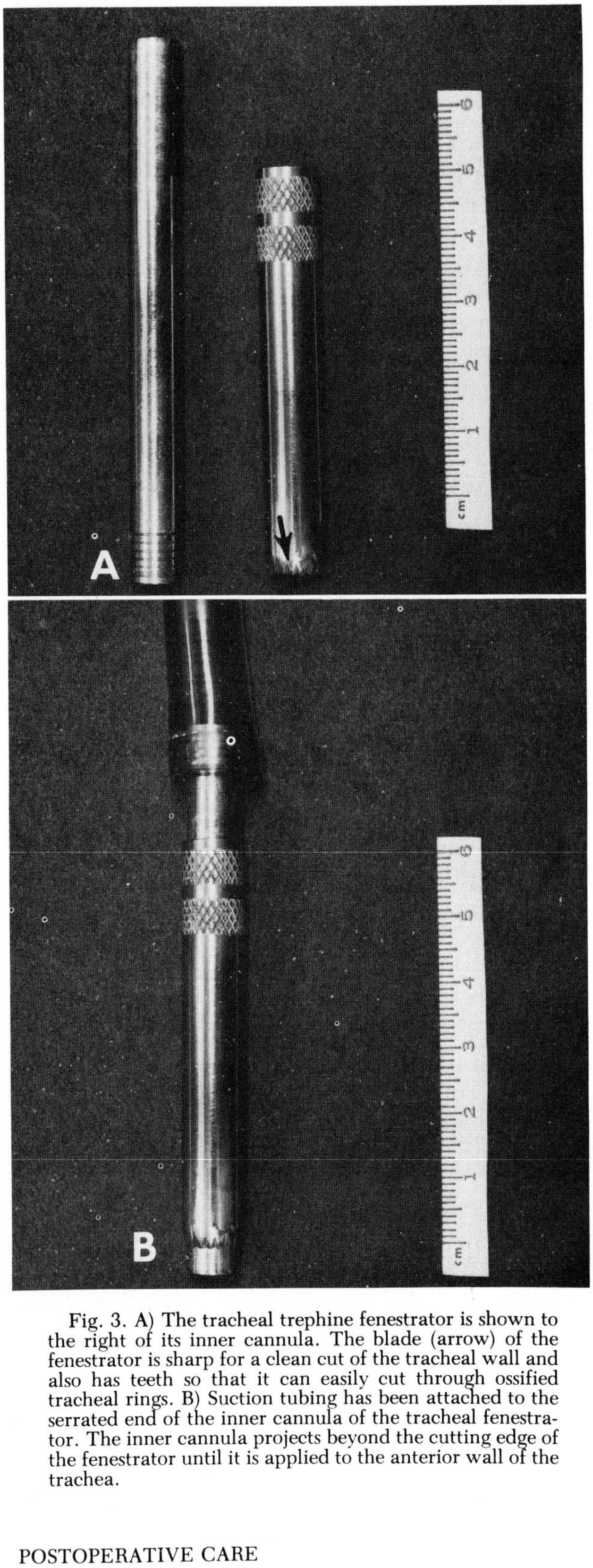

Fig. 3. A) The tracheal trephine fenestrator is shown to the right of its inner cannula. The blade (arrow) of the fenestrator is sharp for a clean cut of the tracheal wall and also has teeth so that it can easily cut through ossified tracheal rings. B) Suction tubing has been attached to the serrated end of the inner cannula of the tracheal fenestrator. The inner cannula projects beyond the cutting edge of the fenestrator until it is applied to the anterior wall of the trachea.

POSTOPERATIVE CARE

The face plate is left in place for seven to ten days or until the silicone tracheal cannula is secured in place and the tracheotomy incision is healed. it is advisable to clean under the face plate twice a day with either peroxide solution or Betadine® solution. A record is made of the groove into which the face plate has been inserted.

The small silicone ring washer replaces the face plate in the same groove when the face plate is removed (Fig. 5 e). The cannula can be shortened to a convenient length at this time simply by cutting it with straight scissors. The ring washer prevents medial displacement of the tube and is much less irritating to the skin surrounding the tracheotomy as compared to the face plate.

The silicone tracheal cannula can be plugged when it is not needed to assist or replace the upper airway. The plug is inserted with a twist and will remain in place by friction. A silk suture can be placed through the plug and around the neck to prevent its being lost when not in use (Fig. 5 e).

Postoperatively, a lateral soft tissue x-ray, preferably a xeroradiograph, of the larynx and trachea is obtained to make certain that the inner flange is in the proper position and firmly against the inner aspect of the anterior tracheal wall (Fig. 6).

LONG-TERM SILICONE TRACHEAL CANNULA

The silicone tracheal cannula has been altered for a long-term tracheotomy by omitting the three barb-like rings adjacent to the inner flange. The shaft of the cannula between the inner flange and the first outer ring has a highly polished surface (Figs. 6 D and 7 A). This surface permits and encourages growth of epithelium both from the trachea and the skin so as to line the tissue of the tracheotomy tract.

Two washers are supplied with the long-term silicone tracheal cannula. These washers can be placed in various positions as shown in Figure 7 B, C. The position of the washer(s) depends on the distance between the anterior tracheal wall and the surface of the anterior cervical skin and are necessary to maintain the position of the inner flange against the anterior cervical tracheal wall. The plug is used in patients who require a tracheotomy intermittently. A patient with sleep apnea, for example, would use this plug during waking hours and remove it at night for sleep.

VALVE FOR THE SILICONE TRACHEAL CANNULA

A special valve (Fig. 8) has been designed. This is attached to the silicone tracheal cannula in those patients with insufficient inspiratory airway and adequate expiratory airway. An example of this is a patient with bilateral vocal cord paralysis in the position of adduction. The housing of the valve mechanism is constructed from a more dense silicone as compared to the silicone tracheal cannula.

The valve is applied to the silicone tracheal cannula by inserting it over the cannula which has been shortened to the desired length (Fig. 8 B, C). It is

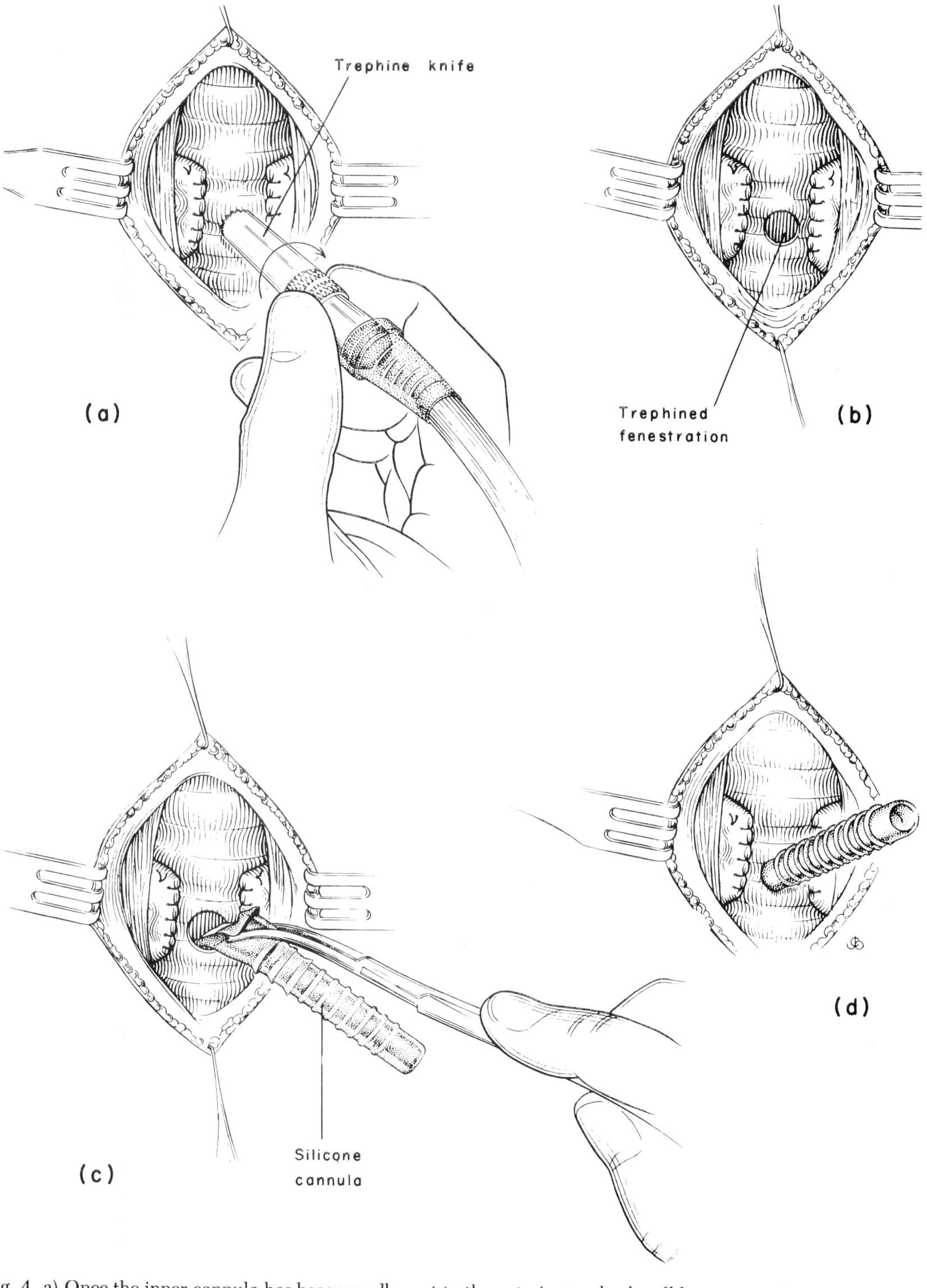

Fig. 4. a) Once the inner cannula has become adherent to the anterior tracheal wall by suction, the outer, or trephine, portion of the tracheal fenestrator is advanced to the tracheal wall. A core of tracheal wall is cut by rotating the fenestrator in a clockwise direction. The suction will prevent this core from falling into the tracheal lumen. b) The anterior tracheal wall has been fenestrated. c) The flanged end of the tracheal cannula is grasped with a curved hemostat and inserted through the fenestrated tracheal wall. d) The flange is now intraluminal.

held in place by four prongs which fit into the groove of the cannula (Fig. 8 C).

The valve mechanism consists of a very thin silicone hinged diaphragm (Fig. 8 D) which opens inwardly during inspiration (Fig. 8 E) and closes against the inside of the anterior aspect of the valve housing during expiration (Fig. 8 F). During forceful expiration such as coughing, the diaphragm of the valve pressure releases by partially extruding from the anterior end of the valve housing (Fig. 8

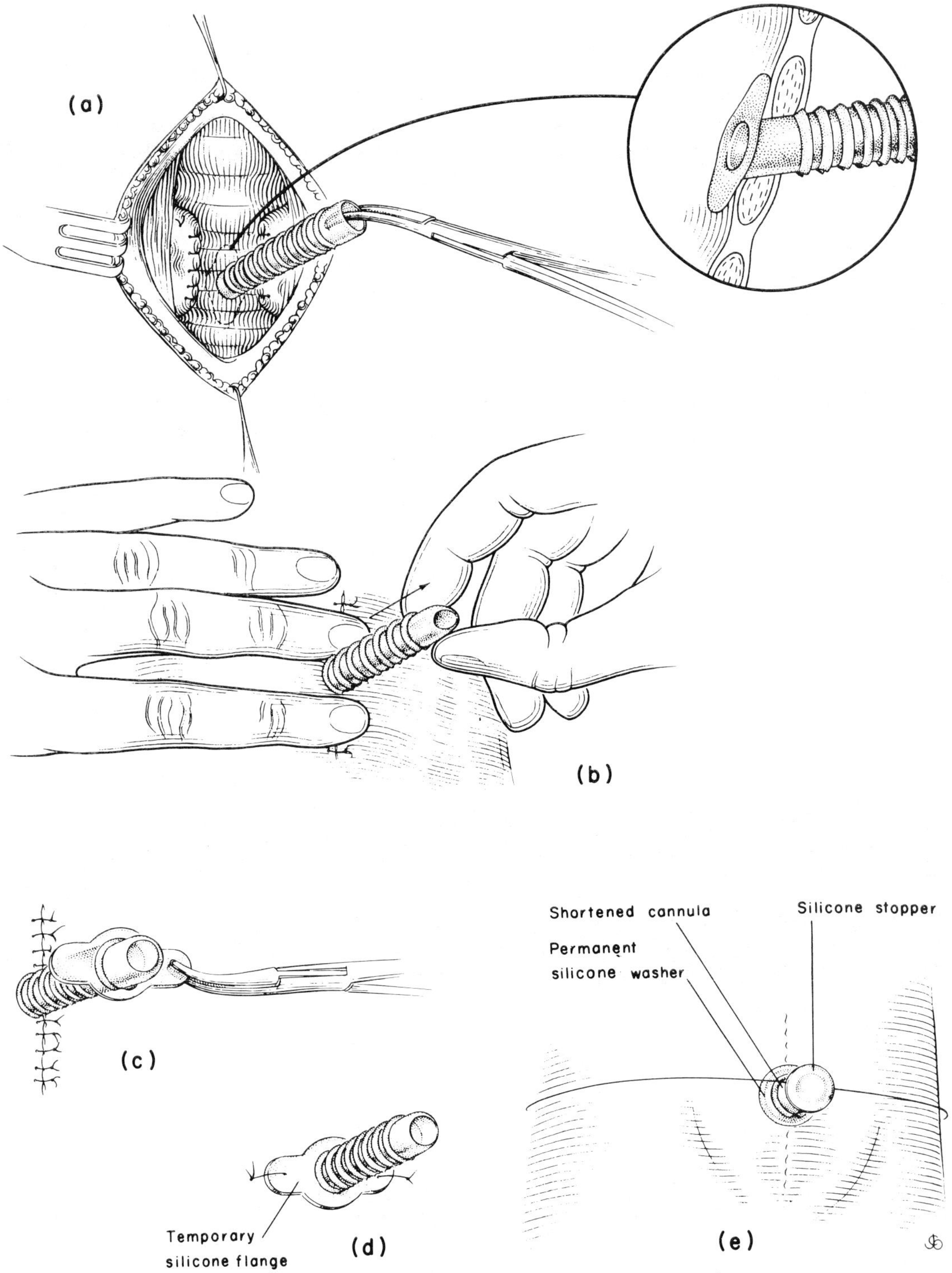

Fig. 5. a, b) The end of the cannula is pulled anteriorly so that the flange fits *snuggly* against the anterior intraluminal tracheal wall. c) Following repair of the incision, the face plate is advanced to the groove adjacent to the skin surface, and d) is secured to the skin with one 3-0 polyethylene suture through each wing. An endotracheal tube can be inserted into the silicone tracheal cannula as the patient recovers from anesthesia. e) The face plate has been removed and replaced by the ring washer. The cannula can be shortened by cutting it in a groove with straight scissors. A silk suture is placed through the plug so that it will not be lost when not in use.

G). The diaphragm of the valve is very easily reengaged into functioning position by placing the end of the index finger against the end of the valve housing.

The silicone tracheal cannula valve has *advantages* over previous tracheotomy valves. During inspiration it allows for sufficient air flow even during strenuous exercise. The valve is silent as it functions in contrast to the very noisy clicking sound of the metallic tracheotomy valves. The valve is easily cleaned using liquid detergent (liquid Ivory®) and then rinsed with clear hot water. It is either air dried or dried with an ordinary towel. The valve is durable and almost indestructible and rarely needs repair.

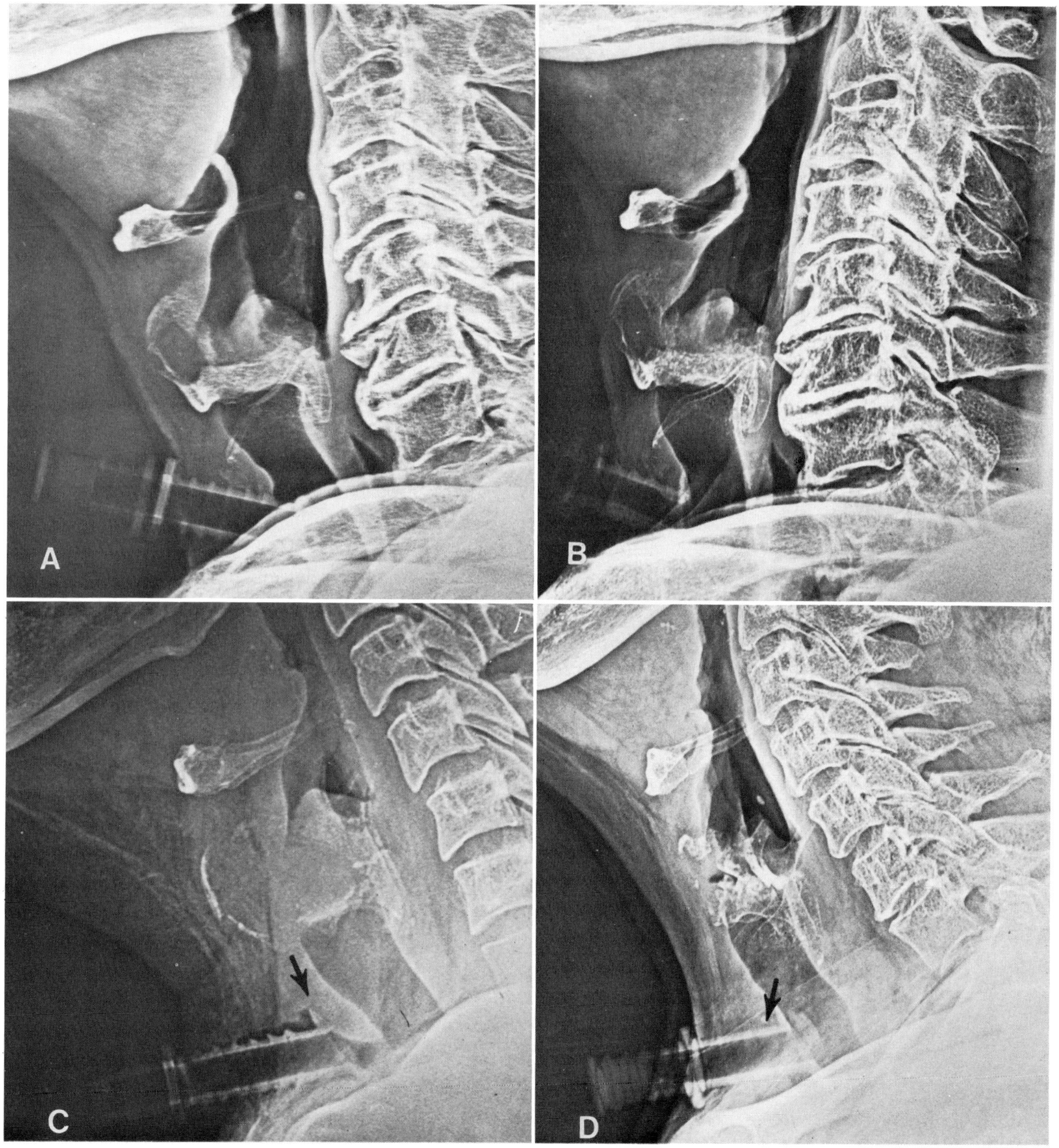

Fig. 6. A) Soft-tissue x-ray or xeroradiograph is taken postoperatively to determine the position of the inner flange and shows it too far intraluminally. B) The cannula was advanced and is now in proper position. C) The flange of the cannula is in the soft tissues (arrow) anterior to the trachea and must be pushed into the lumen of the trachea. D) A xeroradiograph of another patient showing the inner flange fitting snuggly against the anterior intraluminal trachea. Note that there are no ridges on the cannula between the trachea and skin (arrow). This cannula has been designed for long-term use. This x-ray also demonstrates the advantage of the 27° angle of the flange to the long axis of the cannula.

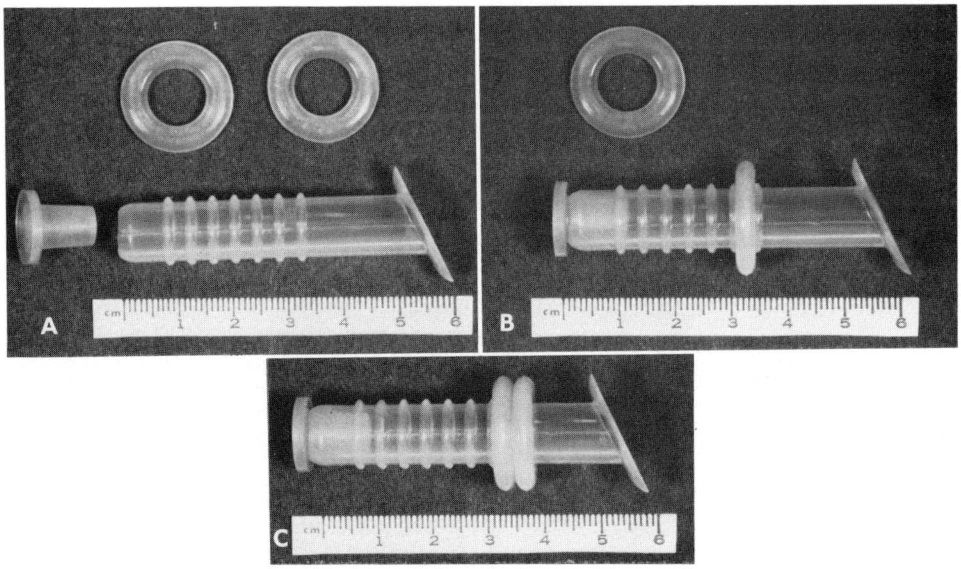

Fig. 7. A) The silicone tracheal cannula for long-term use is shown with two washers and a plug. This differs from the other cannula in that the three circumferential ridges adjacent to the inner flange are omitted. B) The washer is placed in varied positions depending on the distance between the anterior tracheal wall and the skin. In this photograph the washer is placed in the innermost groove. C) Two washers are placed posterior to the innermost ridge when the distance between the trachea and skin is short.

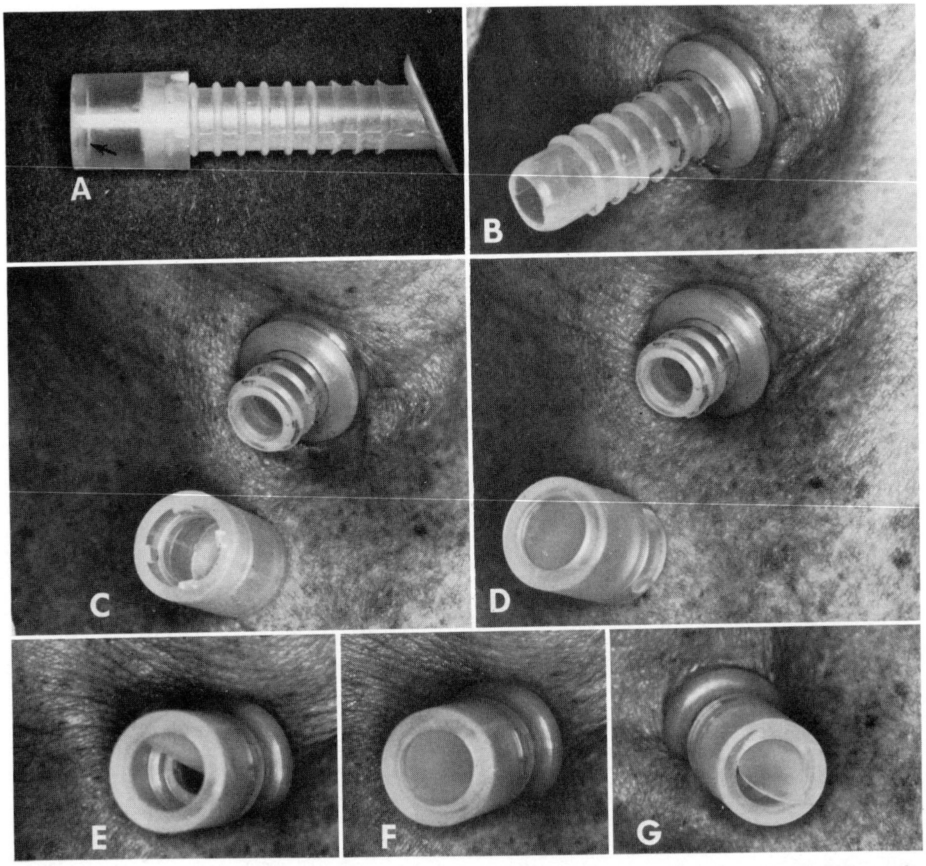

Fig. 8. A) A side view of the valve for the silicone tracheal cannula is shown in this photograph. The outline (arrow) of the hinged diaphragm can be seen inside the valve housing. B) In this case there is a short distance between the anterior tracheal wall and the skin. The two washers are applied posterior to the innermost ridge. C) The cannula is shortened to the desired length (here, two grooves showing) with suture scissors or a number ten surgical blade. The four prongs on the posterior aspect of the valve housing serve to secure the valve to the cannula. D) The hinged diaphragm can be seen inside the anterior aspect of the valve housing. E) The valve has been applied to the cannula. The diaphragm is pulled inward during inspiration. F) During expiration the diaphragm is forced against the valve housing and the expired air is directed to the larynx. G) During forced expiration such as a severe cough the diaphragm is forced through the opening in the anterior aspect of the valve housing. The diaphragm is easily replaced with a touch of the finger.

AN ENDOSCOPIC TECHNIQUE FOR RESTORATION OF VOICE AFTER LARYNGECTOMY

MARK I. SINGER, MD ERIC D. BLOM, PhD

INDIANAPOLIS, INDIANA

Reports of restoration of voice after total laryngectomy include diversion of exhaled pulmonary air through planned or spontaneous fistulae with a variety of modified tracheal cannulas and valves. Limitations of these techniques include aspiration, scar closure of the shunts, wound complications, and failure to achieve voice consistently. We report a two-year experience with an endoscopic method using a unique valved prosthesis eliminating complicated surgical reconstructions, aspiration, and stenosis. Fifty-four of 60 patients (90%) achieved fluent voices with one deglutition problem. Radiation therapy preceded voice restoration in 63% of the patients and radical neck dissection in 72%. The endoscopic procedure, hospitalization and period of speech therapy are short and constitute a cost-effective voice rehabilitation program. The results of this simple method and lack of complications are encouraging.

INTRODUCTION

Restoration of voice after total laryngectomy may occur with diversion of exhaled pulmonary air into the esophagus or hypopharynx. Successful case reports of spontaneous fistulae and planned shunts accompany the history of laryngectomy surgery.[1-3] There are also descriptions of modified tracheal cannulas, flutter valves, reeds, and air bypass devices spanning nearly 100 years.[4-7] Glottic replacement procedures for restoration of laryngeal functions are frequently complicated by aspiration, scar obliteration of the shunts, or breakdown of the operated tissues.

In 1958 Conley et al[8] stated: "The technical problem to overcome consisted of creating a passageway that would permit the free flow of air from the trachea into the esophagus without the passage of food or saliva from the gullet into the trachea. The great inconvenience caused by an inadvertent small pharyngeal or esophageal fistula would unquestionably condemn any such uncontrolled communication." Ogura et al[9] proposed an experimental laryngeal substitute based on observations of satisfactory function of the "simplified" larynx following conservation surgery. Long-term animal results were characterized by life-threatening aspiration pneumonia, obstruction, and rejection of the implanted prosthetic devices.

Recently European and Japanese laryngologists have introduced subtotal laryngectomy with maintenance of some residual laryngeal function, or total laryngectomy with construction of a tracheo-hypopharyngeal shunt for voice restoration.[10-12] The ideal of voice without external fistulae and appliances makes these techniques of interest. The results, however, are inconsistent; and the inconveniences of leakage and stenosis of the shunts require multiple revision procedures for satisfactory function.

The "neoglottic" procedures, as they have been incorrectly labeled, are applied to lesions failing the established criteria for conservation laryngeal surgery. In many cases, they represent extended conservation procedures or narrow field laryngectomies. The local recurrence rate is unacceptable and has been reported as high as 25% in pseudoglottic reconstructions.[13]

The conventional treatment of extensive laryngeal carcinoma often includes radical neck dissection and supravoltage radiation therapy. Primary voice restoration surgery in this population is accompanied by a considerably higher incidence of stenosis, wound breakdown, and mediastinitis than would be expected in patients undergoing laryngectomy alone.[14,15] Delayed voice restoration after laryngectomy is no freer of serious complications, with carotid hemorrhage reported in some instances.[16]

We propose in this paper a simplified method for voice restoration after total laryngectomy.[17,18] It is an endoscopic procedure, and the problems of aspiration and stenosis are eliminated by the use of an inexpensive, miniature, valved prosthesis developed by the authors. The rehabilitation is rapid following the procedure, and the complications are minimal.

METHODS

The series consists of 60 patients treated over a two-year period from February 1978 to February 1980, at the Indiana University Medical Center and Veterans Administration Medical Center, Indianapolis, Indiana. There were 14 females and 46 males, with an age range from 42 to 78 years.

Forty-three patients (72%) had radical neck dissection with four bilateral dissections. Radiation therapy was used either

From the Department of Otorhinolaryngology, Indiana University School of Medicine and the Audiology-Speech Pathology Service, Veterans Administration Medical Center, Indianapolis.

Presented at the meeting of the American Laryngological Association, Palm Beach, Florida, April 14-15, 1980.

REPRINTS — Mark I. Singer, MD, 1633 N. Capitol Avenue, Suite 780, Indianapolis, IN 46202.

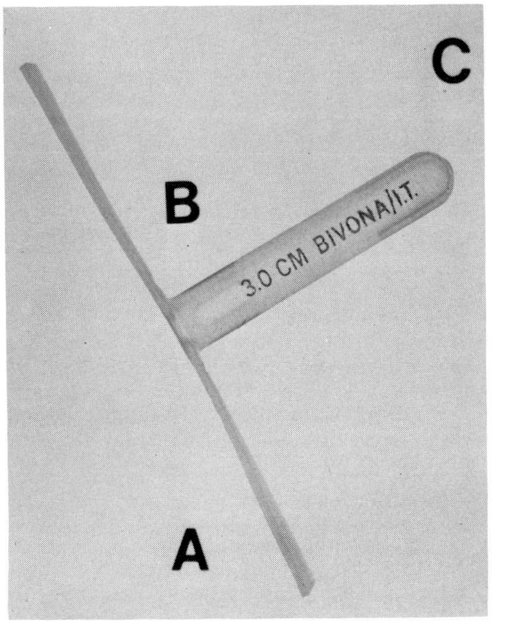

Fig. 1. Blom-Singer voice prosthesis. A - Retention flange; B - Port for air entry; C - One-way valved end.

before the laryngectomy or after, but preceded the voice restoration in 38 patients (63%). The radiation dosage ranged from 4,500 to 7,600 rads mainly delivered by supravoltage equipment.

Thirty-one patients (52%) received both radiation therapy and radical neck dissections and four had staged, multiple flap reconstruction of the pharynx. Only four had developed some functional esophageal voice and the artificial larynx users were not satisfied with their mechanical voice. The earliest the procedure was applied was four weeks after laryngectomy and the longest was 19 years.

All patients were assessed preoperatively by esophageal air insufflation. A catheter (French No. 12) is passed through the nose into the esophagus to the level of the tracheostoma. Air is gently insufflated with the patient at rest, and it leaves the oral cavity producing an esophageal sound. If the air passes into the stomach, the catheter is withdrawn until oral escape is detected. Catheter placement in the oropharynx or superior hypopharynx will result in a breathy whisper and is avoided by further insertion until the esophagus is set into vibration.

When sound is produced, the amount of pressure required is subjectively noted. The patients are then instructed to participate by counting or forming words. The quality of airflow during participatory speech is observed with particular reference to spasm and duration of voice (see discussion).

Voice Restoration Method. The endoscopic procedure is designed to produce a controlled midline tracheoesophageal "puncture." The puncture is stented 36-48 hours until the voice prosthesis is inserted. The site in the stoma is selected for patient accessibility for hygiene, and to eliminate mechanical obstruction to breathing.

The voice prosthesis functions as a one-way valve stent (Fig. 1). It is a hollow tube of silicone, 3 cm long. Thin flanges on either side provide retention. The outside diameter is 5.4 mm (French No. 16). At the proximal end (esophageal side) is a razor-thin slit paralleling the long axis of the tube. It opens as a "duck's bill" with positive air pressure permitting airflow into the esophagus.* It remains closed during swallowing, and performs as a competent one-way valve. The distal end (tracheal side) includes a port on the inferior surface measuring 3.5 x 7.0 mm for exhaled air entry; and the end is open to permit cleaning and to decrease the mechanical resistance to airflow at the stoma.

*Blom-Singer Voice Prosthesis, Bivona Surgical Instruments, Inc, Hammond, Ind.

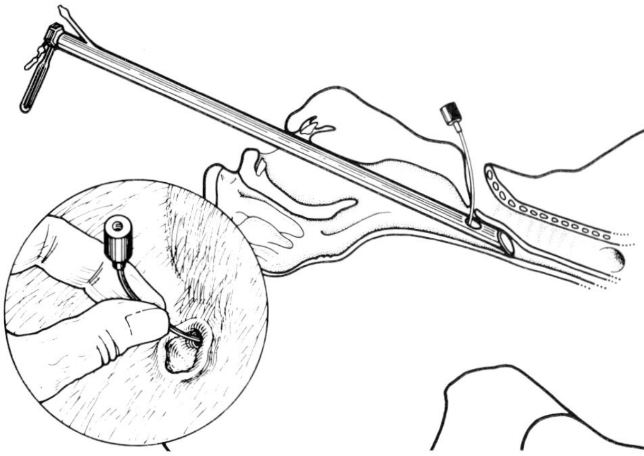

Fig. 2. Perforated esophagoscope in position with posterior tracheal wall puncture. Inset) Puncture at 5 mm from mucocutaneous junction at superior aspect of tracheastoma.

An esophagoscope is placed 2 cm inferior to the tracheostoma. We prefer a modified 7 x 30 cm fiberoptic Holinger esophagoscope, perforated on the beveled surface[19] (Fig. 2). Transillumination of the light through the membranous tracheal wall as well as palpation of the perforation on the endoscope serve to orient the operator.

A trocar is fashioned from a disposable 14 gauge intravenous catheter set, by bending it to form a "C" curve.* This is introduced by the operator through the posterior tracheal wall into the esophagoscope perforation. The puncture is monitored at all times by the endoscopist to prevent a misdirected perforation.

Ideally, the puncture is situated 3 to 5 mm inferior to the mucocutaneous junction of the stoma at the superior aspect (Fig. 2). It must cross the membranous wall of the trachea to prevent the risk of salivary leakage. This level also insures access to the esophagus at a point inferior to the pharyngeal constrictors and Killian's inlet.

The disposable intravenous catheter with wire stylet (60 cm, 24 in) is inserted through the needle and retrieved in the esophagoscope by the endoscopist. The needle is withdrawn and the intravenous catheter is attached to a straight urethral catheter (French No. 14). The tracheal puncture may be dilated with a right-angled hemostat, and the catheter is drawn retrograde into the oral cavity (Fig. 3A).

A loop is completed by drawing the intravenous catheter out of the nose with a second urethral catheter and fixing it to the end of the stent to prevent accidental dislodgement (Fig. 3B). The catheter should rest in the hypopharynx for normal swallowing in the postoperative period.

In the immediate postoperative period, stoma hygiene is maintained by continuous humidification and topical instillation of a 10% solution of acetylcysteine. Analgesics are unnecessary and antibiotics are not used. On the first postoperative day a progressive diet is resumed without difficulty.

On the second day, the stent is withdrawn through the nose, the valved voice prosthesis is inserted, and its flanges are taped to the paratracheal skin. The surgeon and speech pathologist select the proper length prosthesis and insert it in the puncture site immediately after removal of the stenting catheter. It is fixed to dry skin by double-backed adhesive tape. A coating of tincture of benzoin is applied to the skin and flanges, and two reinforcing strips of paper adhesive tape are placed (Fig. 4).

The patient is instructed to occlude the stoma to divert exhaled air through the voice prosthesis into the esophagus, and voice is obtained immediately. The speech pathologist instructs the pa-

*Intracath Intravenous Set, Deseret Co, Inc, Sandy, Utah.

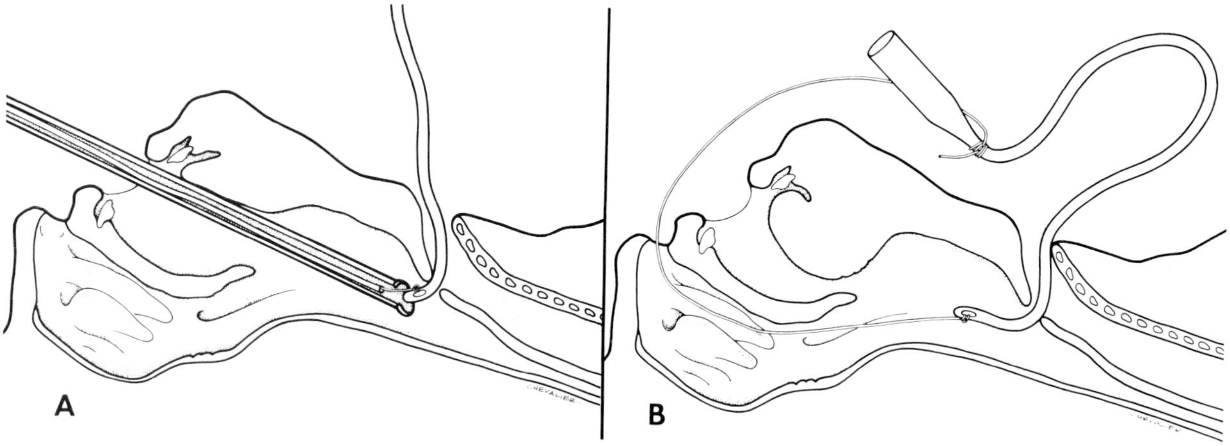

Fig. 3. A) Retrograde placement of catheter for stenting of puncture. B) Stent in place in hypopharynx with pull-out catheter exiting the nose.

tient in proper breath control, articulation, and if necessary, muscle relaxation for satisfactory voice production.

Although the prosthesis remains in place at all times, the patient is instructed on daily removal, cleaning, and replacement as part of his speech therapy. The diet remains unrestricted, and patients are released from the hospital on the average in four to seven days.

RESULTS

Satisfactory communication is regarded as intelligible and fluent to listeners, while nonfluent speakers are classified as failures. From the 60 patients, 54 (90%) achieved fluent voices, and were satisfied with their communication ability.

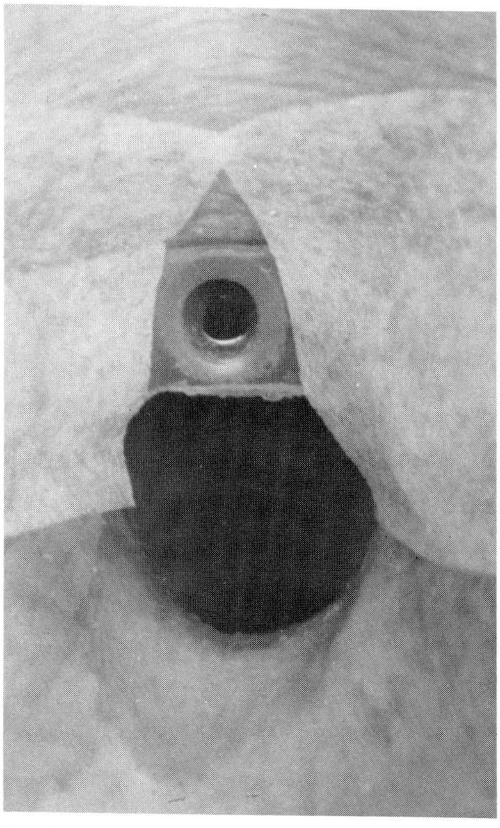

Fig. 4. Voice prosthesis in puncture placed in superior tracheostoma.

No operative complications of infection, wound breakdown, hemorrhage, or aspiration have been noted. Swallowing is reported as normal, and on contrast radiography appears unimpeded. Only one patient developed leakage around the voice prosthesis, and required a second procedure for closure. Five others have developed transient leakage around the voice prosthesis from two to eight months postoperatively. This is successfully eliminated by electrocauterization of the puncture site to enhance stenosis.

The six voice failures were "closed" simply by removing the voice prosthesis. Within one hour the puncture did not leak saliva, and a normal diet could be resumed in six hours. A small mucosal indentation remained on the tracheal wall at 24 hours with no evidence of aspiration.

Inadvertent dislodgement of the voice prosthesis occurred in 15 patients, usually because of lack of attention to adequate installation. The punctures were too stenotic for the patient to reinsert the prosthesis comfortably, but were easily dilated with urethral dilators for reintroduction of the prosthesis.

Twenty-six months is the longest interval that a patient has used the voice prosthesis, and the shortest is two months. There are 6,960 patient days of continuous prosthesis use with an average device life of 60 days. Valve deterioration is indicated by leakage through the prosthesis with resultant coughing.

DISCUSSION

The tracheoesophageal puncture and valved voice prosthesis provide a simple method for voice restoration. The endoscopic midline puncture safely avoids vascular injury, and decreases the risk of salivary leakage into the neck or mediastinum. The puncture is accessible for inspection, patient maintenance, and stenting with the valved prosthesis. A complicated series of stoma fittings, interconnecting tubes, and valves are unnecessary. This technique eliminates the need for skin flaps, dermal or mucosal tubes, and pharyngostoma construction. The contraindications of radical neck dissection, radiation, and postoperative tumor recurrence are avoided.

The surgical procedure and period of hospitalization are short. Speech therapy for prosthesis use and initial voice production is necessary and can be provided by speech pathologists experienced in conventional alaryngeal voice rehabilitation. The time required is also short and represents a cost-effective voice rehabilitation program.

Although this method appears uncomplicated, it is not always "easy" and a number of factors must be considered. A small number of the cases will remain voice failures, and five of the six failure patients in this series had severe pharyngoesophageal spasm with voluntary airflow. This was apparent because of voice failure and resultant gastric distention. The sixth patient had a tight pharyngeal stricture superior to the puncture site effectively preventing airflow.

The voice failures can be predicted preoperatively by the air insufflation test. The test is critical to successful patient selection. Limitation to airflow by this test correlated well with lack of initial voice fluency and the need for reeducation of the pharyngoesophageal muscles for voice production. To date there have been both false positives and negatives, but in limited numbers. We use the test as a relative guide to patient selection, and estimation of time involved for postsurgical rehabilitation.

Other patient selection factors must be considered jointly by the surgeon and speech pathologist. The patient himself should be motivated for voice restoration rather than the family. This is of particular significance among the elderly. The patient must be capable and interested in caring for the stoma and the prosthesis. These functions can rarely be delegated to a family member or visiting nurse.

Candidates should be recovered from the laryngectomy and all adjunctive therapy. They should demonstrate a suitable disease-free interval. Conventional speech therapy may be offered and tried if the patient desires.

The tracheostoma must be of adequate size and not retracted behind the manubrium. Chronic tracheitis and ulceration must be absent before puncture. If the patient customarily uses a tracheal cannula, this is continued following the puncture procedure.

If there is a history of previous unplanned fistulization, stricture, or flap reconstruction, a barium esophagogram is important for preoperative assessment. Dilatations may be required to maintain an adequate lumen for normal nutrition and satisfactory airflow for voice production.

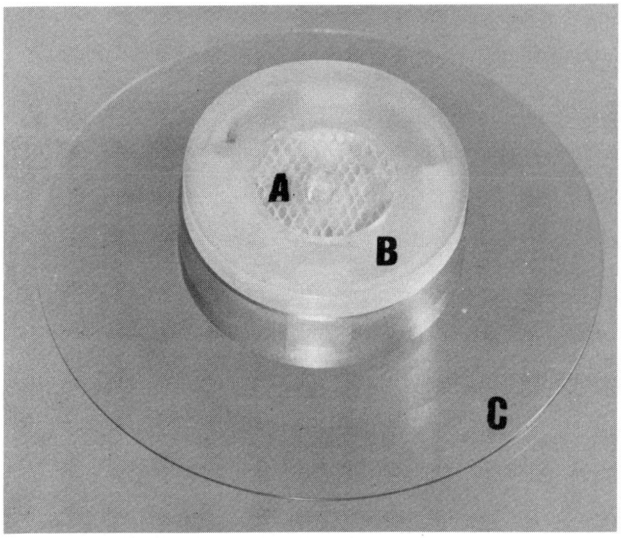

Fig. 5. Respiratory valve for stoma occlusion. A - Adjustable valve diaphragm; B - Disposable valve casing; C - Self-contouring parastomal valve housing.

The patient's general status and medical history are reviewed from the standpoint of anesthetic tolerance. Severe arthritis, visual disturbance, and general unreliability are relative contraindications for this procedure. Chronic obstructive pulmonary disease, diabetes, and alcoholism have not presented significant problems for this method of voice restoration.

The patient's ability to occlude the stoma for voice production varies widely. Careless occlusion allows air escape and decreases the speech intelligibility. Heavy-handed occlusion may distort the tracheoesophageal communication and choke off the voice. Occupational constraints, such as the need to have two hands free, or unclean working conditions, limit the ability to occlude the stoma.

We have developed a light-weight, two-way respiratory valve for use with the voice prosthesis to address these problems* (Fig. 5). It allows two-way airflow at the stoma for breathing and converts to a one-way inspiratory valve with increased breath pressure for voice production. Air is then diverted into the esophagus, eliminating the need for finger occlusion of the stoma. With the increased respiratory demands of exercise, the valve tolerance is adjustable, and the soft diaphragm will evert when expiratory pressure increases during coughing.

The valve fits a housing which is applied to the paratracheal skin, eliminating an indwelling cannula and the potential problems of tracheitis, dilation, and air escape. The valve housing and diaphragm measure 2.5 cm in diameter by 1 cm in width. The optional respiratory valve is intended for use with the voice restoration method and voice prosthesis described in this paper.

*Tabor Plastics, Inc, St. Louis, Mo.

CONCLUSION

In a series of 60 patients after total laryngectomy, 54 have achieved fluent voice without disruption of normal swallowing or respiratory function by the method of endoscopic tracheoesophageal puncture and indwelling voice prosthesis. The low failure rate and freedom from complications have been observed over a two-year period in patients with extensive primary resections, radiation therapy, and varying socioeconomic status.

As a delayed or secondary method for rehabilitation after total laryngectomy, no compromise of conventional cancer surgery or radiation occurs. The need for skin or mucosal tubes, multistaged pharyngostoma construction, and complicated air bypass devices is eliminated. The high risks of radical surgery and radiation therapy are not encountered. The airway requires no protection with a cuffed tracheotomy cannula, and the patient maintains normal swallowing and independent care.

The surgeon and speech pathologist work as a team for the selection and rehabilitation of the laryngectomy patient. It is this interdisciplinary approach to the communication-impaired patient that forms the cornerstone of this voice restoration method. We are encouraged by the results of this simple method and its lack of complications. It appears to represent a safe and effective procedure for alaryngeal voice restoration in a majority of patients who have undergone removal of the larynx.

REFERENCES

1. Gussenbauer C. Ueber die erste durch Th. Billroth am Menschen ausgefuhrte Kehlkopf-Exstirpation und die Anwendung eines kunstlichen Kokokopfes. Arch Klin Chir 1874; 17:343-56.

2. Guttman MR. Rehabilitation of the voice in laryngectomized patients. Arch Otolaryngol 1932; 15:478-9.

3. Kolson H, Glasgold A. Tracheo-esophageal speech following laryngectomy. Trans Am Acad Ophthalmol Otolarygol 1967; 71:421-5.

4. Czerny V. Versuche über Kohlkopfexstirpation. Wien Med Wochenschr 1870; 20:557-61.

5. Brown RG. A simple but effective artificial larynx. J Laryngol Otol 1925; 40:793-7.

6. Briani A. Riabilitazione fonetica di laringectomizzati a mezzo della corrente aerea espiratoria polmonare. Arch Ital Otol Rinol Laringol 1952; 63:469.

7. Taub S. Air bypass voice prosthesis for vocal rehabilitation of laryngectomees. Ann Otol Rhinol Laryngol 1975; 84:45-8.

8. Conley JJ, DeAmesti F, Pierce MK. A new surgical technique for the vocal rehabilitation of the laryngectomized patient. Ann Otol Rhinol Laryngol 1958: 67:655-64.

9. Ogura JH, Shumrick DA, Lapidot A. Some observations on experimental laryngeal substitution in laryngectomized dogs. Ann Otol Rhinol Laryngol 1962; 71:532-50.

10. Arslan M, Serafini I. Reconstrucctive laryngectomy: report of the first 35 cases. Ann Otol Rhinol Laryngol 1972; 81:479-86.

11. Steffieri M, Serafini I. La riabilitazione chirurgica della voce e della respirazione dopo laringectomia totale. 29th National Congress of the Associazione Otologi Ospedalieri Italiana. Bologna: Associazione Otologi Ospedalieri Italiana, 1976:57-111.

12. Amatsu M, Matsui T, Maki T, Kanagawa K. Vocal reconstruction after total laryngectomy: a new one-stage surgical technique. J Otolaryngol Jpn 1977; 80:779-85.

13. Sisson GA, Goldman ME. Pseudoglottis procedure: update and secondary reconstruction techniques. Laryngoscope (In press).

14. Komorn RM. Vocal rehabilitation in the laryngectomized patient with a tracheoesophageal shunt. Ann Otol Rhinol Laryngol 1974; 83:445-51.

Ann Otol 89:1980

NEOGLOTTIC RECONSTRUCTION FOLLOWING TOTAL LARYNGECTOMY

A REAPPRAISAL

BRUCE LEIPZIG, MD

GALVESTON, TEXAS

The purpose of this paper is to analyze the problems and complications which have resulted from neoglottic reconstruction at the University of Texas Medical Branch in Galveston. It has been performed as a primary procedure at the time of laryngectomy on 50 patients. Over 40% of these patients have required a second operative procedure to control major complications of their neoglottis. Aspiration is a nearly constant feature of the procedure, and a significant number of patients do not tolerate it well. Radiation therapy does not appear to increase the number of problems, but the complications are more severe when they do occur, and they are more difficult to control. The indications for surgical neoglottic reconstruction cannot be extended beyond those tumors which are within the confines of the larynx without an increased incidence of major complications. Other relative contraindications to this surgery are poor patient pulmonary reserve, reflux esophageal incompetence, and a "hyperactive" gag reflex. Nine patients with prior treatment which included a total laryngectomy underwent secondary neoglottic reconstruction. In our experience, all have had significant aspiration. About one half of these patients developed speech. The procedure of neoglottic reconstruction must be reviewed critically prior to popular introduction into the surgical armamentarium. A plea for careful study by a small number of experienced surgeons is now in order.

The recent otolaryngologic literature contains several articles attesting to the reliability of the operation and the success of vocal rehabilitation with a one-stage neoglottic reconstructive technique based on that of Staffieri.[1-4] Numerous workshops and presentations seem to promote the operation as a simple procedure to learn and perform. A second modification is now receiving attention as a surgical technique of vocal rehabilitation for previous laryngectomees. The purpose of this paper is to analyze the problems and complications which have resulted from neoglottic reconstruction as a primary procedure following total laryngectomy on 50 patients, and as a secondary procedure for previous laryngectomies on 9 patients at the University of Texas Medical Branch in Galveston during the 3½ years from October 1976 to April 1980. Our initial enthusiasm for this surgical procedure must be tempered by a critical review of our results.

METHODS

Fifty-nine patients have undergone neoglottic reconstruction as described by Staffieri et al,[1] Griffiths and Leipzig,[2] and Leipzig et al[3] at the University of Texas Medical Branch in Galveston since October 1976 (Table 1). Objective analysis of the success or failure of neoglottic reconstruction has been assessed according to three major criteria: 1) the adequacy of cancericidal surgery which is evaluated by the success of local cancer control in the operative field; 2) the ability to swallow food as well as handle one's own secretions without aspiration through the neoglottic tracheoesophageal fistula; and 3) the production of vocal sounds that are acceptable for communication purposes. Further, the role of adjunctive radiotherapy has been evaluated to determine its effect on each of these three criteria.

TABLE 1. PATIENTS UNDERGOING NEOGLOTTIC RECONSTRUCTION

Year	*Primary*	*Secondary*
1976-1977	12	0
1977-1978	18	2
1978-1979	17	7
1979-1980 (6 months)	3	0
Total	50	9

RESULTS

At this time, nine patients have evidenced recurrence of their primary laryngeal cancer as shown in Table 2. Three have recurred locally, ie, at the site of the neoglottic fistula and tracheostoma. Each of these patients had subglottic extension of disease greater than 1 cm below the inferior margin of the true vocal cords on pathologic examination. Each should have had a lower resection of the trachea to prevent recurrence. Six other patients had recurrence of carcinoma; all were at sites metastatic to their original disease and resection. Nineteen patients had subglottic extension of a vocal cord carcinoma that was less than 1 cm in length, and none have recurred in the operative field following total laryngectomy and neoglottic reconstruction (Table 3).

TABLE 2. PATIENTS WITH RECURRENCE OF PRIMARY TUMOR (N = 9)

Site	*No.*
Local (stoma)	3
Regional	3
Distant	3

From the Department of Otolaryngology, Division of Head and Neck Oncology, University of Texas Medical Branch, Galveston.

Presented at the meeting of the American Laryngological Association, Palm Beach, Florida, April 14-15, 1980.

REPRINTS — Bruce Leipzig, MD, Department of Otolaryngology, Division of Head and Neck Oncology, University of Texas Medical Branch, Galveston, TX 77550.

TABLE 3. SUBGLOTTIC EXTENSION AT PATHOLOGIC EXAMINATION

	No. Patients	*Recurrence*
None	28	5
Less than 1 cm	19	1
More than 1 cm	3	3*
Total	50	9

*Local (stoma).

All patients undergoing neoglottic reconstruction, whether primary or secondary, have some difficulty with aspiration. The aspiration is often minor with only a bubble of saliva evident at the neoglottic fistula when the patient attempts to swallow; but in 40% of patients undergoing primary reconstruction, it is a potential threat to life. In order to objectively evaluate this difficulty, each patient was assigned a grade from 1 to 4 as seen in Table 4, with grades 3 and 4 considered major complications, which potentially threaten survival from the operation. Twenty of 50 patients (40%) experienced aspiration to a significant degree (Table 5); 14 of these 20 neoglottic fistulae required revision, and one half of them were closed in order to control aspiration.

Among patients who received a neoglottic fistula metachronous to total laryngectomy, ie, a secondary neoglottic reconstruction, aspiration has been an even more serious problem (Table 5). All of these patients experienced major difficulty, with six of nine patients evaluated as grade 3 and 4 aspirators. Most patients have required or chosen closure of their neoglottis after attempts at revision surgery were unsuccessful to control aspiration.

TABLE 4. COMPLICATIONS OF ASPIRATION

Grade	
1	Bubble on neoglottic fistula
2	Occasional cough, no significant problems
3	Constant cough, worse with eating (ie, potentially dangerous)
4	Pneumonia

The third major area of evaluation is neoglottic speech. A simple objective evaluation of the success of the operation in this area requires, as its only criterion, that the patient be able to communicate primarily with his neoglottic voice. The patient who can make sounds or utter an occasional word or syllable cannot be considered a successful neoglottic speaker. Utilizing this criterion, neoglottic speech was evaluated in each patient (Table 6) with grades 1 and 2 considered as "success." Using these criteria, 25 of 50 patients (50%) who underwent primary neoglottic reconstruction and 4 of 9 patients (44%) who underwent secondary neoglottic reconstruction had successful voice production (Table 7).

TABLE 5. RECONSTRUCTION PATIENTS EXPERIENCING ASPIRATION (N = 50)

Grade	*Primary*	*Secondary*
1	15	0
2	15	3
3	13	4
4	7	2

TABLE 6. EVALUATION OF NEOGLOTTIC SPEECH

Grade	
1	Excellent subjective speech
2	Communicates with voice primarily
3	Occasional word or syllable produced
4	Requires lip reading to understand sounds

TABLE 7. VOICE PRODUCTION FOLLOWING NEOGLOTTIC RECONSTRUCTION (N = 50)

	No. Patients	
Grade	*Primary*	*Secondary*
1	7	2
2	18	2
3	11	4
4	14	1

Radiation therapy is not a contraindication to neoglottic reconstruction. However, when a patient who has had radiation therapy experiences a problem or complication from neoglottic reconstruction, it is more difficult to alleviate or cure the problem. Patients receiving radiotherapy develop voice in about one half of cases: 13 of 27 patients who received some regimen of radiotherapy developed voice; however, 14 (52%) of these patients required revision surgery in order to control a major complication (Table 8). The most common reason for revision surgery was aspiration. Another common reason was spontaneous closure of the neoglottis during radiation treatment. In comparison, 12 of 23 patients who did not receive radiotherapy developed voice, and 8 (34%) required revision to control complications related to their neoglottis. Again, the most common reason for reoperation in this group of patients was for control of aspiration. A similar pattern may be seen among patients who underwent secondary neoglottic reconstruction (Table 8).

DISCUSSION

A critical review of the problems and complications which have resulted has highlighted several

TABLE 8. VOICE PRODUCTION FOLLOWING RADIOTHERAPY (N = 50)

	No. Patients			
	Primary		*Secondary*	
	Voice	*No Voice*	*Voice*	*No Voice*
None	12 (4*)	11 (4*)	2 (2*)	1
Preoperative	2	1*		
Postoperative	10 (6*)	12 (6*)		
Perioperative			2 (2*)	4 (3*)
Full course	1	1*	0	0
Total	25	25	4	5

*Revision required.

TABLE 9. PRIMARY NEOGLOTTIC RECONSTRUCTIONS (N = 50)

Site of Primary Tumor	No. Performed	Success
Glottic larynx	20	14 (70%)
Supraglottis	14	7 (50%)
Subglottis	3	0 (9%)
Pyriform sinus	11	3 (27%)
Vallecula	2	1

areas of concern and contraindication for neoglottic reconstruction. Several problem areas which were not initially apparent to us deserve special consideration.

Patients with subglottic extension of tumor for more than 1 cm below the inferior edge of the true vocal cords should not be considered for neoglottic reconstruction at the time of primary resection and total laryngectomy. Resection of four or five tracheal rings and a low entry into the cervical esophagus make creation of the neoglottic flap technically difficult, and lesser surgery compromises the patient's chance for cure.

Patients whose primary tumor extends beyond the confines of the larynx so that an extended laryngectomy is required, including either a portion of the pharyngeal wall, the vallecula, or the base of tongue, should not be considered for neoglottic reconstruction. To date, 16 of 50 patients have undergone primary neoglottic reconstruction for tumors outside of the larynx (Table 9). Only four of those patients (25%) have had a successful reconstruction according to the criteria of a communicative voice without significant aspiration, as well as a surgical procedure which is cancericidal for local disease. Fifty percent of patients with supraglottic lesions had a successful neoglottic reconstruction, and only among those patients whose tumor was at the level of the true vocal cords was the rate of success comparable to that in the European series (70%). Extensive lesions requiring a large resection of pharynx or tongue make neoglottic reconstruction very difficult. The additional loss of tissue, as well as untoward scarring, lead to gaping of the neoglottic fistula with attendant aspiration.

Aspiration is a nearly constant feature of the procedure and a significant number of patients do not tolerate it well. Many patients have required revision surgery in an attempt to control aspiration, and, among these, half have required closure of the neoglottis. Patients with poor pulmonary reserve do not tolerate even slight aspiration which may predispose to a terminal pneumonia.

Reflux of gastric contents into the esophagus, with possible subsequent aspiration of these gastric contents, should make the cautious surgeon wary of performing neoglottic reconstruction in the patient with esophageal reflux incompetence.

Patients with poor pulmonary function often have difficulty using the neoglottis for speech. A well-constructed neoglottis will remain closed unless considerable pressure is directed through the neoglottis from the trachea. The patient with a low vital capacity will be unable to open his neoglottis or will only be able to use it in a halting fashion (grade 3 or 4 speech). There is no exact volume of air which a patient must be capable of inhaling in order to use his neoglottic fistula; however, patients with severe obstructive and restrictive disease are poor candidates for the procedure.

The adjunctive use of radiotherapy does not appear to significantly increase the risk of complications from neoglottic reconstruction. However, when problems and complications arise, they are harder to control and cure. Patients who have received radiotherapy, either before or after neoglottic reconstruction, have required more revision surgery than those who have not received any radiation therapy (34 vs 52%, $P = 0.05$). More of these patients have required closure of their neoglottis to control aspiration; several have closed spontaneously during radiation treatment. This is sometimes prevented by keeping a piece of black silk suture through the neoglottis. The silk suture is kept in place until radiotherapy is completed, and may serve as a useful guide for occasional office dilatation of the neoglottis in these patients.

Revision surgery has been necessary in 22 of 50 patients undergoing primary neoglottic reconstruction (aspiration in 14 cases, radiotherapy closure in 8). The surgery has been required to control major complications of the neoglottic reconstruction; it has been required more commonly in patients receiving adjunctive radiotherapy than in those who do not receive any radiotherapy.

Secondary neoglottic reconstruction has been very unsuccessful in our experience. All patients experience significant aspiration and less than half have developed communicative voice. The procedure has been fraught with many complications which have been poorly controlled, requiring revision surgery in seven of nine patients to date.

There should be additional critical review of the procedure of neoglottic reconstruction prior to its popular introduction into the surgical armamentarium. Careful study by a small number of experienced surgeons should elucidate indications for a more careful selection of patients and should prepare the surgeon to give better preoperative counseling for neoglottic reconstruction in order to optimize the chance for success.

REFERENCES

1. Staffieri M, Procacini A, Steiner W, et al. Rehabilitation der stimme nach laryngektomie: chirurgische rehabilitation der stimme nach laryngektomie. Laryngol Rhinol Otol Stuttg 1978; 57:477-88.

2. Griffiths CM, Leipzig B. Surgical restoration of voice after total laryngectomy: problems, complications, and revision surgery. In: Bernstein L, ed. Proceedings of the Third International Symposium on Plastic and Reconstructive Surgery of the Head and Neck. New York: Grune & Stratton Inc (in press).

3. Leipzig B, Griffiths CM, Shea JP. Neoglottic reconstruction following total laryngectomy: the Galveston experience. Ann Otol Rhinol Laryngol 1980; 89:204-8.

4. Leipzig B, Griffiths CM. Neoglottic reconstruction following total laryngectomy. Film, American College of Surgeons Motion Picture Library, Chicago, 1979.

≈

NINCDS NOTES*

Dr. Donald B. Tower, NINCDS Director since 1974, has announced that he will retire February 1, 1981. He will end a 28-year career with NINCDS. During his directorship, Dr. Tower reorganized the Institute along program lines, greatly strengthening extramural programs. He also oversaw an extensive survey of neurological and communicative disorders research; seven panels of experts developed a comprehensive long-range plan for research in neurological and communicative disorders. A search committee will begin at once seeking candidates for the NINCDS directorship.

The Department of Health and Human Services has issued regulations dealing with recipients of federal funds who violate the law or fail to honor the terms of previous awards. The "debarment" regulations were published in the Federal Register of October 9, 1980. For copies write to: Office of Scientific and Health Reports, NINCDS.

*This information is prepared monthly by the Office of Scientific and Health Reports, National Institute of Neurological and Communicative Disorders and Stroke, National Institutes of Health, Bldg. 31, Rm. 8A06, Bethesda, MD 20205. (301) 496-5751.

Ann Otol 89:1980

LARYNGOLOGY AND THE NUMBERS GAME

FRANK E. LUCENTE, MD

NEW YORK, NEW YORK

Numbers play a great role in our practice of laryngology, and when used appropriately can be extremely valuable. However, careless or uncritical use may cause them to be an impediment or detriment to clinical practice and teaching. Examples of problems which arise with numbers are readily found in the areas of tumor staging (TNM system), the scientific literature, resident training and communications with third-party agencies. Consideration of these examples reminds us of the need to evaluate our use of numbers frequently.

Numbers dominate our daily lives and pervade our medical thinking. The communications media use numbers in a medical sense to signify the import of a disease or an injury. The government and other third-party agencies ask us to quantify symptoms, findings, and results in order to provide a tangible product with which they might deal. And by academic training, natural inclination, or simple pragmatics we learn to express everything numerically. The advent of computers, machines which function almost exclusively on the basis of numbers, makes our burden in this area even more pressing.

Are there any disadvantages or dangers to our use of numbers? First, the acquisition, computation and application of numbers is time-consuming. Secondly, the process of quantification lengthens and complicates our intellectual work. Thirdly, there is a potential for deleterious redefinition of the doctor-patient relationship if the interposition of numbers and machines between the two persons is not handled carefully.

In looking at numbers in laryngology we encounter four basic questions: Why do we need numbers? Do they mean anything? How accurately do we acquire them? Do we keep them in perspective? Let us consider these questions in regard to several aspects of our specialty: clinical practice, especially tumor staging (TNM system), the scientific literature, residency training and dealing with regulatory agencies.

In the area of clinical practice we encounter the TNM system, a tool used to quantify, classify and give statistical significance to our diagnostic and prognostic approach to cancer. But what are the limitations of this system? What are the unconsidered factors which may overrule, outweigh, or invalidate the considered factors?

For example, with T for tumor, what about the exact size or degree of histological differentiation? What about the characteristics of the border of the tumor and its relationship to surrounding tissue? Is a pushing border different from an infiltrating border? Maybe we should divide T_3s in the supraglottis into several groups. For example, the large anaplastic T_3 with an infiltrating border differs from a small, well-differentiated T_3 with a pushing border. The present T-system also fails to give adequate attention to certain danger areas such as the base of the aryepiglottic fold where a small tumor may readily involve the posterior commissure region. It also risks understaging those iceberg tumors, lesions with a small surface presentation and extensive submucosal infiltration, demonstrated so well by total laryngeal sections of Kirchner[1] and others.

With nodes the TNM system is based on size, number and fixation. However, many of us have seen that the amount of fixation may vary inversely with the experience of the examiner and with his inclination towards surgery. The student, referring physician, or junior resident frequently describes nodes as fixed while the senior attending staff man may be less likely to concur in that diagnosis. This difference in interpretation clouds the literature.

Size, too, is elusive. I recently assembled six round objects and asked three residents and three experienced head and neck surgeons to give the size of each in centimeters. One of the residents gave the best estimates, being off by an average of only 7%. The other two residents were off by 33% and 36%. The attending staff men did slightly better. However, of all 36 measurements offered, 11 were off by more than 30%, even when there was no intervening tissue to hamper palpation. The inaccuracy of these measurements may potentially lead to an inaccurate staging in the TNM system. An additional problem with the N classification is the failure to specify the level of the node.

Although many of the concerns about the TNM system are minor, they raise questions about the accuracy and the value of the TNM system and possibly suggest a conflict between an individualized, patient-oriented approach and the numerical ap-

From the Department of Otolaryngology, Mount Sinai School of Medicine, New York, New York.

Presented at the meeting of the American Laryngological Association, Palm Beach, Florida, April 14-15, 1980.

REPRINTS — Frank E. Lucente, MD, Director, Department of Otolaryngology, City Hospital Center at Elmhurst, Elmhurst, NY 11373.

proach of this system. Are there ways to improve the system and to include factors which are presently ignored? Can we include comorbidity or concurrent disease? Can we list age, sex, marital status, or socioeconomic level, all of which factors may determine therapy and influence survival more than a T or an N or an M?

What about the diagnostic and prognostic role of the patient's symptoms? We are all familiar with the ominous import of pain or respiratory distress in a patient with laryngeal carcinoma, and yet there is no provision for the inclusion of symptoms in the present system. It is particularly important to focus on comorbidity, for our duty is to characterize a lesion in a given patient and to select a therapy and predict an outcome for that patient. Therefore, the inclusion of significant information about concurrent medical diseases is extremely important. Feinstein and associates[2,3] have developed elaborate but useful systems for the classification of comorbid factors and several years ago I suggested the SHAMONT system which added an S for surgeon, H for hospital, A for associate, and O for oncologic facilities to the standard TNM.[4] However, now I would tend to question the applicability of any alphanumeric system.

The value of the TNM system for comparing case series among institutions is also reduced when one considers the fact that in any given year approximately 30,000 new head and neck carcinomas present, and yet the TNM system includes 800 possible categories, perhaps too many categories for so few cases. When one considers the vagaries of measurement within these categories and the nuances of interpretation, one sees that meaningful communication among cancer centers is difficult.

Having considered the role of numbers in our approach to tumor staging, let us direct our attention to three other areas: publications, resident training and third-party involvement in medicine.

The burden to publish continues unabated and some of our publications tend to show an increasing emphasis on statistical significance rather than clinical significance. Series are large, numbers abound, and they are manipulated with ease. But what has happened to the old notion of studying a few patients in depth over a long period and learning from the evolution of disease and the longitudinal evaluation of therapy — characteristics of the medical literature 50 years ago? How often do we hear today of 10 or 20-year follow-up? How often do we see an outdated procedure retracted? Has our research become acquisitive rather than inquisitive? We still need large prospective randomized controlled studies in which the number of variables is minimized and the intrusion of extraneous factors is reduced. They are understandably difficult to produce.

Numbers also have their impact in our training programs with residents being tempted to concern themselves more with acquiring numbers, compiling lengthy operative lists, rather than in studying patients intensively. Perhaps we have all engaged in the easy task of doing a cross-sectional analysis of a large number of patients at one stage of their disease rather than in waiting to report on those patients studied for a longer time. Therefore, we can appreciate the problem of the resident who does not always have the opportunity for such longitudinal studies. However, it is necessary to bring this aspect to their training. In attending daily resident rounds at a teaching hospital, I am often confronted by questions which suggest that the diagnostic or therapeutic decision will be based on the application of probability of a few superficial observations rather than a more time-consuming and intensive analysis and a full appreciation of the history. How difficult it is to teach history-taking and patience.

The final area of concern with numbers is that of governmental and third-party involvement in medicine. Many of us are becoming increasingly aware of the quantity orientation of the city, state, and federal governments. Departmental privileges are granted on the basis of bed occupancy and outpatient volume. Hospitals are reimbursed on the basis of the number of beds occupied. In the surgical line, the only important factor seems to be the number of procedures performed. No attention is given to duration or complexity of procedure, frequency of complications, efficiency of preoperative evaluation, and the results of surgery. One seems to be rewarded for playing the numbers game by admitting a few extra patients, keeping them a few days longer, and scheduling more tonsillectomies and fewer jaw-neck dissections. Once again we see the problem of numbers themselves influencing the practice of medicine.

Having looked at these several areas of numerical involvement, we might wonder about the source of some of these problems. Why do we have an affinity for numbers? Is it because they seem concrete? Are they the foundation of medical science or are they a refuge? Do they possibly have an anesthetic effect — mesmerizing or even seducing the mind? Is it foreseeable that they will dominate our specialty and distract us from those observations which defy quantification and from the intuition, fostered by experience and responsive to serendipity, which influences so much of our therapy? Do we even have areas in which there are no numbers, such as nonverbal communication and the psychosomatic aspects of clinical practice?

As we meet yearly to hear reports of new and exciting advances in science, we might profitably scrutinize any new procedure whose mathematical complexities smack of scientism, a term which means "an exaggerated trust in the efficacy of the methods of natural science to explain . . .

phenomena, to solve pressing human problems, or to provide a comprehensive unified picture of the meaning of the cosmos." We need numbers. We hope that they will be our friends and serve us well, but we should avoid any tendency to use them much as a drunk uses a lamppost, more for support than for illumination.

Even though we may not be able to propose better systems we must be grateful for the occasional opportunity to articulate our discomfort at the imperfections in any system and to suggest periodic reexamination of any tenets which we take for granted or any tools which we use routinely, even something so simple as a numerical system.

REFERENCES

1. Kirchner JA. 100 laryngeal cancers studied by serial section. Ann Otol Rhinol Laryngol 1969; 78:689-709.

2. Feinstein AR. The pre-therapeutic classification of comorbidity in chronic disease. J Chronic Dis 1970; 23:455-68.

3. Feinstein AR, Schimpff CR, Andrews JF Jr, Wells CK. Cancer of the larynx: a new staging system and a re-appraisal of prognosis and treatment. J Chronic Dis 1977; 30:277-305.

4. Lucente FE. Myths in medicine. Trans Am Acad Ophthalmol Otolaryngol 1975; 80:243-6.

≈

SECOND INTERNATIONAL CONFERENCE ON CHOLESTEATOMA AND MASTOID SURGERY

The Second International Conference on Cholesteatoma and Mastoid Surgery will be held March 22-27, 1981 in Tel-Aviv, Israel under the auspices of Tel-Aviv University and Weizmann Institute of Science. For further information contact: Professor J. Sade, P. O. Box 16271, Tel-Aviv, Israel. Telex: 342272 (Kenes) Tel-Aviv.

Ann Otol 89:1980

VOCAL CORD POSITIONING BY SELECTIVE DENERVATION
OLD TERRITORY REVISITED

CLARENCE T. SASAKI, MD
TAKESTUGU IKARI, MD
MASATOSHI HORIUCHI, MD
JOHN A. KIRCHNER, MD
NEW HAVEN, CONNECTICUT

Vocal cord positioning produced by selective laryngeal denervation remains a controversial issue in clinical laryngology. Previous studies fail to arrive at uniform conclusions for two important reasons: 1) failure to mark a reference sagittal plane from which to assess the degree of vocal cord lateralization, and 2) failure to recognize the influence of tracheostomy and respiratory positioning of the vocal cords. The present study makes use of photographic and electromyographic documentation in the assessment of the paralyzed cord. Physiologic inactivation of the cricothyroid muscle by tracheostomy is a key determinant of the lateralized cord observed in acute low vagal and recurrent nerve paralysis. Tracheostomy-related cricothyroid inactivation cannot be ignored as a major determinant of cord positioning in paralysis and should not be overlooked in determining the neuroanatomic site of injury.

INTRODUCTION

The characteristic configuration of the glottis produced by selective denervation is a controversial issue. Numerous studies performed in both animals and in human beings fail to arrive at a consensus of opinion. Conflicting explanations fill the laryngologic literature, creating vague insecurity at the very basis of our clinical judgments. In the beginning Semon[1] invoked sequential injury to neural fascicles within the recurrent laryngeal nerve to explain three stages of paralysis: 1) isolated abductor paralysis, 2) median paralysis, and 3) cadaveric paralysis. Each stage, Semon assumed, resulted from progressive neurofascicular involvement. Further clinical and laboratory observations however, failed to confirm Semon's predictions. Therefore, in apparent desperation more than half a century later, Ellis[2] whimsically ascribed the shape of the glottis to "personal qualities" of the larynx, indicating the level of frustration he experienced in correlating the site of the lesion with the appearance of the paralyzed vocal cord.

Assuming that both abductor and adductor muscles are denervated by injury to the recurrent laryngeal nerve, how is it that such injury classically produces a cord found in the adducted position? To Grossman[3] must go the credit for our present understanding of this phenomenon. In low vagal injury, the median position of the paralyzed cord is unquestionably due to the continued function of the ipsilateral cricothyroid muscle, an extrinsic tensor and adductor of the vocal cord innervated by the intact external division of the superior laryngeal nerve. Grossman's observation is therefore the key to our understanding of the cord paralyzed in the lateral position caused by injury to the vagus nerve above the nodose ganglion, a lesion which, of course, denervates the ipsilateral cricothyroid muscle.

One now had an acceptable neuroanatomic explanation for cord paralysis in either the adducted or the lateralized positions. In short, high vagal paralysis (above the nodose ganglion) produced an adducted cord.

Nevertheless, a number of reports described lateral paralysis due to low vagal injury, an observation inconsistent with the accepted level of neuroanatomic understanding. For example, Lewy and Mathews,[4] reported three cases of "lateral-lying" vocal cord paralysis following intrathoracic surgery. Hofer[5] reported four patients with glottic incompetence due to intrathoracic disease. Kirchner[6] observed glottic incompetence in three patients immediately after cardiovascular procedures. In these and other reports, although tracheostomy had been performed in some patients, its use was not always specified. It was therefore difficult to draw conclusions from published reports, because most of them lacked some essential point of information. Consequently, such observations on the paralyzed larynx exerted an unsettling mood among laryngologists in search of more precise neuroanatomic correlations.

Vocal cord positioning produced by selective laryngeal denervation therefore remains a controversial issue in clinical laryngology. In our opinion, numerous studies failed to arrive at uniform conclusions for two important reasons: 1) failure to mark a reference sagittal plane from which to assess the degree of vocal cord lateralization; and 2) failure to recognize the influence of tracheostomy on respiratory positioning of the vocal cords.

From the Department of Surgery, Section of Otolaryngology, Yale School of Medicine, New Haven, Connecticut. This study was supported by USPHS grant No. R01 HD 09494-05.

Presented at the meeting of the American Laryngological Association, Palm Beach, Florida, April 14-15, 1980.

REPRINTS — Clarence T. Sasaki, MD, Department of Surgery, Section of Otolaryngology, Yale School of Medicine, 333 Cedar Street, New Haven, CT 06510.

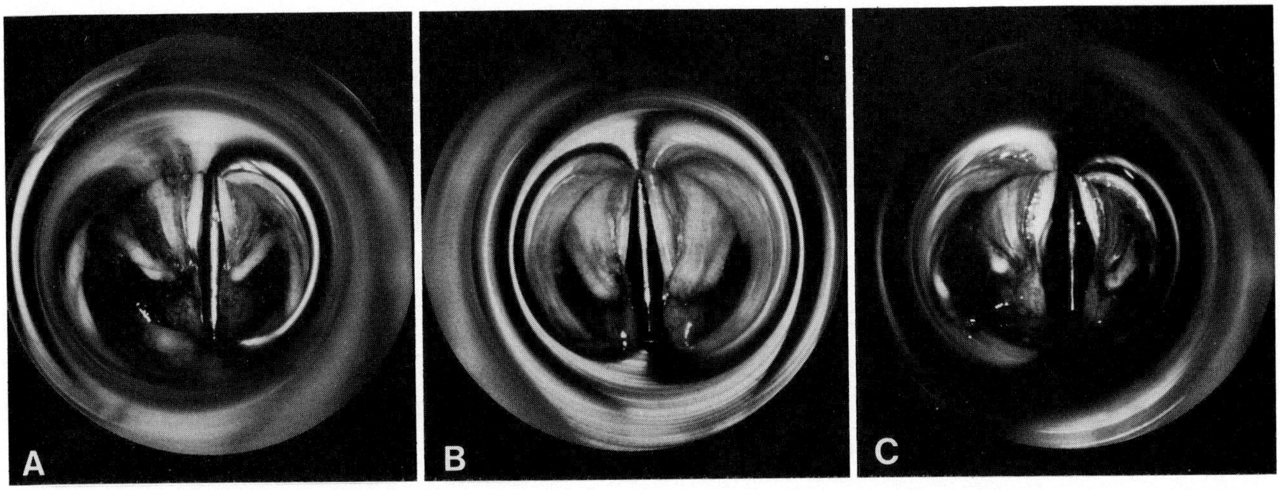

Fig. 1. Kowa photography of the larynx. A) Adducted position; B) intermediate position; C) abducted position. A pin marks the midline. The left cord lies on the left side of each frame.

The authors recognize that lateralized cords may result from muscle atrophy in cases of long-standing paralysis or cricoarytenoid arthritis from prolonged intubation. These are not, however, the situations we wish to address. Rather, it is the configuration of the glottis in acute paralysis that is in question.

Because the principal determinant of vocal cord position in acute low vagal injury is the ipsilateral cricothyroid muscle, its function is key to understanding glottic configuration in paralysis. What factors are capable of inactivating the neurologically intact cricothyroid muscle to cause a paralyzed cord to lateralize from the midline? In this study, the electromyographic activity of the cricothyroid muscle is therefore correlated with vocal cord positioning after selective laryngeal denervation in both tracheostomized and untracheostomized subjects.

METHODS

Ten adult dogs were anesthetized with pentobarbital sodium 25 mg/kg body weight. A constant level of anesthesia was maintained in stage III, plane I. The larynx and trachea in these spontaneously breathing dogs were exposed by a vertical midline neck incision. The right recurrent laryngeal nerve (RLN) was sectioned in four untracheostomized dogs. These four dogs were subsequently tracheostomized and restudied. In a second group of four untracheostomized dogs, the right vagus nerve was sectioned at the thoracic inlet. These four dogs were later tracheostomized and restudied. The remaining two undenervated control dogs were likewise studied before tracheostomy and restudied thereafter.

A Kowa camera was used to photograph the glottis before and after selective denervation. Electromyography (EMG) of the cricothyroid (CT) and posterior cricoarytenoid (PCA) muscles was accomplished with hooked wire electrodes (platinum-iridium 0.051 mm diameter). The electromyographic signal was amplified (DAM 5A, WP Instruments) and displayed on an oscilloscope (Tektronix 564). Oscilloscopic spike activity was photographed with a camera (Grass C-4).

Arterial blood gases, analyzed with a Radiometer PHM 72, were maintained within narrow physiologic limits. Body temperature, measured with a rectal thermometer, was kept at 38 C by warming the anesthetized animal with a heating pad placed beneath it.

Using a pin to mark the midline, we recognize three vocal cord positions, determined by Kowa photography (Fig. 1 A, B, C). 1) The adducted position refers to a median lie, 2) intermediate refers to a lateralized position, and 3) abducted refers to an extremely lateralized position.

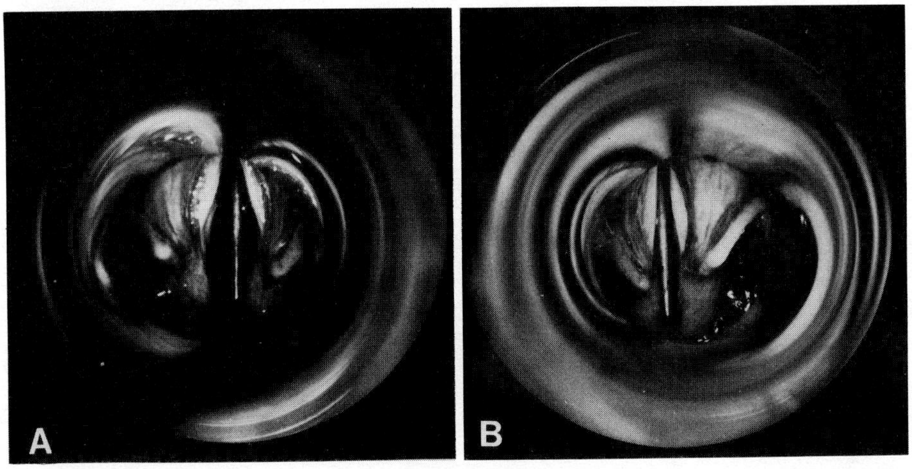

Fig. 2. Neurologically intact larynx *before* tracheostomy. A) Inspiration; B) expiration.

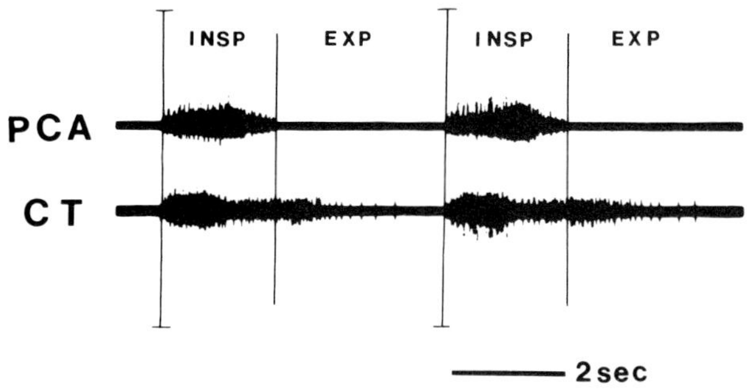

Fig. 3. EMG of right PCA and right CT muscles *before* tracheostomy. Phasic inspiratory activity of PCA produces cord abduction. CT activity on inspiration causes the cord to elongate. Expiratory CT activity causes the cord to adduct.

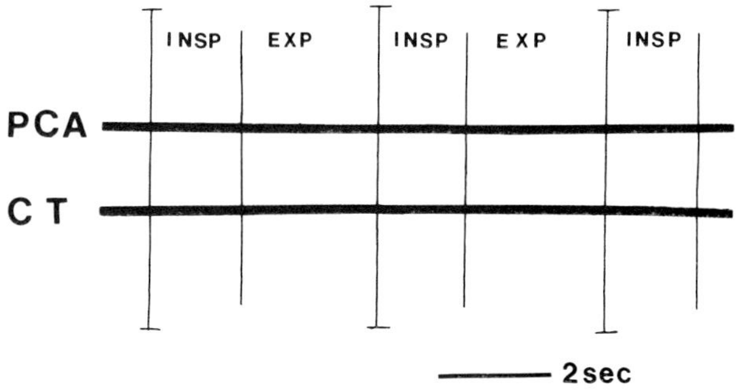

Fig. 5. Tracheostomy abolishes both PCA and CT activity.

RESULTS

Neurologically Intact Larynx Before Tracheostomy (Fig. 2 A, B). On the inspiratory phase of respiration the vocal cords abduct and elongate. While in expiration, the cords close to the median position. The reason for this is of course well-known. The PCA muscle becomes active on inspiration, thus producing cord abduction. On the other hand, the CT muscle acts in both phases of the respiratory cycle accounting for inspiratory elongation and expiratory adduction. In the normal spontaneously breathing dog, the glottis therefore widens on inspiration and narrows on expiration. Note that expiratory narrowing is an active phenomenon, not necessarily due to passive recoil alone (Fig. 3).

Neurologically Intact Larynx After Tracheostomy (Fig. 4 A, B). The vocal cords remain in the intermediate position in both phases of the respiratory cycle. Decreased airway resistance produced by the tracheostomy abolishes physiologic activity of both the PCA and CT muscles. The cords therefore remain practically motionless in both the inspiratory and expiratory phases of spontaneous respiration through the tracheostomy (Fig. 5).

Right Recurrent Laryngeal Nerve Section Before Tracheostomy (Fig. 6 A, B). On inspiration the intact left cord abducts and elongates, whereas the right denervated cord assumes the median position. Inspiratory CT activity causes the denervated cord to adduct on inspiration. In expiration, both cords adduct due to bilateral expiratory CT activity. Thus the denervated cord remains in the adducted position during both phases of the respiratory cycle by continued action of the CT muscle. Note that CT activity responsible for bringing the paralyzed cord to the midline position and keeping it there throughout the respiratory cycle is not tonic activity, but clearly phasic in its pattern of behavior. That is to say, there is clearly an inspiratory burst of activity followed by distinct expiratory spike distribution (Fig. 7).

Right Recurrent Laryngeal Nerve Section After Tracheostomy (Fig. 4 A, B). Both vocal cords assume the intermediate position throughout the respiratory cycle. Tracheostomy abolishes the physiologic activity of both PCA and CT muscles (Fig. 5). In very light anesthesia, during coughing, the neu-

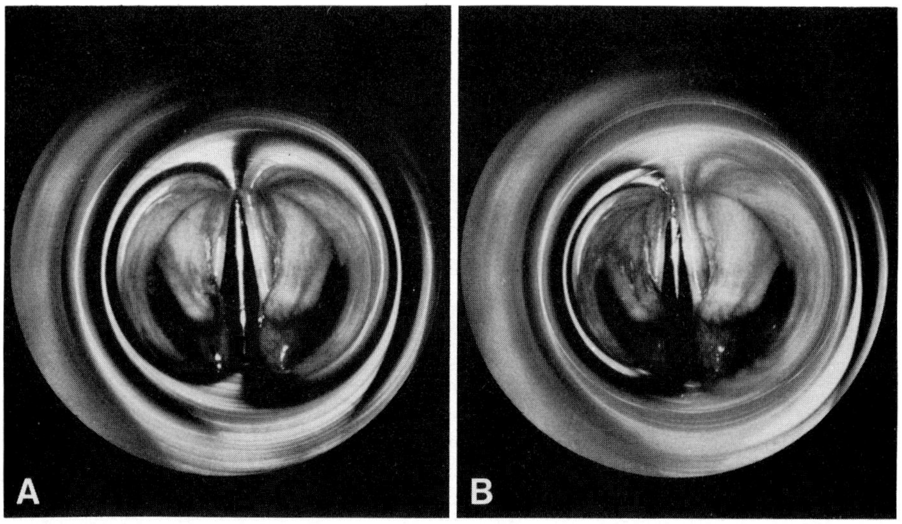

Fig. 4. Appearance of the larynx *after* tracheostomy. A) Inspiration; B) expiration. The left cord lies on the left side of each frame.

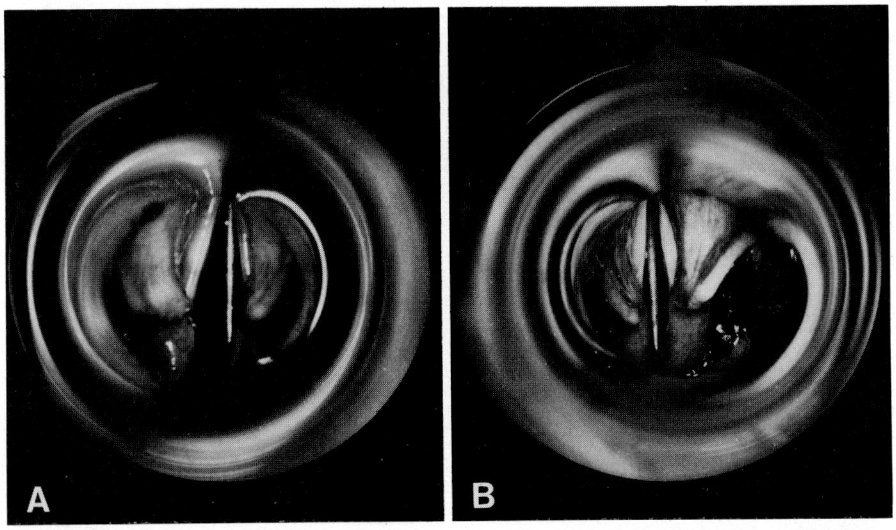

Fig. 6. Right recurrent nerve section *before* tracheostomy. A) On inspiration the intact left cord abducts and elongates. The denervated right cord is adducted. B) On expiration both cords adduct. (An identical pattern is seen after right vagotomy.) The left cord lies on the left side of each frame.

rologically intact cord adducts, but the denervated cord remains in its intermediate position. Due to mechanical disadvantage of this cord, an ineffective cough results (Fig. 8).

Right Vagotomy Before Tracheostomy (Fig. 6 A, B). On inspiration the intact left cord abducts and elongates whereas the right denervated cord assumes the median position. Inspiratory CT activity causes the denervated cord to adduct. On expiration, both cords assume the median position due to bilateral CT contraction. The pattern of vocal cord positioning from vagotomy is therefore identical to that of right RLN section before tracheostomy.

Right Vagotomy After Tracheostomy (Fig. 4 A, B). Both vocal cords assume the intermediate position throughout the respiratory cycle. Tracheostomy abolishes the physiologic activity of both PCA and CT muscles. Again, when coughing is induced, the denervated cord, mechanically disadvantaged, fails to adduct sufficiently to produce an effective diaphragmatic expulsion of air (Fig. 8).

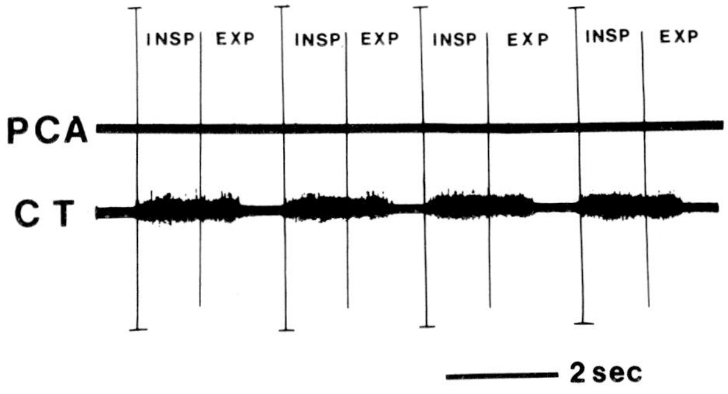

Fig. 7. EMG of the right PCA and right CT muscles *after* right recurrent laryngeal nerve section *before* tracheostomy. PCA is silent because it has been denervated. CT is active on inspiration and expiration.

From these observations it is quite clear that the glottic configuration produced by low vagal injury is identical to that caused by RLN injury. From a clinical standpoint, therefore, the position of the denervated cord does not allow one to readily distinguish between low vagal and recurrent laryngeal nerve interruption. More significant is the effect of tracheostomy on glottic configuration. Precisely how, therefore, does tracheostomy affect the respiratory activity of the laryngeal muscles?

The following explanations are key to an understanding of vocal cord positioning in the presence of tracheostomy. As ventilatory resistance decreases, the inspiratory activity of PCA diminishes (Fig. 9). After three to five minutes of tracheostomized breathing, inspiratory PCA activity disappears. It is therefore apparent that a critical level of ventilatory resistance is essential for continued PCA inspi-

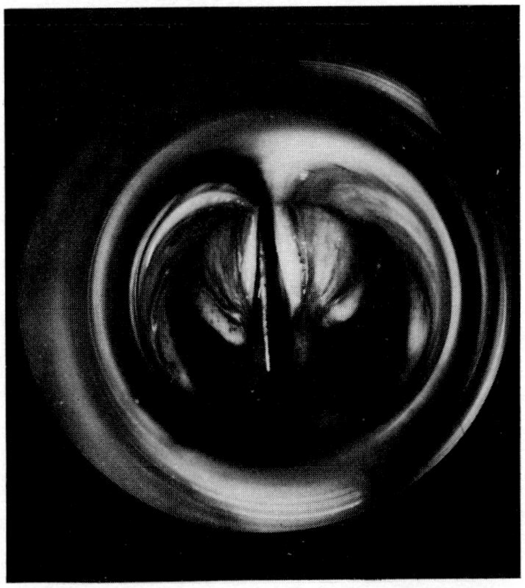

Fig. 8. During a cough, the denervated right cord fails to adduct sufficiently from its lateralized position.

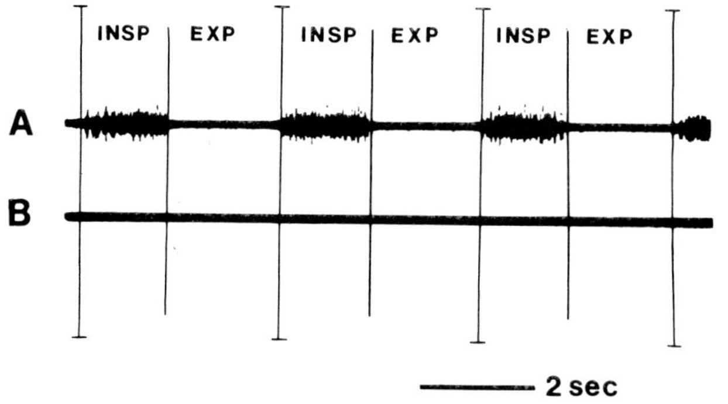

Fig. 9. EMG of the PCA muscle. A) Before tracheostomy; B) after tracheostomy.

ratory contractions.[7] The effect of tracheostomy on CT inspiratory activity is even more striking. Immediately upon reducing ventilatory resistance, inspiratory CT contraction is abolished[8] (Fig. 10).

On the other hand, expiratory CT activity is directly controlled by a rise in subglottic pressure. This evoked response continues for as long as subglottic pressure remains elevated[8] (Fig. 11). The threshold of this pressure-sensitive response is determined by a critical rate of rise in subglottic pressure, measuring 30 cm of water per second in normocapneic, well-oxygenated dogs[8] (Fig. 12). Therefore, when tracheostomy abolishes the critical pressure changes necessary to trigger expiratory CT contraction, it necessarily inactivates this muscle in expiration as well (Fig. 10).

DISCUSSION

Physiologic inactivation of the CT muscle by tracheostomy is therefore an important consideration in the evaluation of the paralyzed cord. Grossman's early observations carry the highest significance only if one recognizes the modifying role of tracheostomy on cord position. The authors suggest that lateralized cord paralysis may result from low vagotomy, if the ipsilateral CT muscle is physiologically inactivated. Although some have speculated that vagal interruption may mysteriously "inhibit" the CT muscle,[9] this suggestion remains unconfirmed by the present data. Rather, the role of tracheostomy is of far greater significance in CT inactivation and should therefore be recognized as a key determinant of the lateralized cord observed in acute low vagal or RLN paralysis. Tracheostomy-related CT inactivation cannot be ignored as a major determinant of cord positioning in paralysis.

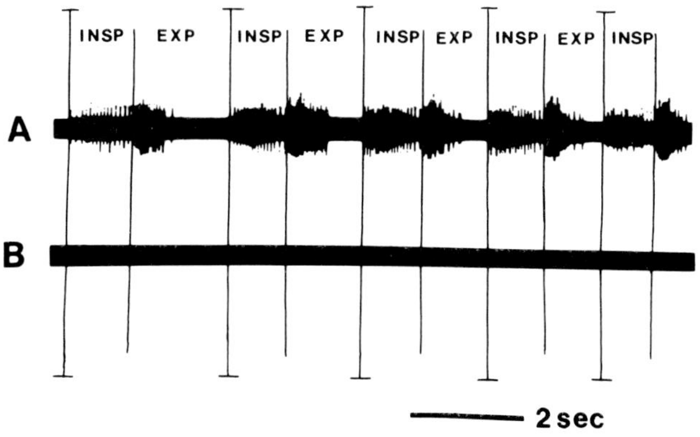

Fig. 10. EMG of the CT muscle. A) Before tracheostomy; B) after tracheostomy.

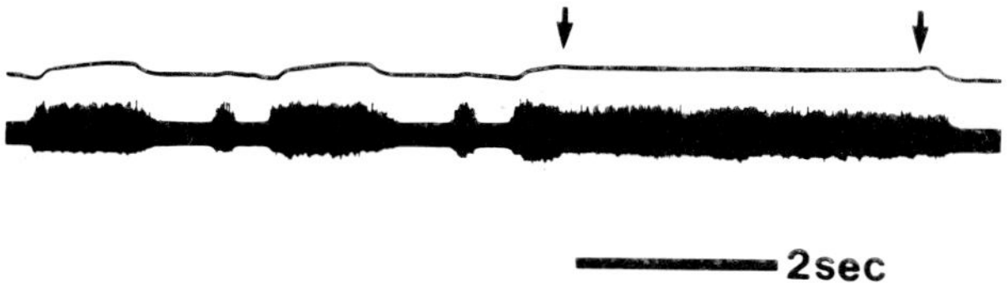

Fig. 11. EMG of the CT muscle (bottom tracing). Subglottic pressure (top tracing). Duration of positive pressure stimulation determines duration of CT evoked activity (arrows).[8]

The authors do not suggest that every case of lateralized paralysis is due to tracheostomy. This, of course, would involve faulty and improper deduction. What we do emphasize is that tracheostomy can and will cause lateralization of a paralyzed cord, and that this should not be overlooked in determining the neuroanatomic site of injury.

We hope these observations will further clarify and strengthen our understanding of basic laryngologic principles by responding to the quest raised by Semon more than a century ago.

The authors do not suggest that every case of lateralized paralysis is due to tracheostomy. This, of course, would involve faulty and improper deduction. What we do emphasize is that tracheostomy can and will cause lateralization of a paralyzed cord, and that this should not be overlooked in determining the neuroanatomic site of injury.

We hope these observations will further clarify and strengthen our understanding of basic laryngologic principles by responding to the quest raised by Semon more than a century ago.

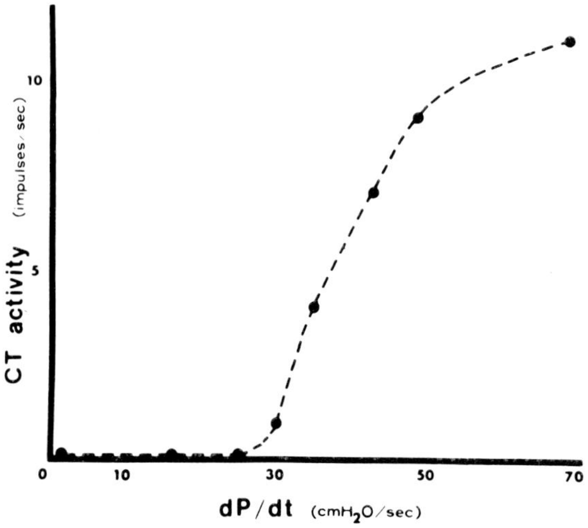

Fig. 12. The threshold of CT elicitation in response to rate of tracheal pressure change measures 30 cm H_2O/sec in a normocapneic, well-oxygenated dog.[8]

REFERENCES

1. Semon F. On the proclivity of abductor fibers of the recurrent laryngeal nerve to become affected sooner than the adductor fibers. Arch Otolaryngol 1881; 2:197-222.

2. Ellis M. Modern trends in diseases of the ear nose and throat. London: Butterworths, 1954.

3. Grossman M. Contribution to the mutual functional relationships of the muscles of the larynx. Arch Laryngol Rhinol 1906; 18:463-71.

4. Lewy RB, Mathews R. Immediate temporary restoration of glottic valve function. Laryngoscope 1965; 75:1348-51.

5. Hofer G. Untersuchungen bei Lahmunger der Motorischen Kehlkopfer. Acta Otolaryngol (Stockh) 1953; 43:100-7.

6. Kirchner JA. Intrathoracic injury to the motor nerve supply of the larynx. Acta Otolaryngol (Stockh) 1977; 83:163-9.

7. Sasaki CT, Fukuda H, Kirchner JA. Laryngeal abductor activity in response to varying ventilatory resistance. Trans Am Acad Ophthalmol Otolaryngol 1973; 77:403-10.

8. Horiuchi M, Sasaki CT. Cricothyroid muscle in respiration. Ann Otol Rhinol Laryngol 1978; 87:386-92.

9. Fukuda H, Kirchner JA. Changes in the respiratory activity of the cricothyroid muscle with intrathoracic interruption of the vagus nerve. Ann Otol Rhinol Laryngol 1972; 81:532-8.

≈

GUIDELINES FOR GRANTS
TRUSTEES OF THE RESEARCH FUND OF THE AMERICAN OTOLOGICAL SOCIETY, INC.

The members of the Board of Trustees of the Research Fund of the American Otological Society have determined guidelines for making grants from the Fund. The following is the formulation of policy.

Grants will be given in the area of otosclerosis: its diagnosis and management, the possible causes and underlying conditions, and an understanding of the disorder that may lead eventually to its prevention or cure.

The present lack of understanding of the disorder and the absence of similar conditions in other animals makes research in this field difficult. A direct approach to the disease may or may not be feasible; therefore, a sound strategy would be to use other approaches, such as the investigation of bone development, growth and repair under various conditions, and the study of other diseases that may be similar to otosclerosis. It is possible that investigations which may seem initially remote from otosclerosis may provide information which will eventually lead to a substantive further understanding of the disease process which underlies otosclerosis. The applicant should describe correlations between proposed research with the clinical pathological entity of otosclerosis.

The policy is to aid and encourage research in the immediate field of otosclerosis and also in adjoining fields, if, in the opinion of the Board, there is a substantial promise that results obtained will be of assistance in the ways indicated, and may lead to the attainment of the objective of the further understanding of otosclerosis.

Applications for a research grant from the Research Fund of the American Otological Society may be obtained from the Office of the Secretary-Treasurer of the Research Fund of the American Otological Society. Write to Robert J. Ruben, M.D., Secretary-Treasurer, Department of Otolaryngology, Albert Einstein College of Medicine, 1300 Morris Park Avenue, Bronx, New York 10461; (212) 430-3036.

All grant requests must be submitted by January 31, 1981.

Ann Otol 89:1980

A SIMPLE METHOD OF LARYNGEAL PHOTOGRAPHY THROUGH THE OPERATING MICROSCOPE
"MACROLENS TECHNIQUE"

EIJI YANAGISAWA, MD
NEW HAVEN, CONNECTICUT

DAVID E. EIBLING, MD
TRAVIS AIR FORCE BASE, CALIFORNIA

MASAFUMI SUZUKI, MD
TOKYO, JAPAN

A simple and inexpensive method of laryngeal photography through the eyepiece of the operating microscope is described. Provided that the operating room is equipped with the microscope, the laryngoscope and the laryngoscope holder, the only essential equipment required is an "aperture-preferred" automatic single lens reflex camera with a 50 mm macrolens. The macrolens of the camera is placed against an eyepiece of the microscope and the laryngeal image is centered and focused via the viewfinder of the camera. The respiration of the patient is temporarily halted. The camera is held still and pictures taken. Kodak high speed Ektachrome® tungsten film ASA 160 is used and push-processed to ASA 320. With practice, one should be able to obtain satisfactory photographs of the larynx suitable for teaching and documentation.

Ever since the first documentation of the successful photography of the larynx by Thomas French in 1882, many different methods of laryngeal photography have been described.[1-9] Recent methods of significant value include direct laryngoscopic photography with the Holinger-Brubaker endoscopic camera;[2,4,9] microscopic photography using the Zeiss surgical microscope with a single lens reflex (SLR) camera attached to a photoadapter and a beam splitter;[6,7] and telescopic photography with a combination of a single lens reflex camera, a telephotolens, a straight or angled telescope, a fiberoptic light transmission sheath and an electronic flash unit.[2,3,5,8]

Although these methods may produce laryngeal pictures of high quality, the expense of the equipment is often prohibitive for the resident or the practicing otolaryngologist who uses it infrequently. The purpose of this paper is to describe a simple and inexpensive method of microlaryngeal photography that utilizes equipment possibly already owned by many otolaryngologists.

EQUIPMENT

The equipment required for this technique is 1) "aperture-preferred" automatic SLR camera; 2) 50 mm macrolens; 3) film; 4) Zeiss operating microscope; 5) laryngoscope; 6) Lewy laryngoscope holder; and 7) light source. Since most of the equipment mentioned above is available in the operating room of most teaching medical centers, the only essential equipment may be an "aperture-preferred" automatic SLR camera with a 50 mm macrolens.

Camera. Any 35 mm SLR camera, which has a built-in match-needle light metering system can be used. However, the periphery of the viewing screen of the camera is usually dark in microscopic photography and it is difficult to read the match-needle of the light metering system. Besides, it may be time-consuming to adjust the exposure. The authors, therefore, use an "aperture-preferred" automatic SLR camera exclusively for this technique. With such an "aperture-preferred" automatic camera, the photographer sets the aperture (f-stop) and the camera automatically sets the correct shutter speed.

The "aperture-preferred" automatic cameras tried by the authors include Nikon FE; Pentax ME; Minolta XG-7, XE-7 and Olympus OM 2. Any "aperture-preferred" camera equipped with a 50 mm macrolens can be used. It is important to mention that a "shutter-preferred" camera cannot be used for this technique.

The Pentax ME camera uses a visible colored light-emitting diode (LED) read-out system which signals under, correct, or overexposure. This is particularly useful in microlaryngoscopy photography in which the periphery of the picture is often dark and the match-needle may not be visible.

Macrolens. A 50 mm macrolens is used. When the macrolens is set at infinity and the microscope is focused with the eyepiece dial at 0, the laryngeal image as seen in the viewfinder of the camera should be in good focus (Fig. 1). The lens diaphragm (f-stop) is set at its maximum aperture

From the Section of Otolaryngology, Department of Surgery, Yale University School of Medicine, the Section of Otolaryngology, Department of Surgery, Hospital of St. Raphael, New Haven, Connecticut, and the Department of Otolaryngology, Keio University School of Medicine, Tokyo, Japan.
Presented at the meeting of the American Laryngological Association, Palm Beach, Florida, April 14-15, 1980.
REPRINTS — Eiji Yanagisawa, MD, 98 York Street, New Haven, CT 06511.

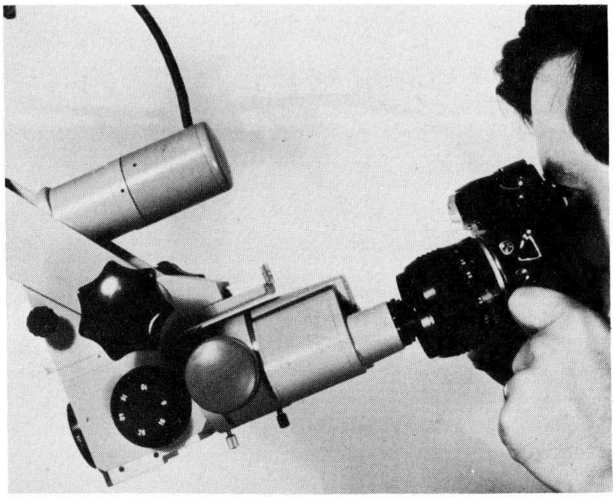

Fig. 1. The macrolens of the camera is placed over an eyepiece of the microscope. The laryngeal image should be in focus via the viewfinder of the camera.

(usually f 3.5) as a smaller aperture does not improve depth of focus in microscopic photography.

The design of the macrolens includes a recessed front housing which enables the lens to be placed directly over the eyepiece of the microscope without direct contact with the lens surface (Fig. 2).

Film. Kodak high speed Ektachrome color film tungsten (3200 K), ASA 160, was chosen after a trial of various color films since it gave the best color results. The film was exposed at ASA 320 and then push-processed as ASA 320. This can be processed by most laboratories for a nominal additional fee or mailed directly to the Kodak laboratory in their special processing envelope, ESP-1.

Laryngoscope. Standard Jako and Dedo laryngoscopes were used in most cases. More recently we have used the Dedo photographic laryngoscope.

Light Sources. Light sources used are 1) the standard laryngoscope light with the microscope light, 2) the standard laryngoscope light with the intensified microscope light using the House-Urban power supply unit, and 3) two Pilling regular light sources connected to each of two fiberoptic light cables of the standard Jako laryngoscope or the Dedo photographic laryngoscope. Every attempt is made to increase the amount of light illuminating the larynx as this allows faster shutter speeds and better photographic results.

The amount of light which falls upon the larynx when transmitted by fiberoptic light depends greatly upon the brightness of the original light source and the total diameter of light-transmitting fibers. The use of the large Jako-Pilling laryngoscope and cables is recommended whenever possible. The bright light sources specifically designed for photography such as Storz (xenon) or Wolf photographic unit, if available, should be utilized. We did not use them in our study.

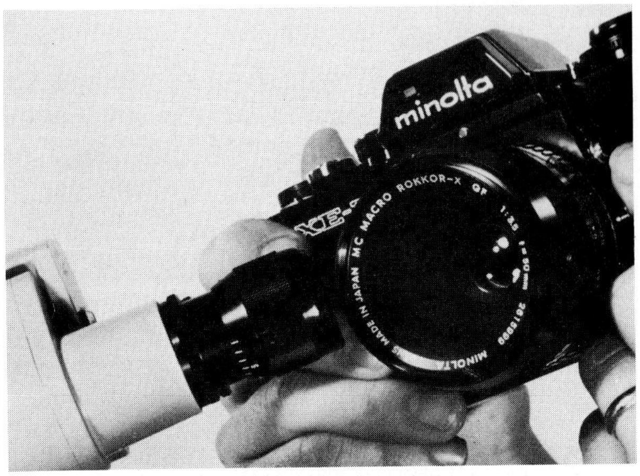

Fig. 2. The recessed front housing of the macrolens prevents direct contact of the lens surface with the eyepiece of the microscope.

TECHNIQUE

With the patient under oroendotracheal general anesthesia the laryngoscope is inserted, positioned, and suspended with the Lewy laryngoscope holder. For an adult patient, a No. 6 endotracheal tube is used.

The larynx is viewed and focused through the eyepieces (12.5 x) of the Zeiss operating microscope with 400 or 300 mm objective lens. If the magnification is set at 25x for a 400 mm lens or 16x for a 300 mm lens, a full-frame view of the vocal cords will be obtained in the camera viewfinder and it will not be necessary to enlarge the laryngeal picture later.

The macrolens is set at infinity and the aperture at maximum (usually f 3.5). The ASA film speed dial of the camera is set at 320 and the exposure compensation dial set at 0 (Fig. 3). The knobs at each joint of the microscope are then tightened to prevent camera movement during exposure.

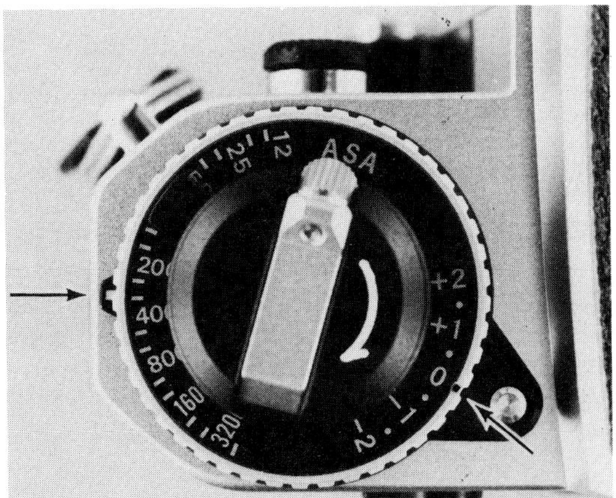

Fig. 3. The ASA film speed dial (left arrow) of the camera (Nikon FE) is set at ASA 320 and the exposure compensation dial at 0 (right arrow).

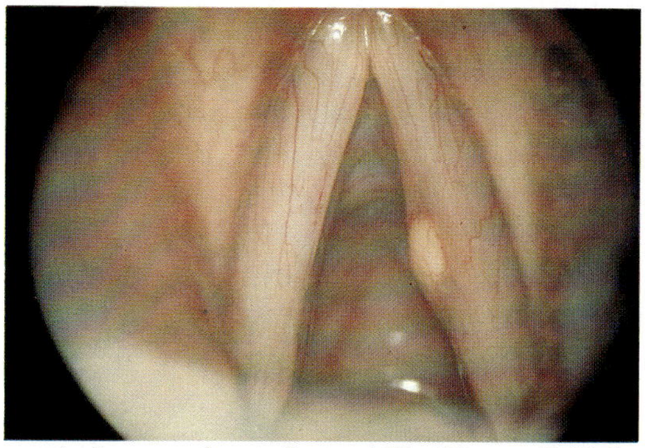

A. Laryngeal cyst: Pentax ME; 400 mm; X 25; f 3.5.

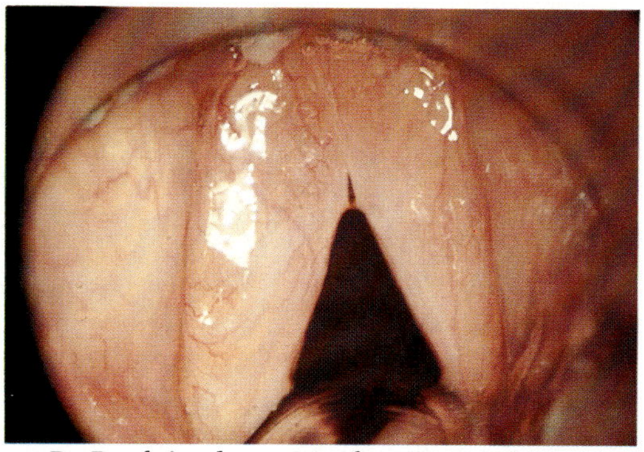

B. Reinke's edema: Minolta XE-7; 300 mm; X 16; f 3.5.

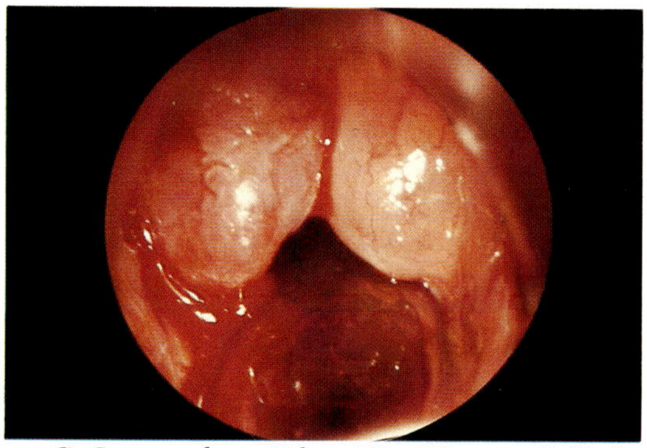

C. Large polyps: Nikon FE; 400 mm; X 25; f 3.5.

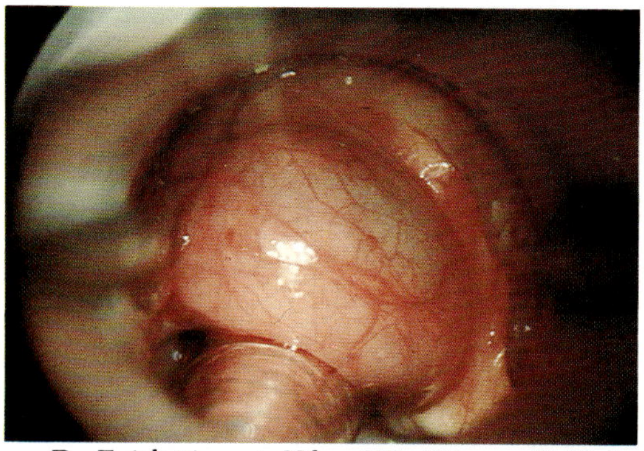

D. Epiglottic cyst: Nikon FE; 400 mm; X 16; f 3.5.

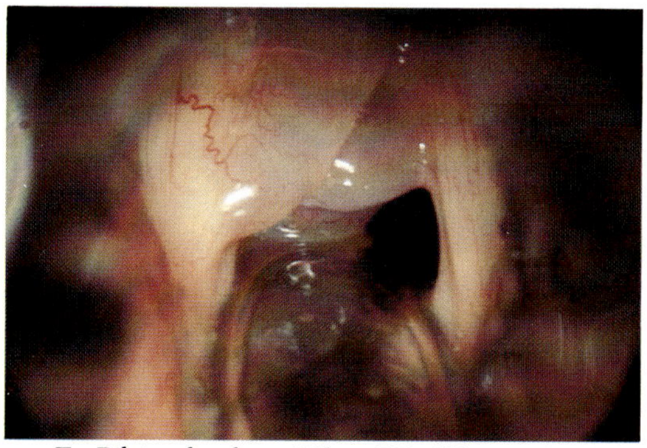

E. Bilateral polyps: Nikon FE; 400 mm; X 25; f 3.5.

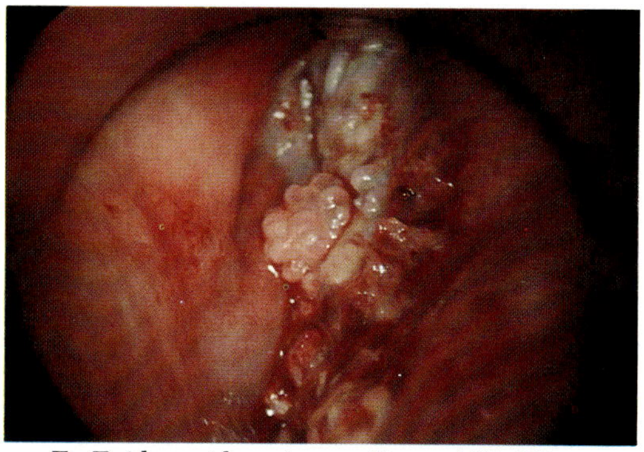

F. Epidermoid carcinoma: Pentax ME; 300 mm; X 16; f 3.5.

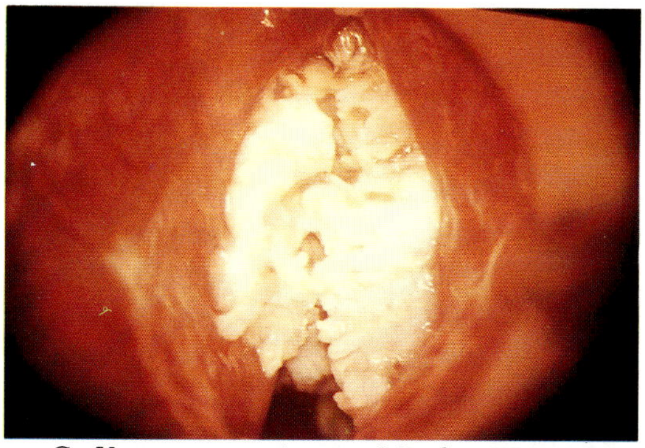

G. Verrucous carcinoma: Minolta XE-7; 400 mm; X 25; f 3.5.

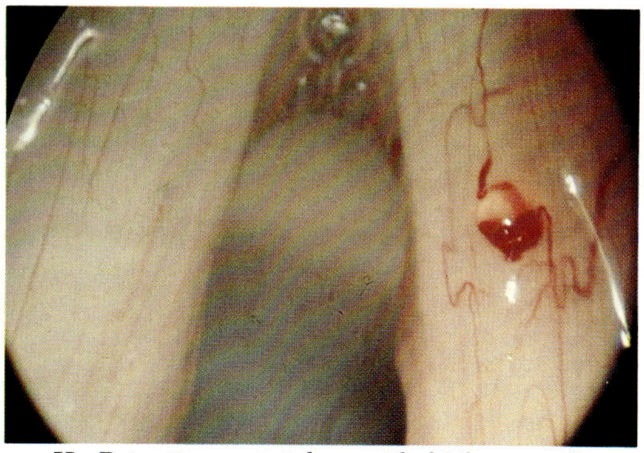

H. Retention cyst taken with high magnification; note the details of the cyst and its blood supply: Pentax ME; 400 mm; X 40; f 3.5.

Fig. 4. Representative photographs taken with the "macrolens technique" with notation of SLR camera, objective lens, magnification, and aperture (f-stop).

The macrolens of the camera is placed against an eyepiece of the microscope and the laryngeal image is centered and focused via the viewfinder of the camera (Fig. 1). Make certain that the subject is in perfect focus as viewed through the viewfinder of the camera. It may be necessary to change the subject-to-microscope distance slightly or turn the macrolens itself in either direction until the subject appears sharpest.

It is important to have an exact alignment of the optical axis of the microscope with the central axis of the laryngoscope.[7] Just prior to taking the picture, the anesthesiologist is asked to halt respiratory movement of the patient temporarily and the pictures are taken. Hold your breath at the moment of shutter release to insure that the camera is held very still. Shutter speeds may be as slow as one-half or one-fifteenth second.

At least three pictures are taken for each laryngeal pathology by bracketing the exposure time. In the "aperture-preferred" automatic camera, this can be accomplished by taking pictures at 0, +1 and −1 of the exposure compensation dial usually located on the top of your camera (Fig. 3).

RESULTS

Satisfactory results were obtained in over 70% of the laryngeal photographs taken. Representative color pictures of various laryngeal conditions taken with the macrolens technique are shown in Figure 4 A-F.

Poor results were mainly due to inadequate illumination and poor focusing. The most common cause was inadequate illumination. It is essential to sufficiently illuminate the larynx either by the laryngoscope light or by the intensified microscope light or by both. The standard laryngoscope light alone was not sufficient for photography. The standard laryngoscopic light with the intensified microscope light using the House Urban power supply provided adequate illumination for photography. Most of the pictures shown were taken using both the laryngoscope light and the intensified microscopic light. Unwanted light reflex from the edges of the laryngoscope can be eliminated by using larger magnification (400 mm objective lens with 25x magnification) or applying a bone wax over the edges of the laryngoscope.

If the power supply to intensify the microscope light is not available, the large Jako laryngoscope with two fiberoptic light cables should be used. Each cable is connected to two separate light sources. The Dedo photographic laryngoscope provided more than an adequate amount of light.

DISCUSSION

Although laryngeal photography with the macrolens technique has long been used in Japan, little has been mentioned in otolaryngologic literature. Since this is a very useful and practical method, we felt that it should be brought to the attention of those who believe that adequate laryngeal photography can only be accomplished with more sophisticated and expensive equipment.

In order to obtain the best possible picture, it is wise to "bracket" the exposure time. It is generally believed that when the "aperture-preferred" automatic camera is used you cannot control the exposure time. This is not true. To intentionally overexpose, turn the exposure compensation dial to the plus (+) side. The +1 represents one full f-stop of overexposure. To intentionally underexpose, turn the dial to the minus (−) side. The −1 represents one full f-stop of underexposure (Fig. 3).

Critical focusing is very important in microscopic photography. It is advisable to "bracket the focus." Since the depth of focus is very shallow in microscopic photography, only a portion of the laryngeal lesion may be in focus. When your focus is not correct, a small lesion may be entirely out of focus. Therefore, for the important pictures, take one picture at the correct focus and two others, one slightly closer to the subject and the other slightly away from the subject. This can be accomplished by turning the focusing dial of the microscope.

Admittedly, one cannot expect to take perfect pictures of the larynx with this simple and inexpensive method. Yet, if all of the steps described in this technique are carefully followed, satisfactory photographs of the larynx can be obtained in the majority of cases. With practice, you should be able to take surprisingly good pictures comparable to those obtained by using more expensive and sophisticated equipment.

SUMMARY

1. The "macrolens technique" is a simple and economical way to photograph the larynx via the eyepiece of the operating microscope.

2. Success of this technique depends upon: a) adequate illumination, b) critical focusing via the viewfinder of the camera, c) stabilization of the patient, the microscope and the camera.

3. This technique is relatively inexpensive and, with practice, good results may be obtained in more than 70% of the cases.

REFERENCES

1. French TR. On a perfected method of photographing the larynx. NY State J Med 1884; 4:655-6.

2. Alberti PW. Still photography of the larynx — an overview. Can J Otolaryngol 1975; 4:759-65.

3. Jako GJ, Strong S. Laryngeal photography. Arch Otolaryngol 1972; 96:268-71.

4. Holinger PA, Brubaker JD, Brubaker JE. Open tube, proximal illumination mirror and direct laryngeal photography. Can J Otolaryngol 1975; 4:781-5.

5. Kleinsasser O. Microlaryngoscopy and endolaryngeal microsurgery. Philadelphia: WB Saunders Co, 1968.

6. Strong MS. Laryngeal photography. Can J Otolaryngol 1975; 4:766-9.

7. Olofsson J, Ohlsson T. Techniques in microlaryngoscopic photography. Can J Otolaryngol 1975; 4:770-80.

8. Berci G, Calcaterra T, Ward PH. Advances in endoscopic techniques for examination of the larynx and nasopharynx. Can J Otolaryngol 1975; 4:786-92.

9. Tardy ME, Tenta LT. Laryngeal photography and television. Otolaryngol Clin North Am 1970; 3:483-92.

≈

INTERNATIONAL SYMPOSIUM ON MAXILLOFACIAL TRAUMA

Symposium to be held November 13-15, 1981 in Detroit is accepting papers for presentation. 20 hours category 1 CME. Wayne State University School of Medicine, Div. of Continuing Medical Education, 9B DRH/UHC, Detroit, MI 48201. (313) 577-1180.

EVOLUTION OF THE CLINICALLY NEGATIVE NECK

E. M. Skolnik, MD

A. H. Katz, MD
R. Mantravadi, MD

S. P. Becker, MD
S. Stal, MD

Chicago, Illinois

A retrospective study was done of 602 patients with primary squamous cell carcinoma of the upper aerodigestive tract and a clinically negative neck (N_o) seen at the University of Illinois Hospital between 1960-1975. There was no uniform policy as to the treatment of N_o neck during this period; therefore in many of the patients, cervical lymph nodes were treated with elective neck dissection and others were followed until they became positive clinically. It was this difference which formed the basis for this study. All the patients were treated surgically; the patients were placed into two groups depending on whether they had radical neck dissection at the same time as resection of the primary. Group 1 consisted of 149 patients and had surgery for the primary only. The 253 patients of group 2 had surgery for the primary and also had a neck dissection. Both groups were analyzed for recurrences in the cervical region. In group 1, 12.9% of the patients developed either ipsilateral or contralateral metastases. Of the group 2 patients, 22% developed palpable nodal disease. The evolution of palpable nodal disease was analyzed by primary site, T-stage, and according to whether the tumor at the primary was controlled. Only 3% of the patients developed lymph nodes when the primary was controlled. The pathology reports of the neck specimens were studied to determine the relationship between a) positive node histology and b) number of nodes positive to the recurrence rate in the neck. Our results showed a 23% failure rate for the histologically positive group and a 21% failure rate for the negative group. The number of positive nodes did not seem to affect the recurrence rate.

INTRODUCTION

The incidence of occult metastatic disease has been well established from analyses of elective neck dissection specimens. It is this knowledge which has fueled the controversy regarding elective neck treatment in the clinically negative neck. The treatment choices available to the head and neck physician range from elective neck dissection or elective neck irradiation to careful observation for evolution of nodal disease.

The question of the benefits of elective neck dissection has yet to be resolved. The arguments for and against elective radical neck dissection (RND) have been carefully reviewed by Nahum et al[1] and the case for elective neck dissection is based upon the following key points:

1. The relatively large incidence of false negative examinations (it varies from 4 to 40% in various studies).

2. Radical neck dissection has a relatively low morbidity and mortality.

3. If the neck must be entered to remove a primary lesion it is better to perform an incontinuity dissection at that time.

4. The cure rate is higher with patients who have clinically negative necks.

5. It is impossible to provide the clinical follow-up necessary to detect the earliest conversion of a neck from N_o to N_r.

6. Allowing neck metastases to develop increases the incidence of distant metastases.

7. The cure rate of radical neck dissection is decreased if gland enlargement occurs or multiple nodes appear.

The case against elective neck dissection is based upon the following key points:[1]

1. The cure rate is not higher if one waits until the neck converts from N_o to N_r.

2. Careful clinical follow-up will allow detection of the earliest conversion from N_o to N_r.

3. Radiation is as effective as radical neck dissection for treatment of the clinically negative neck.

4. Elective neck dissection results in a large number of unnecessary surgical procedures, and radical neck dissection carries a significant morbidity.

5. Elective neck dissection removes a barrier to the spread of disease and also has a deleterious immunologic effect.

The efficacy of elective neck irradiation has been published by various authors,[2-7] but most notably by Fletcher[6] and Million,[3] and Million et al.[2] These authors have advocated that moderate radiation doses, in the range of 5000 rads given over a five-week period, can control subclinical cancer in lymph nodes in over 90% of the cases. Theoretically, this effectiveness was explained on the basis that in the case of N_o stage, the relatively few cancer cells

From the Departments of Otolaryngology and Radiation Oncology, Abraham Lincoln School of Medicine, University of Illinois at the Medical Center, and the Department of Otolaryngology, Northwestern University Medical School, Chicago.

Presented at the meeting of the American Laryngological Association, Palm Beach, Florida, April 14-15, 1980.

Reprints — E. M. Skolnik, MD, Department of Otolaryngology, Abraham Lincoln School of Medicine, P. O. Box 6998, Chicago, IL 60680.

TABLE 1. SURGICAL GROUP 1 — DISTRIBUTION OF PATIENTS WHO DID NOT HAVE RND

Site	T_1	T_2	T_3	T_4	Totals
Glottic	28	36	9	3	76
Supraglottic	8	13	8	4	33
Oral cavity	9	10	2	0	21
Oropharynx	2	0	0	0	2
Totals	47	59	19	7	132

are well oxygenated and thus are more sensitive to lethal injury by radiation.

The status of the cervical lymph nodes is a significant factor in predicting the therapeutic outcome of patients with head and neck cancer.[8] The literature cites changes in survival by 20-40% based solely upon the N-stage at the time of evaluation. In an attempt to influence the cure rate of patients, many authors have recommended elective therapy for the clinically negative necks.[1] The purpose of this paper is to clarify this matter somewhat by reviewing the evolution of the clinically negative neck in head and neck squamous cancers.

MATERIALS AND METHODS

The clinical material for this study consists of 615 patients treated at the Illinois Eye and Ear Infirmary of the University of Illinois from the years 1960 to 1976. All the patients had squamous cell cancers and clinically negative necks at the time of their presentation. The patients were divided into groups based on their initial treatment modality. There were 213 patients who were treated with radiation therapy alone, and 402 patients with surgery.

TABLE 2. SURGICAL GROUP 2 — DISTRIBUTION OF PATIENTS TREATED WITH SURGERY FOR PRIMARY + RND

Site	T_1	T_2	T_3	T_4	Totals
Glottic	11	31	38	6	86
Supraglottic	8	23	28	18	77
Oral cavity	5	30	9	0	44
Oropharynx	1	5	2	0	8
Hypopharynx	7	3	2	0	12
Totals	32	92	79	24	228

A small number of the surgical patients did receive preoperative radiation. These patients were studied in a previous paper[9] where it was established that these doses had no significant effect on local control of the tumors.

In the surgical group there were two further subdivisions. Surgical group one (SG-1) had surgery for the primary and no RND. Surgical group two (SG-2) had surgery for the primary and a concomitant RND. SG-1 consisted of 149 patients and there were 253 patients in SG-2.

TABLE 3. DISTRIBUTION OF GROUP TREATED WITH RADIATION ALONE

Primary Tumor	T-stage* T_1	T_2	T_3	T_4	Totals
Oral cavity	10	20	23	3	56
Oropharynx	3	11	14	9	37
Larynx	0	13	35	5	53
Hypopharynx	0	6	4	6	16
Nasopharynx	6	8	2	7	23
Totals	19	58	78	30	185

*In 2 pts. T-stage could not be determined.

TABLE 4. SURVIVAL ACCORDING TO SITE — SURGERY FOR PRIMARY ONLY (NO RND)*

Site	Total Pts.	Evaluable Pts.	Survival Pts. %
Glottic	83	73	67/73 = 91.7
Supraglottic	33	33	25/33 = 75.7
Transglottic and subglottic	4	3	3/3 = 100.0
Oral cavity	27	21	18/21 = 85.7
Base of tongue	2	2	2/2 = 100.0
Hypopharynx	—	—	—
Total	149	132	115/132 = 87.1

*Min. follow-up - 3 yrs.

These patients have all been analyzed for neck failures. An attempt has been made to clarify the many variables operating here. Neck failures have been analyzed with regard to the T-stage of the primary and control of the primary at the time of the neck recurrence. In addition, in the patients undergoing RND, the relationship between neck failures and the histopathology of the neck failures was evaluated to determine whether the recurrence occurred outside or within the radiation fields.

The treatment plan for the patients in this study was based on the individual needs of each patient and represents the diversity of opinion inevitable in a large teaching institution over 16 years.

The distribution of study material by site and size is shown in Tables 1 and 2 for the surgical cases and Table 3 for the irradiated patients. As is evident by reviewing these Tables, the surgical group that did not have an RND tended to have smaller lesions than the group that did have an RND. This trend is expected in any retrospective study.

RESULTS

In 615 patients 1,230 heminecks were analyzed for recurrence. The 402 patients in the surgical groups were analyzed for survival. The patient's survival was calculated on a three-year basis since 90% of the recurrences appeared within that time frame. The minimum follow-up for the entire group of 615 patients was three years. The survival rate for the two surgical groups is listed by anatomic site and for all stages (Tables 4 and 5). No comparison is intended for these two groups since SG-1 had an overall lower set of T-stages.

The sites of failure of the SG-1 are presented in Table 6. In this group, there were 149 patients initially; however, inadequate records reduced this number to 132 evaluable patients. There were 17 neck recurrences for an overall recurrence rate of

TABLE 5. SURVIVAL ACCORDING TO SITE — SURGERY FOR PRIMARY + RND*

Site	Total Pts.	Evaluable Pts.	Survival Pts. %
Glottic	86	86	49/86 = 57
Supraglottic	82	77	57/77 = 74
Transglottic and subglottic	8	5	5/5 = 100
Oral cavity	49	44	32/44 = 72.7
Base of tongue	12	8	4/8 = 50
Hypopharynx	16	8	6/8 = 75
Total	253	228	153/228 = 67

*Min. follow-up - 3 yrs.

TABLE 6. SITES OF FAILURE FOLLOWING TREATMENT TO PRIMARY ONLY: NO RND (SG 1)

Primary Sites	Total Recurrences In Cervical Region	*Ipsilateral** Uncontrolled	*Ipsilateral** Primary Controlled	*Contralateral** Uncontrolled	*Contralateral** Primary Controlled
Glottic	6/73 = 8.2%	100% (6)	—	—	—
Supraglottic	8/33 = 24.0%	50% (4)	12.5% (1)	25% (2)	12.5% (1)
Oral cavity	3/21 = 14.2%	100% (3)	—	—	—

*Expressed as percentage of total cervical recurrences.

12.9%; 15 (88%) primaries were uncontrolled and two (12%) were controlled. The rate of recurrence of the glottic lesions was 8.2% with all failures being the ipsilateral neck with the primaries uncontrolled.

In patients with primary tumor in the supraglottis, the overall cervical failure rate was 24% and in only two of eight failures were the primary cancers controlled. With the oral cavity lesions, failure in the cervical region was seen in 14.2% of the cases and all were associated with the lack of primary control; however, one was ipsilateral and the other contralateral. Therefore the conversion rate for both the ipsilateral and contralateral cervical lymphatic beds was 1/33 (3%) in patients with controlled primaries.

There were 228 patients suitable for study in the SG-2 group (Table 7). The specimens obtained from this group afforded the advantage to review the histology of the neck nodes and its influence on recurrent disease. The total number of recurrences in the neck was 49 (21.4%). In 29 (59.2%) the primary was uncontrolled.

Associated with glottic lesions there were 19 neck failures (22%). In 11 of these cases, the primary was controlled and in eight the primary was uncontrolled. Thirteen (68.4%) of the neck recurrences were contralateral and approximately half of these were with controlled primaries.

The neck failure rate for supraglottic lesions was 20.7%. None of the operated necks failed when the primary remained controlled. Sixty-two percent conversions were in the contralateral neck and half of these occurred with a controlled primary.

With oral cavity lesions, there were eight (18.1%) neck failures, and no ipsilateral neck failures when the primary was controlled. Of the neck failures in oral cavity lesions, 62.5% were in the contralateral neck, and 80% had primary control. In the base of tongue and hypopharyngeal cancers, all the neck failures were associated with uncontrolled primaries.

In summary of the results of SG-2, there were 49 patients with recurrent neck disease. Twenty of the 49 patients were associated with a controlled primary; within this group of 20 recurrences, 15 were contralateral and five were ipsilateral. Thus the conversion rate in patients with primary control is 15/228 (6.1%) for the contralateral neck and 5/228 (2.1%) for the ipsilateral neck.

The data on neck recurrence were further analyzed concerning the influence of the neck histopathology and subsequent neck failure. Tables 8 and 9 show this relationship for glottic and supraglottic lesions. In the glottic group, there were 13 neck failures in the histologically negative group. In analyzing those failures where the primary was controlled, there were two failures in the histologically positive group including one bilateral failure (three hemi-necks and two patients). In patients with a controlled primary and histologically negative necks there were seven neck failures. Three of these failures were ipsilateral and four were in the contralateral neck. In the supraglottic group, there were seven neck failures in the histologically positive group and nine failures in the histologically negative group. In those patients where the primary was controlled, there were no neck failures in the histologically positive group and five neck failures in the histologically negative group.

Analyzing the rate of contralateral metastasis with the primary controlled, the rate of contralateral neck failures was not influenced by a positive histopathology in the ipsilateral neck. There were ten contralateral neck failures with both glottic and supraglottic lesions when the ipsilateral neck specimen was negative, and only one contralateral neck failure with a positive ipsilateral neck specimen. The neck was not a reliable guide in predicting future contralateral neck disease.

Table 10 shows the site distribution of the micro-

TABLE 7. SITES OF FAILURE FOLLOWING INITIAL TREATMENT IN RND GROUP (SG 2)

Primary Site	Total Cervical References	*Ipsilateral** Uncontrolled	*Ipsilateral** Controlled	*Contralateral** Uncontrolled	*Contralateral** Controlled
Glottic	19/86 = 22.0%	10.5% (2)	26.3% (4)	36.8% (7)	31.6% (6)
Supraglottic	16/77 = 20.7%	37.5% (6)		31.2% (5)	31.2% (5)
Oral cavity	8/44 = 18.1%	37.5% (3)		12.5% (1)	50.0% (4)
Base of tongue	4/8 = 50.0%	50.0% (4)		50.0% (4)	
Hypopharynx	2/12 = 16.6%	100.0% (2)			

*Expressed as percentage of total cervical recurrences.

TABLE 8. SITES OF FAILURE IN GLOTTIC CANCERS ACCORDING TO T-STAGE FOLLOWING INITIAL TREATMENT IN RND GROUP (SG 2)

Site	T-Stage	Total No.	*Ipsilateral* Uncontrolled	*Ipsilateral* Controlled	*Contralateral* Uncontrolled	*Contralateral* Controlled
Glottic (positive nodes in RND spec.)	T_1					
	T_2	2		2*		1*
	T_3	3			3	
	T_4	1			1	
Glottic (negative nodes in RND spec.)	T_1					
	T_2	1				1
	T_3	9	1	2	2	4
	T_4	3	1	1	1	
Total		19	2	5	7	6

*One patient had bilateral neck failure.

scopically positive neck specimens. As expected, the glottic lesions had the lowest number of positive specimens and the hypopharynx and base of tongue had the highest. In Table 11 the histological findings in the radical neck specimens with the cervical failures are correlated. The failure rate was essentially the same when the neck nodes were positive or negative. Further analysis of the neck specimen in Table 12 shows that the number of nodes that were microscopically positive or the extent of the microscopic disease did not influence the cervical failure rate.

The radiation therapy group consisted of 213 patients of whom 187 patients were eligible for study. In all these patients the first and second echelon of lymph nodes were treated with radiation alone and of these 58% were treated with less than 5000 rads and 42% with greater than 5000 rads. It was apparent from the arrangement of the ports that the first echelon of lymph nodes received as much radiation as the primary tumor in 42% of the cases. Thus the dose utilized in the necks in these cases was approximately equal to the dose delivered to the primary. The failures in the radiation group were analyzed according to the location of the recurrence in the neck. Table 13 shows the relationship of the primary status to the site of the neck conversion. There were 35 total neck failures and 26 of these occurred with the primary uncontrolled. Only five neck conversions developed with the primary controlled and of these two occurred within and three outside of the radiation fields. Therefore, the neck conversion rate with the primary controlled for the radiation group was 2/187 (1.1%).

DISCUSSION

The number of patients evaluated in this study (615) compares favorably with the studies of Fletcher[6] in 1972 (187), and Goffinet et al[5] in 1975 (402). In order to develop meaningful statistics, the reviewed cases were staged according to tumor size and a minimum follow-up period of three years was used as a criterion for inclusion in the study.

In patients who had surgery for the primary and no RND (SG-1), the rate of failure in the neck with primary control was less than 2% no matter what the site of the primary. In patients who had surgery for the primary and concomitant RND (SG-2), the rate of failure in the neck with primary control was less than 9% irrespective of the primary site. The failure rate for the ipsilateral neck was 2.1% and for the contralateral neck it was 6.1%. There were more contralateral failures in patients with histologically negative (ipsilateral) neck specimens than in the group with histologically positive neck specimens. This raises a question about the reliability of neck histopathology in predicting future contralateral disease.

In comparing the actual failure rate for patients in SG-1 with the expected neck failures based on Table 10, one finds a significant discrepancy. There were only two neck failures in the untreated necks when the primary was controlled. It is apparent from the distribution of cancers in SG-1 that these are relatively low T-stage lesions. Nevertheless, the failure rate of 1.5% is far below the expected conversion rate based upon a comparison of SG-1 and SG-2. This lends support to the theory that the

TABLE 9. SITE OF FAILURE IN SUPRAGLOTTIC CANCERS ACCORDING TO T-STAGE FOLLOWING INITIAL TREATMENT IN RND GROUP (SG 2)

Site	T-Stage	Total No.	*Ipsilateral* Uncontrolled	*Ipsilateral* Controlled	*Contralateral* Uncontrolled	*Contralateral* Controlled
Supraglottic RND (+)	T_1					
	T_2	1	1			
	T_3	2	1	1		
	T_4	4	1	3		
Supraglottic RND (–)	T_1					
	T_2	3	1		2	
	T_3	2			2	
	T_4	4	2	1	1	
Total		16	6	5	5	

TABLE 10. SITE DISTRIBUTION OF HISTOLOGICALLY POSITIVE ELECTIVE NECK DISSECTION SPECIMENS

Glottic	21/86	24.0%
Supraglottic	27/77	35.0%
Oral cavity	18/44	41.0%
Base of tongue	6/8	75.0%
Hypopharynx	6/8	75.0%

(This data is collected from the SG2 group of 228 patients — see Table 2)

lymph nodes perform a surveillance function when the primary has been controlled.

Examination of Table 12 shows that the number of microscopically positive nodes did not influence the cervical failure rate. The RND is an aggressive form of treatment and an adequate therapy for any amount of microscopic disease. The modified neck dissection should be considered in these patients so that functional and cosmetic structures can be left intact.

TABLE 11. CERVICAL FAILURES AS CORRELATED WITH HISTOLOGICAL FINDINGS IN RND SPECIMENS

Status of Lymph Nodes	*No. Pts.*	*No. Failed*	*% Failure*
Positive nodes	78	18	23.0
Negative nodes	150	31	21.0
Total	228	49	21.5

In the group of patients treated with radiation therapy alone, there were 35 out of 187 patients (18.7%) with neck failures. Most of the failures were in-field and associated with an uncontrolled primary. Additional radiation therapy to out-of-field sites would not have added to primary tumor control. Planned combined therapy should be considered for large lesions in primary sites other than the nasopharynx.

CONCLUSIONS

1. The conversion rate for necks with primary control is not even close to the number predicted based upon percent positive elective neck specimens.

2. Microscopic ipsilateral neck histopathology is not a reliable guide for predicting future contralateral neck conversion.

3. The number of neck failures with primary control is very low with elective RND or elective radiation therapy.

TABLE 12. NUMBER OF LYMPH NODES POSITIVE IN RND SPECIMENS VS FAILURES IN NECK

No. Nodes Positive	*Total No.*	*No. Recurred*	*% Recurrence*
One node +	40	9	22.5
Two nodes	16	4	25.0
Three or more +	22	5	22.7
Totals	78	18	23.0

4. In a series with predominantly T_1 and T_2 lesions, the failure rate in the neck was low with no neck therapy. Radiation therapy is as good as surgery in controlling microscopic neck disease when the primary is controlled.

TABLE 13. CORRELATION OF PRIMARY STATUS AND FAILURE SITE (RADIATION GROUP)

Failure Site	*Status of Primary Disease at the Time of Failure* Uncontrolled	Controlled	*Totals*
In-field*	26	2	28
Supraclavicular nodes	1	2	3
Lower cervical	0	1	1
Posterior cervical	3	0	3
Totals	30	5	35

*Failure occurring within the irradiated field.

5. The number of microscopically positive nodes found in elective RND does not correlate with subsequent neck failures.

6. The most important factor affecting the subsequent neck failure is primary tumor control.

7. Radiation therapy is effective in controlling in-field occult metastasis when the primary is controlled. Low cervical and/or supraclavicular recurrences occur rarely when the primary is controlled; therefore, elective treatment of these areas seems unwarranted.

8. The patients in this study did not have palpable disease anywhere in the neck. In regard to a patient with a head and neck primary and a palpable ipsilateral node and a negative contralateral neck, the conclusions in this study are not applicable and should not be used to plan treatment for the negative contralateral neck.

REFERENCES

1. Nahum AM, Bone RC, Davidson TM. The case for prophylactic neck dissection. Laryngoscope 1977; 87:588-99.

2. Million RR, Fletcher GH, Jesse RH Jr. Evaluation of elective irradiation of the neck for squamous cell carcinoma of the nasopharynx, tonsillar fossa, and base of the tongue. Radiology 1963; 80:973-88.

3. Million RR. Elective neck irradiation for TxNO squamous carcinoma of the oral tongue and floor of the mouth. Cancer 1974; 34:149-55.

4. Bagshaw MA, Thomson RW. Elective irradiation of the neck in patients with primary carcinoma of the head and neck. JAMA 1971; 217:456-8.

5. Goffinet MD, Fletcher GH, Gilbert EH, Weller CA, Bagshaw MA. Irradiation of clinically uninvolved cervical lymph nodes. Can J Otolaryngol 1975; 4:927-33.

6. Fletcher GH. Elective irradiation of subclinical disease in cancers of the head and neck. Cancer 1972; 29:1450-4.

7. Lindberg RD, Barkley H, Jesse RH Jr, Fletcher GH. Evolution of the clinically negative neck in patients with squamous cell carcinoma of faucial arch. Am J Roentgenol 1971; 111:60-5.

8. Spiro RH, Alfonso AE, Farr HW, Strong EW. Cervical node metastasis from epidermoid carcinoma of the oral cavity and oropharynx. A critical assessment of current staging. Am J Surg 1974; 128:562-7.

9. Skolnik EM, Soboroff BJ, Tenta LT, Saberman MN, Jones HC. Preoperative radiation therapy in head and neck cancer. Trans Am Acad Ophthalmol Otolaryngol 1968; 72:937-42.

Ann Otol 89:1980

EXTENDED PARTIAL LARYNGECTOMY

DONALD G. SESSIONS, MD
ST. LOUIS, MISSOURI

This report details the diagnosis and treatment of a patient with a large $T_3 N_0M_0$ laryngopharyngeal cancer by combined surgical excision and planned postoperative irradiation therapy. Surgical excision included a horizontal subtotal supraglottic laryngectomy combined with a vertical hemilaryngectomy and partial pharyngectomy. The patient was reconstructed with a free sternocleidomastoid muscle graft. The results and implications of this therapy are discussed.

Conservation surgery of the larynx refers to surgical removal of malignant tumors involving specific areas of the larynx with preservation of sphincteric, respiratory, and phonatory function. Inherent in this surgical approach is the concept that neither cancer cure nor laryngeal function is sacrificed at either's expense. Previous reports have detailed both operative techniques and the immediate reconstructive procedures which have been employed.[1] Employing strict preoperative criteria, satisfactory long-term results in the treatment of cancer of the larynx have been reported.[2]

Occasionally, an opportunity arises in which the standard preoperative criteria for employing conservation surgical techniques may be enlarged to meet a specific patient need. This report will detail the treatment of a patient with a large supraglottic cancer where the indications for partial laryngectomy were extended.

CASE REPORT

The patient is a 56-year-old white male who presented with a four-week history of hoarseness, sore throat, dysphagia, and odynophagia. He was in good physical condition except for some emphysema.

Examination in the office revealed a large exophytic tumor involving the right aryepiglottic fold, the epiglottis, the right false vocal cord, and the right medial wall of the pyriform fossa. The right true vocal cord could not be seen. There were no palpable lymph nodes in the neck. There were signs of chronic obstructive pulmonary disease.

Direct laryngoscopy confirmed the findings and revealed the right true vocal cord was involved with the tumor. CT scan revealed invasion into the pre-epiglottic space but no cartilage destruction. Laryngogram confirmed the above findings and indicated decreased motion of the right true vocal cord. Pulmonary function studies revealed normal forced vital capacity, mildly decreased forced expiratory volume, and severely decreased minimum midexpiratory flow rate. Arterial blood gases were normal.

Biopsy revealed well-differentiated epidermoid carcinoma. The lesion was staged as a $T_3 N_0M_0$ tumor of the marginal area. The treatment plan involved combined surgery and postoperative irradiation therapy.

Surgical Technique for Resection. The surgical approach included a low collar incision and the raising of an inferior-based thyroid cartilage perichondrial flap. After a horizontal cartilage cut at the ventricular level of the left hemilarynx, the vallecula was entered through a left infrahyoid pharyngotomy. Tumor removal was begun by coming across the left aryepiglottic fold to the anterior commissure. Because the right true vocal cord tumor involved the subglottic area down to just above the cricoid cartilage, a vertical cartilage cut was made in the midline. In order to encompass the lesion, the patient thus underwent a subtotal supraglottic laryngectomy for the superior margin associated with an en bloc right vertical hemilaryngectomy for the inferior and posterior margins and a right partial pharyngectomy for the lateral margin. No neck dissection was performed.

Reconstruction. The resulting defect included the mobile left true vocal cord and the cricoid cartilage. A major portion of the right pyriform fossa was missing. Reconstruction of the defect began with a cricopharyngeal muscle myotomy. A right pseudocord was formed from a large free flap of muscle from the ipsilateral sternocleidomastoid muscle. This was sutured in place between the anterior commissure and the midline of the cricoid cartilage posteriorly. Attempt at marked overcorrection was made. The pharyngectomy was closed by suturing the thyroid perichondrium to the base of the tongue and the lateral pharyngeal wall.

From the Department of Otolaryngology, Washington University School of Medicine, St. Louis, Missouri.
Presented at the meeting of the American Laryngological Association, Palm Beach, Florida, April 14-15, 1980.
REPRINTS — Donald G. Sessions, MD, 517 South Euclid Avenue, St. Louis, MO 63110.

The resected specimen included the epiglottis, both false vocal cords, and the right hemilarynx with its true vocal cord including the arytenoid, en bloc with the pyriform fossa to the lateral pharyngeal wall. Pathologic examination revealed a well-differentiated epidermoid carcinoma involving the superficial laryngeal surface and extending from the epithelial surface of the laryngopharynx around the cartilage of the epiglottis to involve extensively the soft tissue compartment anterior to the epiglottis. The margins of resection of the larynx were free of tumor but the lateral pharyngeal margin showed tumor involving the lateral margin. Vascular invasion was present.

Postoperative Course. The wound healed per primam and the patient underwent 6,000 rads of planned postoperative irradiation therapy to the laryngopharynx and both sides of the neck. He was decannulated without difficulty at four months postoperative. Examination of the larynx revealed a 4 mm glottic chink with good glottic closure. Deglutition was performed with little difficulty. He spoke with a heavy whisper.

Follow-Up. He did well until about 11 months postoperatively, at which time he was admitted for aspiration pneumonia. Direct laryngoscopy at that time revealed some atrophy of the pseudocord. This was treated with a gastrostomy and a cartilage implant reconstruction of the pseudocord. Presently he is decannulated and has a strong voice. He shows no evidence of recurrent disease 16 months postoperatively. Because of some continued problems with glottic incompetence and increased chronic obstructive pulmonary disease it has been elected to leave his gastrostomy tube in for an indefinite period.

COMMENTS

This patient did well following combined subtotal supraglottic laryngectomy, hemilaryngectomy, and partial pharyngectomy associated with full course postoperative irradiation therapy. The complication of late glottic insufficiency resulting in aspiration pneumonia was felt to be due to atrophy of the muscle implant in the reconstructed pseudocord. This occurred at the 11th month postoperative and was treated with a cartilage implant.

Surgical treatment of postsurgical glottic incompetence has centered on Teflon® injection of the pseudocord scar or reconstruction of a new pseudocord. Arnold[3] and Lewy[4] have reported satisfactory results of Teflon injection for an inadequate pseudocord after hemilaryngectomy, but both have pointed out that the procedure is limited by the denseness of the scar. We have noted that if there is tissue space which will accept the Teflon, then this is a very satisfactory approach.

For incompetent glottic insufficiency with a large amount of tissue loss, a pseudocord must be reconstructed. Historically the glottis has been reconstructed with cartilage,[5-9] muscle,[10-14] mucosa,[15-18] and skin[18] with and without laryngeal stents. [15] We have used muscle flaps[14] and cartilage implants.[9,19] Following the use of cartilage implant, if glottic incompetence is still present, the creation of the space in the pseudocord where the cartilage is allows for the future successful injection of Teflon.

This patient did well functionally until the muscle in the reconstructed pseudocord atrophied. In the future, the use of a sternocleidomastoid myocutaneous pedicle flap for this type of reconstruction may well preclude this late complication.

REFERENCES

1. Ogura JH, Sessions DG, Spector GJ, Alonso WA. Roles and limitations of conservation surgical therapy for laryngeal cancer. Can J Otolaryngol 1975; 4:400-2.

2. Ogura JH, Sessions DG. Cancer of the larynx and hypopharynx. In: Anderson R, Hoopes JE, eds. Symposium on malignancies of the head and neck. St. Louis: CV Mosby Co, 1975: 138-44.

3. Arnold G. Vocal rehabilitation of paralytic dysphonia: IX. Technique of intracordal injection. Arch Otolaryngol 1962; 76:358-68.

4. Lewy RB. Glottic reformation with voice rehabilitation in vocal cord paralysis. Laryngoscope 1963; 73:547-55.

5. Payr J. Shildknorpelplastik bei irrepabler Stimmbandlähmung. Dtsch Med Wochenschr 1916; 42:682.

6. Meurman Y. Operative media fixation of the vocal cord in complete unilateral paralysis. Arch Otolaryngol 1952; 55:544-53.

7. Opheim O. Unilateral paralysis of the vocal cord. Operative treatment. Acta Otolaryngol (Stockh) 1955; 75:226-30.

8. Waltner JG. Surgical rehabilitation of the voice following laryngofissure. Arch Otolaryngol 1958; 67:99-101.

9. Ogura JH, Dedo HH. Glottic reconstruction following subtotal glottic-supraglottic laryngectomy. Laryngoscope 1968; 75:865-78.

10. Pressman JJ. Cancer of the larynx: laryngoplasty to avoid laryngectomy. Arch Otolaryngol 1954; 59:395-412.

11. Bailey BJ. Partial laryngectomy and laryngoplasty. Laryngoscope 1971; 81:1742-71.

12. Maran AGD, Hast MH, Leonard JR. Reconstructive surgery for improved glottic closure and voice following partial laryngectomy. Laryngoscope 1968; 78:1916-36.

13. Quinn HJ Jr. A new technique for glottic reconstruction after partial laryngectomy. Laryngoscope 1969; 79:1980-2011.

14. Ogura JH, Biller HF. Glottic reconstruction following extended frontolateral hemilaryngectomy. Laryngoscope 1969; 74:2181-4.

15. Goodyear HM. Hemilaryngectomy method maintaining a satisfactory airway and voice. Ann Otol Rhinol Laryngol 1949; 58:581-5.

16. Som ML. Hemilaryngectomy - a modified technique for cordal carcinoma with extension posteriorly. Arch Otolaryngol 1951; 54:524-33.

17. Conley JJ. The use of mucosal flaps for wound rehabilitation in partial laryngectomy. Arch Otolaryngol 1959; 69:700-3.

18. Conley JJ. Glottic reconstruction and wound rehabilitation. Arch Otolaryngol 1961; 74:21-4.

19. Sessions DG, Ogura JH, Ciralsky RH. Late glottic insufficiency. Laryngoscope 1975; 85:950-9.

Ann Otol 89:1980

ACUTE CRICOARYTENOID ARTHRITIS: LOCAL PERIARTICULAR STEROID INJECTION

GEORGE T. SIMPSON II, MD, MPH
BOSTON, MASSACHUSETTS

AHMAD JAVAHERI, MD
RIVERSIDE, CALIFORNIA

PARVIZ JANFAZA, MD
BOSTON, MASSACHUSETTS

Acute cricoarytenoid arthritis is a frequent complication of rheumatoid arthritis and the most frequent otolaryngologic manifestation of the disease. Over 25% of rheumatoid arthritis cases have discomfort from this problem. Other etiologies can produce cricoarytenoid arthritis. Symptoms range from mild discomfort through hoarseness to complete airway obstruction requiring emergency tracheotomy. Chronic cricoarytenoid arthritis may result in joint ankylosis and vocal fold fixation. Single periarticular triamcinolone injections may bring rapid and dramatic relief of the symptomatology of nonankylosed acute cricoarytenoid arthritis for periods of up to one year if other medical management is adequate. Six cases illustrate the problem and the efficacy of this treatment methodology. Findings, pathology and pertinent literature are discussed. Specific criteria for considering this technique are outlined. This form of therapy has not been described previously.

The cricoarytenoid joint is a true diarthrodial joint with both a synovial lining and fluid-filled space within a fibrous bursa. The joint allows mobility of the arytenoid cartilage. Three movements have been described: a rotatory or rocking movement around the joint axis, a gliding movement parallel to the axis, and a pivoting motion around the posterior cricoarytenoid ligament.[1] These movements are controlled by the antagonistic contractions of the laryngeal musculature and the resultant position of the arytenoid adjusts vocal fold position and vocal quality.

The cricoarytenoid joint is subject to pathologic changes identical with those of diarthrodial joints elsewhere in the body.[2,3] Inflammation of the joint structures can develop with local infectious disease, trauma, or with a systemic illness such as rheumatoid arthritis. Acute inflammatory changes can produce decreased mobility or fixation from local edema and muscle splinting. Chronic inflammation can result in ankylosis, vocal fold fixation, and airway obstruction.

Acute cricoarytenoid arthritis may result from direct extension of such bacterial infections as streptococcal pharyngitis and laryngitis, diphtheria, typhoid fever, syphilis, and tuberculosis. Mumps and probably other viral infections may rarely produce arthritis.[4] Trauma to the joint from intubation of the trachea or esophagus, or endoscopy may produce acute arthritis as may radiation therapy.

Many systemic diseases[2] especially rheumatoid arthritis, osteoarthritis, ankylosing spondylitis gout, Reiter's syndrome, Felty's syndrome,[5] and systemic lupus erythematosus can produce cricoarytenoid arthritis. Radiation therapy may result in chronic arthritis and fixation. Chronic arthritis from any etiology may result in ankylosis. Chronic immobility of the arytenoid from recurrent laryngeal nerve palsy may also produce ankylosis.[2]

The symptoms and physical findings differ in acute and chronic cricoarytenoid arthritis.[2] Exacerbations with acute joint inflammation may obscure the presence of chronic arthritis. There is probably a spectrum of symptoms, physical findings and pathology which includes both acute and chronic cricoarytenoid arthritis.

The symptoms of acute cricoarytenoid arthritis begin with a sensation of fullness, tenseness, or of a foreign body in the throat. Pain soon develops locally and is also referred to the ear. The pain is intensified with speaking, coughing, or swallowing. Hoarseness develops with increasing inflammation. Dyspnea and inspiratory stridor appear as arthritis and fixation progresses. In children and occasionally in adults laryngotracheobronchitis and asthma may be "diagnosed" incorrectly, when in reality, cricoarytenoid arthritis is present.

Examination of the larynx with acute cricoarytenoid arthritis reveals the arytenoids to be red, swollen, and tender to palpation, either directly or by manipulating the larynx (Fig. 1A). The vocal folds may be normal or with intact muscular innervation, the vocal folds will bow laterally with inspiration.

In chronic arthritis, on the other hand, pain usually is minimal or absent. Hoarseness rarely is present and then is only slight. Dyspnea results from bi-

From the Departments of Otolaryngology of Boston City Hospital, Boston University School of Medicine and Tufts University School of Medicine, Boston; and Riverside General Hospital/University Medical Center, Riverside, California.

Presented at the meeting of the American Laryngological Association, Palm Beach, Florida, April 14-15, 1980.

REPRINTS — George T. Simpson, MD, MPH, Department of Otolaryngology, Boston University Medical Center, 720 Harrison Avenue, Boston, MA 02118.

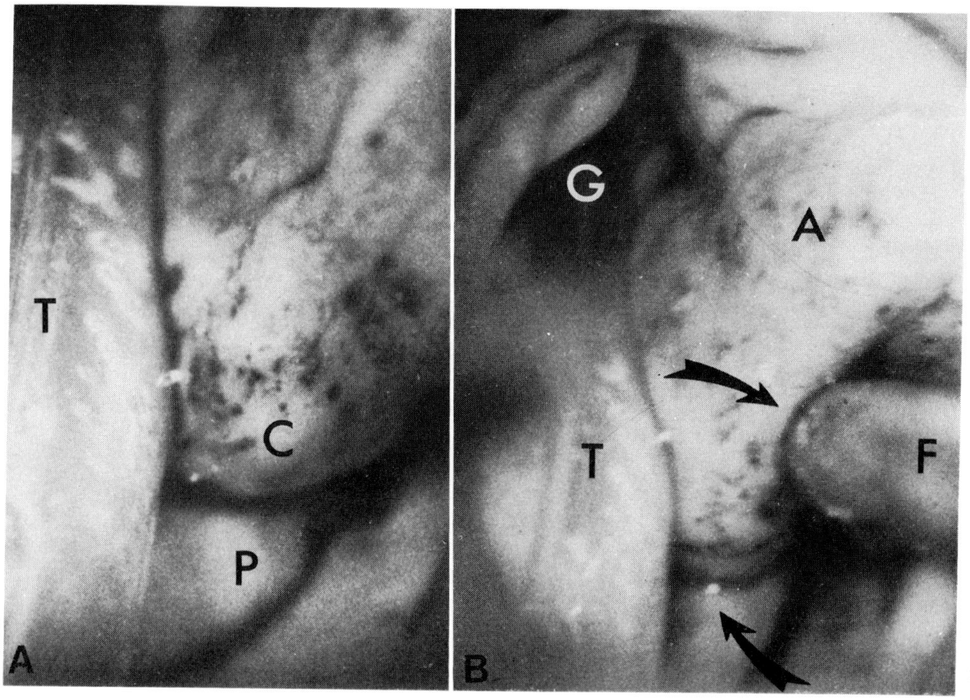

Fig. 1. A) Acute cricoarytenoid arthritis. Note edema and petechiae of inflammation. C - Cricoarytenoid region; P - Posterior pharyngeal wall; T - Endotracheal tube. B) Passive mobility test. Note closed forcep (F) palpating arytenoid (A) mobility (upper arrow). G - Glottic level; T - Endotracheal tube; lower arrow - cricoarytenoid joint level.

lateral fixation, but may not be noted in a bedridden patient. Inspiratory stridor appears with acute exacerbation of the arthritis, respiratory infection, physical exertion, and when the patient is sedated or asleep. Stridor may not be noticed if the patient is inactive, but awake and alert. The inspiratory stridor is frequently mistaken for asthma or chronic bronchitis.

On examination of the larynx with chronic cricoarytenoid arthritis no obvious inflammation is seen. The mucosa over the arytenoids may appear roughened and thickened. The vocal folds are narrowly separated, and bow with inspiration if both arytenoids are fixed. The arytenoids are immobile and found to be fixed to the cricoid on direct palpation.[2]

Therapeutic measures for cricoarytenoid arthritis are of two general types, systemic and local.[2,6] Systemic therapy includes antibiotics for infectious disease, antitoxin for diphtheria; and corticosteroids, antiinflammatory agents and colloidal gold for rheumatoid arthritis. Local measures are directed at correcting the long-term effects of cricoarytenoid fixation, eg, tracheotomy and/or arytenoidectomy for ankylosis and airway obstruction, and vocal fold Teflon® injections for ankylosis with lateral fixation of the arytenoid and vocal fold. No specific local therapy has been suggested for acute or chronic cricoarytenoid arthritis without ankylosis.

The good success we have obtained in treating cricoarytenoid arthritis with a new application or variation of an old technique used for acute arthritis in other diarthrodial joints. Our results to date are promising.

METHODS

Patients. Six patients with rheumatoid arthritis and acute arthritis and inflammatory fixation (without ankylosis) of at least one cricoarytenoid joint were selected for treatment. Three patients had undergone emergency tracheotomy for acute airway obstruction from bilateral vocal cord fixation. All patients had had prolonged therapy with steroid and antiinflammatory agents. All developed acute cricoarytenoid arthritis while on an otherwise satisfactory dosage of these medications.

Technique. Before a muscle relaxant is administered or endotracheal intubation performed, with the patient at a light plane of general anesthesia, direct laryngoscopy is performed. Laryngeal muscle activity is evaluated. Deeper anesthesia and muscular relaxation is attained and a small diameter endotracheal tube inserted or Venturi ventilation established. Arytenoid cartilages are palpated and mobility established (Fig. 1B). A false impression of fixation may result if too large an endotracheal tube is used. If stridor has been present, bronchoscopy may be performed.

Triamcinolone* for injection is prepared in the strength desired (10-40 mg/ml). A 3 or 5-ml Leuer-lock syringe is filled with triamcinolone and attached to a straight laryngeal Teflon injection needle (Fig. 2). One to two milliliters of steroid (10-40 mg) is then injected submucosally in the periarticular regions of the arytenoid eminence(s) (Fig. 3). Postoperative care is as follows any endoscopic procedure.

When arthritis etiology has been established, the procedure can be repeated as necessary for acute relapses as an out-patient technique with local anesthesia and direct or indirect endoscopic technique as is indicated by the preference and experience of the surgeon.

----

*Triamcinolone acetonide: Kenalog®. E.R. Squibb & Sons, Princeton, NJ; triamcinolone diacetate: Aristocort Forte®. Lederele Laboratories, Pearl River, NY.

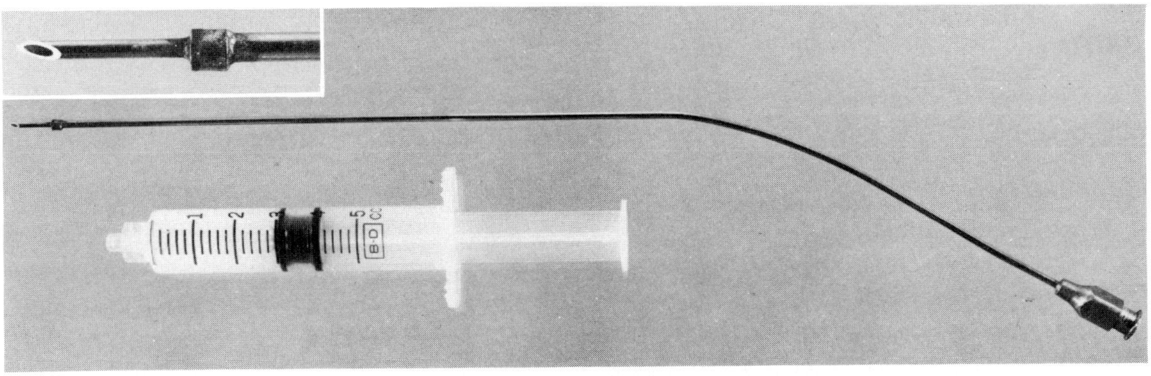

Fig. 2. Injection needle and syringe loaded with triamcinolone. Inset) Injection needle tip.

RESULTS

Six patients have undergone periarticular steroid injections. Their pathology and results of treatment are summarized in Table 1. All experienced dramatic improvement in symptomatology. All tracheotomized patients were decannulated: two within five days of treatment and the other within one month. There were no postoperative complications. One patient died 12 months postoperatively of unrelated causes, without recurrence of severe symptoms. The absence of ankylosis was confirmed at autopsy. One patient developed severe pain without fixation five months after injection. A second injection gave symptomatic relief for an additional eight months. He was then lost to follow-up. One patient required repeat injections for refixation at eight months and remained without symptoms for 1½ years. Two patients developed mild discomfort at four and six months, respectively, after injection, without recurrence of fixation and have had no further injections. One patient had no recurrence of symptoms. Minimum follow-up is six months, maximum 2½ years (Table 1).

DISCUSSION

Cricoarytenoid arthritis has been recognized for over 100 years[7] and intermittently described in textbooks. An almost complete hiatus in discussion concerning this problem existed for much of the early 20th century. In the 30 years preceding the first report of Montgomery et al[8] only one related report had appeared, in 1943.[9]

Montgomery[2] brought awareness of the problem in a series of articles. Both he and Polisar[3] have extensively reviewed the anatomy, pathology and historical literature concerning the cricoarytenoid joint and its progressive inflammatory degeneration. Montgomery first noted the frequency of the problem in rheumatoid arthritis, 26% of patients having symptoms of cricoarytenoid involvement.[2] Many other reports have appeared in the otolaryngologic, medical and anesthesia literature.

A review of this literature revealed that, except for hydrocortisone spray,[10] no local therapy had been described for acute arthritis fixation without ankylosis, or for severe acute arthritis symptoms including pain. Systemic medications are prescribed for local infections and inflammation as well as for systemic diseases. A variety of surgical techniques can be used to manage the complications and sequelae: tracheotomy, arytenoidectomy, arthrodesis, and Teflon injections.

The necessity of performing an emergency tracheotomy four years ago on a hospital nurse of long family acquaintance of one of the authors (GTS) aroused an interest in the symptomatic relief of the severe pain of cricoarytenoid arthritis. Consideration of steroids led to the triamcinolone compounds, approved for local use in intraarticular injection for acute arthritic episodes. The initial injections were performed only for the relief of pain. The resolution of inflammatory fixation, resumption of arytenoid mobility and subsequent decannulation comprised a serendipitous discovery.

While composing this paper, we have discovered a reference in the German literature to a single case of local steroid injection at the cricoarytenoid

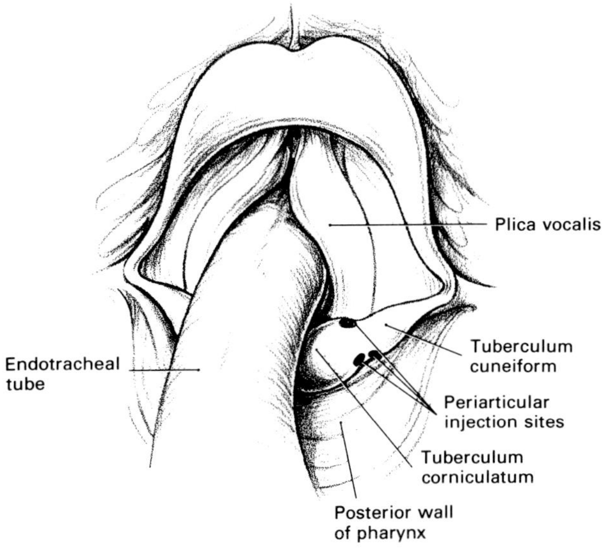

Fig. 3. Diagrammatic illustration of injection sites.

TABLE 1. ACUTE CRICOARYTENOID ARTHRITIS: RESULTS OF LOCAL STEROID INJECTIONS

Patient	*Age (yr)*	*Sex*	*Disease*	*Tracheotomy*	*Recurrence*	*Repeat*	*Follow-up (months)*
1	64	M	RA	Yes	Mild at 6 mo	0	24
2	37	M	RA	No	Fixation at 8 mo; none after 2nd treatment	1 (8)	26
3	42	F	RA	No	Mild	0	18
4	52	M	RA	Yes	Severe pain (5 mo); none after 2nd treatment	1 (5)	13*
5	52	F	Felty's syndrome	Yes	None	0	12†
6	45	M	Gout	No	None	0	12

RA - Rheumatoid arthritis.

*Lost to follow-up.

†Died of unrelated causes; no fixation at autopsy; first patient treated.

joint.[11] This report described a case of complete ankylosis of the cricoarytenoid joints with aphonia following intubation, which was converted to nearly normal mobility and voice using repeated transcutaneous transthyrohyoid membrane injections of fludrocortisone and hyaluronidase under direct microlaryngoscopy followed by repeated passive mobilizations of the joints. In actuality, this "ankylosis" may rather have been a form of inflammatory fixation following trauma, with minimal fibrosis, rather than being a true ankylosis.

Fludrocortisone for parenteral use is not available in this country; only the oral form* is available. Because of its marked effects on sodium retention, its indicated use is only in the treatment of adrenocortical insufficiency and adrenogenital syndrome. For this reason, we believe triamcinolone compounds are distinctly preferable.

Hyaluronidase† hydrolyzes hyaluronic acid, markedly enhancing diffusion of injected substances. It has been a relatively safe compound and has been used to assist absorption of parenteral medications. Its use with local steroid injections around the cricoarytenoid joint may be valid. We have not evaluated this medication for this use; the triamcinolone compounds alone have provided satisfactory results.

As with any technique, a successful result is dependent on careful and proper patient selection. We believe all of the following indications or criteria must be met before giving consideration to the use of the technique we have described:

1. The clinical presence of acute cricoarytenoid arthritis with one or more of these major symptomatic manifestations must be established: inflammatory fixation, airway compromise, or severe pain.
2. The absence of cricoarytenoid ankylosis must be proven by the passive mobility test of Chevalier Jackson, Sr. and W.W. Montgomery.[2]
3. Recurrent laryngeal nerve function must be proven with direct observation of muscular activity.
4. Symptoms have persisted or developed despite careful and adequate medical management of the problem.

Absolute contraindications to this technique (except for the relief of severe pain) include: 1) ankylosis of the cricoarytenoid joint; 2) recurrent laryngeal nerve palsy; 3) other obstructive airway pathology; 4) active infectious inflammation; 5) laryngeal malignancy.

With these criteria fulfulled, the technique can be considered.

Local triamcinolone injections for acute cricoarytenoid arthritis offer a number of advantages:

1. It is therapy delivered locally to a specific involved site.

2. The medication is appropriate, government-approved, and readily available.

3. All instruments are readily available in most operating rooms.

4. No special training is necessary for an experienced laryngologist.

5. Only moments are required to perform the procedure.

6. The technique can be combined with the diagnostic procedure.

7. The injection can be performed under local anesthesia.

8. There is minimal risk.

9. Cost/benefit ratios are excellent, as little or no hospitalization may be necessary.

10. Outpatient treatment is possible.

11. Patient relief is profound.

SUMMARY

A new technique is described: periarticular triamcinolone injections, for specific treatment of

*Fludrocortisone: Florinef®. E. R. Squibb & Sons, Princeton, NJ.

†Hyaluronidase: Wydase®. Wyeth Laboratories, Philadelphia, Penn.

acute cricoarytenoid arthritis and the results of a preliminary clinical trial are reported. The anatomy of the cricoarytenoid joint, and the etiology, clinical manifestations and pathology of cricoarytenoid arthritis are described. Literature discussing the problem and its treatment is reviewed. Specific criteria for patient selection, and indications and contraindications for use of the technique are enumerated. The advantages of the technique for the patient are discussed.

ACKNOWLEDGMENT — We wish to express our appreciation to Ms. Edna Joyner for assistance in the preparation of this manuscript, and to Ms. Marcia Williams for her assistance in preparing the illustrations.

REFERENCES

1. von Leden H, Moore P. The mechanics of the cricoarytenoid joint. Arch Otolaryngol 1961; 73:541-55.

2. Montgomery WW. Cricoarytenoid arthritis. Laryngoscope 1963; 73:801-36.

3. Polisar IS. The cricoarytenoid joint. Laryngoscope 1959; 69:1129-64.

4. Bryer D, Rounthwaite FJ. Cricoarytenoid arthritis due to mumps. Laryngoscope 1973; 83:372-5.

5. Woldorf NM, Pastore PN, Terz J. Rheumatoid arthritis of the cricoarytenoid joint. Arch Otolaryngol 1971; 93:623-7.

6. Jacobs JC, Hui RM. Cricoarytenoid arthritis and airway obstruction in juvenile rheumatoid arthritis. Pediatrics 1977; 59:292-3.

7. Mackenzie M. Diseases of the pharynx, larynx and trachea. New York: William Wood & Co, 1880:347.

8. Montgomery WW, Perone PM, Schall LA. Arthritis of the cricoarytenoid joint. Ann Otol Rhinol Laryngol 1955;64: 1025-33.

9. Myerson MC. Fixation of the cricoarytenoid joints due to streptococcic infection: improvement with the King operation. Arch Otolaryngol 1943; 38:169-70.

10. Copeman WSC. Rheumatoid arthritis and the cricoarytenoid joints. Br J Clin Pract 1968; 22:421-2.

11. Chilla R, Gabriel P. Die Arthritis des Krikoarytanoidgelenkes: uber eine seltene Intubatiousfolge und deren Therapie. Laryngol Rhinol Otol (Stuttg) 1976; 55:389-92.

BLASTOMYCOSIS OF THE LARYNX

JAMES Y. SUEN, MD
LITTLE ROCK, ARKANSAS

STEPHEN J. WETMORE, MD
LITTLE ROCK, ARKANSAS

WILLIAM J. WETZEL, MD
LITTLE ROCK, ARKANSAS

ROBERT D. CRAIG, MD
BARTLESVILLE, OKLAHOMA

Blastomycosis is an uncommon fungal disease which may mimic carcinoma of the larynx. Physical examination may show a granular appearance early in the disease with progression to laryngeal fibrosis. Histologic examination usually shows pseudoepitheliomatous hyperplasia, microabscesses, and giant cells. The broad-based budding yeast organisms may be easily overlooked unless special stains are used. Two cases of laryngeal blastomycosis which were originally treated as carcinoma are reported.

INTRODUCTION

Blastomycosis is a fungal disease which may be mistaken for carcinoma of the larynx.[1-3] Laryngeal involvement is usually a sign of systemic blastomycosis and may occur with or without concurrent pulmonary involvement.

Blastomyces dermatitidis is thought to reside in the soil but only rarely have investigators been able to culture this organism from the soil. Several small epidemics of blastomycosis occurring in North Carolina, Minnesota, and Illinois were carefully studied by epidemiologists, but the source of the organism could not be confirmed by culture techniques.[4] Despite this lack of confirmation, evidence from canine infections as well as analysis of human cases points to soil enriched by bird excreta as the probable ecological niche for this organism.[4] In nature, the fungus *B dermatitidis* grows as a mycelium with dumbbell or lollipop-shaped spores. These become airborne when the mycelium is disturbed and serve as the infecting agents. The spores are usually inhaled into the lungs leading to the pulmonic involvement initially. The organism converts to a budding yeast phase in infected mammals.

Case reports show a 9:1 male predominance.[4,5] Bird hunters seem to be unusually susceptible to the disease.[4] The incidence of blastomycosis is much less than histoplasmosis or coccidioidomycosis, although true incidence figures are not available because it is not a reportable illness in most states.

CLINICAL PRESENTATION

Blastomycosis may present as either an acute pneumonia or as a chronic disease of insidious onset. In epidemics the disease usually presents with an abrupt onset of high fever, productive cough, myalgia, arthralgia, and sometimes erythema nodosum. Usually this form of acute pulmonary infection is self-limited and requires no specific treatment, but occasionally a patient will develop progressive pulmonary or extrapulmonary disease, resulting in death.

The patients with blastomycosis of insidious onset deny symptoms of acute pneumonia and may present instead with a chronic productive cough, blood-streaked sputum, weight loss, malaise, anorexia, low grade fever, and anemia. Chest roentgenographic findings are not diagnostic. Pulmonic infection frequently leads to hematogenous dissemination throughout the body. More than 60% of symptomatic patients have the disseminated form of the disease.

Virtually any organ system may be affected by the disease, with skin as the most frequent site of dissemination. Large verrucous skin lesions or localized chancriform lesions from direct inoculation occur which clinically and sometimes microscopically look like carcinoma. Other body parts involved include the bones, genitourinary system, central nervous system, and upper respiratory system.

Laryngeal Involvement. The most common presenting complaint of patients with laryngeal blastomycosis is persistent hoarseness.[5,6] With early disease one may see an inflammatory stage in which the laryngeal mucosa develops an erythematous granular appearance with multiple gray pinhead microabscesses. This progresses to a grayish, nodular pattern. Ulcerations may develop and are covered by a thin, gray membrane. As the disease progresses, fibrosis occurs, producing fixation of the vocal cords with resulting vocal cord obstruction and eventually laryngeal stenosis. In the far advanced case, multiple laryngocutaneous fistulae may develop.[5]

From the Department of Otolaryngology and Maxillofacial Surgery and the Department of Pathology, University of Arkansas Medical Sciences Campus, Little Rock.

Presented at the meeting of the American Laryngological Association, Palm Beach, Florida, April 14-15, 1980.

REPRINTS — James Y. Suen, MD, Dept. of Otolaryngology, Univ. of Arkansas Medical Sciences Campus, 4301 W. Markham, Little Rock, AR 72205.

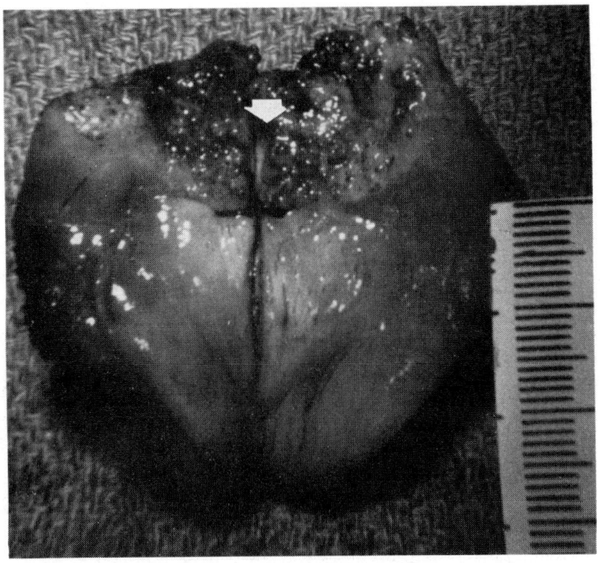

Fig. 1. Epiglottis specimen with ulcerative lesion of the tip. Epiglottis was cut to look at depth of invasion and resutured.

Laboratory Diagnosis. The blastomycosis complement fixation test is unreliable.[7] Most patients with blastomycosis have a negative complement fixation test. Moreover, a positive test is not specific for blastomycosis. The blastomycosis skin test also gives equivocal results even in confirmed cases.[7]

With pulmonary involvement, the diagnosis is usually made by sputum culture and smear. The disseminated lesions are diagnosed by culture and tissue examination. The organism grows in the yeast phase on Sabouraud agar medium at 37 C and plates should be kept four weeks before a negative growth is reported.

CASE REPORTS

Case 1. This white male patient was 53 years old when he presented with a one-year history of sore throats and hoarseness. He had a 40-pack/year smoking history. Indirect laryngoscopy revealed a lesion of the epiglottis, which was thickened, granular, and ulcerative (Fig. 1). He had a 2 cm node in the left mid-jugular area. The initial impression was a T2, N1, M0 squamous cell carcinoma of the supraglottic larynx.

A direct laryngoscopy was performed and a biopsy done. The frozen section diagnosis was squamous cell carcinoma. A supraglottic laryngectomy and bilateral modified neck dissections were carried out. Five months after surgery the patient returned, again complaining of a sore throat. Biopsy of an ulcerated hypopharyngeal lesion revealed pseudoepitheliomatous hyperplasia and occasional granulomata. One year postoperatively the patient returned with bilateral serous otitis media. Biopsies of a nasopharyngeal lesion revealed chronic inflammation. The pathologist decided to review the biopsies and the material from the supraglottic laryngectomy and felt that the original laryngeal lesion was not carcinoma but blastomycosis.

Further questioning of the patient at this time revealed that a skin lesion had been removed from his thigh three years previously and he had been told that it was a fungus infection. His chest x-rays were all interpreted as normal.

The patient was treated with a total dose of 1,800 mg of amphotericin B over five months. In April 1980 the patient was doing well with no significant abnormalities noted on his exam.

Case 2. This 65-year-old white male presented at the University Hospital in August 1974 with a history of hoarseness of six months duration. He had raised chickens and done gardening for years and had a history of excessive smoking. Direct laryngoscopy revealed diffuse granular, edematous changes in most of the endolarynx. Biopsy was interpreted as chronic inflammation with "dysplastic" squamous epithelium. Because of his persistent hoarseness and abnormal-appearing larynx, he had four repeat laryngoscopies over the following two years. The larynx continued to show edema, with granular lesions which were becoming nodular. The repeat biopsies were interpreted as showing inflammation, necrotic debris, and "atypical" or hyperplastic squamous epithelium. Cultures were performed for fungi and tuberculosis and were negative. Tomography demonstrated that the mass on both cords had enlarged and extended both infraglottically and supraglottically.

In September 1976 a presumptive diagnosis of squamous cell carcinoma was made and the patient underwent a full course of radiotherapy (6,500 rads). After treatment the patient continued to have progressive problems with his larynx. He was seen in January 1979 with airway obstruction requiring a tracheostomy. Direct laryngoscopy revealed a small, scarred epiglottis with diffuse nodular and fibrotic changes of the larynx. The vocal cords were partially fixed and difficult to expose because of fibrosis of the larynx. Biopsy at this time revealed inflammatory changes with numerous giant cells and obvious fungi. Review of the preceding biopsies showed occasional fungi resembling *Blastomyces* in each.

His chest x-rays were consistent with a granulomatous process. From August 1973 until 1976 a progressive, bilateral, apical fibronodular pattern with cavitation developed. Hilar and perihilar calcific densities were felt to be secondary to old granulomatous disease, possibly histoplasmosis. From 1976 to 1978 a generalized interstitial fibrosis developed during healing with scarring of the cavitary areas. These changes were consistent with chronic blastomycosis or tuberculosis, or a combined infection, which has been reported.

Fungal serologies for histoplasmosis, blastomycosis, and coccidiomycosis were negative. Urine and prostatic cultures for fungi were negative.

In January 1979 the patient was treated with amphotericin B to a total dose of 1,800 mg over four months. By July 1979 indirect laryngoscopy revealed marked improvement of the larynx and, although there was an adequate airway, there were no obvious lesions but the larynx appeared fibrotic. The vocal cords had nearly normal mobility.

PATHOLOGY

In the first case the tissues from the epiglottis and hypopharynx showed changes typical of infection with *Blastomyces* (Fig. 2A). There was a hyperplastic squamous epithelium which extended in irregular bands through a stroma dominated by chronic inflammatory cells. Collections of acute inflammatory cells formed intraepithelial microabscesses and giant cells were present within these microabscesses (Fig. 2B). Organisms with the morphologic features of *B dermatitidis* were noted frequently. With hematoxylin and eosin (H & E) these organisms appeared as lightly stained, thick-walled structures and were usually within the cytoplasm of giant cells. With periodic acid-Schiff (PAS) or silver methenamine (Gomori) stains, the characteristic 10-15 μm thick-walled ("double contoured") organisms with broad-based budding were easily demonstrated (Figs. 3 and 4).

In the second case the diagnosis was more difficult. The final biopsy revealed pseudoepithelio-

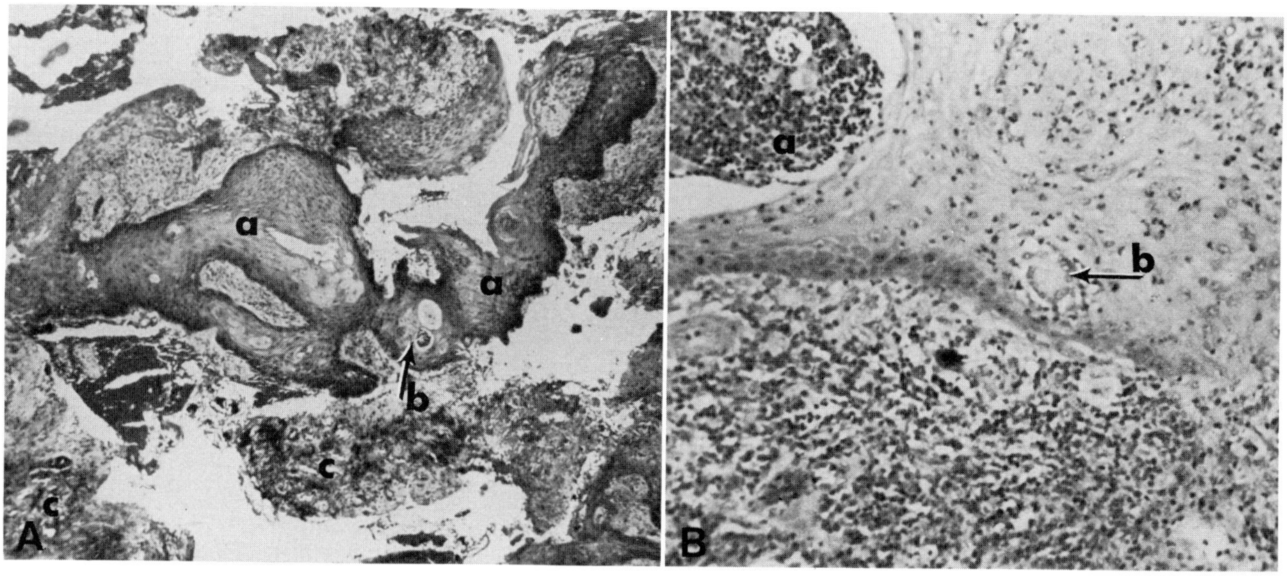

Fig. 2. Pseudoepitheliomatous hyperplasia surrounded by chronic inflammatory cells. A) a - hyperplastic epithelium; b - microabscess; c - chronic inflammatory changes. B) a - microabscess; b - giant cell.

matous hyperplasia, inflammatory infiltrates, and giant cells. The findings were very similar to those in the first case. A search for fungal organisms revealed not only 10-15 μm thick-walled budding fungi characteristic of *Blastomyces* but also numerous 2-3 μm forms which resembled histoplasmosis (Fig. 5). The previous laryngeal biopsies were reviewed and revealed at least one organism on each biopsy. However, microabscesses and giant cells were not apparent and the inflammatory infiltrate was not as marked as in Figure 2A.

The organisms found on all biopsies except the final one were of the large, thick-walled type and no small, histoplasma-like organisms were seen. The fungi were often found in the midst of necrotic debris without surrounding giant cells or inflammatory infiltrates.

DISCUSSION

In the first case the frozen and permanent sections were initially interpreted as squamous cell carcinoma because of the marked pseudoepitheliomatous hyperplasia with atypia. The patient was treated with a supraglottic laryngectomy because the clinical findings also were compatible with cancer. It was a year later, after continued problems resulted in a review of the previous tissue by an astute pathologist, that the *Blastomyces* organisms were noted. Special stains using PAS demonstrated the organisms easily. This patient had normal chest

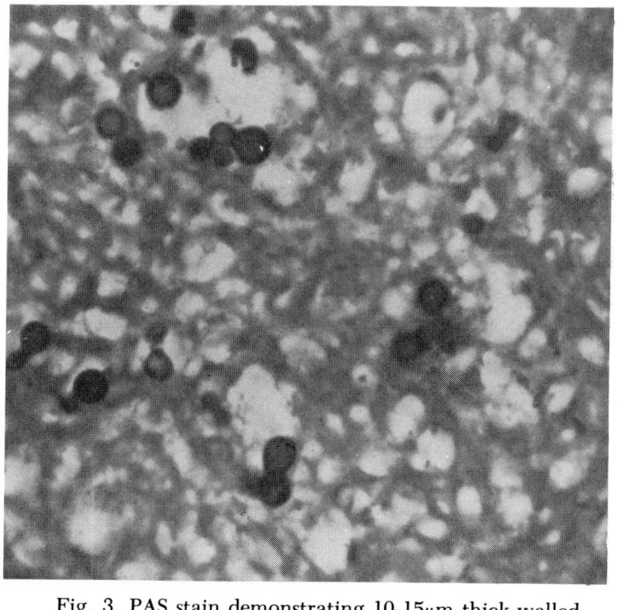

Fig. 3. PAS stain demonstrating 10-15μm thick-walled blastomyces organisms with broad-based budding.

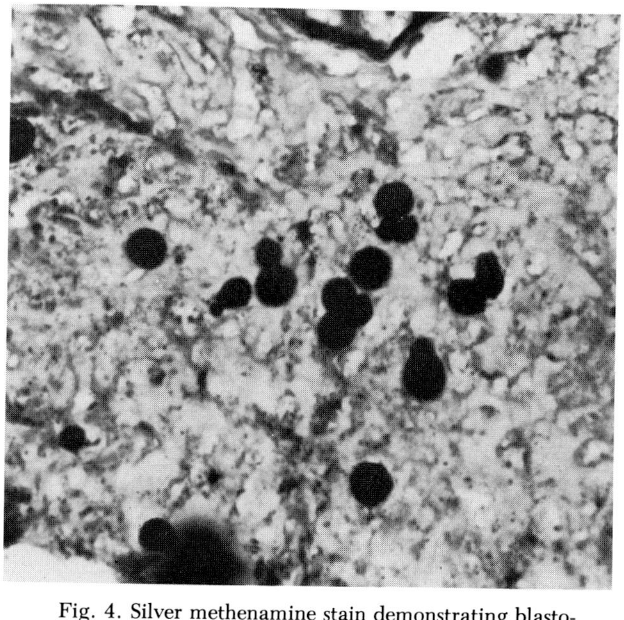

Fig. 4. Silver methenamine stain demonstrating blastomyces organisms.

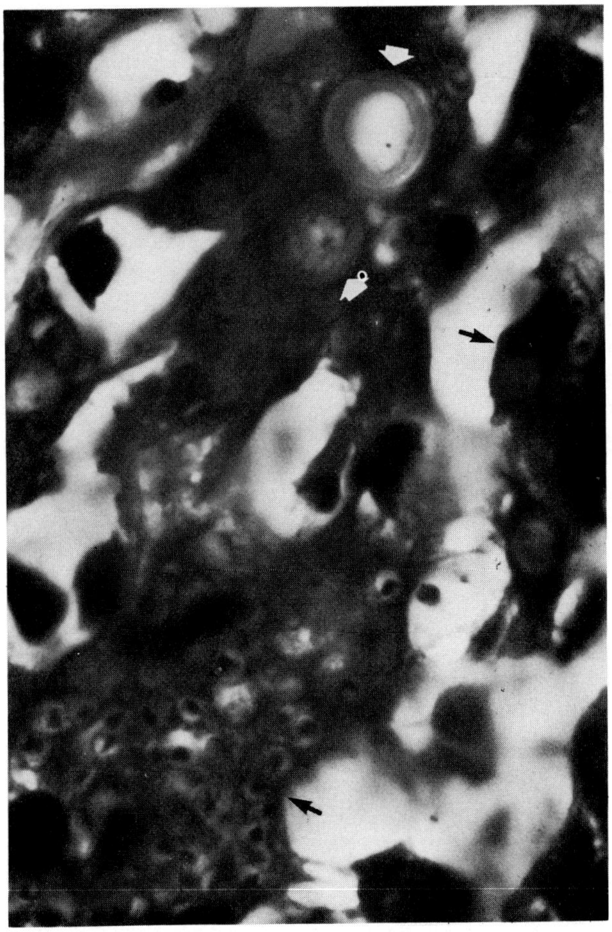

Fig. 5. Two forms of blastomyces organisms (H & E stain): the 10-15 μm thick-walled fungi (white arrows) and the 2-3 μm histoplasmosis-like forms (black arrows).

x-rays, but in all probability he initially had a pulmonary infection with seeding of the skin of his thigh and of his larynx and spontaneous resolution of the pulmonary infection. We cannot rule out primary laryngeal involvement. Primary skin involvement is rare and has been described only in persons who were accidentally inoculated.

In the second case, the problems and diagnosis were more complex. Because of the progressive laryngeal disease and the diagnosis of atypia, it was felt that this patient probably had a verrucous type carcinoma. Rather than do a total laryngectomy without a firm diagnosis, the treating physician elected to administer full course radiation to the larynx. The final diagnosis did not become evident until over four years later when his eighth laryngeal biopsy revealed obvious fungal organisms. This patient had definite pulmonary disease throughout all of his laryngeal problems which was most likely secondary to blastomycosis. In this case the lungs were thought to be the primary site of infection, with secondary involvement of the larynx.

Both cases had findings in almost all of the biopsies which were typical of infection with *Blastomyces* and should have made the pathologist suspect this diagnosis. These suspicious findings were pseudoepitheliomatous hyperplasia, chronic inflammatory changes, microabscesses, and giant cells. When these findings are present with no obvious carcinoma noted, the use of PAS or silver methenamine stains will demonstrate the broad-based budding spores of *Blastomyces* organisms, if present.

The treatment of laryngeal blastomycosis is administration of amphotericin B.[4,8] This drug usually causes nausea, vomiting, chills, and frequently reversible renal insufficiency. Treatment involves intermittent administration of amphotericin B intravenously over several months. Prior to the advent of effective antifungal drugs, disseminated blastomycosis was usually a fatal disease.[4]

SUMMARY

Two patients were presented with blastomycosis of the larynx which had been misdiagnosed as squamous cell carcinoma. The serious clinical consequences of an erroneous diagnosis of squamous cell carcinoma are easily appreciated. Blastomycosis is a progressive and often lethal disease if untreated. One should always consider blastomycosis in patients who continue to have laryngeal problems and the histologic picture reveals pseudoepitheliomatous hyperplasia, chronic inflammatory changes with intraepithelial microabscesses and giant cells.

REFERENCES

1. Fuller TE. Report of a case of blastomycosis of the larynx complicating carcinoma. J Arkansas Med Soc 1936; 33:37-8.

2. Ferguson GB. North American blastomycosis. A review of the literature and a report of two cases primary in the larynx. Laryngoscope 1951; 61:851-72.

3. Pirozzi DJ, Schwarzmann SW, Lewis AD. An unusual case of North American blastomycosis. Arch Dermatol 1978; 114:1370-1.

4. Sarosi GA, Davies SF. Blastomycosis. Am Rev Respir Dis 1979; 120:911-38.

5. Ranier A. Primary laryngeal blastomycosis: a review of the literature and report of a case. Am J Clin Pathol 1951; 21:444-50.

6. Thornell WC. Blastomycosis of the larynx. Ann Otol Rhinol Laryngol 1955; 64:1155-63.

7. Cush R, Light RW, George RB. Clinical and roentgenographic manifestations of acute and chronic blastomycosis. Chest 1976; 69:345-9.

8. Bennett M. Laryngeal blastomycosis. Laryngoscope 1964; 74:498-512.

Ann Otol 89:1980

CONSERVATIVE SURGICAL TREATMENT OF CHONDROSARCOMA OF THE LARYNX

ROBERT W. CANTRELL, MD
ROBERT A. JAHRSDOERFER, MD
JAMES F. REIBEL, MD
MICHAEL E. JOHNS, MD
CHARLOTTESVILLE, VIRGINIA

Chondrosarcoma of the larynx is a rare malignant tumor sometimes encountered by otolaryngologists. Since they are usually of low grade malignancy, total laryngectomy is indicated only in cases of high grade malignancy or where total excision by conservative (partial) laryngectomy is not feasible. This paper reviews chondrosarcoma of the larynx, discusses a patient who developed this tumor, and describes a method of conservative surgical excision and laryngotracheal reconstruction when the tumor involves the cricoid, the most common site of occurrence in the larynx.

Chondrosarcoma of the larynx is a rare form of sarcoma sometimes encountered by otolaryngologists. Since it is usually of low grade malignancy, the methods of treatment applied to most sarcomas, ie, chemotherapy, irradiation, and radical surgery, do not apply. Total laryngectomy may be required for high grade malignant tumors, recurrent lesions, or in those cases where total excision by conservative laryngeal surgery is not feasible. Nearly all laryngeal chondrosarcomas can be managed successfully by excision through laryngofissure, thyrotomy, or partial laryngectomy. This paper reviews laryngeal chondrosarcoma, discusses a patient who developed this tumor, and describes a method of conservative surgical excision and laryngotracheal reconstruction when the tumor involves the cricoid, the most common site of occurrence in the larynx.

INCIDENCE

Approximately 58 laryngeal chondrosarcomas have been reported in the past 80 years,[1-16] and it was not until 1935 that New[13] referred to the malignant tumor of laryngeal cartilage as chondrosarcoma. In most published series chondrosarcomas are grouped with other cartilaginous tumors of the larynx, making the exact incidence difficult to determine, and several cases have been reported more than once. Of the 58 definite cases reviewed, the average age was 58 years (range 33-91) with 43 males and 15 females developing the tumor.

CLINICAL FEATURES

The most common presenting symptom was hoarseness in 40 cases, dyspnea in 14, dysphagia in 2, and an anterior neck mass in 2 cases. Many patients had both hoarseness and dyspnea and several had dysphagia as well. These symptoms had been present from one month to eight years with nearly all being present more than six months. Since most of these tumors grow slowly intraluminally, the signs and symptoms are easily understood and relate to the size and location of the tumor within the larynx.

LOCATION

Seventy-eight percent (45 of 58) of these tumors arose from the cricoid, usually the posterior or posterolateral areas. Nine (15%) arose from the thyroid cartilage, three from the arytenoids and one was reported as arising in the vocal cord. No cases of epiglottic chondrosarcoma were reported.

If the tumor grows externally it is usually firmly attached to the thyroid cartilage. More commonly the external appearance of the patient is unremarkable. Indirect laryngoscopy may show partial or complete vocal cord paralysis due to pressure and size of the lesion. Most often only a subglottic mass covered with mucosa is seen. At this point the differential diagnosis is between benign lesions such as amyloidosis, laryngeal cyst, laryngoceles, neurilemmoma, and fibroma, or malignant lesions such as carcinoma or the various sarcomas.

RADIOLOGIC APPEARANCE

The tumor can be shown by soft tissue x-ray techniques, xeroradiography, tomography, and laryngogram. These are not diagnostic and usually serve only to confirm and document the clinical impression of a mass in the subglottic area. Occasionally x-rays may show calcification.

DIAGNOSIS

Direct laryngoscopy with biopsy is the usual method of diagnosis. Occasionally biopsy of the firm, cartilaginous tumor mass is very difficult.

From the Division of Head and Neck Oncology, Department of Otolaryngology and Maxillofacial Surgery, University of Virginia Medical Center, Charlottesville, Virginia.

Presented at the meeting of the American Laryngological Association, Palm Beach, Florida, April 14-15, 1980.

REPRINTS — Robert W. Cantrell, MD, Department of Otolaryngology, Box 430, University of Virginia Medical Center, Charlottesville, VA 22908.

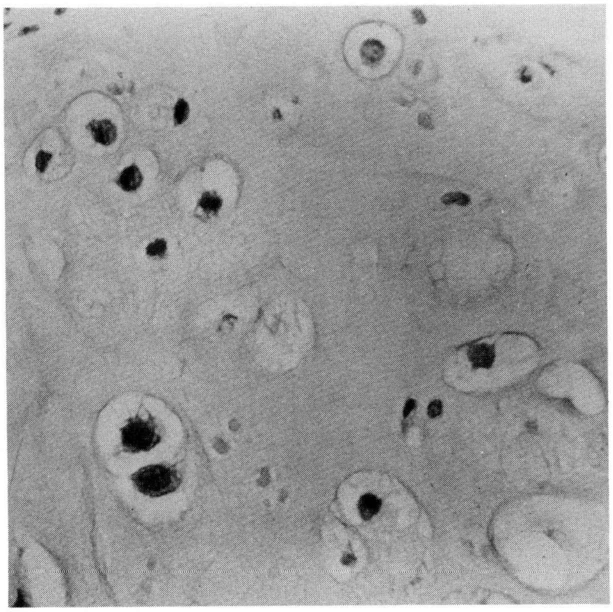

Fig. 1. Photomicrograph of chondrosarcoma. Note binucleated cells. (x400)

Usually, however, a biopsy specimen can be obtained for histological evaluation.

MICROSCOPIC PATHOLOGY

Lichtenstein and Jaffe[17] listed the histological criteria: 1) irregularity in the size of the cells and their nuclei; 2) increased numbers of cells; 3) hyperchromatic nuclei; 4) giant cartilage cells with single or multiple nuclei and/or clumps of chromatin (binucleated cells) (Fig. 1).

Laryngeal chondrosarcomas tend to be diagnosed as benign chondromata and the correct diagnosis is sometimes not made until they recur. It is fortuitous that both lesions are treated the same initially. These tumors can be graded by Broder's classification depending on cellularity, mitoses, and nuclear size. In chondrosarcomas located throughout the body, there is a correlation between classification and metastatic activity. For example, of two series[18,19] totaling 351 cases from all sites in the body, 50% were grade I, 39% grade II, 11% grade III, and none grade IV. Metastases did not occur in any grade I lesions; they occurred in 10% of grade II and 71% of grade III lesions. Five-year survival was likewise correlated (Table 1). It is reasonable to assume these correlations exist for the larynx also.

Most laryngeal chondrosarcomas are low grade malignancies and rarely metastasize. However, 3 of the 58 patients reviewed did develop metastases; 1 patient[15] developed cervical lymph node and pulmonary metastases two years following total laryngectomy necessitated by recurrence of the primary tumor five months after excision via laryngofissure. He also had a tumor embolus in the renal artery which led to a kidney infarct. Another

TABLE 1. SURVIVAL

Grade	*5 yr (%)*	*10 yr (%)*
I	90	83
II	81	64
III	43	29

patient[16] also developed pulmonary metastases 11 months following total laryngectomy necessitated by recurrence of the primary tumor seven months after resection via laryngofissure. The third case[9] was a 71-year-old female who developed a local recurrence 23 years after a local resection. She was treated with a tracheotomy and irradiation but succumbed seven years later (30 years after the primary diagnosis) of laryngeal airway problems. The histological grading of these tumors could not be obtained.

MANAGEMENT

Airway problems must be managed first, and a tracheostomy may be required prior to performing a direct laryngoscopy and biopsy to make the diagnosis. After the diagnosis is established, it must be determined if the tumor is of high or low grade malignancy. Most pathologists can make this determination, given sufficient tissue. If a particular pathologist cannot, the tissue can be sent for review and confirmatory diagnosis at any number of major medical centers. The patient is not harmed by this delay; in fact, he will be much better served. If the tumor is of high grade malignancy, total laryngectomy may be indicated. The number of cases is so small as to make this recommendation debatable. We recommend total laryngectomy for high grade chondrosarcoma.

Fortunately, most (95%) are of low grade malignancy. Laryngofissure and/or thyrotomy with complete excision of the lesion and its base (partial laryngectomy) is required. Seventy-eight percent occur in the cricoid (usually posterior or posterolateral), and many surgeons are reluctant to resect adequate amounts of the cricoid, the keystone of the larynx. This fact may account for the high incidence of recurrence following laryngofissure (generally 60%; 100% in one series of six patients). In spite of this high recurrence rate, most surgeons still prefer laryngofissure and excision since the recurrences, which sometimes occur years later, are local, usually slow growing, and can be managed by further conservative surgery.

Some patients in this series had tumors so extensive that total laryngectomy was required to ensure complete removal.

In this series of 58 patients, 42 had laryngofissure/thyrotomies and/or partial laryngectomies, 10 had total laryngectomies initially (and at least 4 more had total laryngectomies after recurrence), 1 had endoscopic removal of a small tumor, 2 had tumors excised from the external surface of the

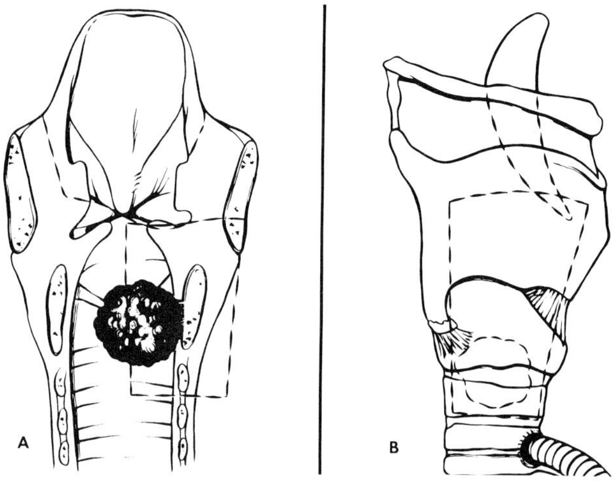

Fig. 2. A) Line drawing of larynx showing tumor location and proposed lines of resection. B) Drawing of proposed resection on exposed larynx.

thyroid cartilage, and 3 had only palliative treatment (two tracheostomies and one gastrostomy). Several patients[6,8,9] had irradiation with no apparent beneficial effect.

CASE REPORT

A 47-year-old white female was referred to the University of Virginia Medical Center on July 19, 1979, for evaluation of a recurrent anterior neck mass and increasing dyspnea. She had had a partial thyroidectomy for goiter 15 years earlier and had done well until two years prior to admission when she noticed the onset of stridor, exertional dyspnea, and a slowly enlarging neck mass. Examination by the local otolaryngologist confirmed a bilaterally enlarged thyroid and a subglottic mass. She was also an insulin-dependent diabetic.

Physical examination was unremarkable except for stridor, dyspnea, a markedly enlarged, firm thyroid and a mass attached to the right posterolateral subglottic area. Both vocal cords moved well.

Admission laboratory studies included a hemogram, urinalysis, chest x-ray, thyroid function studies, and SMA-12; results were all

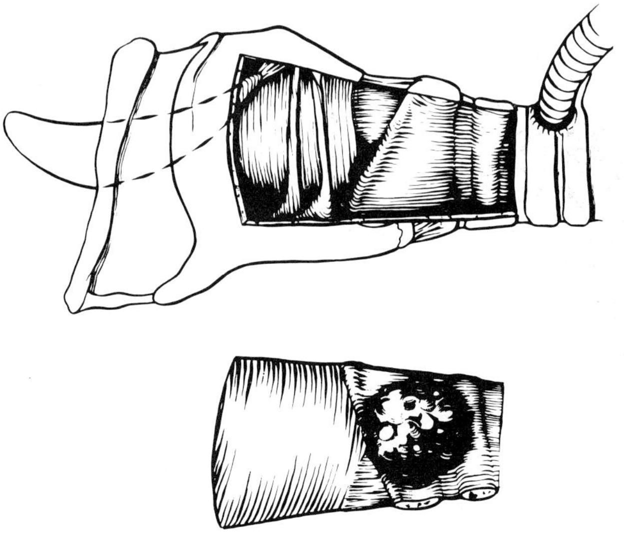

Fig. 3. Drawing of specimen and laryngeal defect.

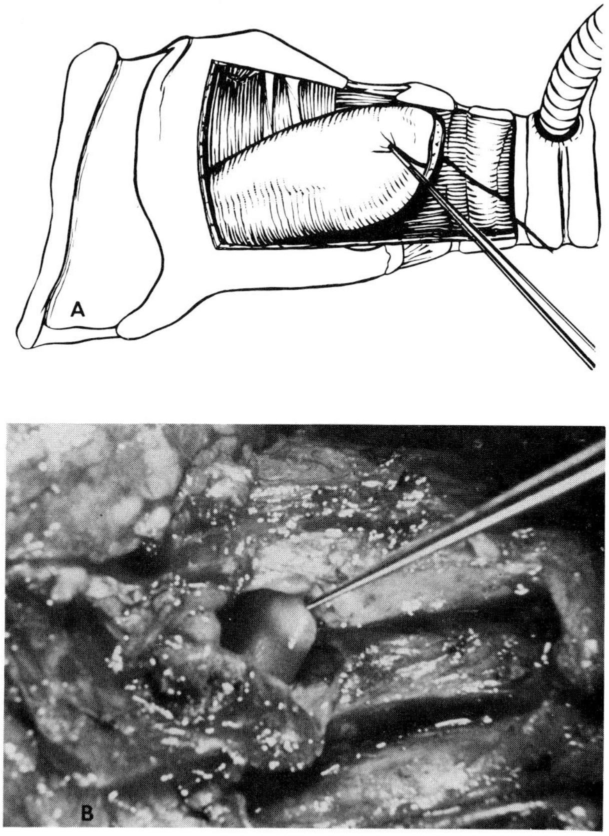

Fig. 4. A) Drawing and B) photograph of epiglottis being retracted after dissection.

within normal limits. A xerogram of the neck confirmed the mass in the subglottic region.

On July 20, 1979, the patient underwent a tracheostomy under local anesthesia, and, under general anesthesia, a direct laryngoscopy and excisional biopsy of the subglottic mass and a total thyroidectomy. The mass was pedunculated, firm, and gritty but did not appear cartilaginous grossly. It was attached to the right posterolateral cricoid and first tracheal ring (Fig. 2A). At this point, we felt we were dealing with a thyroid lesion which had extended into the laryngotrachea.

The thyroid was then approached and upon exposing it, there appeared two large, purplish-tan lobes of tissue measuring 3 x 2 x 2 cm on the left and 5 x 3 x 2.5 cm on the right. There was little or no resemblance to a normal thyroid and the tissue appeared to be growing into the right cricothyroid membrane in the area where the endolaryngotracheal mass previously had been removed.

Histological diagnosis of the subglottic mass was grade I chondrosarcoma, and nodular goiter with Hashimoto's thyroiditis of both thyroid lobes.

Postoperatively the patient did well, was discharged on July 24, 1979, on thyroid replacement therapy, and was scheduled for readmission on August 9, 1979, to undergo definitive laryngeal surgery.

On August 10, 1979, general anesthesia was administered via an endotracheal tube through the tracheostoma and an apron flap was elevated. Upon elevating the flap a 2 cm nodule in the thyrohyoid area was noted. It was similar clinically to the previous thyroid tissue, and frozen section diagnosis confirmed Hashimoto's thyroiditis in this thyroid remnant in the area where one usually finds a thyroglossal duct cyst.

A laryngofissure was performed, carried through the cricoid and first tracheal cartilage. The incisions were carried horizontally between the first and second tracheal rings and just above the

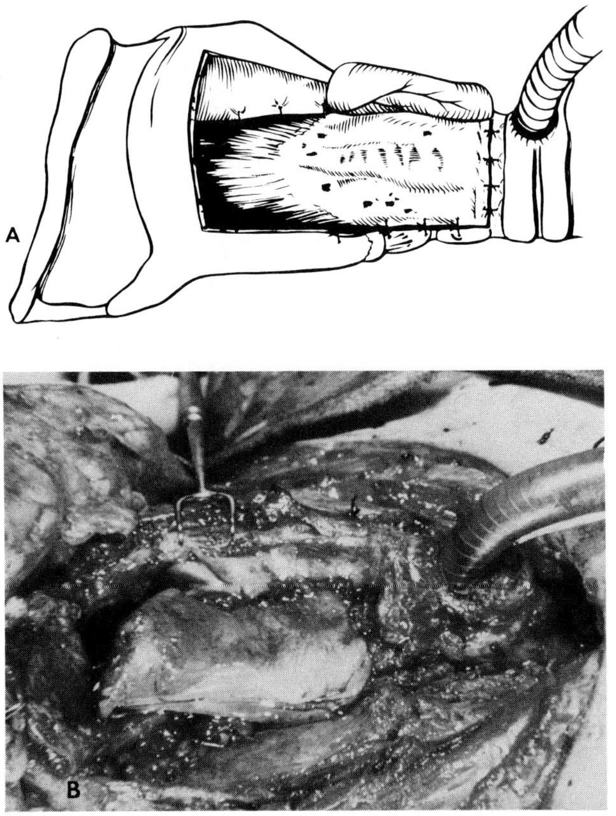

Fig. 5. A) Drawing and B) photograph of epiglottic flap trimmed and sewn in position.

right true vocal cord (Fig. 2B). The incision was then made vertically in the interarytenoid area and carried down through the first tracheal cartilage, veering slightly to the left of midline in the area of the tumor. Frozen section confirmed the margins were free of tumor.

A rather large defect consisting of most of the right thyroid cartilage, the right half of the cricoid, and the right half of the first tracheal cartilage then existed (Fig. 3). To close this, the epiglottis was detached from its left lateral attachments and its base, but its right lateral attachments, including the right aryepiglottic fold, were preserved (Fig. 4A,B). The fold was rotated 180° inferiorly and the mucosa of the lingual epiglottic surface incised in a "T" fashion and elevated. The tip of the cartilage was squared and the mucosa sutured to the remaining laryngotracheal mucosa with submucosal sutures (Fig. 5A,B). A laryngeal stent was placed prior to closure, the cartilage was reinforced by suturing, and a portion of the right sternomastoid muscle was turned over the suture lines and sewn in place (Fig. 6A,B). The apron flap was closed.

The patient did well postoperatively until the fourth day when she coughed vigorously and expelled the stent. This did not delay convalescence and by the seventh postoperative day, her nasogastric tube was removed and she was started on oral feedings without aspiration. She was discharged on the eighth postoperative day with a tracheostomy tube in place.

The patient was seen 12 days after discharge and the tracheostomy tube was replaced with an Olympic® button. She could talk with the button occluded but could not breathe. When seen two months later, she was wheezing, and the Olympic button was replaced with a number six tracheostomy tube. Xerography of the larynx showed distortion of the subglottic area, and she was readmitted for a direct laryngoscopy.

Upon inspecting the larynx directly, a flap of tissue protruding from the right portion of the larynx was noted to be occluding the airway. This was removed by microdissection. After removing this flap, the larynx appeared relatively normal except for the portions of the epiglottis, which was well healed. There was no evidence of tumor.

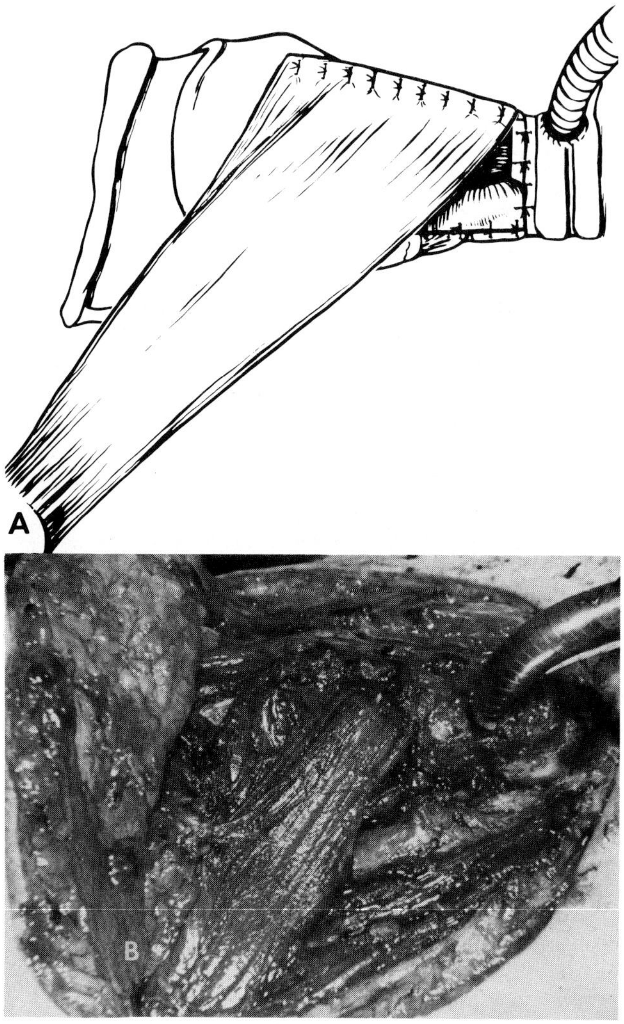

Fig. 6. A) Drawing and B) photograph of portion of sternocleidomastoid muscle sewn in place over epiglottic flap.

Following discharge, the patient was seen in one month and again in three months. Her voice is satisfactory and she has returned to normal activity. She can perform tasks which she has been unable to do for more than a year. Although she has a partial airway, it is not sufficient to allow decannulation. Inspection of the larynx shows insufficient abduction of the left cord on inspiration, but good adduction on phonation with the left cord abutting the epiglottic flap, producing the voice. A laryngoplasty to allow decannulation and tracheostomy closure is planned in June.

Comment. This patient illustrates most of the features of laryngeal chondrosarcoma. The lesion arose from the cricoid; it was slowly progressive for approximately two years, with dyspnea being the main symptom.

The tumor was classified as low grade malignancy and resection via a laryngofissure approach ending with a partial laryngectomy is likely to be curative. Reconstruction with a composite epiglottic flap offers some hope for a relatively normal, functioning larynx, but with removal of more than 50% of the cricoid, the prospect of both normal respiration and normal speech is minimal.

REFERENCES

1. Barocchini LM, McCoy G. Cartilaginous tumors of the larynx. Ann Otol Rhinol Laryngol 1968; 77:146-53.

2. Brandenburg JH, Harris DD, Bennett M. Chondrosarcoma of the larynx. Laryngoscope 1967; 77:752-62.

3. Clerf LH. Sarcoma of the larynx: report of eight cases. Arch Otolaryngol 1946; 44:517-24.

4. Cocke EW Jr. Benign cartilaginous tumors of the larynx. Laryngoscope 1962; 72:1678-1730.

5. Eggleston AA, Wolff D. Histopathology of the ear, nose and throat. Baltimore: Williams and Wilkins, 1947:956-7.

6. Goethals PL, Dahlin DC, Devine KD. Cartilaginous tumors of the larynx. Surg Gynecol Obstet 1963; 117:77-82.

7. Gorenstein A, Neel HB, Weiland LH, Devine KD. Sarcomas of the larynx. Arch Otolaryngol 1980; 106:8-12.

8. Huizenga C, Balogh K. Cartilaginous tumors of the larynx. Cancer 1970; 26:201-10.

9. Hyams VJ, Rabuzzi DD. Cartilaginous tumors of the larynx. Laryngoscope 1970; 80:755-67.

10. Link MR. Chondroma and chondrosarcoma of the larynx. Ann Otol Rhinol Laryngol 1949; 58:70-85.

11. Mansfeld D. Ueber Knorpelgeschwülste des Kehlkopfs nebst Mitteilung eines Falles von Chondroma myxomatodes. Fränkels Arch Laryngol 1909; 22:508-23.

12. Mayoux P, Martin H, Rebattu JP. A propos de deux observations de chondromes du larynx. J Fr Oto-Rhino-Laryngol 1944; 4:127-31.

13. New GB. Sarcoma of the larynx: report of two cases. Arch Otolaryngol 1935; 21:648-52.

14. Putney FJ, Moran JJ. Cartilaginous tumors of the larynx. Ann Otol Rhinol Laryngol 1964; 73:1-12.

15. Sirota JJ, Hurwitz A. Chondrosarcoma of the larynx. Arch Otolaryngol 1952; 56:290-3.

16. Ungerecht K. Multiple Chondrome und Chondrosarkome des Larynx und der Trachea mit chondromyxosarkomatösen Rezidiven. Arch Klin Ohren Nasen Kehlkopfheilkd 1951; 160:158-69.

17. Lichtenstein L, Jaffe H. Chondrosarcoma of bone. Am J Pathol 1943; 19:553-74.

18. Evans HL, Ayala AG, Romsdahl MM. Prognostic factors in chondrosarcoma of bone. Cancer 1977; 40:818-31.

19. Pritchard DJ, Lunke RJ, Taylor WF, Dahlin DC, Medley BE. Chondrosarcoma: a clinicopathologic and statistical analysis. Cancer 1980; 45:149-57.

≈

AFIP TRAINING PROGRAM IN HEAD AND NECK PATHOLOGY

A three-month fellowship is available to residents in training in otolaryngology as well as postgraduate fellows. This fellowship is designed to provide a broad-based understanding of pathology of the head and neck in one of the institutions with the most expertise and experience in this country. The curriculum consists of daily lecture periods discussing the pathology of the head and neck area, examination and discussions of interesting consultation cases, self study material and encouragement to undertake a publishable research project. Facilities for temporal bone dissection are available.

Interested candidates may contact Vincent J. Hyams, MD, Chief, Otolaryngic Pathology, Armed Forces Institute of Pathology, Washington, DC 20306.

AIRWAY OBSTRUCTION IN A HEMOPHILIAC CHILD

JOHN F. STANIEVICH, MD
BUFFALO, NEW YORK

GABRIEL MARSHAK, MD
PITTSBURGH, PENNSYLVANIA

SYLVAN E. STOOL, MD
PITTSBURGH, PENNSYLVANIA

The hemophiliac patient is in constant danger of death from hemorrhage. The danger of bleeding into the submucosal areas of the upper aerodigestive tract, however, does not primarily lie in the blood loss but rather is due to compression and edema of the upper airway. The treatment of choice, in addition to the direct treatment for the specific clotting factor deficiency, is elective nasotracheal intubation, since in most cases this interstitial bleeding, resulting in airway compromise, recedes in four to five days.

The hemophiliac patient is in constant danger of death from hemorrhage. The hemorrhage, which bleeds into the submucosal areas of the floor of the mouth, pharynx and larynx, does not endanger life primarily because of blood loss, but rather due to compression and edema of the larynx and upper trachea, resulting in asphyxia.

A case is presented with review of the literature to illustrate the complexity of the problem and the proper multidisciplinary approach needed for successful management of such cases.

CASE REPORT

A five-year-old black male with severe hemophilia A presented to the emergency room with a two-day history of increasing submandibular swelling without antecedent trauma. Dysphagia, dysarthria and slight hoarseness were noted by the mother. Physical examination revealed an apprehensive youngster in no respiratory distress, with normal vital signs and no fever. The floor of the mouth was tense, ecchymotic and swollen, and a soft mass involving both submandibular and submental triangle was seen. Hemoglobin was 10.1 gm % with hematocrit of 29.5% and the prothrombin time was 87.9 seconds (normal = 26-34 seconds). This patient had less than 1% of the normal levels of factor VIII and also had antifactor VIII antibodies (last titer 1:16). Lateral neck film showed a markedly swollen epiglottis (Fig. 1). He was started on cryoprecipitated factors II, VII, IX and X (Proplex®, Hyland Co.) 50 mg/kg every six hours, but the swelling of his neck and floor of the mouth increased with involvement of the base on the tongue, causing some respiratory difficulty. Because of progression of his symptoms, elective nasotracheal intubation was carried out with inhalation induction and anesthesia (N_2O, O_2, halothane). The base of the tongue valleculae and epiglottis were very ecchymotic and edematous, and the interior of the larynx could not be visualized, so that the intubation was performed with the otolaryngologist guiding the tube and the anesthesiologist listening for breath sounds.

The patient did well postoperatively although his neck swelling increased considerably for one day, in spite of large doses of cryoprecipitated factors II, VII, IX, and X and epsilon aminocaproic acid* (to minimize the risk of fibrinolysis). By the fifth day, the swelling decreased considerably and he was extubated under general anesthesia. The oral cavity, hypopharynx and larynx, except for the vocal cords, showed only minimal ecchymosis.

DISCUSSION

Spontaneous submucosal bleeding in the floor of the mouth, pharynx and larynx is uncommon in hemophilia. Lewis,[1] reporting on the cause of death of 28 hemophilia patients in a series of 310 patients, described only one such case. The outcome of submucosal bleeding in the upper aerodigestive system is unfavorable, as shown by the 12 cases that have been reported in the English literature. One patient died from the rapid development of submucosal pharyngolaryngeal bleeding, which blocked the airway before help could be given.[2] Five[1,3] patients had whole blood transfusion, four of whom sur-

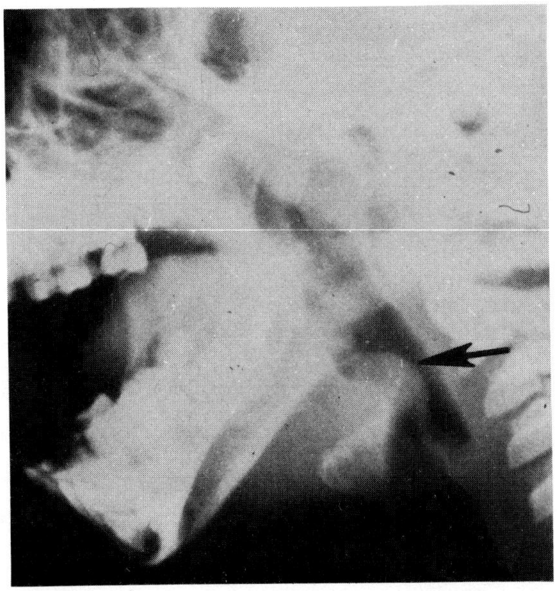

Fig. 1. Lateral neck film showing markedly swollen epiglottis (arrow).

*Amicar®, Lederle Laboratories, Wayne, NJ.

From the Department of Otolaryngology, University of Pittsburgh School of Medicine, Children's Hospital of Pittsburgh, Pittsburgh, Pennsylvania.

Presented at the meeting of the American Laryngological Association, Palm Beach, Florida, April 14-15, 1980.

REPRINTS — John F. Stanievich, MD, Department of Otolaryngology, University of Pittsburgh School of Medicine, Children's Hospital of Pittsburgh, Pittsburgh, PA 15213.

vived and one[1] died of overtransfusion. Five patients had tracheostomy[3,4] to relieve the airway obstruction but four died, and two patients[5,6] survived following oral and nasotracheal intubation.

In most cases, the symptoms and signs of impending airway obstruction in the hemophiliac develop slowly over hours and occasionally, even days. Such patients, complaining of dysphagia, dysarthria or sore throat with or without fever, should be admitted to the hospital. Lateral neck films are very helpful, especially in those cases where, because of the swelling of the floor of the mouth and tongue, the hypopharynx and larynx cannot be properly assessed. The patient should be given the benefit of the direct treatment for the specific clotting factor deficiency. If swelling increases either in the soft tissues of the neck or in the mouth, it is better to provide an alternate airway when this can be accomplished as an elective procedure, rather than wait until the child is in severe respiratory distress. This should be done with inhalation induction and anesthesia without use of muscle relaxants. Intubation in such cases is always difficult and usually accomplished without direct visualization.

Since the interstitial submucosal and subcutaneous bleeding in the hemophiliac resolves in two to five days, we feel that nasotracheal intubation is preferable to tracheotomy because the incision and dissection will result in a wound which may bleed and granulate, thus increasing the need for prolonged hospitalization and replacement of coagulation factors.

REFERENCES

1. Lewis JH. Causes of death in hemophilia. JAMA 1970; 214:1707.

2. Davidson CS, Epstein RD, Miller GF, Taylor FHI. Hemophilia; clinical study of 40 patients. Blood 1949; 4:97-119.

3. Baird KH, Meyer SF. Severe sublingual and paratracheal hemorrhage in hemophilia with recovery following tracheotomy. J Pediatr 1943; 23:90-7.

4. Edwards AR. Death from respiratory obstruction in hemophilia. Med J Aust 1951; 1:227-8.

5. Boyd WHF. Respiratory obstruction in hemophilia recovery after intubation. Lancet 1950; 1:302.

6. McDonald AC, Robson JG, Wapshaw H. Hemophilia with respiratory obstruction. Br Med J 1953; 1:1144-6.

Ann Otol 80:1980

CANDIDA LARYNGITIS IN CHRONIC MUCOCUTANEOUS CANDIDIASIS
ITS ASSOCIATION WITH *CANDIDA* ESOPHAGITIS

JAMES P. DUDLEY, MD ROGER KOBAYASHI, MD HOWARD M. ROSENBLATT, MD
WILLIAM J. BYRNE, MD MARVIN E. AMENT, MD E. RICHARD STIEHM, MD
LOS ANGELES, CALIFORNIA

Four patients with chronic mucocutaneous candidiasis (CMC) underwent esophagoscopy and microlaryngoscopy. Cultures were obtained by biopsy of the larynx and the esophagus. Three of the four patients with laryngeal disease proven by laryngoscopy and culture also had extensive esophageal disease. One patient with a normal larynx by examination and culture also had a normal esophagus. There appears to be a good correlation between the presence of laryngeal and esophageal disease.

Chronic mucocutaneous candidiasis (CMC), a defect in cell-mediated immunity, is characterized by infection of the mucous membranes, skin, hair, and nails.[1] Although these infections may heal without a trace, scarring can be the end result. When extensive infection involves an organ such as the esophagus, the resulting stenosis presents a difficult management problem. Since early treatment prevents extensive esophageal disease and probably limits scarring in the esophagus, early diagnosis of esophageal involvement and prompt treatment is important. Unfortunately the symptoms of disease, such as dysphagia, are not necessarily accurate guides in determining the extent of disease. Because of this, esophagoscopy has been frequently used in the evaluation of CMC patients, even those without esophageal symptoms. Although the same rules of early diagnosis and prompt treatment no doubt apply when the disease involves the larynx, laryngeal examination is apparently infrequently done. In fact, most of the reports of laryngeal CMC have not included a description of the larynx.[2-4] Despite the scarring and hoarseness which may occur with laryngeal involvement, the more life-threathening sequela is that which produces esophageal stenosis. Monitoring the disease as it affects the esophagus would be easier if there were a correlation between esophageal and laryngeal infection. Although esophagoscopy is the definitive procedure to determine the extent of *Candida* involvement, the study of Kobayashi et al[5] provided an opportunity to compare laryngeal and esophageal disease in the same patient and to see if the more easily examined larynx can act in any way as a mirror to the esophagus.

METHODS

Four patients with the diagnosis of CMC ranged in age from 11 to 17. Although dysphagia was present in three of the four patients, hoarseness was not a constant symptom in all four patients. Direct microlaryngoscopy was done at the time of a fiberoptic esophagoscopy. Fungus cultures were obtained by biopsy of the vocal cords and biopsy of the esophageal wall.

RESULTS

Three patients with symptoms of dysphagia had visual evidence of esophagitis and laryngitis, while one patient who had no dysphagia had a normal larynx and esophagus. *Candida albicans* was obtained by biopsy of the esophageal wall and the vocal cords in each of the three patients with obvious esophageal and laryngeal disease. In the one patient with no evidence of disease the organisms failed to grow from the biopsies of the vocal cord and esophagus.

One patient underwent a combined esophagoscopy and microlaryngoscopy following treatment with amphotericin B. There was no evidence of laryngitis in this patient and *C albicans* failed to grow from the laryngeal biopsy. There was minimal esophageal involvement with *C albicans*.

DISCUSSION

In this small group of patients, there appears to be a good correlation between infections of the larynx and the esophagus. Three patients with esophageal disease had visual evidence of laryngitis and biopsy proven *Candida* infection. One patient with no evidence of esophageal disease had a normal larynx. The larynx of a patient who was treated with amphotericin was not infected with *Candida*, and its appearance was normal. Although there was some esophageal disease in this patient, the extent of involvement was minimal. Although esophagoscopy is the procedure of choice to determine how much of the esophageal mucosa is involved, the application of laryngoscopy may prove a useful adjunct in the management of these patients.

From the Department of Surgery, Division of Head and Neck Surgery; and the Department of Pediatrics, Divisions of Allergy and Immunology, and Gastroenterology, University of California at Los Angeles, Los Angeles, California.

Presented at the meeting of the American Laryngological Association, Palm Beach, Florida, April 14-15, 1980.

REPRINTS — James P. Dudley, MD, Division of Head and Neck Surgery, 62-158 UCLA Medical Center, Los Angeles, CA 90024.

REFERENCES

1. Stiehm ER. Chronic mucocutaneous candidiasis: clinical aspects. In: Edwards JE, moderator. Severe candidal infections. Clinical perspective, immune defense mechanisms, and current concepts of therapy. Ann Intern Med 1978; 89:91-106.

2. Chilgren RA, Meuwissen HJ, Quie PE, Hong R. Chronic mucocutaneous candidiasis, deficiency of delayed hypersensitivity, and selective local antibody defect. Lancet 1967; 2:688-93.

3. Wells RS, Higgs JM, MacDonald A, Valdimarsson H, Holt PJ. Familial chronic mucocutaneous candidiasis. J Med Genet 1972; 9:302-10.

4. Leikien S, Parrott R, Randolph J. Clotrimazole treatment of chronic mucocutaneous candidiasis. J Pediatr 1976; 88:864-6.

5. Kobayashi RH, Rosenblatt HM, Carney JM, et al. Candida esophagitis and laryngitis in chronic mucocutaneous candidiasis. Pediatrics (in press).

≈

LURIE LIBRARY FUND

Many inquiries have been made about a memorial fund to which friends and colleagues of Dr. Moses Hyman Lurie could contribute. Shortly before his death Dr. Lurie established a modest fund for the purchase of books in Otolaryngology for the Library at the Massachusetts Eye and Ear Infirmary. The Library Committee of the Infirmary has verified that donations can be made in memory of Dr. Lurie to this fund. Contributions may be sent to the "Lurie Library Fund," in care of Mr. Charles Snyder, Librarian, Massachusetts Eye and Ear Infirmary, 243 Charles St., Boston, MA 02114.

Ann Otol 89:1980

REPAIR OF SUPRAGLOTTIC LARYNGEAL STENOSIS WITH POSTCRICOID INVOLVEMENT

A CASE REPORT

PATRICK J. DOYLE, MD

VANCOUVER, BRITISH COLUMBIA, CANADA

A supraglottic stenosis with postcricoid stenosis was successfully corrected in a single stage procedure by excising the scar tissue and the arytenoid cartilage and the use of mucosal flaps to recover the right side of the larynx and postcricoid area. By obtaining good mucosal approximation without tension the need for a free skin graft or mucosal graft was avoided.

Some patients suffering from posttraumatic laryngeal stenosis present with an associated postcricoid stenosis.

A 23-year-old male was involved in a motor vehicle accident in September 1978. He suffered a fractured mandible and a laryngeal fracture. An immediate tracheotomy was performed and the mandibular fracture repaired by open reduction and wiring. The mandible healed uneventfully but he could not be extubated and was therefore referred to an otolaryngologist two months after the original injury.

He then presented with almost total obstruction of his laryngeal airway, a very weak breathy voice, inability to swallow solids and aspiration of liquids. A direct laryngoscopy was described as showing "extensive synechiae at the glottis and a subglottic granuloma. The granuloma was removed." There was no change in his condition during the ensuing months and he was referred for further evaluation and treatment in April 1979.

Indirect laryngoscopy revealed severe distortion of the supraglottic larynx with displacement of the epiglottis to the left (Fig. 1A). A supraglottic stenosis prevented visualization of the vocal cords. Tomography showed severe distortion of the right side of the larynx. Direct laryngoscopy was performed and the subglottic larynx was examined through the tracheotomy. There was no subglottic stenosis or granuloma present. Scar tissue replaced the right side of the larynx extending to the postcricoid area and causing marked narrowing at the entrance to the esophagus. The right arytenoid was dislocated anteriorly and imbedded in scar tissue.

This patient, therefore, had lost all or part of the three major functions of the larynx, ie, airway, respiratory tract protection, and voice production. He had a supraglottic stenosis with dislocation of the

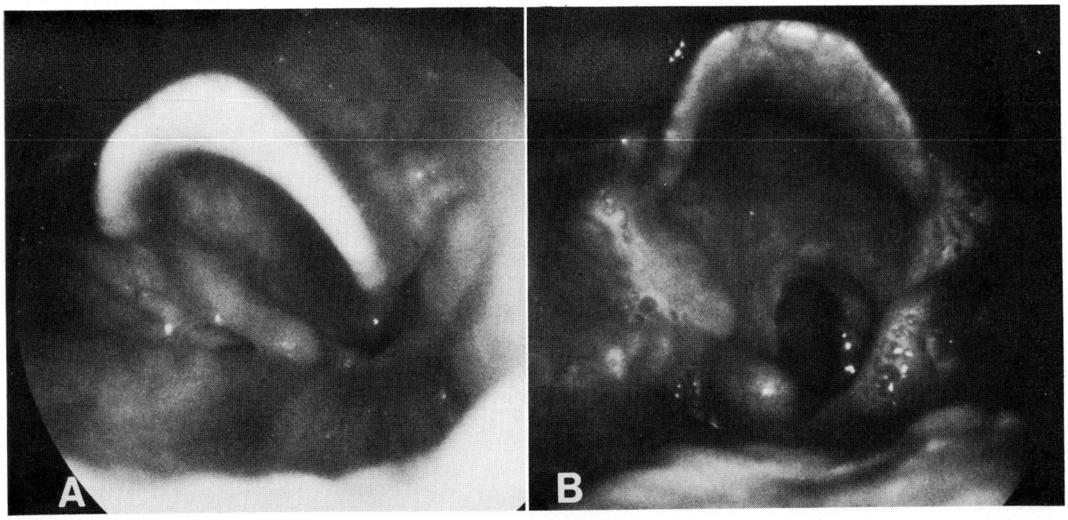

Fig. 1. A) Indirect laryngoscopy, preoperatively. Note severe distortion of the supraglottic larynx, with displacement of the epiglottis, dislocation of the arytenoid and stenosis extending to the postcricoid area. B) Indirect laryngoscopy, five months postoperatively.

From the Division of Otolaryngology, University of British Columbia, Vancouver, Canada.

Presented at the meeting of the American Laryngological Association, Palm Beach, Florida, April 14-15, 1980.

REPRINTS — Patrick J. Doyle, MD, 1081 Burrard Street, Vancouver, B.C., Canada, V6Z 1Y6.

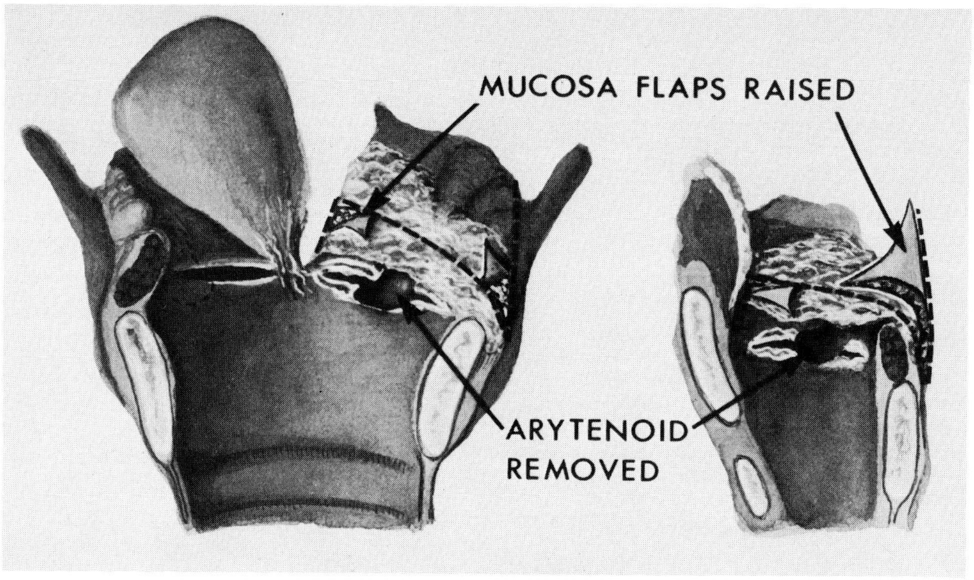

Fig. 2. Diagrammatic representation of the operative procedure. Mucosal flaps were elevated, scar tissue and arytenoid excised, and Z-plasty performed using the mucosa of the medial wall of the larynx and the pyriform sinus.

right arytenoid and narrowing of the esophagus due to scar tissue in the postcricoid area. It was decided to attempt a one-stage repair realizing that there was a possibility that a second stage would be necessary and further that the correction of one function, such as his airway, might increase his problem with aspiration.

A thyrotomy was performed which confirmed the findings on direct laryngoscopy. An incision was then made along the line of scar tissue and mucosal flaps raised superiorly and inferiorly so that we could use the tissue of the pyriform sinus and the mucosa of the wall of the intrinsic larynx to perform a Z-plasty (Fig. 2). The scar tissue was completely excised and the right arytenoid removed. The mucosal flaps were then rotated and the Z-plasty completed without any mucosal tension or remaining raw areas. It was not necessary, therefore, to use either a free mucosal graft or a free skin graft. A nasogastric feeding tube was inserted and the larynx closed over a soft stent. The postoperative course was uneventful. The stent was removed in five days and the larynx healed without the formation of stenosis or granuloma. Indirect laryngoscopy revealed an adequate glottic airway with good movement of the left cord and a minimal glottic defect on phonation. The nasogastric feeding tube was removed ten days after the surgery and the patient allowed to take a normal diet which he did without difficulty. He was extubated five weeks postoperatively. The patient now has no airway problem and no problem with dysphagia or aspiration (Fig. 1B). His voice is somewhat hoarse but he has good volume and no social problem.

Ann Otol 89:1980

RETROSPECTIVE COMPARISON OF CONSERVATIVE AND RADICAL NECK DISSECTION IN LARYNGEAL CANCER

ROBERTO MOLINARI, MD
FAUSTO CHIESA, MD
GIULIO CANTÙ, MD
CESARE GRANDI, MD

MILAN, ITALY

A retrospective comparison of radical and conservative technique for neck dissection in cancer of the larynx was made, starting from analysis of 98 patients operated on with the conservative procedure (128 cervical neck fields at risk of recurrence) at the Istituto Nazionale Tumori of Milan. Furthermore, a series of 162 patients was selected from more than 500 radical neck dissections performed in the past to set up a series as comparable as possible as far as several parameters were concerned. No significant difference was found between radical and conservative neck dissection with regard to the incidence of recurrences in the operative field, either considering the whole series (2.5% versus 1.6%), or cases with histologically proven metastases (9.4% versus 4.5%). Conservative neck dissection seems as safe as radical neck dissection, at least within the limits set in the present study for the indication of the former procedure, ie, nonsuspect nodes or metastatic mobile nodes not greater than 2.5 cm.

A conservative technique for radical neck dissection (RND) was proposed by Suarez[1] in 1963 for cancer of the larynx, but only in 1967 was it rationally systematized by Bocca and Pignataro[2] from the technical point of view. During the last ten years this procedure has been more frequently applied, and its short and long-term results have been the subject of some reports, mainly in Europe.[3-7] Almost all of the authors, considering both survival and neck recurrence rates, concluded quite empirically that conservative neck dissection (CND) is indicated for nonpalpable or palpable mobile nodes not larger than 3 cm.

Nevertheless, many surgeons are perplexed about the possibility of replacing the classical RND with the conservative procedure. A retrospective comparison between these two modalities has been attempted by André et al[6] and Lingeman et al,[7] but for many reasons the conclusions drawn in both papers are improper. In the report of André et al, the surgical procedure used was not the typical CND but rather a simple removal of the lymphatic jugular chain, the so-called anterior triangle dissection;[8] in addition, all cases received systematic postoperative radiotherapy. In the series of Lingeman et al, patients were treated with either the typical conservative procedure or the anterior triangle dissection; moreover, the series included different localizations of the cancer (larynx, mouth, oropharynx, hypopharynx), and also in this series many of the patients received postoperative radiotherapy. It is evident that no objective judgment can be drawn from these treatments on the effectiveness of the typical conservative procedure, basically because the RNDs being compared were performed on previously selected cases, which represented the remainder of the patients who were selected for the conservative procedure.

No prospective clinical trial has yet been carried out. To evaluate whether or not such a trial was necessary, we decided to analyze a rather large series of cases operated on with CND and to compare it retrospectively with a series operated on with RND, as analogous as possible as far as several parameters are concerned.

METHODS

The study started with the analysis of a series of 300 consecutive CNDs performed at the Istituto Nazionale Tumori of Milan during the past eight years for cancer involving mainly the larynx and hypopharynx, but also the oral cavity, the thyroid, the oropharynx, and other sites. In all these cases, the indications for the conservative procedure were almost invariably the following: no palpable nodes in the neck (N0 — prophylactic dissection; palpable but nonsuspect nodes (N1a-2a); palpable nodes suspect to contain neoplastic growth, provided they were mobile and not larger than 2.5 cm. When the size of the nodes was 2.5 cm or more or their mobility was reduced, a radical or modified dissection was performed; the latter cases are not included in the present study.

The CND was always performed en bloc with the primary tumor when it was located in the larynx or hypopharynx; in the case of oral or oropharyngeal cancer, the dissection was done either as a concomitant or a delayed procedure. The patients treated for cancer other than laryngeal are numerous and have several localizations with different biological behavior so that their analyses are more difficult; in addition, the lengths of follow-up are shorter and the number of cases evaluable for survival or recurrence is too small. The present study therefore deals only with cancer of the larynx, since it is the tumor with the best local prognosis and allows the best conditions for judging the control of neck metastases.

From 1972 to 1975, a consecutive series of 119 patients with cancer of the larynx was treated with partial, total, or extended laryngectomy combined with a CND, which was unilateral in 89 cases and bilateral in 30. Twenty-one patients were excluded because of postoperative death (1 patient), death due to intercurrent disease (4 patients), unspecified cause of death (if due to recurrence of the primary tumor or lymph node metastases or to distant metastases, 4 patients), or preoperative or postoperative radiotherapy (12 patients). The series under analysis is

From the Istituto Nazionale per lo Studio e la Cura dei Tumori, Milan, Italy.
Presented at the XII International Cancer Congress, Buenos Aires, Argentina, October 5-11, 1978.
REPRINTS — Roberto Molinari, MD, Istituto Nazionale Tumori, Via Venezian, 20133 Milan, Italy.

TABLE 1. CONSERVATIVE DISSECTION — METASTASES BY CLINICAL STAGING AND HISTOLOGICAL CONTROL (N = 128)

	NO				N1-2a				N1-2b				Total			
	No.			%	No.			%	No.			%	No.			%
N−	67			84.8	19			86.4	20			74.1	106			82.8
N + R−	11	13.9	12	15.2	3	13.6	3	13.6	5	18.5	7	25.9	19	14.8	22	17.2
N + R +	1	1.3			—				2	5.4			3	2.4		
Total	79				22				2				128			

represented by 98 patients who underwent unilateral CND (59 patients), bilateral CND (30 patients), or bilateral dissection that was conservative on one side and radical on the opposite side (9 patients). None of them received radiotherapy. All these patients were followed-up for at least three years. In a previous analysis[9] of neck recurrences after RND, 97% occurred within the third year.

On the whole, we are dealing with 128 CNDs, which means 128 operative cervical fields at risk of recurrence. Incidence and distribution of the metastases detected in the specimens are reported in Table 1. Twenty-two metastases were found in 128 dissections (17.2%). According to the clinical classification of the nodes (TNM, International Union Against Cancer), 12 metastases were detected among the 79 N0 (15.2%), 3 among the 22 N1-2a (13.6%), and 7 among the 27 N1-2b (26%). As a consequence, 15 metastases were detected among the 101 nonsuspect cases (14.8%) and 7 among the 27 patients with suspected nodes (25.9%). The incidence of extranodal spread (N + R +) was 3/22 (13.6%).

To provide a series of cases as analogous as possible to be significantly compared with the CND series, a selection was made from the records of patients who underwent RND for cancer of the larynx from 1965 to 1970. During those years, the indication for the neck operation was exactly the same as today. The cases were selected by taking into account: analogous clinical classification of the primary cancer, analogous composition of the series with regard to the clinical classification of the nodes, identical indication for neck dissection (N0, N1-2a, N1-2b, mobile and not greater than 2.5 cm), and absence of preoperative or postoperative radiotherapy. The only variant was that the accessory spinal nerve was preserved in 70% of the cases. These patients had also been followed for at least three years.

The series at comparison consists of 162 patients operated on with unilateral dissection, which means 162 operative fields at risk of recurrence. For this group, frequency and distribution of metastases detected in the specimens are reported in Table 2. Thirty-two metastases were found among 162 dissections (19.7%): 21 among the 91 cases classified as N0 (23%), 3 among the 46 cases classified as N1-2a (6.5%), and 8 among the 25 cases classified as N1-2b (32%). Twenty-four metastases were, therefore, found among 137 nonsuspect cases (17.5%) versus 8 of 25 cases with suspected nodes (32%). The incidence of extranodal spreading (N + R +) was 25%.

Table 3 compares the incidence of metastases in both series, according to the preoperative clinical classification of the nodes. Some differences in composition may be a consequence of a more careful classification in the CND group, where the choice of the technique depended on characteristics and size of the nodes. Furthermore, the incidence of capsular rupture was higher in the RND group, and this can be explained by a more restrictive interpretation of the concept of mobility in the CND group, which sometimes induced the surgeon to perform a RND even if the node was less than 2.5 cm. In spite of these differences, the series seem reasonably comparable.

RESULTS

Time of Accomplishment. The mean duration of the RND added to the time of the laryngectomy was one hour and ten minutes; this time was longer in the CND, where the mean duration was one hour and 35 minutes.

Surgical Complications. No significant difference was found between RND and CND with regard to postoperative mortality: one postoperative death due to pulmonary complications occurred in both groups (1/119, 0.8% vs 1/162, 0.6%). With regard to major complications, in one CND operated patient, a postoperative pharyngeal fistula gave rise to erosion of the internal jugular vein with subsequent hemorrhage, which required reoperation, ligature, and resection of the vein; the patient recovered with no further complications. One patient who underwent RND developed, in the same conditions, a carotid hemorrhage which required ligature of the artery with consequent hemiplegia. Minor complications occurred in both groups with the same frequency, except for lymphorrhea, which appeared in three patients who underwent RND but never after a CND.

The length of the postoperative course was mainly affected by problems resulting from a pharyngeal fistula in which the incidence was the same in both groups. The mean duration of hospitalization after the operation was 17 days in CND and 18 days in RND patients.

Three-Year Results. During the follow-up (Table 4), six recurrences developed in 290 operative fields at risk (2%), ie, 11% of the 54 detected metastases.

TABLE 2. RADICAL NECK DISSECTION — METASTASES BY CLINICAL STAGING AND HISTOLOGICAL CONTROL (N = 162)

	NO				N1-2a				N1-2b				Total			
	No.			%	No.			%	No.			%	No.			%
N−	70			77	43			93.5	17			68	130			80.2
N + R−	17	18.7	21	23	3	6.5	3	6.5	4	16	8	32	24	14.8	32	19.7
N + R +	4	4.4			—				4	16			8	5.0		
Total	91				46				25				162			

TABLE 3. INCIDENCE OF METASTASES BY CLINICAL STAGE AND TYPE OF PROCEDURE (N = 297)

	Radical		*Conservative*		*Total*	
	No.	*%*	*No.*	*%*	*No.*	*%*
N0	21/91	23.0	12/79	15.2	33/170	19.4
N1-2a	3/46	6.5	3/22	13.6	6/68	8.8
N1-2b	8/25	32.0	7/27	25.9	15/59	25.4
Total	32/162	19.7	22/128	17.2	54/297	18.2

According to the initial clinical classification of the nodes, the overall recurrence rate was 2.5% in the RND group versus 1.6% in the CND group. There were no recurrences in either series in the necks initially classified as nonsuspect but with palpable nodes (N1-2a), and the difference between N0 and N1-2b was very small (2.3% vs 4% after RND and 1.3% vs 3.7% after CND).

According to the findings of the histological control of the nodes (Table 5), the incidence of recurrences was identical after either RND or CND when the nodes were found negative (N-: 0.8% vs 0.9%). In the presence of histologically positive nodes, recurrences appeared in 9.4% of the RND and in 4.5% of the CND group. The absence or presence of extranodal spread affected the recurrence rate as follows: N + R− = 8.3% after RND and 5.3% after CND; N + R + = 12.5% after RND and 0% after CND (only three cases).

TABLE 4. REGIONAL RECURRENCE RATE BY CLINICAL STAGING AND TYPE OF DISSECTION (N = 290)

	Radical		*Conservative*		*Total*	
	No.	*%*	*No.*	*%*	*No.*	*%*
N0	3/91	2.3	1/79	1.3	4/170	2.3
N1-2a	0/46	—	0/22	—	0/68	—
N1-2b	1/25	4.0	1/27	3.7	2/52	3.8
Total	4/162	2.5	2/128	1.6	6/290	2.1

DISCUSSION

The conservative technique requires 25 to 30% more time than RND to be accomplished. This is certainly a worthwhile cost from the functional and cosmetic viewpoint, also considering the absence of an increase in postoperative complications.

The analysis of Tables 1 and 2, which show the distribution of the metastases according to the clinical preoperative classification, raises once more the issue of the fallibility of palpation in evaluating the presence or absence of metastases in nodes not greater than 2.5 cm. False-negative nodes ranged from 15% to 23% (N0 +), whereas false-positive nodes (N1-2b-) were 68 to 74%. On the other hand, this is a particularly important question in view of the indication for associating a neck dissection with laryngectomy. According to the findings of a previous retrospective study[10] on the usefulness of prophylactic dissection in cancer of the larynx, our policy is to perform it systematically in cases other than T1 (and T2, glottic) on one or both sides depending on the site of the primary tumor. In fact, only 40% of late metastases can be cured, so that the availability of less aggressive surgical procedures on the neck nodes, to be safely performed unilaterally or bilaterally en bloc with the laryngectomy, seems to us particularly important. An overall recurrence rate of 2.1% (7.4% among the patients with nodal involvement) confirms the effectiveness of the surgical treatment of neck metastases in cancer of the larynx, using whatever kind of neck dissection en bloc with the primary tumor. In spite of the relatively small number of patients with lymphatic involvement (54 cases), we think that the detailed analysis of the criteria used for selecting the series of RND to be compared with the CND group makes this retrospective comparison quite reliable.

The conservative procedure seems to be as effective as RND, at least when the node metastases are microscopic or not larger than 2.5 cm and mobile. It is noteworthy that three of the four recurrences after RND occurred in clinically negative necks (3/91 = 2.3%): this confirms that the RND series did not include more advanced cases. The absence of recurrences among the cases classified as N1-2a (palpable nonsuspect nodes) in both groups suggests the possible presence of some favorable lymph node reaction (immunological?).

With regard to the histological findings, the absence of nodal microscopic involvement does not prevent the appearance of neck recurrences (one case in both groups). This is probably due to intraoperatory seeding of cancer cells circulating within the lymphatic vessels. Nevertheless, the recurrence rate is decisively higher among the cases with confirmed metastases (7.4% vs 0.8%), but it is not strongly affected by the presence of capsular break (N + R −, 7%; N + R +, 9%). This is in part due to the fact that the neck dissections were performed en bloc with the larynx and mainly because all the

TABLE 5. REGIONAL RECURRENCE RATE BY HISTOLOGICAL STAGING AND TYPE OF DISSECTION (N = 290)

	Radical			*Conservative*			*Total*		
	No.	*%*		*No.*	*%*		*No.*	*%*	
N−	1/130	0.8		1/106	0.9		2/236	0.8	
N + R−	2/24	8.3	3/32 9.4	1/19	5.3	1/22 4.5	3/43	7.0	4/54 7.4
N + R +	1/8	12.5		0/3	0		1/11	9.0	
Total	4/162	2.4		2/128	1.6		6/290	2.1	

nodes considered in the present study were not larger than 2.5 cm and mobile, so that the extracapsular spreading was always only microscopic. No difference was found between CND and RND; if any, recurrences were a little more frequent after RND than CND (9.4% vs 4.5%, respectively, 8.3% vs 5.3% among N+R− cases and 12.5% vs 0% among N+R+ cases), but the difference is not statistically significant, also because only three cases were N+R+ in the CND group. Furthermore, in a few patients who underwent CND, extracapsular spread was clinically noticed during the operation, and the planned surgical procedure was modified (removal of the internal jugular vein or other structures or even RND). If these cases had been included in the study, the above-mentioned differences would probably be annulled.

In conclusion, the CND seems to be as effective as the radical procedure in cancer of the larynx when performed en bloc with the laryngectomy, provided that lymph node metastases, when detected, are not greater than 2.5 cm. Previous studies have proved that the incidence of extranodal spread is an absolute determinant factor when the size of the metastasis increases from 2 to 3 cm.[11,12] As a consequence, the safety limits of the CND still need to be specified: it is probable that an extension of the indications of this procedure to larger nodes will require modified techniques, such as removal of the internal jugular vein or the sternomastoid muscle. However, technical acrobatics can be easily accepted only when a bilateral neck dissection is to be performed to reduce the consequences of the operation. If the node is larger than 3 cm, and mainly if its mobility is reduced (macroscopic extranodal spread), there is no doubt that, in the case of unilateral dissection, the RND yields the best results from the oncological viewpoint.

REFERENCES

1. Suarez O. El problema de las metastasis linfaticas y aligades del cancer de laringe y hipofaringe. Rev Otorrinolaringol (Santiago) 1963; 23:83.

2. Bocca E, Pignataro O. A conservation technique in radical neck dissection. Ann Otol Rhinol Laryngol 1967; 76:975-88.

3. Pignataro O. Indicazioni, limiti e risultati dello svuotamento laterocervicale funzionale nel cancro della laringe. Tumori 1974; 60:585-90.

4. Pignataro O. Indicazioni e limiti dello svuotamento funzionale laterocervicale nel cancro laringeo. Nuovo Arch Ital Otol Rinol Laringol 1977; 5:423-9.

5. Bocca E. Critical analysis of the techniques and value of neck dissection. Nuovo Arch Ital Otol Rinol Laringol 1976; 4:151-8.

6. André P, Laccourreye H, Haguet JF, et al. Comparaison des résultats carcinologiques à long terme entre les évidements cervicaux radicaux et conservateurs. Ann Otolaryngol Chir Cervicofac 1975; 92:113-26.

7. Lingeman RE, Helmus C, Stephens R, et al. Neck dissection: radical or conservative. Ann Otol Rhinol Laryngol 1977; 86:737-44.

8. Silvestre-Begnis C. Cancer de laringe. In: Acta XXVI Congresso Argentino de Cirurgia. Buenos Aires; 1955:578-766.

9. Molinari R, Zingo L. Patogenesi delle recidive di metastasi sul campo di svuotamento laterocervicale per carcinomi orofaringolaringei. Tumori 1969; 55:371-85.

10. Molinari R. Indicazioni, limiti e risultati degli svuotamenti laterocervicali tradizionali nel cancro laringeo. Tumori 1974; 60:573-84.

11. Sancho H, Hauss G, Saravane D. Etude des corrélations histocliniques. Conséquences sur le plan pronostique des adénopathies cervicales métastatiques. Nuovo Arch Ital Otol Rinol Laringol 1977; 5:473-80.

12. Micheau C, Sancho H, Gérard-Marchant R, et al. Pronostic des adénopathies cervicales métastatiques en fonction des facteurs anatomo-pathologiques. Nuovo Arch Ital Otol Rinol Laringol 1978; 6:5-14.

Ann Otol 89:1980

DESTRUCTION AND REGENERATION OF JAWBONE AFTER CRYOGENIC APPLICATION

AN EXPERIMENTAL STUDY

RICHARD KUYLENSTIERNA, MD
PER-GOTTHARD LUNDQUIST, MD   ARTHUR NATHANSON, MD
STOCKHOLM, SWEDEN

On 13 rabbits part of the lateral aspect of the jawbone was frozen with liquid nitrogen in two sessions. The animals were sacrificed 2, 4, 12, and 24 weeks after the cryosurgery. The specimens were analyzed with microangiography according to the Spalteholz technique and with light microscopy. The whole width of the lateral cortex, measuring around 3 mm, was subject to bone destruction two weeks after cryosurgery. New bone formation, on the other hand, was evident in the frozen area and on the undamaged periosteum some distance from the lesion. The same area, 12 weeks after the injury, was completely restored. Bone destruction and regeneration are discussed with special reference to the vascular response to the injury.

INTRODUCTION

Cryosurgery has been proven to be of value in the treatment of several neoplastic bone conditions as well as in superficially growing soft tissue tumors. In the case of oral carcinomas, particularly of the floor of the mouth or the gingiva, their near proximity to bone can render it necessary to include adjacent bone tissue within the cryolesion to insure a radical ablation of the neoplasm.

The effects of low temperatures on soft tissue are rather well understood[1-3] whereas only a few reports have been issued dealing with cryogenically induced effects on bone tissue, often with emphasis on the histopathological appearance and without reference to the vascular response.[4-7] Several investigators have clearly shown that the ultimate extent of the cryolesion in soft tissue is influenced not only by direct thermal influence on the cells, but also by direct and progressive vascular damage.[8,9]

In a previous investigation undertaken by Kuylenstierna et al[10] on the early morphological changes on rabbit mandible after cryosurgery, it was shown that the acute lesion was caused mainly by circulatory events.

A complete arrest of the microcirculation within the cortical bone and adjacent marrow cavity, but without obvious damage to bone or tooth cells, was observed with light microscopy. It was also shown that the circulation in the soft tissue surrounding the bone was disturbed, with signs of thrombosis and extravasation of blood corpuscles.

The aim of the present investigation was to evaluate the subsequent effects on mandibular bone and its surrounding tissue of cryogenic application. Special attention was paid to the microvascular changes after cryogenic trauma and its significance for the remodelling of injured bone. Cryosurgical impact on tooth and nerve tissue as well as on muscle tissue within the area of damage will also be discussed.

METHODS

Thirteen young adult rabbits were operated on under general anesthesia maintained by intravenous injections (35 mg/kg) of Mebumal® (ACO Pharmaceutical Company). The periosteally covered lateral side of the left (in two cases the right) mandible was exposed through a straight incision, slightly above the inferior margin of the jawbone and extending from the angulus approximately 30 mm forward. The soft tissues were retracted with great care in order not to impair the circulation.

Freezing was carried out using a Frigitronic CE-2A cryounit utilizing liquid nitrogen as coolant. The probe tip (with flat surface and diameter of 4 mm and equal to a surface area of 1256 mm^2) was gently placed against the periosteally covered mandibular bone slightly in front of the first molar and under the incisor, approximately 5 mm above the inferior margin of the jawbone (Fig. 1). Freezing was performed in two sessions with a spontaneous thaw in between, a total freezing time of six minutes and a recorded probe tip temperature of − 160 C. The operation was terminated with wound closure using interrupted sutures. The animals were sacrificed 2, 4, 12, and 24 weeks after cryosurgery (Table 1).

Microangiography. A microangiographic technique with India ink infusion was used in the study of the vascular response of the mandibular bone to the freezing and compared with the contralateral *not* frozen mandibular half, according to a technique described by Nathanson.[11]

On the day of sacrifice the animal received 10,000 immunizing units Heparin® (Vitrum), 5 ml Xylocaine® (Astra) 0.5%, and Mebumal intravenously in a dose of 35 mg/kg body weight. The abdominal aorta was exposed and 500-600 ml of 20% India ink solution was slowly infused from a height of 150 cm above the heart level during approximately one hour. The rabbits survived the infusion for about half an hour.

Preparation for Microangiography and Histology. After completion of the India ink infusion, the jaw was removed from the skull and the bone freed from soft tissues except for its surround-

From the Department of Otolaryngology, Karolinska sjukhuset, King Gustaf V Research Group and Södersjukhuset, Stockholm, Sweden. Supported by grants from the Cancerföreningen and the Swedish Medical Research Council (MFR B79-17X-03915-078).

REPRINTS — Richard Kuylenstierna, Department of Otolaryngology, Karolinska sjukhuset, S-104 01 Stockholm 60, Sweden.

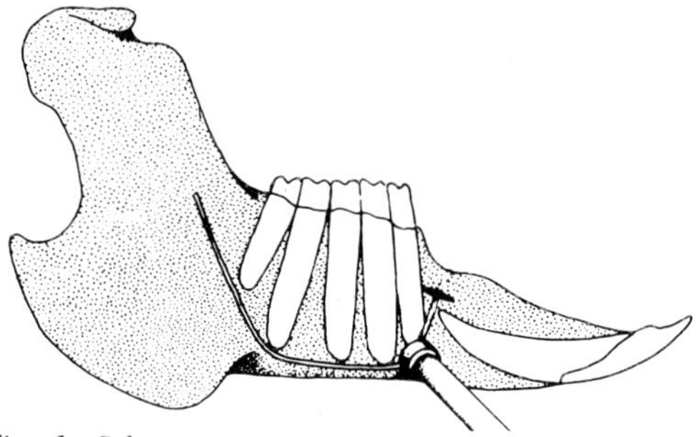

Fig. 1. Schematic drawing demonstrating the lateral aspect of the rabbit mandible and the cryoprobe applied to the bone.

ing periosteal layer. The two halves of the mandible were separated at the midline and each half was fixed with a solution of 10% formaldehyde for one day, decalcified with 5% trichloracetic acid for one week, dehydrated in alcohol and clarified with methylsalicylate according to the technique described by Spalteholtz.[12] After completion of the decalcifying process a central segment of each mandibular half with a width of about 15 mm was sectioned and cut into 0.5-0.9 mm thick slices, which were examined in a stereomicroscope and photographed with a macrophotographic unit.

Alternating sections from the central specimen were put in xylol embedded in paraffin wax and cross sectioned in 5-10 μm thick slices with a sliding microtome (MSE) for ordinary light microscopy. The sections were stained with hematoxylin and eosin, and Mallory's azan method.

RESULTS

Gross Observations. All rabbits fed normally and did not lose weight during the observation period. There were no clinical signs of fracture of the jawbone during that time. Neither were there any signs of infection in the cryosurgically treated area.

Light Microscopy. Two weeks after cryosurgery, bone destruction of the whole lateral cortex could be seen in one case (Fig. 2). In the other two cases, there were more local signs of bone destruction.

Regeneration of new bone, which in one case was abundant and in the other two cases was more limited after two weeks, always started in the marrow cavity between the medial and lateral cortices (Fig. 3). At the margins of the lesion, new bone was formed by the periosteum undamaged by cryosurgery (Fig. 2). New bone also regenerated from dead bone at the bottom of the lesion (Fig. 4). These findings became more conspicuous four weeks after the cryogenic application. The area on the lateral cortex undergoing both destruction and regeneration measured approximately 10 x 10 x 3 mm.

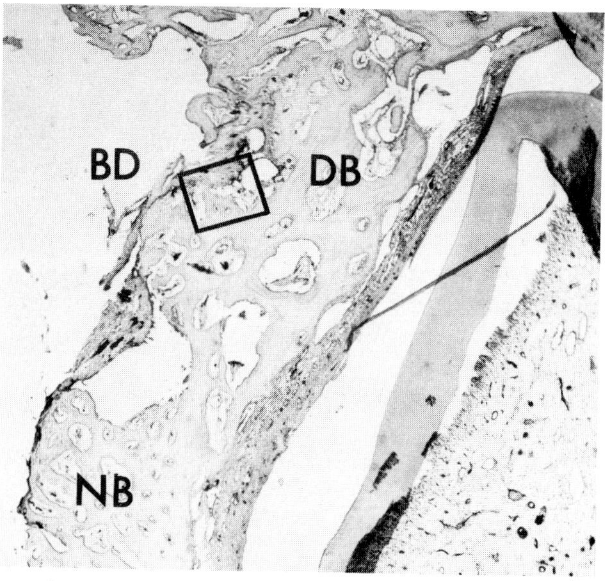

Fig. 2. Cross section of mandible two weeks after cryosurgery showing a large bone defect (BD) with new bone formation (NB) at the margins of the lesion and on dead bone (DB). (The insert is Fig. 4.) (x 22)

Four weeks after cryosurgery the mandibular nerve, which lies beneath the lateral cortex, showed clear signs of degeneration with vacuole formation in two cases, but seemed normal in the third (Fig. 5). No damage was detected in the pulp cavity or in the dentin of the teeth. Nor were any massive bleedings seen in the pulp.

Twelve weeks after cryosurgey, only a minimal impression was detected on the lateral cortex as a trace of the former bone destruction (Fig. 6). Instead the lateral cortex was replaced by new bone already transformed into lamellar bone (Fig. 7) and no trabecular bone was seen. Occasionally some resorption cavities were present and new bone forma-

TABLE 1. PROCEDURES COMPLETED ON EXPERIMENTAL RABBITS

Rabbit No.	*Side Frozen* *Left*	*Right*	*Observation Time (wks)*	*Microangiography*	*Light Microscopy*
13	+		2	+	+
18	+		2	–	+
19	+		2	+	+
7	+		4	+	+
11	+		4	+	+
12	+		4	–	+
17		+	12	+	+
21	+		12	+	+
22	+		12	+	+
14	+		24	+	+
15	+		24	+	+
16		+	24	+	+
20	+		24	+	+

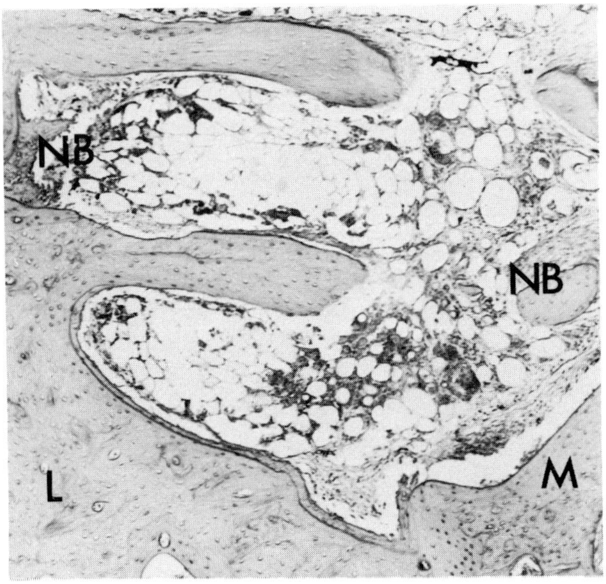

Fig. 3. New bone formation (NB) two weeks after cryosurgery in the marrow cavity on both medial (M) and lateral (L) sides. (x 50)

tion then took place from the periosteum, but more restricted than that originally present. The lateral cortex was, however, in all cases completely restored. Signs of degenerative changes within the mandibular nerve were still present in some specimens, and the muscle tissue overlying the cryosurgical lesion had been completely destroyed and replaced by fat and granulation tissue (Fig. 6). Signs of thrombosis or inflammatory reaction could not be detected in the soft tissues.

Twenty-four weeks after cryosurgery the only histological finding indicating previous damage to the lateral cortex was a limited groove in one specimen, suggesting that the remodelling had ceased before the normal curved mandibular shape had been achieved. No signs of infection of bone resorption were detected in the region treated.

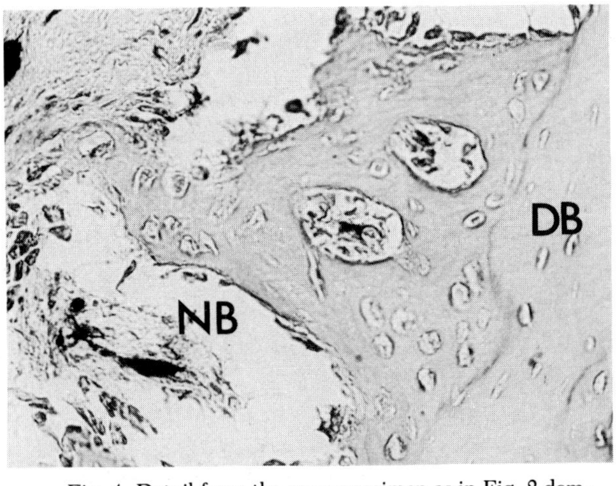

Fig. 4. Detail from the same specimen as in Fig. 2 demonstrating new bone formation (NB) taking place on the dead bone (DB). (x 320)

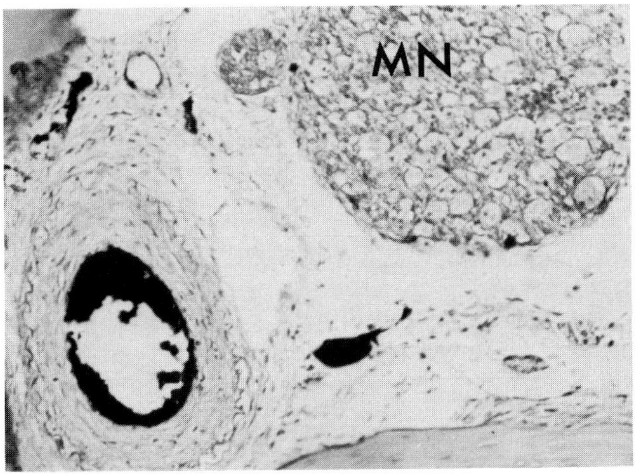

Fig. 5. Patent and seemingly normal-looking alveolar artery (bottom left) and degenerating mandibular nerve (MN) in the mandibular canal, four weeks after cryosurgery. (x 120)

Periosteal bone formation was occasionally seen to an extent corresponding to normal bone turnover. The mandibular nerve exhibited a completely normal appearance similar to that of the control side (Fig. 8). No reduction had occurred in the thickness of the fat and granulation tissues overlaying the cryotreated area. The alveolar artery remained patent and no degenerative change was detected in the walls of the artery throughout the investigation.

Microangiography. Two weeks after cryosurgery the marrow cavity became filled with numerous dilated and tortuous vessels, which started a recanalization of the old haversian canals. The

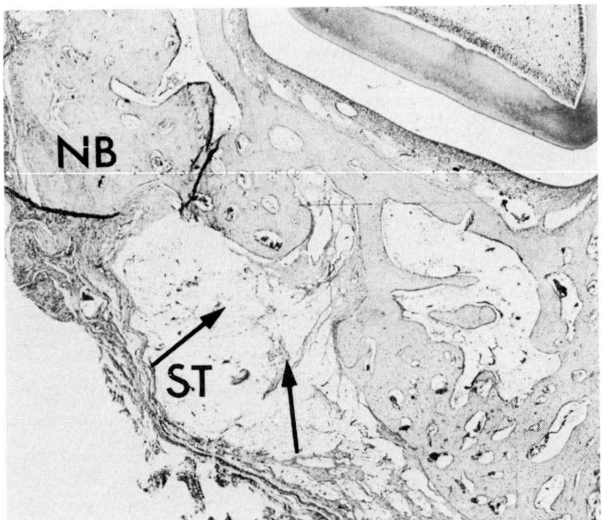

Fig. 6. Lateral side of the mandible 12 weeks after cryotreatment. Arrows indicate a small groove in the bone, which is not yet completely restored. Note the loose appearance of the soft tissue (ST) and the protruding newly formed bone (NB) at the margin of the lesion. (x 17)

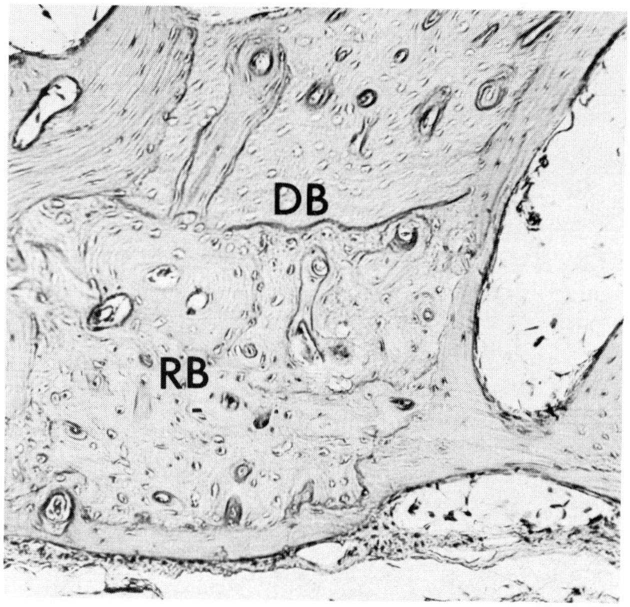

Fig. 7. Restored lateral part of the mandible 12 weeks after treatment. Note remodelling bone (RB) outside dead bone (DB). (x 120)

capillary network in the cortex was, however, sparser than normal two and four weeks after cryosurgery (Figs. 9 and 10).

The vessels in the marrow cavity regained their normal size and number from 12 weeks after treatment, though some specimens showed occasional dilated marrow vessels even 24 weeks after freezing.

After 12 weeks the capillaries of the cortex seemed dilated and tortuous and most of them had a longitudinal course through the jawbone instead of the normally occurring radiating route (Figs. 11 and 12). At the end of the period the cortex capillaries had regained their normal size and course (Figs. 13 and 14).

The vessels in the soft tissues covering the cryo-

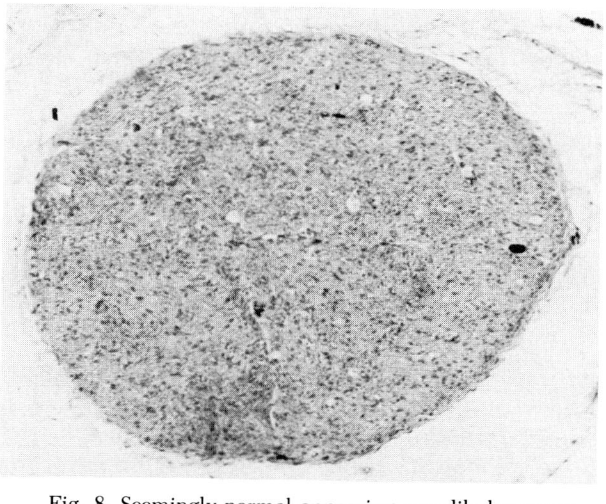

Fig. 8. Seemingly normal-appearing mandibular nerve underlaying the cryotreated area 24 weeks after surgery. (x 80)

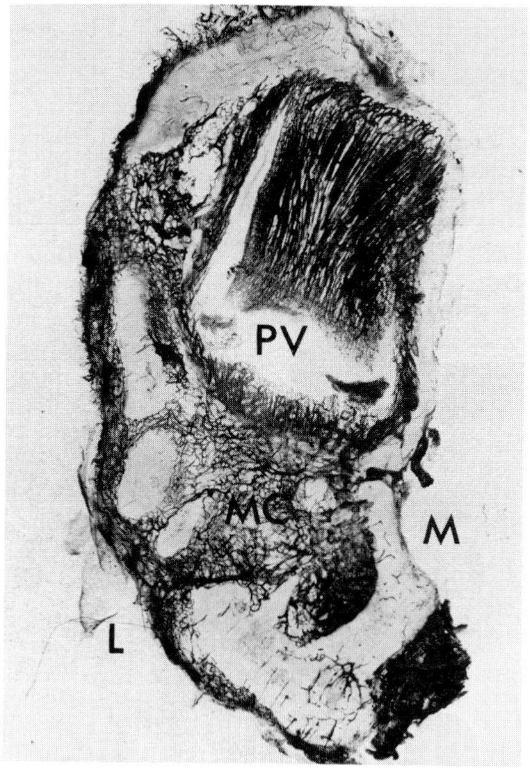

Fig. 9. Spalteholz preparation 570 μm thick of the mandible four weeks after cryosurgery. Note the sparse filling of the intracortical vessels on the lateral side (L) compared with the medial side (M). The vessels in the marrow cavity (MC) are dilated, the pulp vessels (PV), however, are normal in appearance. (x 11)

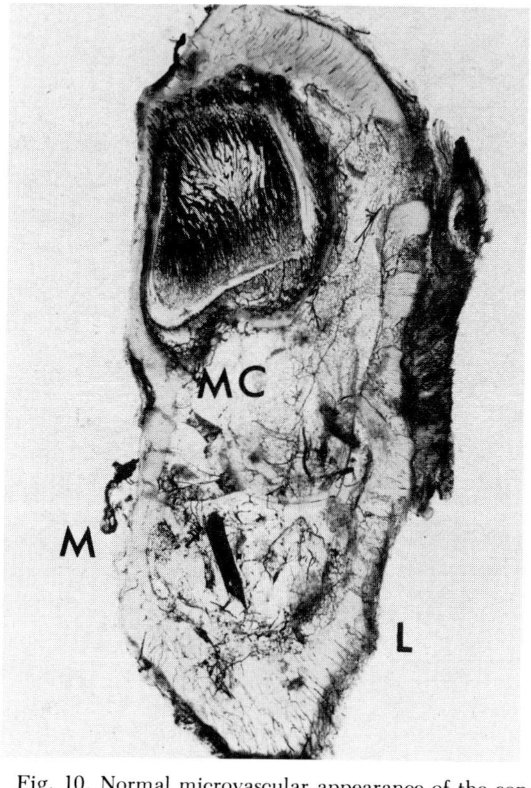

Fig. 10. Normal microvascular appearance of the contralateral side of the same specimen as in Fig. 9, 550 μm thick, same abbreviations as in Fig. 9. (x 11)

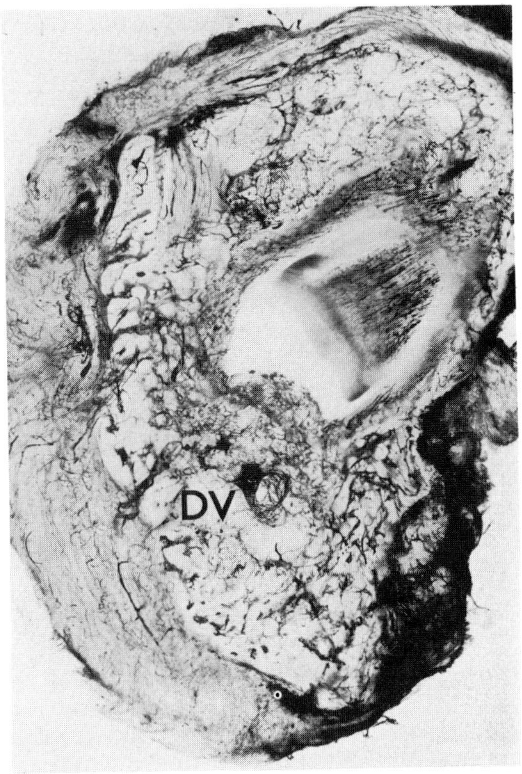

Fig. 11. Vascular architecture 12 weeks after treatment. Note dilated vessels (DV) within the injured lateral cortices. The vessels here have a longitudinal course. The section is 900 μm thick. (x 12)

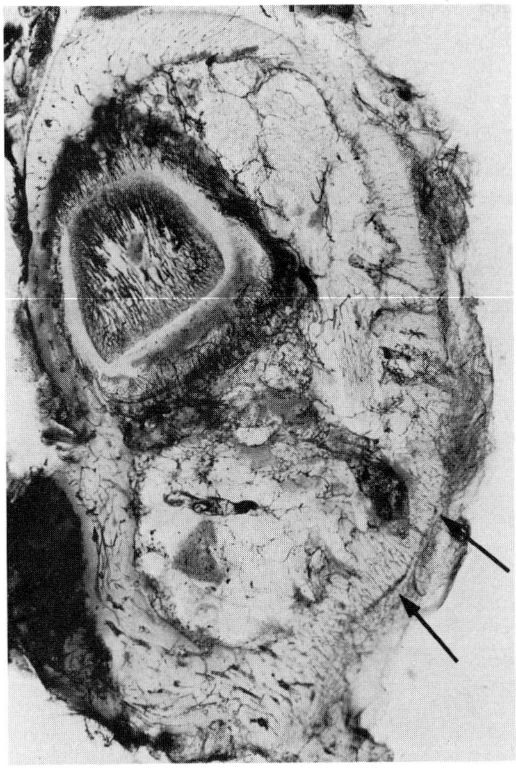

Fig. 12. Normal vascular appearance on the contralateral side of the same specimen as in Fig. 11. Note the slender radiating intracortical vessels on the lateral side (arrows). The section is 630 μm thick. (x 12)

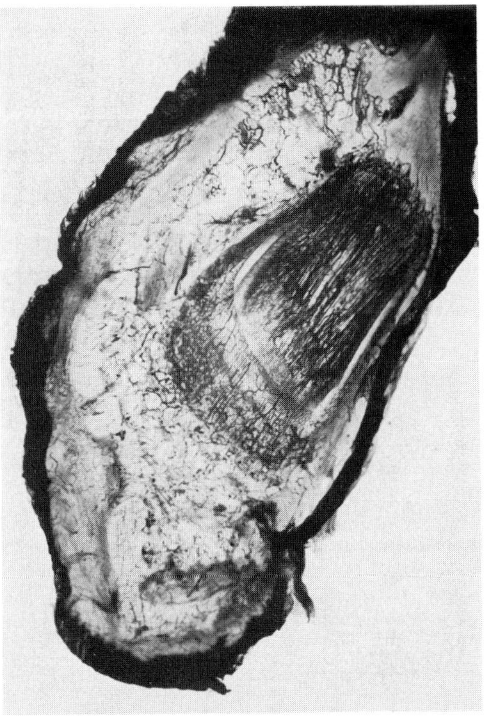

Fig. 13. Twenty-four weeks after cryosurgery the vascular architecture within both cortex and marrow was completely restored to normal, as in this specimen. The section is 750 μm thick. (x 11)

surgically treated area in some cases appeared normal in size and distribution two and four weeks after freezing. After 12 weeks, the soft tissue network in all specimens became very sparse and this was still the picture at the end of the observation period.

The vascularity of the teeth was of normal appearance throughout the investigation.

DISCUSSION

The immediate effects on the microcirculation of cryosurgically treated soft tissues have been described in detail by some authors, eg, Zacarian et al[8] and Whittaker.[9] They have shown that the initially constricted microvessels, particularly the venules, became dilated within hours after cryosurgery, which led to stasis and the development of total arrest of the microcirculation.

The endothelial cells of the vessels became damaged with leakage and hemorrhages into the soft tissues during the thawing phase. The same events take place after cryosurgery on bone tissue.[10]

The cells within the cryotreated area will, of course, succumb, leading to a widespread degeneration, unless the blood circulation is restored in proper time. The vascularity of bone is considerably reduced compared with that of the soft tissues. It is therefore difficult to foresee the final effects on bone microcirculation and regeneration after cryosurgery.

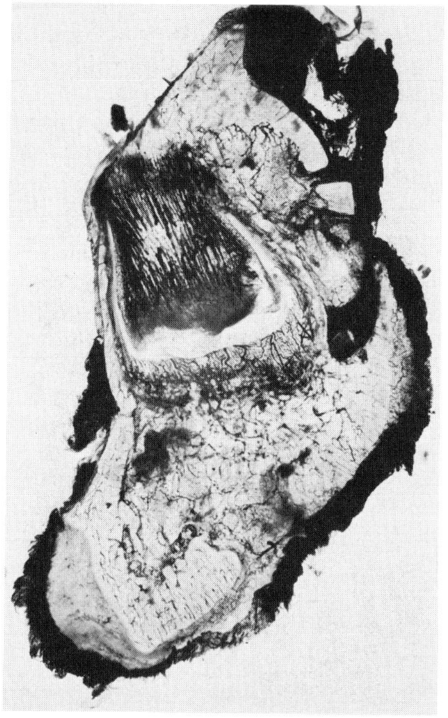

Fig. 14. The contralateral specimen from the same animal as in Fig. 13. The section is 600 μm thick. (x 11)

Cryosurgery is recommended and considered a reliable modality of treatment for bone cysts and even bone tumors.[13-15]

Some authors have reported a high incidence of spontaneous fracture after cryotreatment of bone.[14] Gage et al[16] noticed fractures in 11 of 16 thigh bones 12 weeks after cryosurgery.

The interrelationship between revascularization and regeneration of bone has not been studied in the aforementioned investigations. The present investigation shows hypervascularity and bone regeneration as starting mainly in the marrow cavity two weeks after cryosurgery. The cortex is, at this time, still avascular and demonstrates bone destruction leading to a breakdown of the lateral cortex within two to four weeks. Bone regeneration also originates from the periosteum at some distance from the lesion.

There were no fractures of the frozen mandibles in the present investigation. There are many explanations for this. For instance, did the microcirculatory arrest only comprise a well-defined area in which the medial cortex was *not* included?[10]

Thus the microcirculation within the medial cortex, as well as the pulpal circulation, was not affected. These findings were probably due to remaining patency of the alveolar artery, which is the main artery of the mandible supplying bone, marrow cavity, and teeth. The mucosal circulation on the medial side of the mandible was never affected. The high rate of circulation within the pulp cavity and in the proximity of the alveolar artery might make these richly supplied areas more resistant to cryogenic trauma than other more sparsely circulated areas. Another reason for the resistance of teeth structures to this type of influence is the many bony and enamel layers shielding the pulp cavity from the freezing on the lateral aspect of the mandible.

In the lateral cortex, bone regeneration was apparent two weeks after cryosurgery and a normal thickness was present within 12 weeks. Bone regeneration apparently kept pace with bone resorption. This fact, together with the unaffected medial cortex, gave sufficient stability to the jawbone to prevent spontaneous fractures in spite of the substantial forces created by the rabbit's habit of perpetual jaw grinding.

The first signs of increased vascularity of the marrow cavity could be detected after two weeks. This hypervascularization was even more conspicuous after four weeks. During the same period, there was only a limited revascularization of the lateral cortex. The hypervascularity of the marrow cavity subsided and returned to a normal status in most specimens 12 weeks after cryosurgery while the vessels of the lateral cortex, on the other hand, were dilated and tortuous, resembling the former picture of the marrow cavity. These observations imply that the process of revascularization originates in the marrow cavity and spreads outwards, and not the reverse.

No trabecular bone was formed in the lateral cortex 12 weeks after cryosurgery. The previously formed bone was undergoing remodelling.

Osteogenesis and vascularity have been shown to be closely interrelated.[17,18] Göthman[19] found the liveliest arterial response related to regions where radiopaque callus was heaviest in tibial fractures in the rabbit and monkey. Thorogood and Gray[20] showed, with both light and electron microscopy, that vascularization always preceded osteogenesis in bone grafting. Zuckman et al[21] claimed that though the development of newly formed vessels was a necessary preliminary stage for osteogenesis, it was not sufficient in itself. Cummings[7] emphasized that osteogenesis occurs in bone devitalized by freezing, provided there is ample vascularization and an absence of overwhelming infection.

Our findings indicate that hypervascularization of bone affected by cryosurgery is an expression of a generally increased metabolism due to both resorptive and regenerative processes. These processes kept in step in the present investigation. This may be due to favorable circumstances, for instance, the ceaseless jaw grinding of the test animal, which may enhance and stimulate circulation. Though the experiments are not directly comparable, Cummings[7] had problems with osteomyelitis after reimplantation of frozen mandibular autografts in dogs. This problem never arose in the present investigation probably because of the ample vascularization. Also, the continuity of bone was never mechanically broken.

The extent of soft tissue damage on the lateral side of the mandible exceeded that of the underlying cortex. Two weeks after cryosurgery the muscles were replaced by a sparse network of fibrous tissue interwoven with fat cells. A progressive thickening of this scar tissue was followed at least four weeks after surgery. Microscopically the amount of fat cells within the scar tended to increase. No regeneration of striated muscles was observed during the study. The metabolic rate of muscle tissue is higher than that of denser tissues such as bone, which makes muscle tissue more susceptible not only to the cryogenic impact, but also to the vascular disturbance induced by the surgical trauma.

There are few reports on cryogenically induced lesions of nerve tissue. Barnard[22] found, on the seventh day after freezing the infraorbital nerve in mice, a complete degeneration of nerve fibers in the proximal part of the nerve. This injury was always reversible and 16-24 weeks after the cryogenic application, the nerve fibers were found to be normal with light microscopy. The same author reported a functional blockade of the infraorbital nerve in 27 patients, with a mean duration of 90 days.

In our series, degeneration of the mandibular nerve was a constant finding from 4 to 12 weeks after cryosurgery, and was occasionally found two days after treatment. Twenty-four weeks after treatment the nerve had regained a normal appearance, similar to that of the control side, in two cases where it could be visualized. These findings are thus congruent with those of Barnard.[22] Consequently cryosurgery may be of value in the treatment of neuralgia such as facial pain and temporarily to relieve pain caused by necrotizing incurable tumors.

It is evident from the present investigation that the soft tissue overlying the frozen bone was more damaged and did not regenerate to the same extent as the cryogenically treated bone. These findings are equivalent to those of Gage,[16] who found that cryosurgery was particularly apt when treating oral carcinomas invading bone.

It is our opinion that only tumors with a limited spread into the bone should be treated with cryosurgery. This limitation is due to the necessity to spare one of the bone cortices in order to avoid a spontaneous fracture, and to maintain a framework for new bone formation.

CONCLUSIONS

1. The lateral cortex of the jawbone two weeks after cryosurgery showed bone destruction with a maximum depth of 3 mm. New bone formation was at the same time evident in the frozen area starting from the marrow cavity and from the periosteum at some distance from the lesion. The whole width of the lateral cortex was rebuilt 12 weeks after cryosurgery.

2. The alveolar artery, the pulpal circulation, as well as the microcirculation of the medial cortex of the jawbone, remained intact during the observation period.

3. The outgrowth of new capillaries took place from the marrow cavity extending towards the lateral cortex.

4. There were no signs of inflammation or spontaneous fracture of the cryogenically treated bone.

5. The mandibular nerve in many cases showed signs of degeneration from 4-12 weeks but had regained a normal appearance when studied at 24 weeks.

6. There were no signs of damage to teeth structures in the cryosurgically treated area.

REFERENCES

1. Gill W, Fraser J, daCosta J, Beazley R. The cryosurgical lesion. Am Surg 1970; 36:437-45.

2. Neel MB, DeSanto LW. Cryosurgical control of cancer: effects of freeze rates, tumor temperatures, and ischemia. Ann Otol Rhinol Laryngol 1973; 82:716-23.

3. Farrant J, Walter CA. The cryobiological basis for cryosurgery. J Dermatol Surg Oncol 1977; 3:403-7.

4. Schargus G, Winckler J, Schröder F, Schäfer B. Cryosurgical devitalization of bone and its regeneration: an experimental study with animals. J Maxillofac Surg 1975; 3:128-31.

5. Bradley PF, Fisher AD. The cryosurgery of bone: an experimental and clinical assessment. Br J Oral Surg 1975; 13:111-27.

6. Fisher AD, Williams DF, Bradley PF. The effect of cryosurgery on the strength of bone. Br J Oral Surg 1977-1978; 15:215-22.

7. Cummings CW. Experimental observations of canine mandibular regeneration following segmental removal, freezing and reimplantation. Ann Otol Rhinol Laryngol 1978; 87 Suppl 54:1-11.

8. Zacarian SA, Stone D, Clater M. Effects of cryogenic temperatures on microcirculation in the golden hamster cheek pouch. Cryobiology 1970; 7:27-39.

9. Whittaker DK. Vascular responses in the oral mucosa following cryosurgery. J Periodont Res 1977; 12:55-63.

10. Kuylenstierna R, Lundquist PG, Nathanson A. Early morphological changes on rabbit mandible after cryogenic application. Arch Otorhinolaryngol 1980; 226:35-43.

11. Nathanson A. The early vascularization of an autogenous bone inlay into an artificial defect in the rabbit mandibula. Acta Otolaryngol (Stockh) 1978; 85:135-48.

12. Spalteholz KW. Über das Durchsichtigmachen von Menschlichen und Tierischen Präparaten. 2nd ed. Leipzig: S. Hirze, 1914.

13. Biesecker JL, Marcove RC, Huvos AG, Miké V. Aneurysmal bone cysts. Cancer 1970; 26:615-25.

14. Marcove RC, Weis LD, Vaghaiwalla MR, Pearson R, Huvos AG. Cryosurgery in the treatment of giant cell tumours of bone. Cancer 1978; 41:957-69.

15. Oeseburg MB, Rogge CWL, Koops HS, Oldhoff J. Cryosurgical treatment of aneurysmal bone cysts. J Surg Oncol 1978; 10:9-20.

16. Gage AA, Greene GW, Neiders ME, Emmings FG. Freezing bone without excision. JAMA 1966; 196:770-4.

17. Trueta J, Cavadias A. Vascular changes caused by the Küntcher type of nailing. J Bone Joint Surg 1955; 37-B:492-505.

18. Trueta J. The role of the vessels in osteogenesis. J Bone Joint Surg 1963; 45-B:402-18.

19. Göthman L. Vascular reactions in experimental fractures: microangiographic radioisotope studies. Acta Chir Scand 1961; Suppl 284.

20. Thorogood PV, Gray JC. The cellular changes during osteogenesis in bone and bone marrow composite autografts. J Anat 1975; 120:27-47.

21. Zuckman J, Maurer P, Berbeson C. The effect of autografts of bone and periosteum in recent diaphyseal fractures: an experimental study in the rabbit. J Bone Joint Surg 1968; 50-B:409-22.

22. Barnard JDW. The use of cryogenic nerve blockade in the management of facial pain. Proceedings of the 4th Congress of the European Association of Maxillo-facial Surgery. Venice, 1978.

OTOLARYNGOLOGY AND MEDICINE TODAY IN THE PEOPLE'S REPUBLIC OF CHINA

BRIAN F. MCCABE, MD

In September 1980 the Chinese Medical Association sponsored a lecture tour for a group they termed the "First American ENT Delegation to China." Your Editor and Coeditor were privileged to be members of that delegation. Following is a report of some of our impressions of that fascinating trip.

The delegates were selected through Dr. Samuel Rosen, a long-time friend of that country who was making his eighth trip to China. The complex details of the trip were worked out over a period of many weeks by Mrs. Helen Rosen. These two individuals were highly appropriate to lead the delegation not only for their knowledge of the country but for a special empathy they have for the Chinese people, which is returned with deep respect and obvious affection.

The ten-member medical delegation, consisting of Drs. Samuel Rosen, Beverly Armstrong, Stanton Friedberg, Jerome Goldstein, Brian McCabe, Daniel Miller, Loring Pratt, Robert Schindler, Ben Senturia and John Shea, delivered over 80 lectures in four cities (Shanghai, Peking, Hangchow and Canton) and participated in question and answer panels after each session. At the request of the Chinese, lecturers were selected to cover every aspect of modern otolaryngology with the exception of cosmetic surgery. Audiences ranged from a seminar group of 30 academicians to a group of 550 general otolaryngologists and other interested physicians and health workers. Lectures were somewhat difficult to deliver because of the necessity of compacting a 30-minute talk into 15 minutes, requiring a high degree of precision and selectivity. This was necessary because approximately half the speaking time had to be given over to an interpreter. Audiences in each city listened to every word delivered with rapt attention and were uniformly effusive with praise and thanks.

In general, otolaryngology and medicine as a whole have been isolated from many of the developments in the United States. We were taken on tours of hospitals and clinics in every city. All questions were welcomed and we were taken anywhere we wanted to go and walked the streets with impunity. At its best, otolaryngology is good in China and in certain areas as good as some of the leading institutions in our country. This alone is amazing because for three decades they have had few teachers from abroad to describe the advances occurring in medicine; they have been to a large degree self-taught, mainly through the studious pursuit of information accessible in journals. China is a relatively poor country and cannot afford thousands of journal subscriptions. They circumvent this by acquiring a few copies of a journal each month and then duplicating them for distribution within the country. We were most impressed by their laryngeal cancer surgery and management of carcinoma of the esophagus. Their cure rates in the latter are believed to be the highest in the world. We personally witnessed acupuncture anesthesia and came away convinced of its effectiveness for operations on the neck.

In some areas China is ahead of the West. This is most apparent in preventive medicine. They have somehow been able to rid the country of all mosquitoes and flies without upsetting the ecological balance. Intensive "patriotic wars" have been periodically waged to eliminate the "four pests," mosquitoes, flies, rats, and sparrows. Except in the countryside, cats and dogs are seldom seen for they must be given food which is needed for people.

The greatest single problem facing China today is population control. It is estimated that the Chinese number one billion. Their population had increased by two hundred million in only the past ten years. They have approached birth control with vigor and determination. They point out if they do not do this the population by the year 2080 will be four billion. Their aim is the one-child family, which if effective will reduce the population by the year 2080 to 300 million. The birth control program is conducted on three levels: the government gives couples a monetary bonus if they have one child; if a second child is born the bonus must be returned. If there is a third child a fine is levied. On the city level, families with more than one child are not given any extra food ration coupons for the extra person. Finally, on the the local neighborhood level, a mandatory "block" meeting is held and a family planning official lectures about birth control. The couple with more than one child is held up to the others as unfair and unpatriotic.

Our general impressions of the Chinese people are that they seem well fed and content. Their socialism appears to work primarily because there are incentives at every level of activity. Our most lasting impression was that the Chinese people deeply and sincerely wish a warm and growing friendship with our people.

ENG of the Month

PACEMAKER ARTIFACT ON ENG TRACING

William R. Wilson, MD

Boston, Massachusetts

The electronystagmogram (ENG) of this 76-year-old female, who was referred for diagnostic evaluation of vertigo, demonstrates an electronic artifact secondary to the signal generated by a cardiac pacemaker. The patient had complaints of dizziness, staggering and tinnitus associated with visual "grayouts" lasting 15-20 seconds almost daily for several months. Three years prior to her evaluation, a Medtronic® endocardial pacemaker had been placed in the trabecular system of the right ventricle via the right cephalic vein for correction of a complete heart block.

During the left optokinetic test (Fig. 1A) the upward pen deflections generated by the pacemaker can be seen at regular intervals among the beats of nystagmus. The small artifacts are more easily noted when the eyes are still, as in the erect-sitting position (Fig. 1B). The bodily conductivity of this signal changes and the waveform is altered in size and polarity by the head-hanging position (Fig. 1C). Pacemaker artifact is a single spike but is best characterized by its regularity. On the ENG, the instrument appears to discharge each 0.9 seconds (the actual monitored pacemaker interval in the cardiac lab was 0.858 for a heart rate of 72 beats per minute).

The ENG was entirely normal, including hyperventilation testing. The pacemaker functions normally. She is followed by the medical service and her transitory vestibular symptoms are attributed to hyperventilation-anxiety attacks.

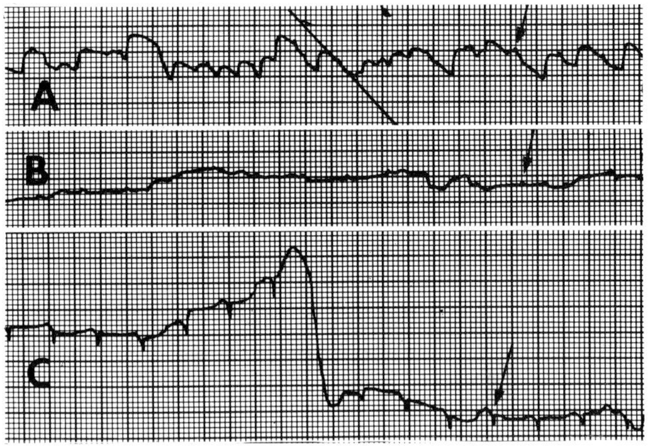

Fig. 1.

The message of this brief report is to caution those interpreting ENGs of the presence of unsuspected artifacts. Eye blinks, especially in the form of blepharospasm, can be a source of confusion, particularly on vertical leads. Cervical and facial muscle tics should also be noted by the ENG technician. Rarely an EKG signal can be seen on the ENG. Causes of external glitches include poor grounding, broken or loose lead wires, and short voltage surges produced by electrical switches or relays.[1] In the future, signals from pacemakers no doubt will become a more common artifact.

From the Department of Otolaryngology, Massachusetts Eye and Ear Infirmary, Boston, Massachusetts.

Reprints — William R. Wilson, MD, Department of Otolaryngology, Massachusetts Eye and Ear Infirmary, 243 Charles Street, Boston, MA 02114.

Acknowledgment — The ENG was performed by Mrs. Elizabeth McHugh, ENG Laboratory, Massachusetts Eye & Ear Infirmary, Boston, Massachusetts.

REFERENCES

1. Barber HO, Stockwell CW. Manual of electronystagmography. St. Louis: CV Mosby Co, 1976:63-9.

BOOK REVIEWS

Auditory Investigation: The Scientific and Technological Basis

Edited by *H. A. Beagley*. Hard cover, black and white illustrations, indexed, referenced, 600 pp, 1980. Oxford University Press, New York. Price $95.00.

The "auditory investigation" in the title of this volume includes the auditory investigation of patients in modern clinical practice as well as auditory investigation in the context of research on the auditory system. The methods and tools of engineering sciences have been increasingly employed in medical investigation and medical practice. This is especially true with respect to auditory investigations which must couple the physical acoustic stimuli with the biological responses at physical, physiological and psychological levels in the sensory system. For this reason persons with training in engineering sciences have contributed and continue to contribute significantly to our understanding of the auditory system. This handbook in the Oxford Medical Engineering Series is intended to help fill the informational gaps between the engineering and biomedical sciences for engineers, for otologists, and for a new breed of audiologists who aspire to become equally conversant in both areas.

The major unifying thread for the book lies in the sequence of electroacoustics (electronics and acoustics) to electrophysiology. Part I includes six chapters on pertinent digital and analog instrumentation for the generation, control, transmission, measurement, and analysis of signals and responses. The breadth of treatment is excellent and the depth is appropriate for most purposes. Many references are provided for the further reading necessary to many detailed, full scale engineering applications.

Part II reviews the sound stimuli commonly used in auditory investigations and the variety of acoustic measurements made for many different purposes. These include threshold and suprathreshold audiometry, measurement of acoustic impedance, tympanometry, and acoustic reflex thresholds. A chapter of "Speech Pattern Audiometry" brings together information on articulation, phonetic and acoustic characterization of speech, the roles of stress, inflection, vowel formant transitions, voicing and voiceless contrast, and temporal factors in a way that demonstrates the difficulties that have been encountered with the standardization of tests using speech.

The methods used for various animal studies and for electrophysical assessment of human hearing are included in Part III, "General Auditory Investigations." The former include measurements of motion of the basilar membrane, the classic cochlear potentials under various conditions, responses from single hair cells and single auditory neurons, and responses in the central auditory pathways. The latter include electrocochleography, brainstem reflexes, auditory nerve and brainstem evoked responses, middle latency responses, responses of cortical origin, and late cortical responses.

This appears to be a very useful book for anyone who plans to become concerned with the electroacoustics and electrophysiology of auditory investigations in basic science or clinical practice. The book should be available in the library of any ENT department that sponsors such investigations, and many young otologists and biomedical engineers will want a personal copy.

DONALD H. ELDREDGE, MD
St. Louis, Mo.

Sedation, Local and General Anesthesia in Dentistry, Third Edition

Edited by *Niels Bjorn Jorgensen* and *Jess Hayden, Jr.* Hard cover, black and white illustrations, indexed, 1980. Lea & Febiger, Philadelphia. Price $27.50

Although written as a dental textbook this book ably covers all of the problems of anesthesia for the ambulatory patient regardless of the specialty involved.

The book is divided into the following sections: 1) Total physical evaluation of the patient as an essential prologue to any type of anesthesia. 2) Sedation relative to local or general anesthesia. This section offers a comprehensive and well-illustrated, documented and detailed study of sedation, analgesia and anesthesia relative to anatomy, technics and side effects. 3) This section deals fully with all equipment in use. It too is fully illustrated. 4) A comprehensive, condensed resumé of the history of anesthesia is very well presented. 5) This section on anatomy, neurophysiology and pharmacology is superb. The illustrations are excellent, being accurate, clear and graphic.

An outstanding quality of the text is its readability. Approaching it as a textbook the reader soon discovers that the style of presentation induces the reader to read with increasing interest. It is difficult to put the book down.

As a final note it must be said that its textbook teaching value and thorough coverage of the subject leaves only the need for practice and clinical training to make the reader proficient in anesthesia. Of course another point of view, which might bc considered as criticism, is that the inexperienced operator may be lulled into a false sense of security by relying solely on this one textbook.

JEROME S. GROSBY, DDS
St. Louis, MO

BOOKS RECEIVED

Basic Industrial Hearing Conservation

By David F. Barr, PhD, and Richard K. Miller. Black and white illustrations, hard cover, glossary, appendix, 125 pages, 1979. The Fairmont Press, Inc., Atlanta, $26.95.

Guide to Noise Control Literature

By Richard K. Miller. Hard cover, 148 pages, 1980. The Fairmont Press, Inc., Atlanta, $24.95.

Concepts in Cancer Care. A Practical Explanation of Radiotherapy & Chemotherapy for Primary Care Physicians

By Jay Scott Cooper, MD, and Donald J. Pizzarello, PhD. Index, black and white illustrations, hard cover, 257 pages, 1980. Lea & Febiger, Philadelphia, $16.50.

Neurological Surgery of the Ear, volume II

By Herbert Silverstein, MD, and Horace Norrell, MD. Black and white illustrations, indexed, hard cover, 396 pages, 1979. Aesculapius Publishing Co., Birmingham, $60.

Otolaryngology, 3 volumes, 2nd edition

By Michael M. Paparella, MD, and Donald A. Shumrick, MD. Volume I: Basic Sciences and Related Disciplines ($70); Volume II: The Ear ($55); Volume III: Head and Neck ($70), hard cover, indexed, black and white illustrations, 3020 pages, 1980. W.B. Saunders Co., Philadelphia, $185 - the Set.

The Voice and Its Disorders, 4th edition

By Margaret C.L. Greene, FCST. Black and white illustrations, indexed, hard cover, bibliography, 446 pages, 1980. J.B. Lippincott Co., Philadelphia, $47.50.

Evoked Potentials

Edited by Colin Barber, MD. Black and white illustrations, indexed, hard cover, 603 pages, 1980. University Park Press, Baltimore, $34.50.

AN APPRECIATION

When a paper is submitted for publication to the ANNALS OF OTOLOGY, RHINOLOGY AND LARYNGOLOGY, the Editor or Coeditor selects two or three reviewers to evaluate the manuscript. One of the reviewers is usually a member of the Board of Editors or the Emeritus Board. However, because of the increasing complexity of the research or clinical observations contained in submitted manuscripts, the second or third reviewer is sought among otolaryngologists and investigators in the United States and Canada and occasionally abroad, who have special knowledge in the particular subject area.

We are happy to list the names of the reviewers who have, during the past year, undertaken the demanding job of carefully and comprehensively assisting us in this time consuming assignment. Our gratitude goes also to those who willingly and generously gave the time necessary to provide the ANNALS with fine book reviews and abstracts of national and international journals. All have been gracious and generous in their response and we thank them.

Ben H. Senturia, MD, Editor
Brian F. McCabe, MD, Coeditor

W.A. Alonso
W. Arnold
R.W. Babin
H.O. Barber
J. Bardach
J.M. Bernstein
H.F. Biller
D. Brackmann
D.P. Bryce
J.R. Chandler
J.D. Clemis
B. Cohen
J.J. Conley
P. Dallos
H. Dedo
A. Duvall
A. Eviatar
J.W. Folkins
I. Friedmann
J.C. Gallagher
R. Goldstein
M.D. Graham
J. Hanson
J.E. Hirsch
J. Holmquist
V. Honrubia
J. Innitzer
A. Jahn
R. Jahrsdoerfer
J. Jerger
H.K. Kashima
A. Katz
R.S. Kimura
D.P. Kuehn
T. Lai
S.S. Lefrak
F.E. LeJeune
M.W. Lowder
R. Maca
M.D. Marcus
F.H. McGovern
G. Mogi
H.L. Morris
E.N. Myers
C.W. Norris
W.R. Panje
M. Payne
D.P. Pascoe
G.R. Popelka
J. Porcaro
B. Proctor
D.F. Proctor
F.W. Pullen
H.R. Senturia
D. Sessions
J. Sheehy
P.A. Shurin
K.H. Siedentop
B. Silver
J.L. Sloyer
P. Sprinkle
J.H. Whicker

AUTHOR INDEX

Aantaa, E., Suppl. No. 68:7
Ahmed, A.R., 428
Alonso, A., Suppl. No. 76:2
Altmann, G., Suppl. No. 68:110
Ament, M.E., 574
Anderson, R.G., 331
Andersson, B., Suppl. No. 68:115
Antunez, J-C. M., Suppl. No. 76:23
Anyanwu, C.H., 129
Aprigliano, F., 391
Ardito, J.M., 401
Arnold, W.J., Suppl. No. 69:4
Assimes, I.K., 406
Axelsson, G-A., Suppl. No. 69:4

Babin, R.W., 262
Bale, P.M., 443
Barsanti, R.G., Suppl. No. 68:281
Batsakis, J.G., 91, 196
Becker, S.P., 551
Beery, Q.C., Suppl. No. 68: 28, 190, 290; Suppl. No. 69:11
Bellucci, R.J., Suppl. No. 74:42
Benitez, L.D., 370
Benjamin, B., 443
Berg, M., Suppl. No. 68:4
Bergstrom, L., 135, Suppl. No. 74:31
Berlin, C.I., Suppl. No. 74:62
Bernstein, J.M., Suppl. No. 68:104, 326; Suppl. No. 69:15
Berzins, I.K., Suppl. No. 68:138, 339
Bess, F.H., Suppl. No. 68:228; Suppl. No. 69:19
Biller, H.F., 103
Binder, W.J., 103
Birck, H.G., Suppl. No. 68:278, 324; Suppl No. 69:23
Birkhan, J.H., 46
Blom, E.D., 529
Blom, P., 75
Blonder, J., 165
Bluestone, C.D., 124; Suppl. No. 68:3, 28, 34, 41, 47, 71, 178, 190, 290, 319; Suppl. No. 69:4, 11, 19
Boeckman, C.R., 434
Boies, L.R., Jr., 225
Bordley, J.E., 84; Suppl. No. 74:3
Brackmann, D.E., Suppl. No. 75
Bradley, W.H., Suppl. No. 69:23
Branefors, P., Suppl. No. 68:117
Brookhouser, P.E., Suppl. No. 74:1
Brooks, D.N., Suppl. No. 68:246; Suppl. No. 69:19
Buchwach, K.A., Suppl. No. 68:324
Buckingham, R.A., Suppl. No. 68:56
Bumsted, R.M., Suppl. No. 72
Burgio, P.A., 325
Bushey, M.J., 459
Bussi, M., 173
Bylander, A., Suppl. No. 68:20
Byrne, W.J., 574

Calcaterra, T.C., 108
Canalis, R.F., 58, 184
Cantekin, E.I., 253; Suppl. No. 68:28, 34, 41, 47, 71, 178, 190, 290; Suppl. No. 69:11
Cantrell, R.W., 567
Cantu, G., 578
Carpenter, A-M., Suppl. No. 68:121; Suppl. No. 69:13
Catanzaro, A., Suppl. No. 70
Cates, K.L., Suppl. No. 68:138
Chiesa, F., 578
Chisin, R., 180
Clemis, J.D., 296
Clopton, B.M., Suppl. No. 66:5, 8
Cohen, S.R., 437, 497
Conner, G.H., 459
Cooper, J.C., Suppl. No. 68:62
Cortesina, G., 173
Corvera, J., 370
Cotton, R.T., 409, 508
Craig, H.B., Suppl. No. 68:172
Craig, R.D., 563
Crispin, M., 165
Cyr, D.G., Suppl. No. 74:63

Dahlberg, T., Suppl. No. 68:117
Daniel, I.D., 198
Dare, B.J., 198
Davis, J.M., 483
Davis, W.E., 318
DeBlanc, G.B., Suppl. No. 68:14
DeLeon, S.Y., 401
Dobie, R.A., Suppl. No. 74:62
Don, M., Suppl. No. 75
Donegan, J.O., 409
Downs, M.P., Suppl. No. 68:168; Suppl. No. 69:27
Doyle, P.J., 576
Doyle, W.J., 49; Suppl. No. 68:28, 34, 41, 47, 71
Draf, W., Suppl. No. 68:303
Dudley, J.P., 428, 574
Dunbar, J.S., 409
Duvall, A.J. III, 335

Egami, T., 147
Egbue, M.O., 129
Eggermont, J.J., Suppl. No. 75
Eibling, D.E., 547
Eisemann, M.L., 271
Eliachar, I., 46
Enomoto, T., 132
Esterly, N.B., 268
Ewertsen, H.W., Suppl. No. 74:28

Faras, A.J., 467
Faw, K.D., 312, 446
Fearon, B., Suppl. No. 74:146
Ferlito, A., Suppl. No. 69:11
Ferrer, J.L., Suppl. No. 68:56
Fiellau-Nikolajsen, M., Suppl. No. 68:223
Fisher, G.H., 72
Fletcher, P., Suppl. No. 74:182
Fraysse, B.G., Suppl. No. 76:2
Frenkiel, S., 406
Freyss, G.E., Suppl. No. 68:196; Suppl. No. 69:19
Fria, T.J., 253; Suppl. No. 68:190, 200
Friedman, E.M., 342
Friedmann, I., Suppl. No. 68:241; Suppl. No. 69:11
Friel-Patti, S., Suppl. No. 74:171

Gacek, R.R., 1, 201, 249
Gal, T.F., 188
Galey, F.R., Suppl. No. 76:23
Galvis, A.G., 124
Gapany-Gapanavicius, B., 180
Gates, G.A., Suppl. No. 68:62; Suppl. No. 69:23
Gebhart, D.E., Suppl. No. 69:23
Geller, K.A., 437, 497
Gerrard, J.M., Suppl. No. 68:153
Giebink, G.S., 479; Suppl. No. 68:138, 161, 339; Suppl. No. 69:15
Gikas, P.W., 162
Ginsberg, I.A., Suppl. No. 77:1, 10, 17, 25
Glasscock, M.E. III, 29, 318
Glydensted, G., 117
Goodman, M.L., 6
Goodwin, R.E., 72
Gorenstein, A., 425
Gottschalk, G.H., Suppl. No. 68:301
Goycoolea, M.V., Suppl. No. 68:121, 249
Graham, M.D., 162, Suppl. No. 68:241
Grandi, C., 578
Greenes, R.A., 100
Griffiths, C.M., 204
Grönroos, P., Suppl. No. 68:357
Gross, N.B., 176
Gussen, R., 157

Halpin, T.C., 450
Hamashima, T., 140
Handler, S.D., 419
Hanson, D.G., 257
Harada, T., 147
Harford, E.R., Suppl. No. 69:19
Hawkins, D.B., 454
Hayes, J.W., 29
Häyry, P., Suppl. No. 68:143
Healy, G.B., 472; Suppl. No. 68:102
Henderson, F.W., Suppl. No. 69:9
Hentzer, E., 121
Herbert, W.I., 437
Herer, G.R., 342
Hermann, G., 20
Herva, E., Suppl. No. 68:357
Herzon, F.S., 81, 388
Hill, J.C., Suppl. No. 69:15
Hill, J.H., 162

Hind, J.E., Suppl. No. 74:136
Hiroto, I., 24, 359
Hixson, P.K., Suppl. No. 74:175
Hodges, G.M., Suppl. No. 68:241
Holinger, L.D., 65, 397
Holmquist, J., Suppl. No. 68:11, 65, 322; Suppl. No. 69:11
Honjo, I., 276; Suppl. No. 68:25; Suppl. No. 69:11
Hook, P.E., Suppl. No. 74:179
Horiuchi, M., 541
Horowitz, F.D., Suppl. No. 68:264; Suppl. No. 69:27
House, W.F., Suppl. No. 76:2
Howie, V.M., Suppl. No. 69, 4, 19
Huber, P.S., Suppl. No. 77:1, 10, 17, 25
Huff, J.S., Suppl. No. 68:138, 161
Hughes, G.B., 318
Hukee, M.J., 335
Hull, M.T., 168
Hussl, B., Suppl. No. 68:79; Suppl. No. 69:4

Ikari, T., 220, 541
Ingelstedt, S., Suppl. No. 68:4, 11
Ingvarsson, L., Suppl. No. 68:275
Ishii, T., Suppl. No. 68:83; Suppl. No. 69:13
Ivarsson, A., Suppl. No. 68:207

Jackson, C.G., 318
Jafek, B.W., 388
Jahrsdoerfer, R., 348, 567
Janfaza, P., 558
Jarlstedt, J., Suppl. No. 68:322
Jauhiainen, T., 366
Jaumann, M.P., Suppl. No. 68:62
Javaheri, A., 558
Javal, E., Suppl. No. 74:103
Jerger, J.F., Suppl. No. 69: 27; Suppl. No. 74:134
Jesteadt, W., Suppl. No. 74:88
Joachims, H.Z., 46
Johns, M.E., 188, 567
Johnson, U., Suppl. No. 68:129
Juhn, S.K., 479; Suppl. No. 68:121, 153, 161; Suppl. No. 69:15
Jung, T.T.K., Suppl. No. 68:153

Kaku, Y., Suppl. No. 68:236
Kamme, C., Suppl. No. 68:275
Kaneko, M., 103
Karjalainen, M., 69
Karma, P., Suppl. No. 68:357; Suppl. No. 69:15
Karr, L.J., Suppl. No. 68:133, 351
Kasantikul, V., 29
Katz, A.H., 551
Kawamoto, K., Suppl. No. 68:236; Suppl. No. 69:13
Keller, G., Suppl. No. 69:9
Keller, M.D., Suppl. No. 69:9
Kern, E.B., 209, 462
Khan, W., Suppl. No. 68:281
Kileny, P., 9
Kimes, K.K., Suppl. No. 68:41, 47
Kinney, S.E., 291
Kirchner, J.A., 541
Klein, J.O., Suppl. No. 68:3, 5, 98; Suppl. No. 69:4, 9, 15
Kobayashi, R., 574
Komiyama, S., 359
Kosinski, D., Suppl. No. 68:104
Kowata, I., Suppl. No. 68:236
Krespi, Y.P., 20
Krzyzek, R.A., 467
Kuehn, D.P., Suppl. No. 74:138
Kumazawa, T., 276; Suppl. No. 68:25, 147
Kuylenstierna, R., 582

Laine, U., 69
Laird, M.A., Suppl. No. 68:172
Lanese, R.R., Suppl. No. 69:9
Langenbrunner, D.J., Suppl. No. 68:285
Larsen, P.K., Suppl. No. 68:271
Laurell, A-B., Suppl. No. 68:129
Lavonen, A., 69
Lawrence, M., 325; Suppl. No. 74:9
Leake, H. III, Suppl. No. 68:264; Suppl. No. 69:27
Leinonen, M., Suppl. No. 68:357
Leipzig, B., 204, 534
Lester, J., 117
Levin, D.L., 268
Lewis, D.M., Suppl. No. 68:278, 344; Suppl. No. 69:15
Lewis, G.B., Jr., 437
Lewis, J.T., 62
Lidén, G., Suppl. No. 68:214; Suppl. No. 74: 22, 53
Lifschitz, W.S., 176
Lildholdt, T., Suppl. No. 68:67
Lim, D.J., Suppl. No. 68:3, 278, 344; Suppl. No. 69:2, 4, 13
Linthicum, F.H., Suppl. No. 76:23
Lippmann, R., Suppl. No. 74:79
Lopez-Rios, G., 370
Lovell, M., 388
Lowell, E.L., Suppl. No. 74:19
Lowell, S.H., 479
Lowery, H.W., Suppl. No. 69:4
Luban, N.L.C., 342
Lucente, F.E., 538
Lundgren, K., Suppl. No. 68:275; Suppl. No. 69:23
Lundquist, P-G., 582
Luotonen, J., Suppl. No. 68:357
Luxford, W.M., 454
Lybolt, J., Suppl. No. 74:158

Maeda, S., Suppl. No. 68:333
Mair, I.W.S., 75
Maisels, M.J., 459
Mäkelä, P.H., Suppl. No. 68:357; Suppl. No. 69:15
Makishima, K., 24, 359
Manac'h, Y., Suppl. No. 68:196
Mann, R., Suppl. No. 68:281
Mantravadi, R., 551
Marshak, G., Suppl. No. 68:316, 572
Matkin, N.D., Suppl. No. 74:50
Matsui, K., 132
McCabe, B.F., 9, 262, 590
McCaffrey, T.V., 209, 462
McCann, G.D., Suppl. No. 76:23
McCloskey, D.E., Suppl. No. 68:285
McDougall, J.C., 425
Meadema, S.J., Suppl. No. 68:344
Meistrup-Larsen, K.I., Suppl. No. 68:271
Melnick, W., Suppl. No. 69:19
Menyuk, P., Suppl. No. 68:257; Suppl. No. 69:27
Menzio, P., 173
Merwin, G.E., 225
Merzenich, M.M., Suppl. No. 74:84
Meurman, O.H., Suppl. No. 68:7
Meyerhoff, W.L., Suppl. No. 68:249; Suppl. No. 69:23
Miller, J.M., Suppl. No. 66:5, 8, 11, 15
Mills, E.L., Suppl. No. 68:161
Mizuhira, V., 377
Mogi, G., Suppl. No. 68:333; Suppl. No. 69:15
Molinari, R., 578
Molino, R., 173
Møller, A.R., Suppl. No. 69:19
Møller, M.B., Suppl. No. 69:19
Montgomery, W.W., 6, Suppl. No. 73; 521
Morehead, D.M., Suppl. No. 74:165
Morehead, K.E., Suppl. No. 74:165
Morehead, W.A., Suppl. No. 74:165
Morgenstern, C., Suppl. No. 68:76; Suppl. No. 69:11
Mora, B., 173
Muenker, G., Suppl. No. 68:308; Suppl. No. 69:11, 23
Murphy, S., 81
Murti, K.G., Suppl. No. 68:178
Myers, A.R., 78
Myers, D., Suppl. No. 68:104
Myers, E.N., 13
Mygind, N., Suppl. No. 68:271

Nadol, J.B., Jr., 251
Nakashima, T., 24, 140, 359
Narcy, P.P., Suppl. No. 68:190
Nathanson, A., 582
Neriah, Z.B., Suppl. No. 68:316
Netsky, M.G., 29
Nilsson, N-I., Suppl. No. 68:129
Nisengard, R., Suppl. No. 68:104
Nodar, R.H., 291
Northern, J.L., Suppl. No. 68:233; Suppl. No. 69:19
Nwafo, D.C., 129
Nylén, O., Suppl. No. 68:115, 117

O'Connell, E.J., 425
O'Connor, A.F., 194
Ogra, P.L., Suppl. No. 68:326; Suppl. No. 69:15
Ogura, J.H., 312
Okano, Y., 13
Okazaki, N., 276; Suppl. No. 68:25
Olson, J.E., 286
Onodera, A., 37
O'Shea, J.S., Suppl. No. 68:285
Ossoff, R.H., 268, 401
Ostfeld, E., 33, 165; Suppl. No. 68:110

Paggi, R.E., Suppl. No. 68:185
Palva, T., 366; Suppl. No. 68:143, 269; Suppl. No. 69:23
Paonessa, D.F., 383
Paparella, M.M., Suppl. No. 67; Suppl. No. 68:121, 249; Suppl. No. 69:4
Papsidero, M.J., 512
Paradise, J.L., Suppl. No. 68:3, 319; Suppl. No. 69:4, 23
Parulekar, S.S., 383
Pashley, N.R.T., 512
Peacor, D.R., 229
Peck, J.E., Suppl. No. 74:70
Pellettiere, E.V. II, 65
Perkins, W.H., Suppl. No. 74:150
Perlman, H.B., Suppl. No. 69:11
Peters, J.F., Suppl. No. 74:59
Peterson, C-M., Suppl. No. 68:115

Pezzullo, J.C., Suppl. No. 68:285
Pfingst, B.E., Suppl. No. 66:1, 8, 11
Philips, B.J., Suppl. No. 74:153
Phillips, D.C., Suppl. No. 68:41, 47, 71
Pickett, J.M., Suppl. No. 74:74
Ploussard, J.H., Suppl. No. 68:133, 351
Pohl, D., 443
Poliquin, J.F., Suppl. No. 70
Pöntynen, S., Suppl. No. 68:357
Poulsen, G., Suppl. No. 68:217
Powell, W.J., 58
Prellner, K., Suppl. No. 68:129; Suppl. No. 69:15
Probst, G., 253
Proud, G.O., Suppl. No. 74:47
Puglese, J., Suppl. No. 68:296
Puhakka, H., Suppl. No. 68:7
Pukander, J., Suppl. No. 68:357

Quenelle, D.J., 62
Quick, C.A., 467
Quie, P.G., Suppl. No. 68:138, 339
Qvarnberg, Y., Suppl. No. 68:269

Rahko, T., 69
Ranney, J.B., 257, Suppl. No. 69:3, 27
Rapin, I., 303
Reddy, R., 417
Regan, J.B., Suppl. No. 68:285
Reibel, J.F., 567
Reichert, T.J., 312, 446
Reiter, D., 78
Renvall, U., Suppl. No. 68:65, 214; Suppl. No. 69:19
Rockette, H.E., Suppl. No. 68:290
Rodriguez, W.J., Suppl. No. 68:281
Rogers, K.D., Suppl. No. 68:319
Rood, S.R., 49
Rosales, J.K., 406
Rose, J.S., Suppl. No. 77:10
Rosenblatt, H.M., 574
Rosner, B.A., Suppl. No. 68:5
Ross, M.D., 229
Ross, S., Suppl. No. 68:281
Rothmann, B.F., 434
Rothstein, F.C., 450
Rowe, L.D., 430
Roydhouse, N., Suppl. No. 68:312; Suppl. No. 69:23
Ruben, R.J., 303; Suppl. No. 69:19, 27; Suppl. No. 74:132
Rubinstein, E., 33
Rudin, R., Suppl. No. 68:11
Rudnick, M.D., Suppl. No. 77:1, 10, 17, 25
Ruth, R.A., 188
Ruuskanen, O., Suppl. No. 68:7
Ryan, A.F., Suppl. No. 70
Rynnel-Dagöö, B., Suppl. No. 69:15
Ryu, J.H., 9, 262

Sabo, D.L., Suppl. No. 68:190, 200
Sadé, J., Suppl. No. 69:4
Saito, Y., 377
Salamat, M.S., 229
Sando, I., 13, 147
Santi, P.A., 335
Sarno, C.N., 296
Sartoris, A., 173
Sasaki, C.T., 220, 541
Sato, M., 37
Saunders, W.H., Suppl. No. 69:23
Schiff, M., Suppl. No. 70
Schiffman, G.D., Suppl. No. 68:351
Schild, J.A., 65
Schram, J.L., Suppl. No. 68:278, 344
Schuknecht, H.F., Suppl. No. 65
Schuller, D.E., 515
Schulz, P., Suppl. No. 68:303
Schwartz, D.M., Suppl. No. 68:211, 296
Schwartz, R.H., Suppl. No. 68:211, 281, 296; Suppl. No. 69:15, 23
Seid, A.B., 409, 508
Sekula, J., Suppl. No. 74:25
Seltzer, S., 497
Senturia, B.H., Suppl. No. 68:3; Suppl. No. 69:4
Seo, I.S., 168
Sessions, D.G., 556
Shea, J.P., 204
Sheehy, J.L., 331
Sherman, J.M., 414
Shibahara, Y., Suppl. No. 68:236
Shrewsbury, D.S., 225
Shugar, J.M., 20
Shurin, P.A., 93; Suppl. No. 69:23
Sibakov, M., Suppl. No. 68:357
Siegel, M.I., Suppl. No. 68:41
Silberstein, E.B., 62
Silverman, S.R., Suppl. No. 74:15
Simon, K., 46
Simpson, G.T. II, 558
Singer, M.I., 529
Skolnik, E.M., 551
Sloyer, J.L., Jr., Suppl. No. 68:133, 351; Suppl. No. 69:15
Smith, D.M., Suppl. No. 68:153
Smith, H.G., 472
Snow, J.B., Jr., Suppl. No. 74:43
Sobol, S.M., 312
Sofferman, R.A., 215
Søhoel, P., 75
Som, P.M., 20, 103
Sooy, F.A., Suppl. No. 74:12
Sørensen, H., Suppl. No. 68:271
Spector, G.J., 312
Spelman, F.A., Suppl. No. 66:1, 5, 8
Spoden, J.E., 279
Stal, S., 551
Stanievich, J.F., 572
Steiner, W., Suppl. No. 68:54
Stern, R.M., Suppl. No. 68:178
Stewart, J., Suppl. No. 68:14
Stiehm, E.R., 574
Stool, S.E., 124; Suppl. No. 68:172, 190; 572
Strife, J.L., 409
Strong, M.S., 472
Stroud, M.H., 312
Suen, J.Y., 563
Sutton, D., Suppl. No. 66:1, 11, 15
Suzuki, J-I., Suppl. No. 68:83
Suzuki, M., 547
Svanborg-Edén, C., Suppl. No. 68:115
Svendsen, P., Suppl. No. 68:65
Szeinberg, A., 165

Tabata, T., 132
Takasaka, T., 37
Takeda, K., 359
Tally, F.P., Suppl. No. 68:102
Taylor, F.H., Suppl. No. 68:319
Teele, D.W., Suppl. No. 68:5, 102
Terry, L.L., Suppl. No. 74:5
Thompson, J.W., 428, 497
Thomsen, J., 117; Suppl. No. 68:271; Suppl. No. 69:23
Tilsner, T., 225
Timonen, M., Suppl. No. 68:357
Tjellström, A., Suppl. No. 68:322
Tom, L.W.C., 419
Tomich, C.E., 168
Tonndorf, J., 353
Toriyama, M., Suppl. No. 68:83
Tos, M., 117, Suppl. No. 68:91, 217; Suppl. No. 69:13
Toupet, M.G., Suppl. No. 68:196
Tucker, G.F., 268, 401; Suppl. No. 74:142
Tucker, H.M., 504
Tuohimaa, P., Suppl. No. 68:7

Ulsø, C., 121
Ulvestad, R.F., 257; Suppl. No. 69:23
Umeda, Y., Suppl. No. 71
Unni, K., 425
Ushiro, K., 276

Van Hattum, R.J., Suppl. No. 74:161
Vap, J.G., Suppl. No. 68:185
Vaughan, C.W., 472
Vauthy, P.A., 417
Victor, S., 198
Virolainen, E., Suppl. No. 68:7
Virtanen, H., 366

Wada, J., Suppl. No. 68:236
Warfel, K.A., 168
Warner, E.D., 279
Warr, W.B., Suppl. No. 74:114
Watanabe, I., 377
Watanabe, K., 241, 377
Watanabe, N., Suppl. No. 68:333
Watson, C.S., Suppl. No. 74:96
Watson, J.D., 489
Watts, S.L., 467
Weber, A.L., 100, 483
Webster, D.B., Suppl. No. 66:15; Suppl. No. 68:254
Webster, M., Suppl. No. 68:254
Weider, D.J., Suppl. No. 68:14
Weisman, R.A., 58, 419
Welzl-Mueller, K., Suppl. No. 68:79
Wenthold, R.J., Suppl. No. 74:121
Weshler, Z., 180
Wetmore, S.J., 563
Wetzel, W.J., 563
White, M., Suppl. No. 74:84
Wicher, K., Suppl. No. 68:104
Wiederhold, M.L., Suppl. No. 68:185
Wiet, R.J., Suppl. No. 68:14, 28; Suppl. No. 69:9
Williams, I., 342
Williams, J.D., 239
Wilson, W.R., 591
Wolf, J.A., 430
Wolfe, J.W., 286
Wood, R.E., 414
Woods, R., Suppl. No. 69:4
Worthington, D.W., Suppl. No. 74:59
Wullstein, H.L., Suppl. No. 69:4, 23
Wullstein, S.R., Suppl. No. 69:4

Yamashita, T., Suppl. No. 68:147
Yanagisawa, E., 547
Ylikoski, J., Suppl. No. 68:143

Zajtchuk, J.T., Suppl. No. 68:185
Zechner, G., Suppl. No. 68:87; Suppl. No. 69:13

SUBJECT INDEX

Acoustic Immittance Findings in Acute Otitis Media. D.M. Schwartz, R.H. Schwartz, Suppl. No. 68, 211.

Acoustic Reflex as Predictor of Middle Ear Effusion. G.E. Freyss, P.P. Narcy, Y. Manac'h, M.G. Toupet, Suppl. No. 68, 196.

Acoustic Reflex Latency Test in Evaluation of Nontumor Patients with Abnormal Brainstem Latencies. J.D. Clemis, C.N. Sarno, 296.

Acoustic Reflex Response During Curare-Induced Weakness. R.A. Ruth, M.E. Johns, T.F. Gal, 188.

Adenoidectomy and Tonsillectomy, Role of in Management of Children with Middle Ear Effusion. J.B. Snow, Jr., Suppl. No. 74, 43.

Adenoidectomy for Otitis Media with Mucoid Effusion. N. Roydhouse, Suppl. No. 68, 312.

Adenoidectomy in Recurrent Otitis Media, Efficacy of. Historical Overview and Preliminary Results from Randomized, Controlled Trial. J.L. Paradise, C.D. Bluestone, K.D. Rogers, R.H. Taylor, Suppl. No. 68, 319.

Adenoidectomy versus Tympanostomy in Chronic Secretory Otitis Media. G. Marshak, Z.B. Neriah, Suppl. No. 68, 316.

Adenoma, Pituitary Presenting as a Sphenoid Sinus Lesion. X-Ray of the Month. J.M. Davis, A.L. Weber, 483.

Airway, Foreign Bodies in. Five-Year Retrospective Study with Special Reference to Management. S.R. Cohen, W.I. Herbert, G.B. Lewis, Jr., K.A. Geller, 437.

Airway Obstruction, Acute, in Epidermolysis Bullosa Dystrophica of Larynx and Trachea. J.W. Thompson, A.R. Ahmed, J.P. Dudley, 428.

Airway Obstruction, Acute, Upper, in Infants and Children. Evaluation by Fiberoptic Bronchoscope. P.A. Vauthy, R. Reddy, 417.

Airway Obstruction in a Hemophiliac Child. J.F. Stanievich, G. Marshak, S.E. Stool, 572.

Airway Obstruction, Upper, in Infectious Mononucleosis. J.A. Wolfe, L.D. Rowe, 430.

Airway Obstruction with Laryngeal Sarcoidosis. R.A. Weisman, R.F. Canalis, W.J. Powell, 58.

Airway Resistance, Laryngeal Regulation of. II. Pulmonary Receptor Reflexes. T.V. McCaffrey, E.B. Kern, 462.

Airway, Upper, Acute, Obstruction, Pulmonary Edema Following Relief of. A.G. Galvis, S.E. Stool, C.D. Bluestone, 124.

Airway, Upper, in Neonates, Acquired Stenosis of. An Increasing Problem. M.J. Papsidero, N.R.T. Pashley, 512.

Airways, Lower and Upper, A Study of the Physiologic Relationship with ^{133}Xe. E.B. Silberstein, J.T. Lewis, D.J. Quenelle, 62.

Allergy, Middle Ear and Nasal, Relation Between. Experimental Study. T. Yamashita, N. Okazaki, T. Kumazawa, Suppl. No. 68, 147.

Ampullary Nerve, Posterior Branch of the Singular Nerve in the Otic Capsule. Y. Okano, I. Sando, E.N. Myers, 13.

Anacusis, Surgical Treatment of Recurrent Perilymph Fistula with. C. Ulsϕ, E. Hentzer, 121.

Anaerobic Bacteria, Cultures for, in Persistent Effusions of Middle Ear. D.W. Teele, G.B. Healy, F.P. Tally, Suppl. No. 68, 102.

Anatomy of the Eustachian Tube in the Rhesus Monkey (Macaca mulatta) and Man: Implications for Physiologic Modeling. W.J. Doyle, S.R. Rood, 49.

Anesthetic Gases, Effect of on Middle Ear Pressure in Presence of Effusion. G.A. Gates, J.C. Cooper, Jr., Suppl. No. 68, 62.

Anomalies, Bronchogenic, Subcutaneous. P. Sϕhoel, P. Blom, I.W.S. Mair, 75.

Anomalies, Developmental, Ear-Related, of Branchial Clefts and Arches I and II. R.J. Bellucci, Suppl. No. 74, 42.

Antibiotic-Resistant Bacteria in Otitis Media with Effusion. D.J. Lim, D.M. Lewis, J.L. Schram, H.G. Birch, Suppl. No. 68, 278.

Antibody Coated Bacteria in Otitis Media with Effusions. J.M. Bernstein, D. Myers, D. Kosinski, R. Nisengard, K. Wicher, Suppl. No. 68, 104.

Antibody Levels, Study of in Children with Purulent Otitis Media. P. Branefors, T. Dahlberg, O. Nylén, Suppl. No. 68, 117.

Antihistamine-Adrenergic Combination. Diagnostic and Therapeutic Studies in Treatment of Childhood Serous Otitis Media. J.S. O'Shea, D.J. Langenbrunner, D.E. McCloskey, J.C. Pezzullo, J.B. Regan, Suppl. No. 68, 285.

Apnea, Reflex, in Infants with Innominate Artery Compression of Trachea. J.M. Ardito, R.H. Ossoff, G.F. Tucker, Jr., S.Y. DeLeon, 401.

Arteritis, Cranial, in Otolaryngology. R.A. Sofferman, 215.

Artery, Innominate, Compression of Trachea in Infants with Reflex Apnea. J.M. Ardito, R.H. Ossoff, G.F. Tucker, Jr., S.Y. DeLeon, 401.

Arthritis, Cricoarytenoid, Acute: Local Periarticular Steroid Injection. G.T. Simpson II, A. Javaheri, P. Janfaza, 558

Arthritis, Cricoarytenoid, Rheumatoid Complicated by Upper Esophageal Ulcerations. W.W. Montgomery, M.L. Goodman, 6.

Audiology, Pediatric, Behavioral Methods in: Past, Present, Future. N.D. Matkin, Suppl. No. 74, 50.

Audiometry, Electrophysiologic. D.W. Worthington, J.F. Peters, Suppl. No. 74, 59.

Audiometry, Impedance. G. Lidén, Suppl. No. 74, 53.

Auditory Brainstem Responses in Children with Otitis Media with Effusion. T.J. Fria, D.L. Sabo, Suppl. No. 68, 200.

Auditory Maturation, Neurophysiological Correlates of. E. Javel, Suppl. No. 74, 103.

Auditory Nuclei Development in Mouse Brainstem. D.B. Webster, M. Webster, Suppl. No. 68, 254.

Auditory Perceptual Learning, Time Course of. C.S. Watson, Suppl. No. 74, 96.

Auditory Science, Research Priorities in — Panel. Suppl. No. 74.
- The Audiologist's View. J. Jerger, 134.
- The Otologist's View. R. Ruben, 132.
- The Physiologist's View. J.E. Hind, 136.

Auditory System, Developing Plasticity of. R.J. Ruben, I. Rapin, 303.

Auditory System, Efferent Components of. W.B. Warr, Suppl. No. 74, 114.

Auditory System, Neurochemistry of. R.J. Wenthold, Suppl. No. 74, 121.

Bacillary Infections (Acute Gram-Negative) of Middle Ear and Mastoid. E. Ostfeld, E. Rubinstein, 33.

Behavioral Methods in Pediatric Audiology: Past, Present, Future, N.D. Matkin, Suppl. No. 74, 50.

Blastomycosis of Larynx. J.Y. Suen, S.J. Wetmore, W.J. Wetzel, R.J. Craig, 563.

BOOK REVIEWS
- Baloh, R.W., Honrubia, V., Clinical Neurophysiology of the Vestibular System, 289.
- Berendes, J., Link, R., Zollner, F., Hals-Nasen-Ohren-Heilkunde in Praxis und Klinik, Bank 5, Ohr (The Ear), 485.
- Birrell, J.F., Paediatric Otolaryngology, 389.
- Gerlings, P.G., Atlas of the Histopathology of Ear Tumors, 389.
- Gregory, H.H., Controversies about Stuttering Therapy, 290.
- Hutchinson, B.B., Hanson, M.L., Mecham, M.J., Diagnostic Handbook of Speech Pathology, 199.
- Iliff, C.E., Iliff, W.J., Iliff, N.T., Oculoplastic Surgery, 389.
- Kelly, J.F., Management of War Injuries to the Jaws and Related Structures, 198.
- Kleinsasser, O., Microlaryngoscopy and Endolaryngeal Microscopy, 486.
- MacKay, I.R.A., Introducing Practical Phonetics, 198.
- McCarthy, P.L., Shklar, G., Diseases of the Oral Mucosa, 485.
- Montgomery, W.W., Surgery of the Respiratory System, Volume 1, Second Edition, 289.
- Newby, H.E., Audiology, Fourth Edition. 289.
- Ordy, J.M., Brizzee, K.R., Sensory Systems and Communication in the Elderly, Volume 10, Aging, 486.
- Rintelmann, W.F., Hearing Assessment: Perspectives in Audiology, 199.
- Rudolph, R., Fisher, J.C., Ninnemann, J.L., Skin Grafting, 288.
- Senturia, B.H., Marcus, M.D., Lucente, F.E., Diseases of the External Ear: An Otologic-Dermatologic Manual, 485.
- Simmons, F.B., Gillam, S.F., Mattox, D.E., An Atlas of Electronystagmography, 288.
- Snow, J.B., Jr., Introduction to Otorhinolaryngology, 290.

Stell, P.M., Maran, A.G.D., Head and Neck Surgery, Second Edition, 288.

Tosi, O., Voice Identification: Theory and Legal Applications, 199.

Ventry, I.M., Schiavettri, N., Evaluating Research in Speech Pathology and Audiology, 486.

Bougienage, Retrograde in Emergency Management of Tracheal Stenosis. I. Eliachar, K. Simon, J.H. Birkhan, H.Z. Joachims, 46.

Brain Abscess, Associated with Bilateral Temporal Bone Cholesteatoma. X-Ray of the Month. A.F. O'Connor, 194.

Brainstem Auditory Evoked Potentials for Detection of Retrocochlear Pathology. S.E. Kinney, R.H. Nodar, 291.

Brainstem Electric Responses, Auditory, and Electrocochleography, in Patients with Pontine Angle Tumors. J.J. Eggermont, M. Don, D. E. Brackmann, Suppl. No. 75.

Brainstem-Evoked Responses, Binaural Interaction in. R.A. Dobie, C.I. Berlin, Suppl. No. 74, 62.

Brainstem Histopathology Following Chronic Scala Tympani Implantation in Monkeys. J.M. Miller, D. Sutton, D.B. Webster, 15. Animal Studies of a Cochlear Prosthesis. Suppl. No. 66.

Brainstem Latencies, Abnormal, with Acoustic Reflex Latency Test in Evaluation of Nontumor Patients. J.D. Clemis, C.N. Sarno, 296.

Brainstem, Mouse, Auditory Development in. D.B. Webster, M. Webster, Suppl. No. 68, 254.

Branchial Clefts and Arches I and II, Ear-Related Developmental Anomalies of. R.J. Bellucci, Suppl. No. 74, 42.

Bronchogenic Anomalies, Subcutaneous. P. Søhoel, P. Blom, I.W.S. Mair, 75.

Bronchoscopy, Flexible, Pediatric. R.E. Wood, J.M. Sherman. 414.

Cancer, Induction of by DNA Viruses. Sixth Daniel C. Baker, Jr. Memorial Lecture. J.D. Watson, 489.

Cancer, Laryngeal, Retrospective Comparison of Conservative and Radical Neck Dissection in. R. Molinari, G. Cantu, F. Chiesa, C. Grandi, 578.

Candida Laryngitis in Chronic Mucotaneous Candidiasis. Its Association with *Candida* Esophagitis. J.P. Dudley, R. Kobayashi, H.M. Rosenblatt, W.J. Byrne, M.E. Ament, E.R. Stiehm, 574.

Cannula, Tracheal, Silicone. W.W. Montgomery, 521.

Capillary Permeability, Characteristics of in Nasal Mucosa. K. Watanabe, Y. Saito, I. Watanabe, V. Mizuhira, 377.

Carcinoid and Mucoepidermoid Carcinoma of Bronchus in Children. J.C. McDougall, A. Gorenstein, K. Unni, E.J. O'Connell, 425.

Carcinoma, Carcinoid and Mucoepidermoid, of Bronchus in Children. J.C. McDougall, A. Gorenstein, K. Unni, E.J. O'Connell, 425.

Carcinoma, Mucoepidermoid, of the Larynx: A Case Report and Review of the Literature. W.J. Binder, P. Som, M. Kaneko, H.F. Biller, 103.

Carcinoma of Human Maxillary Sinus, Establishment of New Cell Line from. T. Nakashima, K. Makashima, I. Hiroto, 24.

Carcinoma of the Larynx, Clear Cell: A Variant of Mucoepidermoid Carcinoma. I.S. Seo, C.E. Tomich, K.A. Warfel, M.T. Hull, 168.

Carcinomas, Mucopidermoid and Acinous Cell, of Salivary Tissues. Pathology Consultation. J.G. Batsakis, 91.

Cell Line, New, from Human Maxillary Sinus Carcinoma, Establishment of. T. Nakashima, K. Makishima, I. Hiroto, 24.

Cerebrospinal Rhinorrhea, Extracranial Surgical Repair of. T.C. Calcaterra, 108.

Chemoreceptor Reflexes. Laryngeal Regulation of Airway Resistance. T.V. McCaffrey, E.B. Kern, 209.

Chemotherapy, Topical, of Recurrent Respiratory Papillomatosis. Preliminary Report. H.G. Smith, G.B. Healy, C.W. Vaughan, M.S. Strong, 472.

Childhood Communication Disorders: Present Status and Future Priorities. Suppl. No. 74.
Introduction. P.E. Brookhouser, 1.

China, People's Republic of, Otolaryngology and Medicine Today. B.F. McCabe, 590.

Cholesteatoma and Chronic Otitis Media. G.O. Proud, Suppl. No. 74, 47.

Cholesteatoma, Bilateral Temporal Bone, with an Associated Brain Abscess. X-Ray of the Month. A.F. O'Connor, 194.

Cholesteatomas, Intramembranous and Mesotympanic, Associated with an Intact Tympanic Membrane in Children. S.M. Sobol, T.J. Reichert, K.D. Faw, M.H. Stroud, G.J. Spector, J.H. Ogura, 312.

Cholesterol Granuloma and Lactoferrin in Idiopathic Hemotympanum. J. Sadé, A. Halevy, A. Klajman, T. Mualem, Suppl. No. 68, 240.

Chondrosarcoma of Larynx, Conservative Surgical Treatment of. R.W. Cantrell, J.F. Reibel, R.A. Jahrsdoerfer, M.E. Johns, 567.

Chondroid Chordoma: Case Report and Literature Review. J.E. Spoden, R.M. Bumsted, E.D. Warner, 279.

Chordoma, Chondroid: Case Report and Literature Review. J.E. Spoden, R.M. Bumsted, E.D. Warner, 279.

Chordoma, Intracranial. X-Ray of the Month. R.A. Greenes, A.L. Weber, 100.

Chordoma, Sphenoocipital Presenting as a Nasopharyngeal Mass: A Case Report. M.L. Eisemann, 271.

Cilia, Atypical, of Human Nasal Mucosa. T. Takasaka, M. Sato, A. Onodera, 37.

Ciliary Ultrastructure, Normal, in Children with Kartagener's Syndrome. F.S. Herzon, S. Murphy, 81.

Cineradiographic Analysis of Eustachian Tube Function: Experimental Study. I. Honjo, N. Okazaki, K. Ushiro, T. Kumazawa, 276.

Clear Cell Tumors of Salivary Glands. Pathology Consultation. J.G. Batsakis, 196.

Cleft Palate Children, Eustachian Tube Function in. W.J. Doyle, E.I. Cantekin, C.D. Bluestone, Suppl. No. 68, 34.

Cleft Palate, Nonhuman Primate Model of, Its Implications for Middle Ear Pathology. W.J. Doyle, E.I. Cantekin, C.D. Bluestone, D.C. Phillips, K.K. Kimes, M.I. Siegel, Suppl. No. 68, 41.

Clerf, Louis H. Lecture, First. Jefferson Medical College. Otorhinolaryngology: A Progress Report. J.E. Bordley, 84.

Cochlear and Middle Ear Disease, Screening Procedure for Detection of. U. Renvall, G. Lidén, Suppl. No. 68, 214.

Cochlear Disorders, Acute: The Combination of Hearing Loss, Recruitment, Poor Speech Discrimination, and Tinnitus. J. Tonndorf, 353.

Cochlear Fluid Balance. A Clinical/Research Overview. A.J. Duvall III, P.A. Santi, M.J. Hukee, 335.

Cochlear Histopathology Following Two Implant Designs for Use in Scala Tympani, Comparison of. D. Sutton, J.M. Miller, B.E. Pfingst, 11. Animal Studies of a Cochlear Prosthesis. Suppl. No. 66.

Cochlear Implants, Operating Ranges for. B.E. Pfingst, F.A. Spelman, D. Sutton, 1. Animal Studies of a Cochlear Prosthesis. Suppl. No. 66.

Coding Considerations in Design of Cochlear Prostheses. M.M. Merzenich, M. White, Suppl. No. 74, 84.

Cognitive Development, Effects of Otitis Media on. F.D. Horowitz, H. Leake III, Suppl. No. 68, 264.

Communication Disorders, Childhood: Present Status and Future Priorities. Suppl. No. 74.

Communication Disorders, Area of, Educational and Training Priorities for Clinicians and Researchers. A Health Science Campus Chancellor's Perspective. F.A. Sooy, Suppl. No. 74, 12.

Communication Disorders: Investigator Training and Support Needs. M. Lawrence, Suppl. No. 74, 9.

Communicative Disorders, Research in, Improving Grant Applications for. D.G. Hanson, R.F. Ulvestad, J.B. Ranney, 257.

Communicatively Disadvantaged Child, Support of Programs for: Role of Private Foundation. L.L. Terry, Suppl. No. 74, 5.

Communicatively Disadvantaged, Priorities in Service Delivery to: Habilitation Needs. S.R. Silverman, Suppl. No. 74, 15.

Communicatively Disadvantaged, Problems of. An Overview. J.E. Bordley, Suppl. No. 74, 3.

Computer-Aided and Graphic Reconstruction of Human Endolymphatic Duct and Sac: A Method for Comparing Menière's and Non-Menière's Disease Cases. J.C.M. Antunez, F.R. Galey, F.H. Linthicum, G.D. McCann, Suppl. No. 76, 23.

Computer Tomography and Translabyrinthine Surgery in Assessment of Acoustic Neurinoma, Comparison of. M. Tos, G. Glydensted, J. Thomsen, J. Lester, 117.

Condylomata and Laryngeal Papillomata, Relationship Between. Clinical and Molecular Virological Evidence. C.A. Quick, S.L. Watts, R.A. Krzyzek, A.J. Faras, 467.

Congenital Lesions and Laryngeal Development. G.F. Tucker, Jr., Suppl. No. 74, 142.

Congenital Malformations of the Ear. Analysis of 94 Operations. R. Jahrsdoerfer, 348.

Cricoarytenoid Arthritis, Acute: Local Periarticular Steroid Injection. G.T. Simpson II, A. Javaheri, P. Janfaza, 558.

Cricoarytenoid Arthritis, Rheumatoid, Complicated by Upper Esophageal Ulcerations. W.W. Montgomery, M.L. Goodman, 6.

Cricoid Split, Anterior, as an Alternative to Tracheotomy Management of Extubation Problem in Premature Child. R.T. Cotton, A.B. Seid, 508.

Cricopharyngeus in the Neonate. T.J. Reichert, K.D. Faw, 446.

Cryogenic Application, Destruction and Regeneration of Jawbone After. Experimental Study. R. Kuylenstierna, P-G. Lundquist, A. Nathanson, 582.

Cupular Dynamics and Second-Order Vestibular Adaptation. R.W. Babin, J.H. Ryu, B.F. McCabe, 262.

Curare-Induced Weakness, Acoustic Reflex Response During. R.A. Ruth, M.E. Johns, T.F. Gal, 188.

Cysts, Maxillary, Treatment of. G.E. Merwin, T. Tilsner, L.R. Boies, D.S. Shrewsbury, 225.

Cysts, Saccular, and Internal Laryngocele in Children. J.O. Donegan, J.L. Strife, A.B. Seid, R.T. Cotton, J.S. Dunbar, 409.

Deafness, Congenital, Pathology of: Present Status and Future Priorities. L. Bergstrom, Suppl. No. 74, 31.

Deafness, Mondini's: Review of Histopathology. M.M. Paparella, Suppl. No. 67.

Decongestant with or without Antihistamine, Effect on Eustachian Tube Function. E.I. Cantekin, C.D. Bluestone, H.E. Rockette, Q.C. Beery, Suppl. No. 68, 290.

Denervation, Selective, Vocal Cord Positioning by. Old Territory Revisited. C.T. Sasaki, M. Horiuchi, T. Ikari, J.A. Kirchner, 541.

Disadvantaged Child, Communicatively, Support of Programs for: Role of Private Foundation. L.L. Terry, Suppl. No. 74, 5.

Discrimination of Synthesized Speech, Effect of Word Speed, Number of Words and Habituation on. T. Rahko, M. Karjalainen, U. Laine, A. Lavonen, 69.

Diverticulum, Tracheal, Congenital. Case Report. S. Frenkiel, I.K. Assimes, J.K. Rosales, 406.

DNA Viruses, Induction of Cancer by. Sixth Daniel C. Baker, Jr. Memorial Lecture. J.D. Watson, 489.

Dysplasia, Mondini: A Clinical and Pathological Study. H.F. Schuknecht, Suppl. No. 65.

Educational and Training Priorities for Clinicians and Researchers in Area of Communication Disorders. A Health Science Campus Chancellor's Perspective. F.A. Sooy, Suppl. No. 74, 12.

Efferent Components of the Auditory System. W.B. Warr, Suppl. No. 74, 114.

Effusion, Effect of Anesthetic Gases on Middle Ear Pressure in the Presence of. G.A. Gates, J.C. Cooper, Jr., Suppl. No. 68, 62.

Electrocochleography and Auditory Brainstem Electric Responses in Patients with Pontine Angle Tumors. J.J. Eggermont, M. Don, D.E. Brackmann, Suppl. No. 75.

Electrophysiologic Audiometry. D.W. Worthington, J.F. Peters, Suppl. No. 74, 59.

Emergency Management of Tracheal Stenosis: Retrograde Tracheal Bougienage. I. Eliachar, K. Simon, J.H. Birkhan, H.Z. Joachims, 46.

Endolymphatic Duct and Sac, Human, Computer-Aided and Graphic Reconstruction of: A Method for Comparing Menière's and Non-Menière's Disease Cases. J.C.M. Antunez, F.R. Galey, F.H. Linthicum, G.D. McCann, Suppl. No. 76, 23.

Endolymphatic Hydrops and Menière's Disease: Clinical-Histopathological Correlations. B.G. Fraysse, A. Alonso, W.F. House, Suppl. No. 76, 2.

Endolymphatic Hydrops with Absence of Vein in Paravestibular Canaliculus. R. Gussen, 157.

Endoscopy and Biopsy in Gastroesophageal Reflux in Infants and Children. B. Benjamin, D. Pohl, P.M. Bale, 443.

Endoscopy of the Pharyngeal Eustachian Tube. M.P. Jaumann, W. Steiner, M. Berg, Suppl. No. 68, 54.

ENG of the Month. Pacemaker Artifact on ENG Tracing. W.R. Wilson, 591.

Epidemiology of Otitis Media in Children. D.W. Teele, J.O. Klein, B.A. Rosner, Suppl. No. 68, 5.

Epidermolysis Bullosa Dystrophica of Larynx and Trachea. Acute Airway Obstruction. J.W. Thompson, A.R. Ahmed, J.P. Dudley, 428.

Epitympanum, Surgical Landmark for Facial Nerve in. R.R. Gacek, 249.

Esophageal Disease, High Incidence of Pulmonary Symptoms in Infants Evaluated for. F.C. Rothstein, T.C. Halpin, 450.

Esophageal Foreign Bodies of Dental Origin, Impacted. D.C. Nwafo, C.H. Anyanwu, M.O. Egbue, 129.

Esophageal Stenosis in Children. Chevalier Jackson Lecture. F. Aprigliano, 391.

Esophageal Ulcerations, Upper, Complicated by Rheumatoid Cricoarytenoid Arthritis. W.W. Montgomery, M.L. Goodman, 6.

Esophagitis, *Candida*, Its Association with *Candida* Laryngitis in Chronic Mucocutaneous Candidiasis. J.P. Dudley, R. Kobayashi, H.M. Rosenblatt, W.J. Byrne, M.E. Ament, E.R. Stiehm, 574.

Eustachian Tube Function and Middle Ear Mechanics, New Impedance Method for Measuring. A. Ivarsson, Suppl. No. 68, 207.

Eustachian Tube Function and Retraction of the Tympanic Membrane. J. Holmquist, U. Renvall, P. Svendsen, Suppl. No. 68, 65.

Eustachian Tube Function, Cineradiographic Analysis of: Experimental Study. I. Honjo, N. Okazaki, K. Ushiro, T. Kumazawa, 276.

Eustachian Tube Function, Effect of Decongestant with or without Antihistamine. E.I. Cantekin, C.D. Bluestone, H.E. Rockette, Q.C. Beery, Suppl. No. 68, 290.

Eustachian Tube Function, Effect of Surgical Alterations of the Tensor Veli Palatini Muscle on. E.I. Cantekin, D.C. Philips, W.J. Doyle, C.D. Bluestone, K.K. Kimes, Suppl. No. 68, 47.

Eustachian Tube Function in an American Indian Population. Q.C. Beery, W.J. Doyle, E.I. Cantekin, C.D. Bluestone, R.J. Wiet, Suppl. No. 68, 28.

Eustachian Tube Function in Children and Adults with Normal Ears, Comparison of. A. Bylander, Suppl. No. 68, 20.

Eustachian Tube Function in Cleft Palate Children. W.J. Doyle, E.I. Cantekin, C.D. Bluestone, Suppl. No. 68, 34.

Eustachian Tube Function in Pathological Ears, Comparative Preoperative Evaluation of. H. Virtanen, T. Palva, T. Jauhiainen, 366.

Eustachian Tube Function, Sonometric Evaluation of, Using Broadband Stimuli. K.G. Murti, R.M. Stern, E.I. Cantekin, C.D. Bluestone, Suppl. No. 68, 178.

Eustachian Tube in the Rhesus Monkey (Macaca mulatta) and Man, Comparison of the Anatomy: Implications for Physiologic Modeling. W.J. Doyle, S.R. Rood, 49.

Eustachian Tube Occlusion Following Oxygen Supply of Middle Ear Mucosa. C. Morgenstern, Suppl. No. 68, 76.

Eustachian Tube, Opening Mechanism of. Clinical and Experimental Study. I. Honjo, N. Okazaki, T. Kumazawa, Suppl. No. 68, 25.

Eustachian Tube, Pharyngeal, Endoscopy of. M.P. Jaumann, W. Steiner, M. Berg, Suppl. No. 68, 54.

Evoked Potentials, Auditory, Brainstem, for Detection of Retrocochlear Pathology. S.E. Kinney, R.H. Nodar, 291.

Evoked Responses, Brainstem, Binaural Interaction in. R.A. Dobie, C.I. Berlin, Suppl. No. 74, 62.

Ewing's Sarcoma of the Mandible. P.M. Som, Y.P. Krespi, G. Hermann, J.M. Shugar, 20.

Extubation Problem in the Premature Child, Management of. Anterior Cricoid Split as an Alternative to Tracheotomy. R.T. Cotton, A.B. Seid, 508.

Eye-Tracking Patterns, Manual Quantitative Assessment of the Eye-Tracking Test. Y. Umeda, Suppl. No. 71, 1.
I. Manual Quantitative Assessment of Eye-Tracking Patterns, 1.
II. Standardization of the Eye-Tracking Test, 7.

Facial Nerve in the Epitympanum, Surgical Landmark for. R.R. Gacek, 249.

Fetal Rat, Otoconial Formation in. M.S. Salamat, M.D. Ross, D.R. Peacor, 229.

Fiberoptic Bronchoscope, Evaluation by. Acute Upper Airway Obstruction in Infants and Children. P.A. Vauthy, R. Reddy, 417.

Fistula, Perilymph with Anacusis, Surgical Treatment of Recurrence. C. Ulsø, E. Hentzer, 121.

Foreign Bodies, Impacted Esophageal, of Dental Origin. D.C. Nwafo, C.H. Anyanwu, M.O. Egbue, 129.

Frequency Analysis in Normal and Hearing-Impaired Listeners. W. Jesteadt, Suppl. No. 74, 88.

Frequency-Gain Characteristics for Hearing Aids, Review of Recent Research on Selection of. R. Lippmann, Suppl. No. 74, 79.

Gas Absorption in Middle Ear. E.I. Cantekin, W.J. Doyle, D.C. Phillips, C.D. Bluestone, Suppl. No. 68, 71.

Gas Composition of Middle Ear During Nitrous Oxide-Oxygen Ventilation. E. Ostfeld, M. Crispin, J. Blonder, A. Szeinberg, 165.

Gastroesophageal Reflux, Endoscopy and Biopsy in, in Infants and Children. B. Benjamin, D. Pohl, P.M. Bale, 443.

Gerbils, Drug-Treated, Normal and Ototoxic, Single Cell Responses in. N.B. Gross, W.S. Lifschitz, 176.

Glottic Closure Reflex: Control Mechanisms. T. Ikari, C.T. Sasaki, 220.

Grand Rounds. Septic Osteoradionecrosis of the Mandible. S.S. Parulekar, D.F. Paonessa, 383.

Grant Applications for Research in Communicative Disorders, Improving. D.G. Hanson, R.F. Ulvestad, J.B. Ranney, 257.

Guest of Honor, Sven Ingelstedt. D.J. Lim, Suppl. No. 68, 1.

Habilitation Model. Language Stimulation Group. P.K. Hixson, Suppl. No. 74, 175.

Haemophilus influenzae, Ampicillin-Resistant Strains of in Otitis Media treated with Trimethoprim-Sulfamethoxazole. R. Schwartz, W.J. Rodriguez, W. Khan, R. Mann, R.G. Barsanti, S. Ross, Suppl. No. 68, 281.

Head and Neck Surgeon: A Guide for Thyroid Disease. R.M. Bumsted, Suppl. No. 72.

Hearing Aids, Frequency-Gain Characteristics for, Review of Recent Research on Selection of. R. Lippmann, Suppl. No. 74, 79.

Hearing Aids, Uses and Abuses of. J.E. Peck, Suppl. No. 74, 70.

Hearing and Sickle Cell Anemia. E.M. Friedman, G.R. Herer, N.L.C. Luban, I. Williams, 342.

Hearing-Impaired, Advances in Sensory Aids for: Visual and Vibrotactile Aids. J.M. Pickett, Suppl No. 74, 74.

Hearing-Impaired and Normal Listeners, Frequency Analysis in. W. Jesteadt, Suppl. No. 74, 88.

Hearing-Impaired, Educational Programming for: Present and Future, Panel. Suppl. No. 74.
Denmark, H.W. Ewertsen, 28.
Poland, J. Sekula, 25.
Sweden, G. Lidén, 22.
United States, E.L. Lowell, 19.

Hemophiliac Child, Airway Obstruction in a. J.F. Stanievich, G. Marshak, S.E. Stool, 572.

Hemoptysis in Children. L.W.C. Tom, R.A. Weisman, S.D. Handler, 419.

Hemotympanum, Idiopathic, Cholesterol Granuloma and Lactoferrin. J. Sadé, A. Halevy, A. Klajman, T. Mualem, Suppl. No. 68, 240.

Hyperplasia of Larynx, Lymphoid, Simulating Neoplasia. E.V. Pellettiere II, L.D. Holinger, J.A. Schild, 65.

IgA Circadian Rhythm, Nasal Secretory: A Single-Dose Suppression Test. P. Menzio, R. Molino, B. Morra, M. Bussi, A. Sartoris, G. Cortesina, 173.

IgA Distribution and Secretory Activity in Immunopathological Study of the Larynx. T. Nakashima, S. Komiyama, K. Makishima, K. Takeda, I. Hiroto, 359.

IgA Distribution and Secretory Activity: Local Immune System of Nasal Mucosa in Inflammation. T. Nakashima, Y. Hamashima, 140.

Immune System, Mucosal: Implications in Otitis Media with Effusion. J.M. Bernstein, P.L. Ogra, Suppl. No. 68, 326.

Immunoelectrophoresis, Countercurrent, Evaluation of, as a Diagnostic Tool in Bacterial Otitis Media. E. Ostfeld, G. Altmann, Suppl. No. 68, 110.

Immunofluorescent Study on Middle Ear Mucosa. G. Mogi, S. Maeda, N. Watanabe, Suppl. No. 68, 333.

Immunoglobuline E-Mediated Disease: Otitis Media in Young Infant. J.L. Sloyer, J.H. Ploussard, L.J. Karr, Suppl. No. 68, 133.

Immunologic Response to Pneumococcal Polysaccharide Vaccine in Infants. J.L. Sloyer, J.H. Ploussard, L.J. Karr, G.D. Schiffman, Suppl. No. 68, 351.

Immunopathological Study of the Larynx. IgA Distribution and Secretory Activity. T. Nakashima, S. Komiyama, K. Makishima, K. Takeda, I. Hiroto, 359.

Impedance Audiometry. G. Lidén, Suppl. No. 74, 53.

Impedance Screening. Integral Part of Hearing Screening. J.L. Northern, Suppl. No. 68, 233.

Impedance Screening for Children. Need for More Research. F.H. Bess, Suppl. No. 68, 228.

Implant Designs for Use in Scala Tympani, Comparison of Cochlear Histopathology Following Two. D. Sutton, J.M. Miller, B.E. Pfingst. Animal Studies of a Cochlear Prosthesis. Suppl. No. 66, 11.

Implantation of Scala Tympani in Monkeys, Chronic Brainstem Histopathology Following. J.M. Miller, D. Sutton, D.B. Webster. Animal Studies of a Cochlear Prosthesis. Suppl. No. 66, 15.

Implanted Ear, Effects of the Flow of Current in the: Design of the Cochlear Prosthesis. F.A. Spelman, B.M. Clopton, B.E. Pfingst, J.M. Miller. Animal Studies of a Cochlear Prosthesis. Suppl. No. 66, 8.

Implants, Cochlear, Operating Ranges for. B.E. Pfingst, F.A. Spelman, D. Sutton. Animal Studies of a Cochlear Prosthesis. Suppl. No. 66, 1.

Induction of Cancer by DNA Viruses. Sixth Daniel C. Baker, Jr. Memorial Lecture. J.D. Watson, 489.

Infectious Mononucleosis, Upper Airway Obstuction in. J.A. Wolfe, L.D. Rowe, 430.

Inner Ear Pathology and Otitis Media. A Review. M.M. Paparella, M.V. Goycoolea, W.L. Meyerhoff, Suppl. No. 6, 249.

Intracanalicular Neurilemmomas: Clinicopathologic Study. V. Kasantikul, M.G. Netsky, M.E. Glasscock III, J.W. Hayes, 29.

Intubation, Endotracheal, Laryngeal Stenosis from. Review of 58 Cases. D.B. Hawkins, W.M. Luxford, 454.

Intubation, Orotracheal, Prolonged in the Newborn. G.H. Conner, M.J. Bushey, M.J. Maisels, 459.

Investigator Training and Support Needs: Communication Disorders. M. Lawrence, Suppl. No. 74, 9.

Jawbone, Regeneration and Destruction of, After Cryogenic Application. Experimental Study. R. Kuylenstierna, P-G. Lundquist, A. Nathanson, 582.

Kartagener's Syndrome, Normal Ciliary Ultrastructure in Children with. F.S. Herzon, S. Murphy, 81.

Keratoacanthoma of the Head and Neck. R.E. Goodwin, G.H. Fisher, 72.

Labyrinthectomy versus Middle Fossa Vestibular Nerve Section in Menière's Disease. A Critical Evaluation of Relief of Vertigo. M.E. Glasscock III, G.B. Hughes, W.E. Davis, C.G. Jackson, 318.

Lactoferrin and Cholesterol Granuloma in Idiopathic Hemotympanum. J. Sadé, A. Halevy, A. Klajman, T. Mualem, Suppl. No. 68, 240.

Language and Learning, Research Priorities in. P. Fletcher, Suppl. No. 74, 182.

Language-Based Learning Disabilities. P.E. Hook, Suppl. No. 74, 179.

Language Deficiency in Children. D.M. Morehead, K.E. Morehead, W.A. Morehead, Suppl. No. 74, 165.

Language Development in Persistent Otitis Media. P. Menyuk, Suppl. No. 68, 257.

Language Stimulation Group. Habilitation Model. P.K. Hixson, Suppl. No. 74, 175.

Laryngeal Cancer, Retrospective Comparison of Conservative and Radical Neck Dissection in. R. Molinari, G. Cantu, F. Chiesa, C. Grandi, 578.

Laryngeal Development and Congenital Lesions. G.F. Tucker, Jr., Suppl. No. 74, 142.

Laryngeal Papillomata and Condylomata, Relationship Between. Clinical and Molecular Virological Evidence. C.A. Quick, S.L. Watts, R.A. Krzyzek, A.J. Faras, 467.

Laryngeal Papillomatosis, Juvenile, Management of, Double-Barreled (Diversionary) Tracheostomy in. H.M. Tucker, 504.

Laryngeal Photography Through the Operating Microscope, Simple Method of, "Macrolens Technique." E. Yanagisawa, D.E. Eibling, M. Suzuki, 547.

Laryngeal Regulation of Airway Resistance. Chemoreceptor Reflexes. T.V. McCaffrey, E.B. Kern, 209.

Laryngeal Regulation of Airway Resistance. II. Pulmonary Receptor Reflexes. T.V. McCaffrey, E.B. Kern, 462.

Laryngeal Sarcoidosis with Airway Obstruction. R.A. Weisman, R.F. Weisman, R.F. Canalis, W.J. Powell, 58.

Laryngeal Stenosis from Endotracheal Intubation. Review of 58 Cases. D.B. Hawkins, W.M. Luxford, 454.

Laryngeal Stenosis, Supraglottic, with Postcricoid Involement, Repair of. Case Report. P.J. Doyle, 576.

Laryngeal Surgery in the Pediatric Patient. B. Fearon, Suppl. No. 74, 146.

Laryngeal Ventricle: Historical Features. R.F. Canalis, 184.

Laryngectomy, Endoscopic Technique for Restoration of Voice After. M.I. Singer, E.D. Blom, 529.

Laryngectomy, Partial, Extended. D.G. Sessions, 556.

Laryngectomy, Total, Neoglottic Reconstruction Following. A Reappraisal. B. Leipzig, 534.

Laryngectomy, Total, Neoglottic Reconstruction Following: Galveston Experience. B. Leipzig, C.M. Griffiths, J.P. Shea, 204.

Laryngitis, *Candida* in Chronic Mucocutaneous Candidiasis. Its Association with *Candida* Esophagitis. J.P. Dudley, R. Kobayashi, H.M. Rosenblatt, W.J. Byrne, M.E. Ament, E.R. Stiehm, 574.

Laryngocele, Internal, and Saccular Cysts in Children. J.O. Donegan, J.L. Strife, A.B. Seid, R.T. Cotton, J.S. Dunbar, 409.

Laryngology and the Numbers Game. F.E. Lucente, 538.

Laryngotracheal Stenosis, Long-Term Stenting for. D.E. Schuller, 515.

Larynx and Trachea, Epidermolysis Bullosa Dystrophica of. Acute Airway Obstruction. J.W. Thompson, A.R. Ahmed, J.P. Dudley, 428.

Larynx and Tracheobronchial Tree, Foreign Bodies in, in Children. Review of 225 Cases. B.F. Rothman, C.R. Boeckman, 434.

Larynx and Tracheobronchial Tree, Papilloma in Children. Retrospective Study. S.R. Cohen, K.A. Geller, S. Seltzer, J.W. Thompson, 497.

Larynx, Blastomycosis of. J.Y. Suen, S.J. Wetmore, W.J. Wetzel, R.D. Craig, 563.

Larynx, Chondrosarcoma of, Conservative Surgical Treatment. R.W. Cantrell, J.F. Reibel, R.A. Jahrsdoerfer, M.E. Johns, 567.

Larynx, Clear Cell Carcinoma of: A Variant of Mucoepidermoid Carcinoma. I.S. Seo, C.E. Tomich, K.A. Warfel, M.T. Hull, 168.

Larynx, Immunopathological Study of. IgA Distribution and Secretory Activity. T. Nakashima, S. Komiyama, K. Makishima, K. Takeda, I. Hiroto, 359.

Larynx, Mucoepidermoid Carcinoma of: Case Report and Review of the Literature. W.J. Binder, P. Som, M. Kaneko, H.F. Biller, 103.

Learning Disabilities, Language-Based. P.E. Hook, Suppl. No. 74, 179.

Literature, Pediatric, Recent, Relevant to Otolaryngology, Commentary on. P.A. Shurin, 93.

Lupus Erythematosus, Systemic, Asymptomatic Nasal Septal Perforations in. D. Reiter, A.R. Myers, 78.

Lymphocyte Morphology in Middle Ear Effusions. T. Palva, P. Hayry, J. Ylikoski, Suppl. No. 68, 143.

Lymphoid Hyperplasia of Larynx Simulating Neoplasia. E.V. Pellettiere II, L.D. Holinger, J.A. Schild, 65.

Lymphoma, Malignant, in Middle Ear Cleft, Primary Presentation of. B. Gapany-Gapanavicius, R. Chisin, Z. Weshler, 180.

Malformations of the Ear, Congenital. Analysis of 94 Operations. R. Jahrsdoerfer, 348.

Mandible, Ewing's Sarcoma of. P.M. Som, Y.P. Krespi, G. Herman, J.M. Shugar, 20.

Mandible, Septic Osteoradionecrosis of. Grand Rounds. S.S. Parulekar, D.R. Paonessa, 383.

Mastoid and Middle Ear, Acute Gram-Negative Bacillary Infections of. E. Ostfeld, E. Rubinstein, 33.

Mastoid Pneumatization and Secretory Otitis Media. B. Hussl, K. W-Mueller, Suppl. No. 68, 79.

Matrix Vesicles, Electron Microscopic Study of in Tympanosclerosis. I. Friedmann, G.M. Hodges, M. Graham, Suppl. No. 68, 241.

Maxillary Cysts, Treatment of. G.E. Merwin, T. Tilsner, L.R. Boies, D.S. Shrewsbury, 225.

Maxillary Sinus Carcinoma, Human, Establishment of New Cell Line from. T. Nakashima, K. Makisima, I. Hiroto, 24.

Menière's and Non-Menière's Disease Cases, A Method for Comparing: Computer-Aided and Graphic Reconstruction of Human Endolymphatic Duct and Sac. J.C.M. Antunez, F.R. Galey, F.H. Linthicum, G.D. McCann, Suppl. No. 76, 23.

Menière's Disease and Endolymphatic Hydrops: Clinical-Histopathological Correlations. B.G. Fraysse, A. Alonso, W.F. House, Suppl. No. 76, 2.

Menière's Disease, Labyrinthectomy versus Middle Fossa Vestibular Nerve Section in. A Critical Evaluation of Relief of Vertigo. M.E. Glasscock III, G.B. Hughes, W.E. Davis, C.G. Jackson, 318.

Middle Ear Analyzer, Otoadmittance, Automatic, Validation of. T.J. Fria, E.I. Cantekin, G. Probst, 253.

Middle Ear and Cochlear Disease, Screening Procedure for Detection of. U. Renvall, G. Lidén, Suppl. No. 68, 214.

Middle Ear and Mastoid, Acute Gram-Negative Bacillary Infections of. E. Ostfeld, E. Rubinstein, 33.

Middle Ear and Nasal Allergy, Relation Between. Experimental Study. T. Yamashita, N. Okazaki, T. Kumazawa, Suppl. No. 68, 147.

Middle Ear Cleft, Primary Presentation of Malignant Lymphoma in. B. Gapany-Gapanavicius, R. Chisin, Z. Weshler, 180.

Middle Ear Defense System, Cells Involved in. M. Goycoolea, M.M. Paparella, S.K. Juhn, A-M. Carpenter, Suppl. No. 68, 121.

Middle Ear Disease in a School for the Deaf, Screening for. S.E. Stool, H.B. Craig, M.A. Laird, Suppl. No. 68, 172.

Middle Ear Disease, Obliterative Fibrotic, in Systemic Vasculitis. J.H. Hill, M.D. Graham, P.W. Gikas, 162.

Middle Ear Effusion, Acoustic Reflex as a Predictor of. G.E Freyss, P.P. Narcy, Y. Manac'h, M.G. Toupet, Suppl. No. 68, 196.

Middle Ear Effusion in Chinchilla, Effect of Prostaglandin on the Composition of. T.T.K. Jung, D.M. Smith, S.K. Juhn, J.M. Gerrard, Suppl. No. 68, 153.

Middle Ear Effusion, Possible Long-Term Consequences of. D.N. Brooks, Suppl. No. 68, 246.

Middle Ear Effusion, Prevalence and Spontaneous Course of. Tympanometry in Three-Year-Old Children. M. Fiellau-Nikolajsen, Suppl. No. 68, 223.

Middle Ear Effusion Problems, Identification of Children at Risk for. M.P. Downs, Suppl. No. 68, 168.

Middle Ear Effusion, Proceedings of the Second International Symposium on Recent Advances in. Suppl. No. 68.

Middle Ear Effusion, Report of Research Conference on Recent Advances in. Suppl. No. 69.

Middle Ear Effusion, Role of Tonsillectomy and Adenoidectomy in Management of Children with. J.B. Snow, Jr., Suppl. No. 74, 43.

Middle Ear Effusion, Surgery of Mastoid in Ears with. J. Holmquist, J. Jarlstedt, A Tjellström, Suppl. No. 68, 322.

Middle Ear Effusion, Use of Short Couse of Prednisone for Treating. Double-Blind Crossover Study. R.H. Schwartz, J. Puglese, D.M. Schwartz, Suppl. No. 68, 296.

Middle Ear Effusions, Hearing Loss in Relation to Physical Properties of. M.L. Wiederhold, J.T. Zajtchuk, J.G. Vap, R.E. Paggi, Suppl. No. 68, 185.

Middle Ear Effusions in Relation to Bacteriological Findings, Biochemical and Immunochemical Characteristics of. S.K. Juhn, G.S. Giebink, J.S. Huff, E.L. Mills, Suppl. No. 68, 161.

Middle Ear, Insertion of Ventilation Tubes into: Results and Complications. Seven-Year Review. W. Draf, P. Schulz, Suppl. No. 68, 303.

Middle Ear Effusions, Lymphocyte Morphology in. T. Palva, P. Hayry, J. Ylikoski, Suppl. No. 68, 143.

Middle Ear Exudate and Serum, Concentration of Penicillin V in, During Treatment of Acute Otitis Media. L. Ingvarsson, C. Kamme, K. Lundgren, Suppl. No. 68, 275.

Middle Ear, Frequency of Pathologic Changes in. R. Rudin, J. Holmquist, Suppl. No. 68, 11.

Middle Ear, Gas Absorption in. E.I. Cantekin, W.J. Doyle, D.C. Phillips, C.D. Bluestone, Suppl. No. 68, 71.

Middle Ear Gas Composition During Nitrous Oxide-Oxygen Ventilation. E. Ostfeld, M. Crispin, J. Blonder, A. Szeinberg, 165.

Middle Ear Inoculation of Nonviable *Streptococcus pneumoniae*, Experimental Otitis Media Following. S.H. Lowell, S.K. Juhn, G.S. Giebink, 479.

Middle Ear Mechanics and Eustachian Tube Function, New Impedance Method for Measuring. A. Ivarsson, Suppl. No. 68, 207.

Middle Ear Mucoperiosteum, Epithelial Changes in or of. Experimental Study. I. Kowata, Y. Shibahara, Y. Kaku, J. Wada, K. Kawamoto, Suppl. No. 68, 236.

Middle Ear Mucosa and Auditory Tube in Nonpurulent Otitis Media. G. Zechner, Suppl. No. 68, 87.

Middle Ear Mucosa, Immunofluorescent Study on. G. Mogi, S. Maeda, N. Watanabe, Suppl. No. 68, 333.

Middle Ear Mucosa, Oxygen Supply of under Normal Conditions and after Eustachian Tube Occlusion. C. Morgenstern, Suppl. No. 68, 76.

Middle Ear Pathology, Nonhuman Primate Model of Cleft Palate and Its Implications for. W.J. Doyle, E.I. Cantekin, C.D. Bluestone, D.C. Phillips, K.K. Kimes, M.I. Siegel, Suppl. No. 68, 41.

Middle Ear, Persistent Effusions of, Cultures for Anaerobic Bacteria. D.W. Teele, G.B. Healy, F.P. Tally, Suppl. No. 68, 102.

Middle Ear Pressure in the Presence of Effusion, Effect of Anesthetic Gases on. G.A. Gates, J.C. Cooper, Jr., Suppl. No. 68, 62.

Middle Ear Pressure, Negative. Variations by Season and Sex. T. Lildholdt, Suppl. No. 68, 67.

Middle Ear Pressure, Observations of. Commentary with Movie. R.A. Buckingham, J.L. Ferrer, Suppl. No. 68, 56.

Mondini Dysplasia: A Clinical and Pathological Study. H.F. Schuknecht, Suppl. No. 65.

Mondini's Deafness: A Review of Histopathology. M.M. Paparella, Suppl. No. 67.

Morphophonemic Processes in Children. J. Lybolt, Suppl. No. 74, 158.

Mother-Child Interaction, Aspects of as Related to the Remediation Process. S. Friel-Patti, Suppl. No. 74, 171.

Mucoepidermoid and Carcinoid Carcinoma of Bronchus in Children. J.C. McDougall, A. Gorenstein, K. Unni, E.J. O'Connell, 425.

Myringoplasty. A Review of 472 Cases. J.L. Sheehy, R.G. Anderson, 331.

Nasal and Middle Ear Allergy, Relation Between. Experimental Study. T. Yamashita, N. Okazaki, T. Kumazawa, Suppl. No. 68, 147.

Nasal Mucosa, Characteristics of Capillary Permeability in. K. Watanabe, Y. Saito, I. Watanabe, V. Mizuhira, 377.

Nasal Mucosa, Human, Atypical Cilia of. T. Takasaka, M. Sato, A. Onodera, 37.

Nasal Mucosa in Inflammation, Local Immune System of: IgA Distribution and Secretory Activity. T. Nakashima, Y. Hamashima, 140.

Nasal Septal Perforations, Asymptomatic, in Systemic Lupus Erythematosus. D. Reiter, A.R. Myers, 78.

Nasopharyngeal Mass, Sphenoocipital Chordoma Presenting as: A Case Report. M.L. Eisemann, 271.

Neck, Clinically Negative, Evolution of. E.M. Skolnik, A.H. Katz, S.P. Becker, R. Mantravadi, S. Stal, 551.

Neck Dissection, Conservative and Radical, Retrospective Comparison of in Laryngeal Cancer. R. Molinari, G. Cantu, F. Chiesa, C. Grandi, 578.

Neoglottic Reconstruction Following Total Laryngectomy. A Reappraisal. B. Leipzig, 534.

Neoglottic Reconstruction Following Total Laryngectomy: Galveston Experience. B. Leipzig, C.M. Griffiths, J.P. Shea, 204.

Neonate, Cricopharyngeus in. T.J. Reichert, K.D. Faw, 446.

Neonate, Infant and Child, Stridor in, Etiology of. L.D. Holinger, 397.

Neonates, Acquired Stenosis of the Upper Airway in. An Increasing Problem. M.J. Papsidero, N.R.T. Pashley, 512.

Neural Elements for Stimulation Through a Cochlear Prosthesis, Estimates of. B.M. Clopton. F.A. Spelman, J.M. Miller, 5. Animal Studies of a Cochlear Prosthesis. Suppl. No. 66.

Neurilemmomas, Intracanalicular: Clinicopathologic Study. V. Kasantikul, M.G. Netsky, M.E. Glasscock III, J.W. Hayes, 29.

Neurinoma, Acoustic, Comparison of Computer Tomography and Translabyrinthine Surgery in Assessment of. M. Tos, G. Glydensted, J. Thompsen, J. Lester, 117.

Neuroanatomical Correlates of Vestibular Function. R.R. Gacek, 2.

Neurochemistry of the Auditory System. R.J. Wenthold, Suppl. No. 74, 121.

Neurophysiological Correlates of Auditory Maturation. E. Javel, Suppl. No. 74, 103.

Newborn, Prolonged Orotracheal Intubation in. G.H. Conner, M.J. Bushey, M.J. Maisels, 459.

NINCDS Role of in Study of Otitis Media with Effusion. J.B. Ranney, Suppl. No. 69, 3.

Nitrous Oxide-Oxygen Ventilation, Middle Ear Gas Composition During. E. Ostfeld, M. Crispin, J. Blonder, A. Szeinberg, 165.

Nystagmus, Block. ENG of the Month. J.E. Olson, J.W. Wolfe, 286.

Nystagmus, Vestibular, Effects of Attention-Requiring Tasks on. P. Kileny, B.F. McCabe, J.H. Ryu, 9.

Obituary. Sven Ingelstedt, Suppl. No. 68, 1.

Oculomotor and Vestibular Abnormalities in Vertebrobasilar Insufficiency. J. Corvera, L.D. Benitez, G. Lopez-Rios, M.T. Rabiela, 370.

Orofacial Embryology, Anatomy and Physiology. D.P. Kuehn, Suppl. No. 74, 138.

Osteoradionecrosis, Septic, of the Mandible. Grand Rounds. S.S. Parulekar, D.F. Paonessa, 383.

Otic Capsule, Branch of the Singular Nerve in. Y. Okano, I. Sando, E.N. Myers, 13.

Otitis Media, Acute, Acoustic Immittance Findings in. D.M. Schwartz, R.H. Schwartz, Suppl. No. 68, 211.

Otitis Media, Acute, Active and Conservative Treatment of. Prospective Studies. Y. Qvarnberg, T. Palva, Suppl. No. 68, 269.

Otitis, Acute, and Penicillin: Short and Long-Term Results. J. Thompsen, K.I. Meistrup-Larsen, H. Sørensen, P.K. Larsen, N. Mygind, Suppl. No. 68, 271.

Otitis Media, Acute, Concentration of Penicillin V in Serum and Middle Ear Exudate During Treatment of. L. Ingvarsson, C. Kamme, K. Lundgren, Suppl. No. 68, 275.

Otitis Media and Inner Ear Pathology. A Review. M.M. Paparella, M.V. Goycoolea, W.L. Meyerhoff, Suppl. No. 68, 249.

Otitis Media and Otitis Media with Effusion, Report of the Ad Hoc Committee on Definition and Classification of. B.H. Senturia, C.D. Bluestone, J.O. Klein, D.J. Lim, J.L. Paradise, Suppl. No. 68, 3.

Otitis Media, Bacterial, Evaluation of Countercurrent Immunoelectrophoresis as a Diagnostic Tool in. E. Ostfeld, G. Altmann, Suppl. No. 68, 110.

Otitis Media, Chronic, and Cholesteatoma. G.O. Proud, Suppl. No. 74, 47.

Otitis Media, Chronic, Secretory, Pathogenesis and Pathology. M. Tos, Suppl. No. 68, 91.

Otitis Media, Complement and Cl_q Binding Substances in. K. Prellner, N-I. Nilsson, U. Johnson, A-B. Laurell, Suppl. No. 68, 129.

Otitis Media, Effects on Cognitive Development. F.D. Horowitz, H. Leak III, Suppl. No. 68, 264.

Otitis Media, Experimental, Following Middle Ear Inoculation of Nonviable *Streptococcus pneumoniae.* S.H. Lowell, S.K. Juhn, G.S. Giebink, 479.

Otitis Media, Experimental, in Chinchillas. D.M. Lewis, J.L. Schram. S.J. Meadema, D.L. Lim, Suppl. No. 68, 344.

Otitis Media in Children, Epidemiology of. D.W. Teele, J.O. Klein, B.A. Rosner, Suppl. No. 68, 5.

Otitis Media in the American Native, Natural History of. R.J. Wiet, G.B. DeBlanc, J. Stewart, D.J. Weider, Suppl. No. 68, 14.

Otitis Media in the Young Infant: An IgE-Mediated Disease? J.L. Sloyer, J.H. Ploussard, L.J. Karr, Suppl No. 68, 133.

Otitis Media, Microbiology of. J.O. Klein, Suppl. No. 68, 98.

Otitis Media, Nonpurulent, Auditory Tube and Middle Ear Mucosa in. G. Zechner, Suppl. No. 68, 87.

Otitis Media, Persistent, Effect on Language Development. P. Menyuk, Suppl. No. 68, 257.

Otitis Media, Pneumococcal, and Pneumococcal Vaccine; Efficacy of Animal Models for Studying. G.S. Giebink, I.K. Berzins, P.G. Quie, Suppl. No. 68, 339.

Otitis Media, Polymorphonuclear Leukocyte Function During. G.S. Giebink, I.K. Berzins, K.L. Cates, J.S. Huff, P.G. Quie, Suppl. No. 68, 138.

Otitis Media, Purulent, Study of Antibody Levels in Childen with. P. Branefors, T. Dahlberg, O. Nylén, Suppl. No. 68, 117.

Otitis Media, Recurrent, Efficacy of Pneumococcal Vaccination Against. Preliminary Results of Field Trail in Finland. P. Karma, J. Luotonen, M. Timonen, S. Pöntynen, J. Pukander, E. Herva, P. Grönroos, M. Leinonen, M. Sibakov, P.H. Mäkelä, Suppl. No. 68, 357.

Otitis Media, Recurrent, Efficacy of Adenoidectomy in. Historical Overview and Preliminary Results from Randomized, Controlled Trial. J.L. Paradise, C.D. Bluestone, K.D. Rogers, F.H. Taylor, Suppl. No. 68, 319.

Otitis Media Secondary to Ampicillin-Resistant Strains of Haemophilus Influenzae, Trimethoprim-Sulfamethoxazole in Treatment of. R. Schwartz, W.J. Rodriguez, W. Khan, R. Mann, R.G. Barsanti, S. Ross, Suppl. No. 68, 281.

Otitis Media, Secretory and Mastoid Pneumatization. B. Hussl, K. W. Mueller, Suppl. No. 68, 79.

Otitis Media, Secretory, Chronic; Adenoidectomy versus Tympanostomy in. G. Marshak, A.B. Neriah, Suppl. No. 68, 316.

Otitis Media, Secretory, Prevalence of, in Seven to Eight-Year-Old School Children. E. Virolainen, H. Puhakka, E. Aantaa, P. Tuohimaa, O. Ruuskanen, O.H. Meurman, Suppl. No. 68, 7.

Otitis Media, Serous, and Type 1 Tympanoplasties in Children. Retrospective Study. K.A. Buchwach, H.G. Birck, Suppl. No. 68, 324.

Otitis Media, Serous, Childhood, Diagnostic and Therapeutic Studies in. Results of Treatment with Antihistamine-Adrenergic Combination. J.S. O'Shea, D.J. Langenbrunner, D.E. McCloskey, J.C. Pezzullo, J.B. Regan, Suppl. No. 68, 285.

Otitis Media with Effusion, Anatomy, Cell Biology, and Pathology. Panel III, D.J. Lim et al., Suppl. No. 69, 13.

Otitis Media with Effusion, Antibiotic-Resistant Bacteria in. D.J. Lim, D.M. Lewis, J.L. Schram, H.G. Birck, Suppl. No. 68, 278.

Otitis Media with Effusion, Auditory Brainstem Responses in Children with. T.J. Fria, D.L. Sabo, Suppl. No. 68, 200.

Otitis Media with Effusion, Definition and Classification. Panel I-A. B.H. Senturia et al., Suppl. No. 69, 4.

Otitis Media with Effusion, Epidemiology and Natural History. Panel I-B. J.O. Klein, F.W. Henderson, M.D. Keller, R.R. Lanese, R.J. Wiet, Suppl. No. 69, 9.

Otitis Media with Effusion, Eustachian Tube and Middle Ear Physiology and Pathophysiology. Panel II. S. Ingelstedt et al., Suppl. No. 69, 11.

Otitis Media with Effusion, Histopathological Study of. T. Ishii, M. Toriyama, J-I. Suzuki, Suppl. No. 68, 83.

Otitis Media with Effusion, Implications of Mucosal Immune System. J.M. Bernstein, P.L. Ogra, Suppl. No. 68, 326.

Otitis Media with Effusion in Children, Identification of. E.I. Cantekin, C.D. Bluestone, T.J. Fria, S.E. Stool, Q.C. Beery, D.L. Sabo, Suppl. No. 68, 190.

Otitis Media with Effusion, Management. Panel VI. T. Palva et al., Suppl. No. 69, 23.

Otitis Media with Effusion, Microbiology, Immunology, Biochemistry and Vaccination. Panel IV. P.L. Ogra et al., Suppl. No. 69, 15.

Otitis Media with Effusion, Nonsurgical Management of. G.H. Gottschalk, Suppl. No. 68, 301.

Otitis Media with Effusion, Proceedings of the Second International Symposium on Recent Advances in. Suppl. No. 68.

Otitis Media with Effusion, Recent Advances in. Introduction. Proceedings of the Second International Symposium. C.D. Bluestone, D.J. Lim, W.H. Saunders, B.H. Senturia, Suppl. No. 68, 2.

Otitis Media with Effusion, Report of Research Conference on Recent Advances in. Suppl. No. 69.

Otitis Media with Effusion, Report of Research Conference on Recent Advances in. Introduction. D.J. Lim, Suppl. No. 69, 2.

Otitis Media with Effusion, Results after Treatment of. G. Muenker, Suppl. No. 68, 308.

Otitis Media with Effusion, Role of NINCDS in Study of. J.B. Ranney, Suppl. No. 69, 3.

Otitis Media with Effusion, Screening and Diagnosis. Panel V. C.D. Bluestone et al., Suppl. No. 69, 19.

Otitis Media with Effusion, Sequelae and Impact. Panel VII. R.J. Ruben et al., Suppl. No. 69, 27.

Otitis Media with Effusions, Antibody Coated Bacteria in. J.M. Bernstein, D. Myers, D. Kosinski, R. Nisengard, K. Wicher, Suppl. No. 68, 104.

Otitis Media with Mucoid Effusion, Adenoidectomy for. N. Roydhouse, Suppl. No. 68, 312.

Otoadmittance Middle Ear Analyzer, Automatic, Validation of. T.J. Fria, E.I. Cantekin, G. Probst, 253.

Otoconial Formation in the Fetal Rat. M.S. Salamat, M.E. Ross, D.R. Peacor, 229.

Otolaryngology and Medicine Today in the People's Republic of China. B.F. McCabe, 590.

Otolaryngology, Cranial Arteritis in. R.A. Sofferman, 215.

Otorhinolaryngology: Progress Report. First Louis H. Clerf Lecture. Jefferson Medical College. J.E. Bordley, 84.

Ototoxic and Normal Drug-Treated Gerbils: Single Cell Responses in. N.B. Gross, W.S. Lefschitz, 176.

Ototoxicity, Aminoglycoside, Following Middle Ear Injection. Suppl. No. 77.
- I. Experimental Approach and Histological Criteria for Evaluating Drug Effects. M.D. Rudnick, I.A. Ginsberg, P.S. Huber, 1.
- II. Quantitative Analytical Procedure. M.D. Rudnick, I.A. Ginsberg, P.S. Huber J.S. Rose, 10.
- III. Comparative Quantitative Analysis. I.A. Ginsberg, M.D. Rudnick, P.S. Huber, 17.
- IV. Influence of Vestibular Stimulation. P.S. Huber, I.A. Ginsberg, M.D. Rudnick, 25.

Pacemaker Artifact on ENG Tracing. W.R. Wilson, 591.

Palatine Tonsils, Papillary Hypertrophy of. T. Enomoto, T. Enomoto, K. Matsui, T. Tabata, 132.

Papilloma of Larynx and Tracheobronchial Tree in Children. Retrospective Study. S.R. Cohen, K.A. Geller, S. Seltzer, J.W. Thompson, 497

Papillomata, Laryngeal, and Condylomata, Relationship Between. Clinical and Molecular Virological Evidence. C.A. Quick, S.L. Watts, R.A. Krzyzek, A.J. Faras, 467.

Papillomatosis, Laryngeal, Juvenile, Double-Barreled (Diversionary) Tracheostomy in Management of. H.M. Tucker, 504.

Papillomatosis, Recurrent Respiratory, Topical Chemotherapy of. Preliminary Report. H.G. Smith, G.B. Healy, C.W. Vaughan, M.S. Strong, 472.

Paravestibular Canaliculus, Course and Contents of. I. Sando, T. Egami, T. Harada, 147.

Paravestibular Canaliculus, Endolymphatic Hydrops with Absence of Vein in. R. Gussen, 157.

Pathologic Changes in the Middle Ear, Frequency of. R. Rudin, J. Holmquist, Suppl. No. 68, 11.

Pathology Consultation. Mucoepidermoid and Acinous Cell Carcinomas of Salivary Tissues. J.G. Batsakis, 91.

Pediatric Literature, Recent, Relevant to Otolaryngology, Commentary on. P.A. Shurin, 93.

Pendred's Syndrome with Atypical Features. L. Bergstrom, 135.

Perceptual Evaluation of Velopharyngeal Competency. B.J. Philips, Suppl. No. 74, 153.

Perceptual Learning, Auditory, Time Course of. C.S. Watson, Suppl. No. 74, 96.

Perilymph Fistula, Recurrent, with Anacusis, Surgical Treatment of. C. Ulsφ, E. Hentzer, 121.

Peroxidase Activity in Tracheal Epithelium, Localization of. K. Watanabe, 241.

Pharyngeal Epithelial Cells, Human, in Vitro, Attachment of *Streptococcus pneumoniae* to. B. Andersson, O. Nylén, C-M. Peterson, C. Svanborg-Edén, Suppl. No. 68, 115.

Photography, Laryngeal, Through the Operating Microscope, Simple Method of, "Macrolens Technique." E. Yanagisawa, D.E. Eibling, M. Suzuki, 547

Physiologic Relationship of Lower and Upper Airways, Study with ^{133}Xe. E.B. Silberstein, J.T. Lewis, D.J. Quenelle, 62.

Pneumococcal Polysaccharide Vaccine, Immunologic Response in Infants. J.L. Sloyer, J.H. Ploussard, L.J. Karr, G.D. Schiffman, Suppl. No. 68, 351.

Pneumococcal Vaccination, Efficacy against Recurrent Otitis Media. Preliminary Results of Field Trial in Finland. P. Karma, J. Luotonen, M. Timonen, S. Pöntynen, J. Pukander, E. Herva, P. Grönroos, M. Leinonen, M. Sibakov, P.H. Mäkelä, Suppl. No. 68, 357.

Pneumococcal Vaccine and Otitis Media, Efficacy of Animal Models for Study. G.S. Giebink, I.K. Berzins, P.G. Quie, Suppl. No. 68, 339.

Pontine Angle Tumors, Electrocochleography and Auditory Brainstem Electric Responses in Patients with. J.J. Eggermont, M. Don, D.E. Brackmann, Suppl. No. 75.

Prednisone, Use of Short Course of for Treating Middle Ear Effusion. Double-Blind Crossover Study. R.H. Schwartz, J. Puglese, D.M. Schwartz, Suppl. No. 68, 296.

Prevention and Treatment of Stuttering. W.H. Perkins, Suppl. No. 74, 150.

Primate Model of Cleft Palate, Nonhuman, Its Implications for Middle Ear Pathology. W.J. Doyle, E.I. Cantekin, C.D. Bluestone, D.C. Phillips, K.K. Kimes, M.I. Siegel, Suppl. No. 68, 41.

Prostaglandin, Effect of on Composition of Chinchilla Middle Ear Effusion. T.T.K. Jung, D.M. Smith, S.K. Juhn, J.M. Gerrard, Suppl. No. 68, 153.

Prostheses, Cochlear Design of, Coding Considerations in. M.M. Merzenich, M. White, Suppl. No. 74, 84.

Prosthesis, Cochlear, Animal Studies of. B.M. Clopton, J.M. Miller, B.E. Pfingst, F.A. Spelman, D. Sutton, D.B. Webster, Suppl. No. 66.

Prosthesis, Cochlear Design of: Effects of the Flow Current in the Implanted Ear. F.A. Spelman, B.M. Clopton, B.E. Pfingst, J.M. Miller. Animal Studies of a Cochlear Prosthesis. Suppl. No. 66, 8.

Prosthesis, Cochlear, Estimates of Essential Neural Elements for Stimulation Through. B.M. Clopton, F.A. Spelman, J.M. Miller. Animal Studies of a Cochlear Prosthesis. Suppl. No. 66, 5.

Pseudodiverticulum, Vallecular, Management of. R.R. Gacek, 201.

Pulmonary Edema Following Relief of Acute Upper Airway Obstruction. A.G. Galvis, S.E. Stool, C.D. Bluestone, 124.

Receptor Reflexes, Pulmonary II. Laryngeal Regulation of Airway Resistance. T.V. McCaffrey, E.B. Kern, 462.

Reflex, Glottic Closure: Control Mechanisms. T. Ikari, C.T. Sasaki, 220.

Research Conference, Report of Recent Advances in Otitis Media with Effusion. Introduction. D.J. Lim, Suppl. No. 69, 2.

Retrocochlear Pathology, Brainstem Auditory Evoked Potentials for Detection of. S.E. Kinney, R.H. Nodar, 291.

Rhesus Monkey (Macaca mulatta) and Man, Comparison of the Anatomy of the Eustachian Tube: Implications for Physiologic Modeling. W.J. Doyle, S.R. Rood, 49.

Rhinorrhea, Cerebrospinal, Extracranial Surgical Repair of. T.C. Calcaterra, 108.

Salivary Glands, Clear Cell Tumors of. Pathology Consultation. J.G. Batsakis, 196.

Sarcoidosis, Laryngeal, with Airway Obstruction. R.A. Weisman, R.F. Canalis, W.J. Powell, 58.

Sarcoma, Ewing's, of the Mandible. P.M. Som, Y.P. Krespi, G. Hermann, J.M. Shugar, 20.

Scala Tympani, Comparison of Cochlear Histopathology Following Two Implant Designs for Use in. D. Sutton, J.M. Miller, B.E. Pfingst. Animal Studies of a Cochlear Prosthesis. Suppl. No. 66, 11.

Scala Tympani Implantation in Monkeys, Chronic Brainstem Histopathology Following. J.M. Miller, D. Sutton, D.B. Webster. Animal Studies of a Cochlear Prosthesis. Suppl. No. 66, 15.

Screening, Impedance. Integral Part of Hearing Screening. J.L. Northern, Suppl. No. 68, 233.

Screening, Impedance, for Children. Need for More Research. F.H. Bess, Suppl. No. 68, 228.

Screening Procedure for Detection of Middle Ear and Cochlear Disease. U. Renvall, G. Lidén, Suppl. No. 68, 214.

Screening Tympanometry in Infants and Two-Year-Old Children. M. Tos, G. Poulsen, Suppl. No. 68, 217.

Sensory Aids for the Hearing-Impaired, Advances in: Visual and Vibrotactile Aids. J.M. Pickett, Suppl. No. 74, 74.

Septal Perforations, Nasal, Asymptomatic, in Systemic Lupus Erythematosus. D. Reiter, A.R. Myers, 78.

Sickle Cell Anemia and Hearing. E.M. Friedman, G.R. Herer, N.L.C. Luban, I. Williams, 342.

Singular Nerve Branch (Posterior Ampullary Nerve) in Otic Capsule. Y. Okano, I. Sando, E.N. Myers, 13.

Sphenoid Sinus Lesion, Pituitary Adenoma Presenting as. X-Ray of the Month. J.M. Davis, A.L. Weber, 483.

Speech Discrimination, Poor, Tinnitus, Hearing Loss, and Recruitment: Combination of in Acute Cochlear Disorders. J. Tonndorf, 353.

Speech, Research Priorities in. R.J. Van Hattum, Suppl. No. 74, 161.

Stenosis, Acquired, of the Upper Airway in Neonates. An Increasing Problem. M.J. Papsidero, N.R.T. Pashley, 512.

Stenosis, Esophageal, in Children. Chevalier Jackson Lecture. F. Aprigliano, 391.

Stenosis, Laryngeal, Supraglottic, with Postcricoid Involvement, Repair of. Case Report. P.J. Doyle, 576.

Stenosis, Laryngotracheal, Long-Term Stenting for. D.E. Schuller, 515.

Streptococcus pneumoniae, Attachment of to Human Pharyngeal Epithelial Cells in Vitro. B. Andersson, O. Nylén, C-M. Peterson, C. Svanborg-Edén, Suppl. No. 68, 115.

Stridor, Etiology of, in Neonate, Infant and Child. L.D. Holinger, 397.

Stuttering, Prevention and Treatment of. W.H. Perkins, Suppl. No. 74, 150.

Suppression Test, Single-Dose: Nasal Secretory IgA Circadian Rhythm. P. Menzio, R. Molino, B. Morra, M. Bussi, A. Sartoris, G. Cortesina, 173.

Synthesized Speech, Discrimination of, Effect of Word Speed, Number of Words and Habituation. T. Rahko, M. Karjalainen, U. Laine, A. Lavonen, 69.

Tectorial Membrane, Attachment of, Revealed by Scanning Electron Microscope. M. Lawrence, P.A. Burgio, 325.

Temporal Bone Cholesteatoma, Bilateral, with an Associated Brain Abscess. X-Ray of the Month. A.F. O'Connor, 194.

Temporal Bone Removal, Extracranial Technique for. J.B. Nadol, Jr., 251.

Thyroid Disease: A Guide for the Head and Neck Surgeon. R.M. Bumsted, Suppl. No. 72.

Tinnitus, Fluctuating, Unusual but Treatable Cause of. J.D. Williams, 239.

Tinnitus, Hearing Loss, Recruitment, and Poor Speech Discrimination: Combination of in Acute Cochlear Disorders. J. Tonndorf, 353.

Tonsillectomy and Adenoidectomy, Role of in Management of Children with Middle Ear Effusion. J.B. Snow, Jr., Suppl. No. 74, 43.

Tonsils, Palatine, Papillary Hypertrophy of. T. Enomoto, T. Enomoto, K. Matsui, T. Tabata, 132.

Trachea, in Infants with Reflex Apnea, Innominate Artery Compression of. J.M. Ardito, R.H. Ossoff, G.F. Tucker, Jr., S.Y. DeLeon, 401.

Tracheal Cannula, Silicone. W.W. Montgomery, 521.

Tracheal Diverticulum, Congenital. Case Report. S. Frenkiel, I.K. Assimes, J.K. Rosales, 406.

Tracheal Epithelium, Localization of Peroxidase Activity in. K. Watanabe, 241.

Tracheal Stenosis, Emergency Management of: Retrograde Tracheal Bougienage. I. Eliachar, K. Simon, J.H. Birkhan, H.Z. Joachims, 46.

Tracheal T-Tube, Silicone, Montgomery, Manual for Care of. W.W. Montgomery, Suppl. No. 73.

Tracheobronchial Tree and Larynx, Foreign Bodies in Children. Review of 225 Cases. B.F. Rothmann, C.R. Boeckman, 434.

Tracheobronchial Tree and Larynx, Papilloma of, in Children. Retrospective Study. S.R. Cohen, K.A. Geller, S. Seltzer, J.W. Thompson, 497.

Tracheotomy, Anterior Cricoid Split as an Alternative to. Management of Extubation Problem in Premature Child. R.T. Cotton, A.B. Seid, 508.

Tracheostomy (Diversionary), Double-Barreled, in Management of Juvenile Laryngeal Papillomatosis. H.M. Tucker, 504.

Translabyrinthine Surgery in Assessment of Acoustic Neurinoma, Comparison of Computer Tomography and. M. Tos, G. Glydensted, J. Thomsen, J. Lester, 117.

Trimethoprim-Sulfamethoxazole in Treatment of Otitis Media Secondary to Ampicillin-Resistant Strains of *Haemophilus influenzae*. R. Schwartz, W.J. Rodriguez, W. Khan, R. Mann, R.G. Barsanti, S. Ross, Suppl. No. 68, 281.

Tympanic Membrane in Children, Intact, Intramembranous and Mesotympanic Cholesteatomas Associated with. S.M. Sobol, T.J. Reichert, K.D. Faw, M.H. Stroud, G.J. Spector, J.H. Ogura, 312.

Tympanic Membrane, Retraction of and Eustachian Tube Function. J. Holmquist, U. Renvall, P. Svendsen, Suppl. No. 68, 65.

Tympanometry in Three-Year-Old Children. Prevalence and Spontaneous Course of MEE. M. Fiellau-Nikolajsen, Suppl. No. 68, 223.

Tympanometry Screening in Infants and Two-Year-Old Children. M. Tos, G. Poulsen, Suppl. No. 68, 217.

Tympanosclerosis. A Theory of Pathogenesis. M. Schiff, J.F. Poliquin, A. Catanzaro, A.F. Ryan, Suppl. No. 70.

Tympanosclerosis. Electron Microscopic Study of Matrix Vesicles. I. Friedmann, G.M. Hodges, M. Graham, Suppl. No. 68, 241.

Tympanoplasties, Type 1, and Serous Otitis Media in Children. Retrospective Study. K.A. Buchwach, H.G. Birck, Suppl. No. 68, 324.

Tympanostomy versus Adenoidectomy in Chronic Secretory Otitis Media. G. Marshak, Z.B. Neriah, Suppl.No. 68, 316.

Ulcerations, Esophageal, Upper, Complication in Rheumatoid Cricoarytenoid Arthritis. W.W. Montgomery, M.L. Goodman, 6.

Vallecular Pseudodiverticulum, Management of. R.R. Gacek, 201.

Vasculitis, Systemic, Obliterative Fibrotic Middle Ear Disease in. J.H. Hill, M.D. Graham, P.W. Gikas, 162.

Velopharyngeal Competency, Perceptual Evaluation of. B.J. Philips, Suppl. No. 74, 153.

Ventilating Tubes, Insertion into Middle Ear: Results and Complications. Seven-Year Review. W. Draf, P. Schulz, Suppl. No. 68, 303.

Ventricle, Laryngeal: Historical Features. R.F. Canalis, 184.

Vertebrobasilar Insufficiency, Vestibular and Oculomotor Abnormalities in. J. Corvera, L.D. Benitez, G. Lopez-Rios, M.T. Rabiela, 370.

Vertigo, Critical Evaluation of Relief of. Labyrinthectomy versus Middle Fossa Vestibular Nerve Section in Menière's Disease. M.E. Glasscock III, G.B. Hughes, W.E. Davis, C.G. Jackson, 318.

Vestibular Adaptation, Second-Order, and Cupular Dynamics. R.W. Babin, J.H. Ryu, B.F. McCabe, 262.

Vestibular and Oculomotor Abnormalities in Vertebrobasilar Insufficiency. J. Corvera, L.D. Benitez, G. Lopez-Rios, M.T. Rabiela, 370.

Vestibular Function, Neuroanatomical Correlates of. R.R. Gacek, 2.

Vestibular Nerve Section, Middle Fossa versus Labyrinthectomy in Menière's Disease. Critical Evaluation of Relief of Vertigo. M.E. Glasscock III, G.B. Hughes, W.E. Davis, C.G. Jackson, 318.

Vestibular Nystagmus, Effects of Attention-Requiring Tasks on. P. Kileny, B.F. McCabe, J.H. Ryu, 9.

Vestibular Stimulation, Influence of. Aminoglycoside Ototoxicity Following Middle Ear Injection. IV. P.S. Huber, I.A. Ginsberg, M.D. Rudnick, Suppl. No. 77, 25.

Vestibular Testing in Children. D.G. Cyr, Suppl. No. 74, 63.

Vibrotactile and Visual Aids: Advances in Sensory Aids for the Hearing-Impaired. J.M. Pickett, Suppl. No. 74, 74.

Vocal Cord Positioning by Selective Denervation. Old Territory Revisited. C.T. Sasaki, M. Horiuchi, T. Ikari, J.A. Kirchner, 541.

Voice Restoration After Laryngectomy, Endoscopic Technique for. M.I. Singer, E.D. Blom, 529.

Word Speed, Number of Works and Habituation Effect on the Discrimination Score of Synthesized Speech. T. Rahko, M. Karjalainen, U. Laine, A. Lavonen, 69.

Xanthogranuloma, Juvenile, Intraoral and Cutaneous. R.H. Ossoff, D.L. Levin, N.B. Esterly, G.F. Tucker, 268.

X-Ray of the Month. Intracranial Chordoma. R.A. Greenes, A.L. Weber, 100.

X-Ray of the Month. Pituitary Adenoma Presenting as Sphenoid Sinus Lesion. J.M. Davis, A.L. Weber, 483.

TYMPANOSCLEROSIS

A THEORY OF PATHOGENESIS

Maurice Schiff, MD
Jacques F. Poliquin, MD
Antonio Catanzaro, MD
Allen F. Ryan, PhD

Supplement 70 — Vol. 89, July-August, 1980, No. 4, Part 2
THE ANNALS OF OTOLOGY, RHINOLOGY & LARYNGOLOGY

Presented at the meeting of the American Otological Society, Inc., Palm Beach, Florida, April 13-14, 1980.

The authors wish to express their appreciation to the Trustees of the Research Fund of the American Otological Society, Inc., for grant support and to the Duaei Ear Foundation for its supplemental financial support.

THE ANNALS PUBLISHING COMPANY
4949 FOREST PARK BLVD.
ST. LOUIS, MISSOURI 63108

TYMPANOSCLEROSIS
A THEORY OF PATHOGENESIS

MAURICE SCHIFF, MD
SAN DIEGO, CALIFORNIA
ANTONIO CATANZARO, MD
SAN DIEGO, CALIFORNIA
JACQUES F. POLIQUIN, MD
SHERBROOKE, QUEBEC, CANADA
ALLEN F. RYAN, PhD
SAN DIEGO, CALIFORNIA

Tympanosclerosis is a disease which affects the tympanic membrane (TM) and middle ear. The locus for the essential pathology is in the connective tissue component of the drum which is the lamina propria. In the middle ear, the pathology is in the basement membrane. In the early stages there is a minimal involvement of the mesenchymal component, usually seen as a small white macula, or scar, in the drum. In advanced disease, the hyalinization of the mesenchymal component together with the attraction of the calcium ion leads to a thick, dense, calcified scar.

The theory of pathogenesis for this disease entity is that the connective tissue component of these structures is stimulated by infection, inflammation, or trauma involving some degree of local immunological hypersensitivity. With severe middle ear infection, the mucosa of the inner surface of the drum becomes permeable, and the ground substance of the lamina propria becomes edematous taking up water together with components of complement from the middle ear disease. The abnormal middle ear secretions contain the immunoglobulin components capable of participating in the process. If there is any damage to the connective tissue, the adsorption and repair permits the body to react immunologically against the destroyed tissue, thereby sensitizing this area.

Experiments were performed with the guinea pig in which the tympanic membrane was removed and the lamina propria isolated and prepared as an immunological antigen. When this material was injected into the rabbits, a high, satisfactory antiguinea pig tympanic membrane antibody was formed (anti-GPTM). It was then possible to remove this anti-GPTM antibody from the serum. The tissue specificity was determined by immunofluorescent staining which showed it to be adsorbed onto the TM, middle ear mucosa, as well as the basement membrane of the respiratory tract. The guinea pigs which were passively sensitized with anti-GPTM antiserum demonstrated the binding of the antibodies on the tympanic membrane when subject to trauma, infection, or cautery. The manifestation was in the anatomical area related to the injury. Complement fixation was, likewise, demonstrated.

Controlled animals which were not traumatized, or were not passively sensitized, included those which were injected with IgG from rabbits not sensitized against GPTM. They showed no fixation of antibody or complement in the TM. Following injury the antibody and complement bound to the TM provide the necessary elements for the subsequent immunopathologic disease entity known at tympanosclerosis.

A tympanosclerosis model in animals has been the result of our research. The fact that tympanosclerosis can be produced experimentally would lead one to conclude that it is a disease entity in its own right. However, due to the fact that it must have an infection or inflammation of the middle ear, or tympanic membrane (TM), preceding this development would strongly indicate that this is not a disease in its own right but is an abnormality of tissue reaction brought about by an immunologic alteration in the local tissue response. In the case of tympanosclerosis, the Koch postulates do not apply.

LITERATURE REVIEW

This abnormality of tissue response, tympanosclerosis, has been observed for many centuries. Quoting from Gibb,[1] the earliest description of a condition which we now recognize as tympanosclerosis was first discussed by Cassebohm[2] in 1734. This essentially involved the discussion of the calcareous deposits in the TM. It was not until more than a century later that a more extensive discussion regarding this problem, particularly as it extends into the middle ear cavity, was described by von Tröltsch[3] in 1869. He described this change and noted the decrease in resilience of the drum and middle ear mucosa and applied to it the term "sclerosis." Politzer,[4] who had done a considerable amount of scholarly work in the problems of the ear, turned his attention to this abnormality of repair in 1883 and gave a more ample description of this problem. Within the next decade, Habermann[5] in 1892, and Walb[6] in 1893, further discussed the problems of this interesting type of sclerosis.

For the first half of the 20th century very little additional information, clarification, or interpretation of this process appeared in the literature. The advent and application of the operating microscope changed not only the technical aspects and improvement of surgery, but once again produced an impetus to the study and management of various pathologic problems, since something now could be done about them. In 1956, Zöller[7] gave his paper on tympanosclerosis and introduced this term into common usage. He was able to clarify some of the

From the Department of Surgery and Otolaryngology, and the Department of Internal Medicine, University of California, San Diego, California, and the Department d'oto-rhino-laryngologie, Centre Hospitalier Universitaire, Universite de Sherbrooke, Sherbrooke, Quebec, Canada.

histologic differences between tympanosclerosis and otosclerosis, demonstrating a bone involvement in the latter and the lamina propria involvement in the former. The fact that surgical treatment could improve the management of middle ear disease prompted Goodhill[8] to discuss some of the problems concerning otosclerosis and other conditions which fixed the footplate and called this pseudo-otosclerosis. House and Sheehy[9] discussed some of the improved surgical treatments in tympanosclerosis in 1960 and then elaborated in a larger case series in 1962[10] with further insights, particularly as related to the ability to use tympanoplastic grafting techniques. In 1961, Harris[11] was able to amplify the characteristics of tympanosclerosis and began to stimulate the quest for answers to the finer questions as to whether or not this process could be invasive or not. Supporting the concept of bony destruction, Zaritskii et al[12] in 1969 noted the necrobiotic changes with the resorption and formation of cavities in the bone. In 1968, Sluchanko[13] pointed out the differences between adhesions which occurred in the middle ear and the processes associated with tympanosclerosis.

Up to this time, the discussion of pathogenesis was limited to those of reemphasis of the cellular reaction to chronic inflammation and the increase in fibrous and hyaline tissue changes. There is uniform agreement, almost totally, that middle ear infections must precede the development of this process.

With the advent of the 1970s, the increased awareness of the immunologic influence and disease formation finds Musta and Chisiu[14] suggesting that the immunocompetence of cellular response was involved in this process. An excellent discussion of this subject matter was presented by Gibb.[1] Not only was this presentation very comprehensive, but his observations are of such significance as to provoke and stimulate an attempt to answer some of the clinical questions within the concept of our theory of pathogenesis. It is unfortunate that the title of the work of Kinney[15] in 1978, took it out of the mainstream of study on tympanosclerosis, since it related to inflammatory ossicular fixation. This work is one of the most comprehensive and largest series to date, containing within it several excellent clinical observations with statistics to confirm his viewpoint.

Working in the Connective Tissue Research Laboratory at the Univeristy of Copenhagen in 1963, one of the authors, MS, has made definitive note of similarities between tympanosclerosis and connective tissue diseases of immunologic origin. At that time, the immunologic, manipulative technology had not developed to its present refinement, and the technology for detection and isolation of sensitive elements at a cellular level had not been well evolved. Within the next decade enormous strides were made in these two areas, permitting the resumption of the quest for a theory of pathogenesis for tympanosclerosis based on immunologic induction and manipulation.

HISTOGENESIS AND THEORIES OF ORIGIN

The histogenesis of tympanosclerosis morphologically is fairly well described and agreed upon by most clinicians. There is invariably a history of previous episodes of otitis media followed by one or more subsequent occurrences which apparently provoke the local tissue response. These are characterized by an increase in the activity of the fibrous layer of the drum with a considerable decrease in the elasticity and/or compliance of the TM. This occurs in the lamina propria or lamina fibrosa. There is a characteristic increase in the amount of collagen laid down together with a subsequent hyaline degeneration in the fibrous stromal layer. This can occur in all the surfaces of the middle ear whether it be on the drum, or ossicles, or on the promontory.

In Sade's[16] excellent study of the nature and development of the mucous glands and cilia in the presence of otitis media, one sees this contrast to the morphologic changes which occur in tympanosclerosis. Tos and Bak-Pederson[17] in a very detailed study actually were able to demonstrate that the amount of secretion not only decreases per square millimeter area, but also that the number of glands decreases progressively with the severity of tympanosclerosis. This appears in the vast majority of cases. Such findings also help explain the clinical observation that only a few ears with tympanosclerosis alone have much drainage.

The open and closed category of this disease refers to the evidence of a perforation or simply involvement in the intact TM as seen visually with no major involvement of the middle ear. This becomes clinically important because the compliance and impedance of the drum can now be measured so accurately with tympanometry that many early cases, particularly the closed type, are detected simply by a flattened impedance curve which correlates histologically with the alterations within the fibrous layer of the drum.

As the disease process progresses and ages, the mass generally tends to attract calcium ions in which a distinct deposit is present in a large number of cases. Gibb[1] commented that even occasional ectopic areas of bone were encountered, but he noted that it had with it an unusual fibrous woven architecture. The two characteristic appearances of the tympanosclerotic mass are those of lamellar layers and those which are firm masses. This probably relates to the manner of lying down this abnormal connective tissue, either by constant stimulation or by repeated lamellar growths. Often the advent of calcium into the mass alters the texture so that lamellar arrangements are discouraged, and firm dense adherent masses are formed. Such findings are confirmed in the scanning electron microscopy and x-ray analyses noted by Lim.* He observed that the plaque of tympanosclerosis does contain very high levels of calcium and that two types of histology appear, one diffuse and the other sporadic, and all the specimens examined appear to be related to a history of otitis media.

It is agreed that tympanosclerosis is preceded by infections of otitis media. The question arises as to the capability of the infections to stimulate fibroblastic activity in general, or a tympanosclerotic response in particular. Plester[18] found only 10% incidence of tympanosclerosis in his large series of 3,000 otologic cases. He noted that in those cases that he operated, "90% had perforations of the eardrum, and the majority of the patients' ears were not infected at the time of surgery and had been free of inflammation for years." From his observations one would appear to conclude that only a minority (10%) of ear infections develop tympanosclerosis.

What is the mechanism involved in this process? If infection alone were the cause, why is not the incidence rate higher? Kinney[15] studied 1,495 chronic ear surgeries with a total of 311 who had tympanosclerosis. This is roughly a 20% incidence rate. Of the group that had this problem, 78% had a history of over ten years' duration. What is of significance, age wise, is that nearly 80% occurred in patients over the age of 30. This would suggest that the incidence among children may be high, but since it takes so long to bring about eventual damage, tympanoclerosis is not frequently seen in the younger age group. The incidence of cholesteatoma, preoperatively, was less than 10%. The presence of a wet ear in tympanosclerosis strongly suggested the presence of cholesteatoma. This indeed proved to be true in his series, showing that 20% were noted to have cholesteatoma, and over half of them had wet ears when first seen.

There were many who concluded that exudative otitis media was a prerequisite to tympanosclerosis. In these cases, they felt a hypervirulent bacteria or virus was the cause. Some concluded that the glue ear from the action of staphylococci and pneumococci during prolonged treatment with antibiotics could bring about this change. Others believed that the lack of the function of the eustachian tube together with a "tubotympanic catarrh" was a cause. Hybasek[19] thought that inflammation activated by a virus as the active "noxa or agent," was the cause implemented "by enzymes and later by antigenic action," which provoked irritation of tissues. His description was predicated on the role of infection and a catarrhal type of otitis media. He felt firmly that cholesterol-type granuloma was necessary to bring about the final stage which was tympanosclerosis. This is not in keeping with the findings of most of the otological community.

Gibb[1] felt quite rightly that tympanosclerosis develops in narrow, or cul-de-sac areas such as the round window, where exudate remains for a long while. In addition to that, these areas do not have ciliary function to eliminate secretions. He theorized that the mucosa would have to be necrotized so that a subsequent mucosa could be laid down and thereby account for the marked thickening of the submucosal connective tissue. There is some support to his observations, particularly in that he has observed the oval window, attic and stapedius tendon to be areas involving a high incidence rate of tympanosclerosis in his series of 138 cases.

Ferlito[20] likewise thought that tympanosclerosis required the presence of the organization of the inflamed tissue. The description given for this type of organization would predicate that granulation tissue was a sine qua non for the development of the collagen and the surrounding exudate. This is not true for many cases which have no granuloma formation in its process. Likewise implicated was the presence of effusion as the first stage of tympanosclerosis. He also felt that stagnant exudate was the "ground for future organization and sclerosis." Schuknecht[21] also noted the development of hyalinized collagen, particularly around the ossicular chain.

In general, the concepts and theories of the origin of tympanosclerosis fall into the following categories: A) infection followed by necrosis and granulation tissue; b) ischemic changes; c) stasis of infected material.

THEORY OF PATHOGENESIS

Our theory of pathogenesis proposes that tympanosclerosis has an immune component which occurs in the TM following an insult or mucosal disruption. The trauma may be mild, such as a myringotomy incision, with or without tubes, which on occasion will show a small chalky patch under the microscope. The other more common traumata to the TM are either by infection, physical trauma, or treatment with cauterizing agents. Sitting beneath all of these stimuli is a possible genetic component which might be involved. This would explain the relative infrequency of tympanosclerosis in the general large population of people, particularly children with otitis media.

Whatever the trauma is, it must be sufficient in nature to be able to create some edema of the epithelium, thereby permitting insult to approach the lamina propria. The most common severe type of tympanosclerosis is the open type, or those with perforations. The closed type has no perforation.

*Lim DJ. Personal communication.

Since tympanosclerosis never occurs on the first insult, it therefore strongly suggests that the following scenario takes place in preparing the local tissue injury to respond in an abnormal manner the next time a similar response is elicited. One of the first things that occurs in the process of injury, regardless of the source, is a reorientation of water. The edema that follows may be microscopic, but if it involves trauma that reaches the connective tissue layer, then the ground substance, which has a strong proclivity for water imbibition, becomes activated. As mucosa becomes inflamed, microscopically the space between the desmosomes becomes greater, and the surface area is now permeable in contrast to the marked and distinct integrity of a normal, untraumatized mucosa. Infection would include inflammation, which is a lower level of activity and can be incorporated into the concept of infection with the exception of the advent of an infecting organism. The same type of tissue changes take place. Following edema is the congestion in the capillary bed and the back pressure leading to release of fluid and cellular components. Whereas the lamina propria is relatively avascular, it contains mucopolysaccharide components such as hyaluronic acid which has a marked proclivity for water imbibition. If the nearby capillaries are leaking fluid, this is very easy to enter and penetrate into the lamina propria. If there is enough fluid present at a microscopic level, the fibrillar components can be stretched and broken asunder.

Studies with special dyes which favor the mucopolysaccharide component in light microscopy demonstrate this increased fluid uptake. Dyes like toluidine blue will show the large increment of blue staining material, which is water loaded under these conditions. With the advent of cellular components, particularly polymorphonuclear leukocytes' response, the autolytic enzymes are now available for the destruction of some of the components of the lamina propria. You now have some of the broken protein and aminoglycans' components which have the capacity to act as a local antigenic stimulation. The reparative process proceeds, the water is once more reabsorbed and taken back into circulation, leaving what amounts to a local concentration of the breakdown product of the lamina propria. This can now be likened unto the stage of preparation of the experimental antigen for this disease entity.

Most of these changes can, theoretically, take place without actual ulceration and physical disruption of the mucosa. However, in many streptococcal infections such as scarlatina, ulceration or even necrosis of the entire drum actually takes place. This leaves a large local deposit of degenerated elements in the TM and probably explains why scarlatina perforations are so often a source for tympanosclerotic development.

The tissue insult lasts for a long period of time. There is a progressive infiltration of monocytes, lymphocytes and plasma cells which now have with them the capacity of making the local tissue immunoglobulin components and initiating the reaction. This is very well demonstrated, even at an electron microscope level, by Lim,[22] in his excellent review. Since many investigators contend that both serous and suppurative otitis media are part of the initiating causes for tympanosclerosis, it is necessary to look back at the early stage of development for a better clarification of the induction of tissue sensitivity. In Lim's[22] summary, he pointed out that the usual concept of allergy as being a cause for the middle ear effusion would have to be mediated by the IgE mechanism. This would call into action the mast cells and basophils, since this immunoglobulin reacts specifically with them. Veltri and Sprinkle[23] have postulated that the immune complex involves the complement response, which indeed seems reasonable, particularly since the polymorphonuclear (PMN) leukocytes are mobilized and active in the process. Such a response indicates that the humoral component is active, and tissue sensitivity is not a part of this response.

Cell-mediated immunity, or delayed hypersensitivity, as suggested by Bernstein and Reisman[25] was the result of mucosal injury with a delayed tissue sensitivity. This was partly based on the fact that the macrophages and lymphocytes, mostly of the T-cell type, were the predominant cells found in the effusion.

From our point of view, it seems most reasonable that both of the processes occur, but there is a difference in their time sequence. The polymorphonuclear reaction is most probable in the acute phase of almost any respiratory infection, and the macrophage plasma cell and lymphocyte are the cells for chronic, or delayed, sensitivity change. The fact that these can be demonstrated in mucosal biopsies is encouraging. The cell most commonly seen with tympanosclerosis is that of chronic infection, ie, macrophage and lymphocyte. Once this local cell population is present simultaneously with the necrotized, or destroyed, or altered lamina propria, the machinery for producing local tissue antibodies is now in motion.

As far as the fibroblast is concerned, it has not been determined whether or not the tissue immune response stimulates the fibroblast to produce more collagen in the already activated ground substance; or does the immune response block the regulator that controls the fibroblast overactivity? This mechanism seems to be more logical, since it would take a long period of time before the dampering mechanism gets a new regulator to tell the fibroblast to stop working (Fig. 1). In contrast, the direct stimulation should stop when the infection is controlled, and the stimulation ceases.

Figure 2 shows a schematic diagram of our induc-

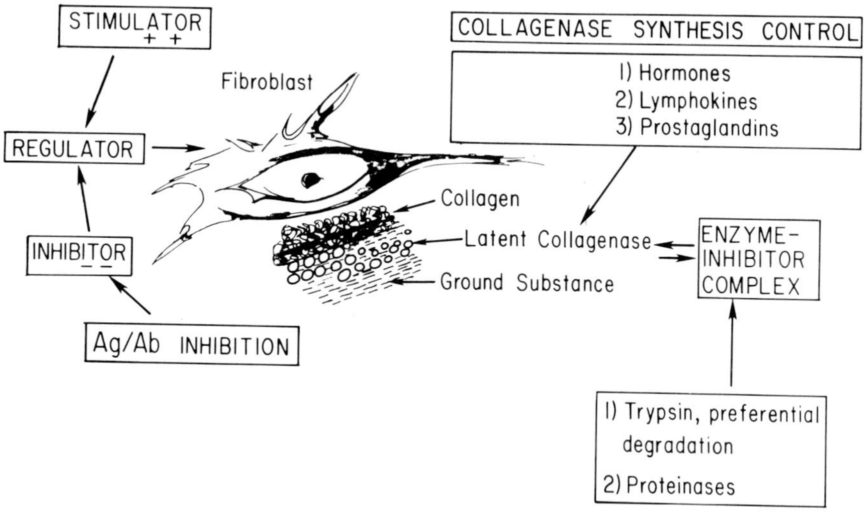

Fig. 1. Diagram of proposed controls in collagen formation from the fibroblast.

tion and development of tympanosclerosis in the guinea pig. Poliquin et al[25] reported the development in detail of our antigenic model against the guinea pig's TM. An antiserum against the connective tissue elements of the guinea pig's TM was raised in rabbits. After absorption against powdered and fresh guinea pig tissues to eliminate nonspecific reactivity, this antiserum was then injected into another guinea pig. After one hour, one drum of the injected animal was subjected to traumatic perforation, bacterial infection, or chemical cauterization. After survival times of 1, 7 or 21 days, antibody deposition in the connective tissue layer of the traumatized drums was demonstrated by immunofluorescence staining. In the myringotomized drums, deposition occurred in a "halo" around the site of the perforation, diminishing in intensity with distance from the myringotomy. Complement was also demonstrated by immunocytochemistry. In the untreated, opposite ears of these animals, no antibody deposition occurred. When normal rabbit serum was substituted for antiguinea pig TM antiserum, no deposition in the membrane was seen after the above types of trauma.

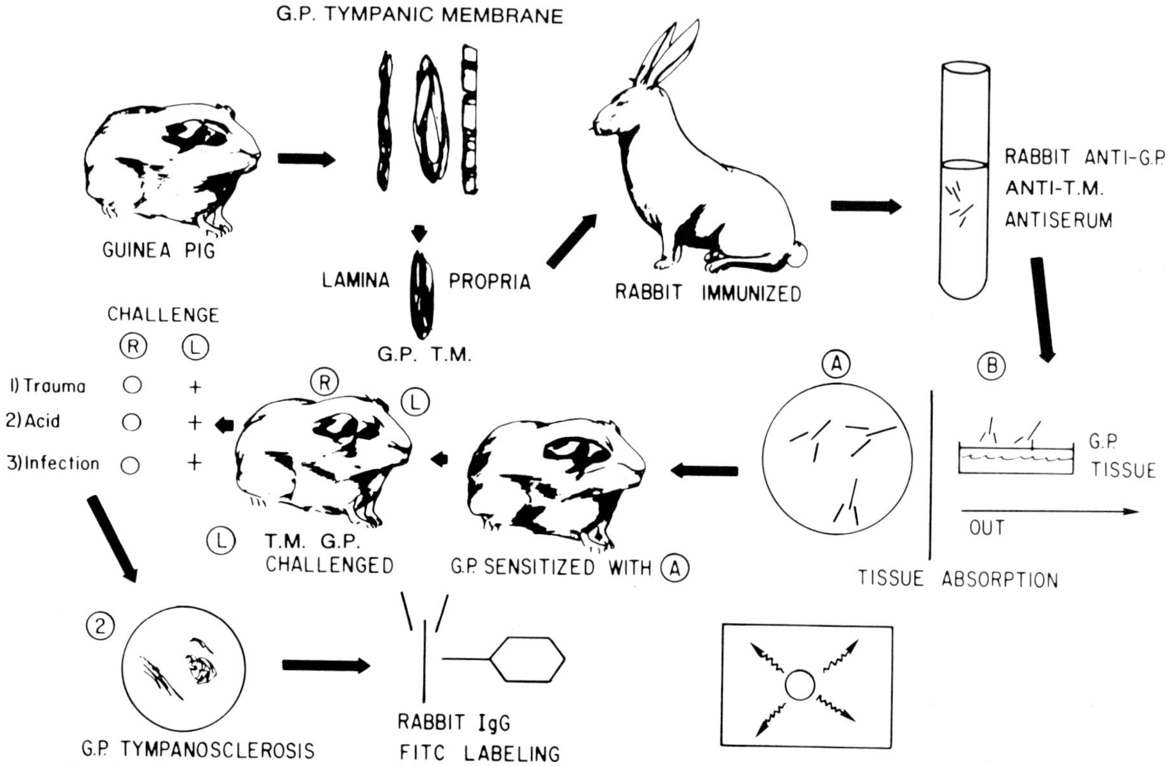

Fig. 2. Schematic of the animal model for the induction and development of experimental tympanosclerosis.

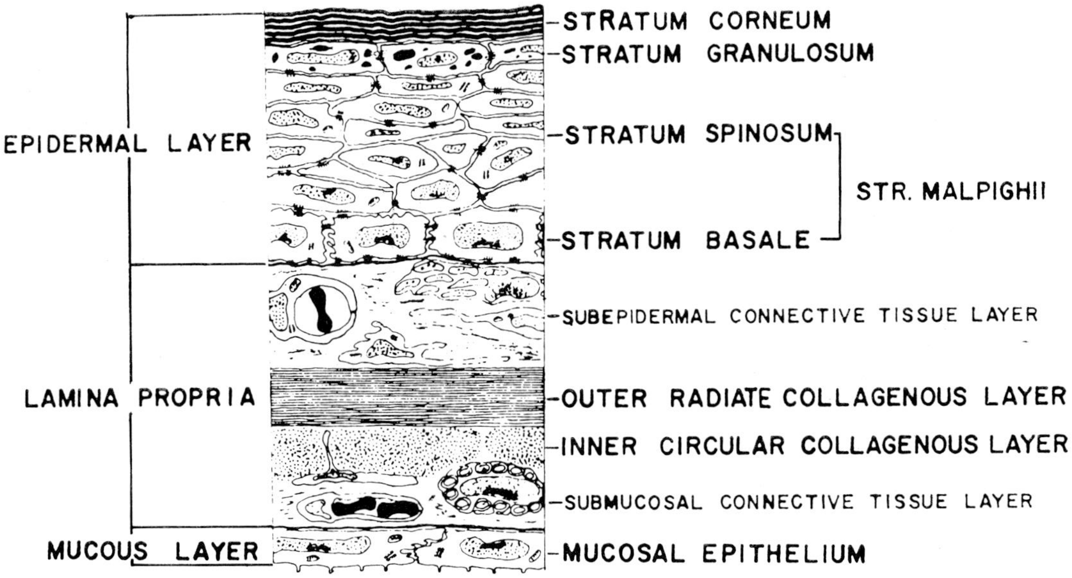

Fig. 3. Cross-sectional view of the tympanic membrane (pars tensa) of the squirrel monkey, schematically represented. Each layer is labeled in drawing. (From Lim.[26] Reprinted with permission.)

In a chronic experiment,* longer survival times were examined in the model described above, utilizing only myringotomy. At three months and six months post-trauma, whitish plaques were observed on the TM at the site of myringotomy. Control subjects, injected with normal rabbit serum rather than antitympanic membrane antiserum, showed little or no plaque formation. The histological appearance of the plaques is described in the following section of this paper.

If antigen becomes bound to the drum, or if the patient develops autoantibodies against the drum, the local tympanic tissue can be sensitized to the development of tympanosclerosis, as demonstrated experimentally. Then, when the second and third time the infection occurs, the pathologic process becomes manifest since this tissue, which has been previously primed, is now challenged.

MICROSCOPY

Light Microscopy. In Figure 3 Lim[26] reconstructed an adaptation from electron microscopy to clarify the structures for light microscopy.

For comparison purposes, examination of Figure 4 shows the normal area of a guinea pig's TM at 400 times magnification. The epithelium and mucosa can be seen as very thin layers in the fiber bundles shown in the dark cross sections. The submucosal and subepithelial areas are difficult to see and appear to be very thin. No separation of the fiber bundles is noted.

The cellular components in Figure 5 or the challenged tympanic area show the marked thickening of the total lamina propria to eight to ten times the thickness of the normal drum. The epithelium on both surfaces is not dramatically changed. However, in the lamina propria the fiber bundles are slightly separated by the activity of the loose connective tissue. The subepithelial and submucosal loose connective tissue is dramatically thickened with calcium lamellae seen in the subepithelial area. It is interesting to note the difference in response between the organized connective tissue, in the fibrous portion of the lamina propria, and the loose connective tissue in the subepithelial layers. All of the hyperplasia which occurred in this material was located in the loose connective tissue layers. This may reflect the mature, cross-linked nature of the collagen in the fibrous portion of the lamina propria versus the less mature collagen in the loose connective tissue.

The extension of this into the electron microscope

*Ryan A, Schiff M, Catanzaro A. An animal model of tympanosclerosis. In preparation.

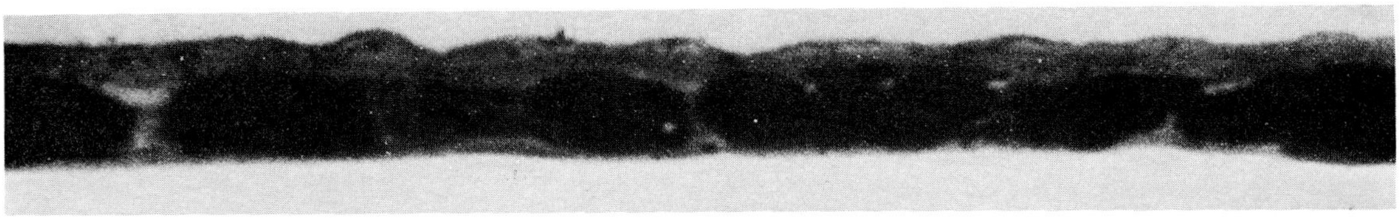

Fig. 4. Light micrograph of the normal tympanic membrane. The discrete bundles of the fibrous layer of the lamina propria are sandwiched between the thin mucosal epithelium and the thicker epidermal epithelium. The loose subepithelial connective tissue contributes minimally to the thickness of the drum. (x400)

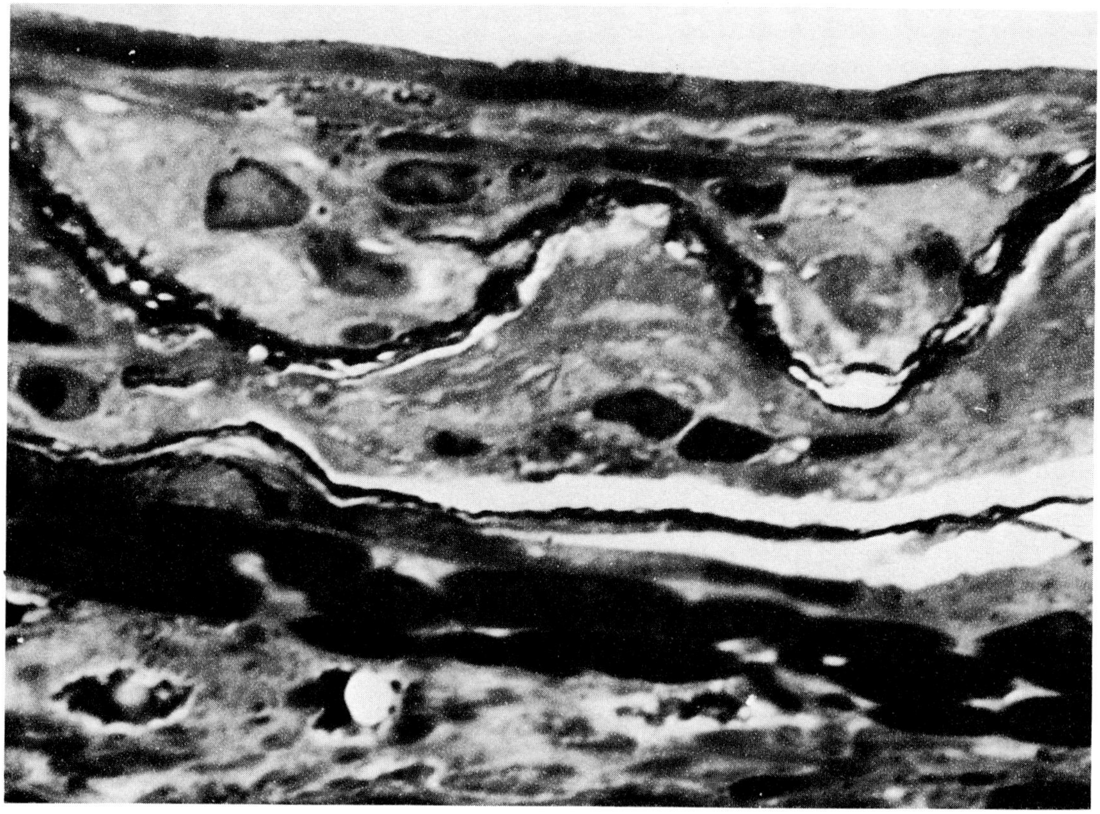

Fig. 5. Light micrograph of guinea pig tympanosclerosis. The fibrous layer of the lamina propria and both the mucosal and epidermal epithelia are largely unchanged. However, both subepithelial connective tissue layers are greatly expanded. Dark bands of calcification run through the subepidermal connective tissue layer. (x400)

shows almost the exact same expansion of these lamina propria components. The proximity of this experimental model to that of the human at an electron microscopic level is, indeed, impressive and is in strong support for the developmental nature of this pathologic process.

Electron Microscopy (EM). The normal EM area of the TM seen in Figure 6 shows that its entire thickness is not very great. Very limited activity in the lamina propria beneath the epithelium and the mucosa is noted. No increase in collagen and no calcification is seen.

In contrast to that is Figure 7 which shows the increased development of the loose connective tissue component with a deposit of lamellar-like lines of calcifying tissue. Normal mitochondria (NM) are seen, and calcifying mitochondria (CM) show precipitation of calcium within them, thus inactivating these organelles for functional purposes. These are very much like the electron microscope studies conducted on human tympanosclerosis. Both the studies of Chang[27] and Sorensen and True[28] show these similar changes in humans in both the cellular and fibrous components, and the amorphous ground substance. The fibroblasts, which have been stimulated during the laying down of new connective tissue, now seem to be irregular cells, more flattened and oval in appearance. Electron-dense autophaged lysosomes were demonstrated which apparently have attracted calcium to them, together with the mitochondria, which were markedly increased in density, some of which have opaque masses of calcium deposits within them. The guinea pig does not have collagen in the same manner as the human TM. The electron microscope studies of both groups of investigators found that the human collagen fibers appeared to be randomly placed and woven in various directions, and they also noted that some of the fibers did not have the characteristic 640 A band. Chang[27] extended his study to an x-ray spectrogram of the calcified material and showed it to be most probably a calcium apatite. One of the interesting observations made with the x-ray defraction technique that he used, showed the intracellular electron-dense material contained more calcium than phosphorus, whereas the extracellular plaques contained more phosphate than calcium. This means that the calcification of tympanosclerosis is distinctly different microchemically than that of normal bone calcification.

One of the changes seen in the electron microscope studies, both by Chang[27] and our group, suggests that the mitochondria have calcium deposits in them, not because the blood calcium serum level is particularly high, but because it is related to the electron-transport function and the ion accumulation. This has been very well laid out in the work of Lehninger.[29] An extension of his thinking might ex-

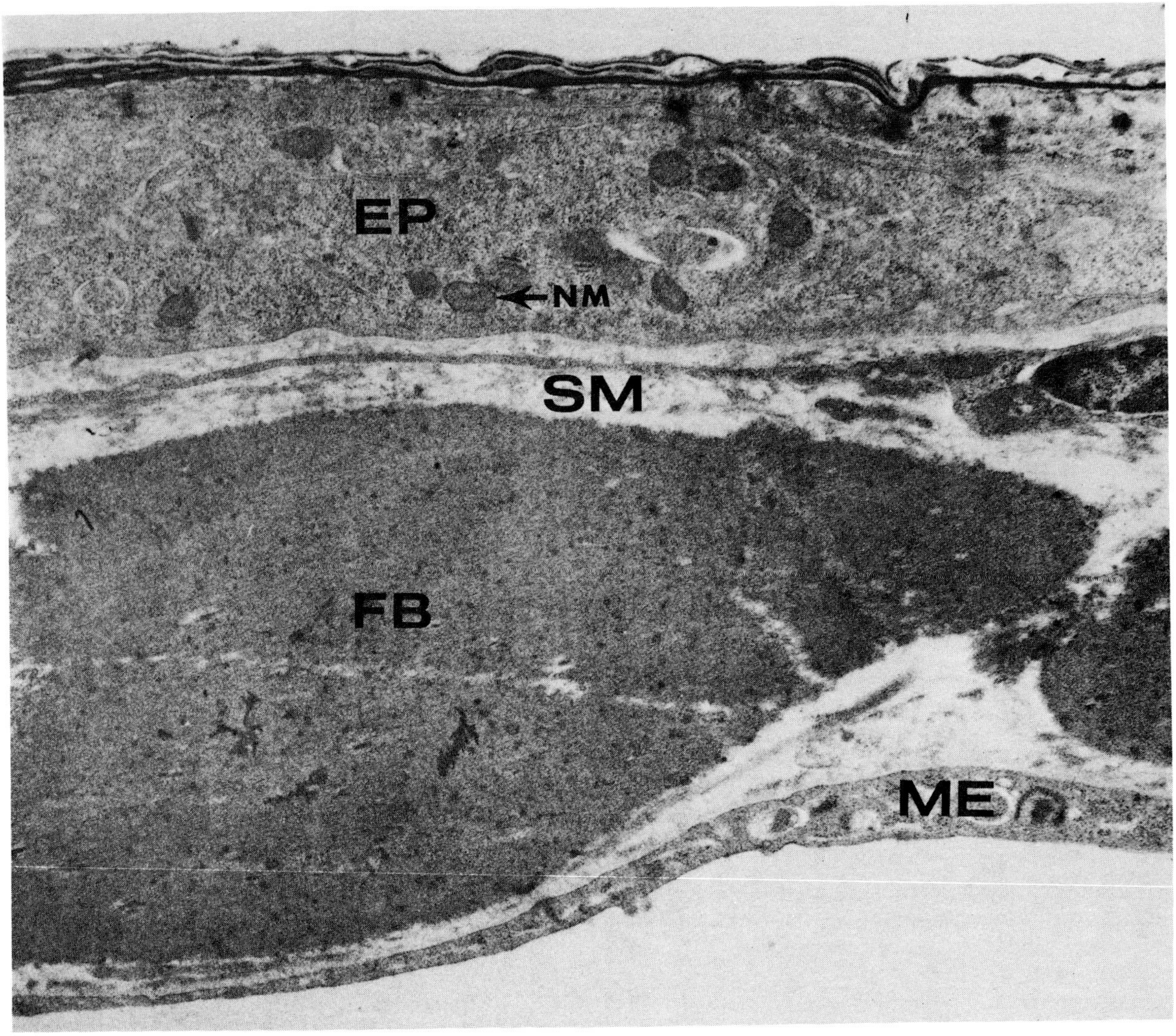

Fig. 6. Electron micrograph of the normal tympanic membrane. The outer epithelial layer (EP) at the top of the figure consists of two cell layers. A thin subepithelial connective tissue layer (SM) separates the epithelium from the fiber bundles (FB) of the fibrous layer of the lamina propria. The mucosal epithelium (ME) is also separated from the fibrous layer by a thin subepithelial connective tissue layer. NM - Normal mitochondia. (x8000)

plain why the calcium concentration is higher intracellularly than extracellularly with reference to the phosphorus. The calcium ions tend to accumulate in degenerating and decomposing tissues, probably because of local alteration of the pH subsequent to the interference with the electron-transport function of the mitochondria by the disease process. Leughthenberger and Fautrez[30] thought that the extracellular deposit of calcium was probably related to the increased synthesis of mucopolysaccharide, particularly the chondroitin sulfate which constitutes a part of the ground substance. The most probable cell to produce these components has been demonstrated as the fibroblast.

The general appearance of tympanosclerosis shows a distinct decrease in cellular activity and cell count. This is apparent functionally with the decrease in the mucous and goblet cells, as well as those within the stroma. The finding of a considerable softening of bones that are enveloped and wrapped in a tympanosclerotic mass probably has its explanation in the fact that not only is the vascular supply lifted from the intimate contact with the bone, but the microchemical changes reported with the degenerating mitochondria suggest that the local environment might prefer a shift in the local demand of calcium for the degenerating tissue. The most proximal source for this would be the contiguous bone enveloped by the tympanosclerotic mass. The study of the collagenase, or similar protease activity of this tissue has not been undertaken yet. Such enzymes have, likewise, the capacity to soften bone by acting on the organic matrix. These factors together with the isolation of the better blood supply to the ossicle itself most probably accounts for the moth-eaten, demineralized appearance of the tympanoslcerotic ossicle. If this is extensive, it can lead to ossicular discontinuity, particularly in the long process of the incus.

It is a well-known fact that when infection oc-

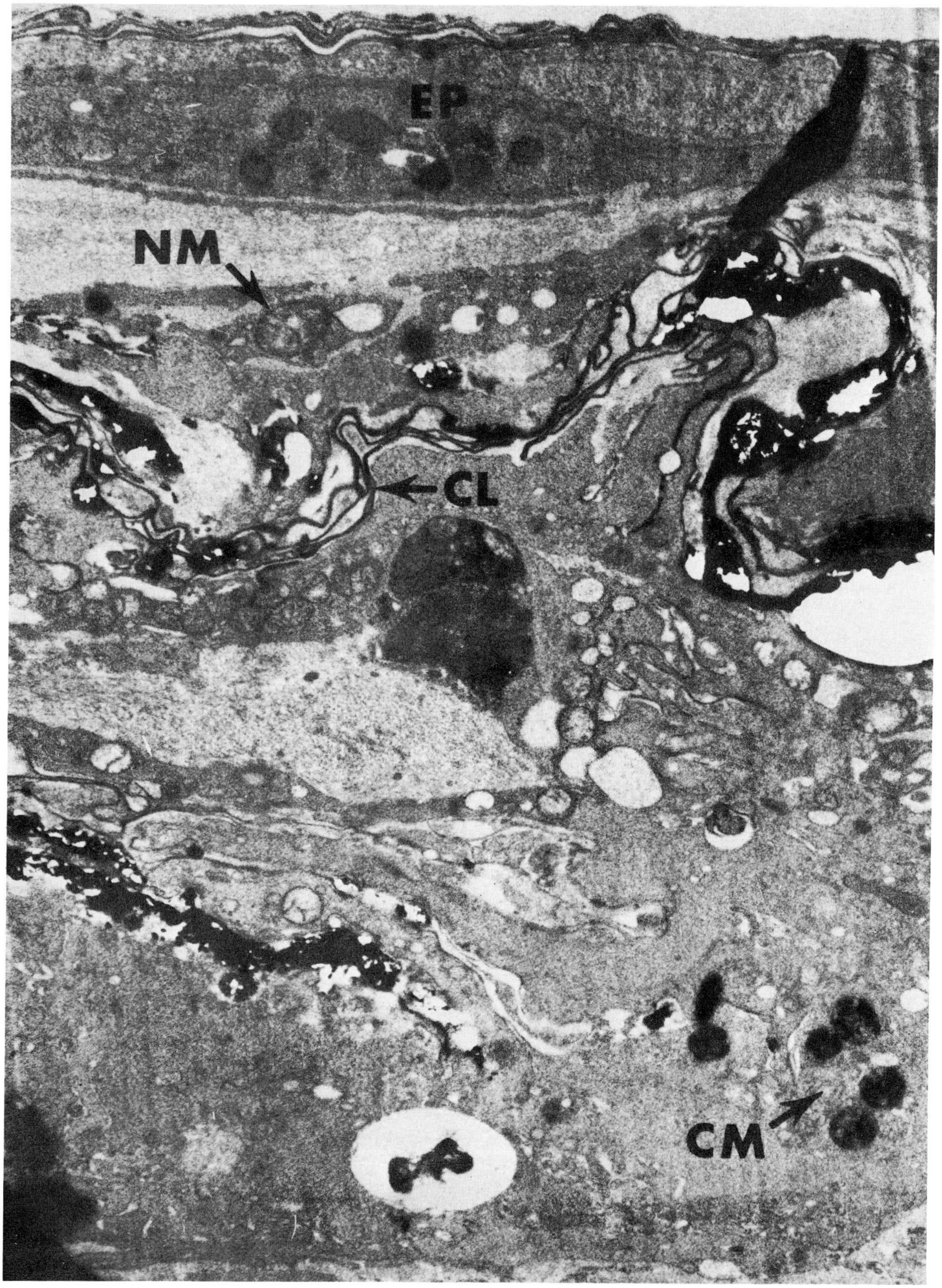

Fig. 7. Electron micrograph of guinea pig tympanosclerosis. The greatly expanded subepidermal connective tissue layer is characterized by calcified lamelae (CL) and calcified mitochondria (CM). Normal mitochondria (NM) are also evident. The epidermal epithelium (EP) is relatively normal in appearance. (x8000)

curs, pH changes occur, and the bone demineralizes. This might explain why one would find a demineralized bone in the early stages of otitic infection. In tympanosclerosis, the inflammatory reaction in the ear has existed for many years, and the availability of the polymorphonuclear leukocyte with its destructive enzymes is not really that close to the bone anymore. The polymorphonuclear leukocytes are present in the early stages of infection, but they are virtually nonexistent in the long-standing tympanosclerosis. It would therefore appear logical that these changes are taking place either by ischemic alterations, or by the interface with tympanosclerosis on the bone in combination.

The ground substance is an important area for the activity demonstrated by this model. In the lamina propria, the subepithelial to submucosal connective tissue layer is the arena where the ground substance interaction appears most important.

The ground substance is made up of a) cells, ie, mast cells, fibroblast, endothelial cells; b) fibrillar components, ie, collagen, reticulin, elastin; and c) acid mucopolysaccharides, ie, hyaluronic acid, chondroitin sulfate A, B, and C. They are maintained in a sol-gel equilibrium which is altered by many factors[31] such as enzymes, ions, hormones and nutrients. The alterations of this occur early in inflammatory changes and the interaction of these factors can alter the nature of the amorphous ground substance to a more organized fibrous state.

DISCUSSION

With the tremendous events in technology, information and knowledge, a reconsideration of many of the clinical aspects of tympanosclerosis in this frame of reference will be presented. It will probably raise as many new questions as we answer.

Incidence and Duration. There are several areas of basic agreement: 1) tympanosclerosis does not occur on the first insult; 2) it takes many years to develop this condition. In the informative study by Harris[11] who showed that there was a 5% incidence rate of tympanosclerosis in a series of over 300 mastoid and tympanoplasty operations, 22% of the cases were in children, and yet none of the children demonstrated tympanosclerosis. In review of 16 of the cases of tympanosclerosis, only 2 were in the 20-30 year age group. All the rest were older. This further emphasizes the fact that it takes a long time to develop clinical tympanosclerosis. House and Sheehy[9] reported a 33% incidence rate. It therefore becomes obvious that the definition is most important. If one refers only to those ears with perforations, which represent over 80% of the tympanosclerotic cases, then these figures remain quite accurate. If one were to redefine the terms from clinical tympanosclerosis, inferring some type of disability to an anatomic consideration, then the incident rate changes. If the chalk marks, or the calcareous deposits in the drum, were included, they would probably double the highest incidences proposed. It is likewise obvious that many subclinical cases are only detected nowadays with the refinement of the tympanometer which is able to measure the impedance and compliance of the TM. Using such an instrument as part of the criteria, this would increase the incidence still further. If we include those ears that have had tubes placed in them and subsequently developed this leukoma, or chalk-white mark, which does not interfere at all with hearing, the incidence would increase greatly.

The comments referable to the development of tympanosclerosis in the TM alone have their application, likewise, to the disease process in the middle ear, since the lamina propria, or fibrous layer, is present between the mucosa and the bone of the middle ear.

In the 138 cases of tympanosclerosis, the location of 24% was in the TM alone, 32% in the middle ear and mastoid, and 44% in both locations.[1]

There were 1,495 chronic ear surgeries reported by Kinney[15] of which approximately 20% had tympanosclerosis, and 80% of these cases were over the age of 30. This further emphasized the fact that it takes a long time to develop this pathologic end state of middle ear inflammation.

Anatomy and Microbiology. It would appear that the pars flaccida would not be involved, since there is no lamina propria in this area in man. However, Lim's electron microscopy study[32] of the pars flaccida showed that this is considerably thicker as a total membrane structure than is the pars tensa. It is true that there is no lamina propria in this area to be organized systematically into tympanosclerosis. However, there is a moderate amount of connective tissue of the more loose type between the two layers of epithelium. When inflammation and edema take place in this area, there is a marked increase in the ground substance with the inflammatory reaction. By the involvement of this edematous tissue in the same chemotactic process, which is initiated by neutrophils in other areas, the calcium ions can likewise be drawn to this area to develop small plaque-like areas of tympanosclerosis in contrast to the large sheets and lamella layers seen in the TM and middle ear. This is based on the premise that the mucosa has become porous enough so that the noxious substances from the infection arrive at the mesenchymal or connective tissue layer and, thereby, are able to induce the sensitizing tissue reaction for the future development of tympanosclerosis.

It is important to note that about 63% of all otitic infections in children were caused by *Hemophilus influenzae.* These organisms have the capacity to create considerable edema in a very short period of time. This is probably due to some toxic effect on the capillary walls permitting such a large outpouring of fluid into the ground substance. In contrast to many other pathogenic organisms, this feature is remarkable.

If one adds to the problems of the *Hemophilus* infection those of the streptococcal organisms with their built-in spreading factor, then the ease and ability to invade into the connective tissue layer becomes obvious. The spreading factor is hyaluronidase and has the capacity to depolymerize the hyaluronic acid and other ground substance components. As these are further depolymerized, the number of molecules increase, and therefore the osmotic pressure is to have even a greater amount of fluid inbibition. If the accompanying neutrophils break down and release their enzymes, the machinery is now in function for the partial destruction of some of the connective tissue elements.

In Zöllner's[7] paper reinstituting the use of the term tympanosclerosis in English for the first time, he presents a classic case of this problem. His patients, like so many others, had scarlet fever in childhood, and both of the ears were now dry, and he proceeded to discuss the anatomic and surgical handling of this massive build-up of tympanosclerosis. It is therefore suggested, from a clinical point of view, that these organisms play an early, major role in the initiation of the events that terminate in the complement cascade which participates intimately with the early inflammatory process. Veltri and Sprinkle,[23] in their several studies have set forth a methodical, logical case for secretory otitis media being an immune complex disease. They also emphasize that some organisms are capable of initiating an immediate damage, and then the organisms are eliminated by antibiotics. The fact that microbial antigens and necrotic debris from the tissue damage are capable of maintaining and perpetuating a middle ear effusion without the presence of bacteria strongly suggests that the immune aspects of this function are seriously implicated. They likewise believe that attacking the middle ear mucosa and supporting structures with lysosomal enzymes found in such ear effusions could result in the type of damage one sees in tympanosclerosis.

Bernstein and Reisman[24] in their study of the role of hypersensitivity in secretory otitis media shifted their emphasis to a cellular immune process noting that the presence of the lymphocytes and the macrophages were the most common cells. The fact that these lymphocytes are predominantly T-cells might very well explain why the tissues became sensitized to the necrotic cellular debris of the lamina propria. The T-cells were able to recognize the debris as "foreign." This allows for the development of a tissue-fixed sensitized area that would react the next time a challenge was presented. This latter description is not much different than part of the experimental work done on our animals. Since both these processes takes place in an orderly sequence from the immediate acute stage to the more prolonged chronic state, it would appear most logical that the cellular-type fixed immunity probably has the essence as a precursor for tympanosclerosis.

Mucosa. Why is there such a large overgrowth of connective tissue, and why does the middle ear react in such a way as to eventually become dry?

One of the interesting characteristics of even advanced tympanosclerosis is the presence of essentially a dry middle ear with almost no discharge in most of the cases. In the 138 cases of tympanosclerosis reported by Gibb,[1] 83% were dry, although perforations were present in 84%. All these perforations were present in the pars tensa of the drum. The fact that they are dry in such a high percentage, and that cholesteatoma is uncommon, both fit well together. This is further confirmed by the work of Kinney[15] who noted that 66% had dry ears, and of the remaining 33% who had mucoid or mucopurulent discharge, 50% of these had cholesteatoma. It becomes apparent that a dry ear and cholesteatoma do not usually go together. In contrast to this, Morgan[33] reported 37% tympanosclerosis in the general ear surgical population, but he found the incidence of cholesteatoma associated with tympanosclerosis, when a perforation existed, at 50%. It would appear, if 50% had cholesteatoma, the incidence or infections of draining ears would be considerably larger than those reported by most otologists. This would strongly suggest that the definition for tympanosclerosis and cholesteatoma, when they coexist, should be looked at and studied with greater scrutiny. As previously noted in Plester's 1971 report of 3,000 tympanoplasties,[18] 10% had tympanosclerosis. Ninety percent of this subgroup had central perforations, and there had been no inflammation or infection of the ear for many ears. In the large majority of these cases, no discharge was present. He also thought that cholesteatoma and tympanosclerosis were strictly a coincidence, not cause-and-effect related.

Place this in contrast to the concept by Hybasek[19] and Ferlito[20] who both thought cholesteatoma was part of the developmental picture. In the cases presented by Harris[11] only 2 of the 16 had cholesteatoma, and these both had some degree of suppuration with it. Also, in the House and Sheehy[9] study, cholesteatoma was not of a high incidence rate in ears with tympanosclerosis.

It is obvious that arriving at an agreement on this problem poses a definite dilemma, most probably in the area of semantics. What is apparent is that most of the cases of tympanosclerosis have been in existence from 10-30 years, and a cholesteatoma active or present for that length of time would have had a considerable amount of bony destruction.

There is usually little bone destruction in tympanosclerosis. The collagenase activity of the cholesteatomatous matrix is well-known.

Why the tympanosclerotic middle ear becomes dry and remains dry, even for such a long period of time, is suggested by the work of Tos and Bak-Pedersen.[17] They showed that as the disease process advances, the activity of the mucous gland is cut down considerably so that the capability of the potential for secretion is slowly eliminated. Sade's[16] work showed the distribution of the secretory cells and cilia in the middle ear. When the promontory and attic areas change their epithelium to either more cuboidal epithelium or squamous metaplasia because of the changes occurring in the lamina propria beneath it, the epithelium is reduced down to the level of greatest biologic energy economics. A good, active blood supply is necessary for secretory activity. Cilia are lost early when nutrition is deprived and the epithelium changes to those requiring less blood. As the thickness of the lamina propria grows, the blood supply is likewise removed from close access. One needs only to lift the epithelium over a tympanosclerotic plaque to see the dearth of bleeding. This is another factor in limiting the amount of nourishment to the mucosa as well as to the glands. Therefore, secretion is decreased.

As noted previously, the presence at the oval window and in the attic and on the stapedius tendon of tympanosclerosis would suggest that this has a combination of anatomic and functional consideration that explain the high incidence in this area. Sade[16] showed that the epithelium in the superior portion of the middle ear is usually nonciliated, the applied implication here being that the normal sweeping and cleansing of the debris is not as easily performed as in the hypotympanic part of the ear. The secretions in the interstices of the oval window, the undersurface of the stapes arch, beneath the fallopian canal, and between the folds of mucosa in and around the ossicles, permits the mucus to remain longer. This is particularly true if the mucus is pathologic with a great increase of viscosity or infections at which time the edema it produces decreases the activity of the glands in that area. The latter is substantiated by the excellent work of Tos and Bak-Pederson[17] in their studies showing the considerable fall in population of secretory glands, and therefore their activity in tympanosclerosis. Their figures are truly impressive when one compares the number of glands per square millimeter area in tympanosclerosis with the number, or density, per square millimeter as compared with other middle ear diseases. It is a fact that many of these secretions that are in stasis contain within them the immunoglobulins and complement factors capable of either activating the immune response at a humoral or cellular level, or participating in the inflammatory response. This may help to explain the high incidence rate in these areas of middle ear.

Bone. Most investigators have found bone from time to time in the tympanosclerotic mass. This represented bone "de nuovo," not a resorbed piece from another origin. Goodhill,[8] in his clear presentation of various types of ossicular chain fixation, noted the effects of tympanosclerosis in both the fixation of the chain as well as in nonotosclerotic disease of the stapes. Others have noted the totipotent capability of a certain fibroblast population which can stimulate osteoblastic production of new bone, even with a considerable intermixture of fibrous components.

This leads to the discussion of otosclerosis and a possible involvement of this disease by a similar mechanism as proposed in this theory of pathogenesis. It is obvious that otosclerosis and tympanosclerosis is not the same. This separation was put to rest long ago by Politzer[4] in 1883. Obviously, not all people who have middle ear infections develop tympanosclerosis. There must be some other factor, most probably the turning on or off of a gene switch to initiate or inhibit development of this condition. A very tantalizing question is raised regarding otosclerosis. There appears to be two types: a) those that have a very definite familial history, in which case the footplate is usually very thick and may have a massive bone growth and b) a second, separate type in which there is no family history of otosclerosis but often a history of an ear infection that was only transient in nature. At surgery, the footplate of a) the former, is dense and white in appearance, whereas the latter b) the fixed footplate has a blue center and appears fixed only in its ligamentous attachment into the oval window. Many of the same connective tissue components that exist in the disease of the lamina propria likewise exist beneath the mucosa on the oval window ligament.

Would it not be reasonable to assume that since such changes as we demonstrated can be made in the TM that a similar infection involving suppurative material in the oval window niche, producing a similar break in the integrity of the mucosa and an involvement of the cartilage, might leave a sensitized area capable of remaining active very slowly and progressively taking many years to develop the otosclerotic fixation similar to that which we have seen in tympanosclerosis? Efforts will be under way to investigate this potential in the near future.

Collagen. Some of the more recent advances in the study of collagen are germaine to tympanosclerosis. Characteristically, there is a large proliferation of connective tissue including amorphous ground substance as well as their fibrillar components such as collagen in tympanosclerosis. This is followed in a later stage by hyalinized degeneration in this tissue, and often calcification. The question arises,

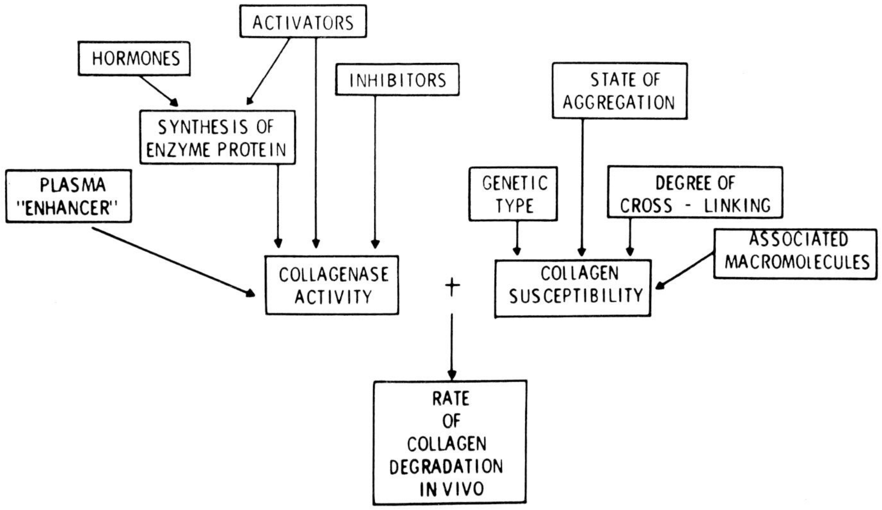

Fig. 8. Diagram of some factors regulating the degradation of collagen. (From Perez-Tamayo.[34] Reprinted with permission.)

why does the collagen accumulate to this extent following its immunologic activation?

There are at present five different known types of collagen. Collagen is not a static substance; it is dynamic and acts as the ground substance. The development of large depots of collagen may be either induced because of increased collagen production, or decreased ability to remove it. The presence of collagen is not immutable. It is not forever. It depends upon the type and degree of cross linkage that has taken place. The best example of this is the huge, thousandfold increase in collagen in the pregnant uterus that lasts for nine months, and in about six months postpartum, the collagen and procollagen units are completely reabsorbed with only a small residual to suggest that the uterus had been pregnant. The removal of collagen is under many controls such as activators and inhibitors of collagenase (Fig. 8). Synthesized enzymes, hormones, and genetic factors as well as the physical state of the collagen itself at a given time are part of the dynamics.

Perhaps tympanosclerosis should likewise be included into the group of diseases with a deficiency of collagen degradation such as cirrhosis of the liver, scleroderma, and osteopetrositis. These other deficiency states have been noted by Perez-Tamayo[34] and certainly are worthy of consideration in this disease, one of whose major characteristics may be failure to degrade and remove excessive collagen.

Certainly, all infections produce an elaboration of ground substance which, if infiltrated with the proper cells, is capable of producing collagen in this matrix. That scars involute, shrink down and almost disappear is part of the normal reparative process in most surgical observations. The medical management of such conditions as otitis media where infection creates considerable edema in the mucosa or beneath it, is likewise resolved by the removal of these substances from the involved structures once the stimulation has ended. The biologic details of the word *resolve* are considerable but are an important part of the reparative process. What is it that turns off the machinery for degrading the collagen and returning the connective tissue to a more normal state? The fact that Perez-Tamayo[34] included scleroderma among these deficiency states makes one strongly think that perhaps the immunologic reactivity that has occurred is capable of turning off the collagenase degradation system, thereby permitting the ground substance and its connective tissue elements to remain and grow slowly without having the feedback circuit to tell this growth to stop as is usually found in normal inflammatory tissue resolution. Activating or inhibiting the regulator for the fibroblast activity would account for the continuous alteration of a collagen. That diseases related to cellular immunity are capable of interfering with enzymatic control of cellular systems is reasonable to imply from other disease pathophysiologic processes. This general area certainly requires a considerable amount of consideration for future investigation.

The role of antitissue antibodies was studied by Kondo et al[35] in scleroderma. Here lymphocytes can release a migration inhibition factor. Only T-lymphocytes were found in the tissue. Lymphocyte mediators can stimulate collagen synthesis. They concluded that the local cell-mediated immune response may be a factor in scleroderma. Hughes et al[36] implied that sensitized cytotoxic lymphocytes and a decline of suppressor T-cells may be responsible for an immune pathogenesis.

The biology of the fibroblast and its secretory collagen is distinctly different in tissue culture from normal dermis and scleroderma, according to Bashey et al.[37] If the biology and the chemistry are dif-

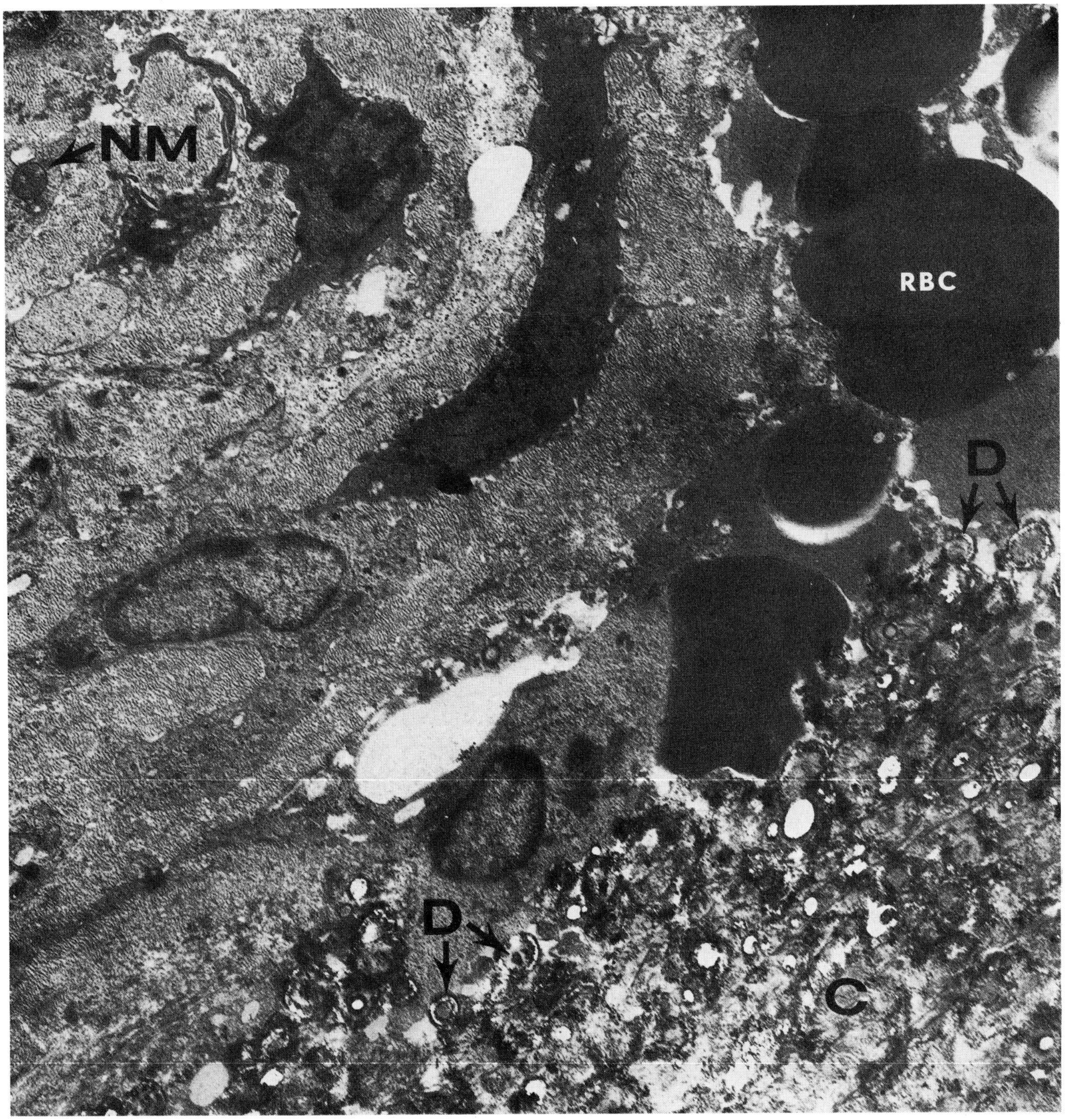

Fig. 9. This human EM picture shows the increased fibrous units together with calcification in the area marked C. RBC - Red blood cell; D - Double ring structures; NM - Normal mitochondria. (x3000)

ferent, that could mean that their potential and susceptibility for destruction are also altered.

In discussing factors that may control collagen resorption, Reynolds et al[38] noted that there are many ways of controlling collagenolytic activity. Collagenases exist in active and latent forms. The latent form is intimately attached to the collagen and can be activated by trypsin or other proteinases. They are activated by causing dissolution of the enzyme-inhibitor complex. The relative concentration of these two components, collagenase and inhibitor, determine the site and extent of collagen resorption. This enzyme, collagenase, is synthesized under control of specific stimuli such as hormones, prostaglandens and lympokines. Polymorphonuclear leukocytes and inflammation can activate collagenase.

Polymorphonuclear leukocytes attack collagen type 1, but not very much type 3. The fibroblast and macrophage release substances capable of attacking both collagen types 1 and 3. Changes during inflammation and healing of the relative proportions of types 1 and 3 collagen are controlled by the collagenase in the tissue, according to Horwitz et al.[39]

Electron Microscopy. Until 1968 no electron microscope studies of note had been performed on the TM. This was a banner year with the two excellent papers by Lim[26,32] and the work of Johnson et al[40] on the ultrastructure and the biochemical observations of the TM. Finally the work by Chang[27] on the EM studies of tympanosclerosis is characterized by degenerating mitochondria with electron-dense masses in fibrocyte-like cells. Also, electron-dense autophaged lysosomes and membrane-bound fragments are among the distended collagen bundles. This is much similar to what we have found in Figure 9 of human tympanosclerosis. It agrees with the animal model considerably.

Friedman[41] who has done much work on tympanosclerosis, stated the following at the Symposium on Histopathology and Pathophysiology of the Middle Ear: "We have been unable to identify tympanosclerosis in experimentally produced infection of the ear of the guinea pig, and these studies are to be renewed stimulated by this symposium."

With our model we have succeeded in inducing these changes in the tympanic membrane of the guinea pig consistent with tympanosclerosis.

CONCLUSION

An animal model for tympanosclerosis has been developed which involves immunologic manipulation. The TM is antigenic. Antibodies can be made to fix in the guinea pig TM when the local injury has occurred. This results in our model of tympanosclerosis. After sensitizing the guinea pig, a proper challenge to the TM elicited a response which fits intimately with the proposed theory of pathogenesis for tympanosclerosis.

Its implication to humans is that tympanosclerosis is an end state of abnormal healing response to a previously sensitized tissue. The theoretical considerations strongly suggest that the prolonged activity of the process is an antigenic blocking of the control mechanism for fibroblastic activity. This involves either excess production or decreased destruction of the new collagen.

With a better understanding of pathophysiology of any disease process, the proper steps for altering, inhibiting, or ameliorating this process can be made possible.

REFERENCES

1. Gibb AG. President's address. Tympanosclerosis. Proc R Soc Med 1976; 69:155-62.

2. Cassebohm IF. Tractatus quatuor anatomici de aure humana, 1734.

3. von Tröltsch AF. Handbuch der Ohrenheilkunde. Leipzig, 1869.

4. Politzer A. A textbook of the diseases of the ear and adjacent organs. Philadelphia: Lea Brothers, 1883.

5. Habermann J. Pathologische Anatomie des Ohres. In: Schwartze H, ed. Handbuch der Ohrenheilkunde. Vol 1. Leipzig: SCW Vogel, 1892:203-302.

6. Walb H. Krankheiten der Paukenhöhle und der Tuba Eustachii. In: Schwartze H, ed. Handbuch der Ohrenheilkunde. Vol. 2. Leipzig: SCW Vogel, 1893:168-298.

7. Zöllner F. Tympanosclerosis. J Laryngol Otol 1956; 70:77-85.

8. Goodhill V. Pseudo-otosclerosis. Laryngoscope 1960; 70:722-57.

9. House WF, Sheehy JL. Tympanosclerosis. Arch Otolaryngol 1960; 72:308-13.

10. Sheehy JL, House WF. Tympanosclerosis. Arch Otolaryngol 1962; 76:151-7.

11. Harris L. Tympanosclerosis — a revived clinicopathologic entity. Laryngoscope 1961; 71:1488-1533.

12. Zaritskii LA, Avramenko LV, Dmitrenko VV. Clinicomorphological changes in adhesive otitis and tympanosclerosis. Zh Ushn Nos Gorl Bolezn 1969; 29:1-8.

13. Sluchanko AP. Fibroblastic processes in the middle ear. Zh Ushn Nos Gorl Bolezn 1968; 28:10-9.

14. Musta O, Chisiu NS. Immuno-competent cells in cold otic diseases (tympanosclerosis, chronic otitis media). Med Interna (Cucur) 1970; 22:1237-41.

15. Kinney SE. Postinflammatory ossicular fixation in tympanoplasty. Laryngoscope 1978; 88:821-38.

16. Sade J. Ciliary activity and middle ear clearance. Arch Otolaryngol 1967; 86:128-35.

17. Tos M, Bak-Pedersen K. Middle ear mucosa in tympanosclerosis. J Laryngol Otol 1974; 88:119-26.

18. Plester D. Tympanosclerosis. J Otolaryngol Soc 1972; 3:325-6.

19. Hybasek I. Relation of otitis media chronica secretorica to tympanosclerosis. Sb Ved Pr Lek Fak Karlovy Univ 1969; 12:135-40.

20. Ferlito A. Histopathogenesis of tympanosclerosis. J Laryngol Otol 1979; 93:25-37.

21. Schuknecht H. Pathology of the ear. Cambridge: Harvard University Press, 1974.

22. Lim DJ. Review: normal and pathological mucosa of the middle ear and eustachian tube. Clin Otolaryngol 1979; 4:213-39.

23. Veltri RW, Sprinkle PM. Secretory otitis media: an immune complex disease. Ann Otol Rhinol Laryngol 1976; 85 Suppl 25:135-59.

24. Bernstein JM, Reisman R. The role of acute hypersensitivity in secretory otitis media. Trans Am Acad Ophthalmol Otolaryngol 1974; 78:120-7.

25. Poliquin JF, Cantanzaro A, Robb J, Ryan A, Schiff M. Antigenicity of the guinea pig's membrane. Otolaryngol Head Neck Surg 1979; 87:852-8.

26. Lim DJ. Tympanic membrane (electron microscopic observation). I. Pars tensa. Acta Otolaryngol (Stockh) 1968; 66:181-98.

27. Chang IW. Tympanosclerosis. Electron microscopic study. Acta Otolaryngol (Stockh) 1969; 68:62-72.

28. Sorensen H, True O. Histology of tympanosclerosis. Acta Otolaryngol (Stockh) 1972; 73:18-26.

29. Lehninger AL. The mitochondrian. Molecular basis of structure and function. New York: WB Saunders, 1964:166-8.

30. Leughthenberger GR, Fautrez J. Nucleinsauren. Stuttgart: G Fisher Verlag, 1966; 3:6-11.

31. Schiff M. The influence of estrogens on connective tissue. In: Asboe-Hansen G, ed. Hormones and connective tissues. Baltimore: Williams and Wilkins, 1966:282-341.

32. Lim DJ. Tympanic membrane. II. Pars flaccida. Acta Otolaryngol (Stockh) 1968; 66:515-32.

33. Morgan WC Jr. Tympanosclerosis. Laryngoscope 1977; 87:1821-5.

34. Perez-Tamayo R. The pathology of collagen degradation. Am J Pathol 1979; 92:508-66.

35. Kondo H. Rabin BS, Rodnan GP. Cutaneous antigen-stimulating lymphokine production by lymphocytes of patients with progressive systemic sclerosis (scleroderma). J Clin Invest 1976; 58:1388-94.

36. Hughes P, Holt S, Rowell NR, Dodd J. Thymus-dependent (T) lymphocyte deficiency in progressive system sclerosis. Br J Dermatol 1976; 95:469.

37. Bashey RI, Jimenez SA, Perlish JS. Characterization of secreted collagen from normal and scleroderma fibroblasts in culture. J Mol Med 1977; 2:153-61.

38. Reynolds JJ, Murphy G, Sellers A, Cartwright E. New factor that may control collagen resorption. Lancet 1977; 2:333-5.

39. Horwitz AL, Hance AJ, Crystal RG. Granulocyte collagenase: selective digestion of type I relative to type III collagen. Proc Natl Acad Sci USA 1977; 74:897-901.

40. Johnson FR, McMinn RMH, Atfield GN. Ultrastructural and biochemical observations on the tympanic membrane. J Anat 1968; 103:297-310.

41. Friedman I. Tympanosclerosis. Ann Otol Rhinol Laryngol 1971; 80:411-3.

THE EYE-TRACKING TEST

Yoshio Umeda, MD

I. MANUAL QUANTITATIVE ASSESSMENT OF EYE-TRACKING PATTERNS

II. STANDARDIZATION OF THE EYE-TRACKING TEST

Supplement 71 — Vol. 89, July-August, 1980, No. 4, Part 3

THE ANNALS OF OTOLOGY, RHINOLOGY & LARYNGOLOGY

CONTENTS

I. Manual Quantitative Assessment of Eye-Tracking Patterns . . . . Page 1

II. Standardization of the Eye-Tracking Test . . . . Page 7

THE ANNALS PUBLISHING COMPANY
4949 FOREST PARK BLVD.
ST. LOUIS, MISSOURI 63108

I. MANUAL QUANTITATIVE ASSESSMENT OF EYE-TRACKING PATTERNS

YOSHIO UMEDA, MD

SAITAMA, JAPAN

Quantitative assessment of the electronystagmogram of the eye-tracking test (eye-tracking pattern) was undertaken in 20 normal subjects and 70 patients with vertigo. The abnormal recordings, contrary to the normal, showed, in varying degrees, remarkable irregularities of eye speed. These irregularities appeared in the form of spikes on the electronystagmogram at the time constant of 0.03 second. We measured the height of the spikes using 40°/sec as a unit and added the units of spikes appearing during a nine-second period to obtain the total index. Total indices ranged from zero (normal) to 40 + (severely abnormal), and their values showed levels of abnormality in the eye-tracking pattern more accurately than the visual analysis in current use.

INTRODUCTION

The eye-tracking test, which consists of recording pursuit eye movements in response to a visual stimulus, is one of the most popular vestibular examinations in current use. In the analysis of the electronystagmograms made in this test of eye-tracking patterns (ETP), however, no standardized methods of quantitative assessment are in general use except for two types of trial analyses using a computer.[1,2] For the purpose of analyzing ETP recorded without the aid of a computer, a simple manual method is preferable.

When compared to normal ETP, abnormal patterns are found to have irregularities of eye speed (Fig. 1, arrows). The author recently found that measurement of these spikes leads to a quantitative assessment of the abnormality of the ETP.

METHODS

SUBJECTS

Twenty normal subjects and 70 patients with vertigo were tested. The details of the vertiginous conditions have been omitted.

MOVING TARGET

The subject was seated on a chair with the head mechanically fixed and asked to follow a moving target at a distance of 70 cm moving in a clockwise circle with a radius of 25.5 cm at a constant rate of 120°/sec. The horizontal component of the eye movement was presented in a sinusoidal curve of 0.33 Hz with a maximum displacement of 20° from the center. The maximum velocity of eye movement was 42°/sec.[3]

RECORDING OF EYE MOVEMENTS

Electronystagmograms of horizontal eye movements were made with electrodes fixed lateral to both outer canthi and to the forehead for a reference ground. The recording was undertaken with the aid of two electronystagmogram channels: the first for eye movement with the time constant of 3.0 seconds and the second for eye speed with the time constant of 0.03 second. In order to obtain the calibration, 10° saccades, from a point 5° to one side of the primary position of the eyes to a point 5° to the other side, were recorded with an amplitude of 1 cm. The recording paper was fed at 1 cm/sec.

DATA ANALYSIS

ETP spikes can be assessed in two different manners, ie, by the frequency of the spikes or by their combined amplitude. The former method is not successful in that an ataxic pattern generally shows fewer spikes than a saccadic pattern, independently of the severity of the disorder. For this reason, the author chose the latter method.

Determination of Measurement Unit. The amplitude of 40°/sec was chosen as the unit for measurement. As shown in Figure 2a, after 10° calibration was determined with the aid of an electrical circuit, the trace of the first channel was shifted to delta waves of 1 Hz with the amplitude of 20° calibration, ie, 2 cm in height. This shift of the first channel brought the amplitude of the second channel to 40°/sec, which was made the basic unit for measuring the height of the spikes.

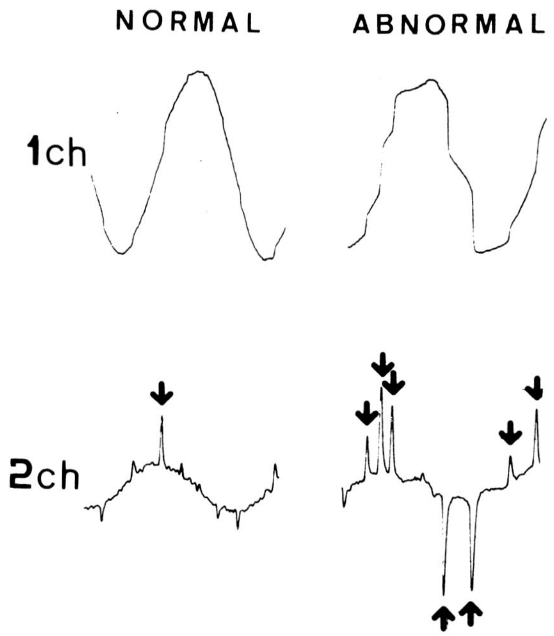

Fig. 1. Eye-Tracking Pattern (ETP). The upper traces (first channel [1 ch]) show horizontal eye movement and the lower traces (second channel [2 ch]) show eye speed. In comparing abnormal ETP with normal ones, we noted apparent irregularities of eye speed in the former (arrows). Measurement of the spikes resulted in a quantitative assessment of the abnormality of the ETP. The spike of the normal ETP (arrow) represents an occasional error.

From the Department of Otolaryngology, Saitama Medical School Hospital, Moro, Saitama-ken, Japan.

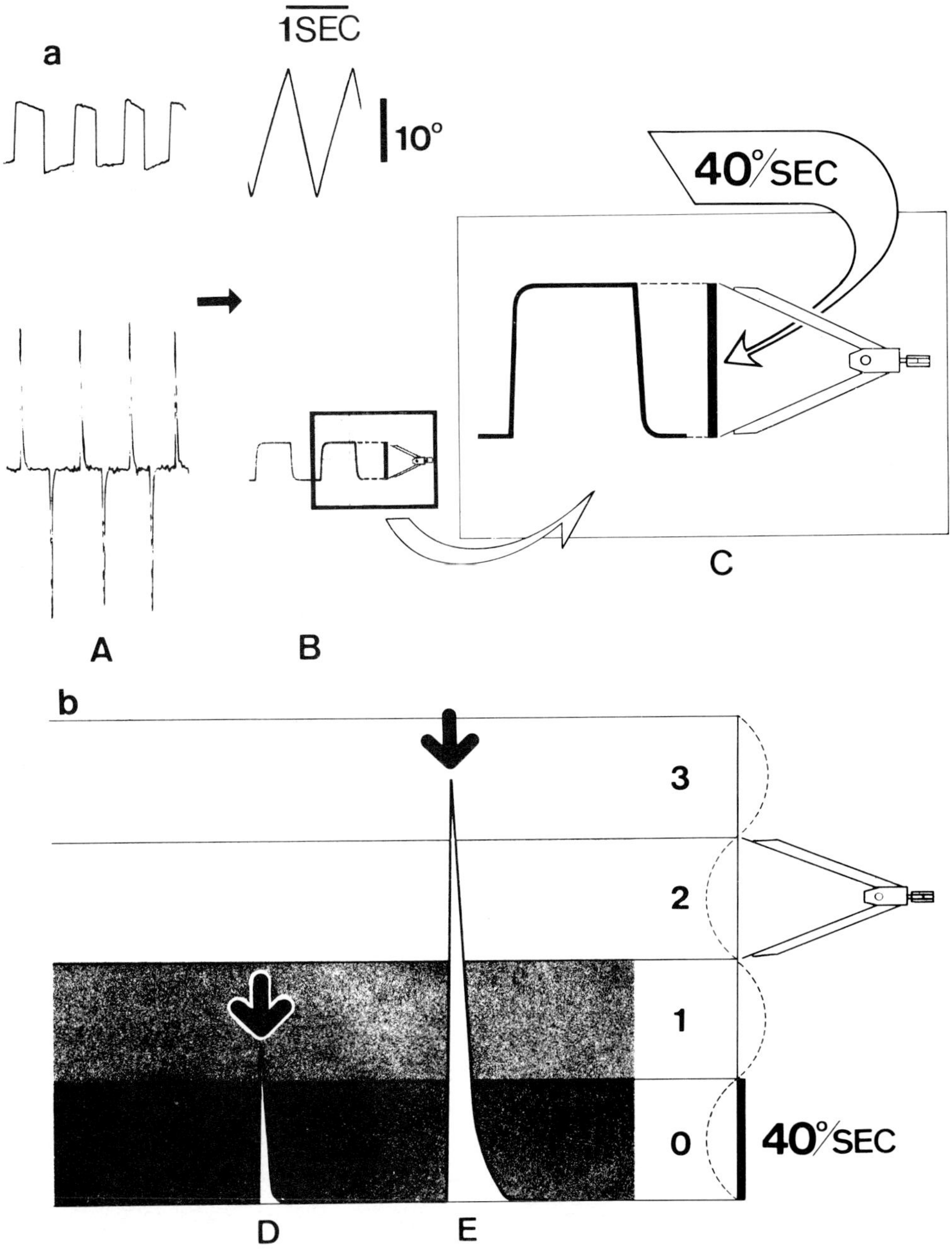

Fig. 2. a) Determination of measurement unit. A - In order to obtain the calibration, 10° saccades were recorded with an amplitude of 1 cm. B - With the aid of an electrical circuit, the trace of the first channel was shifted to delta waves of 1 Hz with the amplitude of 20° calibration, ie, 2 cm in height. This shift of the first channel brought the amplitude of the second channel to 40°/sec. C - 40°/sec was made the basic unit for measurement of the height of the spikes. b) Quantitative assessment of spikes. Measurement of the height of the spikes was based on 40°/sec for one unit. In order to eliminate small spikes (less than 40°/sec) they were assigned to index 0. Spike D was assigned to index 1 and spike E to index 3.

Quantitative Assessment of the Spikes. The spikes were measured from starting point to peak upward and downward (40°/sec represented one unit) with a compass, as indicated in Figure 2. Small spikes of less than 40°/sec, ie, those which did not attain the level of the first unit, were assigned to Index 0. The D spike in Figure 2b was assigned to index 1, and the E spike to index 3.

RESULTS

METHOD OF ASSESSMENT

The method of Figure 2 was applied to the assessment of spikes appearing on three sine waves. The total of the summed values of the spikes was made the total index. For clinical practice, contrasting ETP are shown in Figure 3; the left shows a slight abnormality and has a total index of 6, and the right ETP reveals a severe abnormality and has a total index of 41. This measurement method enables us to assess ETP quantitatively.

CLINICAL APPLICATION AND CLASSIFICATION OF ABNORMALITIES

The total index was calculated for all 70 patients. For the purpose of double checking, the ETP were classified through visual impression, before the

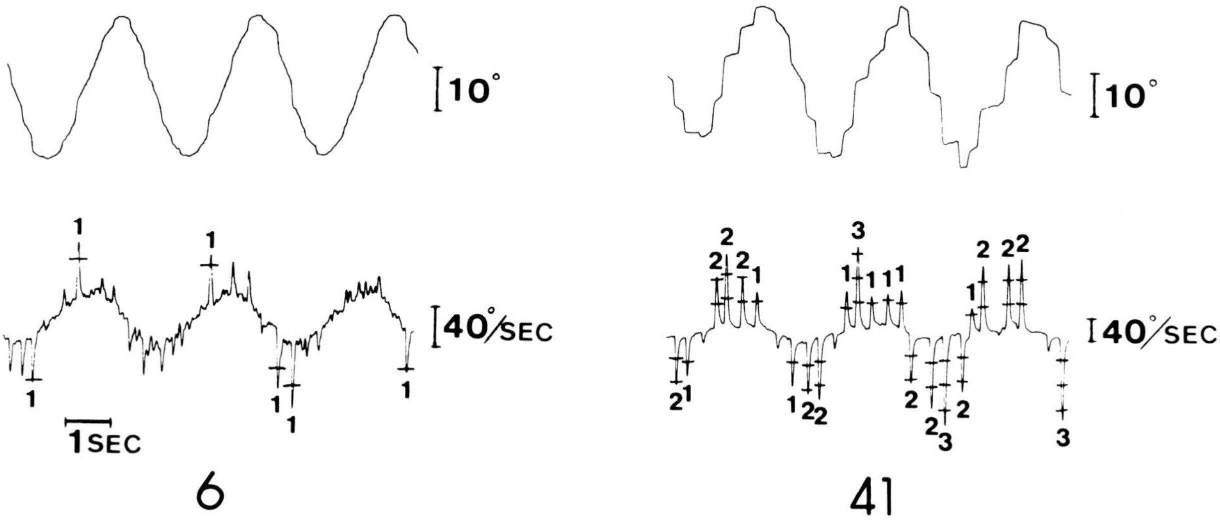

Fig. 3. Method of assessment. The method of Figure 2 was applied to the assessment of spikes appearing on three sine waves, and the total of the summed values of the spikes was made the total index. Left, an ETP with a slight abnormality and total index of 6. Right, an ETP with a severe abnormality and total index of 41. The calibrations are shown by the vertical bars to the right of each tracing: 10° for the eye movement (upper bars); 40°/sec for the eye velocity (lower bars).

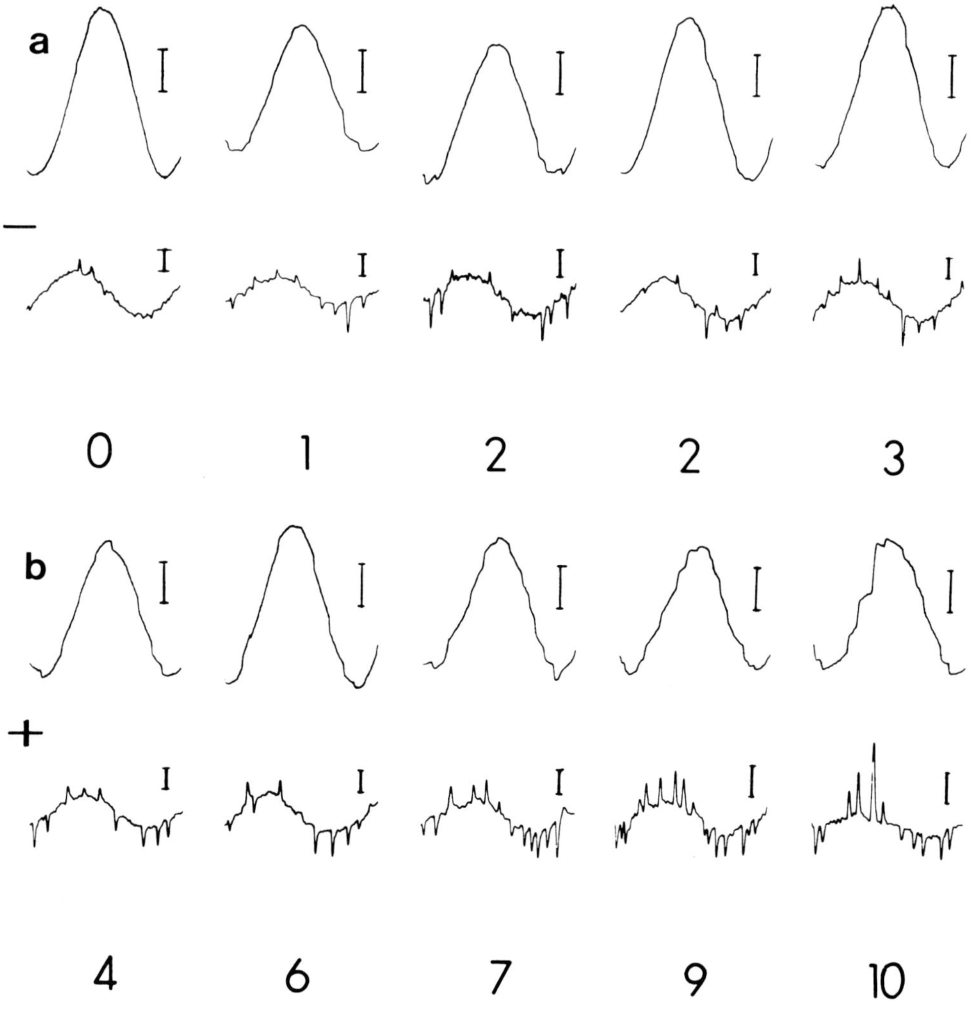

Fig. 4. Classification of abnormalities. Before the quantitative assessment, ETP were classified through visual impression into four groups: a) Normal; corresponded to total indices of 0-3. b) Slightly abnormal; corresponded to total indices of 4-10.

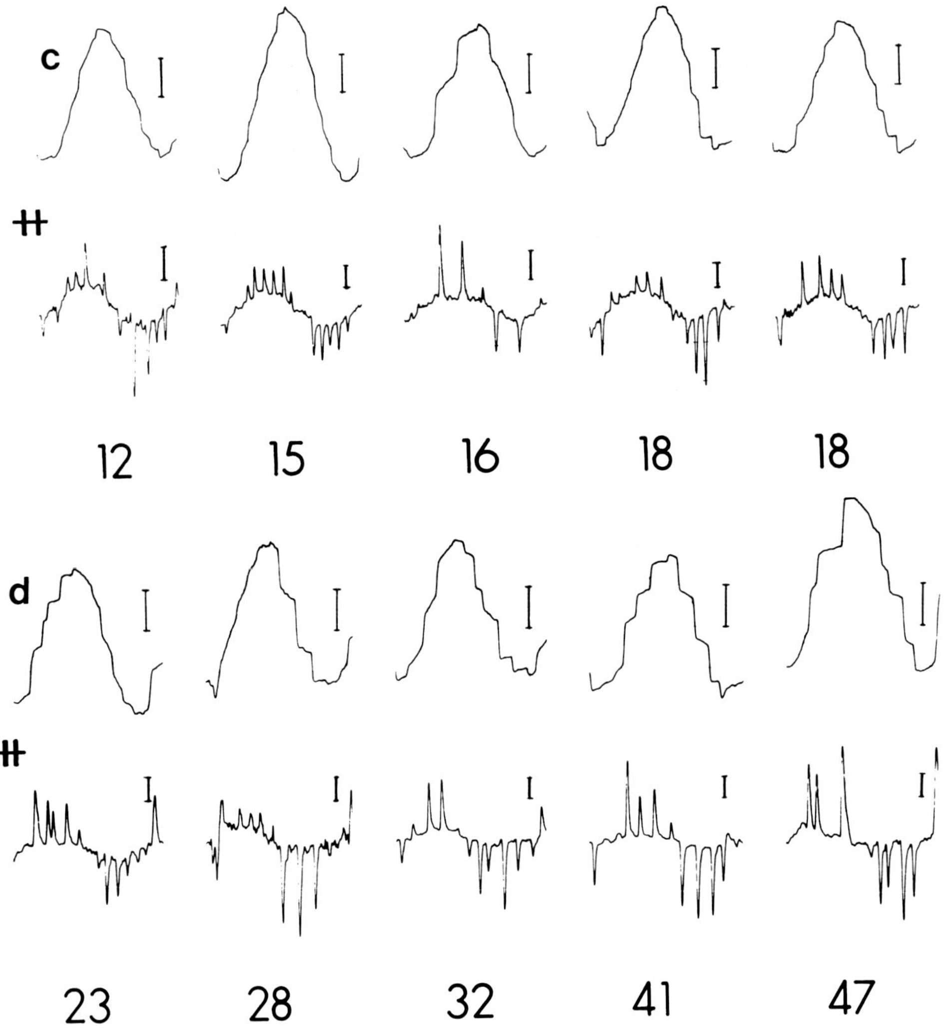

Fig. 4. (Con't) c) Moderately abnormal; corresponded to total indices of 11-20. d) Severely abnormal; corresponded to total indices of 21 or more.

quantitative assessment, into groups: (−) normal, (+) slightly abnormal, (+ +) moderately abnormal, and (+ + +) severely abnormal. It was found that (−) corresponded to total indices of 0-3 in 39 cases, (+) to total indices of 4-10 in 17 cases, (+ +) to total indices of 11-20 in 9 cases, and (+ + +) to total indices of 21 or more in 5 cases. Here, the manual quantitative measurement of ETP was found to be successful. In the control group all ETP were normal, with total indices always below three.

The total indices of all the cases were determined for spikes on three sine waves as shown in Figure 3. For want of space, however, only a part of each ETP is presented as a sample in Figure 4.

ANALYSIS OF A PREVIOUS RECORDING

Visual classifications so far undertaken cannot clearly distinguish borderline recordings. Figure 5 shows the influence of alcohol on the smooth pursuit movement when 100 ml of whiskey was given to a normal subject and her ETP were subsequently recorded. This recording was undertaken three years ago. By the application of the method herein presented, even delicate changes of the ETP could be quantitatively analyzed.

EXCEPTIONAL CASES TO QUANTITATIVE ASSESSMENT

The author also analyzed abnormal ETP other than those of the subjects for this study, and found that the ETP in two different cases did not warrant a quantitative assessment. The first was the ETP of a patient with progressive supranuclear palsy (Steel syndrome) of late stage. In this case the pursuit eye movement was disturbed almost completely and the total index was below three. The second case was the ETP presenting ocular bursts with irregular pauses. In this case (Fig. 6), since the irregularly appearing bursts (left record) were inconsistently superimposed on the ETP, the total index depended on the appearance of bursts. Moreover, as the spikes were not so high, the total index was relatively low for the severity of abnormality.

As a consequence of these conditions quantitative assessment was not applied to one case of severe

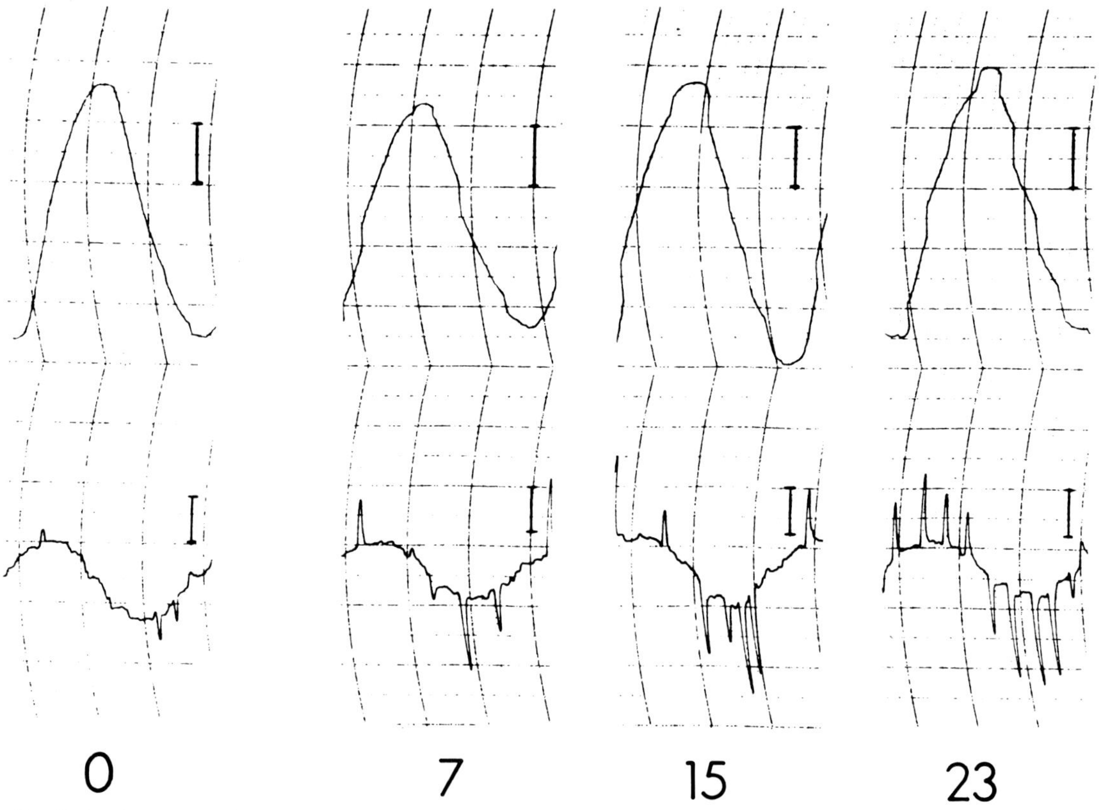

Fig. 5. Application to clinical research: alcohol and ETP. ETP were recorded after 100 ml of whiskey was given to a normal subject. Here, even delicate changes of the ETP could be analyzed quantitatively. Total index 0, before consumption of alcohol; total index 7, 10 minutes after consumption; total index 15, 20 minutes after consumption; and total index 23, 30 minutes after consumption.

ophthalmoplegia and another with burst eye movements.

DISCUSSION

QUANTITATIVE ASSESSMENT OF ETP

So far as we know, the quantitative assessment of ETP has also been undertaken with the aid of a computer in two manners: 1) by measuring the delay of the eye movement for target movement,[1] and 2) by computing 200 eye velocity samples per second.[2] These methods are useful in that they can be applied when computer analysis is commonly utilized in routine vestibular examinations. Until that time, the manual method presented in this paper will be useful.

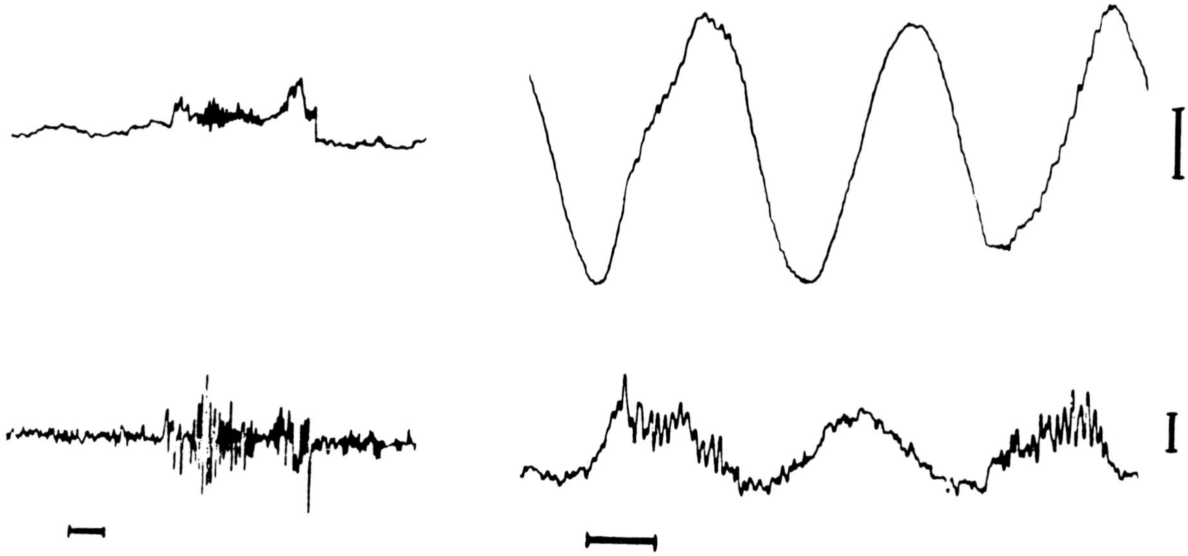

Fig. 6. Exceptional case to quantitative assessment. In this case presenting ocular bursts with irregular pauses (left record: at forward gaze of opened eyes), a quantitative assessment of ETP was meaningless.

UNIT FOR MEASUREMENT

As there were too many spikes to deal with, such small spikes as appeared in nearly normal ETP had to be omitted. In determining the unit for measurement, easy handling of the electronystagmograms is a necessary condition. At present, the electronystagmograph in this country contains an electrical circuit of delta waves of 1 Hz. As mentioned previously in Methods, the eye speed of 40°/sec is automatically obtained by means of the delta waves.

If 20° or 30°/sec were to be used for the measurement unit, too many small spikes would be picked up and the total index would become enormous. Conversely, at the height of 60°/sec, significant spikes would be omitted; at the height of 50°/sec it would be difficult to distinguish a normal from a slightly abnormal level. Consequently, 40°/sec is the most suitable unit for measurement.

SPIKES ON THREE SINE WAVES

ETP are reproductive, but the patterns of sine waves are not exactly reproduced. There are slight differences among them. For example, the ETP on the right side of Figure 3 presents indices of 11, 15,and 15 for the first, second and third sine waves, respectively. The more sine waves assessed, the more accurate the data. However, it is not practical to measure spikes on so many waves. After trial measurements of two, three and four sine waves, it was found that the assessment of three took a moderate amount of time and the resultant total indices were moderate in number.

REMAINING PROBLEMS

Among the many reports on eye-tracking patterns, target speeds are not standardized. In the establishment of a quantitative assessment method, the target speed must also be fixed in order to make a comparison of data from different clinics possible. This problem will be taken up in a subsequent paper.

CONCLUSION

As a method of quantitatively assessing ETP abnormalities, the author suggests a manual measurement of irregularities appearing on the eye speed trace. The measurement was undertaken with the aid of a compass and the abnormalities were expressed in numerals ranging from zero to 40 + .

ACKNOWLEDGMENTS — I wish to thank Professor Jiro Muto, Chief of the Otolaryngological Department of Saitama Medical School, for his unlimited help in this study. To Dr. Tsuneo Akaeda, MD, Akaeda Roppongi Clinic, I wish to express my sincere thanks for his kind advice. My sincere thanks are also due to Miss Etsuko Yoshida, Miss Mikako Ishii and Miss Masae Nozaki for their technical help.

REFERENCES

1. Mizukoshi K, Watanabe Y, Kato I, et al. Computer analysis of the eye-tracking test. Proceedings of 5th Extraordinary Meeting of the Bárány Society. Int J Equilib Res 1975; Suppl:158-62.

2. Baloh RW, Kumley WE, Sills AW, Honrubia V, Konrad HR. Quantitative measurement of smooth pursuit eye movements. Ann Otol Rhinol Laryngol 1976; 85:111-9.

3. Umeda Y, Sakata E. The circular eye-tracking test: I. Simultaneous recording of the horizontal and vertical component of eye movement in the eye-tracking test. ORL 1975; 37:290-8.

II. STANDARDIZATION OF THE EYE-TRACKING TEST

YOSHIO UMEDA, MD

SAITAMA, JAPAN

Standardization of the eye-tracking test, especially of the target velocity, is required for the purpose of comparing abnormalities of eye-tracking patterns recorded in different clinics. In consideration of the results of several good reports on target velocities, we have the following remarks: 1) The maximum velocity of a target which normal subjects can follow without delay of the eye movement is about 20°/sec. 2) When pursuit eye movements of normal subjects are registered with the aid of an electronystagmograph, the eye-tracking patterns will remain normal at target velocities of up to 45°/sec. 3) In order to detect abnormalities of pursuit eye movement with the aid of an electronystagmograph, the target velocity should be as fast as possible, but not exceeding 45°/sec. As an instrument for the examination of pursuit eye movements, for reasons outlined in the text, the Umeda circular eye-tracking test apparatus (amplitude 40°, frequency 0.33 Hz, and target velocity 42°/sec) is ideal. The target amplitude and technical problems in making the apparatus also are discussed.

INTRODUCTION

In a previous paper, the author reported a manual method of quantitative assessment of eye-tracking patterns and emphasized the importance of the standardization of the eye-tracking test.[1] A comparison of abnormalities of eye-tracking patterns recorded in different clinics or countries will be made possible by the standardization of target velocity.

EYE-TRACKING TEST IN CURRENT USE

The upper part of Table 1 indicates the diversity of target movements that have been used in eye-tracking tests with the aid of an electronystagmograph (ENG). In the seven reports shown,[2-8] amplitudes range from 15° to 60° and frequencies from 0.3 Hz to 0.5 Hz. Under these conditions, the maximum velocities of the targets produced a range from 24° to 63°/sec. For clarification, maximum velocities of sine wave targets in relation to amplitude and frequency are shown in Figure 1.

AMPL \ FREQ	0.5 Hz	0.4	0.33	0.3	0.25	0.2
10°	16	13	10	9	8	6
20°	31	25	21	19	16	13
30°	47	38	31	28	24	19
40°	63	50	42	38	31	25
50°	79	63	52	47	39	31

(DEGREE/SEC)

Fig. 1. Amplitude, frequency and maximum velocity. When the target moves in a sine wave, maximum velocity depends on frequency and amplitude. For the eye-tracking test with the aid of an electronystagmograph, maximum velocity should not exceed 45°/sec of visual angle. Velocities of over 45°/sec are shadowed. Numerals indicate maximum velocities in degrees/sec.

In this paper, velocities are presented in degree per second of visual angle, and when the target moved in a sine wave, the approximate value of maximum velocities was calculated by the following formula: π (3.14) x amplitude (degrees) x frequency (Hz). Fractions of 0.5 or more are rounded to one unit; those smaller than 0.5 are dropped. One-third Hertz is presented as 0.33 Hz, but 0.333 Hz was used in the actual calculation.

DISCUSSION OF THE MAXIMUM VELOCITY

In 1930 Dodge et al[9] (Table 1) analyzed the slow phase of optokinetic nystagmus, and eye movements were recorded photographically. They reported that smooth pursuit eye movements were maintained as long as target velocities were less than 40°/sec. The slow phase of optokinetic nystagmus consists of two steps, the first to catch the stimulus immediately after the quick phase of opto-

TABLE 1. MAXIMUM VELOCITY OF THE MOVING TARGET*

Author	*Year*	*Amplitude (degrees)*	*Frequency (Hz)*	*Max. Velocity (degrees/sec)*
Jung[2]	1964	60	0.3	57
Benitez[3]	1970	40	0.5	63
Troost[4]	1972	40	0.3	38
Corvera[5]	1973	20-15	0.5	24-31
Holzman[6]	1973	20	0.5	31
Umeda[7]	1975	40	0.33	42
Shagass[8]	1976	20	0.4	25

Author	Year		*Max. velocity of the target should*
Dodge[9]	1930	*Not exceed*	40°/sec
Westheimer[10]	1954	*Not exceed*	30°/sec
Noorden[11]	1962	*Not exceed*	45°/sec
Robinson[12]	1965	*Be between*	5°-20°/sec
Baloh[13] see text	1976		

*There are several well-analyzed fundamental reports on target velocity (lower part of the table). In practice, however, velocity and mode of target movement are not yet standardized. As a result a diversity of maximum target velocities was found (upper part of the table).

From the Department of Otolaryngology, Saitama Medical School Hospital, Moro, Saitama-ken, Japan.

kinetic nystagmus, and the second to follow the stimulus. These two sorts of eye movement were conducted in the short time of less than one second. On the other hand, actual movement of the target in the eye-tracking test continues for a relatively long time, usually for more than ten seconds. Therefore, use of the slow phase of optokinetic nystagmus is not appropriate for analysis of the pure function of smooth pursuit eye movements.

In 1954, Westheimer[10] used a target making a horizontal sine wave and recorded eye movements photographically. His experiment led to the conclusion that a target at a velocity of more than 30°/sec could not be followed.

In 1962, von Noorden and Mackensen[11] performed experiments with normal subjects with the aid of ENG. The target made a sine wave at an amplitude of 30° with frequencies ranging between 0.25 Hz and 1.6 Hz. Under these conditions, maximum velocities ranging from 24° to 151°/sec were produced. They concluded that the maximum velocity should not exceed 45°/sec for smooth pursuit by normal adult subjects.

The difference between the results of Westheimer (30°/sec) and von Noorden and Mackensen (45°/sec) was due to different methods of analysis. Westheimer used an eye camera and von Noorden and Mackensen used ENG. With the eye camera, abnormalities could be analyzed with the precision of 0.005 second as a unit of time. On the contrary, in the current eye-tracking test using ENG, abnormalities are analyzed by visual judgment of the deformation of eye-tracking patterns with a time constant of one second or more. This long duration of the time constant results in decreased precision in the analysis.

In 1965, more accurate data were described by Robinson.[12] He used the "method of a scleral search coil in a magnetic field" and reported that one could not follow a target without delay of eye movement at velocities of more than 20°/sec.

In 1976, Baloh et al[13] made an excellent study with the aid of a computer. In this experiment, they used a target moving in an amplitude of 36.5° at a constant velocity. For frequencies of 0.1, 0.3, 0.5, 0.7 and 0.9 Hz, velocities of 7.3°, 21.9°, 36.5°, 51.1° and 65.7°/sec respectively, were recorded. The analysis was carried out with 200 samples computed for one second of pursuit eye movements, eg, appropriate analysis revealed the following:

1. Normal subjects could follow a target moving at the velocity of 21.9°/sec without delay.

2. A target with a low velocity of 7.3°/sec could be followed both by normal subjects and patients. At such low velocity, however, patients could not be checked. When the targets moved at high velocities, such as 51.1° or 65.7°/sec, normal subjects could not follow them smoothly, and eye speed could not be kept constant.

3. As a result, a clear distinction between normal subjects and patients was made when the targets moved at the velocities of 21.9° and 36.5°/sec. Moreover, the distinction between subjects was clearer at the higher velocity. The faster the target moved, the more precisely the abnormality was disclosed.

These reports made by our predecessors led us to the following conclusions:

1. The maximum velocity of a target that normal subjects can follow without delay of eye movement is about 20°/sec.

2. When pursuit eye movements of normal subjects are recorded with an ENG, the eye-tracking patterns remain normal at target velocities of up to 45°/sec.

3. In order to detect abnormalities of pursuit eye movement with an ENG, the target velocity needs to be as fast as possible, but not in excess of 45°/sec.

MODE OF TARGET MOVEMENT

As a mode of target movement, a sine wave has been commonly used. But Baloh et al[13] emphasized that a constant velocity target would be ideal. On the other hand, Takemori and Ueno[14] reported that a target drawing an arc was easier to follow than one moving horizontally.

Since 1975, the author has been using the circular eye-tracking test apparatus for the analysis of pursuit eye movements.[7] In this test, the target moves in a clockwise circle (ie, linking *arcs*) with a radius of 20° (40° in amplitude) at a constant velocity with a frequency of 0.33 Hz. These conditions produce a *constant* velocity of *42°sec* for the target, which meets von Noorden and Mackensen's recommendation that the maximum velocity should not exceed 45°/sec. Moreover, horizontal and vertical eye-tracking patterns can be recorded simultaneously with this apparatus. These advantages led us to conclude that the circular eye-tracking test possesses the ideal target movement for the analysis of smooth pursuit function.

METHODS

Velocities of 21° and 42°/sec. In order to confirm the conclusions mentioned at the end of the section, Discussion of the Maximum Velocity, we performed the circular eye-tracking test on 30 patients and 13 normal subjects (Fig. 2a) with the targets moving at velocities of 21°/sec (amplitude 20°, frequency 0.33 Hz) and 42°/sec (amplitude 40°, frequency 0.33 Hz). The analysis was made on the horizontal component. The horizontal component of the circular eye-tracking test with a constant target velocity of 42°/sec is equivalent to a horizontal sine wave with a maximum velocity of 42°/sec.

The velocity of 42°/sec was chosen for the following reason. For standardization of the eye-tracking test, amplitudes and fre-

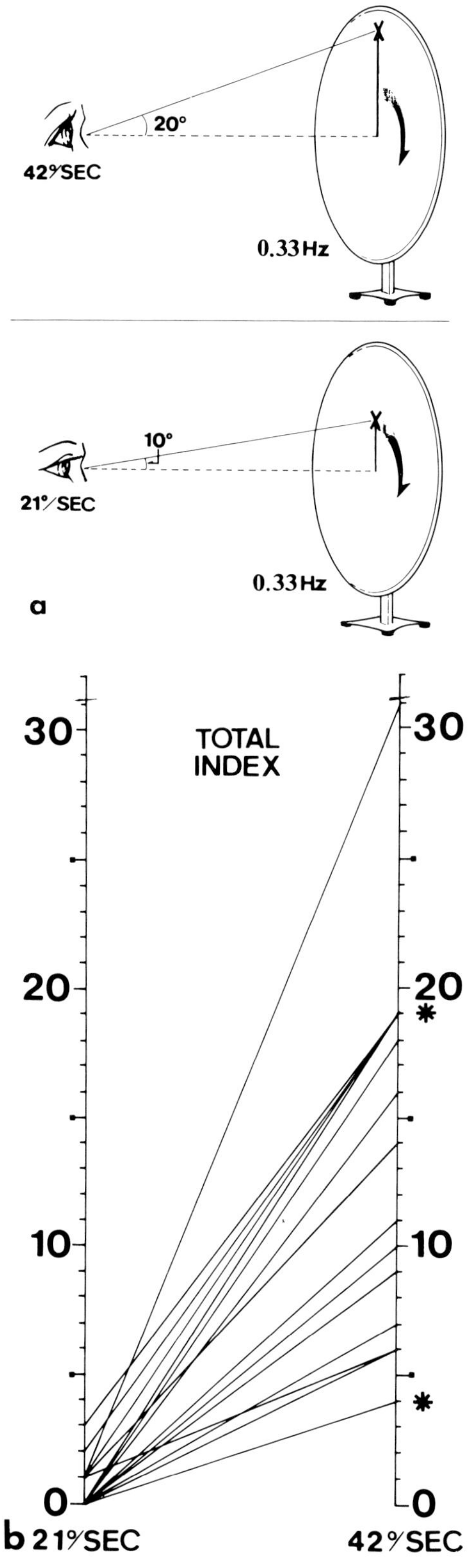

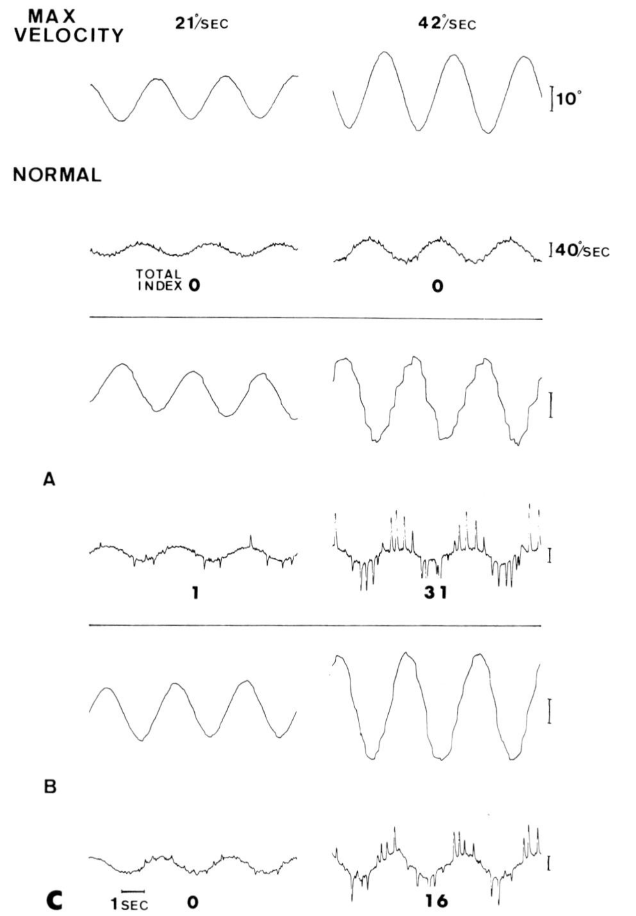

Fig. 2. a) Velocities of 21° and 42°/sec. Upper figure: amplitude of 40° (radius 20°), frequency of 0.33 Hz, and target velocity of 42°/sec. Lower figure: amplitude of 20° (radius 10°), frequency of 0.33 Hz, and target velocity of 21°/sec. b) Analysis of 18 cases with abnormal eye-tracking patterns. In the present study, abnormality could not be clearly detected at a velocity of 21°/sec (left). But when the target moved at 42°/sec, the abnormality appeared quite clearly (right). Numerals are total indices which indicate levels of abnormality. * - In three cases total indices changed from 0 at 21°/sec to 4 at 42°/sec, and in two cases indices changed from 2 to 19. c) Representative cases.

quencies should be presented in simple numerals (Fig. 1). Among the maximum velocities the velocity closest to but not exceeding 45°/sec was 42°/sec.

For comparison, 21°/sec was selected because it is closest to 20°/sec, which is the theoretical value of the velocity at which normal subjects can follow without delay of the eye movement.

With this test, in 18 of 30 patients whose pursuit function was disturbed, abnormalities of the eye-tracking pattern were more evident at 42° than at 21°/sec. Comparative results are shown in Figure 2b. Total indices[1] represent the quantitative assessment of levels of abnormality.

The pursuit function of normal subjects was not disturbed at

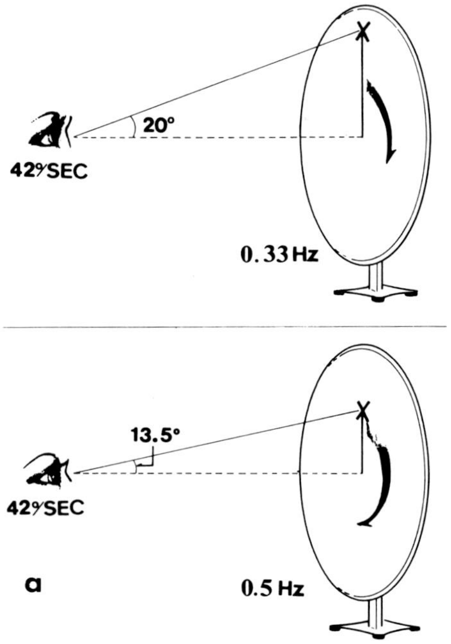

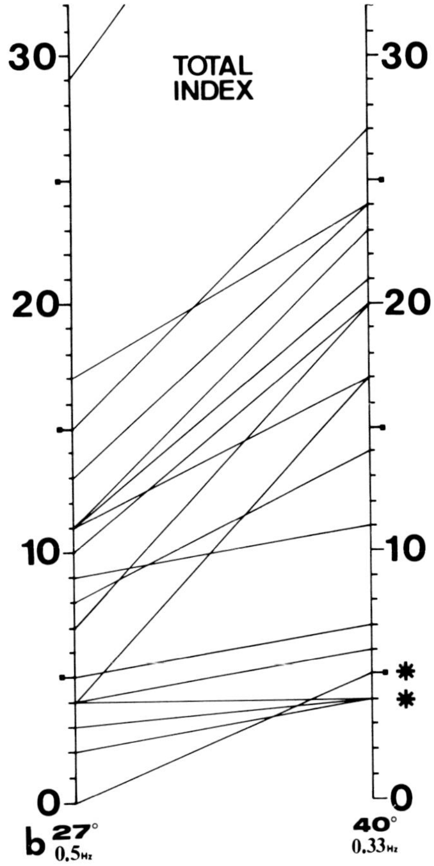

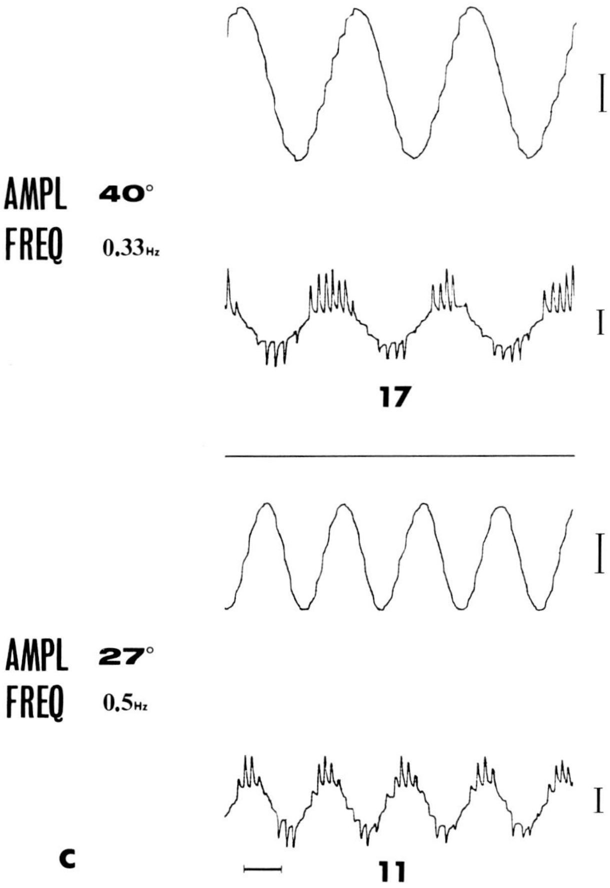

Fig. 3. a) 42°/sec with different amplitudes, 27° and 40°. 42°/sec with an amplitude of 40° and frequency of 0.33 Hz (upper figure) and with an amplitude of 27° and frequency of 0.5 Hz (lower figure). b) At the velocity of 42°/sec, abnormality could be more readily detected at the amplitude of 40° (right) than at 27° (left). * - In two cases, total indices changed from 0 (amplitude of 27°) to 5 (amplitude of 40°) and in two other cases indices did not change (4 with both amplitudes). c) Representative case. The upper record was the horizontal component of the circular eye-tracking test, with an amplitude of 40° and frequency of 0.33 Hz. The lower record was that with an amplitude of 27° and frequency of 0.5 Hz. Numerals indicate total indices. The calibrations correspond to those in Fig. 2b. In the eye-tracking pattern with an amplitude of 27° and frequency of 0.5 Hz, the total index was determined for the spikes appearing during nine seconds, ie, the duration which corresponds to three sine waves with a frequency of 0.33 Hz.

either velocity. Their total indices were within normal limits (three or less). It was interesting that the total indices determined at a velocity of 42°/sec had a tendency to present higher values than those determined at a velocity of 21°/sec (in seven normal subjects the total index was 0 at 21°/sec and 0 at 42°/sec; in three subjects it was 0 at 21°/sec and 1 at 42°/sec; in two subjects it was 0 at 21°/sec and 2 at 42°/sec; and in one normal subject the total index was 1 at 21°/sec and 3 at 42°/sec).

Velocity of 42°/sec with Different Amplitudes. As shown in Figure 1, identical values of maximum velocity can be produced with different amplitudes and frequencies. The circular eye-tracking test was administered to seven normal subjects at the velocity of 42°/sec with different amplitude-frequency combinations: amplitude 27°, frequency 0.5 Hz; amplitude 40°, frequency 0.33 Hz; and amplitude 54°, frequency 0.25 Hz. Many subjects complained of the annoyance of following a target moving

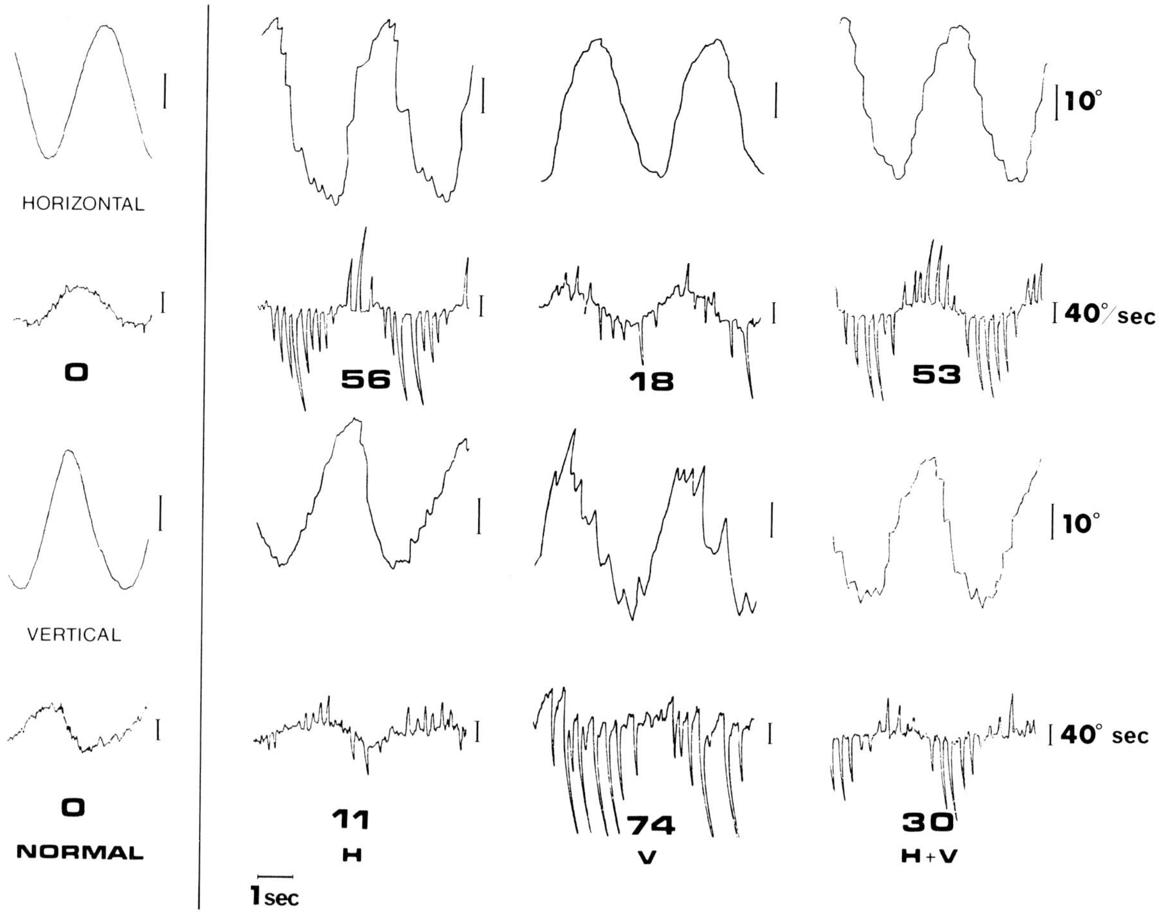

Fig. 4. The circular eye-tracking test. The first trace shows the electronystagmogram of the horizontal component of eye movement (time constant: 3.00 sec), and the second trace shows a differentiated electronystagmogram of the first trace, presenting the velocity of eye movement (time constant: 0.03 sec). The third trace shows the electronystagmogram of the vertical component of eye movement (time constant: 3.00 sec), and the fourth trace shows a differentiated electronystagmogram of the third trace, presenting the velocity of eye movement (time constant: 0.03 sec). Numerals indicate total indices. H -Horizontal component mainly disturbed (a case of horizontal congenital nystagmus). V - Vertical component mainly disturbed (a case of early-stage Arnold-Chiari malformation with vertical nystagmus). H + V - Horizontal and vertical components both disturbed (a case of late-stage Arnold-Chiari malformation, after the decompressive operation, without vertical nystagmus).

with an amplitude of 54°, ie, the visual angle of 27° to all lateral directions, though their eye-tracking patterns were almost normal. For this reason the amplitude of 54° was excluded in our research.

With the conditions of 27° and 40° in amplitude (Fig. 3a), the circular eye-tracking test was given to 30 patients, 20 of whom presented abnormal eye-tracking patterns. In seven abnormal cases, differences between the abnormalities detected under these two conditions were slight; the differences in total indices were three or less. In 13 cases, abnormalities were more evident with an amplitude of 40° and frequency of 0.33 Hz than with an amplitude of 27° and frequency of 0.5 Hz; differences in total indices were four or more (Fig. 3b). These analyses were also made on the horizontal components of the circular eye-tracking test. Figure 3c shows a representative record in which the level of abnormality was higher at 40° than at 27°.

Consequently, in the circular eye-tracking test the target amplitude should be as great as possible up to 54°, at which pursuit is annoying for the subject.

Technical Problems. In order to compare eye-tracking patterns in different clinics or countries, the amplitude, frequency and mode of movement of a target must be standardized. Moreover, it is desirable that an apparatus be simple and inexpensive.

When a visual target of the circular eye-tracking test is set 70 cm in front of the subject, the diameter of the circle increases in proportion to the amplitude: 27° in amplitude, 34 cm in diameter; 40° in amplitude, 51 cm in diameter; 54° in amplitude, 71 cm in diameter. A larger amplitude makes the apparatus bigger, and a bigger apparatus needs a more powerful motor. On the other hand, the time required for one rotation of the motor (circle) consists of seconds: 2 seconds (0.5 Hz), 3 seconds (0.33 Hz), and 4 seconds (0.25 Hz).

The following conditions produce the velocity of 42°/sec:

1. 27° in amplitude, 0.5 Hz in frequency, 34 cm in diameter;
2. 40°, 0.33 Hz, 51 cm;
3. 54°, 0.25 Hz, 71 cm.

Conditions with the amplitudes 27° and 54° should be excluded for the reasons mentioned in the preceding section. Thus, target movement at an amplitude of 40° with frequency of 0.33 Hz, which corresponds to the velocity of 42°/sec resulting from the Umeda circular eye-tracking test, is ideal. Figure 4 shows representative recordings made by this test.

CONCLUSIONS

With the aim of standardizing the eye-tracking test, the author has reviewed the literature and his own experiments. From this, it follows that the target velocity in the eye-tracking test with the aid of an ENG should be as fast as possible up to 45°/sec. For reasons noted, the circular eye-tracking test (amplitude 40°, frequency 0.33 Hz, and velocity 42°/sec) meets this requirement ideally.

ACKNOWLEDGMENT — The author wishes to thank Professor Jiro Muto, Chief of the Otolaryngological Department of Saitama Medical School, for his unlimited help in this study. To Dr. Tsuneo Akaeda, MD, Akaeda Roppongi Clinic, the author wishes to express sincere thanks for his kind advice. The author's thanks are also due to Miss Mikako Ishii, Miss Etsuko Yoshida, and Miss Masae Nozaki for their technical help.

REFERENCES

1. Umeda Y. Manual quantitative assessment of eye-tracking patterns. Ann Otol Rhinol Laryngol 1980; 89 Suppl 71:1-6.

2. Jung R, Kornhuber HH. Results of electronystagmography in man: the value of optokinetic, vestibular, and spontaneous nystagmus for neurologic diagnosis and research. In Bender MB, ed. The oculomotor system. New York: Harper and Row, 1964:428-88.

3. Benitez JT. Eye-tracking and optokinetic tests : diagnostic significance in peripheral and central vestibular disorders. Laryngoscope 1970; 80:834-48.

4. Troost BT, Daroff RB, Weber RB, et al. Hemispheric control of eye movements: II. Quantitative analysis of smooth pursuit in a hemispherectomy patient. Arch Neurol 1972; 27:449-52.

5. Corvera J, Torres-Courtney G, Lopez-Rios G. The neurotological significance of alterations of pursuit eye movements and the pendular eye tracking test. Ann Otol Rhinol Laryngol 1973; 82:855-67.

6. Holzman PS, Proctor LR, Hughes DW. Eye-tracking patterns in schizophrenia. Science 1973; 181:179-81.

7. Umeda Y, Sakata E. The circular eye-tracking test: I. Simultaneous recording of the horizontal and vertical component of eye movement in the eye-tracking test. ORL 1975; 37:290-8.

8. Shagass C, Roemer RA, Amadeo M. Eye-tracking performance and engagement of attention. Arch Gen Psychiatry 1976; 33:121-5.

9. Dodge R, Travis RC, Fox JC. Optic nystagmus: III. Characteristics of the slow phase. Arch Neurol 1930; 24:21-34.

10. Westheimer G. Eye movement responses to a horizontally moving visual stimulus. Arch Ophthalmol 1954; 52:932-41.

11. Von Noorden GK, Mackensen G. Pursuit movements of normal and amblyopic eyes: an electro-ophthalmographic study: I. Physiology of pursuit movements. Am J Ophthalmol 1962; 53:325-36.

12. Robinson DA. The mechanics of human smooth pursuit eye movement. J Physiol 1965; 180:569-91.

13. Baloh RW, Kumley WE, Sills AW, Honrubia V, Konrad HR. Quantitative measurement of smooth pursuit eye movements. Ann Otol Rhinol Laryngol 1976; 85:111-9.

14. Takemori S, Ueno M. An evaluation of eye tracking pattern induced by three different instruments. (In Japanese.) Practica Otologica Kyoto 1975; 68:723-30.

THYROID DISEASE:
A GUIDE FOR THE HEAD AND NECK SURGEON

Robert M. Bumsted, MD

Supplement 72 — Vol. 89, July-August, 1980, No. 4, Part 4

THE ANNALS OF OTOLOGY, RHINOLOGY & LARYNGOLOGY

THE ANNALS PUBLISHING COMPANY
4949 FOREST PARK BLVD.
ST. LOUIS, MISSOURI 63108

THYROID DISEASE: A GUIDE FOR THE HEAD AND NECK SURGEON

ROBERT M. BUMSTED, MD
IOWA CITY, IOWA

Head and neck surgeons are involved in the diagnosis and therapy of thyroid disease with increasing frequency. The surgical techniques utilized for the management of thyroid disease are well known by most head and neck surgeons and will not be discussed in this paper. It is the head and neck surgeons' knowledge of the physiology, medical disorders, and the proper evaluation of the patient with thyroid disease that is most open to criticism. This paper reviews thyroid physiology, basic tests used to assess thyroid function in health and disease, thyroiditis, thyroid carcinomas, and nodules of the thyroid gland. The signs, symptoms, laboratory findings, and the methods of medical and surgical therapy are discussed for each of these disorders. The supplement is not intended to provide expertise, but will provide a general and basic knowledge of thyroid disease.

INTRODUCTION

Otolaryngologists (head and neck surgeons) are involved in the diagnosis and therapy of disorders of the thyroid gland with increasing frequency. This is a natural extension of their expertise in the surgical management of disorders of the head and neck. Surgical procedures are frequently performed by otolaryngologists in the area of the thyroid gland during operations on the larynx and trachea. In addition, their ability to perform standard or modified neck dissections cannot be disputed. Consequently, the otolaryngologist's knowledge of the surgical anatomy in this area should be commensurate with that of any other surgical specialty.

Vocal cord paralysis and airway problems are among the most common complications of operations performed on the thyroid gland. The otolaryngologist is the most adequately trained specialist to manage these complications.

It is the otolaryngologists' knowledge of the physiology of the thyroid and medical disorders that involve this gland that is most open to challenge in their role in the management of patients with thyroid disorders. This paper is not intended to provide expertise, but a general knowledge of thyroid physiology, thyroiditis, thyroid carcinoma, and the management of nodules of the thyroid gland. The management of hyperthyroidism and hypothyroidism is discussed in standard texts and will not be covered here. This paper will be valuable as a basic foundation, should the interested reader decide to pursue the subject in depth.

THYROID PHYSIOLOGY

This discussion of thyroid physiology is not comprehensive, but the basic parameters are presented. The mechanism and control of thyroid hormone production and its known effects will be discussed.

The production and secretion of thyroid hormones is influenced primarily by the thyroid gland itself, the pituitary gland, and the hypothalamus. Thyroid hormones are produced and secreted by the thyroid gland. This is completely controlled by the level of thyroid stimulating hormone (thyrotropin, TSH) which is produced and secreted by the basophil cells of the anterior portion of the pituitary gland. The hypothalamus also plays a role in the secretion of TSH. Thus, the adequate functioning of all these parameters is necessary for normal thyroid gland function. Diseases producing an abnormality of any of these factors may cause abnormal thyroid gland function (Fig. 1).

The primary hormones secreted by the thyroid gland are tetraiodothyronine (T_4, thyroxine) and triiodothyronine (T_3). These compounds are formed by the addition of iodide ions to the amino acid tyrosine. Iodine is selectively trapped by the thyroid gland; however, this is under the total control of

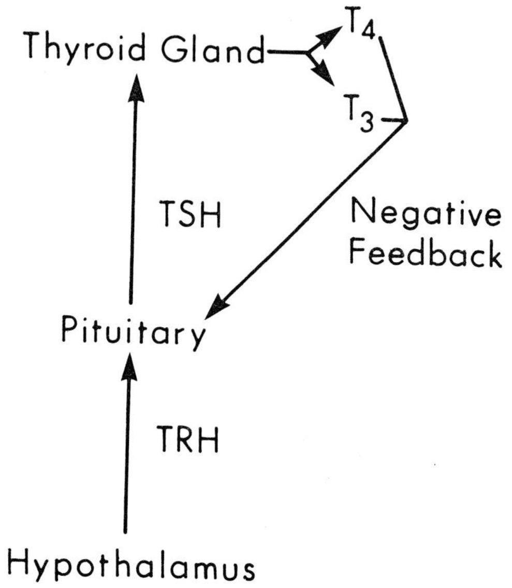

Fig. 1. Thyroid physiology. Schematic diagram illustrating the interrelationship of the thyroid, pituitary, and hypothalamus.

From the Department of Otolaryngology and Maxillofacial Surgery, University of Iowa Hospitals and Clinics, Iowa City, Iowa.

TSH. Once formed, these hormones are stored as thyroglobulin which is the main component of colloid found in the thyroid follicle. Release of these hormones into the circulation is caused by the action of proteolytic enzymes on thyroglobulin, again under the complete control of TSH.

These hormones are essential for normal metabolic function, the development of the body and brain, reproduction, and retardation of some aspects of aging.[1] Presently, many authorities feel that T_4 is a prohormone and the active cellular hormone is T_3. T_4 is apparently converted to T_3 in peripheral tissues in order to exert its effect.[2] Except in unusual cases, the concentration of circulatory T_3 is quite low relative to T_4. In addition, catecholamines may be required for the expression of many of the effects of thyroid hormones.[3]

In serum, thyroid hormones are bound to three circulating serum proteins: thyroxine-binding globulin (TBG), thyroxine-binding prealbumin (TBPA), and thyroxine-binding albumin (TBA). Approximately 75-80% of the hormones are bound to TBG and it is the major determinant of the normal serum levels of T_3 and T_4.[2] The small fraction of hormone which is not bound to protein is called the free fraction and is presumably the metabolically active hormone. Thyroxine (T_4) is 99.97% bound to serum proteins in the blood.[4] Triiodothyronine (T_3) is much less tightly bound to plasma proteins than T_4 (99.66%), but binding is still a significant factor in determining circulating levels of T_3.

Two main factors determine the concentration of circulating thyroid hormone. The first is the level of thyroid hormone production and the second is the concentration of thyroid hormone binding proteins. It is recognized that it is not the total, but the free or unbound thyroid hormone concentration which best correlates with thyroid status.

Thyroid stimulating hormone (TSH) controls iodide uptake, thyroid hormone production and release by the thyroid gland. The production and release of this anterior pituitary hormone is controlled by a negative feedback mechanism of the blood levels of thyroid hormone and thyrotropin releasing hormone (TRH) from the hypothalamus. This hormone (which cannot be measured in serum by a routine clinical method at this time) appears to sensitize the pituitary gland to the negative feedback inhibition of circulating thyroid hormones.[5]

A deficiency of thyroid hormone production may result from disorders in any of the above areas. Diseases of the thyroid gland itself result in primary hypothyroidism. Secondary hypothyroidism is caused by a lack of production of TSH by the pituitary, and tertiary hypothyroidism is secondary to a disorder of the hypothalamus. This deficiency in fetal or neonatal life results in cretinism while onset at an older age produces hypothyroidism.

TABLE 1. THYROID FUNCTION TESTS

- A. Serum thyroxine (T_4)
  1. Protein-bound iodine (PBI)
  2. Competitive protein binding displacement
  3. Radioimmunoassay
- B. Serum triiodothyronine (T_3) — radioimmunoassay
- C. Thyroid binding globulin (TBG) — T_3 uptake
- D. Thyrotropin (TSH) — radioimmunoassay
- E. Thyroid scan and uptake
- F. Thyroid antibody tests
- G. Ultrasonography
- H. Other tests of thyroid function
  1. Cytomil (T_3) suppression test
  2. Thyrotropin-releasing hormone test

Classically, cretinism causes dwarfism, mental retardation, failure to thrive, enlarged tongue, umbilical hernia, thick and dry skin, hyporeflexia, and retarded bone age. Adult hypothyroidism is typically manifest by cold intolerance, dry skin, constipation, weight gain, hair loss, fatigue, retarded mentation, and a slow reflex relaxation phase. Common otolaryngologic manifestations include thyroid gland enlargement, hearing loss, hoarseness, enlarged tongue, and nasal obstruction.[5]

The most common causes of primary hypothyroidism are lymphocytic (Hashimoto's) thyroiditis and radioiodine therapy of thyrotoxicosis. Secondary hypothyroidism is caused by pituitary disorders such as neoplasia, granulomas or infarction. Tertiary hypothyroidism is rare.

Excessive production of thyroid hormones results in hyperthyroidism. Common signs and symptoms include fatigue and weakness, tachycardia, weight loss with increased appetite, a fine tremor, heat intolerance, excessive sweating, brisk reflexes, and lid lag.

The most common cause of hyperthyroidism is Graves' disease which is most likely caused by a disturbance of the immune system.[6] Ophthalmologic disorders (most commonly proptosis) are frequently associated with Graves' disease. Other causes of hyperthyroidism include an autonomous toxic nodule, subacute thyroiditis, pituitary tumors (secreting TSH), excessive thyroid hormone ingestion and rarely tumors secreting TSH-like hormones or hypersecretion of triiodothyronine (T_3) by the thyroid (T_3 toxicosis).[7] These patients have the signs and symptoms of hyperthyroidism with normal thyroxine and elevated triiodothyronine levels.

THYROID FUNCTION TESTS (TABLE 1)

A. AND B. QUANTITATION OF SERUM THYROXINE (T_4) AND TRIIODOTHYRONINE (T_3)

1. Protein-bound iodine (PBI) is the classical method used for evaluation of circulating thyroid hormone. This is a nonspecific test as two thirds of the T_4 molecule is iodine and in normal subjects

80-90% of the PBI is T_4. However, values are often falsely high secondary to iodine contamination from medications containing iodine (expectorants, etc), radiopaque contrast media, and others. This test is still useful for specific problems in thyroid disease such as Hashimoto's or subacute thyroiditis, where thyroidal iodoproteins are present in the circulation in increased amounts. However, it is now largely surpassed by more specific tests.

2. The competitive protein binding displacement assay (Murphy-Patee) is performed by determining the amount of displacement of a radioactive labeled T_4 from a relatively specific binding protein caused by T_4 in an ethanol extract of the patient's serum. The more T_4 present in the patient's serum the more the labeled T_4 is displaced from the binding protein. It is the size, shape, and charge of the T_4 molecule rather than its iodine content which provide the response in this test. It is more specific than the PBI test.

3. Radioimmunoassay is the most recent advance and is based on the same principle as the competitive protein binding assay.[9] It is extremely sensitive and very small quantities (2.5 to 25 μl of serum are required) may be used for this assay. This method is also utilized for the determination of T_3.

C. ASSAY OF THYROID BINDING GLOBULIN (TBG) — T_3 UPTAKE

The amount of circulating TBG is indirectly evaluated by the resin uptake test. In this test, radioactive T_3 or T_4 is added to the patient's serum and mixed. A resin sponge is then added to the mixture which absorbs the unbound fraction of the radioactive T_3 or T_4. The amount of labeled hormone bound to serum proteins is directly proportional to the concentration of unoccupied TBG binding sites; the more sites available, the smaller the quantity of the added labeled hormone absorbed to the resin, and, as usually reported, the lower the value. The resin uptake is a direct reflection of the fraction of the added labeled hormone that is free (nonbound) and is, therefore, lower in patients with TBG excess and higher in patients with TBG deficiency. TBG excess results in an elevated serum hormone concentation but a lower resin uptake. The opposite is true of TBG deficiency.

Analyzing the level of serum T_3 and T_4 in relation to the T_3 uptake gives the most accurate assessment of thyroid function. Multiplication of these two factors (hormone levels and resin uptake) reflects the actual free (metabolically active) hormone concentration. This is frequently called the free thyroxine index or T_7.

Causes of increased TBG (which will increase serum levels of T_3 and T_4 and decrease resin uptake) include pregnancy, oral contraceptives, excess estrogens, cirrhosis (sometimes), infectious hepatitis (sometimes) and occasionally an inherited condition. Causes of decreased TBG (which decreases levels of T_3 and T_4 and increases the resin uptake) include androgens, acromegaly (sometimes), nephrotic syndrome, hypoproteinemic states, and occasionally an inherited deficiency.

D. ASSAY OF THYROTROPIN (TSH)

TSH measurement by radioimmunoassay is now available and is useful in detecting early hypothyroidism secondary to thyroid gland dysfunction. In fact, it is the most sensitive test available for the detection of primary hypothyroidism. TSH is readily and reproducibly detectable at elevated levels (which are seen in early hypothyroidism secondary to thyroid dysfunction); however, it is impossible to differentiate low values from normal values and therefore the test is only used to diagnose hypothyroidism. TRH may be measured in the serum on an experimental basis but is not available at this time as a routine laboratory test.

E. THYROID SCAN AND UPTAKE

Thyroid scanning is usually used to determine if function of the thyroid gland is due to a diffuse or localized increase in function and if the functional activity of a single or dominant thyroid nodule is "cold" (does not concentrate radioactive material), "hot" (concentrates radioactive material) or isofunctional (concentrates similarly to the rest of the gland). The incidence of malignancy is much greater in a cold nodule.

Radioisotope tests of thyroid function are commonly performed with ^{131}I, ^{123}I, and ^{99m}Tc. ^{123}I is preferred to ^{131}I as the radiation dose is lower. ^{99m}Tc provides the lowest radiation dose of the above isotopes and is used primarily for determining functional activity of thyroid nodules rather than glandular uptake. In addition to a lower radiation exposure, the scan may be performed within an hour after injection rather than the following day as required by the iodine isotopes. A disadvantage of this isotope is that an occasional nodule appears "hot" with technetium which is "cold" on iodine scan.[5] Other isotopes reported include ^{75}Se, ^{67}Ga, ^{197}Hg, and ^{99m}Tc-bleomycin. However, frequent deviations from the results of iodine scans markedly limit their specificity and usefulness.

The thyroid uptake test measures the capacity of the thyroid gland to accumulate iodine. The primary problem (which has arisen recently) with the interpretation of the results of this test has been the apparent decrease in the normal range for the 24-hour uptake of iodine. This apparently reflects an increase in the average dietary ingestion of iodine in the United States. As a result of this, discrimination between hypothyroid and normal ranges has become very difficult. Causes of decreased uptake are hypothyroidism, ingestion of substances containing iodine, ingestion of thyroid hormone, TSH deficiency, and the use of medications which inhibit organification of iodine (tolbutamide, reserpine, phenylbutazone, para-aminosalicylic acid, and antithyroid agents). Elevated uptakes are seen in patients with hyperthyroidism and iodine deficiency. At the present time this test is useful only for detecting thyroid hyperfunction.

F. THYROID ANTIBODY TESTS

The tanned red cell agglutination method is a sensitive test for detecting thyroglobulin antibodies. Low titers (less than 1:1000) are seen in a variety of thyroid disorders such as Graves' disease, thyroid cancer, or acute thyroiditis. High titers (greater than 1:10,000) are seen in over 90% of patients with autoimmune (Hashimoto's) thyroiditis. This is the most sensitive test to demonstrate thyroglobulin antibodies.

Another method of detecting thyroid antibodies is to measure antithyroid microsomal antibodies by a complement fixation test. Titers of greater than 1:64 support a diagnosis of autoimmune thyroiditis. This is seen in 98% of patients with this disorder.

Other antibodies demonstrated in patients with thyroid disease include an antibody against a colloid component other than thyroglobulin and an antinuclear component.

All of the above antibodies are generally present in high titer in Hashimoto's thyroiditis, but may be seen in low levels of Graves' disease, asymptomatic relatives of patients with Graves' disease and Hashimoto's thyroiditis, thyroid cancer, and in some apparently normal persons.[10]

G. ULTRASONOGRAPHY

Nodules of the thyroid may be evaluated by ultrasound techniques to differentiate solid from cystic lesions. This is an easily performed, noninvasive technique which provides accurate differentiation of solid and cystic lesions in the 80-90% of lesions.[11,12] This provides additional information (and confirmation of physical findings) which is important in the management of nodules of the thyroid.

H. OTHER TESTS OF THYROID FUNCTION

The cytomil (T_3) suppression test is performed by treating the patient with 75 μg of cytomil per day for one to two weeks and then performing a scan. This test is used primarily to determine if a hyperfunctioning thyroid gland or nodule is autonomous (functioning independently of TSH). The radioisotope uptake of a normal or nonautonomous gland will be suppressed while autonomous glands and nodules continue to concentrate radioactive iodine.[13]

The thyrotropin-releasing hormone test involves the intravenous administration of TRH and measuring the response of the serum TSH 30 minutes later. TRH is a tripeptide which has been purified and synthesized. Patients with primary (thyroid) hypothyroidism have elevated TSH levels and are hyperresponsive to TRH. Secondary (pituitary) hypothyroidism has essentially no response to TRH. Tertiary (hypothalamic) hypothyroidism demonstrates a mild and delayed response. Thus, this test allows the determination of the source of hypothyroidism.[1]

TABLE 2. CLASSIFICATION OF THYROIDITIS*

- A. Inflammatory thyroiditis due to known agents
  - 1. Infectious
    - a. Acute
    - b. Chronic
  - 2. Thyroiditis secondary to other agents
    - a. Trauma
    - b. Radiation
- B. Inflammatory thyroiditis due to unknown agents
  - 1. Subacute (deQuervain's)
  - 2. Invasive fibrous (Riedel's struma)
- C. Autoimmune thyroiditis
  - 1. Struma lymphomatosa (Hashimoto's)
  - 2. Lymphocytic

*Adapted from Strahan et al.[14]

THYROIDITIS (TABLE 2)

Thyroiditis in its present usage includes diseases of the thyroid gland known to be caused by infectious agents and all lesions which have a lymphoid infiltrate. The classification used in this presentation was proposed by Strahan et al[14] (Table 2).

A. Inflammatory Thyroiditis Due to Known Agents

1. Infectious

a. Acute: This occurs infrequently and is most often associated with sepsis. It is more common in females and occurs most frequently in the 20 to 40 age group.[14] It occurs after acute infections of the pharynx and upper respiratory tract. Specific routes of invasion include the bloodstream, direct invasion from contiguous structures, the lymphatics, direct trauma, and a persistent thyroglossal duct.[15]

Streptococcus hemolyticus, *Staphylococcus aureus*, and pneumococcus are the most common bacteria isolated from these cases. This disease may also be precipitated by viral diseases. These include chicken pox, measles, and cat scratch fever.[14]

Patients usually have an abrupt onset of fever, chills, pain (which is frequently referred to the mandible or ear), with marked local tenderness, swelling, and occasional fluctuation of the area of the thyroid gland. Cough, hoarseness and aphasia may be present. Dyspnea occurs in more than half of the patients and tracheotomy may be necessary.[15]

The differential diagnosis includes subacute

thyroiditis, cellulitis, cervical adenitis, perichondritis of the thyroid cartilage, acute hemorrhage into a thyroid adenoma, fulminant malignancy, and rarely Riedel's struma.

Initial therapy is the administration of appropriate antibiotics. Abscess formation is uncommon but does require surgical drainage when present. Steroids may be of benefit in thyroiditis associated with viruses. The usual duration is 7-14 days.[15]

Complications include rupture anteriorly through the strap muscles beneath the skin, posteriorly into the esophagus or trachea, or inferiorly into the mediastinum. Laryngeal edema necessitating a tracheotomy may result. Thyroid function is usually normal after the infection resolves.

b. Chronic: Chronic infectious thyroiditis may be caused by echinococcus, actinomycosis, tuberculosis, or syphilis.

Tuberculous thyroiditis is most commonly caused by disseminated tuberculosis. Rare causes include direct extension from cervical or laryngeal involvement and occurrence as a primary disease. Diffuse enlargement with nodule formation is present on clinical examination.[16] Therapy includes appropriate antitubercular medication, incision and drainage, and occasionally subtotal thyroidectomy in cases which fail to respond to medical management.

Syphilitic thyroiditis most commonly presents as a gumma, although it may appear as a diffuse thyroiditis. It is usually unilateral. The swelling is smooth and nodular, often with cervical lymph node involvement. Diagnosis is by histologic examination of the tissue and serology. The response to antisyphilitic therapy is usually excellent.[14]

2. Thyroiditis Secondary to Other Agents

a. Trauma: Trauma is a rare cause of thyroiditis. However, rupture of the thyroid capsule may permit the entrance of bacteria producing thyroiditis. Therapy is that of infectious thyroiditis.

b. Radiation: Both gamma rays from an external source and beta rays from radioactive iodine cause inflammatory changes in the thyroid. The clinical severity is not necessarily dose-related. Symptoms are erythema, edema, and tenderness. In cases with severe edema, tracheotomy may be necessary. Treatment is symptomatic and the inflammation usually subsides by the twelfth week after completion of therapy.[14]

B. Inflammatory Thyroiditis Due to an Unknown Etiologic Agent

1. Subacute or deQuervain's thyroiditis: This is also known as granulomatous thyroiditis, giant cell thyroiditis, creeping thyroiditis, struma granulomatosa, acute noninfectious thyroiditis, acute simple thyroiditis, pseudogiant cell thyroiditis, and pseudotuberculous thyroiditis. A viral etiology is suspected.[10,14] Clinical aspects which seem to resemble a benign viral infection include the following conditions. It is often preceded by an upper respiratory tract infection and the illness often occurs at the time of an outbreak of a specific viral disease. It has been reported in association with mumps, measles, influenza, the common cold, adenovirus, Coxsackie virus, infectious mononucleosis and cat scratch fever.[10] Frequently a prodromal phase of muscular aches, malaise, and fatigue is present. Leukocytosis rarely occurs and after some weeks or months complete recovery is usual. It is felt that subacute thyroiditis represents a stereotyped inflammatory response to any number of a certain variety of viruses.[17]

Subacute thyroiditis is more common in females (4:1 to 6:1),[14] and usually occurs in the fourth and fifth decades.[18] The onset may be acute but is often mild with sore throat, malaise, odynophagia and dysphagia, with pain and tenderness in the thyroid gland. Initially the gland is tender, although enlargement may not occur until later. The disease may be unilateral in 20% of the cases.[19] The tenderness of the gland is probably the most important diagnostic sign.[18]

Laboratory tests demonstrate a high erythrocyte sedimentation rate, an absent or very low titer of antithyroid antibodies, and a low uptake on thyroid scan. Serum T_4 levels are usually normal but may be elevated due to increased absorption from damaged follicles.[10,18]

Differential diagnosis includes acute infectious thyroiditis, hemorrhage into an adenoma, acute hyperthyroidism, nodular goiter, and carcinoma. Needle biopsy is usually recommended to establish the diagnosis (when in question). However, surgical exploration and biopsy may be necessary to differentiate this disease from carcinoma. At surgical exploration, perithyroiditis is usually present but the capsule of the gland is identifiable and separates from the trachea and adjacent muscles (this distinguishes this disease from Riedel's struma).[15]

Microscopic features include follicular degeneration, variable fibrous replacement, and infiltration of leukocytes, lymphocytes, and plasma cells. The presence of histocytes and giant cells produces a tuberculoid appearance (caseous necrosis is never seen), which is the characteristic feature of subacute thyroiditis.

Treatment is with steroids which do not cure the disease but suppress the symptoms until the illness has run its course. Surgical intervention is used for those patients in whom medical therapy has failed or when carcinoma is suspected.[15]

One of the main features of subacute thyroiditis is its well-defined course which is principally self-limiting and persists no longer than one to three months. Generally there is no subsequent derangement of thyroid function.

2. Invasive fibrous thyroiditis or Riedel's struma: This disease (also known as Riedel's thyroiditis, ligneous thyroiditis, woody thyroiditis, eisenharte strumitis, and chronic productive thyroiditis) is a relatively rare form of thyroiditis which is felt to be an inflammatory process rather than a degenerative or involutionary change.

The incidence is equal in males and females, and is most common in the fourth and fifth decades.[15] Clinical manifestations result from severe pressure secondary to thyroid enlargement and firm fixation to cervical muscles and the trachea. This frequently causes suffocating attacks, stridulous cough, and dyspnea because of the tracheal involvement. The disease is often unilateral and characterized by stony hardness with fixation to nearby tissues on physical examination. Laboratory tests usually demonstrate a normal T_4 and ^{131}I uptake.

Differential diagnosis is principally that of malignant disease and surgical biopsy may be required to establish the diagnosis.[10] Histologic examination demonstrates near total replacement of follicles with fibroblastic tissue without lymphoid infiltration. The characteristic feature is extension beyond the thyroid capsule so that the entire cervical region (carotid sheath, trachea, cervical muscles, and thyroid gland) is involved in diffuse fibrosis.

This disease is believed to be self-limiting with morbidity and mortality usually related to respiratory problems. Surgical therapy is directed only towards the relief of pressure, which may require a wedge resection of the thyroid isthmus and/or tracheostomy. There is no effective medical therapy.

C. Autoimmune Thyroiditis

1. Struma lymphomatosa or Hashimoto's thyroiditis: This disease (also known as Hashimoto's struma, lymphadenoid goiter, autoimmune thyroiditis, and chronic lymphoid thyroiditis) is the most common type of thyroiditis. It is now widely held to be an autoimmune disease based on both cell-mediated and humoral immunity. A variety of circulating antithyroid antibodies have been found in this disease,[20] and the presence of cell-mediated immunity has been reported using several techniques.[10] It is thought to be an inherited disease, as it has a high incidence in close relatives. It also has a close relationship to Graves' disease, as they both may occur in the same individual. Both of these diseases frequently occur in close relatives and antithyroid antibodies are present in both disorders.[20]

Hashimoto's thyroiditis is predominately a disease of women in the fourth and fifth decades.[10] Typically the onset is insidious with gradual enlargement of the thyroid (50% of patients have noted goiter prior to the development of other symptoms). Additional symptoms include fullness and pressure in the throat, dysphagia, hoarseness, and dysphonia.[15] Palpation usually demonstrates a moderately large, nontender, firm, rubbery thyroid.[20] It may be unilateral but is most commonly bilateral.

Serum thyroxine is usually low (hypothyroid) but may be normal (euthyroid). Many patients do have an elevated PBI, but this is due to an excess of non-thyroxine protein-bound iodinated compounds released into the circulation secondary to the inflammation. The ^{131}I uptake is usually normal. A very high titer of serum antithyroglobulin antibodies is frequently present.

Differential diagnosis includes subacute thyroiditis (if tenderness is present), nodular goiter, or carcinoma. Needle biopsy will confirm the diagnosis.

Pathologic features include varying amounts of lymphocytic infiltration with germinal centers and intralobular fibrosis. The most characteristic and significant microscopic feature is the alteration of the epithelium to a distinctly oxyphilic type, with cells larger than normal with abundant cytoplasm and nuclei that may be hyperchromatic.[21]

Treatment is with thyroid replacement therapy and ordinarily the goiter will disapear or become smaller.[20] Surgical treatment may be necessary to relieve pressure symptoms or when carcinoma is a consideration. Three percent of these patients do have thyroid carcinoma. However, McConahey[20] reports that all patients with thyroid cancer have had "easily palpable, suspicious nodules in the thyroid."

2. Lymphocytic thyroiditis: This disease is felt to be caused by the release of an abnormal and ineffective thyroid secretory product resulting in higher than usual levels of thyrotropic hormone causing compensatory changes in the thyroid gland. It occurs predominately in young women, adolescents, and children. Rapid and diffuse enlargement of a previously normal gland is characteristic.

Laboratory tests show the serum thyroxine to be normal or elevated, and uptake is usually normal. Antibodies to thyroglobulin antigens are present but in lower quantities than in Hashimoto's thyroiditis.

Pathologically, extensive lymphocytic infiltration is observed with or without germinal centers. It is distinguished from Hashimoto's thyroiditis by the lack of oxyphilic epithelial changes.

The treatment is the administration of synthetic thyroid hormone on a long-term basis or the goiter may recur. Surgery is rarely indicated.[15]

TABLE 3. HISTOLOGIC CLASSIFICATION OF THYROID CANCER

A. Papillary adenocarcinoma (50-60%)
   1. Pure
   2. Mixed
B. Follicular adenocarcinoma (17-36%)
   1. Pure
   2. Clear cell
   3. Oxyphil (Hürthle) cell
C. Medullary carcinoma (1-7%)
D. Undifferentiated carcinoma (5-15%)
   1. Small cell (compact or diffuse)
   2. Giant (spindle) cell
   3. Mixed
E. Epidermoid carcinoma
F. Other
   1. Lymphoma
   2. Sarcoma
   3. Metastatic

THYROID CARCINOMA (TABLE 3)

Carcinoma of the thyroid presents an extremely broad spectrum of malignancy. Crile and Hawk[22] have compared carcinoma of the thyroid to carcinoma of the skin, which also develops tumors of variable malignancy including the highly malignant melanoma, the moderately malignant squamous cell carcinoma, and the less aggressive basal cell carcinoma. Because of this broad spectrum, several different systems of classification have been proposed.[22-25] To be meaningful, a classification must take into account not only the morphologic characteristics, but also the biologic behavior of the neoplasm. The classification of Bell[23] presented in Table 3 includes such considerations. Also included are a relative range of incidences from review of several series.[24,26-28]

Most pathologists include in the papillary group all tumors containing papillary elements whether or not follicular features are present (if undifferentiated features are also present, they are then classified as undifferentiated). This is based on the morphological characteristics and their biologic behavior as they respond similarly to therapy. To simplify the pathologic classification, thyroid carcinoma may be described as differentiated (papillary, mixed and follicular), medullary, and undifferentiated. In general this order of classification proceeds from the most benign (papillary) to the highly malignant undifferentiated carcinoma.

Malignancies of the thyroid are relatively rare and were estimated to account for 1,150 deaths and 8,100 new cases in the United States in 1976.[29] The overall clinical incidence is twice as common in females as in males and is more common in Caucasians than Negroes. Careful pathological examination of thyroid glands obtained at autopsy from individuals without clinical evidence of thyroid disease has demonstrated a 5.7% incidence of occult thyroid malignancy.[30] Surprisingly, the incidence (in autopsy specimens) is equal in males and females. Though females have a greater incidence of clinical thyroid cancer, the prognosis is consistently better in all thyroid cancers in women compared to men. Age also plays a role in the prognosis of differentiated (papillary and follicular) carcinomas as these tumors are more aggressive and have a greater lethal potential in patients over 40.[23] Differentiated tumors in patients under 21 have an excellent prognosis with nearly the same mortality rate as the general population.[31]

No specific etiology of thyroid carcinoma is known, but several factors do play a role in its development. These include ionizing radiation, long-term thyrotropin (TSH) stimulation, hereditary factors, and sex.

Radiation exposure does produce an increased incidence of thyroid cancer. Studies have shown that up to 2% of patients with an exposure of 500 rads to the thyroid in infancy develop a subsequent carcinoma.[25] A higher incidence is seen in patients who received greater amounts of radiation. Thyroid radiation in patients less than 20 years of age has a far greater risk of inducing neoplasia than a similar dose in adults.[32] Thyroid cancers which develop following irradiation are usually differentiated (most commonly papillary and occasionally follicular).[23]

Long-term TSH stimulation produces hyperplasia, nodule formation, autonomous function, and occasionally malignant changes. Hereditary factors are significant in familial medullary carcinoma which may be inherited as an autosomal dominant with reduced penetrance.[23] Most clinically evident thyroid carcinomas occur in greater frequency in females, although the etiology of this is not clear.

A. *Papillary Adenocarcinoma*

Papillary carcinoma is the most common malignancy of the thyroid. It is a low-grade malignancy and grows slowly. The majority of papillary tumors are found to have some follicular areas on pathologic examination; most authors have shown that as long as a papillary component is present, the clinical behavior is similar to a pure papillary carcinoma.[22,24,33,34] These tumors tend to occur at a younger age than other thyroid malignancies, although they may be seen at any age. The incidence is more common in females than males with a ratio of approximately 3:1.[24]

Papillary carcinoma has a high incidence of lymph node metastasis with most series reporting clinical nodal metastasis in the range of 30-40%.[24] The incidence of occult metastasis has been reported to range from 30-70%.[35-37] Metastases to lymph nodes are most often ipsilateral but occasional instances of bilateral spread will occur.[36] Distant metastases are uncommon.

These tumors also demonstrate a very high incidence of multicentricity (either microscopic multicentric primary foci or noncontiguous dissemination or metastasis of the primary lesion) in the thyroid gland when careful pathologic examination of surgically excised specimens is performed. Various studies have shown this occurs in the range of 32-88%.[26,33,38-40] However, the local recurrence rate in patients undergoing lobectomy alone ranges from 5-7% and Tollefsen et al[33] feel that this laboratory evidence of papillary carcinoma in the opposite lobe is of little clinical significance. They feel this is analogous to the high autopsy incidence of asymptomatic microscopically diagnosed prostatic cancer.

Pathologically, papillary carcinoma is typically unencapsulated and invasive into adjacent thyroid parenchyma. It is composed of papillary projections and neoplastic (but well-differentiated) follicles of varying proportions.

The most common presenting symptom is a "goiter" of varying duration. Approximately 10% of patients present with a neck mass without a palpable lesion in the thyroid.[24]

The treatment of this lesion is quite controversial, both for the thyroid itself and for the lymph nodes in the neck and superior mediastinum. The therapy to the thyroid gland, as recommended by Attie et al,[35] Wilson[41] and Marchetta[42] is total thyroidectomy. The basis for this is threefold: the high incidence of multicentric foci; if the patient develops metastasis, a total thyroidectomy is a prerequisite to the use of therapeutic radioactive iodine; and dissection is easier and can be more adequately performed the first time the surgeon is in the area. Geissinger et al,[26] De Groat,[25] Crile and Hawk[22] and Bell[23] all recommend a complete lobectomy on the side of the lesion and a subtotal resection on the opposite side unless there is clinical evidence of bilateral involvement at the time of surgery. Their rationale for this is the previously mentioned low incidence of local recurrence and the much lower incidence of hypoparathyroidism postoperatively. Tollefsen et al[33] recommend unilateral lobectomy with removal of the isthmus as the surgical procedure unless there is obvious clinical involvement of the opposite lobe.

Mazzaferri et al[43] have reviewed the results of therapy in 576 patients with papillary carcinoma of the thyroid. Their findings indicate that total or near-total thyroidectomy was associated with fewer recurrences and lower mortality. Patients undergoing total thyroidectomy, when compared to all other patients (as a group) receiving less aggressive surgical therapy, demonstrated lower recurrence and death rates. These differences were statistically significant.

Most authors recommend removal of lymph nodes from the tracheoesophageal groove on the side of the lesion and any nodes that are clinically palpable. If these are positive on frozen section, a modified radical neck dissection is performed.[22,23,25,32,41,42] Geissinger et al[26] recommend a standard neck dissection if clinical evidence of nodal involvement is present or if positive nodes are found on frozen sections. Attie et al[35] recommend a modified neck dissection on the side of the lesion in all patients because of the high incidence of metastasis (both clinically and occult). Several authors, including Block et al[37,44] Bell,[23] and Tollefson et al[33] stress the importance of removing the anterosuperior mediastinal lymph nodes as well as those along the course of the recurrent laryngeal nerve on the side of the lesion. This can easily be performed through the cervical incision without splitting the sternum. Metastasis to lymph nodes in the anterosuperior mediastinum occurred in 9% of patients and is always associated with metastasis to cervical lymph nodes.[44] Mazzaferri et al[43] demonstrated that the extent of lymph node surgery in these patients with histologically proven node metastasis had no significant effect on the recurrence or survival rates. "Node picking," modified and standard neck dissection all gave equally effective results.

In conclusion, surgical therapy for papillary carcinoma of the thyroid as recommended by the majority of authors would consist of a total lobectomy on the side of the primary tumor, a subtotal lobectomy on the opposite side (unless there is obvious clinical involvement) with frozen section biopsy of adjacent nodes and the performance of regional lymphadenectomy or a modified neck dissection (leaving the sternocleidomastoid muscle and the spinal accessory nerve). Dissection of the anterior-superior mediastinum must be performed if nodal metastases are present.

All patients are treated with lifelong suppression therapy with thyroid hormone. Thyroid hormone therapy appears to be beneficial only in differentiated tumors (papillary and follicular). Differentiated tumors appearing in prepubertal children and adults over 40 years of age are less likely to respond to thyroid suppression therapy.[23] Thyroid replacement therapy has been demonstrated to significantly lower recurrence and death rates in papillary carcinoma.[43] The mechanism of action is the suppression of TSH production and many of these tumors appear to be dependent upon TSH for further growth.

Radioiodine therapy is recommended postoperatively for all patients who have tumors which will take up ^{131}I and were either inoperable, incompletely excised at the time of surgery, or have distant metastasis.[23] A large majority (almost 85%) of well-differentiated tumors (papillary and follicular) will demonstrate uptake of iodine under the stimulation of myxedema with elevated TSH levels.[23] Thyroid ablation is necessary prior to this therapy, but if a total lobectomy and subtotal lobectomy on the opposite side have been performed, radioiodine ablation of the remaining thyroid tissue is possible.[23] The risks of radioiodine therapy include bone marrow depression, radiation pneumonitis (if pulmonary metastases are present), and leukemia. Tumor response to ^{131}I cannot be determined in advance (even if the tumor has good uptake) as the radiosensitivity of individual tumors varies.

External radiation has been successfully used for alleviation of pain from metastasis. External radiotherapy for local disease is not recommended (unless necessary for palliation) for papillary tumors since dedifferentiation into anaplastic carcinoma has occurred.[41]

Different authors have given varying rates of survival for papillary carcinoma. The survival is by and large excellent, but does progressively decrease over a longer period of time than the usually reported five-year figures. Most deaths from the disease occur more than five years after diagnosis, and most of the deaths occur because of recurrence of local disease rather than distant metastasis.[24] Fransilla[34] reviewed several large series of carcinoma of the thyroid and reported the five-year survival ranged from 73-93%; however, in his series 21% of patients died from papillary carcinoma with a 10- to 20-year follow-up. Wilson[41] reports a 96% five-year survival. De Groat[25] feels the net extra mortality on long-term follow-up is in the range of 10-20%. Woolner et al,[24] in their large series of 541 cases, have divided patients with papillary carcinoma into three groups based on the extent of disease at the time of surgery. Those patients with occult papillary carcinoma (defined as a tumor 1.5 cm or less in diameter with or without nodal metastasis) all survived with a follow-up of 3 to 32 years (there were 146 patients in this group). All the mortality in their series occurred in tumors which were larger than 1.5 cm or tumors which had invaded beyond the thyroid capsule. Mazzaferri et al[43] demonstrated a higher rate of recurrence in patients under 30 years of age, lesions larger than 2.5 cm in diameter, local invasion outside of the thyroid capsule, and in patients who did not receive thyroid replacement and ^{131}I therapy postoperatively.

In summary, the survival rate for papillary carcinoma is good. However, the disease will be the eventual cause of death in 10-20% of patients with long-term follow-up. The prognosis appears to be worse in prepubertal children,[22] patients more than 40 years of age, patients whose tumor is greater than 1.5 cm in diameter and/or has extracapsular invasion, and patients undergoing a limited thyroidectomy.[25,43] The presence or absence of cervical lymph node metastasis has no effect on recurrence or survival if therapy is directed to these metastasis.

B. Follicular Adenocarcinoma

Follicular carcinoma is the second most common carcinoma of the thyroid and is a more lethal disease than papillary carcinoma. It is more prevalent in the older age group (above 40) than papillary carcinoma. The female to male ratio is again approximately 3:1. Most studies report a low rate of lymph node metastasis (ranging from 2-20% positive nodes); distant metastases are more frequent (ranging from 15-65%).[24,34,45] Distant metastases are most commonly skeletal or pulmonary, but many occur anywhere.

Pathologically, follicular carcinoma is characterized by acinar structure formation with various amounts of colloid content in the lumen. There is an absence of any papillary growth pattern. These tumors are almost never multicentric.[22]

Again, the usual presenting sign is most commonly a goiter (usually of considerable duration).[24] It may also present with pressure symptoms (respiratory distress, dysphagia, etc). Occasionally, the initial findings are a neck mass or distant metastasis.

The therapy of follicular carcinoma is again controversial pertaining to the thyroid gland. Marchetta,[42] Wilson,[41] and Geissinger et al[26] recommend total lobectomy on the side of the lesion and subtotal lobectomy on the noninvolved lobe unless there is clinical evidence of involvement (when a total thyroidectomy is performed). Tollefson et al[45] and Crile and Hawk[22] recommend a total lobectomy with isthmusectomy unless both lobes are clinically involved. Most authors perform a modified neck dissection only if there is frozen section evidence of nodal involvement. The majority of authors treat follicular carcinoma the same as papillary: subtotal thyroidectomy (total lobectomy and subtotal lobectomy), unless both lobes are clinically involved, and a modified dissection is performed with evidence of nodal metastasis.

The results of therapy are poorer than those with papillary carcinoma. Results vary widely depending on the duration of follow-up and the method utilized for reporting results. DeGroat[25] feels the net extra mortality is approximately 50% over 10-15 years. Tollefson et al[45] report a determinant five-year survival of 70%, dropping to 42% at 25 years. They also note that when distant metastases are present, the five-year survival (determinant) is 22%. Fransilla[34] reported a relative survival rate (determinant) of 40% at ten years.

In summary, follicular carcinoma is more aggressive than papillary carcinoma, with 50-60% of patients eventually dying of their disease. Increased mortality is associated with distant metastasis at the time of presentation. Some authors[22,24] feel that significant invasion (pathologically) of the thyroid capsule or blood vessels yields a poorer prognosis, but others do not find this to be true.[45]

All cases of follicular carcinoma should be treated with thyroid supression therapy. The indications for postoperative ^{131}I therapy are similar for papillary carcinoma. External radiotherapy is again primarily reserved for the alleviation of pain or palliation.

Hürthle cell carcinoma is listed in the classification presented previously as a type of follicular carcinoma. It is a distinct clinical entity pathologically; however, the clinical course and method of therapy is similar to follicular carcinoma.[46] Microscopically, the Hürthle cells are characterized by large cells with ample acidophilic cytoplasm with a homogeneous or granular appearance. It may be very difficult to predict the biologic behavior of many of the lesions on gross and microscopic examination. Accepted criteria for malignancy are the presence of nondegenerative cytologic abnormalities, invasion of the capsule or blood vessels, and metastasis to lymph nodes.[47] Hürthle cells are also found in Hashimoto's thyroiditis.

These tumors are seen more frequently in females and occur primarily in adults. Cervical lymph node metastases are infrequent and distant metastases occur more commonly than nodal metastases. Mortality is largely attributed to distant metastasis.[46] Results of therapy are similar to follicular carcinoma. These tumors may respond to thyroid suppression, but they do differ from follicular carcinoma in that they rarely take up ^{131}I.[47]

C. Medullary Carcinoma

Medullary carcinoma is reported to comprise 1-7% of all thyroid malignancies.[48-50] These tumors have several distinctive properties: the simultaneous occurrence with other endocrine tumors (pheochromocytoma and parathyroid adenoma or hyperplasia), a form of malignancy that is familial, and biochemical properties that provide for early detection of disease and for monitoring recurrence on the follow-up.[48-50] The cell of origin is the c-cell which is derived from the ultimobranchial body and neural crest.[51] This tumor occurs with almost equal frequency in males and females, and over a wide age range. Most arise spontaneously (80-90%); however, the tumor may be inherited as a Mendelian dominant with reduced penetrance (10%). The familial form of tumor is more commonly associated with parathyroid adenomas, pheochromocytomas, and mucosal neuromata.[50]

The most common presenting symptom is a mass (which is characteristically very firm) in the thyroid gland or a multinodular goiter. Thirty percent of patients have clinically significant diarrhea and occasionally a frank carcinoid syndrome is present.[48,50]

Medullary carcinoma of the thyroid has significant biochemical activity and all tumors seem to produce calcitonin and histaminase. Other products identified include ACTH, prostaglandins, and serotonin.[48] Calcitonin (a hypocalcemic producing agent) and histaminase have been used as biochemical markers for this tumor. Virtually all patients have elevated serum calcitonin by radioimmunoassay. If metastatic disease is present, these levels remain elevated even after the primary lesion is surgically excised. Elevated plasma histaminase after surgical removal may also be an important biochemical clue to persistence.[48]

Microscopically, they are distinguished by polyhedral neoplastic cells arranged in sheets transversed by connective tissue septae which divide the tumor into nests of cells of variable size. This compartmental arrangement, or organoid pattern, together with the presence of a substance characterized as amyloid and the absence of neoplastic follicles and papillary elements, is the diagnostic microscopic feature of the tumor.[50] It is frequently bilateral (60%), even without clinical evidence of this, and in the familial variety it is uniformly bilateral.[50] Cervical lymph node metastasis often occurs early (as high as 50% of patients, even when the tumor is 1 mm or less in size), and distant metastasis occurs later to the lungs, liver, bone, and other organs.[48,49]

Preoperative diagnosis can be established by elevated calcitonin levels, the calcium infusion test, (calcium is infused and the serum calcitonin response to this is measured), or a pentagastrin stimulation test.[52] These tests are worthwhile in patients with a history suggestive of pheochromocytoma or any of the other syndromes associated with medullary carcinoma. It should be performed annually on all family members of a patient with a familial carcinoma. Additional preoperative evaluation of a patient with familial disease includes urinary VMA and metanephrine levels (to rule out pheochromocytoma), and serum calcium and phosphorus (to assess the parathyroid glands). These tests should be performed postoperatively in all spontaneous cases of medullary carcinoma.[48]

There are two radiographic features of medullary carcinoma which may be diagnostic preoperatively. Both the primary and metastatic lesions tend to calcify with a dense, irregular distribution of calcium throughout the tumor mass. Therefore soft tissue x-rays of the neck are indicated. Chest films may also be diagnostic as these tumors tend to metastasize to mediastinal soft structures and produce a widening of the superior mediastinum.[48]

Recommended surgical therapy for this lesion is total thyroidectomy and standard neck dissection with frozen section evidence of cervical lymph node metastasis.[48] A standard neck dissection is recommended for this carcinoma as a higher incidence of recurrence is found when a modified neck dissection is performed.[49,53] This tumor does not take up ^{131}I and rarely responds to thyroid suppression.[48-50] Full replacement doses of thyroid hormone are necessary following total thyroidectomy. Radiation therapy seems useful only for palliation of bone pain,[48] but Hill et al,[50] recommend administering postoperative prophylactic radiotherapy to the neck, supraclavicular areas, and upper mediastinum when nodes in the opposite neck were found to contain tumor. They also treat unresectable or residual tumor with external radiotherapy, but controlled series to demonstrate its effectiveness are not available at this time. Chemotherapy is generally ineffective, but some recent success has been reported with adriamycin.[54]

The prognosis of this tumor is variable and includes rapid demise or long-term survival even in the presence of metastatic disease.[53] Reported survival rates include 55-80% at five years and 57-78% at ten years.[49,50,55] These results may be influenced by the rather high percentage of familial carcinomas (approximately 20-25%) in these series, which are known to have a better survival rate than the more frequent spontaneous medullary carcinoma. Factors associated with increased survival were younger age (less than 50 years), familial disease, and bilateral tumors. It should be noted that all these factors may be related to the familial form of the disease, as they are all characteristic of it. Patients with cervical metastasis at the time of the initial operation had a much poorer prognosis (ten-year survival of 46% as compared to 80%) than patients without metastasis. The most common site of tumor recurrence was locally or in the neck.

D. Undifferentiated Carcinoma

Undifferentiated or anaplastic carcinomas constitute approximately 5-15% of all thyroid carcinomas.[24,56] These tumors occur primarily in later life with a peak incidence in the seventh and eighth decades, but may also be seen at a younger age. Again they are more common in females than males. Many authors feel that most if not all of these tumors arise from preexisting more differentiated thyroid carcinomas.[23,57] The three histologic types of undifferentiated carcinoma are small cell (diffuse or compact), giant cell (or spindle cell), and mixed patterns.

These carcinomas present clinically with a usually obviously malignant thyroid mass with fixation to adjacent neck structures and accompanied by pressure symptoms, cough, dyspnea, hoarseness, vocal cord paralysis, and dysphagia. Widespread metastases are frequently present at the time of the initial examination.[23,58]

The prognosis of this tumor is extremely poor. A recent review of the literature shows that only 14 of 144 cases survived for more than one year after diagnosis and the average duration of life after diagnosis is six months.[42] Local disease is the major cause of death but distant metastases are present in over three fourths of the patients.[23]

Obviously no method of therapy is very successful in this disease. Recently Rogers et al[56] published an early report of a method of therapy using surgical resection and postoperative radiation therapy combined with multiple courses of actinomycin D. Surgical therapy consisted of resection of all gross tumor (if possible) by either a partial or total thyroidectomy with radical neck dissection if positive nodes were found. Patients were then treated with cobalt 60, administering 6,000 rads in six weeks. In the fourth week of radiotherapy, chemotherapy with actinomycin D is given biweekly until toxicity and then repeated every two or three months. Three of six patients treated in this manner are free of disease for more than two years. This study does demonstrate the most promising method of therapy to date, but further analysis is required to establish its true effectiveness. At present our results with this method of therapy have failed to yield the results reported by Rogers et al.

TABLE 4. EVALUATION OF A THYROID NODULE

A. History
B. Physical examination
C. Laboratory
   1. T_4, T_3 uptake
   2. Antithyroid antibodies
   3. Scan
   4. Ultrasound
D. Other tests (based on history and physical)

THE EVALUATION AND THERAPY OF A THYROID NODULE (TABLES 4-8)

Thyroid cancer is a relatively rare disease compared to nodular goiter (which has an incidence of 2-4% in adults), with carcinoma being present (depending on various studies) in 4-17% of these goiters. As it is impractical to remove all goiters, the problem is to select those patients with the greatest probability of carcinoma for surgical therapy. Table 4 presents an overview of the evaluation of a thyroid nodule.

In the initial history important factors include the lack of or presence of symptoms, the period of time the lesion has been present, a past history of radiation exposure, and a family history of thyroid disease. In the physical examination, the patient should be checked for clinical evidence of hyperthyroidism or hypothyroidism, the presence or absence of clinically suspicious neck nodes, a careful examination of the thyroid performed with specific reference to the character of the nodule (its size and consistency), the presence of multiple nodules, and the size, mobility, and character of the entire gland. Indirect laryngoscopy is performed to evaluate recurrent nerve function.

TABLE 5. RISK FACTORS OF MALIGNANCY IN A THYROID MASS

A. Age
B. Radiation exposure
C. Isolated nodule
D. Sex
E. Physical examination
F. Laboratory findings
G. Growth pattern
H. Pregnancy

Laboratory tests are often dictated by the history and physical examination. However, most patients require a serum thyroxine (T_4), a T_3 resin uptake test, antithyroid antibodies, radioactive scan of the thyroid and ultrasonography. A thyrocalcitonin level (calcium infusion or pentagastrin stimulation test) should be determined in all patients with a family history of thyroid carcinoma (if the histologic diagnosis is unavailable) and on patients with symptoms compatible with a pheochromocytoma and/or significant diarrhea. In addition, these patients should have a soft tissue x-ray of the neck.

If the lesion proves to be a functioning (hot) nodule on the thyroid scan, one may attempt to suppress this by giving the patient thyroid hormone for two to three weeks and then repeating the scan. Other methods of evaluation include echography and thermography. Clark et al[59] have been able to differentiate solid lesions from cystic lesions in over 80% of the cases utilizing echography (ultrasonography). Cystic thyroid nodules are rarely malignant, but mixed (solid and cystic) lesions have an incidence of malignancy similar to solid lesions.[13,59]

Following the completion of the history, physical examination and laboratory tests, the problem arises as the the proper therapy. There are many factors to consider in evaluating the risk of malignancy in thyroid nodules (Table 5).

Age: Approximately 50% of isolated thyroid nodules appearing in children are malignant. Multinodularity increases with age and the incidence of cancer in a single palpable nodule decreases with age.[13]

Radiation Exposure: A past history of neck or mediastinal irradiation is significant as there is a high incidence of malignancy in these situations. These malignancies are usually differentiated (papillary and follicular) carcinomas and demonstrate a high incidence of multicentricity.[29] Any palpable nodule on physical examination or cold nodule on thyroid scan must be presumed to be malignant in patients with a prior history of radiation.

The Isolated Nodule: There is a much higher incidence of malignancy in single nodules as compared to multiple nodules. This ranges from 4-33% in different series in the literature.[13]

TABLE 6. DIFFERENTIAL DIAGNOSIS OF A THYROID MASS

1. Benign adenoma
2. Hemorrhage into the gland
3. Lobulation of normal thyroid tissue
4. Lobulation secondary to chronic thyroiditis
5. Primary malignancy
6. Metastatic malignancy
7. Intrathyroid cyst
8. Autonomous nodule
9. Thyroiditis and malignancy
10. Hyperplasia of one lobe
11. Lesion from adjacent structure

Sex: All thyroid disease (including nodules and malignancy) is more common in females than males. Multinodularity is also more common in females, however an isolated lesion occurring in a male is more likely to be malignant.

Physical Examination: A firm to hard consistency of a nodule increases the risk of malignancy. Other physical signs such as adherence to adjacent structures, the presence of cervical nodes, and vocal cord paralysis are highly suggestive of malignancy. Vocal cord paralysis may be caused by benign thyroid disease including goiter, thyroiditis (especially Riedel's), and adenoma, or by extrathyroidal conditions. As previously mentioned, totally (not mixed) cystic nodules rarely contain carcinoma.[13,59]

Laboratory Findings: Carcinomas are nearly always cold nodules on radioiodine scan. Hoffman et al[60] reported a patient who had a hot nodule on scan and was found to have carcinoma; however, other authors make the statement that a hot nodule has never proven to be malignant in their experience.[61] Some series report that up to 25% of cold nodules are malignant.[62] Carcinomas are extremely rare in lesions that are documented to be totally cystic by echography. High titers of antithyroid antibodies may be present in thyroiditis, although lower titers may be found in association with carcinoma and carcinoma may coexist with Hashimoto's thyroiditis.[60]

Growth Pattern: A recent or rapid growth is always an ominous sign and suggests either malignancy or hemorrhage into the lesion.

Pregnancy: The appearance of a nodule during pregnancy has an increased chance of being malignant.[42]

In summary, the incidence of malignancy is increased in the young, males, a single nodule, a past history of irradiation, a firm or hard lesion, recent growth, a cold nodule on scan, and if the patient is pregnant.

The differential diagnosis of a palpable mass or nodule in the thyroid is listed in Table 6.

Crile and Hawk[63] have advocated needle aspiration and/or biopsy of certain thyroid lesions. They use this for diffuse enlargement of the thyroid thought to be thyroiditis, nodules of the thyroid thought to be benign, and cysts of the thyroid or hemorrhage into adenomas in which the diagnosis is suspected because of the sudden appearance or rapid growth of the nodule (a history that rules out the presence of a differentiated or operable carcinoma). They have performed this safely and without significant complication and have been able to make the diagnosis in 96% of the cases. This degree of accuracy was confirmed by Schnürer and Widström with a 93% agreement between cytological and histological diagnosis.[64] It should be repeated, however, that they do not perform a needle biopsy or aspiration if they are suspicious of a differentiated malignancy. Others may recommend needle biopsy and aspiration (for cytology) of all masses, but an experienced pathologist or cytologist is required for accurate diagnosis.

The therapy of thyroid nodules is as controversial as the therapy of thyroid carcinoma. This includes both the medical and surgical treatment.

Available medical therapy includes treatment with thyroid suppression and radioiodine therapy. Most controversial is thyroid suppression in cold nodules. In thyroid suppression therapy, the patient is kept on full thyroid suppression for three to six months and the response is determined by monitoring the change in size of the nodule. If the nodule disappears, the patient is kept on full thyroid suppression for the rest of his life and monitored intermittently by follow-up examination. If the nodule fails to disappear surgery is usually performed. Some authors report that up to 20% regress,[65] others feel that very few (less than 1%) will respond to this therapy,[60,66] while still others report that the nodule will disappear in the majority of patients.[40] Thomas[65] reports that nodules that regress tend to be less than 2.5 cm in diameter, of recent origin, in patients less than 40 years of age, and in females.

In summary, thyroid suppression therapy should probably not be utilized in patients in whom malignancy is suspected clinically by physical examination and in children and males with isolated cold nodules. Some authors would not agree with this and perform a trial of suppression in all patients.

Surgical therapy is also controversial as to the indications for and the extent of the surgical procedure. Some authors recommend a simple lumpectomy (nodulectomy),[63] others recommend a subtotal lobectomy on the side of the lesion,[13] and still others recommend a total lobectomy on the side of the lesion.[60,65] At present a total lobectomy is always utilized at our institution. Advantages of this approach include complete removal of the involved lobe so that further surgery in this area (with a much higher incidence of injury to the recurrent laryngeal nerve) is unnecessary. If permanent sections demonstrate malignancy not identified in frozen section, reoperation is unnecessary provided careful follow-up examinations are performed when a differentiated malignancy is present. Morbidity, mortality, and operating time are essentially the same for nodulectomy, partial and total lobectomy.

TABLE 7. THERAPY OF HYPERFUNCTIONING ("HOT") NODULES

- A. T_3 suppression test
- B. Nonautonomous (suppressible)
  - 1. Thyroid hormone replacement
  - 2. Continued observation
  - 3. Indications for further therapy
    - a. Hyperthyroidism
    - b. Progressive enlargement
- C. Autonomous (nonsuppressible)
  - 1. Hyperthyroidism
    - a. Antithyroid medication
    - b. Radioiodine
    - c. Surgery
  - 2. Euthyroid
    - a. Observation
    - b. Radioiodine
    - c. Surgery

Therapy of Hyperfunctioning ("Hot") Nodules (Table 7)

Up to 25% of solitary thyroid nodules are found to be hyperfunctioning on iodine scan.[67] When hyperfunction of a nodule is present, further evaluation is required to determine if the nodule is autonomous (functioning independently of TSH control and consequently nonsuppressible by the administration of thyroid hormone) or nonautonomous (under TSH control). This is most commonly performed by the administration of triiodothyronine (25 μg TID) for 1-2 weeks and repeating the radioactive iodine scan. This produces two groups of patients, those with autonomous (still hot on repeat scan) and nonautonomous nodules (nonfunctioning on repeat scan).

Therapy of nonautonomous nodules is the administration of full replacement doses of thyroid hormone with continued observation. Progressive enlargement or the development of hyperthyroidism (the nodule has become autonomous) are indications for further therapy as follows.

The therapy of autonomous nodules may be medical or surgical. Toxic (hyperthyroid) nodules may be treated by antithyroid medication, radioactive ^{131}I, or surgery. If hyperthyroidism is present the patient should be returned to a euthyroid state by medical therapy prior to surgery. Nontoxic (euthyroid) nodules may be treated with frequent observation (progressive enlargement or the development

TABLE 8. THERAPY OF HYPOFUNCTIONING ("COLD") NODULES

A. Ultrasonography
B. Cystic lesions
  1. Thyroid hormone suppression
  2. Aspiration and cytology
  3. Observation
  4. Surgery: indications
    a. Progressive enlargement
    b. Compressive symptoms
    c. Cosmesis
    d. Suspicion of malignancy
C. Solid and mixed lesions
  1. Thyroid hormone suppression
  2. Surgery: indications
    a. Failure of suppression
    b. Compressive symptoms
    c. Cosmesis
    d. Suspicion of malignancy

of hyperthyroidism is an indication for further therapy), radioactive iodine, or surgery.

The therapy of "hot" nodules is equally effective by radioactive ^{131}I or surgery. Both eliminate the immediate potential for the development of thyrotoxicosis. Advantages of surgery include the elimination of the requirement of prolonged observation, improved cosmesis if an obvious thyroid mass is present, the avoidance of radiation exposure (especially in younger individuals), and the establishment of a pathological diagnosis. Advantages of radioiodine therapy include the elimination of the morbidity and mortality of a surgical procedure and a less aggressive method of therapy; however, hyperthyroidism may recur at a later date. The method of choice depends upon the condition and desires of the patient, and the philosophy of the physician managing the patient.

Therapy of Hypofunctioning "Cold" Nodules (Table 8)

Cold and isofunctioning solitary thyroid nodules (75% of isolated thyroid nodules) on radioisotope scan may be further subdivided into solid, mixed, and cystic lesions on the basis of ultrasonography. Solid and mixed lesions have a greater risk of malignancy (18%) and adenoma formation (51%) than do cystic lesions (especially if they are less than 4 cm in diameter).[5]

Solitary cold nodules that are cystic on ultrasonography may be treated with thyroid suppression and needle aspiration of the lesion with cytologic examination of the aspirant. When the cytology is not suspicious for malignancy the patient may be treated with long-term thyroid suppression and frequent observation. Progressive enlargement, cosmetic or compressive symptoms, and the suspicion of malignancy are indications for surgical intervention. Cystic lesions less than 3 cm in diameter have less than a 2% incidence of malignancy.[67,68]

Solid and mixed solitary cold nodules have a greater incidence of malignancy and may be treated immediately with surgery or after a failure of regression of the nodule with thyroid suppression therapy. Most authors feel that either a subtotal or total lobectomy is needed for adequate excision of the nodule. Further therapy depends on frozen section diagnosis. If frozen section diagnosis is benign but the permanent sections show papillary or follicular carcinoma, further surgical intervention is generally not indicated unless there is clinical evidence of recurrent disease or the patient is felt to be unreliable for prolonged observation. These patients do need frequent, careful, prolonged follow-up. A medullary carcinoma does require a total thyroidectomy performed as soon as possible after the permanent section diagnosis is made. In patients with multiple nodules surgery is recommended if a nodule becomes clinically suspicious for malignancy.[13]

Therapy of Patients with a History of Radiation Exposure

Patients with an uncertain history of prior radiation exposure are treated in the manner previously outlined. A definite history of prior radiation exposure does place the patient at a greater risk for the development of malignancy and consequently the indications for medical and surgical therapy are modified at our institution.

The National Cancer Institute[29] has recommended that these individuals undergo a periodic examination at least every two years indefinitely. Thyroid scans are not felt to be mandatory unless palpation reveals an abnormality. However, many physicians do prefer to obtain a scan on all of these patients (the present policy at our institution). Patients with a normal examination and scan are reexamined at regular intervals, and a repeat scan is obtained when a palpable change occurs in the thyroid gland. Patients with a normal clinical examination and a "cold" nodule on scan need to be carefully reexamined for the presence of the nodule. If no abnormality is palpated three options of therapy are available: careful follow-up examination, thyroid supression, or surgical exploration. In view of the high percentage (27%) of malignancy of cold nodules on scan without a palpable lesion on physical examination,[69,70] we recommend surgical excision of the thyroid. Any patient with a palpable nodule on physical examination is recommended for a surgical procedure regardless of the findings on scan and ultrasound.

The surgical procedure performed in patients with a definite history of radiation exposure is a total or near total thyroidectomy with a complete lobectomy performed on the side of the lesion. A lobectomy alone is felt to be an inadequate procedure as radiation-induced thyroid tumors are more likely to be multifocal (both papillary and follicular) than spontaneously occurring tumors.[29]

The importance of consultation with an internist with an interest in endocrinology or an endocrinologist in the management of all patients with disorders of the thyroid cannot be overemphasized. Their special knowledge and expertise in this area allows a significant contribution to overall care and management of the patient with thyroid disease. In addition, the potential for the development of a team approach to the care of the patient with thyroid disease is present, with each specialist contributing in his area of knowledge in a climate of respect and trust. This provides for the maximization of patient care with benefits for all physicians involved.

REFERENCES

1. Bartuska DG, Dratman MB. Evolving concepts of thyroid function. Med Clin North Am 1973; 57:1117-32.

2. Larson PR. Test of thyroid function. Med Clin North Am 1975; 59:1063-74.

3. Waldstein SS. Thyroid-catacholamine interrelations. Annu Rev Med 1966; 17:123-32.

4. McMurry JF Jr. Thyroid function testing. Postgrad Med 1975; 57:52-6.

5. Bain J, Walfish PG. The assessment of thyroid function and structure. Otolaryngol Clin North Am 1978; 11:419-43.

6. McKenzie JM, Zakarija M, Bonnyns M. Graves disease. Med Clin North Am 1975; 59:1177-92.

7. Hollander CS. Clinical and laboratory observations in cases of T3 toxicosis. Lancet 1972; 1:609-11.

8. Murphy BEP, Pattee CJ. Determination of thyroxine utilizing the property of protein-binding. J Clin Endocrinol Metab 1964; 24:187-96.

9. Chopra IJ. A radioimmunoassay for measurement of thyroxines in unextracted serum. J Clin Endocrinol Metab 1972; 34:938-47.

10. Volpe R. Thyroiditis, current views of pathogenesis. Med Clin North Am 1975; 59:1163-75.

11. Miskin M, Rosen IB, Walfish PG. Ultrasonography of the thyroid gland. Radiol Clin North Am 1971; 51:125-37.

12. Burke G. The triiodothyronine suppression test. Am J Med 1967; 42:600-8.

13. Wright HK, Burrow GN, Spaulding S, Sheahan DG. Current therapy of thyroid nodules. Surg Clin North Am 1974; 54:277-88.

14. Strahan RW, Calcaterra TC, Ward PH. Thyroiditis: a classification and review. Laryngoscope 1971; 81:1388-400.

15. Shapiro SL. Thyroiditis. EENT Monthly 1973; 52:261-4.

16. Klossen KP, Curtis GM. Tuberculous abscess of the thyroid gland. Surgery 1945; 17:552-9.

17. Volpe R, Row VV, Ezrin C. Circulating oral and thyroidal antibodies in subacute thyroiditis. J Clin Endocrinol Metab 1967; 27:1275-84.

18. Bicknell PG, Bateman AD. DeQuervains subacute thyroiditis. J Laryngol Otol 1974; 88:163-5.

19. Crile G Jr, Rumsey EW. Subacute thyroiditis. JAMA 1950; 142:458-63.

20. McConahey WM. Hashimoto's thyroiditis. Med Clin North Am 1972; 56:385-96.

21. Lindsay S, Dailey ME, Friedlander J, Yee G, Soley MH. Chronic thyroiditis: clinical and pathologic study of 354 patients. J Clin Endocrinol Metab 1952; 12:1578-600.

22. Crile GO Jr, Hawk WH. Carcinoma of the thyroid. Cleve Clin Q 1971; 38:97-104.

23. Bell GO. Cancer of the thyroid. Med Clin North Am 1975; 59:459-70.

24. Woolner LB, Beahrs OM, Black BM, McConahey WM, Keating FR. Classification and prognosis of thyroid carcinoma. Am J Surg 1961; 102:354-87.

25. DeGroat LJ. Thyroid carcinoma. Med Clin North Am 1975; 59:1233-46.

26. Geissinger WT, Horsley JS, Parker FP, Alrich EM. Carcinoma of the thyroid. Ann Surg 1974; 179;734-9.

27. Crocher DW. Thyroid carcinoma. Surgery 1973; 73:671-6.

28. Lohreny FN. Thyroid cancer and its diagnosis, treatment and prognosis. Wis Med J 1973; 72:97-100.

29. National Cancer Institute. Information for physicians on irradiation-related thyroid cancer. CA 1976; 26:150-9.

30. Sampson RJ, Woolner LB, Bahn RC, Kurland LT. Occult thyroid carcinoma in Olmsted County Minnesota: prevalence at autopsy compared with that in Hiroshima and Nagasaki, Japan. Cancer 1974; 34:2073-6.

31. Buckwalter JA, Thomas CG, Freeman JB. Is childhood thyroid cancer a lethal disease? Ann Surg 1975; 181:632-9.

32. Schottenfeld D. Epidemiology of thyroid cancer. Laryngoscope 1978; 88 Suppl 8:55-7.

33. Tollefsen MR, Shak JP, Huvos AG. Papillary carcinoma of the thyroid. Am J Surg 1972; 124:468-72.

34. Fransilla KO. Is the differentiation between papillary and follicular thyroid carcinoma valid? Cancer 1973; 32:853-64.

35. Attie JN, Khafif RA, Steckler RM. Elective neck dissection in papillary carcinoma of the thyroid. Am J Surg 1971; 122:464-71.

36. Pollack RS. Cervical lymph node metastasis of thyroid cancer. Am J Surg 1961; 102:388-94.

37. Block MA, Miller JM, Horn RC Jr. Thyroid carcinoma with lymph node metastasis — effectiveness of total thyroidectomy and node dissection. Am J Surg 1971; 122:458-63.

38. Sloan LW. Of the origin, characteristics and behavior of thyroid cancer. J Clin Endocrinol Metab 1954; 14:1309-35.

39. Underwood CR, Ackerman LV, Eckert C. Papillary carcinoma of the thyroid. Surgery 1958; 43:610-21.

40. Clark RL, White EC, Russell WO. Total thyroidectomy for cancer of the thyroid, significance of intraglandular dissemination. Ann Surg 1959; 149:858-66.

41. Wilson SM. Carcinoma of the thyroid, modalities of therapy. Surg Clin North Am 1973; 53:169-74.

42. Marchetta FC. Carcinoma of the thyroid gland: current therapy. J Surg Oncol 1974; 6:401-8.

43. Mazzaferri EL, Young RL, Oertel JE, Kemmerer WT, Page CP. Papillary thyroid carcinoma: the impact of therapy in 576 patients. Medicine 1978; 56:171-96.

44. Block MA, Miller JM, Horn RC Jr. Significance of mediastinal lymph node metastasis in carcinoma of the thyroid. Am J Surg 1972; 123:702-5.

45. Tollefson MR, Shak JP, Huvos AG. Follicular carcinoma of the thyroid. Am J Surg 1973; 126:522-8.

46. Tollefson MR, Shak JP, Huvos AG. Hürthle cell carcinoma of the thyroid gland. Am J Surg 1975; 130:390-4.

47. Thompson NW, Dunn EL, Batsakis JG, Nishiyama RM. Hürthle cell lesions of the thyroid gland. Surg Gynecol Obstet 1974; 138:555-60.

48. Baylin SB. Medullary carcinoma of the thyroid gland: use of biochemical parameters in detection and surgical management of tumor. Surg Clin North Am 1974; 54:309-23.

49. Chong GC, Beahrs OH, Gizemore GW, Woolner LH. Medullary carcinoma of the thyroid gland. Cancer 1975; 35:695-704.

50. Hill CS Jr, Ibaney ML, Samaan NA, Ahearn MJ, Clark RL. Medullary carcinoma of the thyroid gland: an analysis of the M. D. Anderson Hospital experience with patients with the tumor, its special features, and its histogenesis. Medicine 1973; 52:141-71.

51. Gonzales-Licea A, Hartman WH, Yardley JH. MCT. Ultrastructural evidence of its origin from the parafollicular and its relation to carcinoid tumors. Am J Clin Pathol 1968; 49:512-20.

52. Hennessy JF, Wells SA Jr, Ontjes DA, Cooper CW. A comparison of pentagastrin injection and calcium infusion as provocative agents for the detection of medullary carcinoma of the thyroid. J Clin Endocrinol Metab 1974; 39:487-95.

53. Fierstein J, Sessions DG, Thawley SE, Ogura JH. Medullary carcinoma of the thyroid. Laryngoscope 1976; 86:1594-601.

54. Gottlieb JA, Hill CS Jr, Ibanez ML, Clark RL. Chemotherapy of thyroid cancer: an evaluation of experience with 37 patients. Cancer 1972; 30:848-53.

55. Kaplan EL, Peskin GW. Physiologic implications of MCT gland. Surg Clin North Am 1971; 51:125-37.

56. Rogers JD, Lindberg RD, Hull CS Jr, Gehan E. Spindle and giant cell carcinoma of the thyroid: a different therapeutic approach. Cancer 1974; 34:1328-32.

57. Maddox WA, Knott HW, Dowling EA. Carcinoma of the thyroid: review of fifteen years' experience 1) origin of spindle and giant cell carcinoma and 2) occurrences of thyroid cancer in extopic thyroid tissue. Am Surg 1971; 37:653-60.

58. Nishiyama RH, Dunn EL, Thompson NW. Anaplastic spindle cell and giant cell tumors of the thyroid gland. Cancer 1972; 31:113-27.

59. Clark OH, Greenspan FS, Coggs GC, Goldman L. Evaluation of solitary cold thyroid nodules by echography and thermography. Am J Surg 1975; 130:206-11.

60. Hoffman GL, Thompson NW, Heffron C. The solitary thyroid nodule. Arch Surg 1972; 105:379-85.

61. McKenney JF. Thyroid nodule. Postgrad Med 1975; 57:103-5.

62. Brown L. Kantounis S. The thyroid nodule. Am J Surg 1976; 129:532-6.

63. Crile G Jr, Hawk WA Jr. Aspiration biopsy of thyroid nodules. Surg Gynecol Obstet 1973; 136:241-5.

64. Schnürer LB, Widström A. Fine-needle biopsy of the thyroid gland. A cytohistological comparison in cases of goiter. Ann Otol Rhinol Laryngol 1978; 87:224-7.

65. Thomas CG. Surgery of the thyroid. Med Clin North Am 1975; 59:1247-61.

66. Brooks JR. The solitary thyroid nodule. Am J Surg 1973; 125:477-81.

67. Walfish PG, Miskin N, Rosen IB, Strawbridge HTG. Application of special diagnostic techniques in the management of nodular goiter. Can Med Assoc J 1976; 115:34-40.

68. Crile G Jr. Treatment of the thyroid cyst by aspiration. Surgery 1966; 59:210-2.

69. Refetoff S. Continuing occurrence of thyroid carcinoma after irradiation to the neck in infancy and childhood. N Engl J Med 1975; 292:171-5.

70. Arnold J. ^{99m}Tc-pertechnetate thyroid scintigraphy in patients predisposed to thyroid neoplasms by prior radiotherapy to the head and neck. Radiology 1975; 115:653-7.

MANUAL FOR CARE of the MONTGOMERY SILICONE TRACHEAL T-TUBE

William W. Montgomery, MD

Supplement 73 — Vol. 89, July-August, 1980, No. 4, Part 5

THE ANNALS OF OTOLOGY, RHINOLOGY & LARYNGOLOGY

THE ANNALS PUBLISHING COMPANY
4949 FOREST PARK BLVD.
ST. LOUIS, MISSOURI 63108

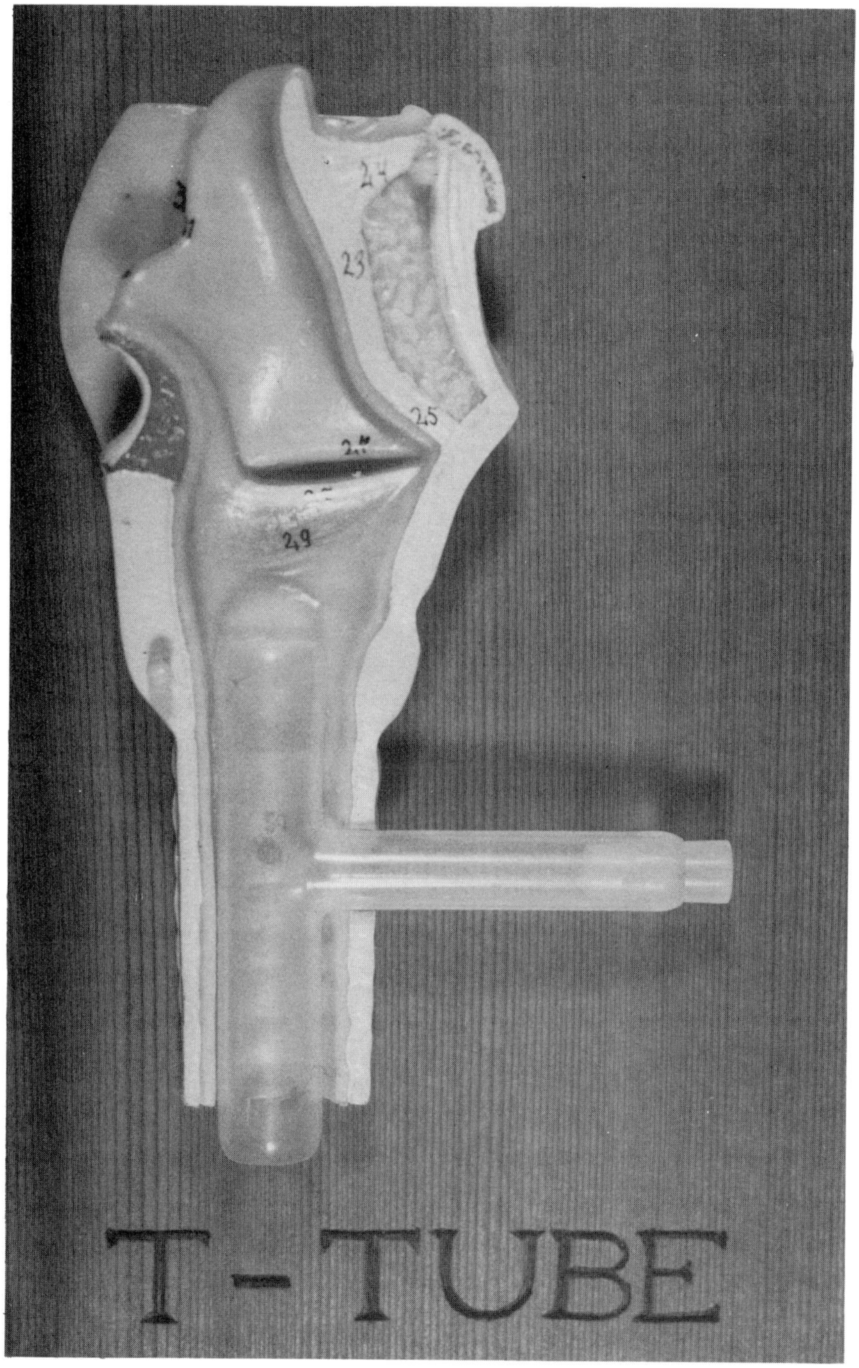

A No. 13 regular T-tube is shown in place. The short intraluminal end faces superiorly (short end up) to the level of the junction of the subglottic cervical trachea.

CONTENTS

Introduction 1

Features 1

Uses 3

Suctioning 3

Insertion 3

Removal 4

Grafting 5

Anesthesia via Tracheal T-tube 5

Preoperative and Postoperative Orders 7

MANUAL FOR CARE OF THE MONTGOMERY SILICONE TRACHEAL T-TUBE

William W. Montgomery, MD
Boston, Massachusetts

INTRODUCTION

We are currently treating a large number of defective tracheas. This number will continue to increase until we learn more about the prevention of injury to the subglottis and cervical trachea.

In 1964, I described a two piece acrylic T-tube stent (Fig. 1). This device was used to support a reconstructed cervical trachea and was the precursor to the silicone tracheal T-tube stent which evolved after considerable laboratory research in 1965.

The silicone tracheal T-tube (Fig. 2) was designed to maintain an adequate tracheal airway as well as to provide support in the stenotic trachea which has been reconstituted or reconstructed. It is supplied with a plug which is inserted and secured in place by a slight twist. The plug remains in place by friction and will not become dislodged even during forceful coughing. The tracheal T-tube is supplied in sizes from 4.5 to 16.0 mm (outside diameter) (Fig. 3A). The infant sizes range from 4.5-6.0 mm while the 8 mm size is used for pediatric patients. Sizes 10-13 mm are best suited for the adolescent and adult female and sizes 12-16 mm are for the adult male trachea. Statistically the most commonly used sizes are 10, 12 and 13 mm. The curvature at the junction of the external and intratracheal portions of the T-tube facilitates cleaning and suctioning. The external portion of the tube can be tilted in an inferior or superior direction to facilitate insertion of suction tubing. Long T-tubes (Fig. 3B) are supplied to treat defects in the thoracic trachea.

This instruction manual has been compiled to assist the doctor, nurse and family with the care of the patient who has a silicone tracheal T-tube in place.

FEATURES OF THE SILICONE TRACHEAL T-TUBE

1. Serves as both a stent and a tracheotomy tube.

2. Silicone initiates little or no tissue reaction. It does not harden with prolonged contact with body temperature and secretions.

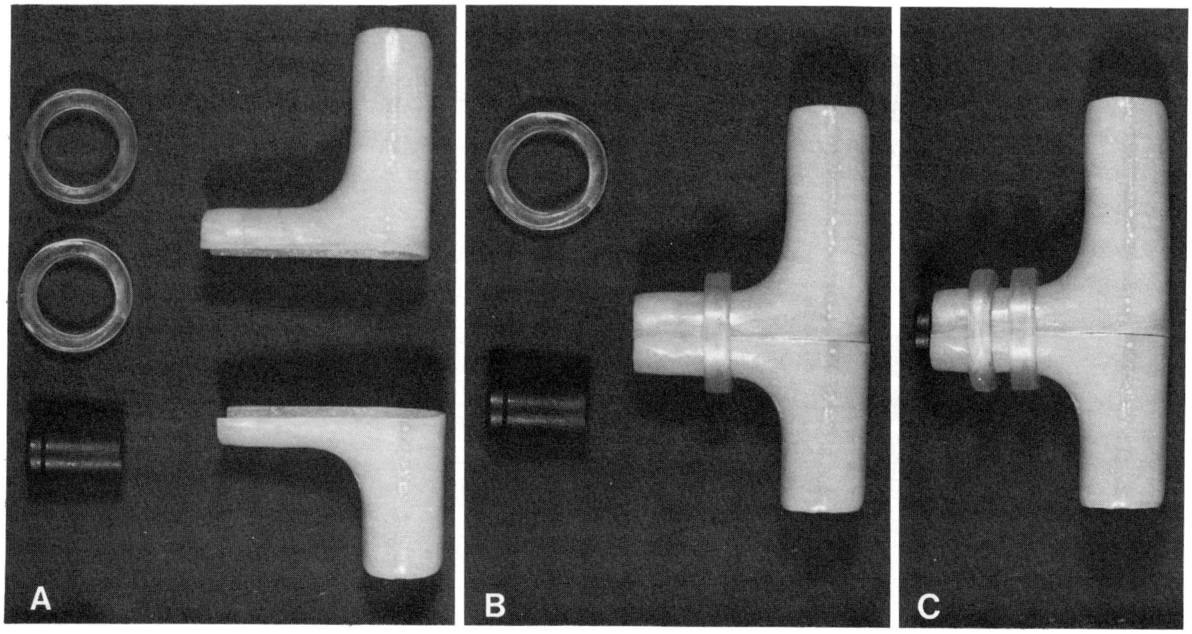

Fig. 1. A) Original tracheal T-tube stent constructed from acrylic. Components are: upper and lower halves of the T-tube, two lock washers and a plug. B) The two halves have been joined after being inserted into the proximal and distal trachea. The first lock washer is applied to the external limb. C) The plug and second lock washer are in place.

From the Massachusetts Eye and Ear Infirmary, Boston, Massachusetts.

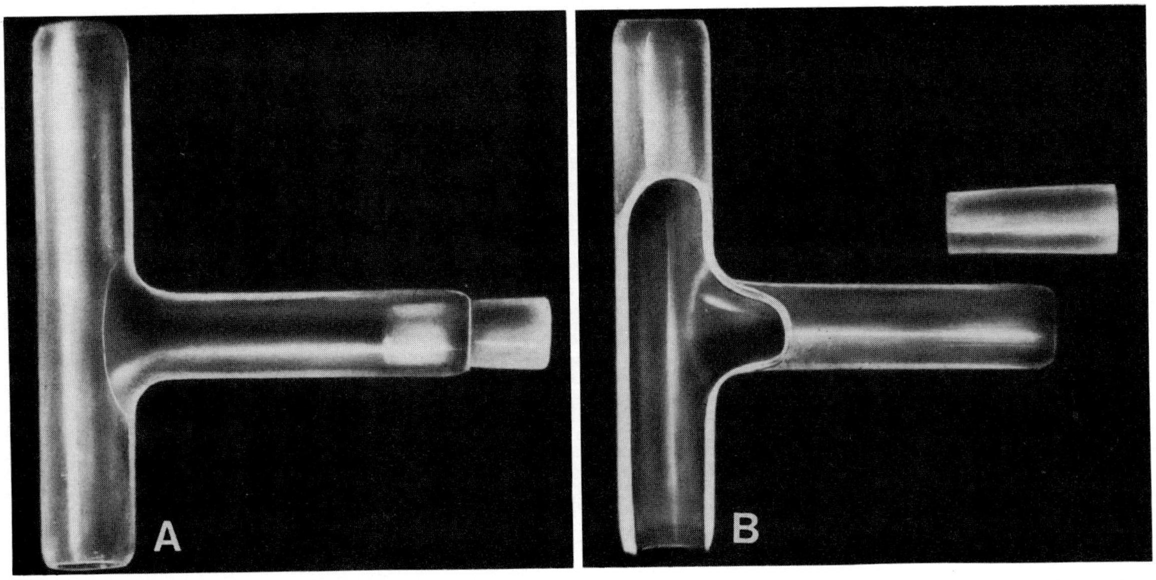

Fig. 2. A, B) The silicone T-tube which serves as both a tracheal stent and a tracheotomy tube. The plug is also made of silicone. The portion of the T-tube which projects from the tracheotomy orifice is of a smaller diameter than that of the intraluminal portion. The two intraluminal portions of the T-tube are of different lengths.

3. The intraluminal portion is of sufficient density and thickness to support a reconstituted or reconstructed stenotic trachea.

4. The intraluminal portion is sufficiently soft so as not to injure the lining or supporting structure of the trachea.

5. The ends of the tube are tapered. Thus, injury does not occur with asynchronous motion between the end of the tube and the tracheal mucosa.

6. Mucus and crusts do not readily adhere to the very smooth surfaces of silicone rubber.

7. The T-tube is widened by the curvature at the junction of its intraluminal and extraluminal portions. This 1) supports the anterior tracheal wall

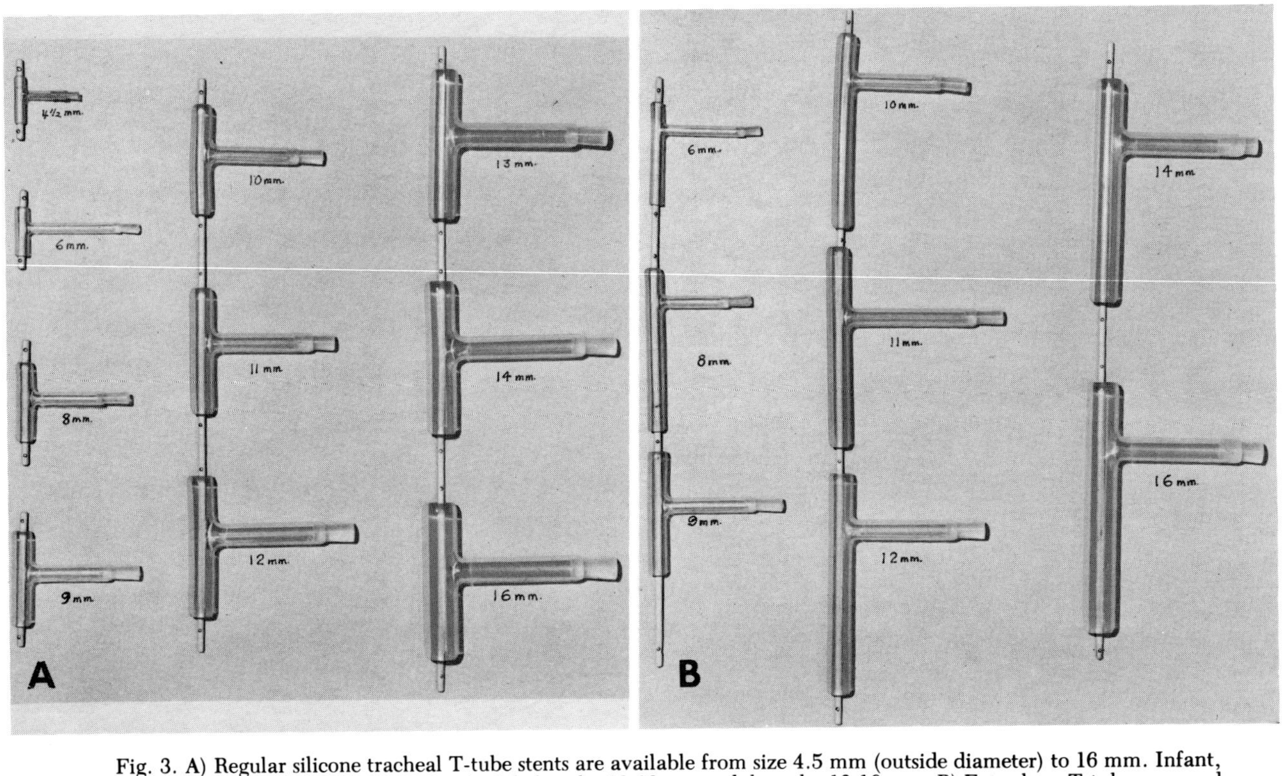

Fig. 3. A) Regular silicone tracheal T-tube stents are available from size 4.5 mm (outside diameter) to 16 mm. Infant, 4.5-6 mm; pediatric, 8 mm; adolescent and adult female, 10-13 mm; adult male, 12-16 mm. B) Extra long T-tubes are used to stent stenosis of the thoracic trachea.

at the tracheotomy site, and 2) facilitates suctioning and cleaning.

8. The extraluminal portion is of sufficient length so that it can be used with an obese neck. This portion of the T-tube can be shortened simply by cutting with scissors.

9. The silicone T-tube is supplied with a plug which is inserted with a slight twist. The plug remains in place by friction and will not become dislodged even with forceful coughing.

10. Frequent changing of the T-tube is not necessary. In cases where the trachea cannot be reconstructed it has remained in place and plugged for more than three years without a change.

11. Most of the time the T-tube remains plugged (one patient $6^1/_2$ years). This allows for normal respiration and phonation while the stent is in place.

USES OF THE TRACHEAL T-TUBE

1. Acute tracheal injuries.
2. Support reconstituted trachea.
3. Support reconstructed trachea.
4. With segmental resection and anastomosis.
5. Support intrathoracic tracheal stenosis.
6. Use with tracheal stenosis when the cervical or thoracic trachea cannot be repaired.
7. Use as a substitute for the cervical trachea when it cannot be reconstructed. Currently there are six such patients with the T-tube in place ranging from 2-7 years. A few patients in this group have over a period of years regenerated a mucosa-lined trachea supported by scar tissue which has remained adequately patent so that a T-tube or a tracheotomy is not necessary.

SUCTIONING OF THE SILICONE TRACHEAL T-TUBE

The external portion of the T-tube can be tilted superiorly or inferiorly to facilitate suctioning (Fig. 4). It is important to select a suction catheter small enough to be easily inserted. As a general rule, most patients require suctioning both superiorly and inferiorly several times a day during the first ten days after insertion of the T-tube. Thereafter, twice daily suctioning is required.

It is not necessary to insert the suction catheter any great distance beyond the ends of the T-tube. This only produces irritation of the tracheal lining and coughing.

TECHNIQUE FOR INSERTING THE SILICONE TRACHEAL T-TUBE

The T-tube should be inserted by the surgeon (Fig. 5). Suction apparatus and a large, narrow, curved hemostat are the needed equipment. Usually the T-tube is inserted in the operating room while the patient is under general anesthesia. It can be in-

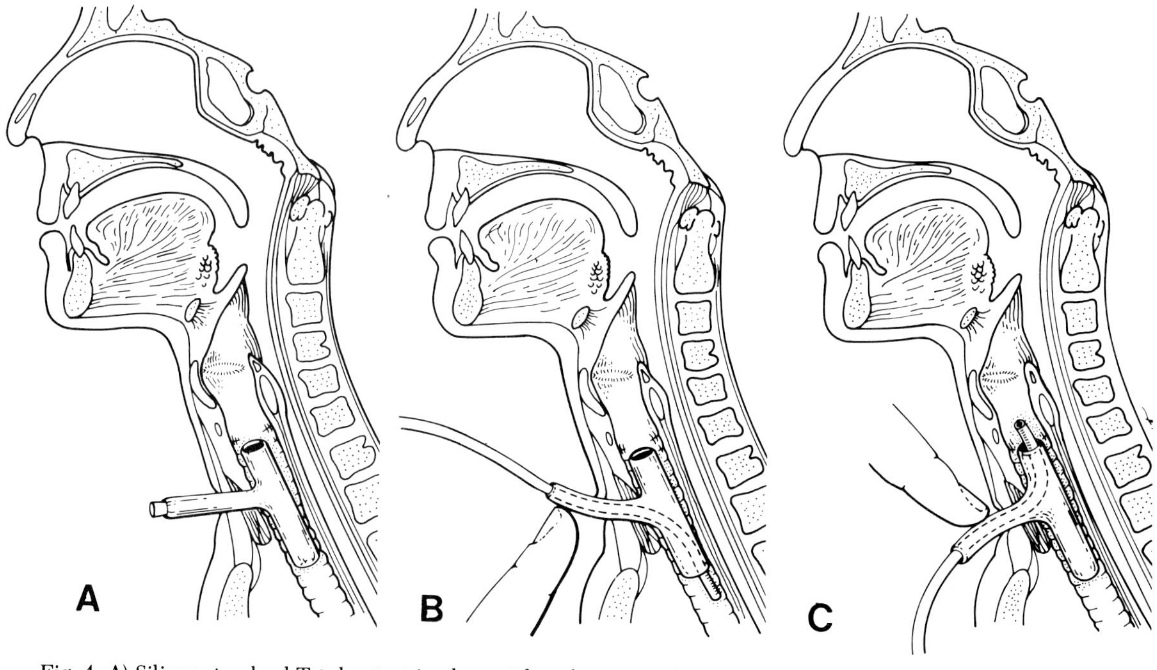

Fig. 4. A) Silicone tracheal T-tube stent in place with a plug inserted into its extraluminal limb. The upper intraluminal limb is usually shorter than the lower, although these can be reversed if additional length is needed superiorly. The junction of the intraluminal and extraluminal portions of the T-tube is designed to facilitate insertion of a suction tubing. B) When suctioning the lower segment of the T-tube and trachea, the extraluminal limb is elevated as the suction tubing is inserted. C) The suction tubing is directed superiorly into the upper intraluminal tracheal limb of the T-tube by bending the extraluminal limb in an inferior direction.

serted in the office or at the bedside in patients who have had the T-tube in place for several months.

REMOVAL OF THE SILICONE TRACHEAL T-TUBE

Most patients have not required a change of the tracheal T-tube prior to its final removal. On occasion, however, it is necessary to remove and replace the T-tube and this should be done:

1. if the intraluminal portion of the T-tube becomes partially obstructed and cannot be cleaned;

2. if the T-tube is not in proper position;

3. as an emergency (by doctor, nurse or relative) if the T-tube becomes obstructed. A metal tracheotomy tube with obturator should be kept on hand to be inserted immediately after emergency removal of the T-tube.

To remove (Fig. 6), the external limb of the T-tube is grasped with the thumb and index finger of the right hand while the index and second finger of the left hand are pressed against the skin above and below the external limb of the T-tube. The T-tube is removed by a steady firm anterior pull. On rare occasions (if the T-tube has been in place for many months) it may be necessary to make a small vertical incision in the skin above or below the external limb of the T-tube to facilitate removal.

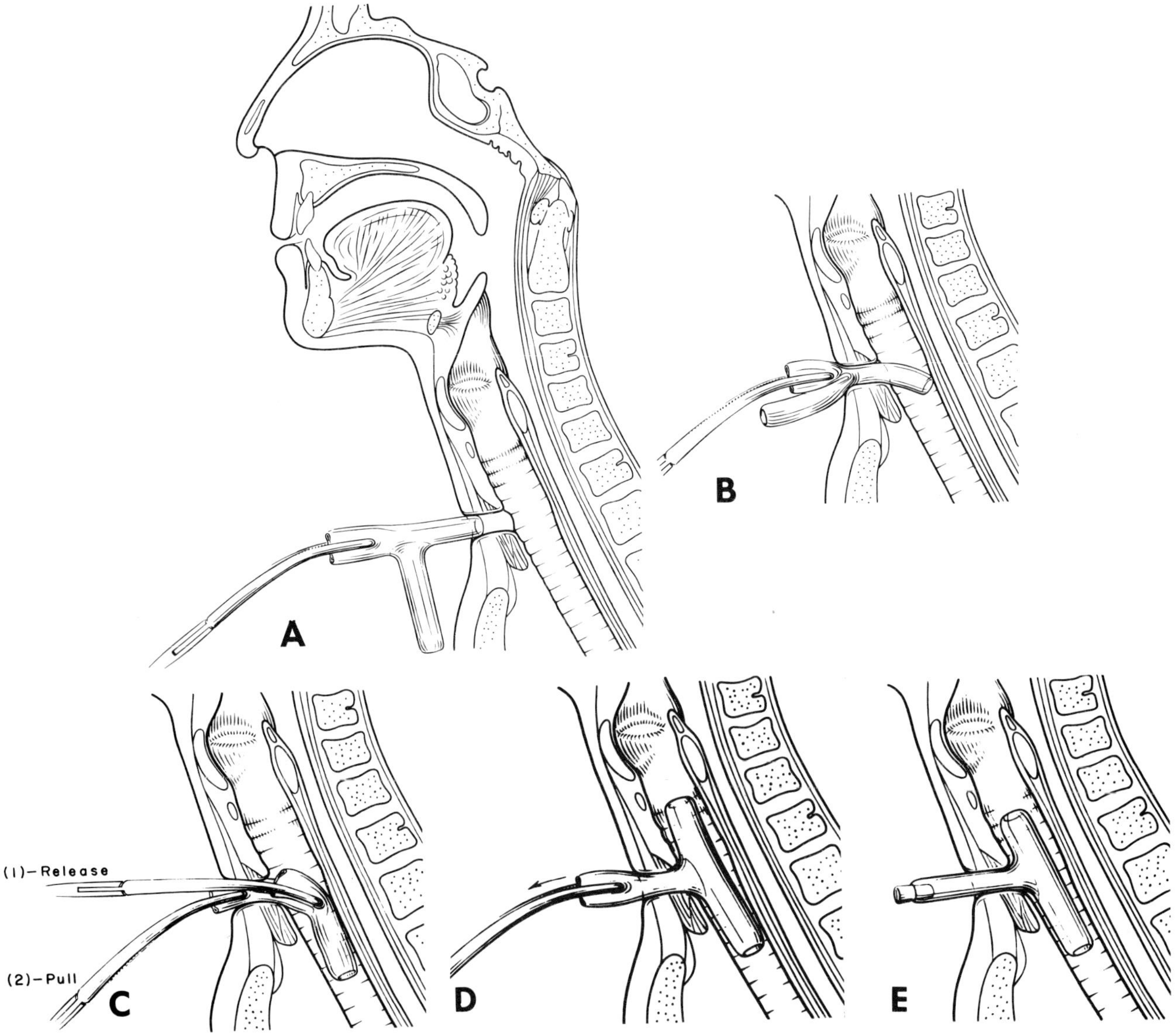

Fig. 5. A) The upper limb of the intraluminal portion of the T-tube is grasped with a hemostat and the lower limb is inserted into the tracheotomy fenestration. B) As the tube is inserted, the lower limb of the intraluminal portion is directed inferiorly into the distal trachea. C) When the entire intraluminal portion of the T-tube is within the tracheal lumen, the external portion of the T-tube is grasped with a second hemostat just before the first hemostat is released. D) An anterior pull on the exterior portion of the T-tube will direct the upper limb of the intraluminal portion into place. E) T-tube is in place and the silicone plug has been inserted.

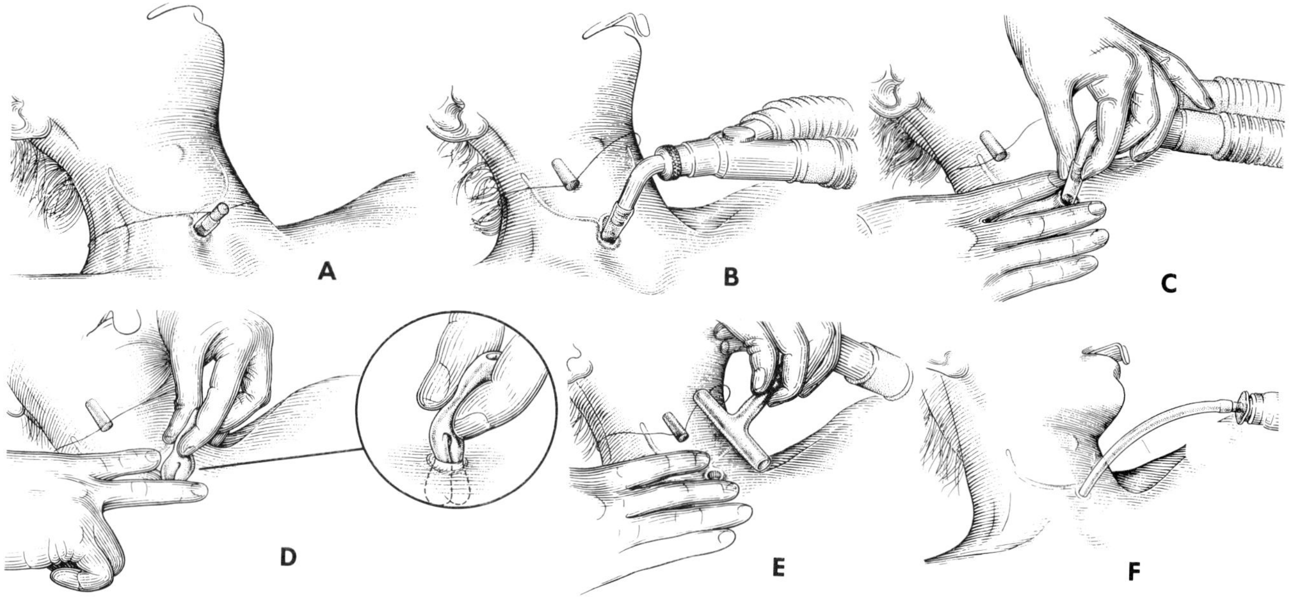

Fig. 6. A) Patient is shown with a silicone tracheal T-tube in place. B) The plug has been removed. Anesthesia is administered via the external limb of the T-tube. C) A finger is placed above and below the external limb to exert pressure in a posterior direction. The exterior limb is pulled anteriorly. D) As the T-tube is pulled from the trachea, the upper and lower intraluminal limbs buckle towards each other. E) The T-tube "springs back" to its proper shape after the intraluminal limbs part from the tracheotomy fistula. F) An endotracheal tube is inserted until the patient has recovered from general anesthesia.

GRAFTS APPLIED TO THE SILICONE TRACHEAL T-TUBE

A split-thickness skin graft is obtained from the supraclavicular region with a half razor blade on a large hemostat or with a small electric dermatome. The graft is usually applied to the patient but on occasion may be applied directly to the T-tube (Fig. 7 B, C). Mucoperiochondrial grafts from the nasal septum have been used successfully. A thin graft is easy to obtain and secure in place. Mucous membrane grafts are obtained from the buccal region being careful to avoid injury to the parotid duct or orifice. The buccal defect is closed either horizontally or vertically depending on the size and shape of the graft obtained (Fig. 7 A).

ANESTHESIA VIA T-TUBE

The loss of anesthesia or air through the upper intraluminal limb of the T-tube while it is in place during surgery has been a problem. A simple solution to this problem is to use the versatile Shiley arterial embolectomy catheter to obstruct the upper

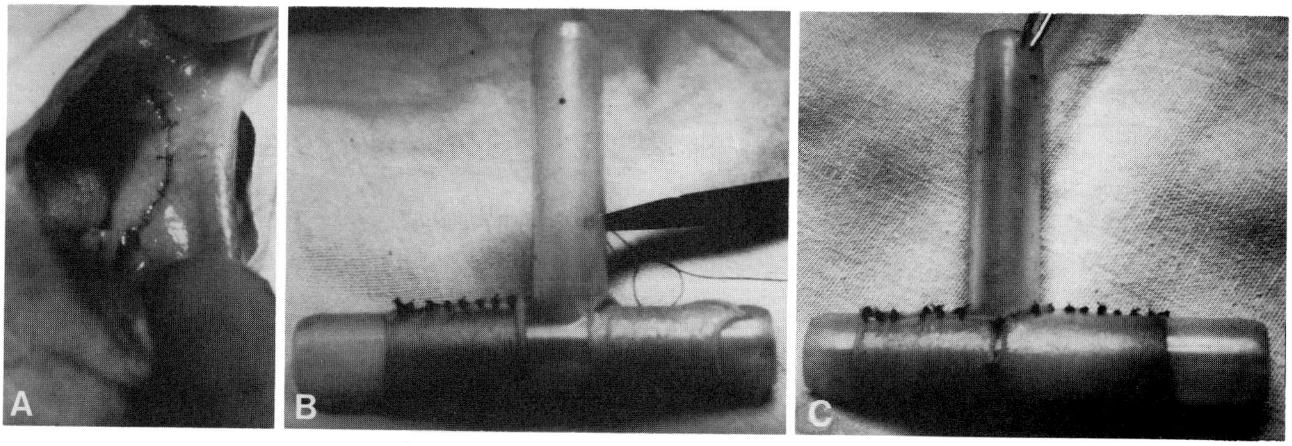

Fig. 7. A) Photograph of the repair following resection of a large buccal mucosal graft. The incisions should avoid the parotid duct papillae and orifice. A 2 x 4 cm mucous membrane graft can be obtained from the nasal septum. There is very little shrinkage with this graft because of its dense submucosal fibrous layer. A split-thickness skin graft is best obtained from the supraclavicular region for it is in the field of operation and void of hair. B) The graft is being sutured to the T-tube. It can be placed at any level. Chromic catgut sutures (No. 4-0) are used to attach the graft to the intratracheal portion of the silicone T-tube. C) Grafts above and below the center of the T-tube have been sutured together. These are used to repair areas void of mucous membrane at the level of the tracheotomy orifice, which is at a lower cervical tracheal level.

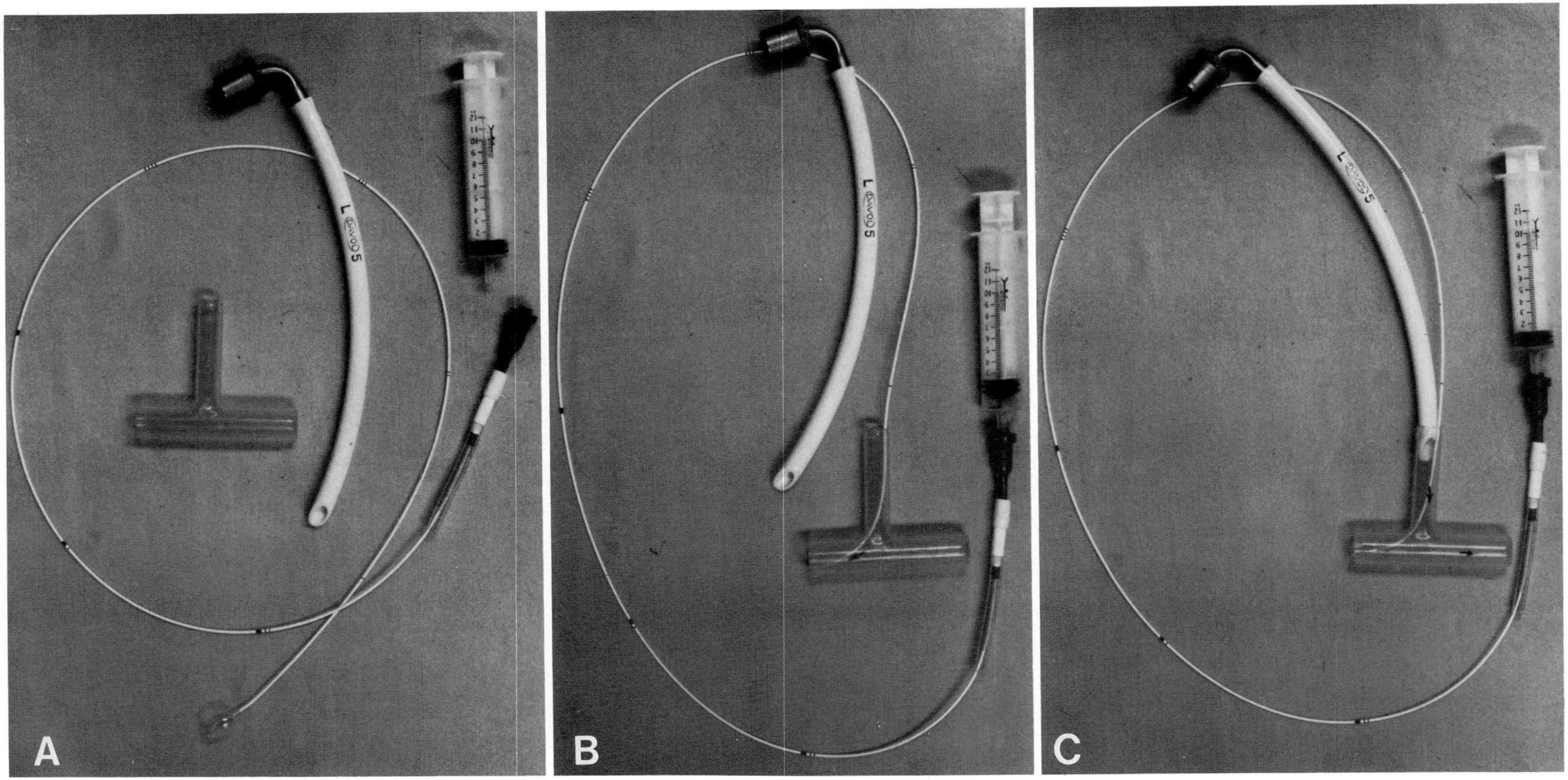

Fig. 8. A) Equipment needed to obstruct the upper intraluminal limb of the T-tube so that anesthesia may be directed to the distal trachea. B) The Fogarty® catheter (Shiley arterial embolectomy catheter) has been inserted into the upper limb of the tracheal T-tube. The catheter has not been inflated and thus much of the anesthetic agent is directed superiorly (arrow). C) The balloon of the catheter is now inflated blocking the upper intraluminal limb of the T-tube. The arrows indicate the direction of air flow.

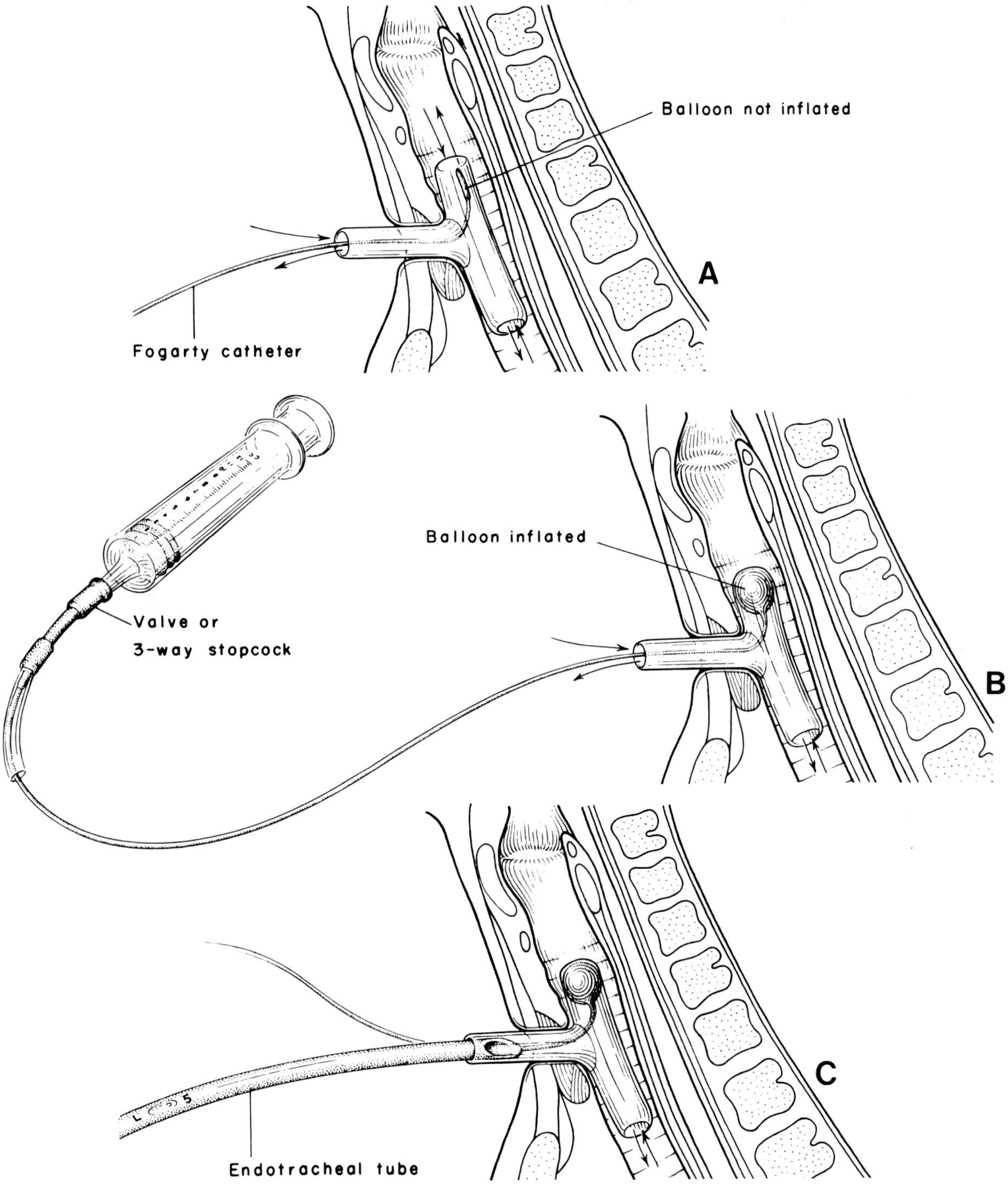

Fig. 9. A) The Fogarty catheter (Shiley arterial embolectomy catheter) has been inserted into the upper intraluminal limb of the T-tube. Arrows indicate the direction of air flow. B) The balloon of the embolectomy catheter has been inflated so as to obstruct the lumen of the upper intraluminal limb of the T-tube. C) An endotracheal tube is inserted into the extraluminal limb of the T-tube. By so doing, a closed system is established with the distal tracheobronchial system.

intraluminal limb of the T-tube (Figs. 8 and 9 A). The endotracheal tube attached to the extraluminal portion of the T-tube is disconnected. The embolectomy catheter is inserted into the upper intraluminal segment and inflated (Figs. 8 and 9 B, C). A closed system between the anesthesia apparatus and the distal trachea is reestablished when the endotracheal tube is attached to the T-tube (Figs. 8 and 9 C). This technique also permits assisted respiration with the silicone tracheal T-tube in place.

PREOPERATIVE AND POSTOPERATIVE ORDERS

Preoperative work-up:

Maxi scan (adult) CBC (child)
Urinalysis
Chest x-ray

Soft tissue x-ray series of larynx and trachea with copper filtration
EKG (adult over 40 years)
Regular diet
Preoperative antibiotics
IV antibiotic started as soon as the preanesthetic IV is inserted

Postoperative care of the T-tube:

1. Antibiotics
   ____________ continue IV ________ hours postoperatively
   ____________ qid po
2. Constant humidity (ultrasonic preferred)
3. External limb of T-tube
   - plugged when recovered from anesthesia if possible
   - if not, humidified air over T-tube
4. Suction at least four times daily upwards and downwards
5. Mucomyst® (10%) ($1\frac{1}{2}$-2 cc) or sodium bicarbonate solution (5%) (2 cc)
   - every four hours, introduce slowly
6. Normal saline solution (2-5 cc)
   - every four hours or 15 minutes after No. 5
7. Clean skin around external portion of T-tube three times a day
   - remove crusts
   - apply Betadine® solution or Aureomycin® (chlorotetracycline HCl) ointment
8. Clean inside of T-tube
   - cotton-tipped applicator dipped in peroxide
   - finish cleaning with dry cotton-tipped applicator

After first 7-10 days:

1. Continue plug in external limb if possible
2. Suction upwards and downwards two to three times a day
3. Mucomyst (10%) or sodium bicarbonate solution (5%) twice daily
4. Continue cleaning of external limb twice daily - inside and outside
5. Continue skin care around T-tube twice daily

Remove and replace T-tube as needed:

1. See instructions
2. Doctor only unless emergency
3. If obstructed, pull out immediately and insert a tracheotomy tube (see Table 1). A tracheotomy tube should be with the patient at all times in case an emergency removal is necessary.

TABLE 1. CORRESPONDING T-TUBE AND TRACHEOTOMY TUBE SIZES

Size T-Tube (mm)	*Size Shiley Tracheotomy Tube*
4.5-6	00
8	0
9	1
10	2
11	3
12	4
13	6
14	6
16	8

CHILDHOOD COMMUNICATION DISORDERS: PRESENT STATUS AND FUTURE PRIORITIES

Supplement 74 — Vol. 89, September-October, 1980, No. 5, Part 2

THE ANNALS OF OTOLOGY, RHINOLOGY & LARYNGOLOGY

Proceedings of a Scientific Dedication Conference Sponsored

by

The Boys Town Institute for Communication Disorders in Children

Omaha, Nebraska

October 5-6, 1978

General Conference Chairman

Patrick E. Brookhouser, MD, FACS

Father Flanagan Professor and Chairman
Department of Otolaryngology and Human Communication
Creighton University School of Medicine.
Director, The Boys Town Institute
for Communication Disorders in Children
Omaha, Nebraska

THE ANNALS PUBLISHING COMPANY
4949 FOREST PARK BLVD.
ST. LOUIS, MISSOURI 63108

CHILDHOOD COMMUNICATION DISORDERS:
PRESENT STATUS AND FUTURE PRIORITIES

COEDITORS

Patrick E. Brookhouser, MD, FACS
Father Flanagan Professor and Chairman
Department of Otolaryngology and Human Communication
Creighton University School of Medicine.
Director, The Boys Town Institute
for Communication Disorders in Children
Omaha, Nebraska

John E. Bordley, MD, FACS
Andelot Professor Emeritus
Laryngology and Otology
Johns Hopkins University School of Medicine
Baltimore, Maryland

PARTICIPANTS

Distinguished Guests and Honorees

Archbishop Daniel E. Sheehan
President
Board of Directors
Father Flanagan's Boys' Home

Reverend Robert P. Hupp
Director
Father Flanagan's Boys' Home

Reverend Matthew E. Creighton, S.J.
President
Creighton University

John E. Bordley, MD
Andelot Professor Emeritus
Laryngology and Otology
Johns Hopkins University School of Medicine

Mr. James Ensign
President
Creighton Omaha Regional Health Care Corp.

Thomas T. Smith, MD
Clinical Professor
Department of Otolaryngology and Human Communication
Creighton University School of Medicine

Guest Faculty

Richard J. Bellucci, MD
Professor and Chairman
Department of Otolaryngology
New York Medical College

LaVonne Bergstrom, MD
Associate Professor
Division of Head and Neck Surgery
UCLA School of Medicine

Charles I. Berlin, PhD
Director
Kresge Hearing Research Laboratory of the South
Professor of Otorhinolaryngology and Biocommunication
Louisiana State University Medical Center

Robert C. Bilger, PhD
Professor
Department of Speech and Hearing Sciences
University of Illinois

Harold Ewertsen, MD
Chief of Auditory Research and Planning
University Hospitals
Copenhagen, Denmark

Blair Fearon, MD
Assistant Professor of Otolaryngology
Department of Otolaryngology
University of Toronto

Paul Fletcher, PhD
Lecturer
Department of Linguistic Science
University of Reading
Reading, England

Janet B. Hardy, MD
Professor of Pediatrics
The Johns Hopkins University
School of Medicine

Joseph Hind, PhD
Professor and Chairman
Department of Neurophysiology
University of Wisconsin
School of Medicine

James Jerger, PhD
Director and Professor of Audiology
Department of Otorhinolaryngology and Communicative Sciences
Baylor College of Medicine

David P. Kuehn, PhD
Department of Speech Pathology and Audiology
University of Denver

Merle Lawrence, PhD
Director
Kresge Hearing Research Institute
Professor of Otolaryngology
University of Michigan
School of Medicine

Gunnar Lidén, MD
Professor
Department of Otolaryngology and Audiology
University of Göteborg
Göteborg, Sweden

Edgar L. Lowell, PhD
Director
The John Tracy Clinic
Los Angeles, California

Michael M. Merzenich, PhD
Associate Professor of Otolaryngology
Director of the Coleman Memorial Laboratory
University of California
School of Medicine

Donald M. Morehead, PhD
Former Director of Research
The Institute for Childhood Aphasia
Stanford University
School of Medicine

G. Paul Moore, PhD
Professor and Acting Chairman
Department of Speech
University of Florida

Michael M. Paparella, MD
Professor and Chairman
Department of Otolaryngology
University of Minnesota Medical School

Sandy Friel-Patti, PhD
UTD/Callier Center
Dallas, Texas

William H. Perkins, PhD
Professor of Speech Communication
Department of Speech Communication
University of Southern California

James M. Pickett, PhD
Professor of Speech Communication Research
Director, Sensory Communication Research Laboratory
Gallaudet College

G. O'Neil Proud, MD
Professor and Chairman
Department of Otolaryngology
University of Kansas Medical Center

Robert J. Ruben, MD
Professor and Chairman
Department of Otolaryngology
Albert Einstein College of Medicine

Jan Sekula, MD
Professor of Otolaryngology
Academia Medyczna
Krakow, Poland

S. Richard Silverman, PhD
Director Emeritus
Central Institute for the Deaf

James B. Snow, Jr., MD
Professor and Chairman
Department of Otorhinolaryngology and Human Communication
University of Pennsylvania
School of Medicine

Francis A. Sooy, MD
Chancellor and Professor of Otolaryngology
University of California Medical Center, S.F.

Luther L. Terry, MD
President
Hearing, Educational Aid and Research Foundation, Inc.
Washington, D. C.

Gabriel F. Tucker, Jr., MD
Head
Division of Otolaryngology and Bronchoesophagology
The Children's Hospital (Chicago)
Professor of Otolaryngology and Maxillofacial Surgery
Northwestern University School of Medicine

Rolland J. VanHattum, PhD
Professor of Communication Disorders
Department of Communication Disorders
State University College at Buffalo

Robert J. Wenthold, PhD
Staff Fellow
Laboratory of Neuro-Otolaryngology
National Institute of Neurological and Communicative Disorders and Stroke
National Institutes of Health

Boys Town Institute/Creighton University School of Medicine Faculty

Patrick E. Brookhouser, MD
Director
Boys Town Institute
Father Flanagan Professor and Chairman
Department of Otolaryngology and Human Communication

David G. Cyr, MA
Coordinator, Vestibular Laboratory
Boys Town Institute
Instructor of Human Communication
Department of Otolaryngology and Human Communication

Peter K. Hixson, PhD
Coordinator, Early Childhood Language Program
Boys Town Institute
Assistant Professor of Human Communication
Department of Otolaryngology and Human Communication

Pamela E. Hook, PhD
Coordinator, Learning Disabilities Program
Boys Town Institute
Assistant Professor of Human Communication
Department of Otolaryngology and Human Communication

Eric Javel, PhD
Research Associate, Auditory Physiology Laboratory
Boys Town Institute
Assistant Professor of Human Communication
Department of Otolaryngology and Human Communication

Walt Jesteadt, PhD
Research Associate, Psychoacoustics Laboratory
Boys Town Institute
Assistant Professor of Human Communication
Department of Otolaryngology and Human Communication

Richard Lippman, PhD
Research Associate, Communication Engineering Laboratory
Boys Town Institute
Assistant Professor of Human Communication
Department of Otolaryngology and Human Communication

John Lybolt, PhD
Coordinator, Speech Pathology Services
Boys Town Institute
Assistant Professor of Human Communication
Department of Otolaryngology and Human Communication

Serge A. Martinez, MD
Director, Medical/Surgical Services
Boys Town Institute
Associate Professor of Otolaryngology
Department of Otolaryngology and Human Communication

Noel D. Matkin, PhD
Director, Language and Learning Center
Boys Town Institute
Professor of Human Communication
Department of Otolaryngology and Human Communication

Daniel F. Mouney, MD
Staff Otolaryngologist and Coordinator of Otolaryngologic Research Programs
Boys Town Institute
Instructor of Otolaryngology
Department of Otolaryngology and Human Communication

James E. Peck, PhD
Coordinator, Audiological Services
Boys Town Institute
Assistant Professor of Human Communication
Department of Otolaryngology and Human Communication

Jon F. Peters, PhD
Research Associate, Clinical Sensory Physiology Laboratory
Boys Town Institute
Assistant Professor of Human Communication
Department of Otolaryngology and Human Communication

Betty Jane Philips, EdD
Associate Director for Clinical Programs, Language and Learning Center
Boys Town Institute
Professor of Human Communication
Department of Otolaryngology and Human Communication

Bruce Warr, PhD
Research Associate, Neuroanatomy Laboratory
Boys Town Institute
Professor of Human Communication
Department of Otolaryngology and Human Communication

Charles S. Watson, PhD
Director, Human Communication Research Laboratories
Boys Town Institute
Professor of Human Communication
Department of Otolaryngology and Human Communication

Don W. Worthington, PhD
Director, Audiology and Vestibular Sciences
Boys Town Institute
Professor of Human Communication
Department of Otolaryngology and Human Communication

CONTENTS

Childhood Communication Disorders: Present Status and Future Priorities. Introduction. P.E. Brookhouser, MD, FACS 1

Problems of the Communicatively Disadvantaged. An Overview. J.E. Bordley, MD, FACS 3

Support of Programs for the Communicatively Disadvantaged Child: Role of the Private Foundation. L.L. Terry, MD 5

Communication Disorders: Investigator Training and Support Needs. M. Lawrence, PhD 9

Educational and Training Priorities for Clinicians and Researchers in the Area of Communication Disorders. A Health Science Campus Chancellor's Perspective. F.A. Sooy, MD 12

Priorities in Service Delivery to the Communicatively Disadvantaged: Habilitation Needs. S.R. Silverman, PhD 15

Panel — Educational Programming for the Hearing-Impaired: Present and Future. Chairman: E.L. Lowell, PhD 19

The United States. E.L. Lowell, PhD 19

Sweden. G. Lidén, MD 22

Poland. J. Sekula, MD 25

Denmark. H.W. Ewertsen, MD 28

Pathology of Congenital Deafness. Present Status and Future Priorities. L. Bergstrom, MD, FACS 31

Ear-Related Developmental Anomalies of Branchial Clefts and Arches I and II. R.J. Bellucci, MD 42

Role of Tonsillectomy and Adenoidectomy in the Management of Children with Middle Ear Effusion. J.B. Snow, Jr., MD 43

Chronic Otitis Media and Cholesteatoma. G.O. Proud, MD 47

Behavioral Methods in Pediatric Audiology: Past, Present, Future. N.D. Matkin, PhD 50

Impedance Audiometry. G. Lidén, MD 53

Electrophysiologic Audiometry. D.W. Worthington, PhD, J.F. Peters, PhD 59

Binaural Interaction in Brainstem-Evoked Responses. R.A. Dobie, MD, C.I. Berlin, PhD 62

Vestibular Testing in Children. D.G. Cyr, MA 63

Uses and Abuses of Hearing Aids. J.E. Peck, PhD 70

Advances in Sensory Aids for the Hearing-Impaired: Visual and Vibrotactile Aids. J.M. Pickett, PhD 74

Review of Recent Research on the Selection of Frequency-Gain Characteristics for Hearing Aids. R. Lippmann, PhD 79

Coding Considerations in Design of Cochlear Prostheses. M.M. Merzenich, PhD, M. White, PhD 84

Frequency Analysis in Normal and Hearing-Impaired Listeners. W. Jesteadt, PhD 88

Time Course of Auditory Perceptual Learning. C.S. Watson, PhD 96

Neurophysiological Correlates of Auditory Maturation. E. Javel, PhD 103

Efferent Components of the Auditory System. W.B. Warr, PhD 114

Neurochemistry of the Auditory System. R.J. Wenthold, PhD 121

CONTENTS

Panel — Research Priorities in Auditory Science. Chairman: M. Lawrence, PhD . . . 132

The Otologist's View. R. Ruben, MD . . . 132

The Audiologist's View. J. Jerger, PhD . . . 134

The Physiologist's View. J.E. Hind, PhD . . . 136

Orofacial Embryology, Anatomy and Physiology. D.P. Kuehn, PhD . . . 138

Laryngeal Development and Congenital Lesions. G.F. Tucker, Jr., MD . . . 142

Laryngeal Surgery in the Pediatric Patient. B. Fearon, MD . . . 146

Prevention and Treatment of Stuttering. W.H. Perkins, PhD . . . 150

Perceptual Evaluation of Velopharyngeal Competency. B.J. Philips, EdD . . . 153

Morphophonemic Processes in Children. J. Lybolt, PhD . . . 158

Research Priorities in Speech. R.J. Van Hattum, PhD . . . 161

Language Deficiency in Children. D.M. Morehead, PhD, K.E. Morehead, W.A. Morehead . . . 165

Aspects of Mother-Child Interaction as Related to the Remediation Process. S. Friel-Patti, PhD . . . 171

Language Stimulation Group. Habilitation Model. P.K. Hixson, PhD . . . 175

Language-Based Learning Disabilities. P.E. Hook, PhD . . . 179

Research Priorities in Language and Learning. P. Fletcher, PhD . . . 182

CHILDHOOD COMMUNICATION DISORDERS: PRESENT STATUS AND FUTURE PRIORITIES

INTRODUCTION

PATRICK E. BROOKHOUSER, MD, FACS
OMAHA, NEBRASKA

The ability to communicate is perhaps the most essentially human of man's endowments and is, of course, the keystone of the learning process by which a child acquires the knowledge required to play a meaningful role in adult society. Yet, the sequential development of intellectual and neuromotor skills necessary to utilize the complex symbol system which forms the basis of language and speech is taken for granted by most parents and clinicians.

More than 10,000,000 children from birth to the age of 21 in the United States suffer from a disease or disability which impairs their communicative ability. These disorders range from obvious anatomical deformities, such as microtia or cleft palate, to such subtle problems as central auditory processing deficits. Gradually, the need for a coordinated multidisciplinary approach to the evaluation and habilitation of the communicatively impaired child has become apparent to clinicians and educators, but many barriers stand in the way of implementation of such a model.

Rapid progress toward making such a comprehensive program available to fill the needs of children with communication disorders across the country has been impeded by diverse factors. Various disciplines involved in the management of childhood communication disorders have somewhat artificially defined their respective spheres of competence to the exclusion of specialists with closely related interests. Areas of overlap have become the subject matter for controversial "turf" battles among the national leadership of professional organizations claiming to represent the "interest" of practicing clinicians. Typically, clinicians providing care and treatment for the communicatively impaired are geographically and administratively separated from researchers interested in the same problems, thus providing little opportunity for creative interaction on a regular basis. Meager financial resources targeted to support research and patient care have been further fragmented among competing agencies each attempting to pursue its own priorities without the benefit of a coordinated plan.

In 1972, the Board of Directors of Father Flanagan's Boys' Home surveyed the most pressing needs of children and identified communication disorders as an area of concern which had received far too little attention from the private sector, as well as from governmental funding agencies. As a result, the Boys Town Institute for Communication Disorders in Children was established in Omaha, Nebraska. This new facility was designed and constructed adjacent to Creighton University's Health Sciences Schools and primary teaching hospital to accommodate the Institute's programs.

The charge given to the Boys Town Institute planning team was:

> To develop a nationally oriented clinical educational and research resource dealing with complex problems of hearing impairment, speech and language disorders, learning disabilities and related problems of human communication.
>
> To develop and implement model programs for the diagnosis, evaluation, treatment and habilitation of youngsters with communication disorders.
>
> To develop and implement programs of basic and applied research to further the knowledge and understanding of human communication disorders and to design new techniques and methods for the management of children with these problems.

The commitment made by Boys Town's Board of Directors to establish and provide substantial operating support for the Institute represents one of the largest efforts of its kind ever undertaken by the private sector.

Many leading physicians, audiologists, speech/language pathologists, educators of the deaf, and researchers gave unselfishly of their time and efforts by coming to Omaha to provide advice and counsel during the Institute's developmental phases. In addition to the special honorees at the dedicatory conference, Drs. John E. Bordley of Baltimore and T. T. Smith of Omaha, the following deserve our special recognition:

Bobby R. Alford, MD, Houston, Texas

Raymond T. Carhart, PhD,† Evanston, Illinois
Leo E. Conner, EdD, Queens, New York
Frederick L. Darley, PhD, Rochester, Minnesota
Leo G. Doerfler, PhD, Pittsburgh, Pennsylvania
Victor Goodhill, MD, Beverly Hills, California
Janet B. Hardy, MD, Baltimore, Maryland
William G. Hardy, PhD,† Baltimore, Maryland
Joseph E. Hind, PhD, Madison, Wisconsin
Merle Lawrence, PhD, Ann Arbor, Michigan
Edgar L. Lowell, PhD, Los Angeles, California
Gunner O'Neil Proud, MD, Kansas City, Kansas
Herbert F. Schliesser, PhD, Lincoln, Nebraska
S. Richard Silverman, PhD, St. Louis, Missouri
Catherine Smith, PhD, Portland, Oregon
Mrs. Spencer Tracy, Los Angeles, California

The Scientific Dedication Conference for the Boys Town Institute for Communication Disorders in Children entitled "Childhood Communication Disorders: Present Status and Future Priorities" represents an initial attempt at providing an interdisciplinary information exchange involving physicians, clinicians, educators, health planners, and researchers with interests in human communication and its disorders. More opportunities to build bridges among the various clinical and research disciplines must be provided in the future to insure continued progress toward solving the vexing problems confronting the communicatively impaired.

†Deceased.

PROBLEMS OF THE COMMUNICATIVELY DISADVANTAGED
AN OVERVIEW

JOHN E. BORDLEY, MD, FACS
BALTIMORE, MARYLAND

The article traces the attitude of various cultures through the centuries toward the hearing and speech handicapped. It outlines the early efforts to develop rehabilitative techniques for such handicaps, and describes a number of the pioneers in the field of education for the "deaf and dumb." The emergence of the opposing philosophies for training the hearing handicapped, the oral school and the signing school, and the influence these two had on the development of education for the deaf is described. The part played by basic research and the development of new instrumentation during the past 50 years in the solution of many of the problems of disordered communication is reviewed. Finally, the philosophic aims are described that led to the establishment of the Boys Town Institute for communicatively handicapped children.

By developing a system for free communication, man has achieved a method to exchange information to recall and to retell his experiences and discuss new ideas. Modern civilization owes its step-by-step development to the data base compiled through thousands of years as the result of man's intercommunication. Many of his solutions to problems were originally passed on as folk tales around the campfires of primitive man. Very early, man became so dependent upon this ability to communicate that those individuals deprived of the opportunity to develop normal communication were considered deviants and were not accepted in the mainstream of society, and indeed with some reason; because the frustrations arising from an otherwise normal child's inability to communicate leads to behavior so violent that children of normal intelligence have been adjudged insane. In Biblical times Hebrew laws stated that the "deaf without speech will be denied all legal rights." Centuries later Justinian went even further and wrote into his legal code a ruling that "the deaf without speech shall be classified with the lunatics and are without legal rights or obligations."

While the world's attitude toward the communicatively handicapped has improved through the centuries since Justinian, we should remember that as late as the enlightened 20th century in this country a number of states continued to support institutions operated for the care of the deaf and insane.

The first record of an attempt to rehabilitate a communicatively handicapped individual was in the 16th century when Pedro Ponce de Leon, a Spanish monk, taught a deaf young nobleman to speak so that he could legally claim his inheritance. This success was an inspiration for the teachers that were to follow. In the 17th century another Spanish monk, Bonet, published a book on the use of signing for the education of the deaf and in 1660 Bonet's system was taken to Scotland by Dalgano, a teacher interested in the problems of the deaf. In 1690 a Swiss teacher named Amman, while in Amsterdam, published a book on methods to instruct the deaf in lip reading; his ideas were shortly adopted by the teachers in Germany interested in the instruction of the deaf. So began a rivalry between signing and oral education for the deaf, which has done so much to retard the progress of deaf education up to the present time. In 1770 the Abbé l'Epee, who had learned Spanish in order to translate Bonet's book, was commissioned by the French king to set up a state school for the deaf and dumb in Paris. This was the first official recognition that the deaf might be rehabilitated through education. In 1807 the next important milestone was reached when the Danish parliament passed a bill making education of the deaf compulsory. Unfortunately, that law set the age for the beginning of education at seven years, which delayed the development of our present concept of the necessity for very early instruction.

Organized instruction of the hearing handicapped was late in its beginning in this country. Charles Green of Boston, probably the pioneer educator here, studied for two years in England under the Braidwoods, returning to this country at the beginning of the 19th century to introduce oral instruction of the deaf. In 1815 a young minister in Massachusetts, Thomas Hopkins Gallaudet, went to Europe for the purpose of studying the methods of instruction for both signing and oral communication. The Braidwoods refused his application to study the oral method under them when they learned that he planned to go to Paris later to study signing under the Abbé Secard. The Abbé welcomed him for a year's study, following which he returned to Hartford and opened the American Assylum for the Deaf, where the signing method

From the Department of Laryngology and Otology, Johns Hopkins University School of Medicine, Baltimore, Maryland.
REPRINTS — John E. Bordley, MD, Department of Laryngology and Otology, Johns Hopkins Hospital, Baltimore, MD 21205.

was introduced. Years later Gallaudet's name was given to the only college ever organized for teaching the deaf. In 1872 Alexander Graham Bell from Scotland opened his school in Boston, where the opposition to the oral method of teaching was so strong that he changed its name to the School for Vocal Physiology and Elocution, a neat cover for his intended activities. He persuaded an otologist, John Blake, to work with him in order to amplify his knowledge of the ear and auditory physiology. Bell was probably the first to recognize the importance of enlisting public interest in the problems of the communicatively handicapped and he gave most of the money he had received with the Volta Award for his work on the telephone to establish the Volta Bureau for "the increase and diffusion of knowledge of the deaf." This became in fact one of the first information centers.

Of course, the early schools for the deaf cared for only a fraction of those suffering from communication disorders, but they did lead to the subsequent development of special education in our public school systems directed at first to the problems of the deaf and later to the broader field of human communication. Until after World War I these educational efforts contributed exclusively to the habilitation or rehabilitation of those suffering communication disorders, and to the enlistment of public concern for such handicaps. However, they failed to contribute to the study of the causes of communication disorders or to their early recognition. They did not attempt to develop techniques for the restoration of hearing or plans for the prevention of communication disorders. Probably the first organized effort to study such problems was begun in 1918 by an otologist in St. Louis, Max Goldstein, who founded the Central Institute for the Deaf in which he planned for interaction between otologists and teachers, and he provided space for research. In the 1930s the Ewings in England reported their work on the early identification of deafness in children and later still Mrs. Spencer Tracy spelled out the role of the parent in deaf education. Since the 1930s the availability of the antibiotics and the development of new electronic techniques have made possible important advances in the surgery for the relief of deafness; and our research laboratories through their efforts have provided us with basic new understanding of the processes of hearing, language acquisition, and speech development. This same period has seen the birth of audiology and its contributions to the development of techniques for early recognition of communication disorders. Most of the advances in the field of human communication have been achieved since the 1950s and have contributed much toward a more scientific approach to the problems of human communication.

However, the real work is only beginning; as yet we do not know how we hear. Many more disciplines must become involved in the field of human communication, many changes must be made in our surgical efforts to restore hearing, and much must be learned about the epidemiology of deafness, and the other forms of communication disorders while the whole field of prevention lies ahead. We have just begun to experiment with new ideas in special education; the teaching machines are only in their primitive development. Real activity in the field of speech was delayed until the 1930s, perhaps because of lack of understanding of the role that hearing and language play in its development, but under such leaders as Fairbanks, Travis, Johnson, Koepp-Baker, and a number of others speech education has kept pace with deaf education. The acquisition of language, and the rate of learning, those two keystones to man's ability to communicate, were not even appreciated until the 1950s.

In spite of all the achievements in the past, we have in this country today over a million children with hearing defects — 500,000 of which have serious difficulty in comprehending normal speech. There are more than 100,000 children of normal intelligence with hearing so distorted that special education is required to learn to speak. Each year an estimated 10-15% of the children entering school have a degree of learning disability which can result in serious problems in language acquisition and about 20% of the children entering school suffer from speech defects. Recent studies have shown that children with normal IQs suffering from communication disorders cannot learn by our present methods of teaching as well as normal children and as a group are undereducated as compared with the norm. They have illiteracy rates as high as 25-30% and the average academic achievement is only about fifth-grade level. We do indeed have a "silent minority" that needs and deserves much more of our time, effort, and resources to bring it into a truly normal society.

We are meeting today to dedicate a new institute. Its basic support is and will be from the private sector. It is planned as a place where the educator, the basic scientist, the sociologist, the audiologist, the otologist, the neurologist, the geneticist, and the medical engineer will sit down together with these children to study them and to design orderly long-range programs for their rehabilitation and education. It has available to it the diagnostic services of medical center laboratories, diagnostic and research facilities for hearing, speech and special education. Here the theorist, the practitioner, and the educator will consult together and plan both clinical and basic research. But above all this institute is dedicated to the service of children suffering from communication disorders. The goal here has been to develop a new national resource for the study of human communication and it is hoped that it represents a significant step forward in our quest to solve the problems of communication disorders.

SUPPORT OF PROGRAMS FOR THE COMMUNICATIVELY DISADVANTAGED CHILD: ROLE OF THE PRIVATE FOUNDATION

LUTHER L. TERRY, MD
WASHINGTON, DC

In comparison to its support of life-threatening diseases, the Federal government has given little support to preventing and alleviating communicative disorders. The very fact that they are not life threatening, means that communicative disorders can remain an uncomfortable, costly, and debilitating factor throughout the lives of millions of children and adults. In view of the magnitude of the problem and the lack of Federal support, responsible leaders are going to have to turn to the general public for support. Foundations, corporations and individuals can provide support for training and organizing services. Such support may well provide them with an opportunity to assist in an area which has touched their families or them personally. Research, training and service programs for the communicatively disadvantaged child are urged to seek finanical support from private foundations.

This new facility is a great tribute to the foresight and zeal of the Boys Town, Dr. Brookhouser and all of those who participated in the planning and execution of this wonderful program. It is important to have an appropriate modern facility in which to work, but from what I have observed this is not only a fine modern building but is clearly an outstanding program to serve the children of our society in an area which badly needs that service. The public can thank Dr. Brookhouser and all of his associates for having made this development possible.

In commenting on the role of private support for programs for the communicatively disadvantaged child I could point to this development, say that this is a beautiful example of what the private sector can do, and then I could sit down. However, I have never been known to resist the opportunity to make a speech so I shall exercise my prerogative and make some comments on the subject.

Those of us who have been aware of the 13 million persons in our society who have hearing disabilities or deafness have been disturbed about the lack of public concern for these people. Money has poured out of our governmental and public sectors to support education, training and care for cancer, heart disease and many of our other illnesses and disabilities. I do not wish to deprecate these actions. It is true that heart disease and cancer constitute some of our major causes of disability and death. Surely, we must continue to support that work. But at the same time it is distressing to see how little concern and support have arisen to aid our citizens who have communicative disorders. One point which is commonly overlooked in this regard is that the vast majority of instances of heart disease and cancer are progressively fatal illnesses and the patient does not survive for long periods of time; on the other hand, communicative disorders and deafness are usually not fatal conditions and the patient may be expected to live a normal life span. This fact alone makes it more imperative that our society take appropriate steps to aid these persons with their problems in order that they may live, not only a more comfortable life, but that they are able to participate in the mainstream of our society and gain the satisfaction of having contributed to the society in which they live. This is important to each and every one of us.

The commitment of the Boys Town Institute to serve children is especially important. When persons get up into my age bracket they will often have otosclerosis or other degenerative processes which will diminish their hearing acuity. They can be a trial and tribulation to the spouse and their colleagues, but they are of an age and degree of maturity which allows them to take personal actions to cope with the problem. Too, there is often much that can be done to assist these elderly persons without complicated educational or medical procedures. Often evaluation will show that a proper hearing aid is a solution to the problem. Furthermore, modern technology has developed instruments which are unobtrusive and more reliable over a longer period of time. Other types of therapy are commonly straightforward and do not require a long-continued team approach to correct the problem. With the communicatively disadvantaged child it is a different proposition. It is not only important that the child is seen at the earliest appropriate age but the process is more complicated and prolonged requiring the collaboration of a team of experts in education and medical therapy. After all, the assistance given that child can determine the development of that person as a participant in our society or a severely disabled person who is a miserable individual to himself and his family and a public burden for the rest of his life.

As one looks at the past and the present cir-

From the Hearing and Educational Aid and Research Foundation, Inc., Washington, DC.
REPRINTS — Luther L. Terry, MD, HEAR Foundation, P. O. Box 57171, West End Branch, Washington, DC 20037.

cumstances of this problem, one can get very disturbed. We have done too little for too long in facing this common disability.

The Federal government has taken a degree of responsibility to cope with the problem and many states have developed commendable programs. But in general, the public and private response has been far from adequate. One could cite the few outstanding examples such as Gallaudet College and Preparatory School, Washington, DC. The new buildings and facilities at Gallaudet are wonderful, but after all, this institution is merely an education and demonstration program and has little impact on the total service problem. Its primary contribution is the training of leaders from the deaf world but also from the hearing world. There are a few states which have developed outstanding institutions but here too, the effort is often long delayed, is not appropriately available, and doesn't serve to cope with the problem in its entirety.

Many of us have been pleased with the development of a Communicative Disorders Program in the National Institute of Neurological and Communicative Disorders and Stroke (NINCDS) and even to have the term "communicative disorders" incorporated into the Institute title is a plus. It is encouraging to have awards and grants available through this program. In addition to the individual Research Project grants, there are Teacher-Investigator Awards, Research Career Development Awards, Individual Research Service Awards for postdoctoral fellows, Institutional Research Service Awards, and Broad Problem Research Program Projects. As a matter of fact, I believe the Boys Town Institute has three or four grants from this source and that there are other grant applications in the process of review. When one sees the number of grant programs in the NINCDS it sounds quite impressive. However it is generally felt that the sums available to support the programs are far from adequate and only a portion of the approved grants can be funded. There appears to be a particular shortage of funds available to support good clinical research programs.

I should also mention that there are several other areas of the Federal government which have an interest in communicative disorders and have some funds for appropriate programs. The Rehabilitation Services Administration, PHS, the Department of Labor, the Environmental Protective Administration, OSHA, and other agencies at the Federal level have interests in this subject area and may very well provide some support for programs related to communicative disorders. No doubt there are others I have not mentioned.

In many states there are programs for the communicatively disadvantaged but these programs are almost all directed toward service and even in this area are woefully inadequate.

I mention these areas of potential support for research and services which are available at the Federal and state levels to serve as a background for my other remarks. There is a lot of potential support available, but each agency has interests in its special mission and one must be aware of those interests before actually applying for grant or contract support. But overall, the message that I wish to get across is that there is a real inadequacy of funds for research and almost a complete lack of support for service programs.

The message is loud and clear. There is not now nor is there likely to be in the immediate future, adequate public agency support for developments in the communicative disorders. In light of this fact, the responsible leaders in the field are going to have to turn to the general public to support many of the needed programs. Some support can be obtained from established foundations and institutions, but there is a rising interest on the part of individuals who can afford and have an interest in supporting research and especially service for the communicatively disadvantaged.

At the moment there are only a handful of private organizations with a high priority interest in the area. The Kennedy Foundation is well-known for its broad interests in retarded individuals. I was proud to see Sargent Shriver and Eunice Kennedy Shriver honored at this meeting for their contributions. The Tracy Clinic is well-known and highly respected but here too the contribution is limited in relation to the national need. Probably one of the most prominent organizations, especially in the support of research, is The Deafness Research Foundation of New York. This foundation has been active in the field for some years and has provided vital support for many programs related to hearing disabilities and deafness. Over half of their grants were for projects which were clinically oriented. This Foundation allocated about $530,000 to program and supporting services in 1977. I understand that the number of requests for grant support has substantially increased in recent years and the funds available have shown a modest increase.

Recently the National Hearing Association of Oak Brook, Illinois has been established under the presidency of Dr. George E. Shambaugh, Jr. This Association has sponsored state of the arts conferences and workshops on various aspects of hearing disabilities. I am not aware of the magnitude of their support in this field but it is a new organization which is expected to make a contribution to research and service in relation to deafness. I do not mean to infer that they are the only programs, but they are prominent examples.

I have been involved recently in the establishment of a new foundation located in the Washington area which is devoted to the problems of hearing disabilities and deafness. The organization, The

Hearing, Educational Aid and Research Foundation, Inc (HEAR) was established about two years ago and is just beginning to get into operation. The HEAR Foundation was established in memory of Mabel Hubbard Bell, the wife of Alexander Graham Bell; and their grandson, Dr. Melville Bell Grosvenor, is one of the founders and a member of the Board of Directors. The Board is yet small and consists of a prominent group of civic leaders, persons in the field of deafness education and two physicians — Dr. John Bordley one of our Honored Guests at this conference was one of the founders and I am serving as a part-time President and member of the Board. We feel that we are very fortunate to obtain the services of Dr. George Fellendorf who has been Executive Director of the Alexander Graham Bell Association since 1962, as our Executive Director. Dr. Brookhauser is a member of our Educational Advisory Committee.

Mabel Hubbard Bell had normal hearing from birth until she had an attack of scarlet fever at the age of four. She lost all of her hearing and her family later took her to Dr. Bell when they were desperately seeking assistance for her at the time when Dr. Bell was doing much of his work on sound transmission. He apparently saw more in her than an experimental subject, for some years later he married her and they produced a family of normal-hearing children.

The HEAR Foundation will devote its activities toward the problems of hearing disabilities and deafness. Particular emphasis will be placed on the problems in childhood. We expect to support programs designed to improve present therapy and rehabilitation, primarily on a demonstration or training basis, and to provide scholarships, fellowships and loans to physicians and other professional personnel showing unusual promise in the problems of hearing and the correction of deafness. The Foundation plans on making an annual Mabel Hubbard Bell award for outstanding work in the field of deafness. The award may be for work in the field of basic research or in clinical application. We have a Medical Advisory Committee and an Educational Advisory Committee which are expected to provide the Board of Directors with direction and guidance in its programs.

The HEAR Foundation has recently, in collaboration with the American Speech and Hearing Association, the Alexander Graham Bell Association and the Better Hearing Institute, been awarded a contract from the Environmental Protection Agency to establish a "National Information Center for Quiet." This project represents our joint concern for noise in our environment, the cumulative damage which it imposes on hearing, and methods of abating such noises. We are also discussing with the Rehabilitation Services Administration and the Department of Labor, other problems of noise in industry and in our general environment. We hope to work with them in the abatement of unnecessary noises in our working and living environment and the employment of hearing-deficient persons in industry. Our program in relation to our commitment to hearing problems in childhood is in the process of development. We do expect to make a significant contribution to this problem over the next few years. We do not expect to conduct research and service programs as a direct staff activity; rather, we plan to support and stimulate programs and persons who can make a contribution in the field. We have a special interest in training teachers and medical care personnel to appreciate the broad problem and to contribute in that manner.

There are many other organizations, both large and small which I have not had an opportunity to mention. The organizations and private philanthropies can be important to you and the development of your programs. Look for the individuals, the personal interests of persons of substance in your community, your area and your region. Many of these interests will be more inclined to help good organizations of service and research near home, and there are a lot of small personal sources, as well as established foundations looking for appropriate programs to support. Every person of advanced age who is having hearing difficulties is interested in the problem. Many of them have considerable resources which can be devoted to the support of meritorious research and service without economic jeopardy to their families or estates. The same is true for many adults who have problems in their children or their grandchildren.

When you are aware of the sources of support from the Federal government and from the state and local resources, you can evaluate the areas of unmet need and concentrate your efforts for support from local and regional individuals and small private foundations. This is your greatest prospect for those program needs which are not provided for in our Federal or state programs.

You know and I know that "Uncle Government," whether he be Federal or local, is not going to meet your needs and reasonable requirements. Many of us hate to go to persons or institutions as beggars, but remember that in many instances you are doing those persons a favor when you provide them with an outlet for their resources which would not, otherwise contribute to welfare and advancement of our society. After all, there is no one who gets greater satisfaction than the person who can afford and has made a significant contribution to the society in which he lives. Don't take his contribution and walk away. You have responsibility to let him know what his dollars have done and that there has been a proper recognition of the donor. This not only assures a donor of your appreciation for his support but creates a desire to make further and probably greater contributions in the future.

There are many trite expressions such as, "It is more blessed to give than to receive," or "God loves a cheerful giver," etc. Trite they may be, but they would not have survived through generations had there not been a kernel of substance and truth in them.

COMMUNICATION DISORDERS: INVESTIGATOR TRAINING AND SUPPORT NEEDS

MERLE LAWRENCE, PhD

ANN ARBOR, MICHIGAN

There are very few "simple problems" left in the area of communication disorders, but that does not mean that there are unsolvable problems. However, in pursuit of these, present day research often requires extensive technical procedures which require teams of investigators trained in different areas. Among these should be the otolaryngologist, but, in this country, there are few involved and there is a paucity of disease-oriented research. In the 1950s and 1960s, the NIH training grant provided funds for bringing doctor of philosophy researchers into clinical departments to set up laboratories and work intimately with the medical doctor. Basic research training is still essential during residency and the number of postresidency fellowships ought to be increased. The familiarity with clinical problems introduced into the research effort should improve the possibility for the conduction of disease-oriented research in addition to the present day emphasis on basic research.

Not too long ago, research was, more or less, a personal endeavor. It arose from the curiosity of an individual who sought, by any methods he could devise, to answer the questions he raised. Generally, the individual was an academician who, through his teaching, saw the need for new knowledge and so he became involved in research which was accepted as an essential part of his scholarly activity. He asked about whatever interested him, and his genius lay in the way he sought his answers, limited only by the technological achievements of the time.

Now the researcher finds himself in the peculiar spot of facing the fact that the era of the simple problem is over and that technological advances have resulted in the necessity that individuals with very different educational backgrounds engage in research on different aspects of the same problem.

This is particularly apparent in the area of communication disorders, which, more precisely defined, refers to disorders of speech and hearing, two extremely complicated processes. The neuromuscular processes called into play in the creation of speech are equally as complicated as the mechanochemical processes of hearing. Obviously, research in these areas involves considerably diverse disciplines, and when it comes down to the question of research training, it becomes necessary to be quite specific as to the field of specialization. One cannot be an expert in medicine, electronics, computers, acoustics, biochemistry, electron microscopy, etc. Consequently, in this country, we find a paucity of disease-oriented research, and instead a more basic science approach to problems in the communication disorders.

When one reads the world literature in the area of the communication disorders, one is impressed by the fact that in the foreign countries most of the research is done by medical doctors (MD) whereas in the United States this research is done mostly by doctors of philosophy (PhD). One is impressed by the observation that the foreign MDs are much more involved than are the MDs of this country. Of course, in Europe an essential part of obtaining acceptance in academic medicine is a well-done research thesis. Following this, many of the European MDs continue spending a considerable portion of their time in the laboratory, motivated by the fact that the nature of medical practice mitigates the drive for increased earnings through private practice.

Communication disorders are primarily medical problems, but it is not essential that an MD do all the research. However, in the provision of research training and financial support there should be orientation toward the goal of eventually solving the disorder with which the human patient is afflicted.

In a survey[1] published in 1974 by the National Association of the Deaf, the following statistics are given for the causes of deafness in those persons who could not hear or understand speech and who lost that ability prior to 19 years of age. Of the population responding, 35% ascribed their deafness to an illness (spinal meningitis, scarlet fever, measles, whooping cough and others), 7.6% to an accident or injury, 31.8% were born deaf (inherited or mother had rubella), and 24.6% reported cause unknown or did not respond. To this list for the older population must be added presbycusis, ototoxicity and overstimulation.

Each of these is amenable to attack in the research laboratory. And with greater emphasis on prevention, the future could see the number of deaf reduced. The role of hyperlipoproteinemia, congen-

From the Kresge Hearing Research Institute, University of Michigan School of Medicine, Ann Arbor, Michigan.

REPRINTS — Merle Lawrence, PhD, Kresge Hearing Research Institute, University of Michigan School of Medicine, Ann Arbor, MI 48104.

ital deafness as secondary to inherited organ dysfunction such as the thyroid, and the mechanisms of the detrimental effects of toxins and noise, may see elucidation in the near future. Added to this should be the continued enhancement of our understanding of voice production and laryngeal control along with surgical methods for reinnervation of the larynx and possibly replacement of an entire larynx.

Of great importance is the researcher in specialities unrelated directly to medicine. The work in auditory electrophysiology, psychoacoustics, biochemistry, and other basic areas contributes to the fund of information needed to provide the data for eventual prevention and treatment of communication disorders. But the medical synthesis of these data is the essential goal. Obviously, support for the basic, often seemingly unrelated, research must continue unabated.

The technological advances of the future are unpredictable, but a few things can be foreseen. The combined transmission and scanning electron microscope opens up new fields for exploring the inner relationship of the cells, blood vessels and neurons of the organ of Corti. The computer offers fantastic possibilities for aids to hearing, for perfecting the speech of the deaf, for analysis of vocal abnormalities, for improving objective audiometry, and for enhancing x-ray images of larynx and ear.

The selection of the appropriate animal model seems to be a hopeful approach. Work in the Michigan laboratories has demonstrated that the Patas monkey (*Erythrocebus patas*), who lives in the very arid environment of sub-Saharan Africa and has little water available to him shows marked hearing loss to low doses of dihydrostreptomycin. Like other desert animals, this monkey probably has an efficient kidney with minimal excretion. By contrast, the pigtail monkey (*Macaca nemestrina*), living in the lush, forest environment of Sumatra and the Malay peninsula with heavy annual rainfall, has a much higher daily water intake and remains, like other species of laboratory animals, unaffected by similar dose levels of dihydrostreptomycin.

As mentioned earlier, because of the very fundamental difference in the approach to the administration of medical care in this country as opposed to that in the countries where the provision of medical care is on a more socialistic basis, we see the MD in those countries more extensively involved in research. In this country, we continue to have a problem of orienting the MD and PhD toward the same goals. The mutual exchange of ideas and research application is weak, and herein lies a great opportunity to strengthen this relationship to the benefit of the communicatively disabled.

In the 1950s and 1960s, the National Institutes of Health (NIH) training grant provided a means for bringing PhD researchers into clinical departments to set up laboratories and to work intimately with the house officer and staff; this work often led to basic disease-oriented research.

Support was provided for the recruitment of basic scientists into programs that formerly had limited numbers of specialists. A biochemist, for example, interested in membrane transport would never pick Reissner's membrane as the tissue upon which to conduct his research. But in order to understand how the ear works, it takes a biochemist to concentrate on this problem. Such individuals have to be enticed into the field, and this necessitates research salary money, because the individual is often working outside the department of his basic discipline.

A deterrent to the progress of disease-oriented research in the future is the loss of the opportunity for bringing these various talents together. The program project grant does not create the same atmosphere the otolaryngology training grant created. The training program, as originally conceived, was just beginning to gel at the time of its curtailment. There are today many former trainees who went through such programs, producing good research themselves, and who are now department chairmen without funds necessary to support the activities they were trained to promote. It is not the quantity of trainees that is of greatest concern, it is the quality of trained specialists.

In this connection it is interesting to look at some of the information revealed by the manpower survey[2] supported by NIH and carried out by the American Council of Otolaryngology. This survey, completed in 1973, was carried out by questionnaire with complete anonymity of the department of individual, so presumably, no defense of the trainees' eventual professional pursuits entered into the response.

Of the 86 (out of 106) programs responding, 21 required research experience of all their residents. Keeping in mind that only 61.3% of all known otolaryngologists responded for a total of 2,734, 459 of these indicated they had had research training in NIH-supported programs. One hundred and forty-six, or 32%, are now either geographic or academic full-time faculty members. Not all of these individuals received stipends, but they did receive research training. As of the time of that report, of the 273 respondents reporting that they had received NIH training stipends, 13 are department chairmen, 5 are full professors, 26 are associate professors, 59 are assistant professors and 66 are instructors. The remaining 104 have no faculty appointment or their rank is unknown.

That 32% of those who went through NIH supported programs went into academic positions does not indicate a flooding of the market; it indicates a replacement of faculty with high quality teacher-investigators. Although fellowships and teacher-investigator awards may appear to be an adequate substitute, they imply a more isolated research environment and are no substitute for the research training integrated into an ear, nose and throat residency program.

This manpower survey contains a special section on the research otolaryngologist. It first points out that the otolaryngologist doing research has special problems because of his lack of specialization in a basic science. Those who indicated in the general questionnaire that they devoted 10% or more of their time to either clinical or basic research were sent a follow-up research questionnaire. There were only 118 otolaryngologists in this category, of whom 62 completed the follow-up questionnaire and 13 deleted themselves. In addition 31 names of known researchers and 12 foreign-trained otolaryngologists engaged in full-time teaching and research were identified for a total of 148, from which 96 responses were received.

Half of the respondents received at least part of their research funds from federal agencies and, for the most part, this research was done in collaboration with basic scientists or clinicians.

The majority of these otolaryngologists, 75 in number, planned either to continue their level of research activity or increase it. The report states: "In addition to the area of clinical research where the medical doctor trained in otolaryngology is indispensable, otolaryngologists develop and perfect new surgical techniques and help to transfer unsolved problems in patient care into hypotheses on which the basic scientist may work."

> "The 85 part-time research otolaryngologists who answered the research questionnaire represent approximately 3% of the 2,734 US otolaryngologists who returned the general questionnaire. When this figure is adjusted to the otolaryngology universe, there are an estimated 110 otolaryngologists seriously involved in research in this country. The addition of the 12 foreign-trained otolaryngologists contributing full time to research makes a pool of only 122 otolaryngologists involved in research. It would appear from these figures that the pool of research otolaryngologists will require enlargement to meet the needs of research in the immediate future."

I thoroughly support the recommendations listed in this survey.

> It is recommended that the number of post residency fellowships be increased. These fellowships are important as they provide the only support for the advanced research training of those otolaryngologists interested in a career of research, either basic or applied. It is necessary to train a proportion of otolaryngologists in research because their knowledge of clinical problems allows for an input of ideas which cannot be contributed by PhDs or MAs. Such trainees will also be well-equipped to assume the responsibility for directing a department at a later time.
>
> Efforts should be made to convince the Congress and the Department of Health, Education, and Welfare of the urgent need for continued long-term Federal support of our training programs.

We must do all we can to bring the needs of the communicatively disabled into the public eye. We should publicize our research advances, and solicit funds to support the laboratory programs.

The essential ingredient in a research effort is a well-trained and industrious investigator. The problem boils down to: first, training the inspired individual, and second, providing him with a well-equipped and stable environment in which he can work. This Boys Town Institute for Communication Disorders in Children can do much to promote research and to bring to public attention the need for support in this area.

REFERENCES

1. National Association of the Deaf. The deaf population of the United States. Silver Spring: 1974.
2. American Council of Otolaryngology. Report on Manpower Resources on Needs in Otorhinolaryngology, Bethesda, Md.: Department of Health, Education, and Welfare; DHEW Pub. no. (NIH) 77-1298, 1975.

EDUCATIONAL AND TRAINING PRIORITIES FOR CLINICIANS AND RESEARCHERS IN THE AREA OF COMMUNICATION DISORDERS

A HEALTH SCIENCE CAMPUS CHANCELLOR'S PERSPECTIVE

FRANCIS A. SOOY, MD

SAN FRANCISCO, CALIFORNIA

Philosophical but practical current discussion of trends in education which could have a profound effect on the future of communicative sciences.

Communicative disorders comprise a broadly diversified group of clinical and psychological problems related directly or indirectly to most medical and psychological disciplines as well as major segments of the physical and biological sciences. It is the diversity in this writer's opinion which makes it so difficult to establish priorities for education and research in these important areas.

Historically, research and training programs in communicative disorders have evolved in three major areas: 1) general college campuses and universities, 2) health science colleges and universities, and 3) government and industry. Within these broad classifications there are two largely nonmiscible components: 1) clinical disciplines, and 2) laboratory disciplines.

As the chief administrative officer of a major health science university, there is little question that closer association between these elements not only results in a more meaningful educational experience but also improvement in the quality as well as quantity of research and training. Cooperation in training and research no matter how useful or well intentioned is extraordinarily difficult to achieve, due in part to the reluctance of faculty to leave the security of their peers for the uncertainty of a new educational milieu. General campus scientists are difficult to recruit to health science campuses, although recent trends toward higher salary scales in the health sciences may ameliorate the problem to some extent. Even the relatively short step from a basic science department to a clinical department is unsettling.

Let us look at some of the trends in education which could have a profound effect on the future of communicative sciences. Enrollment figures for the University of California's eight general campuses which select their students from the top 12.5% of California high school graduates increased 15% between 1971 and 1978. They are projected to increase no more than 2% in the next seven years. This reflects in a general way the declining number of young people in our society, and with it the disappearance of new resources for educational programs, the so-called "steady state."

At the other end of life's spectrum the United Nations Organization projects a 100% increase in the world population over 60 years of age in the next 29 years, an increase of 291,000,000 seniors. Harry Nelson writing in the *Los Angeles Times*[1] states "The growing proportion of elderly may be the secret time bomb which will challenge the financial stability and perhaps the moral integrity of Americans as the United States considers having a comprehensive health plan for everyone in the nation." He goes on to point out that in Sweden those 70 years and older comprise 10% of the population but use 50% of the health care facilities. Those 80 years of age and older comprise 2.5% of the population but represent 25% of the hospital utilization costs.

It is thus not unreasonable to suppose that there will be increasing pressure on the training and research programs in communicative disorders to solve the problems of the elderly. This in turn, if successful, will add new pressures to those factors contributing to the cost of medical care such as: 1) new medical and surgical procedures, 2) increasingly expensive technology, 3) increased number of employees per patient, and 4) a rising public expectation of what medicine can accomplish. This in turn can have a negative effect on funding for research and training. Another ingredient during the period 1960-1975, the number of medical students, interns and residents in US schools has doubled while in the same period the number of graduate students has increased four-fold. It is this important group of young scientists, many without patient care involvement, who will need isolation from the rising tide of concern over the total costs of health care.

Of even more concern is the relative decline since 1965 in the support of biomedical research as a per-

From the University of California, San Francisco Medical Center, San Francisco, California.

TABLE 1. FINANCIAL IMPACT AS RESULT OF STATE SUBVENTION OF LOCAL PROPERTY TAX LOSSES FOR 1978-1979

	9 Campuses	*UCSF Total*
Budget*	1,800,000,000	225,000,000
State funds	767,000,000	62,000,000
Prop. 13 cuts†	58,000,000	4,400,000

*Excludes E.R.D.A. Laboratories.

†Prop. 13 - Proposition 13.

cent of national health expenditures, the absolute decline in support of research training since 1974, and the erosion of Federal support for both research and teaching in schools of medicine since 1965. I am frequently asked "What was the effect of the Jarvis-Gann initiative (Prop. 13) on the University of California?" Table 1 illustrates the financial impact as the result of state subvention of local property tax losses for 1978-79. The extent and severity of future funding constraints is unclear at this time, but it is certain to continue. With the unquestioned stringencies in state support which is already with us and the expectation of similar reductions from the Federal side, private support of research and training assumes an extraordinary importance. A major undertaking such as the Boys Town Institute for Communication Disorders in Children is a far-sighted and extremely valuable addition to the country's biomedical resources.

The private sector cannot, however, assume a major portion of the state and Federal shortfall. Is there then any course which will utilize our existing resources more effectively and be responsive to the changing needs of those we serve? I am convinced that the answer is unequivocally, "Yes," and that the solution lies in close cooperative programs crossing departmental lines, school lines and between universities both local and distant. In essence, the answer lies in joint programs permitting distinguished faculty to retain the security of their peers and yet to challenge with their special skills some of the new frontiers of science and medicine. The number of such programs in the communicative sciences is very small if speech pathology and audiology are valid indicators.

Only 8% or these graduate programs are in health science institutions (17 of 212), and only 4% are at the doctoral level (8 of 17). Conversely of 119 medical schools, eight doctoral programs in speech and hearing represent only 7% of the total.[2] Thus one may assume there is a large reservoir of isolated talent in speech and hearing sciences and medical sciences that could be mutually supportive. There is seldom much controversy over the worthiness or value of cooperative efforts but they so often fail on the details.

The individual objections to cooperative programs can usually be classified under one or more of the seven cardinal sins. These are: 1) pride, 2) covetousness, 3) lust, 4) anger, 5) gluttony, 6) envy, and 7) sloth. Programs once established can falter or fail on similar frailties. Essential factors for successful cooperative arrangements are:

1. The principals should be secure professionals of recognized distinction;

2. The consortia wherever possible should include students at all appropriate levels;

3. Multiple sources of funding may offer more security than single source funding;

4. It is more blessed to give than to receive.

An example of an interuniversity program is the doctoral program in speech and hearing sciences, a joint effort between the University of California, Santa Barbara and University of California, San Francisco, in which the course work is concentrated on the Santa Barbara campus and the clinical and research experience on the San Francisco campus. The Maxillo-Facial Anomalies Clinic, an inter-school program between medicine, dentistry and nursing is involved in the long-term diagnosis and management of craniofacial anomalies. Included are orthodontists, plastic surgeons, audiologists, pediatricians, speech pathologists and nurses. An extremely valuable interdepartmental program is the Reading and Language Development Clinic, staffed by pediatricians, psychologists, audiologists, speech therapists, neurologists, classroom teachers and related students. It deals with complicated problems involving children with educational difficulty and is immensely popular with our students.

Recently while reading an account of the First Crusade, 1096-1099,[3] I was impressed with the similarity between Pope Urban II's efforts to unite the Christian world behind such a worthy cause and the problems encountered in academic administration with cooperative programs. First, by the year 1000 AD the population of Europe exceeded the ability of agriculture to support it (reduced resources). Secondly, there was an abundant supply of ambitious younger sons of noble rank whom the laws of primogeniture excluded from an inherited livelihood (nontenured faculty).

Urban II preached the Crusade throughout Europe, fanning the fires of popular fervor, but in addition he offered other inducements:

1. To the barons, all the land they could conquer in the East (tenure);

2. To the serfs, freedom from feudal obligations and remission of their sins (a better title);

3. To the clergy, release from monastic discipline (no more committees);

4. To the merchants, profits (fee for service).

The academic comparison continues: Many who were ill-prepared or ill-equipped dropped by the wayside. Others such as Baldwin of Bulogne, and Bohemund of Sicily carved out their own empires at Edessa and Antioch — and built large castles to protect their holdings. When the Crusade finally succeeded with Godfrey's foothold atop the North wall of Jerusalem on July 14, 1099, and the capture of the Holy City, the crusaders promptly slaughtered all the inhabitants (getting rid of the dead wood)!

Let me quote in part from Saladin the Great's words to his son al-Zahir after he had recaptured Jerusalem some 90 years later and shortly before his death, "Beware of bloodshed; do not trust in that, for spilled blood never sleeps. Strive to gain the hearts of thy subjects and watch over all of their interests, for thou art appointed by God and by me to look after their welfare." Administrators take heed.

REFERENCES

1. Nelson H. Los Angeles Times, June 19, 1978.

2. Medical education: institutions, characteristics and programs. Association of American Medical Colleges: June 1977.

3. Elias A. Aramco World Magazine, 1979.

PRIORITIES IN SERVICE DELIVERY TO THE COMMUNICATIVELY DISADVANTAGED: HABILITATION NEEDS

S. RICHARD SILVERMAN, PhD

ST. LOUIS, MISSOURI

The bewildering patchwork or organization and organizing principles involved in the delivery of services to the communicatively disadvantaged requires an amalgam of effort. Also helpful would be a clearer understanding of magnitudes, characteristics and habilitation needs of certain subgroups such as the language disabled, the multiply handicapped and the moderately handicapped. Since this conference is concerned primarily with scientific contribution, it is suggested that we are in a transition from intuitive approaches to habilitative procedures to those derived from scientific investigations. This is pointedly documented in the area of language which cuts across all types of communicative disorders, as well as in such areas as early identification, sensory aids, career education, parent guidance, media use and mental health. It is important, too, for scientists to communicate clearly with their many publics.

On first turning my attention to preparation for the topic assigned me, "Priorities in Service Delivery to the Communicatively Disadvantaged: Habilitation Needs" I thought I would focus my remarks on the organization of delivery of services. This approach suggested itself because I believe that our success in habilitation may depend as much on how we organize ourselves to do our work as on our clinical and laboratory discoveries. Scrutiny of delivery of services that are available reveals a bewildering patchwork of organizations, organizing principles and their expression in purposes, sponsorship and support. A compelling future priority is to seek some amalgam of effort particularly as we face the hard facts of costs, manpower requirements, standards, evaluation, social pressure and a host of other issues. I decided not to take this tack, as important as it undoubtedly is, because I felt it was somewhat tangential to the central theme expressed in the subscript of the conference brochure, "Scientific Dedication Conference."

I then thought that an appropriate approach would be a discussion of magnitudes, characteristics and habilitation needs of those subgroups of the larger general population of communicatively disadvantaged who in the future should command more attention than they are now getting. These include especially the language-disabled, the multiply handicapped, and, surprisingly enough, the moderately handicapped. Table 1, for example, shows the additional handicapping conditions coincident with hearing impairment compiled in 1973 by the Office of Demographic Studies at Gallaudet College. Clinicians are familiar, too, with the moderately handicapped child, frequently misdiagnosed, who falls in the cracks of the service delivery system. I soon abandoned this strategy because I am convinced that the subject requires more visible and concentrated treatment than I or the conference was prepared to give it. Perhaps organization of service delivery and characteristics, pertinent for habilitation, of the population to be served are each suitable subjects for full conference consideration. We are likely to be stimulated along these lines by the panel that follows this presentation.

In my opinion the primary service to be delivered, the fundamental habilitation "need," is the development, improvement and, where indicated, maintenance of communication in those in whom it is disordered regardless in what organizational or therapeutic setting the service is rendered. And the implicit focus of this conference is the current or potential contribution of scientific research to the satisfaction of that need.

In that spirit I submit this proposition: More than at any other period in the history of this field we find ourselves in transition from intuitive approaches to habilitative and instructional procedures largely determined by experience to procedures derived from scientific investigations. The transitional phenomenon is strikingly illustrated in an area as fundamental as any for our service tasks namely, language, the stuff of communication by whatever mode it is expressed or received.

We have been challenged to assess our intuitive approaches to the language problem by the theories and findings growing out of the work of students of linguistics, of child development and of the psychology of learning who have merged their interests and methods into the discipline of psycholinguistics. In historical retrospect of the past 20 years or so we find that initially child-language studies were dominated by grammatical formalism. Investigators studied how children acquire and internalize gram-

From the Central Institute for the Deaf, St. Louis, Missouri.

REPRINTS — S. Richard Silverman, PhD, Central Institute for the Deaf, 818 South Euclid Ave., St. Louis, MO 63110.

TABLE 1. PERCENT OF HEARING-IMPAIRED STUDENTS WITH SPECIFIED ADDITIONAL HANDICAPPING CONDITIONS BY AGE GROUP, UNITED STATES: 1971-72 SCHOOL YEAR*

Additional Handicapping Conditions	*Age (yr)* 1-5	6-10	11-15	16+
None	61.4	56.2	55.2	59.6
Brain damage	3.6	3.5	3.5	3.2
Cerebral palsy	1.6	2.1	2.4	4.2
Epilepsy	0.6	0.6	0.7	0.6
Heart disorder	2.1	3.2	1.8	0.8
Mental retardation	2.4	3.9	7.2	8.6
Orthopedic	1.2	0.6	0.7	0.7
Perceptual/motor	1.5	3.7	3.0	1.0
Emotional/behavioral	3.2	5.2	5.0	3.7
Severe visual	2.9	3.9	3.4	2.7
Other	2.2	2.2	2.8	2.7
Blank/unknown	17.3	14.5	14.1	12.3

**Additional handicapping conditions among hearing impaired students: United States: 1971-1972.* Data from the Annual Survey of Hearing Impaired Children and Youth. Washington, DC: Gallaudet College, Office of Demographic Studies, 1973.

matical forms such as questions, passives, and negatives. This led to attempts to write content-free grammars of emerging child language. These were essentially based on distribution of words within children's utterances and made no reference to what their reasons for speaking might be. Equivalence of form rather than differences in meaning was the center of attention.

Rigid formalism came to be questioned with the recognition that it is necessary to study the context in which an utterance is produced in order to understand the meaning the child is trying to express. For example "baby water" may mean "the baby wants water," "the baby is in the water," "the baby spilled the water," etc. This suggested that we need to be concerned with the "semantic rules" that relate words or sentences to things and events.

Even this conceptualization had some gaps. The notion has developed that a complete description of what children are doing when they speak includes not only the actual forms produced and their context but the social use of that speech. Is the utterance a request for information? A casual comment? Or what? Does it take account of the knowledge the hearer shares or does not share with the speaker? Otherwise said, it is the sociolinguistic aspect of communication. Thus the forms, the content or intended meaning and the special uses of speech have emerged as a tripartite focus of most current child-language study.

These investigations of normal language development have begun to influence our thinking if not our management and instructional practices. Evidence of application and results are not at hand probably because of the recency of findings, the issues related to them and the undetermined significance they may have for language acquisition and instruction of hearing-impaired or learning-disabled children. For example, in the approach of generative grammar, language is characterized by acquisition of increasingly complex rules which approximate the rules of adult language. How a child accomplishes this is not clear but it has been suggested that frequent parental expansion of a child's telegraphic speech may be fundamental. It appears from this that language learning is accomplished by imitation of adult structures with appropriate and timely reinforcement and in its more extreme form, as in the case of language-delayed children, by a programmed "behavior modification" approach. On the other hand, there is evidence that children respond to the imitation task in a manner more or less consistent with their present level of grammatical rules and that listening to increasingly complex utterances is a basis for the rules that govern the child's language production. These approaches may not be mutually exclusive and the emphasis on one or the other may depend on the child's language development at a given time.

Concurrent with this notion and perhaps stimulated by it is interest in what I have referred to as the "subtle interweaving of language and thought." The argument is advanced that cognitive development both precedes and enables language development. The aim here is to extract the child's cognitive understanding underlying language performance and to specify the nonlinguistic tasks. The possibility that cognitive strategies are universal in the sense that there are linguistic universals is a hypothesis that merits consideration.

The possible implications for the education of hearing-impaired children, for example, of research in the development of language of hearing children should command our serious and earnest attention. It is conceivable that they may influence, among other things, our modes of communication, the timing, sequencing and structuring of language imput, our concepts of "correctness" of language production at various levels in a child's development and our assessment of language competence and achievement. We may thus be led to hierarchical development as a point of departure for dealing with language disorders rather than pervasive remediation.

Of course, there are other significant areas related directly to habilitative services that point to our state of transition from the intuitive to the scientific. Among these are early identification, audiologic assessment, speech and sensory aids all of which are included in the conference agenda.

Failing prevention of successful medical and/or surgical treatment of disorders, measures need to be instituted based on an understanding of its consequences for the affected individual. In a basic scientific sense we need to understand both normal and pathological transformation of signals at the cochlear (and retinal), neural, perceptual, and linguistic levels and their relation to learning. In a broader applied sense we must concentrate on the prevention of intellectual, psychological and social pathology. We do this by recognizing the potential benefits of shaped sensory and motor experience for a plastic, maturing nervous system. The benefits are more likely to be realized if significant deviation is detected as early in a child's life as possible.

Detailed consideration of procedures aimed at detection and specification of deafness in neonates, infants and young children are beyond the scope of this paper. These include episodic testing by observers, programmed movement-detection transducers in the crib of a neonate associated with tones, and the monitoring of "high risk" children. Whatever turns out to be the method or methods of choice it is fortunate that the search per se has underlined the need for and the value of early detection and follow-up. This, along with public education of all concerned with infants, should improve our screening and identifying score.

Not only are we making progress in detection of deafness, but as we follow a screened-out or identified child, increasingly refined assessment of the nature and degree of hearing loss is within reach: the middle ear by impedance testing, the inner ear and the neural transmission and central nervous system by evoked response methods. We are also learning that more attention is required of audiologists to those items of assessment, in addition to the audiogram, that may be pertinent to remedial and educational management such as perception of patterns, ability to use minimal acoustic cues, asymmetrical auditory processing (dichotic listening), attentiveness to sound, differential sensitivity to signal frequency (frequency resolution), intensity and duration, and combined audiovisual processing. The significance of procedures and measures such as these for hearing aid selection, for auditory training, and for amplification combined with nonauditory communication and sensory aids is still an open question as is the confidence with which we can recommend education and modes of communication based on them. The need to be alert too, whenever possible, to assess handicaps additional to hearing impairment is also important.

As mentioned previously we are intrigued by empirical-descriptive studies that suggest stages at which hearing children induce the phonologic, syntactic and semantic rules of language. Of interest to us, too, is the hypothesis that human beings inherit, rather than learn, some abilities for perceiving speech sounds. Human infants that have not yet begun to speak are able to perceive speech sounds that are not differentiated in the language they eventually speak. This suggests a theory of attrition of potential communication skill if there is no environmental stimulation of genetically determined capability. How much this capability can be modified is probably determined by the kind and amount of environmental stimulation and the time of life or "optimum period" during which it is provided.

The spectrograph and speech synthesizer are enabling us to learn more about the relation of speech perception to speech production. The identification of the acoustic variants that influence speech perception and the fine-grained description of the acoustic parameters of speech production should be important baseline considerations for all who espouse optimum use of residual hearing.

How the abundant talents and vigorous interest of investigators in allied fields are being applied to our problems is no better illustrated than in the search for sensory aids. Currently, there is an extraordinary increase in this activity that engages engineers, speech scientists, psychologists and neurophysiologists. Sensory aids are being designed to extract and transmit features of speech that are likely to facilitate speech perception and, hence, speech production. An impressive effort has gone into the coding of stimuli particularly auditory. The emphasis has been on making available crucial information-bearing elements of signals to the part of the auditory channel that may possibly detect and process them. Clever methods of frequency transposition, insertion of discriminable surrogate signals and various patterns of amplification in association with particular training regimes are being attempted. Here too the evidence for special methods of coding are not overwhelmingly convincing but impressionistic and anecdotal evaluation encourages continued efforts in these directions. Also we shall watch with interest the attempts to adapt finger spelling to phonetic correspondence and to expand and to refine syntactical features of the language of signs.

It becomes clearer as we ponder these alternatives for sensory input whether to the skin, the eye, or the ear or some combination of these that we need to ask more fundamental questions such as the effects of a particular strategy on the operation of short term memory, of the storage of rules of sequential probabilities of linguistic units and chunks, of bisensory processing of information, of the place of immediate, delayed, ambiguous or distorted feedback over any sensory system and of carry-over from structured training regimes with devices to everyday communication. Worthy of note also is the demonstrated value of another class of aids namely the teletype and the promise of the picturephone. We shall continue to learn, too, about implantation of electrodes in the inner ear to transmit an electrical signal to the auditory nerve of postlingually profoundly deaf persons.

In the interest of time I have directed most of my attention to those areas that nicely illustrate not only the intuitive-scientific transition but also those concerns that have traditionally and distinctively commanded the attention of the research community concerned with aural-oral communication. Of course, we are intensely interested in the improvement of media use, in the heartening developments in career and postsecondary education, in the growing interest in models of personality development and their import for mental health of communicatively disadvantaged persons, and in evaluating varying emphases in parent-child programs. These fields of inquiry are not as clearly focused as those I have cited but they certainly point to habilitation needs.

In our state of transition which may last longer than some of us care to predict it is prudent to keep in mind that intuitive approaches based on experience occupy an important place in our professional efforts. However, they should not be indifferent to scientific advances. They should complement them. And given the great open spaces between scientifically determined facts that have been demonstrated to be applicable to habilitation the converse should also apply. Nature sometimes does produce lesions that are not reproducible in the laboratory.

Finally it is not out of order to suggest in this scientific dedicatory context that it is essential for investigators or their spokesmen to engage in a sustained effort to contribute to the understanding and appreciation of the research but who have a substantial stake in its pursuit and in its outcomes. These include especially the families of children, administrators, staff, government, and financial supporters. Too often these potential "consumers" of the research "product" are critical of the choice and level of problems chosen for investigation, are impatient with the pace with which applicable results are achieved, are bewildered by the language in which research is communicated, are irritated by a posture of superior intellect and cultivated detachment assumed by researchers and are skeptical of value received for dollars invested, especially tax dollars.

Improvement of communication about research with the many publics concerned with the communicatively disadvantaged should establish a climate of mutual respect for purposes, methods and integrity of all who are involved whether producers or consumers. In the language of the Conference title the present status of this activity requires that it be placed high in any list of future priorities.

Prominent among the needs from the point of view of research are:

1. Continuing effort to sort out from research findings those that apply to practice.

2. Reexamination of principles that apply to organization of delivery of service.

3. Pragmatic description of populations to be served.

4. Improvement of communication between producers and consumers of research.

CHAIRMAN: EDGAR L. LOWELL, PhD, LOS ANGELES, CALIFORNIA

PANEL — EDUCATIONAL PROGRAMMING FOR THE HEARING-IMPAIRED: PRESENT AND FUTURE

THE UNITED STATES

EDGAR L. LOWELL, PhD
LOS ANGELES, CALIFORNIA

Educational programming for the hearing-impaired in the United States is going to be substantially influenced by the individualized education program (IEP) which is a key concept of the Education For All Handicapped Children's Act, or as it is more commonly referred to, Public Law (PL) 94-142. This is undoubtedly one of the most significant pieces of legislation affecting the handicapped ever passed in this country.

Basically, it guarantees the right of all handicapped children to receive a free and appropriate public education. The term "appropriate" is defined in the regulations in the statement: "Free appropriate public education means special education and related services which: . . . Are provided in conformity with an individualized education program . . ." Thus the IEP is the key to compliance with the requirement of an appropriate education for each handicapped child.

The IEP must be a written statement that is developed in a meeting which includes the following participants:

1. A representative of the public agency, other than the child's teacher, who is qualified to provide, or supervise the provision of, special education.

2. The child's teacher.

3. One or both of the child's parents.

4. The child where appropriate.

5. Other individuals at the discretion of the parent or agency.

The IEP must contain;

1. A statement of the child's present level of performance.

2. A statement of annual goals, including short term instructional objectives.

3. A statement of the specific special education and related services to be provided the child and the extent to which the child will be able to participate in regular educational programs.

4. The projected dates for initiation of services and the anticipated duration of the services.

5. Appropriate objective criteria and evaluation procedures, and schedules for determining, on at least an annual basis, whether the short term instructional objectives will be achieved.

The term "related services" as used in the definition means transportation and such developmental, corrective, and other supportive services as are required to assist a handicapped child to benefit from special education. Among these are included such services as audiology, speech pathology, psychological services, early identification and assessment of disabilities in children, and parent counseling and training.

The law requires that parents have an opportunity to participate in the formulation of an IEP and if they feel that the school is not planning and providing an appropriate education, they have a right to inspect and review all educational records related to the identification, evaluation, educational placement, and provision of a free appropriate education for their child.

They also have the right to obtain an independent educational evaluation at public expense if they disagree with the evaluation obtained by the school district and they have the right to request an impartial hearing to determine if the child is receiving an appropriate education.

These impartial hearings must be conducted by trained hearing officers who must not have a vested interest in the case and are not employees of the school involved. Decisions of the hearing officers can be appealed to the state education agency and

From the John Tracy Clinic, Los Angeles, California.
REPRINTS — Edgar L. Lowell, PhD, Director, The John Tracy Clinic, 806 W. Adams Blvd., Los Angeles, CA 90007.

ultimately to the courts if the issue cannot be otherwise resolved.

Individualized education plans are not a new concept. In selected areas such programs have been prepared for students for some time. They were mentioned in the Elementary and Secondary Education Act of 1965 and the Education Amendments of 1974, which required that programs and services be based on the individual needs of handicapped persons. However, it was not until PL 94-142 that the law contained the specific requirements for developing an IEP and describing the content, the persons responsible, and the date by which IEPs were to be developed.

There are some additional features of PL 94-142 which are worthy of note. The law requires: 1) multifaceted nonculturally biased evaluation, and 2) that handicapped children be educated in the "least restrictive environment," which means that they are educated to the maximum extent appropriate with children who are not handicapped. Again, "appropriate" is the key word.

Special classes, separate schooling or other removal of handicapped children from the regular educational environment can occur when the nature or severity of the handicap is such that education in regular classes without use of supplementary aides and services cannot be achieved satisfactorily. An extreme interpretation of this provision suggested "mainstreaming" for all handicapped children. It is unlikely that total mainstreaming would ever be appropriate, but we undoubtedly will be seeing more handicapped children in regular classrooms. There is considerable discussion over what environment should determine a child's placement. It is argued that a normal-hearing regular classroom placement for a young profoundly congenitally deaf child with little language may be more restrictive for the child than placement in a special and segregated classroom or school.

That, very briefly, is where our educational programming for the hearing-impaired is at the present. As to the future, it will be determined as we gain more experience with the new law.

Because of the undefined terms in the law, "appropriate education," "least restrictive environment," and the fact that parents have guaranteed procedural safeguards with access to local and state hearings, and ultimately the courts, it is likely that the future will see a clarification of these undefined terms through precedent-setting legal decisions.

The law provides some financial support for this increased service program, but that too is being phased in. The mechanisms for insuring compliance are not satisfactorily in place. In fact, some states do not as yet have approved state plans, and in fact, may not be planning to submit them.

It is an understatement to suggest that professionally we were not ready to implement fully the provisions of PL 94-142, even though the law was passed in 1975 and the initial IEPs were not required until October 1977.

Generally speaking, we were not prepared to provide multifaceted nonculturally biased tests to young deaf children. That is a desirable objective but somewhat beyond the state of the art at this time. Possibly PL 94-142 will serve as a stimulus for the development of such instruments.

Our regular classroom teachers were certainly unprepared to cope with mainstreamed handicapped children. In a survey[1] of 1,726 regular classroom teachers, only 21% felt they were adequately prepared to teach mainstreamed handicapped students, and while 80 to 90% favored the offering of in-service and graduate courses to build competence for effective mainstreaming, only 50 to 60% indicated they would be willing to enroll in an in-service level course and only 30 to 40% would commit themselves to a graduate level course.

Very few of our school districts were prepared to provide the array of related services specified, particularly when these had to be delivered in many different regular schools rather than in the centralized special education schools and programs.

Despite the fact that informed parents are required for meaningful participation in the IEP conference, little provision has been made to insure that parents have the experience and background to become meaningful participants as undoubtedly intended in both the letter and spirit of the law.

It is of interest to speculate on the origin and motivation for this sweeping piece of legislation, particularly because, historically, innovation in special education has tended to come from the private sector where we now have a legislative branch of government providing rules; in fact we have rather precise specifications for the way in which educational programming for the hearing-impaired will take place.

It is possible to discern two converging forces that may have been responsible for the governmental involvement. One was undoubtedly the growing awareness that many handicapped children were not receiving an appropriate education, or in some cases any education at all. The other force grew out of the experiences of other minority groups in the fight to obtain their constitutional rights. In the case of the black minority, we have seen how special legislation has been required to insure blacks the rights guaranteed them under the constitution.

PL 94-142 may be viewed as a similar piece of legislation for the handicapped. It can be traced to two important legal cases: the Pennsylvania Association for Retarded Children (PARC) vs the

Commonwealth of Pennsylvania, and Mills vs the Board of Education of the District of Columbia. The PARC decision established that all retarded children have a right to a free public education and the Mills decision included all handicapped children and ruled that if sufficient funds are not available to finance all of the services and programs that are needed and desirable for the handicapped, then the available funds must be expended equitably and thus some services must be denied to all children if they are denied the handicapped; that is, it is forbidden to discriminate against the handicapped as a group by denying them services on the basis of their handicap.

It would appear that rather than have educational programming determined by the courts, a number of states passed laws incorporating provisions of both PARC and Mills that in effect became the forerunners of PL 94-142.

A major question remains as to how PL 94-142 will succeed. Will education programming provide the laudable goals of the law or will we see compromises and evasions as states and local education agencies attempt to stay in compliance in order to be eligible for federal support; but without the necessary tools, personnel, and resources to comply with the intent of the law? Will parents make full use of their new due process guarantees and become active participants in educational programming for their children?

Future educational programming for the hearing-impaired in the United States promises to be a very interesting affair. If we can meet the challenge offered by the legislators, it will undoubtedly be of great benefit to the hearing-impaired.

REFERENCES

1. Flynn JR, Gacka RC, Sundean DA. Are classroom teachers prepared for mainstreaming. Phi Delta Kappan 1978; 59:562.

PANEL — EDUCATIONAL PROGRAMMING FOR THE HEARING-IMPAIRED: PRESENT AND FUTURE

SWEDEN

GUNNAR LIDÉN, MD

GÖTEBORG, SWEDEN

The goal of educational programming for the hearing impaired is that habilitation shall start as early as possible but not later than an age of one year. In order to accomplish this goal, the medical diagnosis of hearing impairment must be made early. In this way, educational programming can be structured in different steps.

The identification of hearing-impaired infants is based on the observations of the parents, the pediatricians at the maternity hospital and the well baby clinics, the otologists, and the audiologists. The final diagnosis will be made at the university or regional audiology centers where a team consisting of otologist, audiologist, social worker, psychologist and preschool teacher for hearing-impaired or deaf children will evaluate the child.

Every woman who leaves the maternity hospital with a child gets a brochure giving the parents information about the normal development of hearing and speech behavior. In this way we alert the parents to observe the child's hearing.

Screening of neonates is not performed in Sweden. Instead we focus on high-risk babies. The main source of referrals to the university or regional audiology centers is the pediatrician at a maternity hospital. He checks the child's history. If any of the factors displayed in Table 1 are applicable, the child is referred to such a center. The mother is called to schedule an appointment for the child when he or she is about four months old. Among the different causes of hearing impairment heredity and viral infection top the list as seen in Table 1. The other factors are less important. The dominant type of heredity is of course the only one which the maternity hosptial can discover. Sporadic deafness of a recessive type might be discovered by our second source of referrals, the well baby clinics. In Göteborg with a half million inhabitants we have 63 well baby clinics. Ninety-four percent of the children up to six years of age are regularly controlled there. A nurse from a well baby clinic pays the first visit to the home when the child is about one month old. At this occasion the brochure about the ear and hearing is discussed as well as the family history of hearing impairment. Between seven and nine months of age, the child's selective attention to sounds is tested by the pediatrician or the nurse with a high-pitched jingle bell at about 40 dB SPL measured at a distance of 20 cm, ie, 8 inches. The investigation begins by getting eye contact with the baby. A red gripper or a red pencil is held in front of the child. While he is looking at it, reaching for it, or putting it in his mouth, the bell is rung behind the child's head. If he hears the sound he stops whatever activity he is engaged in and perhaps looks up. At about seven months of age, the normal child can break the visual contact and look for the sound source. The attention test is not only a test for hearing but also says something about the child's general and mental development. If the child does not respond to the sound or does not localize the sound source, the history related to speech and hearing is simultaneously analyzed and the child will be referred to the university or regional audiology center for further diagnostic work.

The otologist at the county hospitals or in private practice, as well as the parents, can also refer children suspected of hearing impairment, independent of age, to the audiology center.

When the mother with the four-month-old child comes for investigation, the procedure at the audiology center is as follows. The otologist starts with the history and asks for the parent's opinion about the child's hearing and reaction to sounds and to voices. It is important to know how the child uses his voice. If there is suspicion of hearing loss, we try to get an etiological diagnosis if possible. We take blood tests for rubella, toxoplasmosis, and megalocyte virus. X-ray of the cochlea is first done at an age of four. After otoscopy and a general observation of the child's communicative development, the audiologist makes a more comprehensive audiological evaluation. A pure tone audiogram including air-conducted and bone-conducted signals is obtained by a respiration audiometry technique[1] or with observation audiometry. Later in life between the ages of one and three years, visual reinforcement audiometry is used.[2] During these investigations the children are tested with warble tones, either via a loudspeaker, insert earphones or bone vibrator. Next, the discomfort threshold is determined. This is done by observing the blink reflex

From the Department of Audiology and Otolaryngology, Sahlgren's Hospital, University of Göteborg, Göteborg, Sweden.

REPRINTS — Gunnar Lidén, MD, Department of Audiology and Otolaryngology, Sahlgren's Hospital, University of Göteborg, Göteborg, Sweden.

TABLE 1. HIGH RISK CRITERIA USED BY THE MATERNITY HOSPITAL

Priority	*Criteria*
1.	Family history of hearing impairment
2.	Rubella or some other viral disease during the first half of pregnancy
3.	Multiple malformations particularly of the face and ears
4.	Immaturity (birth weight less than 2,500 gm)
5.	Serum bilirubin more than 20 mg% for newborns, not diagnosed as immaturity
6.	Serum bilirubin more than 15 mg% for newborns with the diagnosis of immaturity
7.	Anoxia or neurological symptoms of cerebral origin for more than 24 hours
8.	Congenital infections
9.	Diabetes mellitus in the mother
10.	Hypoglycemia

threshold, which is about 5-10 dB below the discomfort threshold. Whisper and spoken voice tests are always employed, and sound localization ability is also checked. The stimuli are presented through the loudspeakers or the earphones, depending on the age of the child. With these techniques, it is possible to get a reliable audiogram at as early an age as four months.

Another promising technique which seems to be gaining importance is brainstem audiometry. In our center we have only limited experience with this procedure in this age range.

As soon as the degree of deafness is determined, and preferably before one year of age, we initiate the next procedure, which is to fit and evaluate the child's performance with a hearing aid. This procedure is based on the results of aided and unaided tone audiometry with determination of the discomfort threshold.[3]

Otological and audiological follow-up of the hearing-impaired children is performed twice a year during all preschool grades. Impedance audiometry is often employed when serous otitis is suspected. The hearing aids are checked by examining the relationship between acoustic gain and aided and unaided tone thresholds.[4] Earmolds are changed at least once a year.

The next step for the parents, after the degree of deafness is determined, is to talk to the social worker about some welfare benefits which they may be entitled to depending on their child's hearing loss and handicap. A hearing loss of more than 55 dB HL re ISO entitles the family to a subsidy of $4,000 a year until the child reaches 18 years of age.

The educational training part of the habilitation program known as home guidance starts immediately after the clinical investigation is finished. A preschool teacher for hearing-impaired children visits the child one or more times a week for the dual purpose of stimulating the child's speech and language development and counseling the parents.

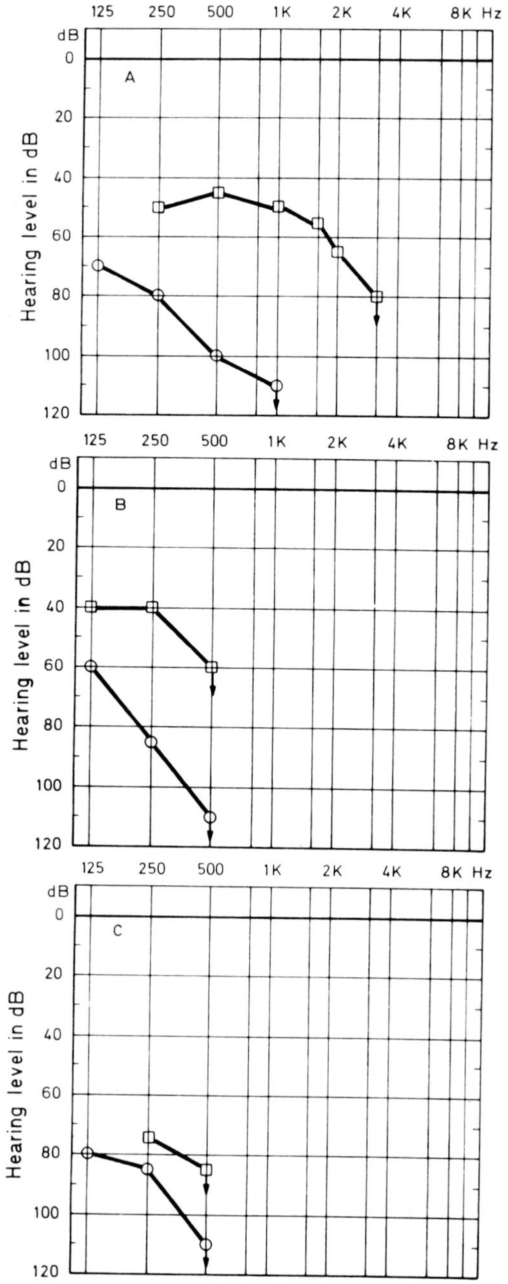

Fig. 1. Unaided (bottom curve in A,B,C) and aided (top curve) tone thresholds in right ear in three types of deaf children. (From Lidén and Kankkunen.[4] Reprinted with permission)

The home guidance service tries to make natural and efficient communicators of the parents. It is also helpful in eliminating emotional disturbances and psychological crises in the parents during the early years after diagnosis. According to our experience, it is also very rewarding to ask a psychologist outside the center for help with crisis therapy.

At such an early age as one year, prediction of the child's ability to acquire language and develop speech is difficult with the commonly used psychological methods. Aided tone audiometry tells how hearing residuals can be utilized with amplification. There seems to be a rather good correlation between the ability to utilize amplification and language development during the first three years of life.[4] Figure 1 shows aided tone audiograms in three deaf children (A,B,C) with similar unaided tone audiograms. In A the aided audiogram shows that amplification can be utilized better than the unaided audiogram predicts. The child also started to use his voice early and speech improved gradually. Type C showed no amplifiable hearing residuals. The speech and language development was extremely slow. Tomography of the inner ear in this case and many others with type C aided audiogram revealed malformed cochleas.

The task of making educational decisions has become more complex in recent years as controversies have arisen concerning both method of teaching severely hearing-impaired children (auditory-oral versus total communication) and the nature of the educational environments in which they may best learn (mainstreaming within regular schools versus special educational schools for the hearing-impaired children). Furthermore the parents of the hearing-impaired child are increasingly influenced by the growing strength of parents' association of hearing-impaired children.

Ten years ago the majority of the profoundly hearing-impaired children having an audiogram type A were trained only with auditory-oral methods. However, today a strong wind is blowing for using total communication from the early start even in this group of children. Preschool teachers are especially educated in total communication. The parents are also advised to participate in manual sign courses.

At an age of about four, hearing-impaired children are integrated in special preschools for normal-hearing children. These preschools have a reduced number of normal-hearing children and are especially equipped. Each group consists of 4 hearing-impaired and 12 normal-hearing children. A preschool teacher for hearing-impaired or deaf children belongs to the staff. There are also some units available for multihandicapped and for psychologically disturbed children who cannot be integrated among the normal-hearing children.

At an age of seven, formal schooling within Sweden's comprehensive school system is begun. Decisions pertaining to the educational placement of hearing-impaired children are made during the year preceeding school entry by a group of people representing residential schools for the deaf, hard-of-hearing classes, preschool teachers, a psychologist and an audiology center. The decisions are based on the communicative, psychosocial and cognitive-perceptual behavior of the child. Depending on these factors, the child is placed in special schools for the deaf, in classes for hard-of-hearing children, or in classes for normal-hearing.

The comprehensive school system of Sweden requires nine years of education. At the special schools for the deaf, the children get one more year. Gifted hard-of-hearing or deaf children can continue their education in secondary school (gymnasium). However, very few profoundly hearing-handicapped take university degrees.

Later in life hearing-impaired persons can join rehabilitation courses for adults and/or courses for continuing education for hearing-impaired adults.

REFERENCES

1. Kankkunen A, Lidén G. Respiration audiometry. Scand Audiol 1977; 6:81-6.

2. Lidén G, Kankkunen A. Visual reinforcement audiometry. Acta Otolaryngol (Stockh) 1969; 67:282-92.

3. Lidén G, Kankkunen A. Hearing aid procedure in young deaf and hard of hearing children. Scand Audiol 1973; Suppl 3:47-54.

4. Lidén G, Kankkunen A. Acoustic amplification for young deaf and hard of hearing children. In: Fant G, ed. International symposium on speech communication ability and profound deafness, 1970, Stockholm. Washington: Alexander Graham Bell Assoc for the Deaf, 1972:63-73.

PANEL — EDUCATIONAL PROGRAMMING FOR THE HEARING-IMPAIRED: PRESENT AND FUTURE

POLAND

JAN SEKULA, MD

KRAKÓW, POLAND

In Poland, a country with 35 million inhabitants, there are over 600,000 persons with bilateral impairment of the hearing necessitating hearing aids and training in speech or in substitute systems of communication. It has been assumed that in the age group 0-19 years (preproductive) there are 50,000 deaf; in the age group 20-49 years there are 122,000; in the age group 50-64 (productive) there are 95,000, and in the age group over 60 (postproductive) there are 342,000, so that these people form almost 1.8% of the whole population of Poland (Table 1). This percentage coincides with the data from other European countries. From the social, economic and medical points of view the preproductive and productive age groups require an intensive campaign for the treatment of deafness as well as hearing and speech rehabilitation.

Among the chief institutions caring for the deaf in Poland (Table 2) are the Ministry of Health and Social Welfare, the Ministry of Education,[1,2] and the Polish Association of the Deaf through its various centers, with the collaboration of the Cooperative Society of the Disabled and social organizations such as the Association for the Campaign against Disability, the Society of Friends of Children, and the Polish Mental Health Association.

The diagnosis and treatment of deafness are carried on in a system of out-patient and hospitalized medical care under the auspices of the Ministry of Health and Social Welfare. Children with defective hearing, deafness, or disturbances in communication are sent to a health service consulting unit, where an otolaryngologist makes the first diagnosis by simple diagnostic methods. Some of those with impaired hearing or deafness are then sent to the consulting unit for rehabilitation of hearing and speech and some (the majority) to the Otorhinolaryngological (ORL) Departments of the Academies of Medicine or to the well-equipped Otolaryngological Departments of the District Hospitals.

TABLE 1. DATA ON THE DEAF REQUIRING HEARING AIDS, SPEECH TRAINING OR SUBSTITUTE COMMUNICATION SYSTEMS

Age	*No.*	*Employment*
0-19	50,000	Preproductive
20-49	122,000	Productive
50-64	95,000	Productive
>65	342,000	Postproductive

In these departments a careful differential diagnosis of deafness and disturbances in speech is made by methods based on apparatus for tonal audiometry, speech audiometry, electric response audiometry (ERA), and impedance audiometry, in collaboration with a pediatrician, a neurologist, a radiologist, a psychologist and a psychiatrist. Small children present a special problem, since the assessment of hearing by conventional audiological methods, especially those which are based on behavioral reactions, meets with considerable difficulty or is even impossible. It should be emphasized that in these cases, in which speech disturbances may be provoked by deafness or some disorder of the motor aphasia type, mental deficiency or a disturbance of mixed type, ERA finds a practical application.

In accordance with the generally accepted international terminology we distinguish three levels of impaired hearing, and the appropriate therapeutic and rehabilitation procedure.

Children with lesions caused by congenital defects of the external and middle ear, inflammations and posttraumatic lesions are admitted to hospital wards for treatment — mainly surgery.

Children with lesions caused by malformation and damage to the inner ear, auditory pathways

TABLE 2. INSTITUTIONS CARING FOR THE DEAF

Ministry of Health and Social Welfare	*Polish Association of the Deaf*	*Ministry of Education*
National Health Service ORL Consulting Units	Consulting Units for Rehabilitation of Hearing and Speech	Special Kindergarten Special Primary School
Academies of Medicine ORL Departments	Compensatory Courses for Secondary School	Primary Vocational School for the Deaf
Rehabilitation Center	Training Productive Centers	Secondary or Technical School for the Deaf

From the Department of Otolaryngology, Copernicus Academy of Medicine, Kraków, Poland.

and centers leading to impaired hearing, disturbances in speech and communication with those surrounding them are sent to consulting units for hearing and speech rehabilitation.

Children with lesions caused by the changes mentioned to such a degree that they are unable to develop, to understand speech, or to communicate in any way with those around them, and who often have complications in the form of lesions of the central nervous system, are sent to special schools for tuition.[3] Organizational changes in diagnosis and therapy are not anticipated in the near future, but we shall endeavor to modernize diagnostic and therapeutic methods and apply them widely.

The rehabilitation of deaf children is organized and supervised by the Polish Association of the Deaf. This is an organization of those incapacitated by deafness, an "association for higher service" aimed at ensuring help and care for the deaf in all vital matters. The statutes of the association[4] lay down the obligations of rehabilitating the deaf in all fields of physical and mental work accessible to them and of helping them to raise their general standard of education and occupational qualifications. In order to fulfill these aims the association organizes and carries on consulting units for hearing and speech rehabilitation for all those with defective hearing in Poland, as well as organizing and superintending training and productive centers.

The consulting unit for hearing and speech rehabilitation is at present a diagnostic-rehabilitation center for children. Its work is based on the cooperation of an otolaryngologist with audiological training, a psychologist, and a logopedist, with the active cooperation of the child. In children of preschool or school age sent to the consulting unit the following are done:

1. Hearing, logopedic, and psychological tests are made.

2. Developmental rehabilitation of hearing and speech is carried out with the use of hearing aids when there are vestiges of hearing, as well as tuition in speech and communiction by lip-reading, the lingual-sign system, and oral speech with the finger alphabet (sign language). Cooperation with the kindergartens and schools for the deaf is maintained, as well as with the parents.

3. The degree of disability in hearing and speech is assessed, and children of school age are qualified for tuition in a) schools with the normal hearing, b) with the hard of hearing, c) for the deaf, and d) for the deaf with additional defects in the locomotor system, sight, or the central nervous system.

At present there are 14 consulting units for rehabilitation of hearing and speech in Poland,[5] but only some children benefit by them — mainly those in urban districts. In future, in accordance with the new administrative division of Poland into 49 provinces, it is anticipated that 49 consulting units will be organized. Of these, ten will fulfill a superior regional role with a wider sphere of work in diagnostics, rehabilitation, consultation, and training. They will be situated in towns where there are medical schools and will work in close collaboration with the ORL departments of these. In future these 49 consulting units will care not only for all deaf children but also for all those with defective hearing in their districts.

The duties of providing education and help for children with developmental defects and disturbances, including deaf children, are undertaken by the Ministry of Education which prepares programs for tuition in kindergartens and special schools as well as for vocational training. Deaf children, after a period of hearing and speech rehabilitation in early childhood, either go to special kindergartens or remain under the care of the rehabilitation unit until they are of school age.

The next stage in the education of the deaf child takes place in a special primary school for a period of seven to nine years, with a syllabus approximating that obligatory in normal schools. After the primary school the pupil may receive occupational training and general education in a primary vocational school for the deaf, and has a choice of 50 occupations and 17 schools in Poland. The program of instruction lasts from three to four years. The most talented have opportunities of receiving secondary education after a compensatory course and after passing the entrance examination to a technical school. Instruction is given by teachers and tutors in collaboration with psychologists, sociologists, and logopedists, under the care of an ear, nose and throat specialist.

We hope that in the future the results of the researches now being carried out by our team within the framework of the five-year program accepted and financed by the United States Department of Health, Education and Welfare[6] will influence the efficacy of rehabilitation of those with hearing disabilities in Poland.

The studies have as their subject the following aspects of rehabilitation in the deaf young:

1. evaluation of the pathophysiological state of the organ of hearing and equilibrium in the deaf young qualified for complex rehabilitation, medical team supervised by an otolaryngologist;

2. the effectiveness of occupational rehabilitation of the deaf young, supervised by an industrial psychologist;

3. the effectiveness of the process of rehabilitation of speech and hearing, supervised by a teacher of the Polish language;

4. the interests of the deaf young as a factor in general rehabilitation, supervised by a surdopsychologist; and

5. factors favoring the release of the activity of the deaf pupil in the process of learning, supervised by a teacher of mathematics.

A total of about 250 pupils of both sexes will have been studied during the fulfilment of the five-year research program. These pupils will be taught in three selected vocational schools:

1. institution for the training of the disabled; primary textile technical school;

2. special teaching and training center; primary technical school;

3. teaching and training center for the deaf; primary technical school.

The deaf young rehabilitated in these institutions are trained as weavers, knitters, locksmiths, leather-workers, and cabinet-makers or joiners.

We believe that more detailed information on those occupations which are most suitable for the deaf and more precise definitions of the factors deciding the efficacy of rehabilitation are essential, not only from the cognitive aspect, but also as a contribution to the better organization of tuition and training of the deaf both in Poland and in other countries.

REFERENCES

1. Ministry of Education (Institute of Vocational Training). Syllabus for special vocational schools. Warsaw, March 1978.

2. Ministry of Education. Principles of special education. Warsaw, 1976.

3. Stasinowski S. Vocational training for deaf children in the Institute for Deaf-Mutes and the Blind. Warsaw, 1970.

4. The Polish Association of the Deaf. Statutes, Warsaw, 1977.

5. Borkowska-Gaertig D. Assumptions for the organization, equipment and working principles of hearing and speech rehabilitation consulting units in Poland (typescript). Warsaw, 1977.

6. Complex Rehabilitation of the Deaf Young. Research Program 19-P-58348-F-01-HEW. SRS, Washington, DC. Report No. 1, 1978.

PANEL — EDUCATIONAL PROGRAMMING FOR THE HEARING-IMPAIRED: PRESENT AND FUTURE

DENMARK

HAROLD W. EWERTSEN, MD
COPENHAGEN, DENMARK

In 1950 a law was passed by the Danish parliament entitled Measures for Deaf and Hard of Hearing Persons in Denmark. This law permitted every Danish citizen with a hearing impairment to have an examination, hearing aids, training and education free of charge, regardless of the handicapped person's age, income or property. It was estimated that around 10,000 persons in Denmark would need audiological treatment, but it soon became apparent that there were many more. Today we know that 2 1/2% of the population need hearing aids, ie, 150,000 persons.

On the map of little Denmark (population 5 million), the circles indicate the three state hearing centers established later on in 1951 (Fig. 1). The triangles indicate audiology clinics established in collaboration with the ENT clinics of the county hospitals. In Denmark we feel that audiology is teamwork, and we have no independently operating audiologists.

In Figure 2 is a partial view of the Copenhagen center which has a staff of 48 persons, consisting of five qualified ENT specialists, one medical doctor under training, four speech and hearing pedagogues, one engineer, five electrotechnicians, nine audiology assistants, six earmold technicians, secretaries and clerks. The center has around 24,000 consultations per year, 4,400 involving children.

More than 90% of all deliveries in Denmark take place in public hospitals. If there is any suspicion of inherited disorders, rhesus incompatibility, diseases during pregnancy, shortage of oxygen, etc, the child is registered in the "risk-group" and is followed more closely than other children. All babies are seen by health nurses who visit the homes at least five times in the first year. If the parents suspect abnormal hearing, the health nurse administers aureopalpebral reflex and performs the Swedish BOEL test, which is a kind of EWING test to measure the audiovisual reflexes. At five months of age, all children have to see the family doctor, and if he, the health nurse, or the parents suspect hearing loss, the child is referred to one of the 15 audiology clinics or to the special Children's Clinic in Copenhagen for examination.

Despite all these precautions, the children average about two years of age before their hearing handicap is discovered. However, the prophylactic work has reduced the number of hearing-handicapped children considerably. If the disorder cannot be corrected otologically, the child is supplied with hearing aids on both ears. The child and the parents are then trained by the special Children's Clinic under the direction of a psychologist. The parents have the opportunity to discuss all aspects of their child's development and future. A training program is set up, and the child is followed once a week in the beginning, and later on once a month, either through visits to the clinic or visits by travelling teachers, who currently adjust the training program. The key for this program is: total communication by means of hearing aids, lipreading, gestures, and sometimes sign language. There are hours of music by means of drums, organs, and other vibrating instruments in order to teach the rhythm of the language to the children. The parents are trained in the Wedenberg method, which means loud talk directly into one of the child's ears. The hearing aid has been removed from this ear while the other remains. This method gives a very good contact between child and parent, and the teachers find that it also gives a better articulation than any other method.

When the child is three years old, he or she is integrated in a kindergarten with normal-hearing children, but still has three or five hours per week of language training by a speech and hearing therapist, who every day goes from kindergarten to kindergarten in the district where hearing-handicapped children are integrated. The hearing-handicapped child is seen by the ENT specialist every half year or every year in the audiology clinic. The hearing aids are monitored, and if necessary new earmolds are made.

At the age of five years, a board of specialists discusses every child in the area, concerning language development, hearing loss, support from the parents; and then the board decides in which of three different kinds of school the child should be placed: 1) a normal class as the only child wearing a

From the State Hearing Centre, Copenhagen, Denmark.

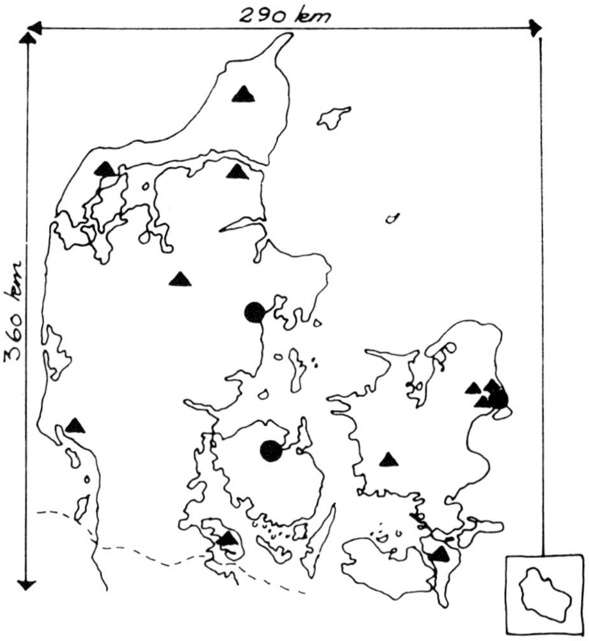

Fig. 1. Map of Denmark (population 5 million) with indication of the audiology clinics. ● Three state hearing clinics, established 1951. ▲ Audiology clinics, established in collaboration with ear, nose and throat clinics of the county hospitals.

hearing aid, 2) a special class with three to six hard-of-hearing schoolmates in a school for normal children (Fig. 3), or 3) enrollment in a special school for handicapped children only. Table 1 summarizes enrollment figures for these three types of schools.

The children with hearing aids who are integrated in ordinary classes get special hours of support. For instance, the teacher of geography will spend one hour with the child and explain to him what is going to be taught and discussed in the class during the following week, so that the child is prepared to benefit from the education of his class. The following week the teacher will check to see that the hearing-handicapped child really has understood the past week's work. The children integrated in normal classes have to follow the program made for that level of ordinary school children.

The special classes are placed in so-called "teaching centers," of which we have 13 all over Den-

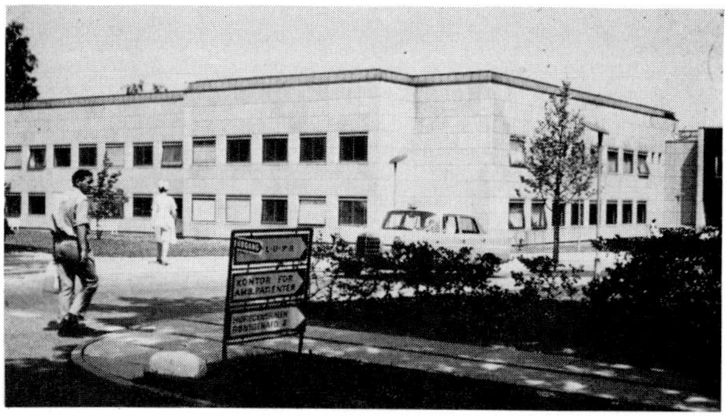

Fig. 2. Part of the hearing center in Copenhagen.

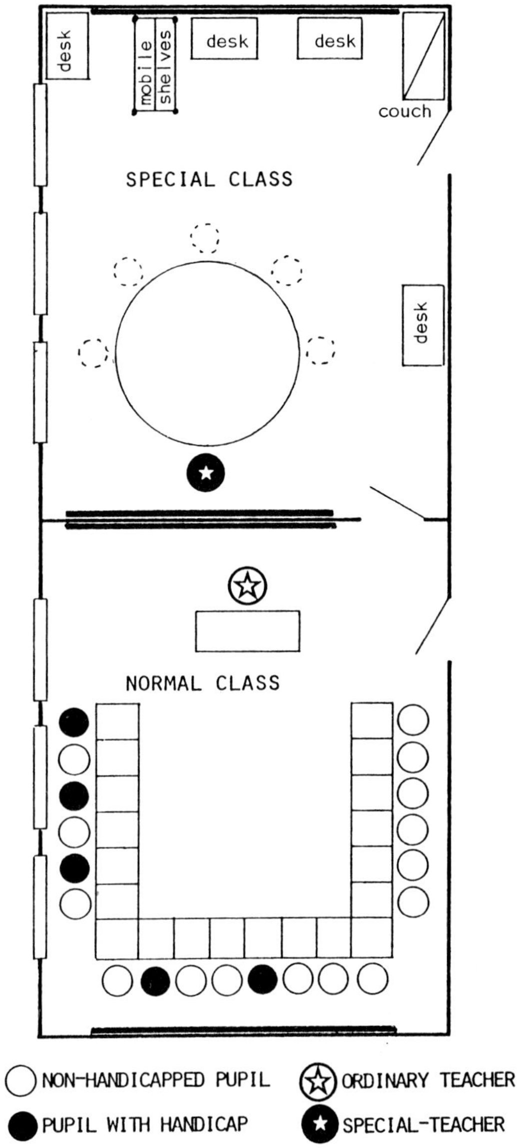

Fig. 3. Arrangements for a special class in a teaching center and for children integrated in a normal class (twin school principle).

mark, so the child can be transported by school bus from his home to the center every day. Only a few pupils from some islands stay in a foster home from Monday to Friday. The special classes are placed alongside normal classes for children of the same age. The teaching centers have special teachers and facilities for medical examination, physiotherapy, and occupational therapy.

Special Schools for the Deaf. We have five such special schools for profoundly deaf children and for children with handicaps other than hearing impairment. Until now there has not been a comprehensive annual evaluation required for the language development of these children; we think this fact has to be remedied in the near future.

School is compulsory from 7 to 17 years, and during the last years the children have to consider

TABLE 1. EDUCATIONAL PROVISIONS FOR DANISH SCHOOL CHILDREN WITH HEARING AIDS IN 1977 (N = 1,873)

Integrated in normal classes	1196
Teaching centers	237
Special schools	440

TABLE 2. EDUCATIONAL PROVISIONS FOR DANISH HANDICAPPED CHILDREN IN 1977 (N = 100,000)*

Integrated in normal schools	75,000
Special classes in normal schools	15,000
In special schools	10,000

*From a population of 800,000 schoolchildren.

which job they would choose after school; they are allowed to stay one week in various jobs to find this out. The children who are deaf or have a profound hearing loss are referred to a special college, where they can stay from 17 to 19 years of age. The purpose of this college is to make the children, who have been living in rather protected surroundings, fit for life in the outside world. They are trained in language, and they go to various factories, work shops, etc, for a longer period in close cooperation with vocational counsellors for the hearing-handicapped. At the age of 19 the young people go out into daily life to start their own living. Some of them have the opportunity to get "protected work," if they cannot get along on their own.

In 1977 there were 800,000 school children in Denmark. Unfortunately, it is not until the normal child is seven years old that he has his hearing tested by screening audiometry. The tests are given at ages 7, 10 and 13, or when the school doctor finds it necessary. In the near future we are going to institute a hearing testing program for kindergarten children. As shown in Table 2, 100,000 of the children were suffering from various handicaps; 75,000 of these were integrated in a normal school; 10,000 got their education in special schools; and 15,000 were placed in special classes integrated in ordinary schools. Each school has a board of five to seven members chosen among parents of the school children. In schools with special classes, the board is supplemented with two parents of handicapped children.

Special Teachers. We have around 500 speech and hearing therapists, who first were ordinary teachers in normal schools after completing five years in a teachers' college. They must work for at least two years in ordinary schools before they are allowed to attend the Royal Danish High School for special teachers, where they are educated and trained for 1 1/2 years. These teachers are responsible for the training and education of schoolchildren with speech defects or hearing handicaps, and moreover, they take care of adults who have developed hearing problems later in life. The teachers pay great respect to the individual child. However, they do not find it possible to have an individual educational program for each child because so many factors influence this situation: intelligence, degree of hearing loss, friends, support from the parents, etc.

In other words, the Danish community offers various educational programs and it is our task together with the parents to fit the child into the proper program for his individual handicap. We are careful not to force the children into too rigid a program concerning formal capacities. We try to avoid frustrations and to work with and develop the child's innate capacities. The main purpose is to make the children happy and harmonious human beings, who as adults will be able to find their appropriate place, and live with their handicap among other people.

PATHOLOGY OF CONGENITAL DEAFNESS
PRESENT STATUS AND FUTURE PRIORITIES

LAVONNE BERGSTROM, MD, FACS
LOS ANGELES, CALIFORNIA

The pathology of congenital hearing loss is as varied as the etiologies. Severe external ear anomalies, such as microtia, and middle ear defects have a significant incidence of accompanying inner ear aplasias, more often of the vestibular than of the cochlear end-organs. Classic inner ear aplasias are discussed, including Michel, Mondini, Alexander and Scheibe. A case illustrating close resemblance between a genetically induced Scheibe malformation and rubella inner ear deformities is presented. A variety of ear disorders acquired during intrauterine or neonatal life, including cytomegalic inclusion disease, hypoxia, erythroblastosis fetalis and later-onset genetic disorders are also discussed. Illustrative case histories are presented as well as priorities for future investigations into the pathology of congenital and genetic hearing loss.

The pathology of congenital deafness has some unique aspects, but also reflects the diversity of the many etiologies of hearing loss in general. Congenital ear pathology may be genetic, as in hereditary disorders and chromosomal defects, or may result from a defect in embryogenesis which may be sporadic or of nonhereditary and often unknown etiology, although it may form part of a syndrome. Defects in embryogenesis may also result from teratogens or acquired injuries to the intrauterine environment. Acquired sensorineural hearing loss in early infancy may be difficult or impossible to distinguish from that which is truly congenital if etiology cannot be ascertained, since the functional difficulty will be similar.

CONGENITAL CONDUCTIVE HEARING LOSS

Congenital defects of any compartment of the ear may cause significant hearing loss. Those involving external ear and canal usually cause partial hearing loss, but anomalies and profound sensorineural impairment of the same or the opposite ear may occur in 12 to 47% of aural atresia cases.[1-3] In another series polytomography of 63 ears showed that 9 had isolated external canal atresia, 4 had isolated middle ear anomalies, 34 combined external canal and middle ear anomalies; 2 had anomalous external and inner ear structures and 5 had deformities of all three compartments. The remaining nine microtic ears were either otherwise normal or may have had defects not detectable by radiography.[4] The middle ear abnormality found most frequently in most series of aural atresia cases is fused, deformed malleus and incus.[5,6] Absence of the stapes (19 of 57 ears) and of all ossicles (11 of 57 ears) was fairly common.[7] Aplasia of the middle ear was present in 12 of 89 ears and was the fourth most common defect found.[5] A variety of other middle ear defects involving ossicles, nerves, muscles, windows and vascular structures have been described and tabulated by Gill,[5] Hough,[8] and Sando and Wood.[9] Atresia confined to the osseous portion of the external canal occurs in ring defects and long-arm-deletion defects of chromosome 18, and middle ear structures appear normal by polytomography. As yet there is no surgical or autopsy report to complete our knowledge of this entity.[10]

Congenital conductive hearing loss is also associated with other external ear anomalies and a variety of syndromes. In some instances the inner ear is also congenitally abnormal. It is interesting that the vestibular portion of the labyrinth appears to be more frequently involved than the cochlea in these instances. Because they are probably underreported, the incidence of either congenitally fixed stapes or fixed malleus is not known, but they are probably more common than the more severe middle ear aplasias seen in individuals with auricular or cranial defects. Ritter[11] has described findings in three cases of bony malleus fixation. Two had fairly mild hearing losses with fixation to the epitympanic walls along the axis of rotation of the malleus and incus. The epitympanum in each case was somewhat poorly pneumatized. In the third case the hearing loss was more severe, with bony fixation laterally, perpendicular to the axis of the ossicular cog. Some exemplary case histories follow.

Case 1. A male infant was the product of a complicated pregnancy. A diagnosis of Apert's acrocephalosyndactyly was made shortly after birth. Audiometry several years later showed bilateral conductive hearing loss which was felt to be congenital, since tympanic membranes were normal. At age nine he underwent exploratory left tympanotomy. A thick, fixed stapes footplate was removed with good hearing result. There was no rush of perilymph.

In a previously reported case, a severe perilymph leak occurred.[12] A subsequent temporal bone study showed congenital stapes footplate fixation by underdifferentiated cartilage in an area of incomplete annular ligament development.[13] Other areas of the primary endochondral capsule were also abnormal, suggesting disturbed maturation or

From the Division of Head and Neck Surgery, University of California at Los Angeles School of Medicine Center for Health Sciences, Los Angeles, California.

REPRINTS — LaVonne Bergstrom, MD, Room 32-34, Rehabilitation, 1000 Veteran Avenue, Los Angeles, CA 90024.

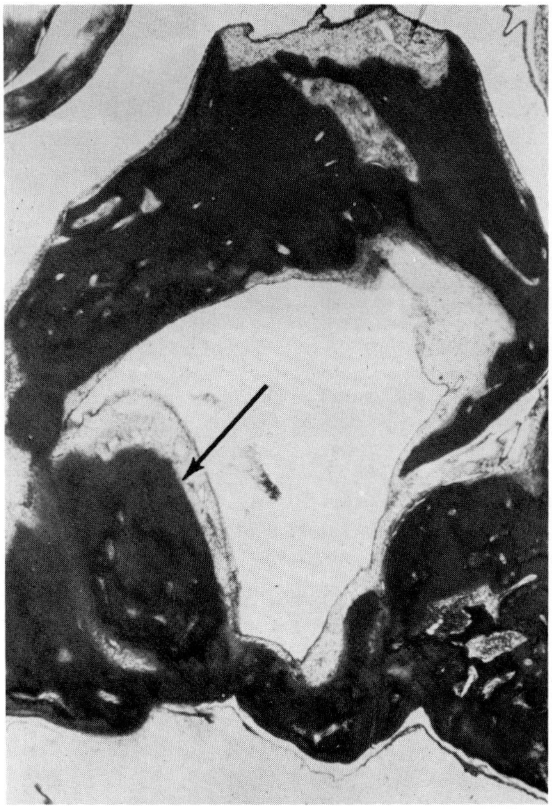

Fig. 1. Deformed stapes in Pierre Robin patient. Note the crowding in the oval window. Arrow points to an exostosis on the footplate (x25). (From Bergstrom et al.[14] Reprinted with permission.)

resorption. The bony facial canal was widely dehiscent at the pyramidal turn. The endolymphatic sac was large, surrounded by thickened fibrous tissue, but the cochlear aqueduct was normal. Saccular otoconia and hair cells were partly absent, but other vestibular end-organs were normal. The cochlea had been artifactually damaged and could not be completely evaluated, but normally developed sensorineural elements could be identified.

Case 2. A male neonate died of respiratory complications of glossoptosis and micrognathia (Pierre Robin syndrome), and of multiple severe cardiac defects. Study of both temporal bones showed narrow epitympanum with crowding of enlarged malleus and incus. The oval windows were narrow and the stapes superstructure abnormally large. In one ear the footplate contained a large exostosis, and a tiny persistent stapedial artery was present (Fig. 1). Vestibular structures and the contents of the internal auditory canal were normal, but unfortunately neither cochlea had been included in the specimens.[14]

Another study showed thickened stapes crura and footplate, minor architectural abnormalities of vestibular organs and unilateral cochlear scala communis and underdeveloped modiolus. The internal auditory canal was small and the facial canal lacked bony covering over a large area.[15]

Case 3. A male neonate succumbed from respiratory obstruction due to micrognathia and glossoptosis associated with mandibulofacial dysostosis of Treacher Collins. He also had bilateral microtia and atresia. Both ears were studied and the findings reported by Sando et al.[16] A bony mass extending from the promontory to the lateral osseous wall of the ear divided the mesotympanum into two compartments. There was neither malleus nor incus. The stapes was monopod in one ear and the footplate fixed (Fig. 2A). In the opposite ear the oval window was filled with connective tissue surrounding a bony structure that might have been a hypoplastic footplate. A bony bar extended to the oval window from its attachment to the lateral wall of the tympanum. The facial nerve exited directly from the geniculate ganglion area through the temporal squama to a subcutaneous position (Fig. 2B). The left lateral semicircular canal was hypoplastic. The cochlea was normal (Fig. 2C).

Other reports have described less severe but generally similar findings at surgery or autopsy. Atresia or narrowing of the ear canal occurs; all the ossicles may be present but deformed; the base of the skull may be grossly abnormal allowing middle cranial fossa contents to be inferiorly displaced; attic and antrum may be missing; the bulge of the horizontal semicircular canal may be absent or malpositioned. Facial nerve anomalies are frequent. Severe lethal visceral defects may be present.[17,18]

Case 4. A male neonate had aural atresia, palatal, ocular, facial, vertebral, cardiac and renal anomalies and died of complications resulting from the visceral anomalies. The right temporal bone was studied. The middle ear contained exudate, effusion and debris. The malleus and incus were oriented along an axis parallel to the cochlear modiolus (Fig. 3A). Only vestigial stapes superstructure was found, and the oval window was slit-like, containing a rudimentary footplate with a small area resembling annular ligament (Fig. 3B). There was bone dust and a great deal of artifact in the inner ear, but there was a mild Mondini aplasia of the cochlea (Fig. 3C).

The patient's clinical findings were compatible with Goldenhar's syndrome.[19] Others have reported aural atresia, ossicular abnormalities and abnormal semicircular canals and vestibule.[20,21] These cases suggest a continuum of severity of involvement of the middle ear as craniofacial structures are more severely dysmorphic. There is a rather low incidence of mild cochlear anomalies but a surprising incidence of vestibular anomalies, especially of the horizontal semicircular canal.

Case 5. A female neonate was born having muliple cranial, rib, and extremity fractures and died of respiratory complications. The diagnosis was osteogenesis imperfecta, congenita form. The temporal bone showed the characteristic osteopenia and osteoporosis. The middle ear, neural, and labyrinthine spaces were normally formed. The posterior crus of the right stapes was fractured with signs of tissue growth around the ends of the fragments, suggesting that the fracture had been present for some time, possibly since the prenatal period (Fig. 4).[14]

Others have reported similar findings,[22-29] while at surgery still others have found soft, bulky footplates in some instances combined with attenuated stapes crura, sometines with only a fibrous attachment to the footplate.[28,30,31] This case demonstrates that the temporal bone may be caught up in systemic chondral or osseous dysplasias which may cause ossicular, labyrinthine, and neural problems. Other examples are achondroplasia, osteopetrosis, dyschondrosteosis, craniometaphyseal dysplasia and diastrophic dwarfism.[32-36]

CONGENITAL SENSORINEURAL HEARING LOSS

The findings in three classic inner ear aplasias,

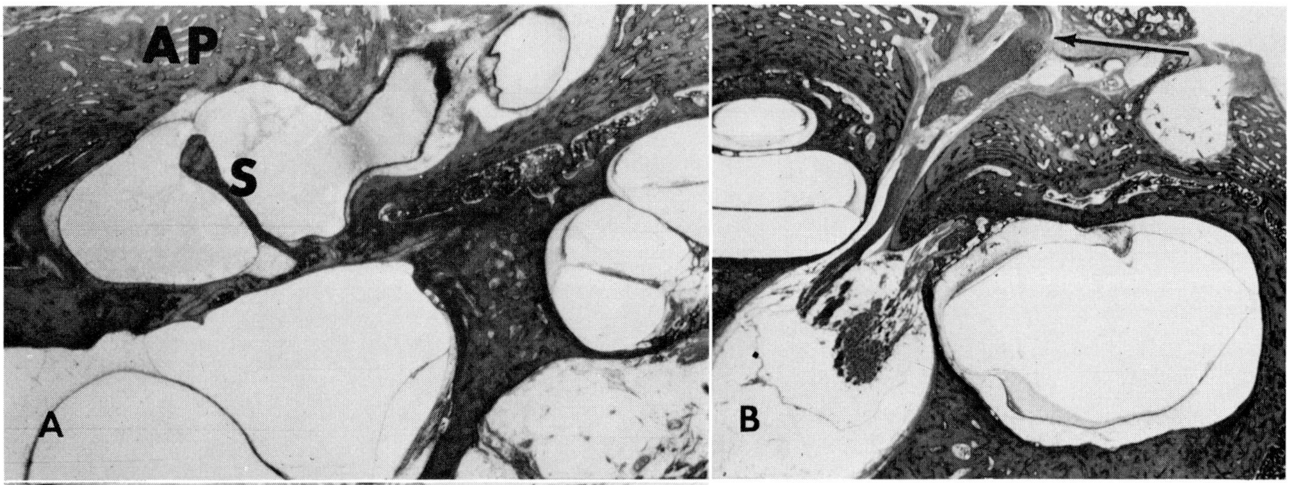

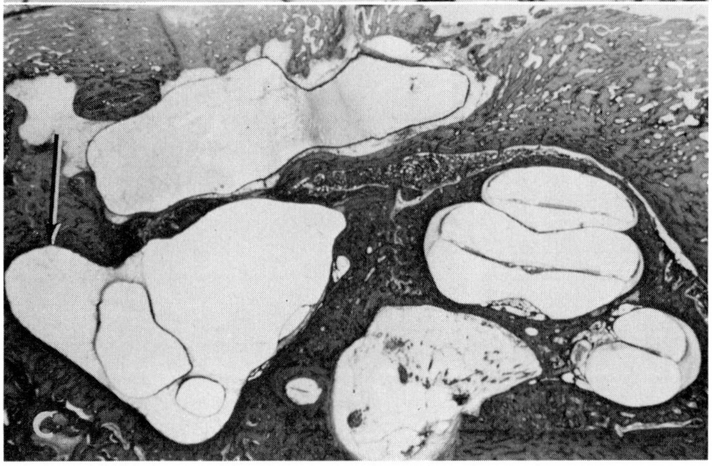

Fig. 2. Temporal bone findings in mandibulofacial dysostosis. A) Monopod stapes (S) is only ossicle in middle ear. An atresia plate (AP) is present. B) Facial nerve (arrow) exiting directly through lateral surface of temporal bone without making a geniculate turn. C) Hypoplastic left horizontal semicircular canal (arrow). Cochlea is normal. From Sando et al.[16] Reprinted with permission.)

the Michel, the Mondini and the Scheibe cochleo-saccular aplasia, are fairly well established. The Michel aplasia is the rarest, estimated to occur in a frequency equal to or less than 1 in every 100 profoundly congenitally deaf individuals.

Case 6. A three-year-old female showed no response to sound on any audiometric test subsequent to hearing loss first being confirmed at age two. Family and prenatal history were negative, and except for mild esotropia, physical examination was normal. Temporal bone polytomography showed bilateral complete absence of labyrinthine spaces, but the middle ear appeared entirely normal (Fig. 5).

In Michel's original description, the stapes and stapedial tendon were absent. The statoacoustic nerve is said to be absent.[37] In the case described above, the internal auditory canal appeared normal, and the fallopian canal ran a normal course. The eighth nerves probably were atrophic. Other cases detected radiographically have shown greatly reduced height of the petrous pyramid, or the petrous bone has contained simple cystic spaces which contain no primordial or differentiated inner ear structures, and the internal auditory canal is absent.[2,37,38] Thalidomide during the early prenatal period may produce aplasia of the inner ear, facial nerve, and varying degrees of external and middle ear aplasia. In some instances the inner ear may be partly developed.[39-41] Near-total aplasia of the inner ear has been reported in the Klippel-Feil syndrome.[42-43]

Classic Mondini or Mondini-Alexander aplasia involves the cochlea, but associated otic defects have been found in many cases studied subsequently, and the definition of the aplasia has been broadened. The cochlea has fewer turns than usual; in some instances only the basal coil is developed. The modiolus is often hypoplastic, and interscalar septae between the middle and apical coils may be absent, forming a scala communis or cloaca. The organ or Corti may be underdeveloped or normally developed, and hair cell and neural atrophy may be seen. The endolymphatic sac and duct may be dilated or may end blindly, and hydrops may be seen. Varying degrees of hypodevelopment of the vestibular labyrinth have been reported. Associated anomalies of oval and round window have been reported.[37,44-50]

Case 7. A 20-year-old male had been known to be deaf in his left ear since age three. He died of failure of his only kidney. Other congenital defects included absence of part of the bladder and right testicle, pulmonic stenosis and ventricular septal defect. The right temporal bone was normal. The left endolymphatic sac and duct were hypoplastic, the sac ending blindly within the temporal bone. The cochlea had only two turns, a normal organ of Corti but profound neural and spiral ganglion atrophy. The cochlear modiolus contained fewer than average neurovascular foraminae which were surrounded by an increased amount of

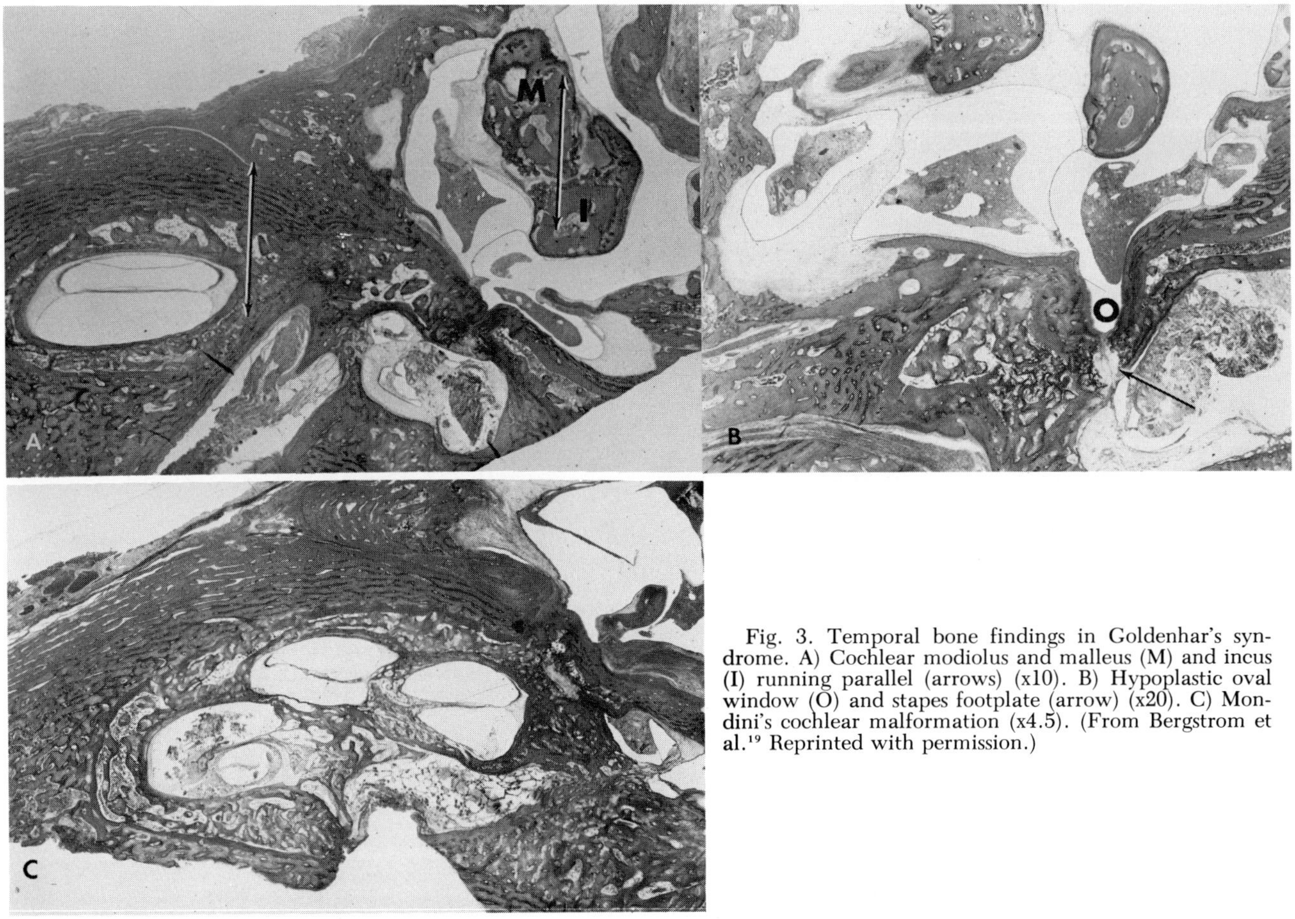

Fig. 3. Temporal bone findings in Goldenhar's syndrome. A) Cochlear modiolus and malleus (M) and incus (I) running parallel (arrows) (x10). B) Hypoplastic oval window (O) and stapes footplate (arrow) (x20). C) Mondini's cochlear malformation (x4.5). (From Bergstrom et al.[19] Reprinted with permission.)

bone (Fig. 6A). This feature is unusual for Mondini malformation. More typical features are seen in Figure 6B.

Cochleosaccular aplasia of Scheibe is probably the most common entity causing severe to profound sensorineural hearing loss. It is an interesting type of pathology because it is seen in a variety of diseases, many of which are genetic in origin. However, certain viral diseases, of which rubella is the prototype, produce a close phenocopy in the ear. In some inbred strains of laboratory animals, regressive changes leading to cochleosaccular degeneration, thought to be of genetic origin, have been associated with endolymphatic hydrops of the cochlear duct. In contrast, in known viral infections, Reissner's membrane is usually in normal or somewhat depressed position. However, late in the course of genetic cochleosaccular degeneration, Reissner's membrane may collapse, making the differential diagnosis difficult where clinical information is incomplete.[51] The pathologic changes are generally confined to the cochlea and saccule. In the cochlea there is atrophy of the stria vascularis, degeneration of the organ of Corti, and retraction and rolling up of the tectorial membrane in the limbus or inner sulcus. The tectorial membrane may be sheathed in flattened epithelial cells. The cochlear changes are most severe in the basal coil, lessening in intensity toward the apex. The saccular macula and otoconia are degenerated and the saccular wall collapsed, except often the lumen is maintained just under the reinforced area of Perlman.[46] Other changes which may be seen are PAS-positive strial deposits seen in several syndromes, most notably in the cardioauditory syndrome of Jervell and Lange-Nielsen.[52] Neural and spiral ganglion atrophy, probably secondary to loss of hair cells and supporting cells, may also be seen.[53]

Case 8. A neonate died from the sequelae of multiple anomalies of brain, palate, eye, lungs, thymus, and gastrointestinal tract. A karyotype had shown a partial deletion of the long arm of a D group chromosome. There was a maternal and paternal family history of several relatives, each of whom had one or more of the more minor anomalies he had. One family member had trisomy 21. The mother also had hyperemesis gravidarum during the first five months of pregnancy, treated with dicyclomine hydrochloride-doxylamine succinate. The temporal bone findings have been previously reported.[14] There were minor middle ear anomalies that would not have affected hearing. Both inner ears showed cochleosaccular degeneration (Fig. 7A, B), and the left cochlear aqueduct was absent, being replaced by a parallel structure which communicated with the round window niche on the tympanic side of the round window membrane. Reissner's membrane was depressed onto the organ of Corti.

Case 9. An infant died at five months of age of pulmonary edema. She had the full-blown congenital rubella syndrome, and the disease had been well documented by appropriate laboratory tests. She had had several audiometric tests, and her best response had been at 80 dB to white noise. The findings have previously been reported by Hemenway et al.[54] The left stapes was fetal in form and development, and a small area was fixed to the oval window by cartilage (Fig. 8A). The inner ear showed cystic dilatations in the stria vascularis, collapse of Reissner's mem-

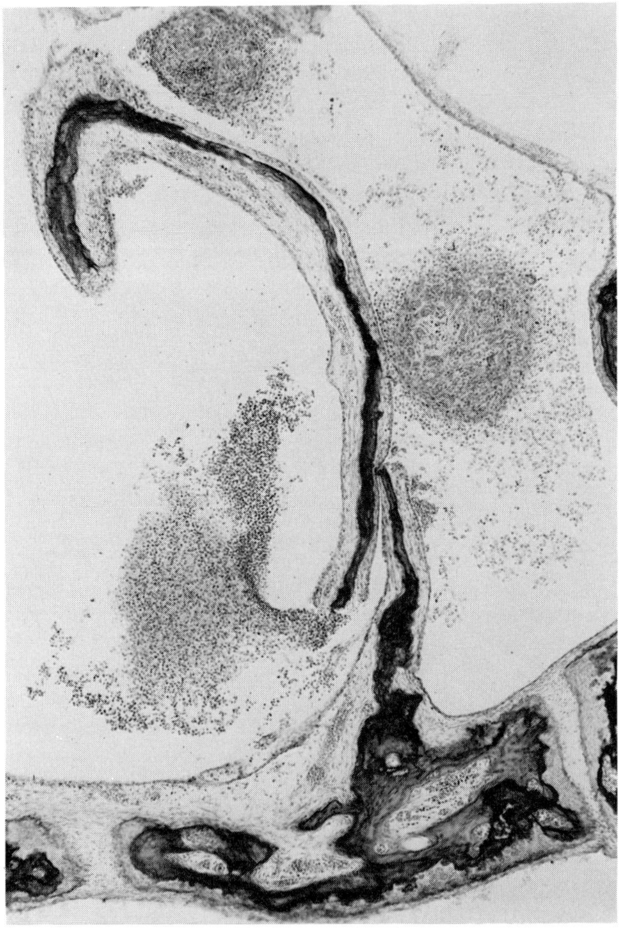

Fig. 4. Congenitally fractured right stapes in neonate who died of the complications of osteogenesis imperfecta (x40). (From Bergstrom et al.[14] Reprinted with permission.)

brane, eosinophilic precipitate in the scala tympani, and severe loss of first and second row hair cells concentrated at 8-15 mm from the basal end of the cochlea with less severe hair cell loss in other areas. In general the findings were those of cochleosaccular degeneration (Fig. 8B, C).

These last two cases had differing etiologies, unusually well established. Both were young infants, so that the effects of secondary degeneration over time should have been minimized. Their middle ear findings were dissimilar. Yet their inner ear pathologies were strikingly similar, although the one had a genetic disorder and the other was due to a viral infection. Viruses can modify the genetic information contained within the cell. Many viruses are transmitted across the placental barrier. Some viruses, including rubella, rubeola, and herpes zoster, among those having the capability of affecting the inner ear, can remain dormant in the body for years and then seem to resurrect and cause further injury. These viruses have the capability to become slow viruses. The possibility might be considered that viral etiology underlies what has heretofore been believed to be genetic cochleosaccular aplasia, perhaps even in inbred, predisposed laboratory animals.

Gussen[55] has recently advanced the interesting

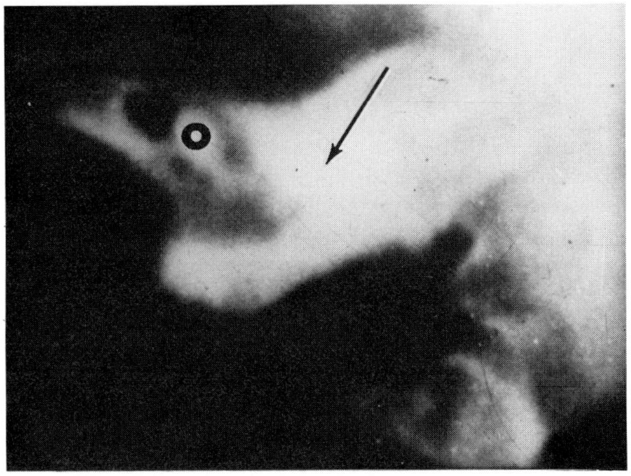

Fig. 5. Polytomographic x-ray of Michel aplasia of the inner ear. A normal ossicle (O) is seen in the middle ear, but solid bone (arrow) fills the area where the inner ear failed to develop. (From Black FO, Bergstrom L, Downs M, Hemenway WG. Congenital deafness. Boulder: Colorado Associated University Press, 1971. Reprinted with permission.)

theory that the primary injury in cochleosaccular degeneration might result from detached otoconia floating from the saccule through the ductus reuniens to the stria vascularis of the cochlea, thus impairing its function.

Case 10. A 67-year-old female died of renal failure, pneumonia and pulmonary embolus. She had never developed speech and probably had been deaf since birth. The inner ears showed cochleosaccular degeneration bilaterally as well as nerve and spiral ganglion atrophy (Fig. 9A). In the basal coil of the right cochlea there were clumps of dark purple, doubly refractile crystalloid bodies enmeshed in fibrous tissue extending from the stria vascularis to Reissner's membrane (Fig. 9B). Reissner's membrane was in fairly normal position throughout both cochleas, and the stria vascularis was atrophic and in some areas cystic.

The pathology in this case resembles that shown by Gussen.[55] Congenital hearing losses may result from prenatal and perinatal acquired problems. It is possible that maternal virus infections other than rubella may damage or interfere with the development of the ear. One of the best established of these is cytomegalovirus, which may cause neurologic deficits, microcephaly, hydrocephaly, ocular findings, and signs of ongoing infection up to many months postnatally. The author has examined three infants having well-documented cytomegalovirus and deafness. The pathology as it affects the ear has been studied both by light and electron microscopy. Cytomegalic inclusion bodies have been seen in the endolymphatic spaces along the stria vascularis and neuroepithelial and epithelial membranes (Fig. 10). There were usually destructive changes in the endorgans and in some instances eosinophilic precipitates. Inflammatory exudate surrounded nerves. The changes do not resemble those in congenital rubella.[56,57] By transmission electron microscopy, viral particles could be seen in epithelial cells of semicircular canal cristae.[57] Erythroblastosis fetalis due to Rh incompatibility between an Rh-negative mother and her Rh-positive infant, if severe or in-

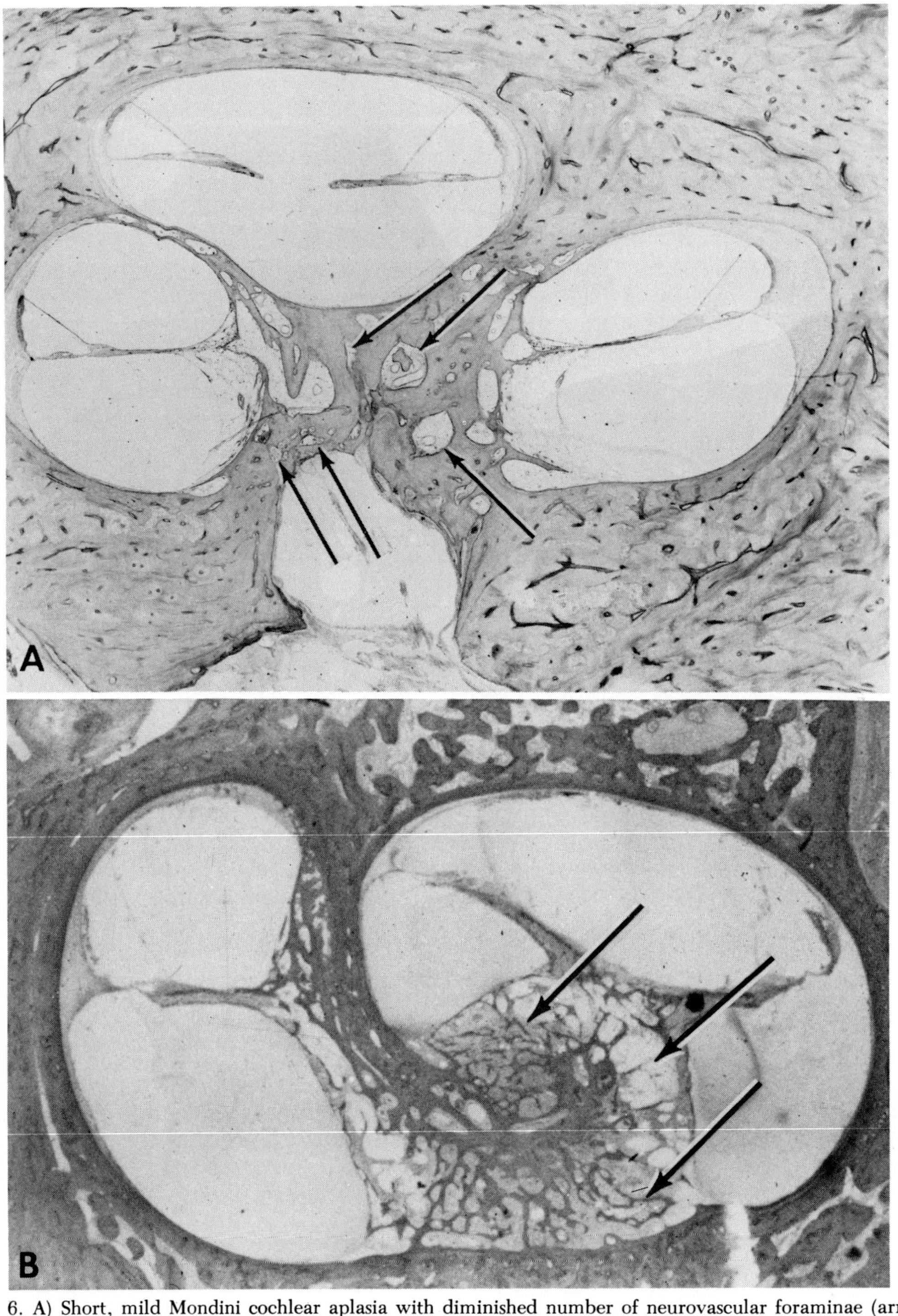

Fig. 6. A) Short, mild Mondini cochlear aplasia with diminished number of neurovascular foraminae (arrows). B) Typical Mondini cochlea with malformed modiolus and poor bone deposition (arrows). (x20)

adequately treated, may cause hearing loss.[58] The overwhelming weight of evidence seems to be that, at least by light microscopy, the lesion is not in the inner ear or auditory nerve but that deposits of bile pigments are seen in the basal nuclei, including the cochlear nuclei. There is injury and loss of cells in the cochlear nuclei.[59-62] Dublin has pointed out that in none of the pathologic cases had audiometry been done.[62]

Hypoxia and prematurity, each separately or in combination with other neonatal problems such as erythroblastosis fetalis, have also been implicated in congenital hearing loss.[63] Extensive studies of the pathology in infants dying of hypoxia have shown no significant temporal bone pathology, as studied by light microscopy, but a paucity of cells in the dorsal and ventral cochlear nuclei.[62,64] Dublin[62] feels that the pathologies of erythroblastosis fetalis and hypoxia are identical, and probably hypoxia causes loss of cochlear nuclei cells. An interesting

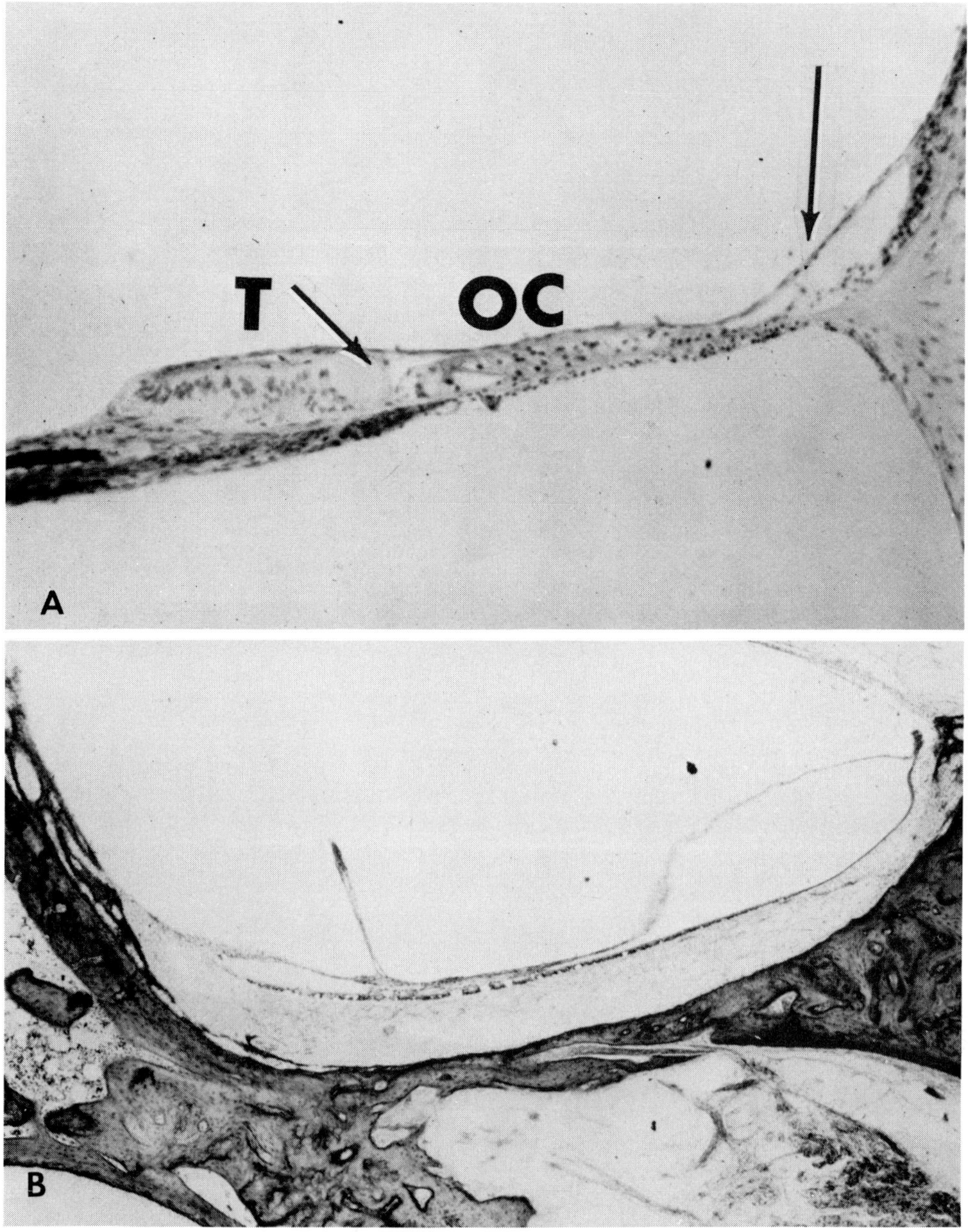

Fig. 7. Genetic cochleosaccular dysplasia showing A) depressed Reissner's membrane (arrow), encapsulated tectorial membrane (T) and compressed organ of Corti (OC) (x100). B) Collapsed saccular wall with degeneration of otolithic membrane and neuroepithelium (x40). (From Bergstrom et al.[14] Reprinted with permission.)

case has been presented by Lindsay[46] of a young man who was markedly hypoxic at birth. He had a steeply sloping sensorineural hearing loss well documented. He died of postoperative complications at age 20. The temporal bone was entirely normal. Unfortunately, the brain was not available for examination.

Congenital disorders may lie dormant for years and the gene expression may become evident in late childhood or adult life. There are a variety of degenerative syndromes, mostly of recessive inheritance, many of neuroectodermal origin, in which various mixes of ocular, spinocerebellar, cutaneous, and aural involvement occur. In only a few is the temporal bone pathology known, and it tends to be either neural or cochleosaccular degeneration.[65,66]

Progressive renal disease and hearing loss, the prototype of which is Alport's dominantly inherited syndrome, has a similar onset and if untreated, a brief, fatal course in males and a more benign one in females. Various types of inner ear pathology have been reported or in some instances none has been seen by light microscopy.[67] It is possible that there are a variety of distinct hereditary nephropathies, some of autosomal recessive inheritance, resembling Alport's. Their pathology is unknown.[19]

In many instances, isolated genetic hearing loss is of later onset, is usually dominantly inherited, but

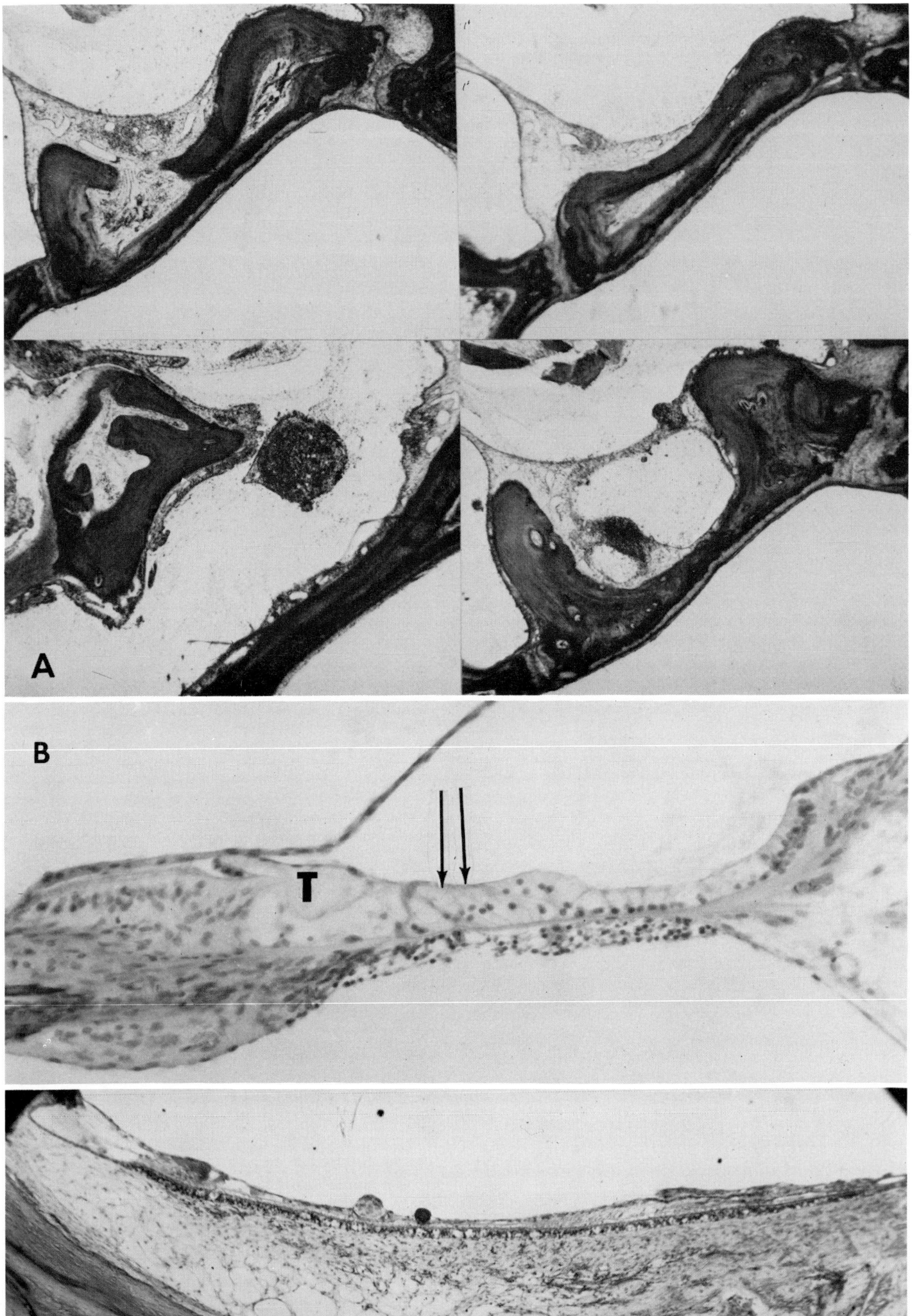

Fig. 8. Prenatal rubella. A) Stapes footplate fixation, also showing fetal form of stapes (x25). B) Encapsulated tectorial membrane (T) and organ of Corti showing degenerated hair cells (arrows) (x100). C) Collapse of saccular membrane onto degenerated otolithic membrane (x40). From Hemenway et al.[54] Reprinted with permission.)

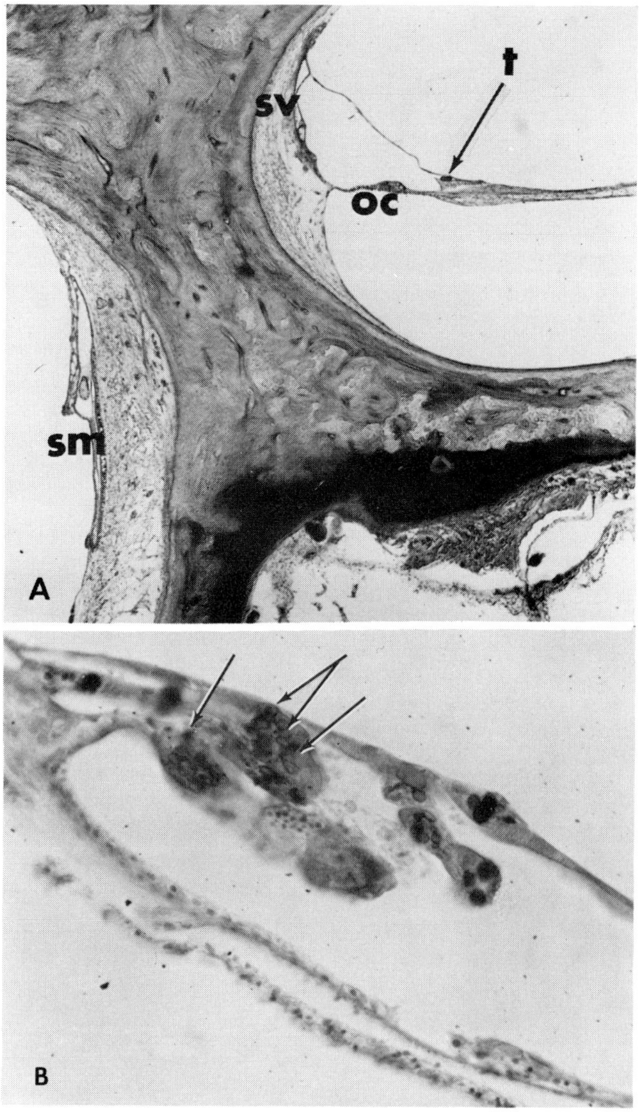

Fig. 9. A) Cochleosaccular degeneration in a congenitally deaf 67-year-old female. Note cystic degeneration of stria vascularis (SV), degenerated organ of Corti (OC), atrophic tectorial membrane (T) in the cochlea, and collapse and degeneration of saccular membrane (SM) (x25). B) Doubly refractile crystalloid bodies (arrows) enmeshed in a scar comprised of degenerated stria and Reissner's membrane in the basal cochlear coil (x400). (From Bergstrom et al.[19] Reprinted with permission.)

may be autosomal recessive or X-linked. A variety of audiometric patterns are seen. Paparella et al[68] have described the temporal bone pathology in several patients. Onset of symptomatic hearing loss may be in late childhood. An early basin-shaped sensorineural hearing loss gives way to a flat loss. The primary pathology appears to be stria vascularis atrophy with secondary hair cell loss and atrophy of the organ of Corti.

Primary neural atrophy as a cause of early deafness, possibly congenital hearing loss, probably is extremely rare. Hypoxia and erythroblastosis may represent this entity. Another exemplary case is presented below.

Case 11. A 58-year-old male died of complications following surgical repair of a luetic, aortic aneurysm due to acquired syphilis some 30 years earlier. The left ear had been known to be deaf since about age three. Temporal bone examination showed good preservation of the organ of Corti and hair cells. However, there was marked loss of spiral ganglion cells and nerve fibers to the apical coil (Fig. 11). Diminished population in other coils was believed to be within normal limits for the patient's age. No other pathology was present, and the cause of the hearing loss could not be determined.[69]

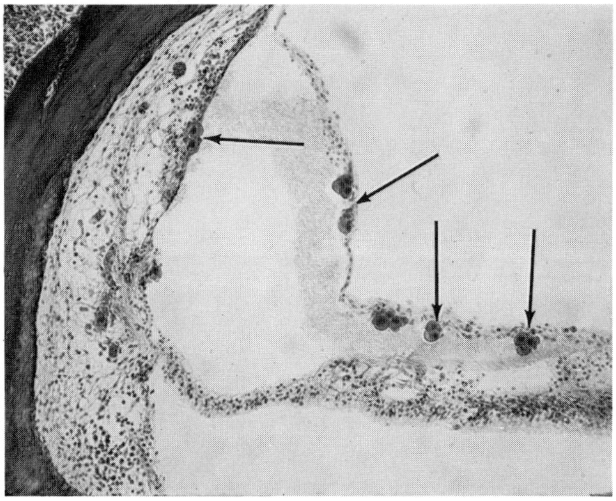

Fig. 10. Pathology in cochlea due to congenital cytomegalovirus infection. Cytomegalic inclusion bodies (arrows) are seen in the stria vascularis and along Reissner's membrane. (From Myers and Stool.[56] Reprinted with permission.)

Syndromes in which sensorineural hearing loss occurs and for which the pathology is known have been collated.[69]

FUTURE PRIORITIES

Our ability to diagnose and treat scientifically patients who have congenital or genetic hearing losses is severely limited by the paucity of existing pathologic material. Unfortunately, it is becoming more difficult to obtain temporal bone specimens, since the percentage of autopsies performed is dropping even in teaching hospitals. Furthermore, specimens from accident and coroners' cases are virtually impossible to obtain in some jurisdictions. However, the situation would be greatly improved if otologists and other clinicans would make concerted efforts to obtain temporal bone pledges.

Our methods of studying ear disease need to be extended to include more frequently the use of preservatives that will permit both light and electron microscopy. Where petrous pyramid polytomography is normal, more surface preparations should be obtained.* Specimens from middle ear surgery should, where possible, be studied in temporal bone pathology laboratories rather than in surgical pathology laboratories, where there is often little interest in and understanding of the specimens submitted. Anomalous ossicles could be photographed both in situ and after removal from the ear.

*Investigational polytomographic study of temporal bone specimens is underway at the University of California at Los Angeles.

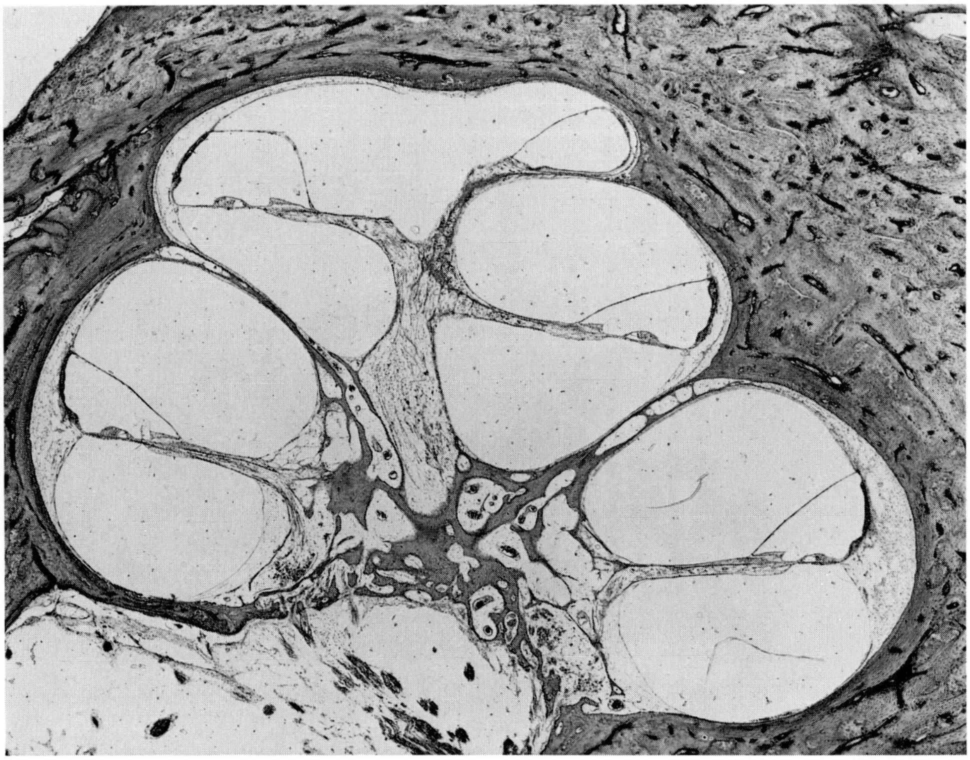

Fig. 11. Unilateral temporal bone pathology in patient deaf in ear since early childhood. Note preservation of the organ of Corti and hair cells and severe neural atrophy (x5). (From Schuknecht H, Bergstrom L. Can J Otolaryngol 1975; Suppl 2:11. Reprinted with permission.)

There has been very little systematic pathologic study of the entire auditory system. There needs to be more correlation between the neuropathologist's findings and those of the otopathologist. The otopathologist and neuropathologist should study each other's material together.

Studies of experimental embryology of the normal and pathologic isolated animal ear in tissue culture as exemplified by Friedmann et al,[52] Ruben et al,[18] and others should be exploited to their fullest for the knowledge they will add to congenital pathology in human ears. Postnatal correlative studies of the biochemistry, virology and immunology of inner ear fluids of genetically defective ears in animals should also be performed. We should continue to refine present methods of examining the ear during life with the idea of developing methodology that will virtually allow us to "look" at the inner ear noninvasively.

Finally, clinicians must assure that each patient has been thoroughly evaluated by painstaking history, perusal of prenatal and postnatal records, detailed examination, complete audiometry, and judicious use of consultations, laboratory and x-ray tests, in order to make pathologic specimens as meaningful as possible.

REFERENCES

1. Naunton R, Valvassori GE. Inner ear anomalies; their association with atresia. Laryngoscope 1968; 78:1041-9.

2. Potter GD. Inner ear abnormalities in association with congenital atresia of the external auditory canal, including a case of Michel deformity. Ann Otol Rhinol Laryngol 1969; 78:598-604.

3. Bergstrom L. Congenital and acquired deafness in clefting and craniofacial syndromes. Cleft Palate J 1978; 15:254-61.

4. Jafek BW, Nager GT, Strife J, Gayler RW. Congenital aural atresia: an analysis of 311 cases. Trans Am Acad Ophthalmol Otolaryngol 1975; 80:588-95.

5. Gill NW. Congenital atresia of the ear. J Laryngol Otol 1969; 83:551-87.

6. Schuknecht HF. Reconstructive procedures for congenital aural atresia. Arch Otolaryngol 1975; 101:170-2.

7. Harada O, Ishii H. The condition of the auditory ossicles in microtia. Plast Reconstr Surg 1972; 50:48-53.

8. Hough JVD. Malformations and anatomical variations seen in the middle ear during the operation for mobilization of the stapes. Laryngoscope 1958; 78:1337-79.

9. Sando I, Wood RP II. Congenital middle ear anomalies. Otolaryngol Clin North Am 1971; 4:291-318.

10. Bergstrom L, Stewart JM, Kenyon B. External auditory atresia and the deleted chromosome. Laryngoscope 1974; 84:1905-17.

11. Ritter FN. The histopathology of the congenital fixed malleus syndrome. Laryngoscope 1971; 81:1304-13.

12. Bergstrom L, Neblett LM, Hemenway WG. Otologic manifestations of acrocephalosyndactyly. Arch Otolaryngol 1972; 96:117-23.

13. Lindsay JR, Black FO, Donnelly WH Jr. Acrocephalosyn-

dactyly (Apert's syndrome): temporal bone findings. Ann Otol Rhinol Laryngol 1975; 84:174-8.

14. Bergstrom L, Hemenway WG, Sando I. Pathological changes in congenital deafness. Laryngoscope 1972; 82:1777-92.

15. Igarashi M, Filippone MV, Alford BR. Temporal bone findings in Pierre Robin syndrome. Laryngoscope 1976; 86:1679-87.

16. Sando I, Hemenway WG, Morgan WR. Histopathology of the temporal bones in mandibulo-facial dysostosis (Treacher Collins syndrome). Trans Am Acad Ophthalmol Otolaryngol 1968; 72:913-24.

17. Maran AGD. The Treacher Collins syndrome. J Laryngol Otol 1964; 78:135-51.

18. Ruben RJ, Toriyama M, Dische MR, Bransilver B, Daly JF. External and middle ear malformations associated with mandibulo-facial dysostosis and renal abnormalities: a case report. Ann Otol Rhinol Laryngol 1969; 78:605-24.

19. Bergstrom L, Thompson P, Wood RP III. New patterns in congenital otonephropathies. Laryngoscope 1979; 89:177-94.

20. Kirkham T. Goldenhar's syndrome with inner ear defects. J Laryngol Otol 1970; 84:855-6.

21. Miyamoto RT, Hamaker RC, Lingeman RE. Goldenhar syndrome: associated with submandibular gland hyperplasia and hemihypoplasia of the mobile tongue. Arch Otolaryngol 1976; 102:313-4.

22. Altmann F. Uber den feineren Bau des schläfenbeines bei der Osteogenesis Imperfecta Congenita und Tarda. Monatsschr Ohrenheilkd Laryngo-Rhinol 1935; 69:448-70.

23. Wullstein H, Ogilvie RF, Hall IS. Van der Hoeve's syndrome in mother and daughter. J Laryngol Otol 1960; 74:67-83.

24. Ogilvie RF, Hall IS. On the aetiology of otosclerosis. J Laryngol Otol 1962; 76:841-96.

25. Opheim O. Loss of hearing following the syndrome of van der Hoeve-De Kleyn. Acta Otolaryngol (Stockh) 1968; 65:337-44.

26. Hall JF, Røhrt T. The stapes in osteogenesis imperfecta. Acta Otolaryngol (Stockh) 1968; 65:345-8.

27. Bretlau P, Jørgensen MB. Otosclerosis and osteogenesis imperfecta. Arch Otolaryngol 1969; 90:4-10.

28. Patterson CN, Stone HB. Stapedectomy in van der Hoeve's syndrome. Laryngoscope 1970; 80:544-58.

29. Zatjchuk JT, Lindsay JR. Osteogenesis imperfecta congenita and tarda, a temporal bone report. Ann Otol Rhinol Laryngol 1975; 84:350-8.

30. Kosoy J, Maddox HE III. Surgical fingings in van der Hoeve's syndrome. Arch Otolaryngol 1971; 93:115-22.

31. Flintoff WM, Karmody CS, Rabuzzi DD. Osteogenesis imperfecta of the stapes: an histological study. J Otolaryngol 1976; 5:37-41.

32. Schuknecht HF. Pathology of sensorineural deafness of genetic origin. In: McConnell F, Ward PH, eds. Deafness in childhood. Nashville: Vanderbilt University Press, 1967:69-90.

33. Suga F, Lindsay JR. Temporal bone histopathology of osteopetrosis. Ann Otol Rhinol Laryngol 1976; 85:15-24.

34. Nassif R, Harboyan G. Madelung's deformity with conductive hearing loss. Arch Otolaryngol 1970; 91:175-8.

35. Kietzer G, Paparella MM. Otolaryngological disorders in craniometaphyseal dysplasia. Laryngoscope 1969; 79:921-41.

36. Walker BA, Scott CI, Hall JG, Murdoch JL, McKusick VA. Diastrophic dwarfism. Medicine 1972; 51:41-59.

37. Ormerod FC. The pathology of congenital deafness. J Laryngol Otol 1960; 74:919-50.

38. Valvassori GE, Naunton RF, Lindsay JR. Inner ear anomalies: clinical and histopathological considerations. Ann Otol Rhinol Laryngol 1969; 78:929-38.

39. Jørgensen MB, Kristensen HK, Buch NH. Thalidomide-induced aplasia of the inner ear. J Laryngol Otol 1964; 78:1095-101.

40. Phelps PD. Congenital lesions of the inner ear, demonstrated by tomography. Arch Otolaryngol 1974; 100:11-8.

41. Takemori S, Tanaka Y, Suzuki JI. Thalidomide anomalies of the ear. Arch Otolaryngol 1976; 102:425-7.

42. McLay K, Maran AGD. Deafness and the Klippel-Feil syndrome: 3 cases. J Laryngol Otol 1969; 83:175-84.

43. Marcus RE. Recognition and diagnosis of hereditary deafness with tomographic correlations. Trans Am Acad Ophthalmol Otolaryngol 1969; 73:409-19.

44. Altmann F. The inner ear in genetically determined deafness. Acta Otolaryngol (Stockh) 1964; Suppl 187:6-39.

45. Sugiura S, Nomura Y. Histological findings in a case of Mondini anomaly of the inner ear. Ann Otol Rhinol Laryngol 1970; 79:1139-42.

46. Lindsay JR. Inner ear pathology in congenital deafness. Otolaryngol Clin North Am 1971; 4:249-90.

47. Adkins WY, Gussen R. Temporal bone findings in the third and fourth pharyngeal pouch (DiGeorge) syndrome. Arch Otolaryngol 1974; 100:206-8.

48. Black FO, Spanier SS, Kohut RI. Aural abnormalities in partial DiGeorge's syndrome. Arch Otolaryngol 1975;101: 129-34.

49. Fitch N, Lindsay JR, Srolovitz H. The temporal bone in the preauricular pit, cervical fistula, hearing loss syndrome. Ann Otol Rhinol Laryngol 1976; 85:268-75.

50. Adkins WY, Gussen R. Oval window absence, bony closure of round window and inner ear anomaly. Laryngoscope 1974; 84:1210-24.

51. Lindsay JR, Matz GJ. The differentiation of acquired congenital from genetically determined inner ear deafness. Ann Otol Rhinol Laryngol 1966; 75:830-43.

52. Friedmann I, Fraser GR, Froggatt P. Pathology of the ear in the cardio-auditory syndrome of Jervell and Lange-Nielsen. J Laryngol Otol 1968; 82:883-96.

53. Fisch L. The aetiology of congenital deafness and audiometric patterns. J Laryngol Otol 1955; 69:479-93.

54. Hemenway WG, Sando I, McChesney D. Temporal bone pathology following maternal rubella. Arch Klin Exp Ohren Nasen Kehlkopfheilkd 1969; 93:287-300.

55. Gussen R. Saccule otoconia displacement into cochlea in cochleo saccular degeneration. Arch Otolaryngol 1980; 106:161-6.

56. Myers EN, Stool S. Cytomegalic inclusion disease of the inner ear. Laryngoscope 1968; 88:1904-15.

57. Davis GL. Cytomegalovirus in the inner ear, case report and electron microscopic study. Ann Otol Rhinol Laryngol 1969; 78:1179-88.

58. Goodhill V. The nerve-deaf child: significance of Rh, maternal rubella and other etiologic factors. Ann Otol Rhinol Laryngol 1950; 59:1123-47.

59. Crabtree N, Gerrard J. Perceptive deafness associated with severe neonatal jaundice; report of 16 cases. J Laryngol Otol 1950; 64:482-506.

60. Gerrard J. Nuclear jaundice and deafness. J Laryngol Otol 1952; 66:39-46.

61. Goodhill V. Clinical pathological aspects of kernicterus nuclear "deafness." J Speech Hear Disord 1956; 21:407-10.

62. Dublin WB.Fundamentals of sensorineural auditory pathology. Springfield: Charles C Thomas, 1976:108-13, 190-5.

63. Abramowicz M, Kass EH. Pathogenesis and prognosis of prematurity. N Engl J Med 1966; 275:938-43, 1001-7, 1053-9.

64. Hall JG. The cochlea and the cochlear nuclei in neonatal asphyxia. Acta Otolaryngol (Stockh) 1964; Suppl 194:8-93.

65. Denny-Brown D. Hereditary sensory radicular neuropathy. J Neurol Neurosurg Psychiatry 1951; 14:237-52.

66. Hallpike CS. Observations on the structural basis of two rare varieties of hereditary deafness. In: de Renck AVS, Knight J, eds. Myotatic, kinesthetic and vestibular mechanisms. Boston: Little, Brown, 1967:285-94.

67. Myers GJ, Tyler HR. The etiology of deafness in Alport's syndrome. Arch Otolaryngol 1972; 96:333-40.

68. Paparella MM, Hanson DG, Rao KN, Ulvestad R. Genetic sensorineural deafness in adults. Ann Otol Rhinol Laryngol 1975; 84:459-72.

69. Bergstrom L. Some pathologies of sensory and neural hearing loss. Can J Otolaryngol 1975; 4 Suppl 2:1-28.

EAR-RELATED DEVELOPMENTAL ANOMALIES OF BRANCHIAL CLEFTS AND ARCHES I AND II

RICHARD J. BELLUCCI, MD

NEW YORK, NEW YORK

Published in a book entitled *Symposium on Diagnosis and Treatment of Craniofacial Anomalies.*

Bellucci RJ. Ear-related developmental anomalies of branchial clefts and arches I and II. In: Converse J, ed. Symposium on Diagnosis and Treatment of Craniofacial Anomalies. St. Louis: CV Mosby, 1979:512-6.

ROLE OF TONSILLECTOMY AND ADENOIDECTOMY IN THE MANAGEMENT OF CHILDREN WITH MIDDLE EAR EFFUSION

JAMES B. SNOW, JR., MD
PHILADELPHIA, PENNSYLVANIA

Evidence for the clinical effectiveness of adenoidectomy or tonsillectomy and adenoidectomy in the management of children with persistent middle ear effusions is incomplete and what evidence there is in the literature is not convincing. In the first year after tonsillectomy and adenoidectomy there is less otitis media. The beneficial effects of tonsillectomy and adenoidectomy on the incidence of otitis media declines in the second year after the operation. The prevailing opinion is that adenoidectomy is not indicated in the vast majority of children in whom a middle ear effusion has persisted for six weeks or more in spite of antibiotic therapy. Factors favoring an adenoidectomy would be persistent nasal obstruction, persistent purulent rhinorrhea and persistent adenoiditis. The role of tonsillectomy is even less clear, but the decision regarding tonsillectomy is made by most clinicians on the basis of the amount of intercurrent or chronic tonsillitis rather than on the basis of the middle ear effusion per se.

The question to be examined in this essay is the role of 1) adenoidectomy and 2) tonsillectomy and adenoidectomy in the management of middle ear effusion in children.

Prior to the mid-1950s, children with persistent middle ear effusion were treated with adenoidectomy and bilateral myringotomies and aspiration. Following Armstrong's reintroduction of ventilation of the middle ear with tympanostomy tubes, adenoidectomy and myringotomies with insertion of tympanostomy tubes became the most widely practiced treatment.[1] In the 1960s, the concept that long term ventilation of the middle ear with tympanostomy tubes was sufficient treatment for patients with effusion of the middle ear was introduced. The immediate results of this form of treatment are impressive with a return of the middle ear toward normal and restoration of the hearing to normal. The problem results from extrusion of the tympanostomy tubes, often after only a few months, and the prompt recurrence of the middle ear effusion. With repetition of the myringotomy and insertion of a tympanostomy tube, the disease process can be kept under control, but unfortunately this procedure requires a general anesthetic in children and may be required several times during the course of childhood.

The question may be more precisely stated: Does adenoidectomy or tonsillectomy and adenoidectomy done in conjection with myringotomies and insertion of tympanostomy tubes reduce the chance of recurrence of middle ear effusion after extrusion of the tympanostomy tubes? Certainly, from the experience in many patients, middle ear effusion does frequently recur after adenoidectomy or tonsillectomy and adenoidectomy following extrusion of tympanostomy tubes. Is the incidence of recurrence of middle ear effusion less in patients who have had an adenoidectomy or tonsillectomy and adenoidectomy than in patients who have had no adenoidectomy or tonsillectomy and adenoidectomy?

The answer to this question is confounded by our lack of precise understanding of the etiology of middle ear effusion. The role of cleft palate, infection in the middle ear, infection in the pharynx, allergy, middle ear secretory activity, eustachian tube obstruction, eustachian tube lymphatic obstruction, adenoid hyperplasia, tonsillar hyperplasia, adenoiditis and tonsillitis are not completely understood. Therefore the theoretical basis for the beneficial effect of adenoidectomy or tonsillectomy and adenoidectomy is uncertain. Evidence for the clinical effectiveness of adenoidectomy or tonsillectomy and adenoidectomy is incomplete in the literature and what is present in the literature is not convincing. The literature has few reports of prospective, randomized studies of the efficacy of adenoidectomy or tonsillectomy and adenoidectomy in middle ear effusion. Parenthetically this situation among operations is not unique to tonsillectomy and adenoidectomy. Nevertheless the literature bears careful consideration in order to study the problem in the future.

LITERATURE REVIEW

In 1963 McKee reported a study of 413 children ranging in age from 2 to 15 years. These children had histories of three or more throat infections or acute respiratory infections with cervical lymphatic adenitis in the previous 12 months.[2] Children with recurrent otitis, sinusitis, exacerbation of rheumatic fever or renal disease and "frequent and severe tonsillitis over a period of several years despite continuous antibiotic therapy" were excluded because

From the Department of Otorhinolaryngology and Human Communication, University of Pennsylvania School of Medicine, Philadelphia, Pennsylvania.
REPRINTS — James B. Snow, Jr., MD, Department of Otorhinolaryngology and Human Communication, University of Pennsylvania School of Medicine, 3400 Spruce St. G 1, Philadelphia, PA 19104.

it was considered unethical to withhold tonsillectomy and adenoidectomy from these children. During the first year after the operations, the children who had the tonsillectomy and adenoidectomy had 0.17 episodes of otitis media while the children without the operations had 0.33 episodes. In the second year after the operations, the children who had the operations had 0.14 episodes of otitis media while the children without the operations had 0.17 episodes. The difference was 0.16 episodes per child during the first year and 0.03 during the second year for an overall reduction in otitis media of one fifth of an episode for two years. This difference is small but statistically significant. It is notable that these children were selected because of sore throat and youngsters with recurrent otitis media were excluded.

In another study also reported in 1963, McKee compared the results of adenoidectomy with tonsillectomy and adenoidectomy in children selected in the same way.[3] At one year, he demonstrated that adenoidectomy reduces very slightly the incidence of otitis media in this group of children with a low incidence of recurrent otitis media prior to the operation.

Mawson et al[4] studied 404 children between the ages of 3 and 12 years who were randomly assigned to tonsillectomy and adenoidectomy or medical management. Thirty percent had two or more episodes of earache or otitis media in the year prior to the randomization. During the first year after the operations, 62% of the two to four years age group had less than two attacks of earache or otitis media against 83% of the controls. In the four to seven years age group, 77% of the children receiving the operations had less than two attacks of earache or otitis media compared to 75% of the controls. In the 8 to 12 years age group, 92% of the children who received the operations had less than two attacks of earache or otitis media compared to 80% of the controls. In the second year even more similar rates were found in the two groups. No significant difference was found in the incidence of otitis media.

In 1967 Roydhouse[5] reported a study of 552 children in which the same criteria of selection were used as in McKee's studies. Again children whose main complaints were relative to the ears were excluded. During the first year after tonsillectomy and adenoidectomy, the children had 0.19 episodes of otitis media while the children without the operations had 0.29 episodes. In the second year after the operations, the children had 0.09 episodes of otitis media while the children without the operations had 0.07 episodes. The difference was 0.10 episodes per child during the first year and –0.02 episodes during the second year for an overall reduction in otitis media of less than 10% for two years.

Rynnel-Dagöö et al[6] reported in 1978 a controlled, randomized study of 76 children with recurrent otitis media, frequent upper respiratory tract infections or nasal obstruction. The children were randomly assigned to adenoidectomy or no adenoidectomy. Those with middle ear effusions were treated with myringotomies and aspiration with tympanostomy tubes being inserted if the aspiration demonstrated tenacious fluid. The group that had the adenoidectomy had less nasal obstruction at one year after the operation than the group that did not have the adenoidectomy, but the incidence of nasal obstruction was the same in the two groups after two years. They were not able to demonstrate any statistically significant difference between the two groups in the incidence of purulent otitis media or middle ear effusions during the two years following randomization. Likewise no difference in hearing loss was present after two years.

Lemon[7] studied adenoidectomy with myringotomy and aspiration versus myringotomy and aspiration alone and found a 3% recurrence of middle ear effusion in six months in the patients who had had an adenoidectomy and a 40% recurrence rate in those who had not had the adenoidectomy.

In general it may be stated that in the first year after tonsillectomy and adenoidectomy there is less otitis media than in the period prior to the operation. The magnitude of this difference is small both in Mawson et al's[4] and Rynnel-Dagöö et al's[6] studies in which the incidence of otitis media prior to operation was fairly high and in McKee's[2,3] and Roydhouse's[5] studies in which the incidence of otitis media prior to operation was low. The beneficial effects of tonsillectomy and adenoidectomy decline in the second year after the operations although Mawson et al demonstrated a persistent substantial difference in the second year. Although Rynnel-Dagöö et al were not able to demonstrate a beneficial effect of adenoidectomy on the incidence of purulent otitis media or middle ear effusion or on the magnitude of the hearing loss at two years, Lemon[7] demonstrated a much lower rate of recurrence of middle ear effusion after adenoidectomy.

Does adenoidectomy or tonsillectomy and adenoidectomy done in conjunction with myringotomies and insertion of tympanostomy tubes reduce the chance of recurrence of middle ear effusion after extrusion of the tympanostomy tubes? For the purpose of seeking an answer to this question, these studies are not as helpful as they might have been because the incidence of middle ear disease accepted for inclusion in the studies was low. If the operations were efficacious, the potential reduction in the incidence of otitis media and middle ear effusion would be small. Indeed, higher incidences of middle ear disease were reasons for exclusion from some of these studies prior to randomization and for withdrawal from the control groups after randomization. Also these patients were not studied with tympanometry.

A major problem in such studies is the lack of documentation of the severity of the problem prior to the operative intervention. It is now well recognized that even in control groups the incidence of the problem declines in individuals under careful observation as compared to the historical account of the problem prior to the entrance into the study.

In the past, serous or secretory otitis media was defined as a sterile middle ear effusion. It is now known that 11 to 60% of middle ear effusions formerly diagnosed as serous or secretory contain infectious bacterial agents. There is evidence that antibiotic therapy promotes the resolution of the middle ear effusions diagnosed clinically as acute otitis media.[8] Likewise there is evidence that prophylactic chemotherapy can reduce the incidence of acute otitis media.[9]

The microbiologic environment of the nasopharynx in middle ear effusions is similar to that in acute otitis media.[10] Adenoidectomy, tonsillectomy and treatment with conventional chemotherapeutic agents have been only partially effective in eradicating these pathogenic bacteria from the nasopharynx.

All of this information suggests that bacterial infection, whether acute or indolent, is a major factor in the etiology and pathogenesis of middle ear effusions. The efficacy of tonsillectomy and adenoidectomy in the management of middle ear effusions has not been answered by the studies so far reported, and comparison of the efficacy of these operations with other forms of treatment for middle ear effusion such as antibiotic therapy, antimicrobial chemotherapy, sympathomimetic amine therapy, antihistamine therapy and insertion of tympanostomy tubes remains to be carried out.

Olson et al[11] have found in a study of the efficacy of pseudoephedrine in the treatment of children with middle ear effusions no difference in the rate of resolution in the control group receiving a placebo and in the group receiving pseudoephedrine. Approximately 60% cleared in both groups. A National Institute of Neurological and Communicative Disorders and Stroke (NINCDS) contract for the study of the efficacy of a combination of a sympathomimetic amine and an antihistamine has been awarded to the Children's Hospital of Pittsburgh. It is hoped that this well-designed study will give us important new information on the efficacy of this widely practiced form of therapy for middle ear effusion.

Persico et al studied 276 children with middle ear effusion, all of whom received ampicillin therapy and 160 of whom received prednisone orally for 10 to 14 days.[12] Within two weeks 53% of the group receiving prednisone were otoscopically, tympanometrically and audiometrically back to normal while only 17% of the group receiving only ampicillin were back to normal. Thirty-eight percent were in need of further treatment at the end of the antibiotic therapy as compared to 37% in the corticosteroid group. Ten percent of the prednisone group showed no improvement compared with 45% of the ampicillin alone group.

Similar studies are needed for the role of pneumococcal immunization, antibiotic therapy, antibiotic or antimicrobial chemotherapeutic prophylaxis, tympanostomy tube insertion, adenoidectomy, and tonsillectomy and adenoidectomy.

In 1971 Paradise and Bluestone initiated a study in Pittsburgh of the efficacy of tonsillectomy and of adenoidectomy. The subjects are randomly assigned to the operation or medical management. Recruitment of study patients has been a problem. The number of children who met the criteria for tonsillectomy is small. Parents of approximately 75% of the children allow random assignment. Preliminary data suggest that children with middle ear disease treated with adenoidectomy show few differences in morbidity from those treated without adenoidectomy. Subsequent morbidity is substantial in both groups.

A multiinstitutional study of the efficacy of adenoidectomy and tonsillectomy and adenoidectomy has been planned through a grant to the Department of Epidemiology of the University of Pittsburgh from NINCDS. The report that was developed from this planning grant has been considered by an ad hoc committee assembled by NINCDS. The ad hoc committee has recommended that studies of the efficacy of adenoidectomy and tonsillectomy and adenoidectomy in the treatment of patients with otitis media are needed and that the efficacy of insertion of tympanostomy tubes should be studied in conjunction with these studies. The point I would make is that the treatment of middle ear effusions should be studied rather than studying the operations.

The problems involved in studying the efficacy of adenoidectomy and tonsillectomy and adenoidectomy in the treatment of middle ear effusions are many. The criteria for the selection of patients is debatable. If the criteria are sufficiently restrictive to obtain a fairly homogeneous study group, the numbers in one institution or even in multiple institutions tend to be too small for a statistically significant difference to be demonstrated. If the criteria are broad enough to encompass a larger number of study subjects, the results lack sufficient specificity to be of value in the decision-making process for an individual child with a specific clinical problem.

Smaller numbers of study subjects could be employed by allowing the child to serve as his own control. After a period of documentation of the incidence and severity of the clinical problem, the operation could be performed and the status of the patient could be determined by prolonged follow-up. The flaw in this design is the tendency for a given child to improve over time without any treatment, and this approach introduces a bias in favor of the treatment under consideration. This problem is fundamentally biostatistical. We need an innovative solution to this dilemma from biostatisticians.

The problem is further confounded by the fact that there are a number of forms of treatment which are in no way mutually exclusive which may be efficacious. Not only do we need a determination of the efficacy of each, we need to know when and how they should be applied in conjunction with each other.

The current state of the art would suggest the following approach to the management of children with middle ear effusions. Bearing in mind the high incidence of pathogenic bacteria in middle ear effusions which do not appear to be acute purulent otitis media, antibiotic therapy, probably with ampicillin for 10 to 12 days, should be considered in children with middle ear effusions who have not recently had antibiotic therapy.

Allergic management should be considered in each child.

In children in whom the middle ear effusion persists after a trial of antibiotic therapy, a six-week trial of a sympathomimetic amine and an antihistamine is in order. If the effusion persists, operative intervention should be considered. In this consideration, the vast body of opinion would concur that myringotomies with insertion of tympanostomy tubes should be carried out. It is at this point that the role of adenoidectomy should be considered. The prevailing opinion is that adenoidectomy is not indicated in the vast majority of children with the first episode of middle ear effusion that has persisted for six weeks in spite of antibiotic and sympathomimetic amine and antihistamine therapy. Factors favoring an adenoidectomy at this point would be persistent nasal obstruction, persistent purulent rhinorrhea and persistent adenoiditis.

In children who have not had an adenoidectomy or tonsillectomy and adenoidectomy who have recurrence of middle ear effusion after extrusion of multiple tympanostomy tubes, the same factors favor adenoidectomy; however, no firm clinical rule is apparent at this time. The role of tonsillectomy is even less clear, but the decision regarding tonsillectomy is still made by most clinicians on the basis of the amount of intercurrent or chronic tonsillitis rather than on the basis of the middle ear effusion per se.

In 1971 I tried to discuss the current state of the art regarding tonsillectomy and adenoidectomy.[13] How different this essay is from that one. A great deal of conservatism regarding adenoidectomy for middle ear disease has occurred in the last 15 years. However we are just as much in need of definitive studies now as we were then.

REFERENCES

1. Armstrong BW. A new treatment for chronic secretory otitis media. Arch Otolaryngol 1954; 59:653-4.

2. McKee WJE. A controlled study of the effects of tonsillectomy and adenoidectomy in children. Br J Prev Soc Med 1963; 17:49-69.

3. McKee WJE. The part played by adenoidectomy in the combined operation of tonsillectomy with adenoidectomy. Second part of a controlled study in children. Br J Prev Soc Med 1963; 17:133-40.

4. Mawson SR, Adlington P, Evans M. A controlled study evaluation of adeno-tonsillectomy in children. J Laryngol Otol 1967; 81:777-90.

5. Roydhouse N. A controlled study of adenoidectomy. Arch Otolaryngol 1970; 92:611-6.

6. Rynnel-Dagöö B, Ahlbom A, Schiratzki H. Effects of adenoidectomy. A controlled two-year follow-up. Ann Otol Rhinol Laryngol 1978; 87:272-8.

7. Lemon AN. Serous otitis in children. Laryngoscope 1962; 72:32-44.

8. Laxdal OE, Merida J, Jones RHT. Treatment of acute otitis media: a controlled study of 142 children. Can Med Assoc J 1970; 102:263-8.

9. Perrin JM, Charney E, MacWhinney JB, McInerny TK, Miller RL, Nazarian LF. Sulfisoxazole as chemoprophylaxis for recurrent otitis media: a double-blind crossover study in pediatric practice. N Engl J Med 1974; 291:664-7.

10. Lundgren K, Rundcrantz H. Microbiology in serous otitis media. Ann Otol Rhinol Laryngol 1976; 25:152-5.

11. Olson AL, Klein SW, Charney E, et al. Prevention and therapy of serous otitis media by oral decongestant. Pediatrics 1978; 61:679-84.

12. Persico M, Podoshin L, Fradis M. Otitis media with effusion: a steroid and antibiotic therapeutic trial before surgery. Ann Otol Rhinol Laryngol 1978; 87:190-201.

13. Snow JB. Current status of the tonsil and adenoid problem. J Okla State Med Assoc 1971; 64:47-52.

CHRONIC OTITIS MEDIA AND CHOLESTEATOMA

G. O. PROUD, MD
KANSAS CITY, KANSAS

Cholesteatoma may arise because of a number of events, but serous otitis media appears to be the precursor in the majority of instances. Whether one enters into conservative, simple excision of the keratotic mass or a more extensive modified radical mastoidectomy or radical exteriorizing procedure will depend upon whether the cholesteatoma is in a very small "pearl-like" mass, confined to a limited area, or whether it is dispersed to the point where total eradication is all but impossible.

The purpose of this presentation is to introduce some thoughts on three aspects of chronic ear disease and cholesteatoma. First some comments will be made upon the etiology of cholesteatoma, second a number of reasons for failure of temporal bone surgery to accomplish its goals will be discussed, and third a plea will be offered for conservatism in the surgical assault upon cholesteatoma in certain instances and a more radical approach in others.

ETIOLOGY OF CHOLESTEATOMA

Taking first things first, the etiology of cholesteatoma has not been clearly established. McGuckin presented good evidence to demonstrate that the keratotic mass may, in some instances, arise in the epithelium of the external auditory canal and invade, in secondary fashion, the middle ear cleft and mastoid process.[1] In fact, McGuckin proposed that the term "otitis media" is a misnomer in the absence of purulence, and he suggested that the mesotympanum may remain essentially healthy unless secondary infection chances to intervene. Careful, prolonged observation of patients with the surgical otoscope in the outpatient clinic tells one that he is probably correct in his assumption, but he gave only lambent treatment to the fact that middle ear effusion coexists with or precedes the "sodden keratotic mass." He relied upon repeated cleansing, by suction, of the diseased canal skin and declared that surgical intervention is seldom required. He stated that such cleansing was sufficient to cure many patients for all time. His theory is an attractive one, but in many instances the canal skin appears so healthy and the site of cholesteatoma emergence so far distant from the skin that one is led to conclude that his theory of origin can be applied to but a few patients.

The thought that cholesteatoma may be of congenital origin and arise in the epitympanic recess has been so well documented by Virchow that the concept appears to be factual and not born of theory alone.[2] Cholesteatoma which arises in this fashion is uncommonly deceptive and dangerous, for it may remain asymptomatic and unrecognized for many years while its erosive mischief is at work. Fortunately, again, the congenital type is probably a rare one.

The suggestion that cholesteatoma arises by migration of external auditory canal epithelium through an attic perforation was submitted by Tumarkin.[3] His thesis carries some allure when cholesteatoma is first seen in a perforation of the membrane of Shrapnell; however, careful observation will establish the fact that most cholesteatomata first presents in pockets in the posterosuperior segment of the pars tensa immediately overlying the long crus of the incus.

On occasions one sees the appearance of cholesteatoma following the development of a marginal pars tensa or pars flaccida perforation due to trauma. In the "misguided" healing process the epithelium invades the tympanum or epitympanum. Sometimes iatrogenic maneuvers such as placing a graft on the lateral aspect of a perforation during a myringoplasty operation may give rise to cholesteatoma when epithelium is buried or grows beneath rather than over the surface of the graft.

The greater number of cholesteatomata, however, appear to arise in response to prolonged serous otitis media. As the latter disease process progresses there comes a time when a retraction pocket develops in the posterior marginal area of the pars tensa. Eventually the pocket becomes adherent to the long crus of the incus and becomes progressively more difficult to reduce by inflation or myringotomy. Later still, the fluid vanishes from the mesotympanum, and at this point the hearing may return to normal. The physician, consequently, relaxes his vigilance assuming that the condition has abated, but often assiduous patient follow-up will reveal that the pocket continues to deepen, and the lenticular process of the incus disappears. Auditory acuity may remain good as nature's own myringo-

From the Department of Otorhinolaryngology, University of Kansas School of Medicine, Kansas City, Kansas.
REPRINTS — G. O. Proud, MD, Department of Otorhinolaryngology, University of Kansas Medical Center, Rainbow Blvd. at 39th St., Kansas City, KS 66103.

stapediopexy has been accomplished. Eventually the pocket or invagination deepens, becomes a sac and invades the tympanum, the epitympanum, the aditus ad antrum, and, at length, the mastoid process. If at some point secondary infection appears, attended by pain or discharge, the patient may return for care.

Just how many pursue this course and how many are self-limited it is impossible to say, for the nomadic pattern of American life makes patient follow-up a singularly difficult assignment. Surgical exploration of the mastoid and epitympanum while fluid is still present in the middle ear and for a time after it disappears usually reveals granulomatous and polypoid tissue surrounded by glue-like xanthachromic fluid in these areas while the mesotympanum ordinarily remains healthy in appearance. Apparently the retraction pocket develops as some sort of reaction to this inflammatory process, perhaps through cicatrix formation. The inciting factor or factors responsible for the inflammation remain unknown.

THE RADICAL MASTOIDECTOMY

Once cholesteatoma is entrenched its surgical excision is indicated. Again and again we hear the old refrain, "The goals of modern otologic surgery are a dry, trouble-free ear, a closed system and improved hearing." The public and our pediatric and medical colleagues have come to expect such an end result. The pity is that such an outcome is so difficult to achieve. We exist, today, in a world of "otologic madness." We seem to be driven to attain the goals just mentioned at any price, and this philosophy can lead to deep regret. One should remember that on occasions a so-called "radical" mastoidectomy may be the most "conservative" procedure that one can perform. When cholesteatoma is extensive, scattered and deeply imbedded, the radical mastoidectomy is the safest operation of the day. The concept of doing a closed procedure with a "second look" in two years carries the threat of peril, for intracranial complication may supervene before the look is taken. Even in the case where the cholesteatoma is an isolated, easily excised "pearl," the hazard of doing a closed procedure may persist, and recurrence may not become apparent for eight or more years. Diminution of hearing, vertigo, otalgia or supra-auricular pain after an apparently good result all are warning alarms heralding recurrence and extension of cholesteatoma and eventual tragedy. In the face of such symptoms revision to an exteriorized radical mastoidectomy is indicated. The amount of deep-seated disease obscured by an innocent-appearing neomembrane is amazing.

To the question, "Is the situation created by performing a radical mastoidectomy inevitably a safe one?", the answer is an unequivocal, "No!" In the healing process a fibroepithelial membrane lines the bowl and middle ear. A cicatricial web may form pockets anywhere in the cavity sealing off the mastoid cavity from the middle ear or vice versa. Even a total stricture may form. In either event entrapment of cholesteatoma, not seen or incompletely removed at surgery, may occur. Nothing defeats one more handily than does entrapment. Such a patient is again in danger, and minor or major revision is indicated, perhaps more than once, until exteriorization is achieved. The patient must in a sense become married to his physician and return at regular intervals to be certain that the ear remains open and as dry as possible.

Yes, the "radical" operation, despite the problems of drainage and the necessity for life-long care, is a good procedure, but what of the hearing? Ordinarily it will be poor, but it will usually be poor before the operation is undertaken. Even when the auditory acuity is serviceable in the preoperative state the postoperative hearing result may be a bad one. Cholesteatoma is stealthy, and as it erodes the ossicles it may interpose itself between a major ossicle and the stapes rendering so-called "cholesteatoma hearing." Naturally the keratotic mass cannot be left behind.

THE CONSERVATIVE APPROACH, A PARADOX

Having introduced an adjuration for an open, exteriorizing attack, the thought that one can, on occasions, be conservative in his approach appears at first blush to be a schizophrenic one. When the cholesteatoma seems to be a limited affair, confined to the epitympanum or posterior margin of the pars tensa, one may be justified in doing a transcanalicular excision of it, leaving the healing process to its own devices. The conservation or gain in hearing may be most gratifying, and, if the patient is followed carefully, this may be all that is required to prevent further extension of the invasive keratotic mass. It is a far cry from an open excision of cholesteatoma and closure with a graft to the limited procedure just described. The latter seldom leads to difficulty, whereas the former may well do so. There is much to be said in favor of the modified radical mastoidectomy as well, for here one does create a mastoid bowl, and the only closed area is the tympanum. Here the postoperative tympanic membrane is thin, and trouble within the mesotympanum or epitympanic recess may be detected early before erosion becomes extensive. Grafts, on the other hand, frequently become quite thick, and observation of entrapped disease through them becomes a difficult task.

Whether one enters into open exteriorizing procedures or employs a more limited and conservative approach the patient must remain under observation for an indefinite period of time. Each problem must be evaluated with regard to the extent and location of the cholesteatoma, and the surgeon's talents deserve equal consideration. All of this, of course, adds to the challenge of temporal bone surgery.

In actuality, what is sorely needed is some procedure or treatment which will interrupt or abort serous otitis media before the retraction pocket develops. Transmyringal grommet insertion serves to improve hearing while the grommet is in place and unobstructed by dried secretion, but proof that the process can be cured by their insertion is wanting. With repeated insertion of grommets after extrusion, eventually the mesotympanum becomes more and more shallow to the point where another insertion is impossible.

If one tries to carry the field by direct assault through a surgical attack on the mastoid and epitympanum, in the early stages, the polypoid and granulation tissue can be excised, but recurrence is frequent and troublesome.[4]

REFERENCES

1. McGuckin F. Concerning the pathogenesis of destructive ear disease. J Laryngol Otol 1961; 75:949-61.

2. Virchow R. Demonstration von Perlgeschwulsten im Felsenbein, Berlin. Klin Wschr. 1889; 26:236.

3. Tumarkin A. Attic cholesteatoma. J Laryngol Otol 1958; 72:610-19.

4. Proud GO, Duff WE. Mastoidectomy and epitympanotomy. Ann Otol Rhinol Laryngol 1976; 85 Suppl 25:289.

BEHAVIORAL METHODS IN PEDIATRIC AUDIOLOGY: PAST, PRESENT, FUTURE

NOEL D. MATKIN, PhD
TUCSON, ARIZONA

A pediatric audiologic test battery consisting of both behavioral conditioning approaches and electrophysiological techniques has been developed and refined during the past decade. At present, a high rate of success can be anticipated in identifying and describing various degrees, types and configurations of pediatric hearing loss. Further, progress has been seen in the development of a battery of materials which are linguistically appropriate for assessing the utilization of residual auditory function among young hearing-impaired children. It is obvious, however, that clinical research is still needed to assure expansion and refinement of existing materials and techniques used for discrimination testing. Further, methodology must be developed for objective analysis of a youngster's auditory response behaviors if additional handicapping conditions are to be identified at an early age. Finally, a major challenge in the future is to analyze through systematic clinical investigation the potential contribution that can accrue with the administration of central audiologic test procedures designed both to identify and to classify various auditory-based language and learning disabilities.

INTRODUCTION

During the past decade, a significant change in the pattern of referrals to pediatric audiology clinics has become evident. Specifically, many children are now being referred during the preschool years, often with parental concern regarding hearing status in that "the child is not talking." Of those youngsters who are identified as hearing-impaired, substantial numbers subsequently are found also to be multihandicapped. Further, with the national thrust toward early intervention, many children with marked developmental delays are being referred from preschool programs to assure that such youngsters have adequate hearing sensitivity to benefit from remediation. Finally, increasing numbers of school-age children having normal audiograms are now being referred for audiologic evaluation with such teacher complaints as " the child does not seem to listen," "the child does not pay attention," "the child has difficulty with auditory comprehension," etc. In short, the types of youngsters being scheduled for comprehensive pediatric audiologic assessments have changed significantly in the past decade. As a consequence, the premise that the majority of children can be successfully evaluated by making minor modifications in the adult test protocol has proven to be untenable in many instances.

The major responsibilities of a pediatric audiologist during an initial audiologic evaluation should be viewed as multifaceted: first, to obtain a reliable assessment of auditory status (which entails far more than obtaining a pure tone audiogram) and then to communicate an effective interpretation of findings to parents, teachers and clinicians, as well as to the referring physician. Another responsibility of equal importance is to screen a youngster's cognitive, motor, linguistic, and social development so that appropriate referrals can be made at the earliest possible time, thus assuring comprehensive rather than fragmented service delivery. What is being suggested is that clinicians who work with young children must not only be competent in the various aspects of clinical audiology, but must also be insightful as to early childhood development and to the importance of effective parent education, guidance, and counseling. A decade ago, few universities with training programs listed even a single course in child audiology. Today, pediatric audiology is viewed as core curriculum in many graduate training programs, certainly a major step forward.

AUDIOLOGIC EVALUATION OF PERIPHERAL IMPAIRMENTS

In 1968, Matkin et al presented a preliminary critique of an auditory test battery for use with pediatric cases.[1] At that time, the shortcoming of relying upon unconditioned behavioral responses to broadband stimuli such as speech, music and assorted noisemakers presented via loudspeakers was highlighted. Subsequent clinical investigation, as well as a recent article by Coleman and Pelson,[2] confirmed the danger of misclassifying hearing status on the basis of an informal unconditioned approach. So the recommendation was made a decade ago that the pediatric audiologist must develop a battery of behavioral conditioning techniques which successfully could be utilized with a broad spectrum of children representing very different cognitive and motor developmental levels. At present, there appears to be wide acceptance of the necessity to utilize such a battery as outlined in Table 1 if one is to maintain a high success rate

From the Language and Learning Center, Boys Town Institute, and the Department of Otolaryngology and Human Communication, Creighton University School of Medicine, Omaha, Nebraska.

REPRINTS — Noel D. Matkin, PhD, Department of Speech and Hearing Science, Speech Building, Room 105, University of Arizona, Tucson, AZ 85721.

TABLE 1. AUDIOLOGIC PEDIATRIC TEST BATTERY FOR PRESCHOOL CHILDREN

Conditioned Play Audiometry
Tangible Reinforcement Operant Conditioned Audiometry
Visual Reinforcement Audiometry
Supplement With:
 Impedance Study
 Sound Field Localization Study

when assessing the auditory sensitivity of young children. In addition to the conditioning techniques initially described which can be used either during air conduction or bone conduction testing, earphone or sound field testing, aided or unaided testing, the merits of supplementing such behavioral measures with an impedance study as well as the assessment of sound field localization at both faint and average conversation levels have been recognized.

Electrophysiological measures, such as brainstem-evoked response audiometry, are then viewed as viable alternatives to the behavioral test battery. It must be recognized, however, that obtaining auditory response data from a youngster under sedation through the utilization of electrophysiological techniques often reveals little about a child's functional use of hearing for integrating and processing auditory information during optimal periods of language learning. As pediatric audiologists have increased their success in obtaining detailed information regarding auditory sensitivity during the very early years and then have followed such children's development over time, it has become apparent that two youngsters with very similar audiograms may function very differently in terms of their utilization of residual hearing. Thus, the need for a developmentally based battery of auditory discrimination materials has been recognized. Unfortunately, with the exception of such studies as those of Leepa and Rintelman,[3] Schwartz,[4] Hieber et al,[5] and Erber and Alencewicz,[6] limited research and clinical investigation have been undertaken in this critically important area. The obvious challenge is to identify and develop appropriate materials for clinical utilization which contain stimuli within the child's linguistic and/or nonlinguistic auditory repertoire.

Despite present limitations, it does appear that many clinicians recognize the critical importance of assessing not only auditory sensitivity but also the ability of the child under study to process information presented at suprathreshold levels. Certainly one of the challenges in the future is to further standardize and refine an auditory discrimination test battery for children so that realistic levels of expectation can be established at a relatively early age by better understanding the limitations imposed by a particular auditory impairment.

Clinical experience further suggests that the presence of additional handicapping conditions may be identified at a much earlier age if attention is focused on the child's response behavior as well as upon the intensity level needed to obtain a minimal response level. Consideration of whether or not the behavioral conditioning technique used is age-appropriate and of other issues such as the number of conditioning trials initially required, the maintenance of the conditioned bond over time, the child's ability to transfer such conditioning across various auditory test signals, as well as the youngster's reaction time, all yield information which in my judgment should be routinely recorded and analyzed when recommendations for additional evaluations are considered. The need for objectifying such clinical observations is apparent.

TABLE 2. A PARTIAL LIST OF RECOMMENDED MEASURES FOR CENTRAL AUDIOLOGIC TESTING WITH CHILDREN

Monosyllabic Words
 Low-Pass Filtered
 Time Compressed
 Unfiltered in
  Noise Competition
  Speech Competition
Staggered Spondees
Binaural Fusion-Spondees
Competing Sentences
Alternating Sentences
Dichotic Listening
  C V Syllables
  Words
  Sentences
Masking Level Differences
  Pure Tones (500 Hz)
  Speech
Pitch Pattern Recognition
  Hummed Response
  Tapping Response

CENTRAL AUDIOLOGIC TESTS

As mentioned earlier, referrals to audiology for assessment of normal-hearing children suspected of having deficits in central auditory processing are increasing. A review of the literature reveals that a number of different procedures have been designated for clinical utilization, either as screening measures or as diagnostic tests.[7] In many instances such measures are based on modification of audiologic tests which have been used for some years with adult patients suspected of having either brainstem or cortical lesions. Table 2 illustrates a partial listing of measures which have been recommended for use either singly or as a test within a central audiologic test battery for children.

While the potential role of the pediatric audiologist in assessing normal-hearing children with deviant auditory behavior undoubtedly will expand in future years, I would like to express two major concerns. First, while central auditory tests have been used with the adult population in an attempt to identify specific sites of lesion within the central auditory pathways, the interpretation of similar tests with children having either minimal or no detectable neurological symptomatology must be questioned. In other words, the question must be raised as to whether one should be evaluating a child with specific auditory learning problems in terms of site of lesion or instead in terms of type of auditory dysfunction. Secondly, it is naive to use such tests without considering the youngster's performance on auditory processing measures as used by a language or learning disabilities specialist and the relationship to academic performance. In other words, deviant response patterns on a central audiologic test battery in and of themselves have little meaning without considering the implications for educational and remedial programming. Thus central audiologic testing should be viewed not as a specialty evaluation but as a component of a multidisciplinary team assessment.

A multidisciplinary pilot study currently being conducted at the Boys Town Institute indicates that a number of research needs should be considered if central audiologic testing is to become a routine audiologic procedure in future years. First, each central audiologic test should be evaluated in terms of the auditory processing task (or tasks) being tapped and the influence of the child's mode of response upon the performance score. Also, developmental performance data for average children in terms of both their score and reaction time must be established for reference. Another area of research need is that the sensitivity and the specificity of each central audiologic test as a screening measure should be determined relative to the type of learning disability under study. In addition, the correlation of various central audiologic and auditory processing tests as diagnostic measures should be established relative to various types of learning disabilities. (As an aside, I am suggesting that the term "learning disabilities" should be viewed as a generic rather than as a specific classification.) Finally, patterns of response on a battery of central audiologic tests should be established relative to various learning disabilities groups.

REFERENCES

1. Matkin ND, Hartford E, Murphy B. A preliminary critique of an auditory test battery for pediatric cases. Unpublished presentation, American Speech and Hearing Association Convention, 1968.

2. Coleman RO, Pelson RO. Marked high frequency hearing loss in children. A problem in early identification. J Speech Hearing Dis 1977; 42:335-9.

3. Leepa ME, Rintlemann WF. Articulation function and test-retest performance of normal-hearing children on three speech discrimination tests: WIPI, PBK 50, and NU Auditory Test No. 6. J Speech Hearing Dis 1976; 41:503-19.

4. Schwartz D. The usefulness of the WIPI-A speech discrimination test for preschool children. Unpublished master's thesis, Central Michigan University, 1971.

5. Hieber TF, Matkin ND, Skalka E, Gerling IJ. The sound effects recognition test (SERT). St. Louis: Auditec, 1980.

6. Erber NP, Alencewicz CM. Audiologic evaluation of deaf children. J Speech Hearing Dis 1976; 41:256-67.

7. Keith RW, ed. Central auditory function. New York: Grune and Stratton, 1977.

IMPEDANCE AUDIOMETRY

GUNNAR LIDÉN, MD
GÖTEBORG, SWEDEN

After a review of the development of acoustic impedance measurements, the principles of tympanometry, static compliance and measurements of the middle ear reflexes are described. The interpretation of tympanometry is done by analyzing three essential features: pressure, amplitude and shape. The influence of high probe tones on the shape of the tympanogram and the possibility of analyzing the stiffness-mass relationship are pointed out. Impedance screening has supplemented tone screening on 5,886 seven-year-olds in five separate investigations from 1972 to 1978. In the last and most conclusive investigation on 1,027 children, the otologist found 6% pathological ears. Stapedius reflex threshold testing (ipsilateral stimulation), criterion level 110 dB SPL rated 7.8% of the ears as abnormal. Tympanometry resulted in 6.5% pathological ears and tone screening at 0.5 kHz 1.9%. Based on these results the following screening procedure is recommended: tone screening at 0.5 and 4.0 kHz supplemented by tympanometry. A middle ear pressure of ≤ -150 mm H_2O, or a flat tympanogram and/or tone screening levels ∓ 20 dB HTL at 0.5 kHz and/or 4.0 kHz are considered at indicative of ear pathology. Children failing the screening test should have a repeat test after four to six weeks at school and only those who do not pass at this time should be referred to an otologist.

INTRODUCTION

Thirty years ago, Metz presented his pioneering work on clinical measurements of acoustic impedance of the ear which enabled both static and dynamic acoustic impedance to be determined.[1] Instrumentation and techniques have advanced considerably since. In order to eliminate some of the technical difficulties in the Metz bridge, Zwislocki introduced the probe-tone technique for absolute impedance measurements.[2] Advanced laboratory analyses of the function of the middle ear have been accomplished with this and similar equipment. I only need to remind you of some of the works by Zwislocki,[3] Møller,[4] Dallos,[5] and Lilly.[6]

The next step towards progress in clinical measurements was the introduction of the mechanical acoustic impedance bridge by Zwislocki in 1963,[7] and the electroacoustic bridge by Terkildsen and Scott-Nielsen in 1960.[8] Both of these bridges have since become commercially available. The former has been replaced by Grason-Stadler oto-admittance meter.

The clinical importance of acoustic impedance measurements, or impedance audiometry as it is usually called nowadays, has increased enormously during recent years. The basic impedance test battery includes tympanometry, static compliance and the measurement of the middle ear reflexes. Although each of these tests provides diagnostic information about the function and integrity of the auditory mechanism, a combination of the results of all three gives a more complete clinical picture and can be recommended strongly.

The principles underlying impedance audiometry as well as its clinical usefulness are well documented. It will suffice then, to give a survey of some of its clinical applications, thus saving time for discussing where we stand today in the ues of impedance audiometry for screening middle ear disease in school children.

Tympanometry. Tympanometry is an objective method for evaluating the mobility of the tympanic membrane and the functional condition of the middle ear. Tympanometry displays changes in eardrum compliance as the air pressure is altered in the external ear canal. Depending on the construction of the measuring instrument, the tympanogram can either indicate a change in the impedance or in the admittance, which is the inverse of impedance. The tympanogram has its impedance minimum pointing downwards or its corresponding admittance maximum upwards.

Tympanograms are interpreted by analyzing three essential features: pressure, amplitude (static acoustic impedance or compliance) and shape. The presence of even moderate underpressure in the middle ear usually abolishes the stapedius reflex. Thus tympanometry should always precede other impedance tests. Until recently, tympanometry has most commonly been performed with a 220 Hz probe tone frequency. Three types of curves are well established (Fig. 1 A-C). The most common is the V-shaped curve with normal amplitude of the peak indicating good mobility of the middle ear system and maximum flow of acoustic energy at atmospheric pressure. A peak at negative pressure reflects underpressure in the middle ear, indicating eustachian tube blockage. The third type shows a flat or relatively flat curve commonly found in perforated tympanic membrane, serous otitis media, and chronic adhesive otitis. With the use of high frequency probe tones (800 Hz) two more clinically useful types of tympanograms can be recognized

From the Department of Audiology and Otolaryngology, Sahlgren's Hospital, University of Göteborg, Göteborg, Sweden.

REPRINTS — Gunnar Lidén, MD, Sahlgrenska Sjukhuset, Department of Audiology, 413 45 Göteborg, Sweden.

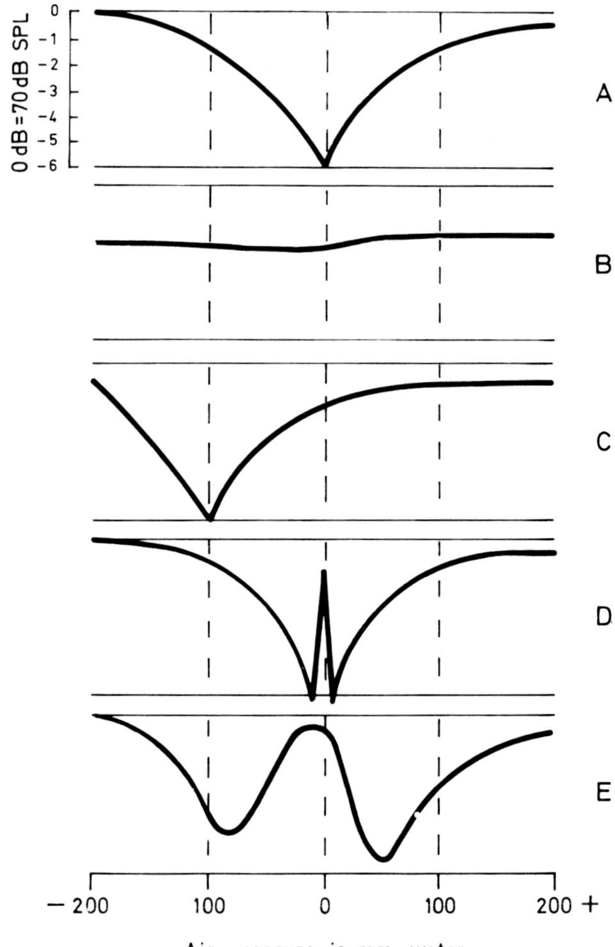

Fig. 1. Five types of tympanograms indicating normal and pathological middle ear mechanism. Probe tone frequency 800 Hz. A) Compliance of the eardrum is greatest at ambient air pressure. B) Virtually no change in the compliance of the drum with a change in air pressure. C) Indicative of negative pressure in the middle ear. D) Eardrum has an atrophic scar. E) Result of ossicular discontinuity.

(Fig. 1 D, E).[9-11] The sharp W curve appears when the eardrum has an atrophic scar or is very hypermobile. The soft undulating W tympanogram is the result of ossicular discontinuity. Patients who have had a stapedectomy with a steel wire replacement show the same type of board and deep undulating notching pattern (Fig. 2).

Some clinicians question the value of high frequency tympanometry. Feldman, however, points out its value in connection with static acoustic impedance measurements.[12] The presence of a healed eardrum perforation may mask the occurrence of stapes ankylosis in such measurement by turning high acoustic impedances into low ones. Thus, from a diagnostic viewpoint it is important to obtain a high frequency tympanogram, preferably with 800 Hz, before measuring static acoustic impedance. With this exception, the sharp W tympanogram is of minor clinical interest because it can also be found in subjects with normal-looking but very

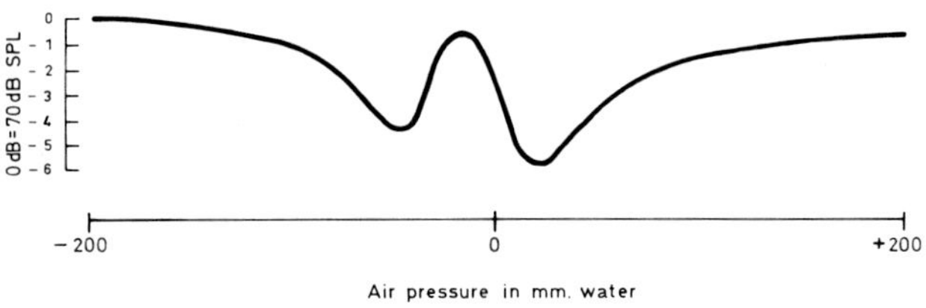

Fig. 2. High frequency tympanogram (800 Hz) in a stapedectomized ear (steel wire and perichondrium).

mobile eardrums. The broad, smoothly undulating tympanogram, which changes its directions with induced negative and positive air pressure changes, is easy to separate from the sharp double peak tympanogram and is important as it indicates interruption of the ossicular chain.

Another advantage with high frequency tympanometry is the possibility of analyzing the stiffness-mass relationship of the ear. A discontinuity of the ossicular chain lowers the resonant frequency of the middle ear and makes the transmission system mass-controlled. Externally applied negative or positive air pressure changes in the ear canal increase the stiffness factor and, if sufficiently close to the resonant frequency shifts the direction of the tympanometric curve. This can be demonstrated with an 1720 oto-admittance meter in combination with a computer.[13] The G, B and Y tympanograms with a 660 Hz probe tone are converted into resistance (R), reactance (X) and acoustic impedance (Z) in the plane of the drum. Figures 3 and 4 show this conversion in a normal hearing subject and in a patient with complete ossicular interruption, respectively. Figure 4a shows how the B tympanogram has an undulating pattern and Figure 4b the corresponding acoustic reactance on the X curve. As can be seen, the X tympanogram is positive close to ambient air pressure in the ear canal but becomes negative with changes in air pressure in either a negative or positive direction. There is a change from mass to stiffness control when the reactance curve passes through the resonant point, zero, and turns from positive to negative. This phase shift is displayed in tympanograms as a change in direction. As a rule, the larger the distance between the zero crossings of the reactance curve, the more undulating and broad the tympanogram will be. Small differences between the zero crossings will give sharp W tympanograms. The irregular shape of the high frequency tympanogram due to the change of sign in acoustic reactance close to resonance has diagnostic value, especially in cases with an intact tympanic membrane, conductive loss and unclear diagnosis.

Static Compliance. Compliance, or mobility of the middle ear, is demonstrated by the amplitude of a tympanogram. It can also be measured separately and expressed in absolute units of volume, impedance or admittance. The measurement unit usually employed is volume, expressed in cubic centime-

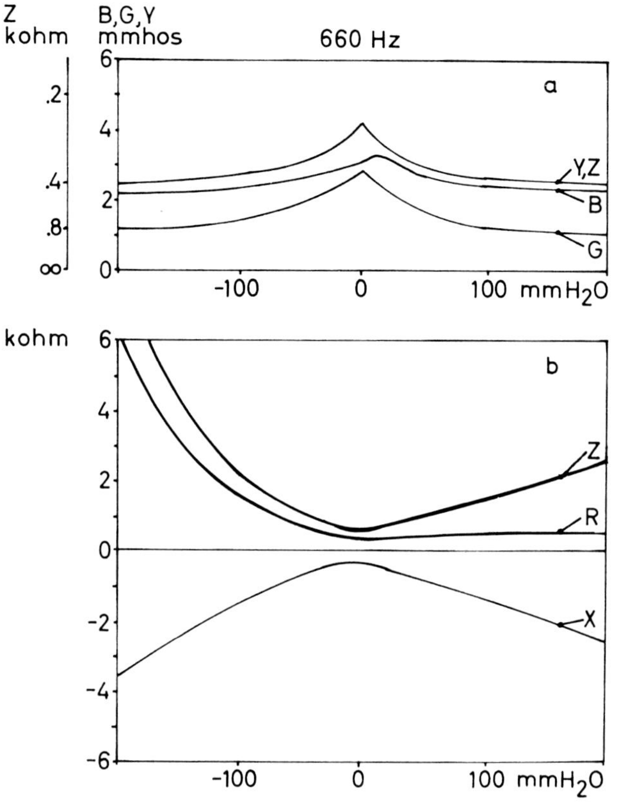

Fig. 3. Normal subject. Probe tone 660 Hz. a) G and B curves. Y and Z calculated. b) Impedance values in the plane of the drum. (From Lidén et al.[13] Reprinted with permission)

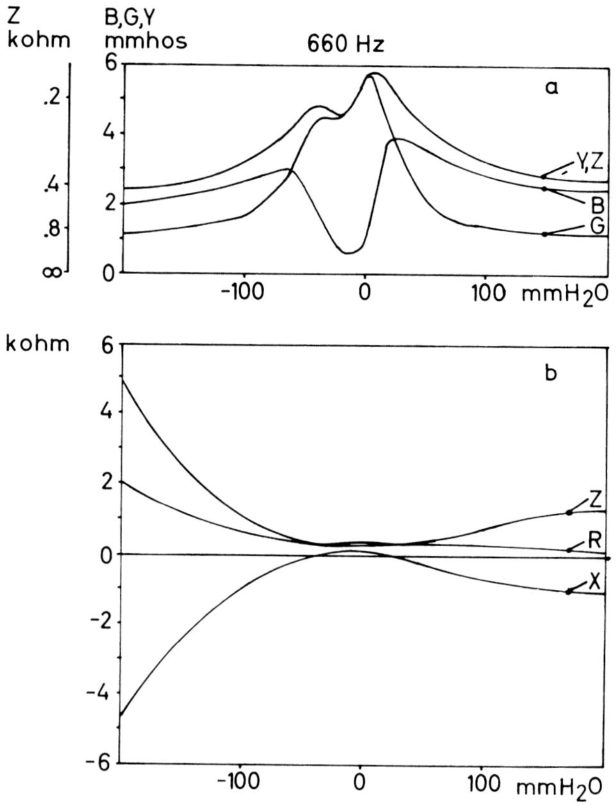

Fig. 4. Ossicular interruption. a) G and B curves. Y and Z calculated. b) Corresponding impedance values in the plane of the drum. (From Lidén et al.[13] Reprinted with permission)

ters. Low compliance values indicate high impedance. There is a considerable overlap between compliance findings for subjects with normal ears and those with middle ear pathologies. The static compliance measure thus is considered the least reliable test in the impedance battery.

As already mentioned, the presence of an overlooked healed perforation of the tympanic membrane in a patient with a conductive hearing loss presumably due to stapes fixation will turn expected high acoustic impedances into low ones and thus obscure the diagnosis. In cases with an intact tympanic membrane and conductive hearing loss, very low acoustic impedance values indicate disruption of the ossicular chain.

The static compliance measure can be used as a physical volume test in order to evaluate the intactness of the tympanic membrane. A large volume in a case with a flat tympanogram usually indicates a perforated tympanic membrane or an open ventilating tube. Normal or low physical volumes are common in serous otitis media.

Intra-aural Muscle Reflexes. Among the impedance tests the intra-aural muscle reflexes have the greatest diagnostic value. These measurements are primarily based on electroacoustic recordings of the activity of the intra-aural muscles as manifested by the sound-reflecting properties of the tympanic membrane. The tensor tympani muscle reflex elicited by air-jet stimulation is of minor importance compared to the acoustic stapedius reflex.

The acoustic stapedius reflex test should, if possible, be employed with both ipsilateral and contralateral stimulation. Cutaneous or tactile stimulation should not be forgotten if there is no response to acoustic stimulation.

The clinical usefulness of the acoustic stapedius reflex is based on the answer to two simple questions: 1) Is the acoustic reflex present or not? and 2) If the reflex is present, what is its threshold? Since middle ear pathology precludes tympanic membrane compliance changes, the acoustic reflex can be expected to be absent in ears with conductive hearing loss regardless of the size of the air-bone gap. Conversely, and from a practical clinical viewpoint, the presence of an acoustic reflex excludes middle ear pathology in ears with normal tympanograms.

The determination of acoustic reflex thresholds can be used as an objective recruitment test in ears with sensorineural hearing loss. As long as the loss is less than about 60 dB HL and the reflex is elicited within the normal stapedius reflex range of 75-95 dB HL, there is a high probability that the hearing loss is of cochlear origin. An elevated stapedius reflex threshold or a nonelicitable reflex in an ear

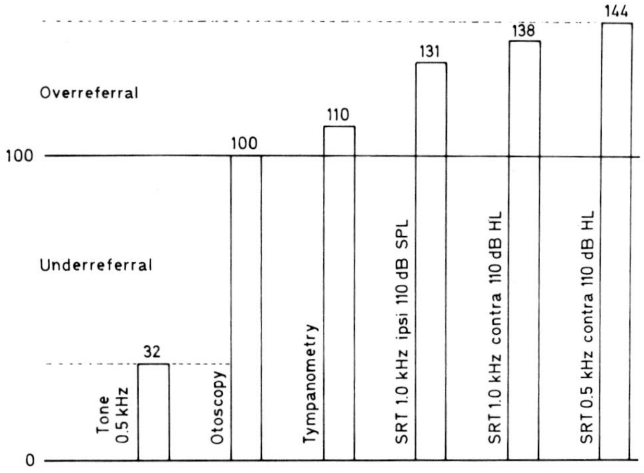

Fig. 5. Comparison between different screening methods and otoscopy.

TABLE 1. CLINICAL APPLICATIONS OF IMPEDANCE AUDIOMETRY

Tympanometry
- Determines mobility of tympanic membrane and functional condition of middle ear, using
  - Pressure
  - Amplitude — static compliance
  - Shape
  - Probe tone frequency
  - Diagnostic application

Intra-aural muscle reflexes
- Measure and record intra-aural reflex activity
- Differentiate between conductive pathologies
- Differentiate between conductive and sensorineural hearing loss
- Objectively test recruitment
- Differentiate between cochlear and retrocochlear hearing loss
- Investigate suspected brainstem lesions
- Estimate hearing threshold and dynamic range
- Detect malingering and psychogenic deafness
- Localize paralysis of the seventh nerve
- Test eustachian tube function
- Verify patulous eustachian tubes
- Identify normal-hearing carriers of genes for deafness
- Identify the tonic tensor syndrome
- Test trigeminal motor function

Impedance audiometry for screening

with normal tympanogram has high significance in the cochlear-retrocochlear evaluation. A pathological stapedius reflex decay test gives further support to retrocochlear pathology.[14]

By using crossed and uncrossed acoustic reflexes, an evaluation of suspected brainstem lesions is possible. These measurements are a great step forward in neuroaudiological diagnosis which will help to strengthen the position of clinical audiology in medicine.

The wide range of clinical application of the intra-aural reflexes has been summarized in Table 1.

Impedance Audiometry and School Screening. Impedance audiometry for screening middle ear disease in school children has attracted considerable interest in recent years. It has been emphasized that tone screening is unreliable and results in too many false negatives.[15] Our goal has been to find a screening procedure which coincides better with otoscopic findings and which does not overlook subjects with sensorineural hearing loss. On a research basis we supplemented pure tone screening with impedance audiometry. The results of pure tone screening were classified as pathological if hearing thresholds were elevated >20 dB HL re International Standards Organization (ISO) 1964 at two or more frequencies. In order to arrive at an impedance criteria which minimizes both false positives and false negatives, five different studies, each using different criteria, were accomplished. During the first four years we used a single impedance and tone screening, but repeated screening, according to Brooks, was adopted during the last two years.[16] During the last mentioned period, tone screening was shortened to include only 0.5 and 3.0 kHz. In spite of this, the test battery was still considered too time-consuming for screening purposes. However, we found it very difficult to decide which of the impedance tests should be excluded and what criteria should be recommended. Finally, after finishing the fifth and last study, we feel confident in making such a recommendation. The following review will tell how we reached this conclusion.

One of our first studies in 1972 comprised 206 ears of randomly selected ten-year-olds.[17] The impedance screening was performed with a Madsen impedance meter ZO-61. The stapedius reflex threshold (SRT) was measured by contralateral stimulation. The tympanogram was classified as abnormal when the maximum compliance occurred at an underpressure of ≤ -80 mm H_2O or if no compliance maximum could be identified, ie, a flat curve. The stapedius reflex threshold was considered abnormal when higher than 95 dB HL at 500 Hz. Our reference points at that time were adults in whom ± 25 mm H_2O pressure and stapedius reflex thresholds ranging from 75-95 dB HL were considered normal. Based on these criteria we found 1.5% pathological ears with screening audiometry, 8% with otoscopy, 12% with tympanometry and 35% with stapedius reflex testing.

The high percentage of pathological values with impedance audiometry compared to otoscopy encouraged us during 1973-1974 to expand the first investigation to a larger population of 1,600 ears on 800 nonselected seven-year-olds. We also moved the pressure criterion to ≤ -150 mm H_2O. Abnormal stapedius reflex thresholds criteria were set at 100, 105 and 110 dB HL. This investigation resulted in 6.5% pathological ears with screening audiometry, 9.8% of the ears had middle ear pressure ≤ -150 mm H_2O, and in addition 2% had flat tympanograms. Depending on the stapedius-reflex threshold criterion selected, we got from 13 to 33% abnormal ears. During 1975-1976 we routinely screened 7,180 ears on nonselected seven-year-olds with only tym-

TABLE 2. REPEATED SCREENING AUDIOMETRY (0.5 AND 3.0 kHz) AND IMPEDANCE AUDIOMETRY IN COMPARISON WITH CLINICAL ASSESSMENT ON 2,054 EARS ON 1,027 NONSELECTED SEVEN-YEAR-OLDS

			Failures (%)					
			Screening 1		*Screening 2*		*Clinical*	
Methods	*dB*	*kHz*	*RE*	*LE*	*RE*	*LE*	*RE*	*LE*
Tone	> 20	HL 0.5	4.4	2.1	3.3	1.5	1.9	1.8
Threshold	20	HL 3.0	2.2	3.4	1.3	1.6	1.2	1.7
SRT CL	≥110	HL 1.0	15.4	15.6	11.4	11.3	8.2	7.6
SRT IL	≥110	SPL 1.0	14.9	14.7	10.8	11.1	7.8	7.4
Pressure	≤ −150 mm H_2O		7.9	8.8	6.1	7.6	5.2	5.3
Flat tympanogram (FT)			1.3	1.3	1.5	0.7	1.3	1.0
Pressure	≤ −150 mm H_2O & FT		9.2	10.1	7.6	8.3	6.5	6.3
Otoscopy							6.0	5.6
Serous otitis without effusion							3.2	2.6
Serous otitis with effusion							1.6	1.9
Wax							0.8	0.5
Various							0.4	0.6

RE - Right ear; LE - Left ear; HL - Hearing level; SRT - Stapedius reflex threshold; SPL - Sound pressure level; CL - Contralateral; IL - Ipsilateral.

panometry and a pure tone sweep check test. The distribution of air pressure in the middle ear showed that 90% of the ears had pressure ≥ −150 mm H_2O, and the results were in very good agreement with the 1973-1974 investigation on 1,600 ears. If a flat tympanogram was used as a single indicator of middle ear pathology, we found 2.3% pathological ears in the 1975-1976 investigation compared to 2% the year before. Only 74% of those with flat tympanograms also had abnormal tone screening.[18]

Brooks has shown very convincingly that most children have a stable middle ear function or only an occasional isolated episode of serous otitis media. Only a minority of the school children being screened have persistent middle ear trouble. The best single indicator of this group, according to Brooks, is the absence of middle ear muscle reflexes at two repeat tests separated in time by about six weeks. With this approach in mind, we revised our 1976 screening program to include tympanometry, stapedius reflex threshold measurements at 0.5, 1.0 and 2.0 kHz and screening audiometry as 0.5 and 3.0 kHz. The impedance screening was performed with a Madsen impedance meter (MZS-76) using contralateral stimulation. The criteria were kept as before. If a child failed any one of these tests, a repeat test was done at school four weeks later. Those who failed the second screening were referred to the Otoaudiological Department for complete clinical evaluation to take place a couple of weeks later. Due to a mishap only 366 children had two complete repeat tests at school which could be used in the final evaluation of the 1976-1977 study. Based on the results of this investigation, we were willing to agree with Brooks that two repeat screening tests diminished the number of false positives referred to the otologist. At the first screening 27% of the children failed one or more of the tests. Four weeks later the children were more healthy, leaving 12.5% of the children for a final clinical investigation which was performed two weeks later. At the final investigation 9.6% of the children failed. The results of screening and of otoscopy of the 1976-1977 study were reported in 1977 in Nashville at the Symposium on Impedance Screening for Children.[19] The otologist found 6.5% of the children to have pathological ears, tympanometry gave 5.2% abnormal subjects, the stapedius reflex threshold test (criterion ≥110 dB HL) 7.6% failures and tone screening at 0.5 kHz 2.7% failures. The crucial question as to whether the stapedius reflex test or the middle ear pressure should be used singly or in combination was not solved in this investigation and needed further evaluation using stapedius reflex testing with ipsilateral stimulation.

Due to the courtesy of Madsen,* the 1977-1978 screening program could be repeated with an impedance meter allowing both ipsilateral and contralateral stimulation.[20] The complete testing program with two repeat screenings at school has been carried out with 1,027 children seven years of age. The results are shown in Table 2. The experienced otologist found 6% pathological ears, the stapedius reflex using ipsilateral stimulation and a criterion of ≥110 dB SPL gave 7.8% failures and tympanometry 6.5%. Tone screening at 0.5 kHz resulted in only 1.9% abnormal ears. It should be mentioned that a complete audiogram was obtained at the time of referral, and only the frequencies 4.0 and 8.0 kHz gave a higher percentage of abnormal values than 0.5 kHz. They were 2.1 and 3.2 respectively.

If we transform the percentage figures of the abnormal impedance and tone screening values into the number of patients and relate them to the otoscopic findings normalized to 100, we can easily see how the different tests are ranked. Figure 5 shows that the overreferral to an otologist is about 30-40% for stapedius reflex threshold testing using a 110 dB borderline for pathology. Ipsilateral measurements at 1.0 kHz are somewhat better than contralateral ones according to this study. Tympano-

*Madsen Electronics, Oakville, Ontario, Canada.

metry looks, however, superior with only about 10% overreferrals. Tone screening at 0.5 kHz gives, however, an underreferral of about 70%.

The results of our study have been computerized. Different criteria and correlations have been carefully analyzed. Based on this information we consider tympanometry with the determination of the middle ear pressure as the method of choice for impedance screening. An analysis of the tone screening results suggest that 4.0 kHz replace 3.0 kHz.

In Sweden, then, we are now ready to recommend tympanometry together with tone screening at 0.5 and 4.0 kHz as a mass screening procedure. The accepted borderlines for ear pathology are middle ear pressure values of ≤ -150 mm H_2O or a flat tympanogram and/or hearing threshold values higher than 20 dB re ISO, 1964 at 0.5 kHz and/or 4.0 kHz.

SUMMARY

After a review of the development of acoustic impedance measurements, the general principles of impedance audiometry consisting of tympanometry, static compliance and measurements of the middle ear reflexes are described. The interpretation of tympanometry is done by analyzing three essential features: pressure, amplitude and shape. The influence of high probe tones on the shape of the tympanogram as well as their clinical applications are discussed. The possibility of analyzing the stiffness-mass relationship is pointed out. The wide range of clinical applications of tympanometry and intra-aural reflexes is summarized in Table 1.

Impedance screening has supplemented tone screening on 5,886 seven-year-olds (11,772 ears) in five separate investigations from 1972 to 1978. In the last and most conclusive investigation of 1,027 children, the otologist found 6% pathological ears. Stapedius reflex threshold testing (ipsilateral stimulation), criterion level 110 dB SPL rated 7.8% of the ears as abnormal. Tympanometry resulted in 6.5% pathological ears and tone screening at 0.5 kHz 1.9%. Based on these results the following screening procedure is recommended: tone screening of 0.5 and 4.0 kHz supplemented by tympanometry. A middle ear pressure of ≤ -150 mm H_2O,or a flat tympanogram and/or tone screening levels >20 dB HTL at 0.5 kHz and/or 4.0 kHz are considered as indicative of ear pathology.

REFERENCES

1. Metz O. The acoustic impedance measured in normal and pathological ears. Acta Otolaryngol (Stockh) 1946; Suppl 63.

2. Zwislocki J. Some impedance measurements on normal and pathological ears. J Acoust Soc Am 1957; 29:1312-7.

3. Zwislocki J. Some measurements of the impedance at the eardrum. J Acoust Soc Am 1957; 29:349-56.

4. Møller A. Tranfer function of the middle ear. J Acoust Soc Am 1963; 35:1526-34.

5. Dallos PJ. Dynamics of the acoustic reflex: phenomenological aspects. J Acoust Soc Am 1964; 36:2175-83.

6. Lilly DJ. Some properties of the acoustic reflex in man. J Acoust Soc Am 1964; 36:2007-8.

7. Zwislocki J. An acoustic method for clinical evaluation of the ear. J Speech Hearing Res 1963; 6:303-14.

8. Terkildsen K, Scott-Nielsen S. An electroacoustic impedance measuring bridge for clinical use. Arch Otolaryngol 1960; 72:339-46.

9. Lidén G, Peterson JL, Björkman G. Tympanometry. Arch Otolaryngol 1970; 92:248-54.

10. Lidén G, Harford E, Hallén O. Tympanometry for the diagnosis of ossicular chain disruption. Arch Otolaryngol 1974; 99:23-9.

11. Lidén G, Harford E, Hallén O. Automatic tympanometry in clinical practice. Audiology 1974; 13:126-39.

12. Feldman AS. Acoustic impedance-admittance measurements. In: Bradford LJ, ed. Physiological measures of the audio-vestibular system. New York: Academic Press, 1975:87-146.

13. Lidén G, Björkman G, Nyman H, Kunov H. Tympanometry and acoustic impedance. Acta Otolaryngol (Stockh) 1977; 83:140-45.

14. Andersson H, Barr B, Wedenberg E. Intra-aural reflexes in retrocochlear lesions. In: Hamberger CA and Wersäll J, eds. Nobel symposium 10: disorders of the skull base region. Stockholm, Almqvist-Wiksell, 1969.

15. Eagles EL, Wishik SM, Doerfler LG. Hearing sensitivity and ear disease in children. A prospective study. Laryngoscope 1967; 1-274.

16. Brooks D. School screening for middle ear effusions. Ann Otol Rhinol Laryngol 1976; 85 Suppl 25:223-8.

17. Renvall U, Lidén G, Jungert S, Nilsson E. Impedance audiometry as screening method in school children. Scand Audiol 1973; 2:133-7.

18. Renvall U, Lidén G, Jungert S, Nilsson E. Impedance audiometry in the detection of secretory otitis media. Scand Audiol 1975; 4:119-24.

19. Lidén G, Renvall U. Impedance audiometry for screening middle ear disease in schoolchildren. In: Harford E, Bess F, Bluestone C, Klein J, eds. Impedance screening for middle ear disease in children. New York: Grune & Stratton, 1978; 197-206.

20. Lidén G, Renvall U. Criteria for impedance screening for schoolchildren. Scand Audiol 1980; 9:121-6.

ELECTROPHYSIOLOGIC AUDIOMETRY

DON W. WORTHINGTON, PhD

JON F. PETERS, PhD

OMAHA, NEBRASKA

The utility of the brainstem evoked response (BER) as a test of peripheral auditory sensitivity in infants and young children is discussed. Two cases are presented to illustrate the application of this technique in multiply handicapped children.

Audiometric procedures based on patients' voluntary responses have proven to be satisfactory for the assessment of auditory function in the majority of individuals. There are, however, certain populations such as malingerers that cannot be satisfactorily tested. In addition, even the best trained staff utilizing a pediatric test battery[1] cannot effectively evaluate approximately 5 to 10% of the children.

In order to evaluate these difficult populations, diverse attempts have been made to develop indirect measures of auditory function. The ultimate goal is to eliminate all reliance on the patient's behavior from the testing procedure and thus achieve a true objective test of hearing. These measures have included but not been limited to physiological variables such as conditioned electrodermal response, cochleopapebral reflex (eyeblink reflex), heart rate, respiration, impedance-admittance and the auditory evoked potentials (AEP). As the body of literature relevant to these procedures is too vast to permit detailed citations, recent reviews[2-6] should be consulted. Although each of these measures has been clinically utilized at one time or another, only the AEP and impedance-admittance[7] have shown sufficient clinical productivity to be currently employed. However, neither procedure is a stand-alone test and both should be interpreted only in conjunction with results from other measures of auditory sensitivity.

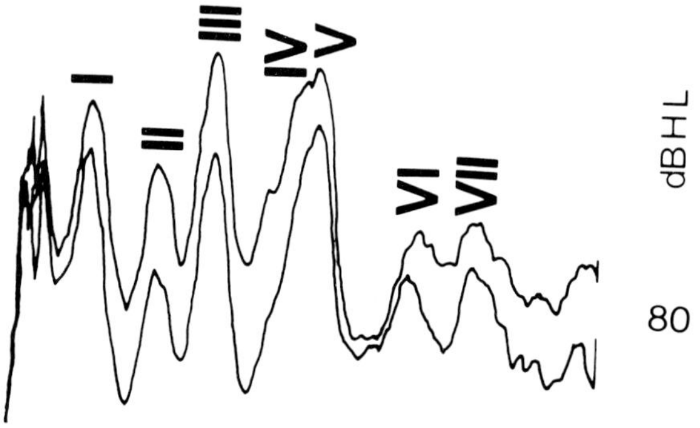

Fig. 1. Typical BER recorded from a subject with normal hearing consisting of a series of seven waves (I-VII) occurring in the first 10 msec following a brief click. In this and all subsequent figures the parameters are: vertex positive up; N = 1024; sweep time = 10.24 msec; gain = 100,000; bandpass = 100-3000 Hz; intensity levels are in dB HL re normal hearing population; rate = 12 rarefaction clicks per second.

The excellent monograph by Davis[4] compares and contrasts the clinical utility of each of the AEP components. He concluded, and other clinicians and researchers agree, that of these components the brainstem evoked response (BER) is the most powerful measure presently available for clinical use. Since we agree with this conclusion, the remainder of this text will focus on the BER and its clinical applicability.

The BER, as originally described in man by Jewett and Williston,[8] consists of a series of seven waves occurring in the first 10 msec following the onset of a brief click or tone pip as seen in Figure 1.

Presently available clinical and research evidence *suggests* that these waves may have the following origins: 1) nerve VIII; 2) cochlear nucleus; 3) superior olivary complex; 4) midbrain; 5) inferior colliculus; 6) medial geniculates and 7) possibly the auditory radiations.[9-12]

The monotonic increase in wave V latency with progressive decreases in stimulus intensity is highly reproducible both within and between subjects as seen in Figure 2. As a result, the latency intensity function for wave V is considered to be a reliable reflection of auditory sensitivity. Figure 3 shows the percentage occurrence of "measurable" waves in the BER as a function of intensity. It clearly shows the occurrence of wave V is stable down to threshold levels in normal hearing populations.

Galambos and his associates[13-15] have also shown that the BER provides direct information about neural maturation. Since this neural maturation proceeds at different rates in the peripheral and central auditory pathways in infants,[16-19] progressive changes occur in both the latency and morphology of the BER. Adult morphology and latency is generally obtained by about 18 months postterm.

In addition, the BER is generally thought to be unaffected by the patient's state (awake, asleep or

From the Department of Otolaryngology and Human Communication, Boys Town Institute/Creighton University, Omaha, Nebraska.

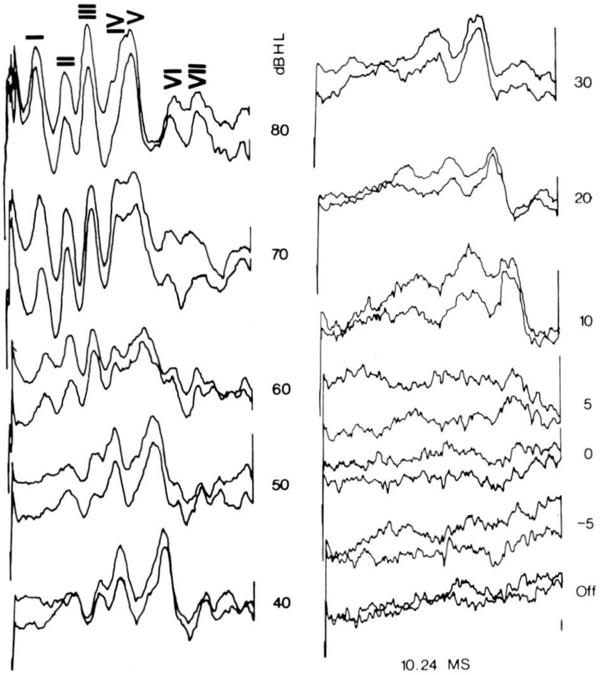

Fig. 2. Progressive increase in latency of all components of the BER as a function of decreasing stimulus intensity. (From Worthington DWW, Peters JF. Ear and hearing, vol 1. Baltimore: Williams and Wilkins, 1980. Published with permission.)

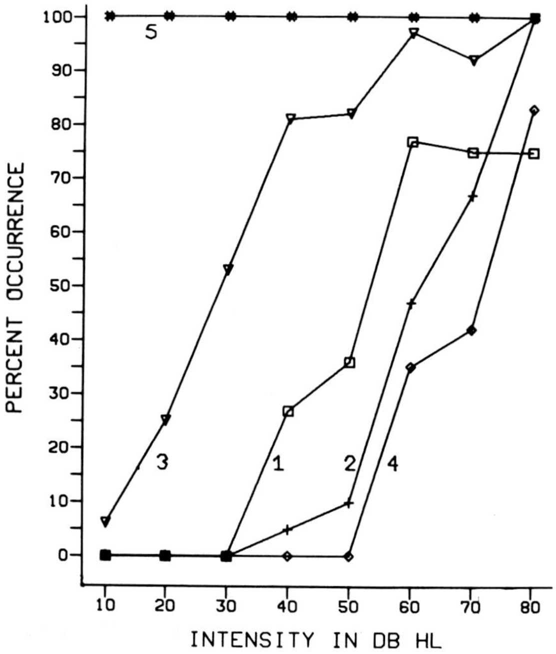

Fig. 3. Percentage occurrence of each BER component as a function of stimulus intensity. N = 34 ears.

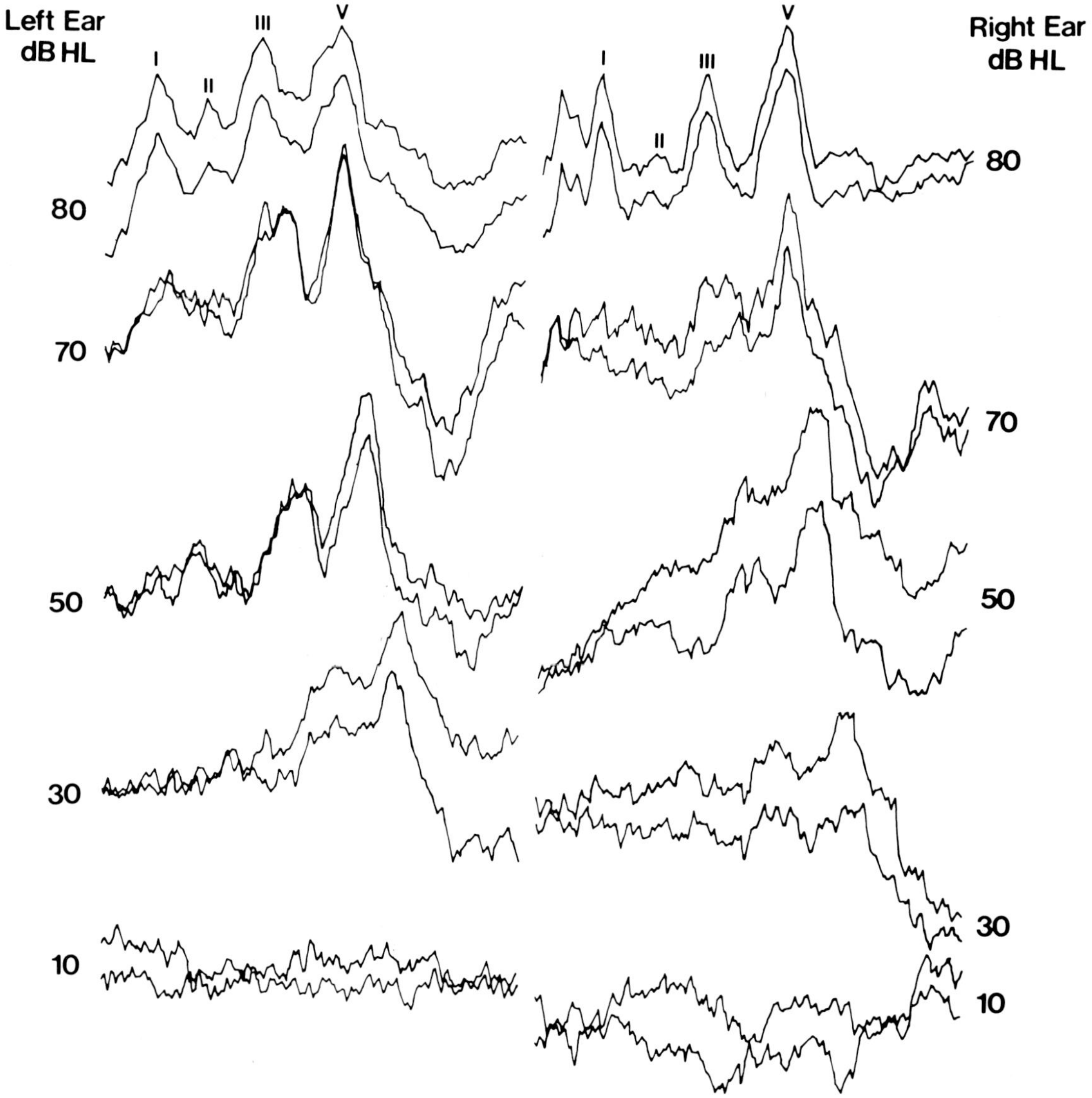

Fig. 4. (Case 1) BER obtained following monaural stimulation at the levels indicated.

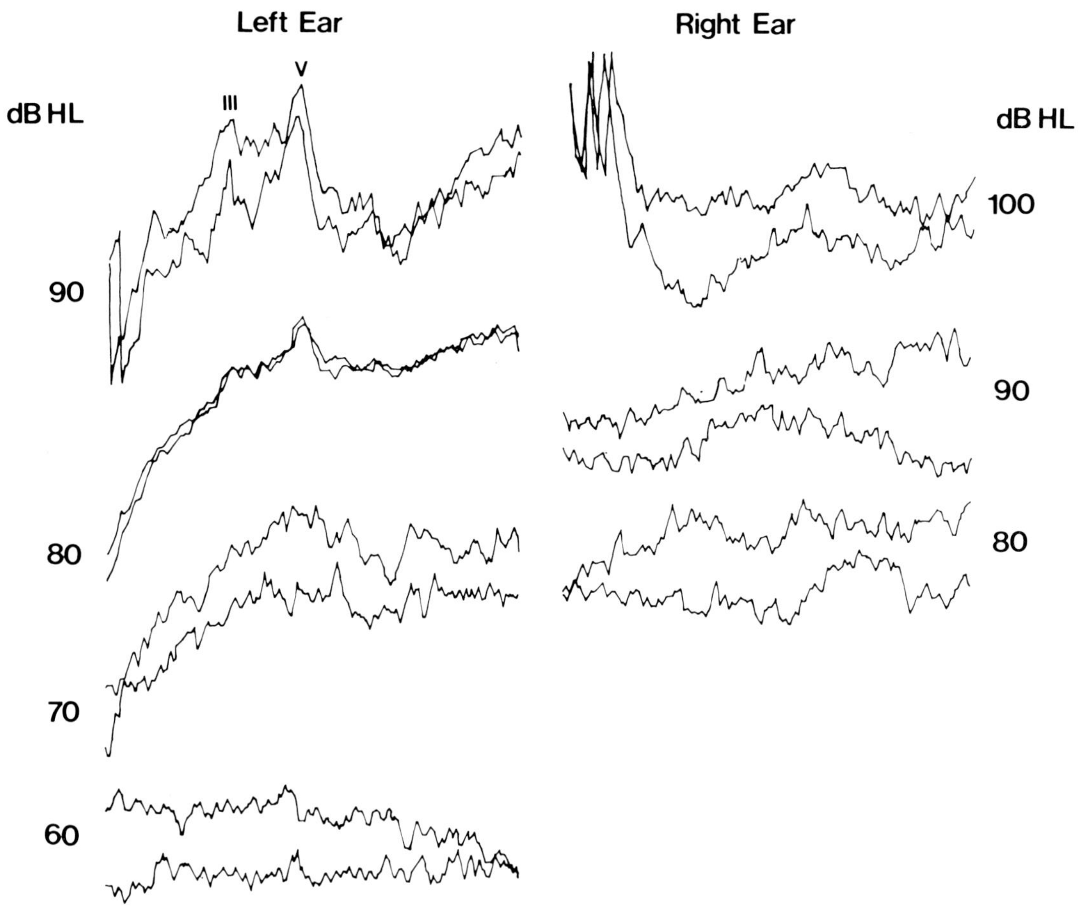

Fig. 5. (Case 2) BER obtained at levels indicated.

sedated) and can be utilized with any age range; electrode placement does not require surgical procedures; response can be isolated to each ear with little or no masking unless high intensity levels are employed; rapid click rates (up to approximately 88 per second) can be utilized to decrease evaluation time; and the possibility for testing at specific frequencies is rapidly becoming available.

All of these factors combine to make the BER well suited for evaluating difficult-to-test children such as the severely retarded or autistic child and the infant at risk for a hearing loss. The BER has also proven valuable in evaluating such clinical problems as suspected neuropathology involving the auditory pathways, nonorganic and/or compensation cases and true psychogenic losses.

The value of the BER as a clinical tool is best illustrated with case discussions.

CASE REPORTS

Case 1. This five-year-old female was the product of a normal pregnancy and delivery. Her seizures, which began at six months of age, are presently controlled by phenobarbital (30 mg 3½ times per day) and Dilantin® (50 mg 2½ times per day). Although her initial motoric skills were not significantly delayed (walked without support at nine months), her parents suspected problems by 12 months since she was not babbling or utilizing any speech utterances. She was evaluated at that time and diagnosed as mildly retarded of unknown etiology. Her inability to cooperate in subsequent hearing evaluations resulted in audiological reports ranging from estimates of normal sensitivity to a profound hearing loss. Thus, she was referred for BER evaluation.

The BER exam was conducted under halothane anesthesia as previous attempts to sedate her for medical examinations resulted in severe paradoxical reactions. Figure 4 shows replicable BER recorded down to 30 dB HL from the left and the right ears. The interwave and wave V latencies for these responses were within normal limits. This information, in conjunction with an impedance study, confirmed the fact that no more than a mild high frequency hearing loss was present. Educational planning could be accomplished without consideration of amplification.

Case 2. A seven-year-old female was diagnosed as a Cornelia de Lange syndrome with mental retardation, retarded growth, and pulmonary stenosis. She was also prone to bouts of serous otitis media. The ENT examination showed the left tympanic membrane to be normal and the right tympanic membrane to be retracted but with no apparent effusion.

Figure 5 shows BER elicited following monaural stimulation of the left and right ears. The replicable BER seen on the left as 80 and 90 dB HL occurred with normal wave V latencies. Only a questionable response was seen on the right at 100 dB HL. These responses are consistent with a severe sensorineural loss on the left and a profound sensorineural loss on the right. On the basis of this evaluation, a decision was made to place trial amplification on the left ear. Subsequent definitive improvements in the child's behavior have been noted by both the parents and her teacher in the Deaf-Blind Program.

Although the BER is definitely a clinically effective objective test of auditory sensitivity, it is not a stand-alone procedure. It is essentially a high frequency phenomena and is significantly affected by different audiometric configurations[20] and presence or absence of conductive pathology and neuropathology which may or may not be related to auditory function. Above all, it is not a test of auditory processing.

REFERENCES

1. Matkin ND. Behavioral methods in pediatric audiology: past, present, future. Ann Otol Rhinol Laryngol 1980; 89 Suppl 74:50-2.

2. Bradford LJ, ed. Physiological measures of the audio-vestibular system. New York: Academic Press, 1975.

3. Jerger J, ed. Modern developments in audiology. New York: Academic Press, 1973.

4. Davis H. Principles of electric response audiometry. Ann Otol Rhinol Laryngol 1976; 85 Suppl 28:1-96.

5. Ruben RJ, Eberling C, Salomon G, eds. Electrocochleography. Baltimore: University Park Press, 1976.

6. Reneau JP, Hnatiow GZ. Evoked response audiometry: a topical and historical review. Baltimore: University Park Press, 1975.

7. Lidén G. Impedance audiometry. Ann Otol Rhinol Laryngol 1980; 89 Suppl 74:53-8.

8. Jewett D, Williston JS. Auditory evoked far fields averaged from the scalp in humans. Brain 1971; 94:681-96.

9. Buchwald JS, Huang CM. Far field acoustic response: origins in the cat. Science 1975; 189:382-4.

10. Starr A, Achoy LJ. Auditory brainstem responses in neurological disease. Arch Neurol 1975; 32:761-8.

11. Starr A, Hamilton AE. Correlation between confirmed sites of neurological lesions of far-field auditory brainstem responses. Electroencephalogr Clin Neurophysiol 1976; 41: 595-608.

12. Stockard JJ, Rossiter VS. Clinical and pathological correlates of brain stem auditory response abnormalities. Neurology (Minneap) 1977; 27:316-25.

13. Motokoff B, Schulman-Galambos C, Galambos R. Brain stem auditory evoked responses in children. Arch Otolaryngol 1977; 103:38-43.

14. Hecox K, Galambos R. Brain stem auditory evoked responses in human infants and adults. Arch Otolaryngol 1974; 99:30-3.

15. Schulman-Galambos C, Galambos R. Brain stem auditory-evoked responses in premature infants. J Speech Hear Res 1975; 18:456-65.

16. Hecox K. Electrophysiological correlates of human auditory development. In: Cohen LB, Salapatek P, eds. Infant perception: from sensation to cognition, vol 2: Perception of space, speech and sound. New York: Academic Press, 1975.

17. Salamy A, McKean CM, Buda FB. Maturational changes in auditory transmission as reflected in human brain stem potentials. Brain Res 1975; 96:361-6.

18. Salamy A, McKean CM. Postnatal development of human brain stem potentials during the first year of life. Electroencephalogr Clin Neurophysiol 1976; 40:418-26.

19. Starr A, Amlie RN, Martin WH, Sanders S. Development of auditory function in newborn infants revealed by auditory brain stem potentials. Pediatrics 1977; 60:831-9.

20. Coats AC, Martin JL. Human auditory nerve action potentials and brain stem evoked responses. Arch Otolaryngol 1977; 103:605-22.

BINAURAL INTERACTION IN BRAINSTEM-EVOKED RESPONSES

ROBERT A. DOBIE, MD CHARLES I. BERLIN, PhD

NEW ORLEANS, LOUISIANA

Published in *Archives of Otolaryngology*.

Dobie RA, Berlin CI. Binaural interaction in brainstem-evoked responses. Arch Otolaryngol 1979; 105:391-8.

VESTIBULAR TESTING IN CHILDREN

David G. Cyr, MA
Omaha, Nebraska

Vestibular evaluation in the pediatric population has in the past taken several forms. For the most part, the pediatric vestibular evaluation has been more subjective than objective. One of the primary reasons for this has been the obvious difficulties encountered in trying to conduct a standard, adult electronystagmography (ENG) procedure on a pediatric patient population not capable of performing in a manner conducive to a good ENG recording. The purpose of this paper is to suggest certain modifications of the standard adult ENG battery for use with young children and infants. Discussion consists of modifications in the areas of various ocular movement tests including sinusoidal pursuit, calibration, optokinetics and gaze testing. In addition, procedures relative to peripheral vestibular output from perrotational and caloric stimulation are discussed. Topics also include the use of a closed-loop caloric irrigator and simultaneous caloric irrigation as viable alternatives to standard, alternate water irrigation when testing the vestibular output of a young child or infant.

Evaluation of the vestibular system in patients presenting with dizziness, disequilibrium, or vertigo has, at least in theory, become more effective with the use of electronystagmography (ENG). However, the degree of effectiveness is highly dependent upon the age of the patient being evaluated.

The ENG procedure, as we know it today, initially gained widespread acceptance for its effectiveness in the evaluation of an alert and usually cooperative adult population. As a product of that success, virtually all of the normative data reported in the literature were compiled from adults, and consequently only a limited amount of information is available specifically related to ENG findings in young children and infants.

Although there are only minimal data available relative to ENG procedures with children, there does exist a fair amount of literature reported in the fields of pediatrics, physical therapy, occupational therapy, neurophysiology, pediatric otolaryngology, and child neurology dealing with various methods (other than ENG) of evaluating the pediatric vestibular system.[1-4] For the most part, although there are a few exceptions, that literature primarily concerns itself either with reflexive response to postural change, perrotatory and postrotatory stimulation, or ice water calorics. Virtually, nothing has been reported in the literature in terms of adapting the standard adult ENG procedure and applying it to young children or infants. We are of course making the assumption that the ENG procedure is *the* tool best suited for pediatric vestibulography. Tha assumption may or may not be appropriate to make.

This paper will not discuss the obvious importance of an appropriate medical examination including laboratory and x-ray studies, case history, etc, as that has been stressed by several authors in the past.[1,2,5] Rather, the scope of this paper will deal primarily with a few suggested modifications of the standard adult ENG battery as applied to young children and infants. Although the time allotted does not permit an in-depth evaluation of all of the currently used procedures in pediatric vestibular examination (excluding ENG), I would like to mention an area that I feel is extremely important and should be recognized: namely, early life vestibular reflex testing following changes in body posture.

Briefly, based upon the premise that a mature central nervous system (CNS) is essential to a child's development of posture as well as to the development of his gross and fine motor coordination (visual figure-ground skills, eye-hand coordination, etc), efforts have been made to identify immaturity within this system through the use of such procedures as visual-evoked potentials,[6] nerve conduction studies[7] and through the utilization of various body, head and limb reflexes in response to postural changes. Those reflexes, which appear to be somewhat dependent upon gestational age, include tonic neck (both symmetrical and asymmetrical), head and neck righting, body righting over head, hopping, buttress, parachute, doll's eye, etc. The above mentioned reflexes, as well as the methods and criteria for their evaluation, are most impressively presented by Eviatar and Eviatar.[8] I urge you to review that publication for an interesting summary of a most significant area of pediatric vestibular evaluation.

Along these same lines of investigation, de Quiros[9] has reported interesting data from a longitudinal study which incorporates the previously mentioned reflexes as they relate to later life-learning disabilities. The author notes that the absence of these early life reflexes (at appropriate ages) is related to language and/or learning difficulties during the school years. Immature, delayed, or inappropriate CNS function, as indicated by the abnormality or absence of these reflexes, may have a significant impact upon a child's abilities in

From the Boys Town Institute for Communication Disorders in Children and Creighton University School of Medicine, Omaha, Nebraska.

communication areas such as reading, writing, language coding and organization, etc. As a result, many of the children in de Quiros' study who were followed over a period of several years and were found to have some sort of language or learning disability at school age, failed to show appropriate postural reflexes at an early age.[10] Dr. de Quiro's most recent publication should prove to be interesting reading for those involved with language, learning, and/or vestibular function of children.

There also exists a good deal of published data dealing with vestibular response in infants and young children to rotational stimulation and stimulation by ice water.[1,4,8] In the latter area, the vestibular response to ice water stimulation in infants was usually measured by nystagmic duration which is a questionably effective means of quantifying vestibular system activity.[11] In addition, the temperature of the ice water stimulus is difficult to control. Even minor changes in water stimulus temperature can make a significant difference in the resultant response within the vestibular endorgan. Also, an ice water stimulus can feverishly drive the vestibular system in a manner far different from everyday physiologic vestibular functioning and as a result, is probably not a very effective means of determining actual vestibular response to subtle changes in posture or acceleration. The lack of pediatric research utilizing a more controlled caloric stimulation and an objectively measured nystagmic response is likely due to the difficulty in adapting the standard adult ENG procedure for use with this younger population.

Before discussing certain modifications of the standard ENG battery for use with children, we should briefly deal with the question, "Why do an ENG on a young child or infant?" Gates wrote, "It is not unusual in neuro-otological practice to discover patients with unrecognized vestibular defects that occurred in childhood."[5] As far back as 1938, Still[12] stressed the importance of identifying vestibular disease in childhood and described some of the resultant psychological sequelae. Since that time, there has emerged a large body of literature dealing with the incidence of childhood vestibular disorders such as pediatric benign paroxysmal vertigo,[13-15] vertiginous epilepsy,[16-18] etc. However, little has been written regarding objectively measured vestibular response in children with unilateral or bilateral sensorineural hearing loss; postviral disease such as measles, mumps, and meningitis; head trauma; monitoring vestibulotoxic medications given in the treatment of pneumonia or meningitis, etc. The pediatrician, for instance, may want to know that the reason that an 18-month-old postmeningitic child can no longer walk effectively is because of bilateral peripheral vestibular involvement or for some other sequela of the meningitis. Eviatar and Eviatar wrote, "Children with congenital deafness occasionally present with delay in the acquisition of postural control and, if tested appropriately, abnormal vestibular function may be demonstrated."[8] It has not been a common occurrence to hear reports that a child with bilateral profound hearing loss will have difficulty walking in the dark at night, based upon the assumption that deaf children are more fearful and cautious in the dark since they have lost that ever so important and heavily relied upon input from both the visual as well as from the auditory system. In actuality, the reason may well be the fact that the child has bilateral vestibular disease secondary to whatever affected the auditory system. In addition to the already absent visual input, absence of vestibular input makes the child rely very heavily on his proprioceptive system to maintain balance. This, of course, is very difficult for him to do.

Use of the standard ENG procedure in adults and older children can be quite effective in defining whether a vestibular system is functioning inside or outside of the normal range and, on many occasions, can specify site of lesion in terms of being either peripheral or central. However, it cannot alone effectively specify the actual pathology. The physician also must rely heavily upon the case history and symptoms in order to place a diagnosis on the patient. A child can rarely effectively communicate history or symptoms; thus, it would seem particularly important to supplement reflex testing, medical examination, etc, with an objective measurement of vestibular function within this young population. Therefore, I would like to suggest to you a few modifications of the standard ENG battery for use with children under the age of five years.

OPTOKINETICS

Optokinetic (OKN) tracking can be measured in very young children with a drum that fits over the child's head or one that fills a good portion of the child's visual field. I would suggest that in OKN testing one not use a hand-held drum; it doesn't work very well with young children. We occasionally use projected cartoon characters on the wall and this is a fairly good procedure for use with three-year-olds but again, below that age level it is difficult to obtain a good OKN response. Instead, we use an overhead OKN drum (Tracoustics model RN238B) (Fig. 1A) for use with our little ones and we find it works very effectively.

Let me digress for just a moment to discuss an issue which is probably going to be receiving significant attention in the future. At this point, there is a real question in my mind as to whether we are really testing the OKN system when we utilize a hand-held type of drum, or whether in fact we are actually testing the visual pursuit system. I do not think that you can effectively test the OKN system unless you utilize a stimulus that fills the patient's entire

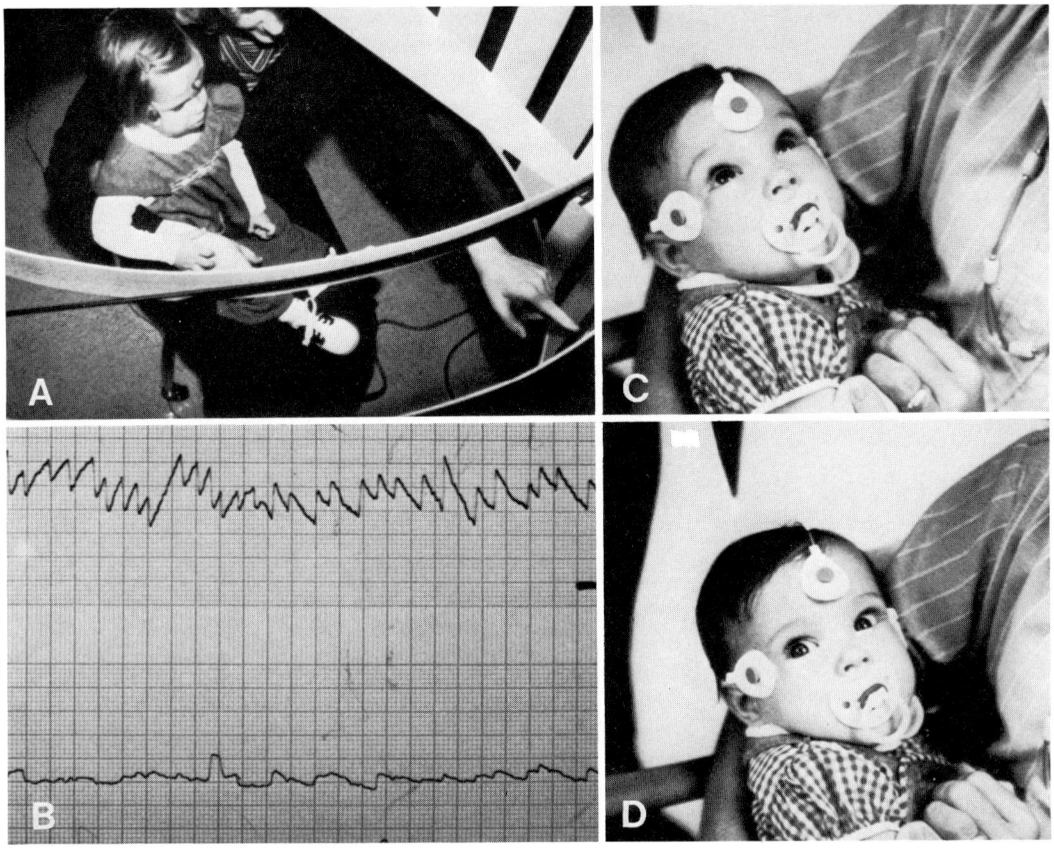

Fig. 1. A) Over-the-head optokinetic (OKN) drum utilized with infants and young children. B) Symmetrical recording of a normal OKN response on an 8-month-old child. C) Infant in mother's arms while seated in a rocking chair. The child's eyes are fixed on a bright object held overhead and we can inspect for nystagmus in center gaze. D) Child's head rotates around her eyes as the mother rocks in the chair. We can inspect for doll's head tracking in this manner to note problems associated with visual motor defects or ocular muscle palsies. (From Cyr DG. Audiology: An Audio Journal for Continuing Education; June 1980. New York: Grune and Stratton. Published with permission.)

visual field such as that of an all-over-the-head drum. Hand-held drums probably measure the visual pursuit system rather than the OKN system, at least in part.

Several reports have been presented indicating that the OKN tracing cannot be obtained in a child under four or five months of age. For the most part, those reports have relied upon an OKN stimulus that did not fill the child's entire visual field. Since the visual pursuit system is not myelinated until the fourth or fifth month of life, I suspect that this system plays an important part in the response or lack of response generated during this attempted OKN test. Utilizing an overhead OKN drum, we have been able to demonstrate OKN responses much earlier than four months of age. Again, I suspect that the reason for this is that overhead drums that fill the visual field specifically test the OKN system while the OKN stimuli that do not fill the visual field are more involved with the visual pursuit system rather than the OKN system. Figure 1B represents a normal OKN response from an eight-month-old child.

CALIBRATION, GAZE AND OCULAR DYSMETRIA

Calibration of the recording unit as well as gaze testing can be accomplished with the use of a standard light bar if the child is at least 3½ years old (Fig. 2A). For very young children, we use a lamp calibrating system (Tracoustics model RN257) (Fig. 2C) which consists of two painted lamp shades mounted on a horizontal bar. Each of the lamp shades is painted with cartoon characters and we have the option of sound, light, or motion with each of the lamp shades. We have found this device to be very effective with children down to approximately six months of age.

These lamps are mounted in such a way that we can alternate the light, motion, and/or sound back and forth between lamps. The child's eyes will follow the motion or lighting back and forth and will create a calibration tracing from which we can figure a calibration factor.

We can also use this unit for gaze testing (Fig. 2B) by holding the child's head still and having her watch the lighted and sound-producing cartoon on the lamp shade. We, of course, do not use the motion for gaze test as that will create an unwanted optokinetic response.

Figure 2D shows a calibration recording on an eight-month-old child. You can notice approxi-

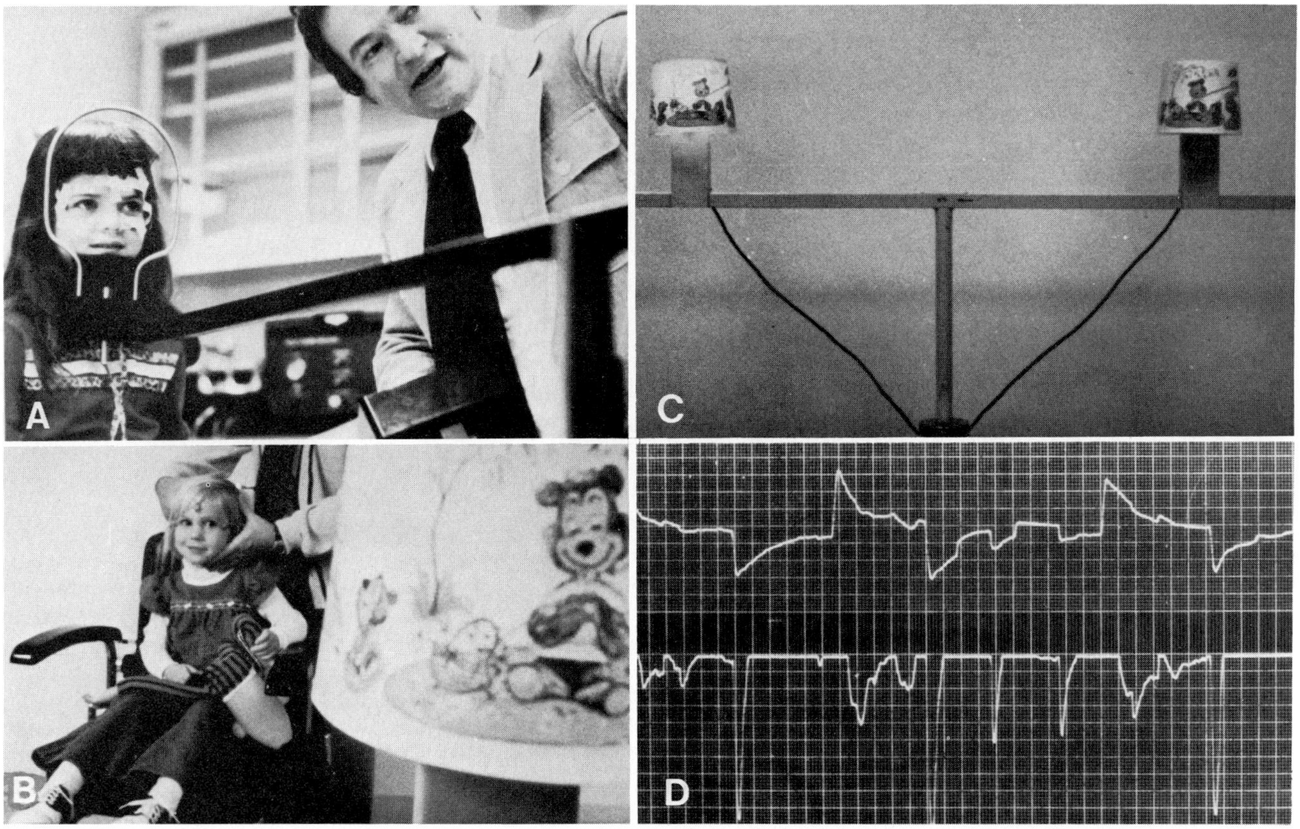

Fig. 2. A) Standard calibration/gaze light bar that can be utilized with children from approximately three to four years of age. B) Child's head is being held in position for the gaze test and the calibration test. C) Modified light bar with lighted, moving characters. D) Calibration recording from an 8-month-old child. Note the approximate deflection of 16 mm for a 20° eye deflection. From this record we can obtain a calibration factor from which we can later measure the nystagmic response. Also note the absence of ocular dysmetria in this recording. (From Cyr DG. Audiology: An Audio Journal for Continuing Education; June 1980. New York: Grune and Stratton. Published with permission.)

mately 16 mm of pen deflection with horizontal eye deflection to the right and to the left. The child was placed at a specific distance from the light bar so that the alternating lamp shades produced a 20° eye deflection. The record may not be as clear as we would get with an adult, but nevertheless it does give us a good idea of the approximate deflection in millimeters from which we can get a calibration factor to work with. You can see from Figure 2D that I have utilized the AC method of amplification on the recorder. We, of course, prefer to utilize a DC recording if at all possible since it is fairly easy to miss ocular dysmetria if only the AC mode is used. With children, however, we are forced to utilize the AC amplification mode and rely on a good visual inspection to detect the presence of dysmetria. We have utilized this particular procedure for calibration, gaze testing, and detection of ocular dysmetria with infants down to as early as four months of age with fairly good success.

Sinusoidal eye tracking can be accomplished using a modified "doll's head" maneuver with the infant or youngster in the parent's arms. The parent holds the child in a rocking chair in a horizontal and perpendicular position while the child's eyes are fixed on a lighted toy directly above him (Fig. 1C). We utilize this procedure in very young infants to get some idea of center gaze. It is important to be able to rule out pathologic gaze nystagmus that is caused by drugs or by a lesion as opposed to the benign, ocular nystagmus that is seen in a fair percentage of the pediatric population. The benign, congenital ocular nystagmus is not pathologic from the standpoint that rarely does it cause difficulties with balance or with visual tracking.

Now let me get back to this rocking chair procedure specifically used with inspection of the visual tracking system. Remember that the child is lying in the arms of the mother who is sitting in a rocking chair. The child's eyes are fixed on a lighted object directly above him.

As they rock back and forth, the head rotates around the eyes from right to left to right to left, etc, as seen in Figure 1D. This creates a sinusoidal tracing on the ENG recorder. Although this may be a rather gross method of ocular tracking, it can provide an inspection of potential problems associated with disconjugate eye movement, ocular muscle pathology, or other visual pursuit pathologies that may affect the remainder of the ENG recording. Since the visual pursuit pathways are not myelinated until the fourth or fifth month of life, it is

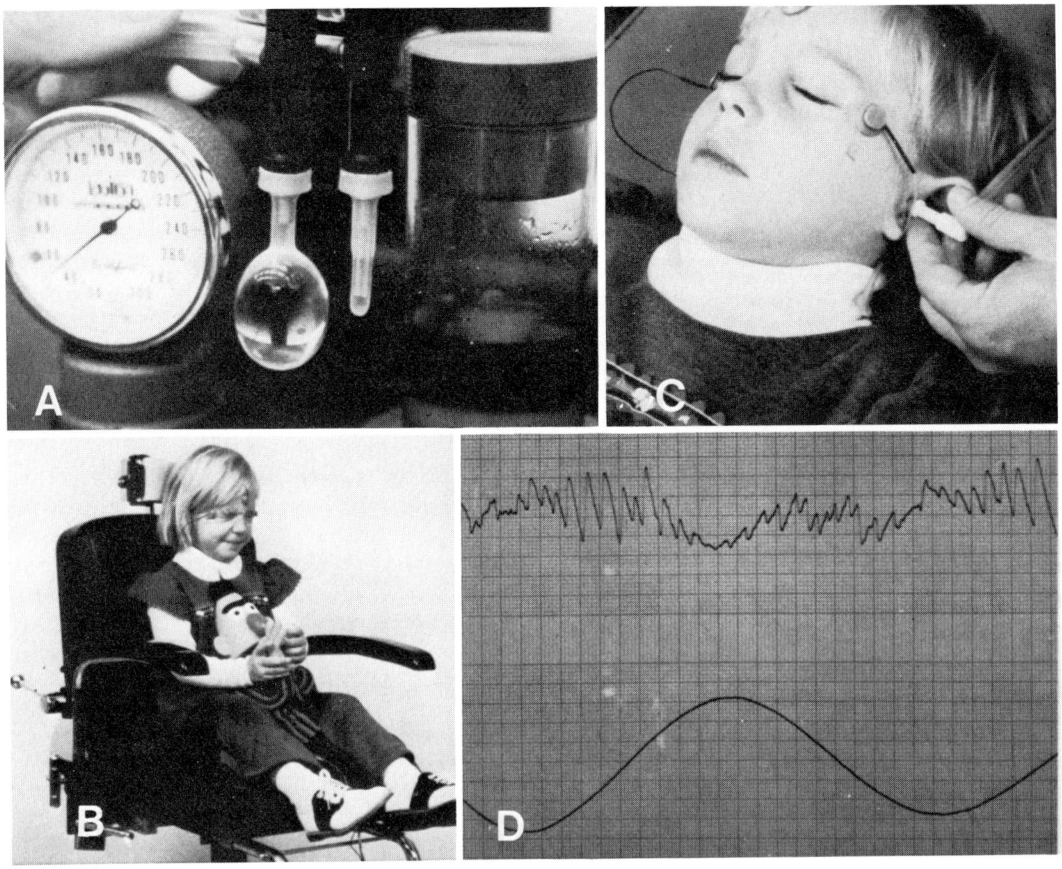

Fig. 3. A) Deflated and inflated balloon probe on the closed-loop irrigator. B) Standard position of a child in the torsion swing chair with eyes closed and head ventroflexed 30°. C) Probe placed in the child's ear canal. D) An abnormal response with rotation to the left compared to a normal nystagmic response with rotation to the right. The lower portion of the recording traces the chair motion (swings up are to the right and swings down are to the left). (From Cyr DG. Audiology: An Audio Journal for Continuing Education; June 1980. New York: Grune and Stratton. Published with permission.)

difficult to perform this type of test until approximately that age.

POSITIONAL TESTS

Position*al* or position*ing* tests can be performed in a darkened room with the young child or infant on a table or in the parent's arms. Although testing in a darkened room may not be as effective as testing with eyes closed, it will sufficiently negate central visual suppression in most cases to permit a nystagmic recording. Blindfolding may also be used but may be more frightening to the child.

PERROTATIONAL TESTS

Vestibular test results can also be obtained using a torsion swing chair in a darkened room or with the child blindfolded (Fig. 3B). The child sits upright in the chair or on the parent's lap if one is testing an infant. The chair then rotates in a 180° horizontal arc. A right-beating nystagmic burst is recorded when the chair swings to the right and a left-beating nystagmic burst is produced when the chair swings to the left. The number of beats that occur in each direction are then counted at a number of points in time. In a normal system, at a given point in time, an approximately equal number of nystagmic beats should occur with movement to the left compared with movement to the right. From our experience, the results must be cautiously interpreted, however, as they do not always agree with caloric results. If for instance, a normal nystagmic burst is identified with acceleration in both directions, a unilateral peripheral weakness cannot necessarily be ruled out, even though the trace would seem to indicate normal function bilaterally. However, if there exists a marked asymmetry when accelerating in one direction compared with the other direction, a unilateral peripheral weakness is predicted and usually supported with subsequent caloric irrigation. You must remember, however, that it is possible to show an increased response on the torsion swing test with rotation in the same direction as that of a concurrent spontaneous nystagmus. That is to say, if a child has a right-beating, direction-fixed spontaneous nystagmus, rotation of the chair to the right will add onto the spontaneous nystagmus, while rotation to the left will negate the spontaneous nystagmus. As a result, the chair recording will show a weakness on the left compared to the right even though the reverse may be true. Ruling out a true unilateral peripheral weakness versus a spontaneous nystagmus is a very difficult task for this test procedure. The test is effective, however, in determining the presence or absence of vestibular output such as that of bilateral weaknesses.

Figure 3D illustrates a weakness on the left ear. With rotation to the right there is good right-beating nystagmus and a poor response with motion to the left. One must remember to keep the child's head ventroflexed 30° in order to get a good recording. This incidently was a unilateral weakness on a 3-year-old, probably secondary to a longitudinal temporal bone fracture.

CALORIC TESTING

In my opinion, probably the most effective method of caloric irrigation with young children and infants is the utilization of a closed-loop caloric irrigator.

Figure 3A illustrates the Brookler-Grams closed-loop irrigator. This device is simply a closed balloon system that fits into the ear canal; air pumps the balloon up and water circulates through the balloon at a fixed flow rate. The balloon fits into the ear as shown in Figure 3C. The closed loop irrigator incorporates a closed water system attached to an ear probe with an inflatable silicone balloon on the end. The probe is placed into the ear canal, water inflates the balloon with a preset amount of pressure. The balloon fills the ear canal, and is held in place fairly securely even if the child should rapidly move. Approximately 200 cc of water circulate inside the balloon for 45 seconds at a fixed flow rate at temperatures of 28.5 and 45.5 C. This, of course, is a slight intensity increase compared to the standard water caloric temperatures. We selected these increased levels to overcome the mass and insulation properties of the silicone balloon. This produces a caloric response almost identical to a standard water irrigation and does it in a relatively safe and painless fashion.

Another method of caloric irrigation that we commonly use consists of utilizing the closed-loop irrigator with simultaneous, binaural, bithermal irrigation (SBB test).[19] The caloric-induced vertigo that is experienced by the patient with standard unilateral stimulation, is minimal or nonexistent with the SBB test if the two inner ear systems are fairly equal in sensitivity. The neural discharge from one labyrinth will cancel the discharge from the simultaneously stimulated opposite labyrinth and theoretically, since no information travels up the medial longitudinal fasciculus, vertigo sensations are not induced. This situation is much less frightening to the child than standard unilateral stimulation. Simultaneous, binaural, bithermal caloric testing also takes the worry out of calibrating between presentations since both ears are being compared under the same degree of recorder sensitivity. This negates the argument that ice water testing, measured by nystagmic duration, is more feasible than measurement of slow phase intensity from a minimal, controlled caloric stimulation. It should be noted, however, that the SBB test only indicates that the vestibular systems are equal; they may be equally active, equally hyperactive, or equally hypoactive. We then have to go back and test at least one ear to insure that there is function from the system.

This procedure has been effective with young children in that we do have an opportunity to check for symmetry between the two systems without creating sensation of vertigo and the vegetative symptoms which are sometimes associated with vertigo. Once we have determined symmetry, we will go back and retest one of the ears to insure that there is indeed output from the peripheral system and that they are not, for instance, bilaterally equally hypoactive.

Two relatively new methods of vestibular evaluation have been recently introduced as potential supplements to or replacements for the standard ENG battery, with the feeling that even in adults ENG evaluates only a small portion of the entire vestibular system. These tests attempt to measure vestibular activity closer to threshold rather than driving the system to its limits with standard caloric testing. Those two procedures include a piezoelectric balance platform and a low frequency harmonic angular accelerating chair. Both of these procedures, although very promising, require a cooperative patient and rarely can be performed on children under the age of five years.

In summary, vestibular evaluation in the cooperative adult patient appears to be markedly improving at the present time. However, these methods have not been satisfactorily developed for use with young children. It is our impression, however, that the previously mentioned modifications can be made in the standard adult ENG procedure. At present, the primary weakness of this method is the obvious lack of normative data available. It will be our major area of concern in the upcoming months to conduct normative studies utilizing the previously mentioned modifications in an effort to help develop a pediatric ENG battery for the evaluation and measurement of vestibular function in children.

REFERENCES

1. Beddoe GM. Vertigo in childhood. Otolaryngol Clin North Am 1977; 10:139-44.

2. Eviatar L, Eviatar A. Vertigo in children: differential diagnosis and treatment. Pediatrics 1977; 59:833-8.

3. Eviatar L, Eviatar A, Naray I. Maturation of neurovestibular responses in infants. Dev Med Child Neurol 1974; 16:435-46.

4. Mitchell T, Cambon K. Vestibular response in the neonate and infant. Arch Otolaryngol 1969; 90:40-1.

5. Gates G. Vertigo. In: Strome M, ed. Differential diagnosis in pediatric otolaryngology. Boston: Little Brown, 1975:75-92.

6. Watanabe K, Iwase K, Hara K. Maturation of visual evoked responses in low-birthweight infants. Dev Med Child Neurol 1972; 14:425-35.

7. Moosa A, Dubowitz V. Assessment of gestational age in newborn infants: nerve conduction velocity versus maturity score. Dev Med Child Neurol 1972; 14:290-5.

8. Eviatar L, Eviatar A. Neurovestibular examination of infants and children. Adv Otorhinolaryngol 1978; 23:169-91.

9. de Quiros J. Neuropsychological fundamentals in learning disabilities. Noveta: Academic Therapy Publications, 1978.

10. de Quiros J. Language disorders and learning disabilities: implications of early vestibular impairment. Presented at the American Speech and Hearing Association, San Francisco, Nov, 1978.

11. Jongkees L. The caloric test and its value in evaluation of the patient with vertigo. Otolaryngol Clin North Am 1973; 6:73-93.

12. Still G. Common happenings in childhood. London: Oxford University Press, 1938.

13. Basser LS. Benign paroxysmal vertigo of childhood. Brain 1964; 87:141-52.

14. Chutorian AM. Benign paroxysmal vertigo in childhood. Dev Med Child Neurol 1972; 14:513-5.

15. Koenigsberger M, Chutorian A, Gold A, Schvey M. Benign paroxysmal vertigo in childhood. Neurology (Minneap) 1970; 20:1108-13.

16. Alpers BJ. Vertiginous epilepsy. Laryngoscope 1960; 70:631-7.

17. Behrman S. Vestibular epilepsy. Brain 1955; 78:471-86.

18. Behrman S, Wyke BD. Vestibulogenic seizures. Brain 1958; 81:529-41.

19. Brookler K. The simultaneous binaural bithermal: a caloric test utilizing electronystagmography. Laryngoscope 1976; 96:1241-50.

USES AND ABUSES OF HEARING AIDS

JAMES E. PECK, PhD
OMAHA, NEBRASKA

The view is expressed that many hearing-impaired individuals are not deriving maximum benefit from amplification or are not using amplification at all because of failure of professionals to keep in mind certain uses and abuses. Some of the specific uses are for minimal and profound hearing losses, adaptation with special earmold modifications, chronic or recurrent conductive losses, part-time use, and binaural listening. Some specific abuses include: unrealistic expectations, overlooking the role of motivation, pressuring persons to try/wear amplification, overamplification, Y cord, inappropriate binaural fittings, and failure to alternate a hearing aid between ears in symmetrical hearing losses.

Hearing aids help many thousands of persons every day. Yet many hearing-impaired persons are not receiving maximum help from their amplification and others are not using amplification at all. This paper is a brief outline of some uses and abuses of hearing aids.

USES

Intermediate Hearing Losses. Hearing aids find their major use in amplifying speech signals to those with intermediate hearing losses, that is, a broad range of losses, say between 40 dB and 90 dB HTL (ANSI, 1969). However, the years have seen increasing amplification benefit to persons with more or less hearing loss, as well as to a wider group of other hearing-impaired persons with special problems.

Minimal Hearing Losses. Persons with mild or even minimal hearing impairment often can derive help from hearing aids. If a person has significant communication demands coupled with a strong motivation to use a hearing aid, we should not impose a fixed minimum decibel level of hearing loss in considering a hearing aid for that person.[1]

Profound Hearing Losses. Similarly, the person with profound hearing impairment often can derive considerable benefit from a hearing aid.[2] Many children with profound early-life hearing impairments utilize acoustic cues from hearing aids to note presence or absence of a signal, to detect spectrum, timing and intensity cues regarding sentence type and emotional content, to monitor their own vocal level, and (within limits) to improve speech discrimination ability, particularly when combined with speechreading. In short, the degree of hearing loss should not dictate one's hearing aid needs or candidacy.

Special Arrangements. The advent of the Contralateral Routing of Signal (CROS) hearing aid introduced the concept of the open or nonoccluding earmold. The classic example of the CROS fitting was the case of the unilateral hearing loss in which the impaired ear was unaidable.[3,4] A hearing aid microphone was placed on the hearing-impaired ear and the signal was routed to the contralateral hearing ear and delivered through an open earmold. It soon became apparent, however, that the open earmold had excellent low-frequency suppression characteristics giving way to fittings called high-frequency CROS and Ipsilateral Routing of Signal (IROS).[5,6] IROS is a conventional fitting in that the entire unit is all on one side, but an open earmold is used to "vent" low frequencies. Additional virtues of the open mold soon were recognized, such as: 1) allowing persons to take advantage of their natural hearing in frequency regions for which they had good hearing, 2) minimizing the sensation of "pressure" from the hearing aid, and 3) being a more comfortable, cooler fitting. The combination of high-frequency emphasis circuitry and the nonoccluding earmold has allowed hearing aid fittings for cases previously considered difficult or impossible.

Natural extensions of the CROS concept were the Bilateral-CROS (BiCROS) and Multi-CROS aids. These arrangements are for the person with a bilateral hearing loss who has only one aidable ear. In the classical BiCROS, microphones are placed at each ear and their signals are directed to the only aidable ear through conventional closed earmold.[7] Going one step further, the Multi-CROS arrangement adds flexibility by allowing the user to activate just one microphone, or the other, or both, depending on the background noise conditions. For example, if there is an interfering noise on the left side, the user can listen just through the right side microphone. If, on the other hand, the noise is on the right side, the user can listen just through the left-side microphone. Finally, if the background level is similar to each side, the user can listen through both microphones.

From the Department of Otolaryngology and Human Communication, Boys Town Institute/Creighton University School of Medicine, Omaha, Nebraska.

The CROS concept has two other applications. One, termed Power CROS, is a fitting for the severely impaired person who wishes to use ear level amplification but is troubled by excessive acoustic feedback. Power CROS minimizes the feedback in two ways, by separating the microphone and receiver, and by employing a standard closed earmold.

The other CROS fitting is for the person who cannot tolerate a closed earmold for medical reasons. Consider the person with chronic otitis externa or otitis media and drainage. Typically, the physician will prohibit a closed earmold for this patient, yet the person may have a substantial hearing loss. With its open earmold, the CROS arrangement may permit utilization of amplification with controlled feedback while maintaining an open ear canal.

Chronic or Frequently Recurrent Conductive Hearing Loss. Usually the individual experiencing conductive hearing loss is not considered a hearing aid candidate, yet not every middle ear problem is amenable to medical treatment. Despite the most diligent medical care, some people have chronic or frequently recurring middle ear problems. Whereas for years the prevailing opinion seemed to be that hearing aids were not for "nerve deafness," it now seems that a reverse idea has taken hold, namely, that hearing aids are not for conductive losses. Of course, neither opinion is true. Hearing aids are designed to help people receive speech, regardless of the location of the hearing problem. Thus, the need for amplification should not be determined by the type of the disorder, but rather by the amount of communicative difficulty the person experiences.

Part-time Use. Akin to the foregoing section is the concept of the part-time user. For some reason, when it comes to hearing aids, we tend to think in terms of full-time use, yet in many other areas of special aids or prostheses, the concept of part-time use is well accepted. Think of persons who use glasses for reading, or a cane when their arthritis acts up. Simply stated, a hearing aid need not be worn 100% of the time to offer 100% help.

Binaural Listening. The superiority of binaural over monaural reception is well established, and most hearing-impaired listeners experiencing communication difficulties have bilateral impairments.[8,9] Thus, it is reasonable to approach amplification from the standpoint of attempting to reestablish the normal binaural auditory input. Binaural hearing aids can help many listeners maintain the more normal situation of receiving speech comfortably in both ears.

The insightful clinician will realize that a number of these areas overlap. The person with a minimal or mild loss may be a good part-time hearing aid user. The individual with a chronic or recurrent middle ear problem may have a minimal or mild loss. The person with chronic otitis media and drainage may require an open mold fitting. The individual using an open mold or CROS arrangement may only need amplification part-time. Finally, many of these people may have significant bilateral losses and perform better with two aids than with one. To put it another way, determining hearing aid candidacy requires considering several dimensions rather than just the audiogram.

Tinnitus. Tinnitus is an all-too-frequent concomitant of hearing loss. Not only is it distressing, but tinnitus also is an interference, causing a less favorable signal-to-noise ratio. No small number of hearing aid users has commented that a hearing aid helps both by making speech louder and by "drowning out" the annoying ear-ringing.

ABUSES

Unrealistic Expectations. Many times, hearing aid use gets off to a painful start or continues as a dismal disappointment because of unrealistic expectations[2] of the user, the user's relatives, a hearing aid dealer or even a professional. Frustration and disappointment almost always follow high expectations, and hearing aid benefit usually suffers. Hearing aids are never replacements for normal ears. Ideally, the levels of expectations should match the individual's hearing ability. Thus, for moderate hearing losses, the expectation might be for considerable speech understanding, whereas for profound childhood losses, the expectation might be for alerting to sound and supplementing speechreading.

Professional Attitude. A corollary to the above is an underappreciation of what a hearing aid can do. Frequently, the attitude from professionals is negative, whereas habilitative and rehabilitative energies are best positive, insofar as possible. The orientation should be one of improved function rather than need as perceived by the professional.[2] The improper attitude toward hearing aids is reflected in patients' reports that someone, a doctor, an audiologist, a speech pathologist, said that, "You can get along without one." The more appropriate orientation, I suggest, should be, "You might get along even better with one." There is small risk to trying a hearing aid, since by Federal mandate, all hearing aids are dispensed on a 30-day trial.

Overlooking Motivation. Already alluded to is the factor of motivation. Ross et al suggest that there is no single more important determiner of hearing aid success than motivation.[1] I suspect many clinicians have seen patients who had been considered ideal hearing aid candidates, yet who totally rejected a hearing aid, even after a trial. Close questioning often reveals that many such patients had a negative attitude and little motivation at the outset, and thus were not ideal candidates at all. While the audiological aspects are important, clinicans must be cautious not to restrict their thinking just to test results. Rather, strong consideration must be given to the nonaudiological aspects, such as the person's communication demands, his own estimate of the problem and, particularly, his motivation.

Pressuring the Hearing-Impaired Person. Hearing loss causes stress, not only to the hearing-impaired person, but also to those in close contact with that person. As a result, hearing-impaired individuals are often unduly pressured to use amplification. This is especially true in the case of the older population. Many times older people grudgingly allow themselves to be brought to hearing clinics, half hoping that the session will at least pacify the family. The older person may perceive few communication problems and may be less demanding of his communicative performance than younger people. Also, the presbycusic patient may have auditory discrimination difficulties beyond those associated with the peripheral hearing loss, making amplification considerably less helpful. Thus, if the person won't try an aid or won't wear the one he has, he may be badgered and berated, or made to feel stubborn and inadequate. Again, hearing aid success is enormously dependent upon the attitude of the person, and failure to recognize these feelings probably retards hearing rehabilitation.

Acoustic Environment. At any given moment, the benefit a hearing aid user derives from his hearing aid depends directly on the acoustic environment in which he finds himself. Noise and reverberation have a major impact on hearing aid benefit.[10]

The hearing aid user and his family, coworkers and friends must be made aware of the strong influence of the background listening conditions on understanding with a hearing aid. Otherwise, the user may become frustrated with the aid, the family may become disgusted with the user's lack of patience, coworkers may be offended by the user's lack of response, and so on. What bewilders the user and others around him is that everyone else seems to be doing just fine. Unfortunately, what they do not understand is that even slight unfavorable changes in the listening conditions can cause the hearing aid user to lose track of the message.

The matter is so much worse for children. Whereas the adult who loses hearing already has the system of his language well in hand, the very young child with hearing loss is faced with the task of acquiring a complicated communication system. In other words, the child has less redundancy to fill in cues obliterated by noise or reverberation. Thus, special education facilities for hearing-impaired children should include quiet, nonreverberant rooms and amplification units that provide the best possible signal-to-noise ratio, such as FM systems.

Overamplification. During the past few years, there has been a growing awareness that hearing-impaired persons often have been fitted with more amplification than they needed. There had been a preoccupation with "correcting the person back to normal," rather than providing just enough gain and output to make a typical speech signal comfortably loud. Recent studies suggest that the desired gain should be equal to about one half of the individual's overall pure tone levels.[11] The point here is not to suggest a method of arriving at the proper gain or maximum output. Rather attention is focused on the observation that hearing aids are often found to be too loud, even though they seemed fine in the quiet test environment.[12] Ways to help guard against overamplification are to use realistic sound levels in the clinical situation and to let the prospective user wear the hearing aid for a short while in the lobby, coffee shop, on the street, etc, where he is exposed to typical background noise levels.

Y-Cord Arrangements. As mentioned earlier, binaural hearing is a goal to be sought in habilitating or rehabilitating the auditorily impaired. At least some binaural advantage usually can be obtained with body aids as well as with ear-level instruments.[13] Unfortunately, in the case of body-borne units, there is a persisting notion that the Y-cord arrangement provides binaural or stereo reception. The Y-cord body aid splits the signal from one microphone and delivers it to the two ears. A single cord exits from the aid and divides, one leg going to one ear and another leg going to the other ear. The cord has a "Y" appearance, giving rise to the name. It is true that the Y-cord system gives two-ear stimulation, but since there is only one microphone pickup, the reception is not truly binaural. True binaural hearing derives from separate signal pickups, one for each ear. Studies have shown that Y-cord is no better than monaural amplification for speech discrimination,[8] although there may be occasions when Y-cord systems are appropriate. The concern here is that by giving the false impression of binaural-stereo listening, the Y-cord may delay providing a genuinely binaural arrangement.

Binaural Amplification.. Abuses in binaural amplification include sins of omission and of commission. A sin of omission is failure to strive for binaural amplification, when there is reasonably similar hearing function between the two ears. Of course, a person may reject a binaural system for financial, psychological or other reasons. As suggested above, any hearing aid fitting is likely doomed if the correct attitude is missing.

A sin of commission is fitting two hearing aids when the person is not a binaural candidate, either audiologically or communicatively. Probably most clinicians have seen patients with two aids who have major differences between the ears, in thresholds, tolerance or speech discrimination ability. Such users may perform better with a monaural fitting to the more aidable ear than with a binaural fitting. In other words, aiding the poorer ear may actually detract from the overall performance through some sort of inhibitory effect.

Another abuse is fitting binaurally the person who has seriously limited financial resources. Even if performance might be better with two aids, the patient is not well served, if purchasing two aids would impose a serious financial burden.

Failure to Alternate Hearing Aid. When a person has two equally aidable ears, but rejects a binaural fitting, it may be well to alternate the single hearing aid between the two ears. It seems that in many monaural fittings, one ear is arbitrarily selected to receive the amplification.

I have a growing suspicion that such a fitting (particularly in moderate or worse losses) prevents a certain degree of auditory training that accompanies hearing aid use. My suspicion arises from my own personal experience with one-ear users who either originally had similar speech discrimination scores or, who never had any form of speech discrimination or tolerance testing. I have been impressed that with surprising frequency these users have markedly better speech discrimination ability and tolerance on the aided side. Certainly, further investigation is needed to support my hypothesis.

I feel that it is important to have each ear become accustomed to amplification for several reasons. First, the usually aided ear could, for some reason, lose a great deal of hearing. Second, that ear could develop a medical condition contraindicating hearing aid use. Third, the person's situation may change, such that he or she may want to try binaural amplification. If the opposite ear were accustomed to an aid, any of these situations could be met by merely utilizing amplification on that opposite side.

Hearing Aid as a Crutch. Occasionally audiologists hear the concern that a hearing aid may become a "crutch." This is a most unfortunate attitude, which implies that the person will become dependent on the aid instead of on his or her own resources. It is as though use of the aid would cause the ear to become atrophied or lazy by letting the aid do the work. Probably the reverse is closer to the truth. Failure to stimulate the hearing mechanism may permit a reduction in effective functioning, as suggested above. Careful counselling should help dispell this harmful notion of the "hearing aid crutch." However, a word of caution: Voicing this concern may be a smokescreen for other negative feelings toward hearing aids that may need to be dealt with.

Hearing Aids to Prevent Hearing Loss. Happily we are seeing the decline of the idea that using a hearing aid will prevent further hearing loss. Still, now and again we hear this comment. The idea is a natural analogy made to disorders in which exercises and stimulation are crucial to prevent further deterioration. A hearing aid will never prevent additional loss of hearing, although it may help to keep the entire auditory system functioning as efficiently as it can. The point here is that persons should not be stampeded off to buy amplification based on false premises, such as preventing them from going deaf.

To conclude, the user's benefits will be maximized when he or she fully understands the limitations, as well as the capabilities, of amplification.

REFERENCES

1. Ross M, Barrett LS, Trier TR. Ear-level hearing aids for motivated patients with minimal hearing losses. Laryngoscope 1966; 76:1555-61.

2. Ross M. Changing concepts in hearing aid candidacy. Eye Ear Nose Throat Mon 1969; 48:27-34.

3. Harford E, Barry JA. A rehabilitative approach to the problem of unilateral hearing impairment: the contralateral routing of signals (CROS). J Speech Hear Disord 1965; 30:121-38.

4. Harford E, Dodds E. The clinical application of CROS: a hearing aid for unilateral deafness. Arch Otolaryngol 1966; 83:455-64.

5. Green DS, Ross M. The effect of a conventional versus a nonoccluding (CROS-type) earmold upon the frequency response of a hearing aid. J Speech Hear Res 1968; 11:638-47.

6. Green DS. Non-occluding ear molds with CROS and IROS hearing aids. Arch Otolaryngol 1969; 89:512-22.

7. Harford E. Bilateral CROS: two-sided listening with one hearing aid. Arch Otolaryngol 1966; 84:426-32.

8. Harris JD. Monaural and binaural speech intelligibility and the stereophonic effect based upon temporal cues. Laryngoscope 1965; 75:428-46.

9. Licklider JCR. Basic correlates of the auditory stimulus. In: Stevens SS, ed. Handbook of experimental psychology. New York: John Wiley and Sons, 1951.

10. Ross M. Classroom acoustics and speech intelligibility. In: Katz J, ed. Handbook of clinical audiology. Baltimore: Williams and Wilkins, 1972.

11. Keith RW, Siniger L. Changing concepts in hearing aid selection. Hear Instr 1978; 29:6-8, 34.

12. Walden BE, Schuchman GI, Sedge RK. The reliability and validity of the comfort level method of setting hearing aid gain. J Speech Hear Disord 1977; 42:455-61.

13. Ross J, Hunt MF, Kessler M, Heniges MP. The use of a rating scale to compare binaural and monaural amplification with hearing impaired children. Volta Rev 1974; 76:93-9.

ADVANCES IN SENSORY AIDS FOR THE HEARING-IMPAIRED: VISUAL AND VIBROTACTILE AIDS

J. M. Pickett, PhD

Washington, DC

An informal sketch is given of the background and current status of research on electronic aids designed to convert speech into visual or tactile patterns in order to alleviate problems of speech reception and speech production by the hearing-impaired. The functions and problems of the major types of such aids are briefly described and literature references are given.

My aim is to describe the most important types of sensory aids that employ vision and touch to try to alleviate the problem of difficult or nonexistent speech communication. There have been quite a number of devices and research efforts in this field. First I will discuss the idea of using visual or tactile feedback as a means of speech training for profoundly deaf children. Then I will go on to the notion of providing visual cues in an aid for receiving speech from other people. Finally, I will discuss the sense of touch as a possible sensory substitute for the ear for the profoundly deaf. More detailed summaries and many reprinted papers in this field will be found in Levitt et al.[1]

All of these devices rely on the technology of speech analysis which began its development at the Bell Laboratories in the middle 1920s. The first modern device was built just after World War II, based on the use of the sound spectrograph, which was developed for the military by Bell. In 1945 Bell wanted to test the idea of setting up a real-time sound spectrograph for the deaf, to display the spectrum of speech. Figure 1 shows a diagram of this first visible speech translator, as it was called. On the right side of the figure is a microphone and a set of filters spanning a range from low to high frequencies; a phosphor belt was passed under lights responding to the outputs of the filters, causing patterns of light to appear and remain on the belt as it moves across from right to left. The pattern shown represents the spectrum changes in time for the phrase "we show speech." The high frequency consonants are on top and the vowel formants in the lower-frequency half, near the bottom.

There is now a new version of visible speech, the speech spectrum display (SSD) manufactured by Spectraphonics, Inc. A TV monitor screen is used as the display and a standard spectrogram is painted on the display and can be held there for the speaker to use to try to correct his own speech. At the Center for Communication Research they are engaged in testing the SSD with children in the Rochester School for the Deaf.

Figure 2 shows the SSD and its display of a spectrogram; it will be seen that the pattern is very clear.

This kind of display presents a lot of important information about speech and it is currently somewhat costly. Some workers in the field have felt that perhaps the analysis should try to separate certain important aspects of voice production and display only those. A good example is the voice pitch trainer. Figure 3 shows a pattern of voice pitch on the display. The trace goes across the screen in time and up and down with the pitch of the voice. This shows two display examples. On the left is registered the pitch of the vowels in a three-syllable utterance. This is with normal intonation with a slight rise on the last syllable and then a fall in the voice pitch. Next to this is the same utterance spoken by a deaf child who has the voice production fault, which is very common, of skipping up into falsetto (in the last syllable) and going out of a normal pitch range. Devices like this are currently used to some extent in speech training of deaf children to try to get their voice pitch in the proper range, to teach them to use the proper changes in voice pitch, and to control their pitch in a normal way. The Center for Communication Research makes a new version of this kind of voice pitch trainer using a TV monitor for the display and with arrangements for showing differences between the pattern of the trainee and a model pattern.

The programming of materials for training, using this type of device, can be controlled by a small computer system. There is one such project at Bolt, Beranek and Newman, Inc. They arranged a voice pitch cartoon game on a display screen which is illustrated in Figure 4. In the top half the game starts when the pupil begins to phonate and one of the balls comes up and starts going across the screen in

From the Sensory Communication Research Laboratory, Gallaudet College, Washington, DC.

Reprints — J. M. Pickett, PhD, Sensory Communication Research Laboratory, Gallaudet College, 7th Street & Florida Avenue, N.E., Washington, DC 20002.

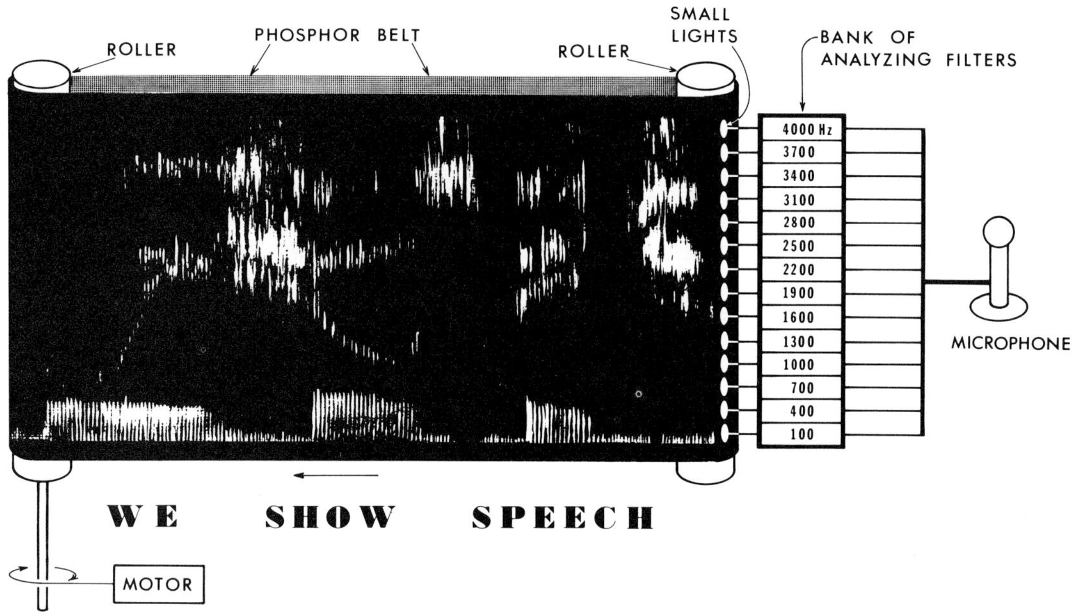

Fig. 1. Diagram of the first Bell Laboratories visible speech translator which analyzed speech by means of a set of filters and displayed the analysis on a moving phosphorescent belt. (Reprinted with permission from Pickett JM. Sounds of speech communication. Baltimore: University Park Press, 1980:35.)

time and up and down with the pupil's voice pitch. The game is to control pitch to get the ball through the hole in the wall; when you do that successfully the ball drops into a basket and a smile lights up on the cartoon face. If you miss, the ball hits the wall, goes back into the starting bin and a frown comes instead.[2]

There are a number of other types of voice training instruments and they are in use to some extent in schools and in speech therapy clinics. One general finding is that it is often difficult to get the training, which is usually successful in the presence of the display, to extend to everyday spontaneous speech.

For voice abnormalities such as hypernasality and repositioning of the tongue after oral surgery, Samuel Fletcher of the University of Alabama, Birmingham, has developed two speech production displays. One detects nasality and displays this on a simple indicator. Another uses an artificial palate to sense the pattern of tongue contact on the hard palate. A group in Japan under S. Hiki has also developed and manufactured a display of tongue contact

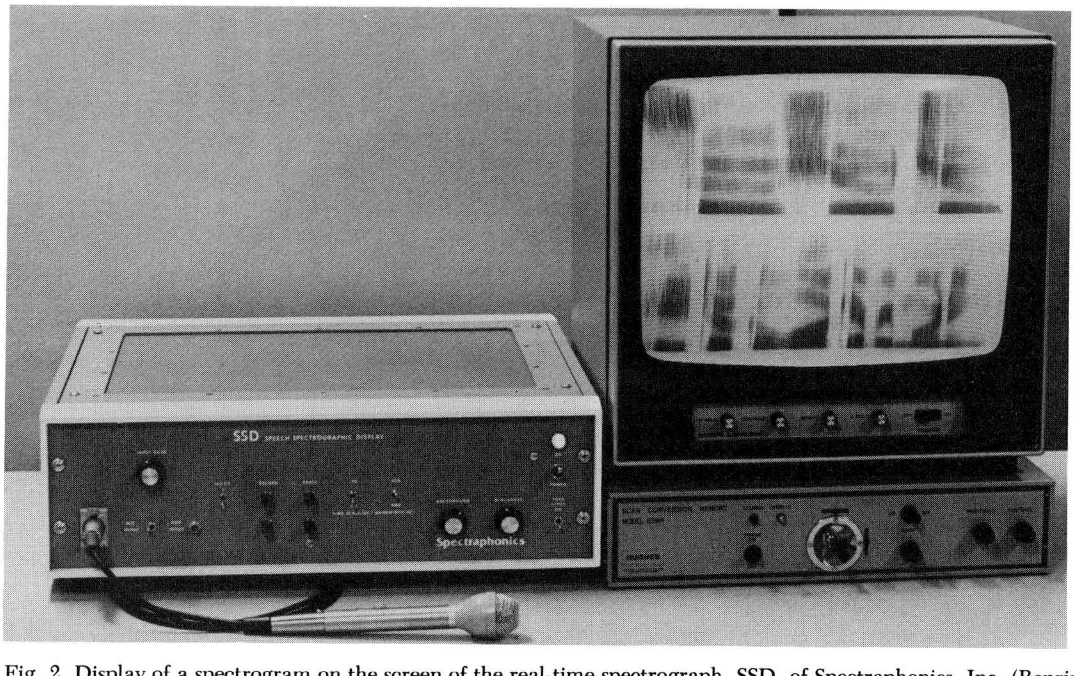

Fig. 2. Display of a spectrogram on the screen of the real-time spectrograph, SSD, of Spectraphonics, Inc. (Reprinted with permission from the Center for Communication Research, Rochester, NY.)

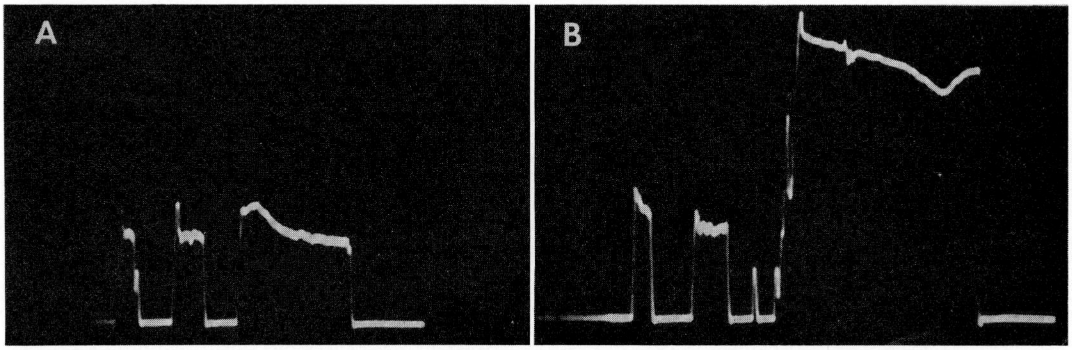

Fig. 3. Displays of voice pitch in time. Two patterns are shown, A) the normal one and B) the same utterance with an abnormal pitch skip. (Reprinted with permission from Risberg A. Visual aids for speech correction. Am Ann Deaf 1968; 113:178-94.)

and used it for training the tongue positions for consonants spoken by deaf children.*

Here at Boys Town Institute a new approach to voice training is being explored using a small electronic word recognizer. The technology of speech understanding by machines is rather highly advanced now and it is possible to build a fairly inexpensive device to recognize spoken words if you are willing to constrain the word set to a small set and the machine is only required to recognize words produced by one talker. The machine has a pattern in it corresponding to a normal utterance of the word; a comparison is made between the stored pattern and the pattern of a new utterance of the word. If the difference is too large it says NO. If the differences are small and within certain limits it says YES. You could use such a machine as a voice production trainer and Richard Lippman here in the Institute is testing this with a simple speech recognizer.

In addition to visible speech indications for speech training visual indicators have also been developed as a means of aiding lipreading. As you know, some of the features of speech are very difficult to lipread. It happens that some of these can be detected acoustically and displayed. A deaf engineer, Hubert Upton, invented such a system for himself, called the Upton eyeglass speechreader. This arrangement uses eyeglasses which are shown in Figure 5 with a small projector mounted so as to send light patterns down to a tiny mirror mounted on the inside of the eyeglass. The mirror reflects the projected light patterns back into the eye of the viewer. If someone is talking to the wearer and he looks directly at the talker's face, the light patterns appear to be near the talker's mouth. The patterns are formed by a small pocket-worn analyzer about the size of a large hearing aid. Features like the plosiveness of consonants and the low frequency murmurs of the nasal consonants turn on certain light-bars in the display.

We did some tests of the Upton eyeglass device as an aid to lipreading and we found that it provided some improvement over lipreading alone.[3] The use of such a device seems most appropriate for persons who are deafened late in life and have a need to get just a modicum of what they cannot get by lipreading.[4] Given a normal knowledge of spoken language a small improvement over a mediocre level of reception can provide increases in speech understanding that are highly useful. It takes a considerable motivation to wear such a device and put up with the flashes of lights that are in your visual field, but Upton himself has been wearing one for about 12 years, and he reports that there is no interference.

*Hiki S. Personal communication, 1980. The training apparatus is the Electropalatograph Model DP-01 and the artificial palate Model SP-01, both manufactured by Rion Co., Ltd., Export Division, No. 7-7, Yoyozi 2-chome, Shibuya-ku, Tokyo 151, Japan.

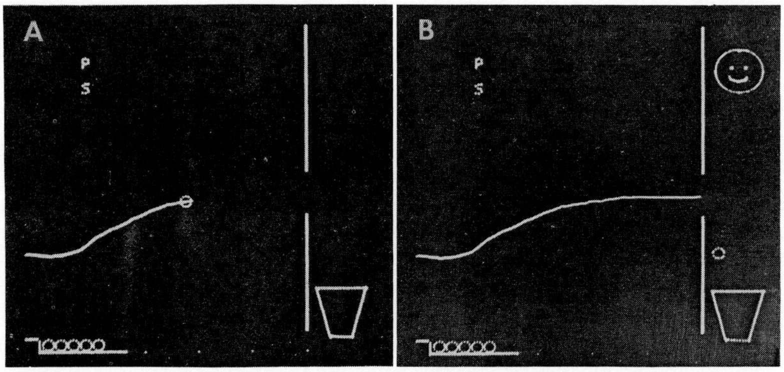

Fig. 4. Displays A & B from a computer-controlled voice pitch game designed by Bolt, Beranek and Newman. (Reprinted with permission from Bolt, Beranek and Newman, Cambridge, Mass.)

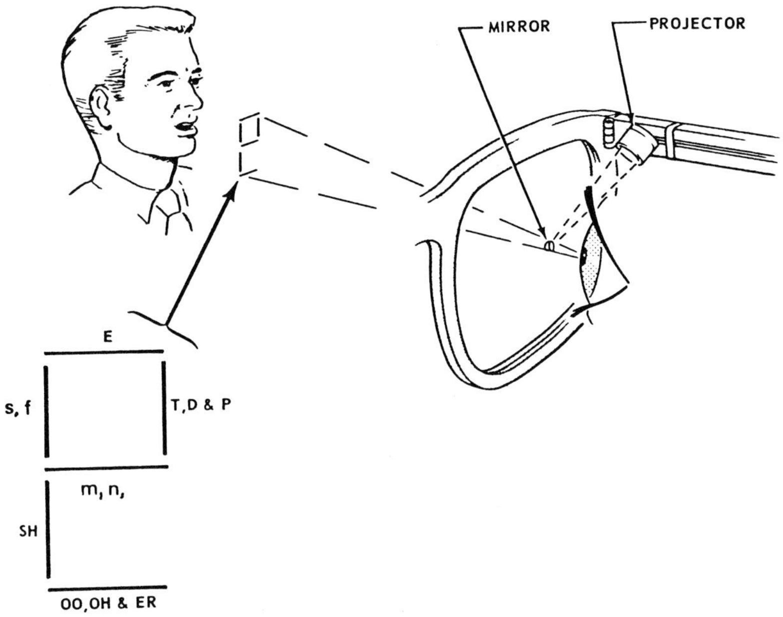

Fig. 5. The Upton eyeglass speech reader. (Reprinted with permission from Bell Helicopter News.)

Tactual speech is our third area of sensory substitution. Particularly for profoundly deaf persons, can we find a way to transform speech to patterns of vibration applied to the skin? The first attempts, in the 1920s, used single vibrators. More recent approaches have been very similar to that of the Bell Laboratories' visible speech, that is, to try to present the spectrum of speech on an array of vibrators on the skin. Figure 6 shows one of these tactual analyzers in a schematic form. There is a microphone, a ten-channel analyzer, and ten vibrators, each of them corresponding to one frequency range of speech coming into the analyzer. The frequency channels are similar to those used for voice vocoders, but instead of producing sound there is a vibrator as the output of each channel. The results with tactual vocoders working on this principle have been rather disappointing. It takes a very long training to be able to sense the different patterns on the skin. Several different schemes of this type, presenting ten or more channels of tactile information have been tried, with limited success and only with long training. Some workers say "That's the way it is; the normal-hearing child takes a long time to learn to perceive speech correctly and we shouldn't expect anything faster with tactile speech." There is a somewhat different philosophy on the part of some workers researching tactile speech. They feel that too much information is presented in vibratory form in these devices and that

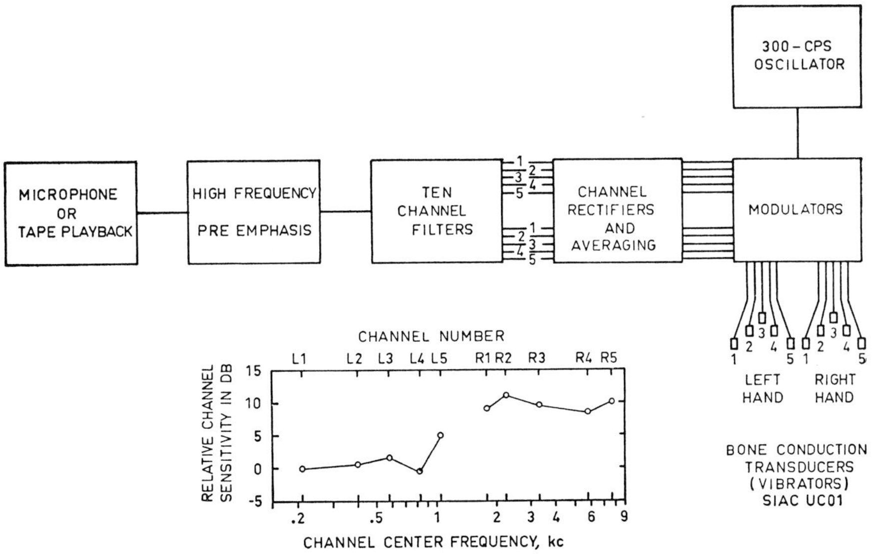

Fig. 6. Scheme of a tactual vocoder. (Reprinted with permission from Pickett JM. Communication of speech sounds by a tactual vocoder. J Speech Hear Res 1963; 6:207-22.)

some kind of more natural tactile differences or different qualities of a few tactile sensations should be used systematically. One good example of this approach was developed and studied at the Central Institute for the Deaf (CID) where there is a tactile speech device which uses only three stimulators, each providing different types of tactile sensation: 1) electrical, 2) vibratory, and 3) spread versus compact. Instead of trying to present a lot of spatial information there are just two alternatives: either the sensation is spread out or it is compact and localized. The tests at CID show that persons with normal hearing and normal language experience can learn to complement lipreading very successfully with this simple tactile display.[5]

There is a more natural system using tactile sensations for speech communication called Tadoma. It was originally developed as a speech therapy method for deaf children. The child would put his hand on the teacher's face so he could feel vibrations of the larynx with the lower fingers, feel the jaw open and close, and feel some of the air flow differences at the mouth. Currently this scheme is used mostly by deaf-blind people as a means of speech communication, and with some success. There is a possibility in the future that some kind of electronic Tadoma method could be developed that would produce natural kinesthetic stimuli from speech signals but wouldn't require the placement of the hand on the speaker's face.

In summary, some devices already developed and available, such as the Upton eyeglass aid and the CID three-feature tactile aid, are now good supplements to lipreading, and could be very useful to the adult who really needs them and will work hard to supplement lipreading beyond what he can get through his hearing aid or by watching the speaker. In another area, the possibility of complete sensory substitution for communication is still in the research stage, but progress is being made. Technologically almost anything is possible now but further study is needed on the more natural tactile codes that are easy to learn and that ethically could be put on a deaf infant.[6]

REFERENCES

1. Levitt H, Pickett J, Houde R, eds. Sensory aids for the hearing-impaired. New York: Institute of Electrical and Electronics Engineers, 1980 (in press).

2. Nickerson R, Stevens KN, Rolling AM. The BBN computer-based system of speech training. Proceedings of the Research Conference on Speech-Processing Aids for the Deaf. Washington, DC: Gallaudet College, 1977 (in press).

3. Pickett JM, Gengel RW, Quinn RJ. Research with the Upton eyeglass speechreader. In: Fant G, ed. Proceedings of the Speech Communication Seminar Stockholm. Stockholm: Almquist and Wiksell, 1974.

4. Gengel R. Research with Upton's visual speechreading aid. Proceedings of the Research Conference on Speech-Processing Aids for the Deaf, Washington, DC: Gallaudet College, 1977 (in press).

5. Scott R, DeFilippo C, Sachs RM, Miller JD. Evaluating with spoken text a hybrid vibrotactile-electrotactile aid to lipreading. Proceedings of the Research Conference on Speech-Processing Aids for the Deaf, Washington, DC: Gallaudet College, 1977 (in press).

6. Pickett JM. On somesthetic transforms of speech for deaf persons. In: McPherson DL, ed. Advances in prosthetic devices for the deaf: a technical workshop. Rochester: National Technical Institute for the Deaf, 1978;184-8.

REVIEW OF RECENT RESEARCH ON THE SELECTION OF FREQUENCY-GAIN CHARACTERISTICS FOR HEARING AIDS

RICHARD LIPPMANN, PhD

OMAHA, NEBRASKA

Following the Harvard master hearing aid study in 1947 there was little research on linear amplification. Recently, however, there have been a number of studies designed to determine the relationship between the frequency-gain characteristic of a hearing aid and speech intelligibility for persons with sensorineural hearing loss. These studies have demonstrated that a frequency-gain characteristic that rises at a rate of 6 dB/octave, as suggested by the Harvard study, is not optimal. They have also demonstrated that high-frequency emphasis of 10-40 dB above 500-1000 Hz is beneficial. Most importantly, they have demonstrated that hearing aids as they are presently being fit do not provide maximum speech intelligibility. Percent word correct scores obtained with the best frequency-gain characteristics tested in various studies have been found to be 9 to 19 percentage points higher than scores obtained with commercial aids owned by subjects. This increase in scores is equivalent to an increase in signal-to-noise ratio of 10 to 20 dB. This is a significant increase which could allow impaired listeners to communicate in many situations where they presently cannot. These results demonstrate the need for further research on linear amplification aimed at developing practical suggestions for fitting hearing aids.

There has been a significant amount of research aimed at determining the potential usefulness of different forms of acoustic signal processing in hearing aids. This research has focused on systems which provide linear amplification, frequency lowering, and nonlinear processing such as amplitude compression or clipping. In this paper a review of recent research on linear amplification is presented.

Research on linear amplification is important both because it can be directly applied to the problem of fitting existing commercial aids and because it can assist in the development of aids which include more complex types of signal processing. Such complex aids can only be properly evaluated if they are compared to the best linear system for a given impaired person. This best linear system can serve as a common reference or bench mark by comparing the performance of this system to that of other more complex types of processing. The best linear system also allows the limitations of linear amplification to be determined and aids in the design of more complex aids. Such aids can be designed by using this linear system as a building block to which more complex forms of processing are successively added.

Unfortunately, we presently do not know how to choose the best linear system for a given person, even though this has been the goal of much research. This research is reviewed in the remainder of this paper.

In this review the term *frequency-gain characteristic* refers to the acoustic gain in sound pressure from sound source to eardrum obtained with an aid relative to the acoustic gain that exists in some other reference condition. An aid with a flat frequency-gain characteristic will thus not necessarily provide acoustic gain from sound source to eardrum that is independent of frequency. It will, however, provide an acoustic-gain characteristic that is identical to that which exists under the reference condition. One important reference condition is the *orthotelephonic* condition[1] in which the listener faces the source at a distance of one meter in a free field. A frequency-gain charactieristic measured relative to the orthotelephonic gain is also referred to as the *functional gain*[2] of an aid. In practice the functional gain or orthotelephonic response is fairly easily obtained by taking the decibel difference between aided and unaided free-field thresholds. The orthotelephonic condition is an extremely important one because it takes into account the significant acoustic gain provided by concha and ear canal resonances, the acoustic coupling between the sound source in an aid and an individual listener's ear, and the placement of the microphone used in an aid on the listener. Unfortunately, other reference conditions and measurement procedures which ignore one or more of these factors have often been used. When this is done only the *nominal response* of an aid has been measured. Such a response is obtained, for example, when the reference condition is defined solely in terms of measurements made on an acoustic coupler or in terms of voltage applied to the sound source used.

One of the first studies on fitting hearing aids was performed at Harvard in 1947.[3] This was the most complete study to be performed up to that time and for many years after and it had a great influence on the research that followed. Characteristics of this study are presented in Table 1. The results of this study indicated that the best aid for the majority of

From the Communication Engineering Laboratory, Boys Town Institute, and the Department of Otolaryngology and Human Communication, Creighton University School of Medicine, Omaha, Nebraska. The preparation of this manuscript was supported by the Boys Town Institute for the Communication Disorders of Children and by a Biomedical Research Development Grant from the National Institutes of Health.

TABLE 1. CHARACTERISTICS OF THE HARVARD MASTER HEARING AID STUDY[3]

Systems
Nominal response: -12, -6, 0, 6, 12 dB/octave HP and LP filtering
Subjects — 18
20% - Moderate to severe sensorineural loss. Sharply sloping audiograms
80% - Mild to severe conductive or mixed loss. Rising, flat, or gently sloping audiograms
Speech Tests
PB word lists - Male talker. In quiet or static noise

HP - High pass; LP - Low pass; PB - Phonetically balanced.

impaired listeners would be one that passed a fairly limited range of frequencies (300-4000 Hz) and had a nominal frequency-gain characteristic (measured using earphones and a 6 cc coupler) which was flat or which rose at a rate of 6 dB/octave.

Recent research has not substantiated the conclusions of the Harvard study. This may primarily be caused by a change over the years in the population of persons who use hearing aids, and also by the limited number of frequency-gain characteristics included in the Harvard study. Most persons who presently wear hearing aids have sensorineural instead of conductive losses because most conductive losses can presently be corrected with surgery. By contrast only 20% of the subjects in the Harvard study had sensorineural losses. Also, many of the frequency-gain characteristics that have recently been investigated were not included in the Harvard study.

The first of a group of recent studies on linear amplification was performed by Jesper Barfod[4] in Denmark in 1972. Characteristics of this study are presented in Table 2. The purpose of this study was to determine whether high-frequency emphasis could increase the intelligibility of speech presented to persons with sharply sloping high-frequency losses. In this study "high-frequency emphasis" referred to an increase in gain of 0 to 68 dB above a frequency of 250 to 1500 Hz. The results of this study were that scores were highest for a nominal response which included 40 to 60 dB of high-frequency emphasis. Scores obtained with the best high-frequency emphasis characteristic tested were 19 percentage points higher than scores obtained with the nominally flat characteristic. After a post hoc analysis of his data Barfod suggested that the best frequency-gain characteristic would be one which amplifies the speech peaks in each frequency region

TABLE 2. CHARACTERISTICS OF THE STUDY PERFORMED BY BARFOD[4] IN 1972

Systems
Nominal response: High-frequency emphasis of 0-68 dB above 250 to 1500 Hz
Subjects — 15
Mild to moderate sensorineural losses. Sharply sloping audiograms
Speech Tests
CVC — Male talker. In speech-shaped noise

CVC - Consonant-vowel-consonant.

TABLE 3. CHARACTERISTICS OF THE STUDY PERFORMED BY PASCOE[2] IN 1975

Systems
1. Flat functional gain
2. Mirror audiogram
3. Flat coupler gain
4. 6 dB/octave rise in coupler
5. Commercial aid simulation
Subjects — 8
Mild to moderate sensorineural losses. Gently sloping audiograms
Speech Tests
HF and PB word lists — Male/female talker. In quiet and speech-shaped noise

HF - High frequency.

to be as loud as they are for a normal-hearing listener.

In 1975 Pascoe[2] performed a study whose purpose was to determine the importance of maintaining the normal field-to-eardrum transfer function when fitting an aid and also to determine whether mirroring the audiogram would provide the best frequency-gain characteristic. Such a characteristic would cause the thresholds of an impaired listener when measured in free-field with the aid on to be normal. Pascoe included only older persons with gradually sloping high-frequency losses and characteristics of his study are shown in Table 3. This study demonstrated that the acoustic gain provided by the concha and ear canal is important. Scores obtained with the system that had a flat functional response were 6 percentage points higher than scores obtained with the system that had a flat coupler response (62 vs 56%). This study also demonstrated the importance of mirroring the audiogram. Scores obtained with the system that mirrored the audiogram were: 11 percentage points higher than scores obtained with the system that had a flat coupler response (73 vs 62%), 7 percentage points higher than scores obtained with a system with the 6 dB/octave rising response suggested in the Harvard study (73 vs 66%), and 19 percentage points higher than a system with a response that simulated the response of a commercial hearing aid (73 vs 54%).

In 1976 Skinner[5] performed a series of experiments designed to determine whether a system that mirrored the audiogram would also be best for subjects with sharply sloping noise-induced losses. Characteristics of this study are presented in Table 4. Scores were highest for the system which provided roughly 22 dB of high-frequency emphasis.

TABLE 4. CHARACTERISTICS OF STUDY PERFORMED BY SKINNER[5] IN 1976

Systems
1. Flat functional gain
2. Mirror audiogram with maximum gain or 11, 22, 33, 44 dB
Subjects — 6
Mild to moderate sensorineural losses. Sharply sloping audiograms
Speech Tests
HF word lists — Male/female talker. In quiet

TABLE 5. CHARACTERISTICS OF THE STUDY PERFORMED BY LIPPMANN[6] IN 1978

Systems

1. Flat functional gain
2. Mirror audiogram
3. Restore normal loudness to 10% speech levels
4. Bands of filtered speech at MCL

Subjects — 5

2 - Moderate to severe sensorineural loss. Flat audiograms.

3 - Moderate to severe sensorineural loss. Sharply sloping audiograms.

Speech Tests

CVCs, words, sentences — Male/female talker. In quiet and speech noise.

This system on the average yielded scores that were 8 percentage points higher than scores obtained with a system with flat functional gain. Although a system that mirrored the audiogram was not tested by Skinner, her results suggest that the extreme high-frequency emphasis that this would require would not be useful for the subjects studied. In a post hoc analysis of her data Skinner suggested that the relative performance of the different systems studied was primarily determined by 1) the audibility of speech spectral energy in different frequency regions (especially 2 to 6.3 kHz), 2) the proximity of speech spectral energy to the threshold of discomfort, and 3) the balance of speech spectral energy between the low (0.5 to 1 kHz) and high (2 to 4 kHz) frequency regions. On the basis of these factors Skinner suggested that the best frequency-gain characteristic should amplify speech peaks at each frequency to be midway between thresholds and discomfort levels at that frequency. Such a characteristic would make most speech sounds audible but not uncomfortably loud. It would also be similar to the characteristic suggested by Barfod[4] which amplifies speech peaks in each frequency region to be as loud as they are for a normal-hearing listener.

As part of a study on multiple-channel amplitude compression, Lippmann[6] in 1978 performed a series of experiments aimed at determining which of the linear systems suggested by previous research and preliminary research would be best for subjects with both flat and sharply sloping audiograms. Characteristics of this study are presented in Table 5. The systems studied included one that mirrored the audiogram as suggested by Pascoe[2] and one that restored normal loudness to the 10% peak speech levels as suggested by Barfod.[4] In addition, a functionally flat system and one that amplified bands of filtered speech to each subject's most comfortable level was included. The high-frequency emphasis provided by the three fitted systems used in this study was 30-60 dB for the subjects with sloping losses and 10-20 dB for subjects with flat losses. These three systems yielded scores that were significantly higher both in quiet and in noise than scores obtained with the system that had a flat functional gain. For the subjects with sloping losses the

TABLE 6. CHARACTERISTICS OF THE STUDY PERFORMED BY LEVITT[7] IN 1978

Wearable Master Aid

Systems

Nominal response: −6 to +12 dB/octave HP and LP filtering

Subjects — 27

Mild to severe sensorineural loss. Gently sloping audiograms.

Speech Tests

CVCs, VCs, words, sentences — Male/female talker. In quiet and speech noise.

average increase in scores was 29 percentage points (68 vs 39%) and for the subjects with flat losses the increase was 12 percentage points (53 vs 41%). Furthermore, although the three fitted systems yielded scores that were roughly equivalent, subjects with sharply sloping audiograms preferred the system that amplified bands of speech to a most comfortable level and provided the least amount of high-frequency emphasis. An analysis of the results of the consonant confusions exhibited by the subjects in this study and of the location of the speech spectral energy relative to each subject's residual dynamic range suggested that intelligibility is highest when most speech energy in each frequency region is audible but not uncomfortably loud.

Levitt,[7] in a study designed to develop a protocol for the prescriptive fitting of a wearable master hearing aid, performed experiments with a wearable aid that had frequency-gain characteristics which were very similar to those tested in the Harvard study.[3] Characteristics of Levitt's study are presented in Table 6. In the main part of this study frequency-gain characteristics of the wearable aid were changed adaptively on the basis of scores obtained with nonsense syllables in six test sessions. Scores obtained with the resulting systems were then compared to scores obtained with other reference systems. Differences in scores were greatest for the nonsense syllable test. For this test the best fitted system provided scores that were: 5 percentage points higher than scores obtained with a nominally flat system (75 vs 70%), 5 percentage points higher than scores obtained with a system that had a nominal response which rose at a rate of 6 dB/octave (75 vs 70%), and 9 percentage points higher than scores obtained with each subject's own aid (75 vs 66%). For the other word and sentence speech tests that were used these differences were not significant.

TABLE 7. RESULTS FROM STUDIES IN WHICH A SYSTEM WITH A 6 dB/OCTAVE RISING RESPONSE WAS EVALUATED*

Study	*6 dB/octave*	*Best MHA Characteristic*	*Materials*
Pascoe (1975)[2]	66%	73%	HF word list
Levitt (1978)[7]	70%	75%	CVs, VCs

MHA - Master hearing aid; CV - Consonant-vowel; VC - Vowel-consonant.

*Percent correct scores from studies which included a system with a coupler response that rose at a rate of 6 dB/octave. The score obtained with this system in each study is compared to the score obtained with the master hearing aid set to the best characteristic tested.

TABLE 8. RESULTS FROM STUDIES IN WHICH A SYSTEM WITH A FLAT RESPONSE WAS EVALUATED*

Study	*Flat*	*Best High-Frequency Emphasis*	*Materials*
Barfod (1972)[4]	31%	50%	CVC
Pascoe (1975)[2]	62%	73%	HF word list
Skinner (1976)[5]	72%	84%	HF word list
Lippmann (1978)[6]	40%	59%	CVC

*Percent correct scores from studies which included a system with a functional (Pascoe,[2] Skinner,[5] and Lippman[6]) or nominal (Barfod[4]) flat response. The score obtained with this system in each study is compared to the score obtained with the master hearing aid set to the best characteristic tested.

TABLE 9. RESULTS FROM STUDIES IN WHICH A SUBJECT'S OWN AID OR A SYSTEM WHICH SIMULATED AN AID WAS EVALUATED*

Study	*Hearing Aid*	*Best MHA Setting*	*Materials*
Barford (1972)[4]	54%	65%	CVCs
Pascoe (1975)[2]	54%	73%	HF word list
Levitt (1978)[7]	66%	75%	CVs, VCs

*Percent correct scores from studies which performed tests with each listener's own aid (Barfod,[4] Levitt[7]) and from a study which included a system with a response that simulated the responses of a commercial aid (Pascoe[2]). The score obtained with each subject's own aid or with the aid-simulation system in each study is compared to the score obtained with the master hearing aid set to the best characteristic tested.

On the basis of the above recent studies there are a number of questions that can be answered. First, "Is a frequency-gain characteristic that rises at a rate of 6 dB/octave, as suggested by the Harvard study, best?" In Table 7 results of studies that addressed this question are presented. As can be seen, scores with the best master-hearing-aid setting in each study were higher than scores with the 6 dB/octave system. The increase in scores of 5 and 7 percentage points obtained with other systems demonstrates that the 6 dB/octave system is not best.

A second question that can be answered is "Is high-frequency emphasis beneficial?" In Table 8 results of studies which addressed this question are presented. As can be seen, scores with systems that include high-frequency emphasis are 11 to 19 percentage points higher than scores obtained with systems with flat frequency-gain characteristics. Given this result it is important to know what amount of high-frequency emphasis was used in these studies. This information is presented in Figures 1 and 2. In these figures the best frequency-gain characteristics averaged over subjects in each study are presented for subjects with gently sloping audiograms (Fig. 1) and for subjects with sharply sloping audiograms (Fig. 2). In these figures functional gains have been normalized to pass through 0 dB at 500 Hz. In both figures the functional gain of the best master hearing aid characteristic tested in each study and averaged over subjects is presented. In all studies high-frequency emphasis of 10-20 dB above roughly 750 Hz was best for subjects with gently sloping audiograms. High-frequency emphasis of 20-40 dB above roughly 750 Hz was best for subjects with sharply sloping audiograms. It is interesting to note the similarity of the average best frequency responses obtained in very different studies.

A third question that can be partially answered from recent studies is, "Do hearing aids as they are presently fitted provide percent word correct scores that are as high at possible?" In Table 9 results of studies which addressed this question are presented. As can be seen, an increase of 9 to 19 percentage points has been obtained in those studies in which the best master hearing aid setting was compared to

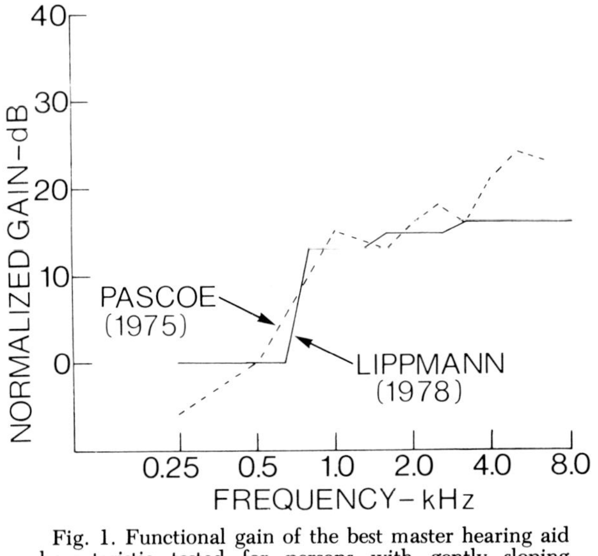

Fig. 1. Functional gain of the best master hearing aid characteristic tested for persons with gently sloping audiograms. All functional gains are normalized to pass through 0 dB at 500 Hz. Solid line is the average response for two subjects in the study of Lippmann[6] and dashed line is the average for all subjects in the study of Pascoe.[2]

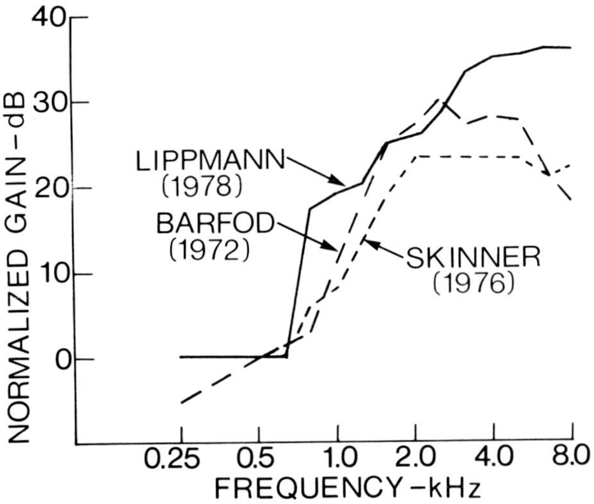

Fig. 2. Functional gain of the best master hearing aid characteristic tested for persons with sharply-sloping audiograms. All functional gains are normalized to pass through 0 dB at 500 Hz. Solid line is the average response for three subjects in the study if Lippmann,[6] long-dahsed line is the average for all subjects in the study of Barfod[4] and short-dashed line is the average for all subjects in the study of Skinner.[5] We have computed the responses for Barfod[4] using an average free-field to coupler response transform for the earphones used.

each subject's own aid or to a system which simulated a typical commercial aid. This result demonstrates the practical importance of research on fitting hearing aids. A significant improvement in speech recognition could be obtained if hearing aids were fitted as in the above studies. This improvement could allow many impaired persons to communicate in situations in which they presently can't.

Although these studies have answered a number of questions, there are still many questions left unanswered. We still do not know how, either empirically or theoretically, to determine the best frequency-gain characteristic for an individual listener. We do not know whether this characteristic should vary in different acoustic environments. We do not know how sensitive speech scores are to perturbations in the frequency-gain characteristics. These questions must be answered by future research.

Some of the results of the above studies provide practical input to the audiologist who fits hearing aids. First, it appears that the best frequency-gain characteristic for an individual listener should probably amplify speech spectral energy at each frequency region to be audible but not uncomfortably loud. To choose a frequency-gain characteristic that will do this it is necessary to take the characteristics of speech, of the aid (as it will be worn), and of the listener's residual hearing, into account. This necessitates free-field testing using the earmold and aid that the listener will use. In addition, it suggests that testing with a variety of speech materials should also be performed and that judgment of the quality of speech as well as percent word correct scores should be used in fitting aids. The above studies also indicate that a properly fitted hearing aid can significantly increase speech reception for impaired listeners. It is thus essential to determine how hearing aids should be properly fitted and if necessary, to develop fitting procedures that an audiologist could use.

ACKNOWLEDGMENTS — The manuscript was typed by Mrs. Carole Dugan.

REFERENCES

1. French NR, Steinberg JC. Factors governing the intelligibility of speech sounds. J Acoust Soc Am 1947; 19:90-119.

2. Pascoe DP. Frequency responses of hearing aids and their effects on the speech perception of hearing-impaired subjects. Ann Otol Rhinol Laryngol 1975; 84 Suppl 23:5-40.

3. Davis H, Stevens SS, Nichols RH, et al. Hearing aids — An experimental study of design objectives. Cambridge: Harvard University Press, 1947.

4. Barfod J. Investigations on the optimal corrective frequency response for high-tone hearing loss. The Acoustics Laboratory, Technical University of Denmark, Report No. 4, 1972.

5. Skinner MW. Speech intelligibility in noise-induced hearing loss: effects of high-frequency compensation. Thesis, Washington University, St. Louis, 1976.

6. Lippmann RP. The effect of amplitude compression on the intelligibility of speech for persons with sensorineural hearing loss. Thesis, Massachusetts Institute of Technology, Boston, 1978.

7. Levitt H. Development of a protocol for the prescriptive fitting of a wearable master hearing aid. Final Report on Contract No. NIH-N01-NS-4-2323 for National Institute of Neurological and Communicative Disorders and Stroke, 1978.

CODING CONSIDERATIONS IN DESIGN OF COCHLEAR PROSTHESES

MICHAEL M. MERZENICH, PhD   MARK WHITE, PhD

SAN FRANCISCO, CALIFORNIA

Some basic considerations in design of multichannel auditory nerve array stimulators and sound processors for an electrical stimulation cochlear prosthesis are briefly reviewed. Considerations specific to the design of strict auditory nerve array simulation-based prostheses are discussed, as are considerations for production of channel vocoder-based and more purely information-based prostheses.

SOME CODING CONSIDERATIONS IN DESIGN OF MULTICHANNEL AUDITORY NERVE ARRAY STIMULATORS

In most investigators' vision of cochlear implants, they are imagined to replace the lost function of a disabled auditory system through simulation of the function of the normal cochlea. In fact, the simulation is necessarily in several important respects a crude one.[1] It is perhaps more appropriate to regard cochlear implant prostheses as creating a new, limited sensory repertoire, using the resources (possibly deteriorated) of the existing auditory nervous system. The potential development (and usefulness) of these kinds of devices are in one sense limited by an obviously imperfect ability to mimic normal auditory nerve array coding. At the same time, it is not bound by invariant cochlear-to-auditory nerve coding translations of sound to nerve discharge patterns imposed by the normally operating system.

In the development of these devices (as with other sensory substitution devices), investigators are faced with a choice between a) employing nerve discharge pattern simulation models; or b) developing a "new" information-based code. In the case of auditory implant prostheses, the practical choice between these alternatives cannot be made now, and perhaps not for many years. In favor of adopting a simulation approach, the recognition value of recorded speech might be of sufficient importance to justify adopting a more information-limited model. While nonsimulation devices are of potentially endless variety, any practical nonsimulation based prosthetic device would, of course, be constructed in a directed attempt to encode speech as intelligible. There are strict requirements of coding that the central nervous system doubtless demands be followed for the efficient encoding of speech as intelligible manifest in the speech descrimination literature.

Before considering possible configurations of such auditory substitution devices for lost audition, it is helpful to consider the limitations (from one point of view) and lack of normal imposed limitations (from another point of view) of a potential multielectrode prosthetic device.

CONFIGURATION OF SIMULATION-BASED PROSTHETIC DEVICES

A simulation-based (or any other) auditory prosthesis electrode driving system has two basic components, ie, a nerve stimulator, stimulating the auditory nerve array according to a given mimicking translation algorithm; and a sound (speech) processor. We shall consider some possible elementary designs of these devices for a practical simulation-based prosthesis.

Nerve Stimulator. Simulation-based multichannel nerve array stimulators must control excitation of auditory nerve fibers as a function of position across the nerve array, ie, *there must be some distributed, predictable control of nerve stimulation.* This is probably only achievable (with acceptable control) with the use of a series of bipolar stimulating elements, each individually exciting a restricted sector of the auditory nerve array.[1]

With such an array, each element (bipolar pair) can simulate the distributed auditory nerve response generated by a single fixed-frequency oscillator (eg, on the output stage of a frequency spectrum vocoder). Some obvious coding limitations of this "vocoder-simulation" model have been discussed by Merzenich et al.[1] Most significantly: 1) In modelling the excitation generated by a fixed frequency oscillator (ie, the neural response to a single tone) the *detailed* spatial pattern of excitation cannot be easily duplicated by a single electrode; 2) the normal asymmetric spread of activity[2,3] as a function of I cannot be easily duplicated; 3) the temporal encoding of stimulus period of lower frequency stimuli is seriously degraded.

A second distributed simulation strategy is to effect a *strict* nerve pattern discharge simulation.[4,5]

From the Departments of Otolaryngology and Physiology, Coleman Memorial Laboratory, University of California at San Francisco, San Francisco, California. This work was supported by NIH Contract N01-NS-7-2367, NIH Grant NS-11804, Hearing Research, Inc, and the Coleman Fund.

REPRINTS — Michael M. Merzenich, PhD, Department of Otolaryngology, Coleman Memorial Laboratory, HSE 863, University of California at San Francisco, San Francisco, CA 94143.

TABLE 1. POTENTIAL ACCOMPLISHMENTS AND LIMITATIONS OF A SIMULATION-BASED COCHLEAR ELECTRICAL STIMULUS PROSTHESIS*

Response Characteristic	*Sound Stimulation Normal Cochlea*	*Electrical Stimulation Channel Vocoder Simulation*	*Does It Matter?*
A) Spread of excitation across the auditory nerve array as a function of I	Asymmetrical growth with tonal stimulation favors spread toward base by about 2:1 up to 45-50 dB; at higher levels, excitation spreads very rapidly toward cochlear base.[2,3,6,9]	Spread of excitation vs I is roughly symmetrical, can reproduce equivalent rates of spread (ie, in both directions) vs I. When excitation spreads to adjacent channels, excitation pattern is irregular.	Simulation of the spread of response (length and position of electrically excited sector) is probably not crucial.†
B) Distribution of response magnitudes within excited region	At low sound levels, there are high discharge rates in the centers of excitation patterns and successively lower rates apical and basal to this hot center (see above cited studies).	All neurons excited by any channel are driven at similar mean firing rates. It is difficult to simulate normal internal spatial pattern structure (rate vs position) in detail.	Probably not; but uncertainty∮
C) Detail, distribution of activity within nerve array	30,000 lines of information to CNS, great overlap, redundancy	Limited number of stimulus channels (practical limit of probably 16-24 channels)	Probably not∳
D) Representation of stimulus period by temporal discharges of auditory nerve fibers	Excellent representation to 1-2 kHz; good to 3-4 kHz; gone by 6-7 kHz[10,11]	Excellent representation to about 200 Hz; degraded at higher frequencies; gone at 800-1000 Hz	Perhaps a fundamental limitation. No known solution§
E) Stochastic, random discharge of units	Successive discharge occurrence not dependent upon time of preceding discharge (beyond the absolute refractory period[11]	All or none driving to each brief stimulus pulse predominates. Fibers track stimulus rates together. Above maximum firing rates, next spike occurrence determined by fibers' absolute refractory periods	Consequences unknown. On given channels, no obvious solution with use of brief biphasic pulses‖
F) Relative time of occurrence of discharges as a function of cochlear place	7-10 msec travel time delays in response genesis, from base to apex.[11,12] Relationship of time of discharge vs cochlear position (and its variance vs cochlear position) is highly predicted.	Interchannel delays are simulatable; intrachannel delays can be controlled to some extent (but only symmetrically) by manipulation of stimulus waveform.	Probably crucial. Devices may rise or fall on the effectiveness of this simulation. ◊

*Characteristics A, B, D, E, and F relate to intrachannel considerations. Characteristics A, C, and F relate to distribution of activity evoked by the electrode array across the nerve array. The Table applies most directly to a channel vocoder simulation device with nonoverlapping channel stimulation.

†The speech detection threshold is about 40-50 dB SPL. At these levels, excitation patterns are relatively discrete, so that simulation of the rapid spread to the base observed at higher stimulus levels may be unnecessary. In a simulation device in which driving is effected with a strict nerve array simulation speech processor, it would be included in the simulation in any event, ie, different electrodes would be driven to reproduce the best facsimile of the overall excitation pattern. The relatively symmetrical excitation (simulating the modestly asymmetric peak of auditory excitation patterns) produced by bipolar electrodes is probably of no real consequence. With further development of stimulation arrays, a more and more sophisticated nerve array discharge pattern can presumably be effected.

∮Given a 16 or 24 channel array, a relatively detailed simulation of the nerve array representation of the speech waveform can be generated.[5] A crude *intrachannel* excitation pattern simulation is possible (by appropriate temporal distribution of stimuli of different amplitudes), but would invariably be somewhat crude if nonsimultaneous stimulation (producing complex field interactions in a large array) were to be avoided without serious limitation of maximum channel output rates and temporal resolution.[8,13]

∳A high-intelligibility representation of speech is achieved with an optimized 12-channel channel vocoder driving fixed frequency oscillators.[14,15] The described multichannel simulation-based prosthesis models generate a simulation of auditory nerve patterned discharge to fixed frequency oscillators of such a channel vocoder. Success or failure of these devices rides with the question as to whether simulation of fixed frequency oscillator responses encode necessary and sufficient information. Ultimate numbers of channels are limited by: Field interactions when electrodes are simultaneously stimulated. If no simultaneous stimulation is allowed, channel output rates (and temporal resolution) are inversely related to channel number.[8,13] When bipolar electrode elements have an intercontact spacing of less than about 0.5 mm, threshold for scala tympani stimulation is rapidly elevated.[1,7]

§Speech can be filtered at 300 Hz without losing intelligibility.[14] In unpublished studies with implanted patients, it appears that the relationships between time of discharge of neurons in different cochlear loci is more important than simulated "phase-locking" per se. There is no obvious remedy for the relatively limited phase-locking generated with pulsatile electrical stimulation.

‖It is difficult to assess the significance of an artificial disturbance of synchronizing of input delivered into the central nervous system. Response properties of central auditory (inferior colliculus) neurons driven by long trains of electrical stimuli do not appear to be very different from normal,[16,17] but psychophysical studies indicate dramatic effects dependent upon synchronizing of input. Some manipulation is possible simply by changing stimulus waveform, as indicated below.

◊ Firing simultaneity can be affected across a stimulated nerve sector by changing stimulus waveform, eg, pulse duration (the farther away from the bipolar electrode, the farther out the fiber lies on the strength-duration curve). Such patterns of relative synchronicity vs position have maxima at the electrode site (as they do in the normal cochlea). Faithfulness of simulation is untested; it is likely of crucial importance in development of simulation-based prostheses (and intrachannel control may be far more appropriate to effect this temporal distribution than interchannel control). Evidence suggesting the significance of such control will be the subject of a full report from this laboratory.

The requirements for the stimulation necessary to effect such a simulation are basically the same as required for vocoder output simulation. That is, restricted, highly controlled excitation must be effected by each channel of a multichannel electrode array. In one described model of this type,[5] each channel (short-length sector of auditory nerve) was stimulated either "on" or "off" (potentially simplifying stimulator design. In this kind of "true simulation" model, the attempt is to simulate as accurately as possible the complete distributed excitation of the auditory nerve array generated by corresponding sound stimuli in a normal ear. Thus, in a "vocoder-simulation" model, considerations in electrode element position and sound processing strategy are principally based on speech psychophysics; while in a strict simulation of eighth nerve spatiotemporal pattern discharge, principal considerations in electrode placement and sound processor design are based on coding studies of auditory nerve fiber discharge in the normal mammalian ear.

Most investigators who have attempted to construct multichannel cochlear prostheses are pursuing the "vocoder-simulation" model (although at least most are not stimulating the nerve array in a way in which it is possible to actually effect it).

Any of these simulation-based devices share basic fundamental design and coding limitations. Some of these are outlined later (Table 1).[1-17]

Speech Processor. Several kinds of speech processors might drive nerve array stimulators. For simulation-based prosthetic devices, two would appear most likely. Both are varieties of "channel vocoders."[14] First, a classic frequency spectrum vocoder could drive electrodes that individually model the driving output of fixed frequency oscillators. Second, a nerve array model simulator output could drive sectors of the auditory nerve to reproduce a complete or abbreviated facsimile of the predicted normal nerve array response. Again, such a model would be based on patterned distribution of excitation across the auditory nerve array.[2,3,5,6] A relatively simple model of this type has been developed by Kiang et al.[5] A device of this kind would be somewhat more difficult to construct than a channel vocoder, but could more faithfully represent higher-stimulus-level excitation patterns, and may have very significant advantages over simple frequency spectrum channel vocoder simulation.

CAN THESE SIMULATION MODELS ACTUALLY BE IMPLEMENTED?

All information necessary to implement these device models is now available. With ideally positioned bipolar electrode pairs, each with interelectrode spacings of about 1 mm[1,7,8] a series of restricted sectors of nerve, each 1, 2, of 3 mm long could be brought under excitation control. Studies of excitation patterns generated by bipolar electrodes in cats would allow an estimate of the suprathreshold nonoverlap boundaries. A physiological method for defining the nonoverlapping boundary condition noninvasively (by estimating electrode excitation patterns) using BSER recording in cats should be applicable in man.[18] (It might also be possible to define the nonoverlapping boundary condition psychoacoustically.)

Tests in animals and cadaver material suggest that appropriate multielectrode arrays can be safely implanted 20-25 mm into the scala tympani in man[4,19]* and that applicable electrodes driven at the top of the required dynamic range are probably within practical "safe" limits. Cochlear damage induced by electrical stimulation itself is probably only effected at levels of current above that required for operation of these devices.[20,21]

In practice, problems of achieving optimal electrode placement, and/or the variability in cochlear dendrite survival can produce about a 2-3x variation in threshold (from roughly 80 to about 300 μamp for 100 μsec/phase biphasic pulses) for different elements of a long multielectrode array. Discrete excitation of surviving ganglion cell soma can be effected in dendriteless cochlear regions of deaf animals.[7] However, where degeneration is patchy, because of differences in threshold some spatially inappropriate stimulation might occur.

Controllable multichannel excitation cannot be easily effected with use of "monopolar" electrodes, or with simple tested electrode arrays employing "common grounding" schemes.[8,13]

In summary, given present knowledge, *these simulation models can now be implemented with use of appropriate bipolar scala tympani multielectrode arrays.*

WILL THEY WORK?

Some of the obvious coding accomplishments and limitations of these simple simulation algorithms are tabulated in Table 1. Several features of response can be only crudely simulated (if at all). The relevance of all of these factors re coding of speech is not completely clear (Table 1). But given these simple stimulators, and given appropriate simulation based speech processors, it should be possible to establish some significant discrimination of speech with these devices.

COMPLEX COCHLEAR SIGNAL INTERACTIONS; SIGNAL TO NOISE PROBLEMS

In a complete simulation model, two-tone suppression effects and distortion product generation would be included (probably unnecessarily). They are possible to simulate. The operational attenuation of the response to noise in the presence of a behaviorally relevant signal (by the olivocochlear bundle or however) in the normal cochlea could not be easily simulated.

NONSIMULATION BASED PROSTHESIS

A true cochlear prosthesis optimist (there are many) might point out that electrical auditory nerve stimulation is, in a sense, *more* controllable than sound stimulation. Cochlear mechanics, transduction and characteristics of the hair-cell ganglion cell synapse follow strict rules of spatial and tem-

*O'Reilly B. Unpublished observations.

poral coding. As pointed out earlier, some of those coding rules can't be followed. But, with electrical stimulation, none must be. It is in this sense that a cochlear electrical stimulation prosthesis is potentially an auditory substitution device. Of course, use of any nonsimulation approach is conditioned by several factors. First, the speech recognition advantages of a simulation-based prosthesis would count heavily in favor of this approach, even if significantly higher discrimination could be effected with a nonsimulation prosthesis. Second, the nervous system has its own rules re the form of information it receives. They are poorly understood. But they will dictate what nonnormal coding will or will not work. Third, any prosthesis must be based on the coding of features of speech necessary for coding it as intelligible (imposed by its structure).

HOW CAN WE DECIDE BETWEEN THESE (OR OTHER) CODING POSSIBILITIES?

We can only decide between these coding possibilities by extensive psychophysical testing with appropriate model stimulators and sound processors in implanted human volunteers. The task is a very large one (especially when the domain of nonsimulation stimulators and speech processors is entered). Our strategy is to decide between these approaches (various facets) by a long series of directed psychophysical studies, driving computer-modeled stimulators with computer-modeled speech processors.[13,22] Given the possibilities, it should be possible to gain significant speech discrimination capabilities in at least a fraction of the profoundly deaf.

BUT WILL ANY ELECTRICAL STIMULATION PROSTHESIS WORK, GIVEN THE STATUS OF THE NERVE AND AUDITORY NERVOUS SYSTEM IN CANDIDATE PATIENT POPULATIONS?

There is a serious question as to whether or not significant speech discrimination can be effected in patients in whom nerve survival is partial and/or patchy. On the basis of nerve survival at the time of implantation, good speech discrimination in an "ideal" simulation-based prosthesis (electrodes arrayed across the speech frequency range) might be expected in 20-40% of the postlingually deaf. It is encouraging that we can discretely excite the invariable few surviving ganglion cells in "dentriteless" regions of severely degenerated cochleas.[7] But of what use such evoked, limited input might be must await appropriate psychophysical testing.

REFERENCES

1. Merzenich MM, White M, Vivion MC, Leake-Jones PA, Walsh SM. Some considerations of multichannel electrical stimulation of the auditory nerve in the profoundly deaf: interfacing electrode arrays with the auditory nerve array. Acta Otolaryngol (Stockh) 1979; 87:196-203.

2. Kim DO, Molnar CE. A population study of cochlear nerve fibers: comparison of spatial distributions of average-rate and phase-locking measures of responses to single tones. J Neurophysiol 1979; 42:16-30.

3. Evans EF. Place and time coding of frequency in the peripheral auditory system: some physiological pros and cons. Audiology 1978; 17:369-420.

4. White MW, Walsh SM, Schubert EA, Merzenich MM. Speech and stimulus processing considerations in the design of a prosthesis for the profoundly deaf. In: Leisman G, ed. Human factors in the design and development of prosthesis. New York: Pergamon Press, 1979.

5. Kiang NYS, Eddington DK, Delgutte B. Fundamental considerations in designing auditory implants. Acta Otolaryngol (Stockh) 1979; 87:203-19.

6. Tsuchitani C. Neural encoding of auditory information. In: McPherson DL, ed. Advances in prosthetic devices for the deaf. Rochester: National Technical Institute for the Deaf, 1978.

7. Merzenich MM, Jones P, Walsh S, Vivion M. 3rd Quarterly Progress Report, NIH Contract N01-NS-7-2367. Neural Prosthesis Contract Program, Bethesda: National Institutes of Health, 1978.

8. Merzenich M, White M. Cochlear implant. The interface problem. In: Hambrecht T, Reswick J, eds. Functional electrical stimulation: applications in neural prostheses. New York: Marcel Dekker, 1977.

9. Pfeiffer RR, Kim DO. Cochlear fiber responses: distribution along the cochlear partition. J Acoust Soc Am 1975; 58:867.

10. Anderson DJ, Rose JE, Hind JE, Brugge JF. Temporal position of discharges in single auditory nerve fibers within the cycle of a sine-wave stimulus: frequency and intensity effects. J Acoust Soc Am 1971; 49:1131-9.

11. Rose JE, Brugge JF, Anderson DJ, Hind JE. Phase-locked response to low frequency tones in single auditory nerve fibers in the squirrel monkey. J Neurophysiol 1967; 30:769-93.

12. Bekesy G von. Experiments in hearing. EG Weaver, ed. New York: McGraw Hill, 1978.

13. White MW. Design considerations of a prosthesis for the profoundly deaf. Thesis, UC Berkeley, Berkeley, Ca., 1978.

14. Flanagan JL. Speech analysis. Berlin: Springer-Verlag, 1972.

15. Carhart R. Minimum stimulation requirements for intelligibility. In: Merzenich M, Schindler RA, Sooy FA, eds. Electrical stimulation of the acoustic nerve in man. San Francisco: Velobind Inc, 1974:171-8.

16. Merzenich MM, Michelson RP, Pettit CR, Schindler RA, Reid M. Neural encoding of sound sensation evoked by electrical stimulation of the acoustic nerve. Ann Otol Rhinol Laryngol 1973; 82:486-504.

17. Merzenich MM. Intracochlear electrical stimulation with a bipolar electrode in animals and man. In: Merzenich M, Schindler RA, Sooy FA, eds. Electrical stimulation of the acoustic nerve in man. San Francisco: Velobind Inc, 1974.

18. White MW, Merzenich MM, Vivion MC. A non-invasive recording technique for evaluating electrode and nerve function in cochleas implanted with a multichannel electrode. In: McPherson DL, ed. Advances in prosthetic devices for the deaf. Rochester: National Technical Institute for the Deaf, 1978.

19. Schindler RA, Merzenich MM, White MW, Bjorkroth B. Multielectrode intracochlear implants. Arch Otolaryngol 1977; 103:691-9.

20. Merzenich MM, O'Reilly BF, Walsh S, Wong-Riley M, Leake-Jones P, Vivion M. 6th Quarterly Progress Report, NIH Contract N01-NS-7-2367. Neural Prosthesis Contract Program, Bethesda: National Institutes of Health, 1979.

21. Walsh SM, Merzenich MM, Schindler RA, Leake-Jones PA. Some practical considerations in development of multichannel scala tympani prosthesis. Audiology 1980; 19:164-75.

22. Eddington DK. Speech discrimination in deaf subjects with cochlear implants. J Acoust Soc Am 1979; 65 Suppl 1:103.

FREQUENCY ANALYSIS IN NORMAL AND HEARING-IMPAIRED LISTENERS

WALT JESTEADT, PhD

OMAHA, NEBRASKA

Recent studies of frequency analysis in listeners with normal hearing and in those with sensorineural hearing losses are reviewed and compared with related physiological data. These studies suggest that it is now possible to obtain detailed audiological or psychoacoustic data for human listeners that closely parallel physiological data obtained in eighth nerve recordings from animals. Implications of these developments for future research with impaired listeners are discussed.

The auditory system has a remarkable ability to resolve and analyze acoustic events in terms of frequency. Studies of frequency analysis in listeners with normal hearing have occupied a central position in auditory research since the time of Ohm and Helmholtz. Recent efforts in a number of laboratories to obtain detailed psychoacoustic data for listeners with sensorineural hearing loss also have focused on various aspects of frequency analysis.[1-6] Physiological data suggest that frequency analysis is a peripheral process that may be largely complete at the level of the eighth nerve.[7] We might expect, therefore, to find impaired frequency analysis in listeners with sensorineural hearing loss because it occurs at the same level as the lesion. Data from recent studies to be reviewed here confirm this expectation and indicate that detailed measures of frequency analysis may lead to a better understanding of the nature of sensorineural hearing loss.

Recent studies of frequency analysis reflect several important related trends in psychoacoustics and can best be understood in the context of those trends. The first of these is toward greater reliance upon physiological research as a source of ideas for new experiments and insights concerning existing data. We now use constructs derived from physiological data the way we once used constructs derived from circuit theory, communication theory, and information theory. The latter areas continue to have an important impact on our work, but there are many more references to basilar membrane mechanics and distributions of eighth nerve responses in the recent psychoacoustics literature than there are to square law devices and ideal detectors. This is particularly true in studies of frequency analysis because the frequency resolving power of the auditory system is the principal feature for which there is a clear correspondence between psychophysical, physiological, and anatomical data. Our current understanding of basilar membrane mechanics and the frequency selective tuning of single neurons in the eighth nerve allows us to account for many frequency analysis phenomena to a first approximation.

The second trend is toward greater theoretical interest in data obtained from impaired listeners. These data may allow us to parcel out closely related processes that cannot be observed independently in normal auditory systems and may therefore provide unique tests of theories of frequency analysis. They probably would not play such an important role were it not for the increased interest in physiological data. Our ability to relate data from normal and impaired listeners at a theoretical level depends in part upon our understanding of the differences in physiology associated with the impairments.

The third trend is toward greater emphasis on the relations among measures of frequency analysis and the relations between these measures and measures of temporal analysis, cochlear nonlinearities, and other theoretically related phenomena. This is evident in recent studies by Leshowitz and Lindstrom,[3] Wightman et al[5] and Festen et al.[8] One motive for this work is to demonstrate that many measures of frequency analysis are converging operations[9] that measure the same fundamental property of the auditory system. Another is to test predictions concerning relations between different properties of the system. Perhaps the most important incentive is the need to obtain a sufficient range of data for impaired listeners to be able to interpret abnormal results. Otherwise, it is often impossible to move beyond the circular conclusion that the results are different because the listener is impaired. In attempting to test theories of frequency analysis using impaired listeners, we are in effect attempting to solve equations with multiple unknowns, because we do not fully understand the nature of the im-

----

From the Department of Otolaryngology and Human Communication, Boys Town Institute/Creighton University School of Medicine, Omaha, Nebraska. This work was supported by the Boys Town Institute for Communication Disorders and by grants NS-14709 and 1-S08-RR09003 from the National Institutes of Health.

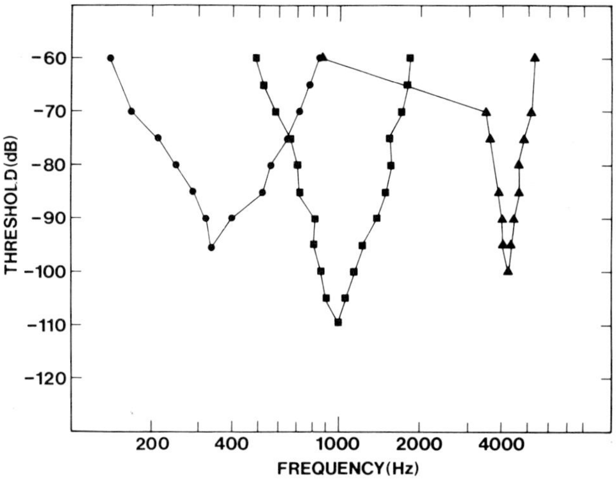

Fig. 1. Representative tuning curves for single neurons in the cat's auditory nerve. Characteristic frequencies were selected to match as closely as possible the probe tone frequencies in Figure 2. (Redrawn from Kiang et al[18].)

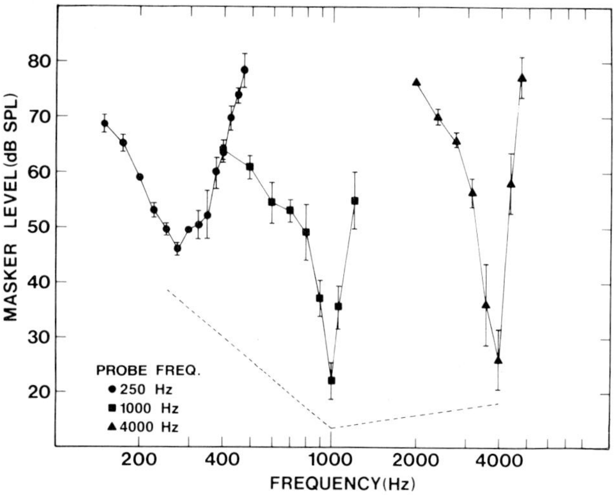

Fig. 2. Example of psychophysical tuning curves obtained with forward masking for listeners with normal hearing. The three functions are for probe frequencies of 250, 1000 and 4000 Hz. The data are means and standard errors for four subjects. Each subject was tested at 10 dB SL.

pairment. To be successful, we must solve a number of equations simultaneously.

A review of the entire literature concerning frequency and temporal analysis in normal and impaired listeners is well beyond the scope of this paper. This review will emphasize recent studies in two areas: measurement of psychophysical tuning curves in normal and impaired listeners and measurement of suppression. Frequency analysis is assessed in both of these areas in terms of the frequency selectivity exhibited in masking. This is an indirect measure, in that masking represents a failure of frequency selectivity, but for studies of impaired listeners it is a particularly appropriate one. Many listeners with sensorineural hearing losses describe problems that we might rephrase in terms of abnormal masking. Difficulty with speech perception in noise is one example.

PSYCHOPHYSICAL TUNING CURVES

Wegel and Lane[10] published the first comprehensive data that describe the masking of one tone by another. Masking patterns obtained by fixing the frequency and level of the masker and varying the frequency of the signal are generally asymmetric, showing more masking of high frequencies by low frequencies than of low frequencies by high. Masking patterns have been measured in listeners with sensorineural losses in several studies[11-16] and have been found to be more asymmetric than in listeners with normal hearing. This result has generally been described as abnormal upward spread of masking. The asymmetry in masking patterns for normal listeners can be accounted for in part by the asymmetry in the excitation pattern produced by the traveling wave on the basilar membrane.[17] The origin of abnormal upward spread of masking observed in listeners with sensorineural losses is less clear.

To answer questions of this kind, we must have psychophysical or audiological measures that more closely parallel physiological measures of auditory function. By changing the tonal masking experiment slightly, it is possible to obtain masking patterns analogous to tuning curves recorded from single neurons in the eighth nerve.[18] Eighth nerve tuning curves can be thought of as threshold functions or audiograms for individual neurons. Several important features of tuning curves are apparent in the examples taken from Kiang et al,[18] shown in Figure 1. Each neuron has a single frequency to which it is most sensitive, high frequency neurons have proportionally narrower tuning curves (sharper tuning), and high frequency neurons show more asymmetry. These features all reflect the fact that the response of each neuron is determined by the activity at a specific location on the basilar membrane; and the location of maximum activity, the peak of the traveling wave, is determined by the frequency of the stimulus.

To obtain a psychophysical measure analogous to physiological tuning curves, we must structure the task so that the same relationships hold. This can be done by using a fixed low level (10 dB SL) tone as the signal. Presumably, only a limited number of neurons will respond to such a signal. We then use a tonal masker in which frequency is varied systematically and we adjust the level of the masker until it just masks the fixed signal. This is presumably equivalent to the point at which the neurons tuned to the signal frequency also begin to respond to the activity generated by the masker. Masking patterns of this type were first obtained for listeners with normal hearing by Small,[19] Vogten,[20] and Zwicker[21] using simultaneous maskers and a number of different psychophysical methods. Figure 2 shows three psychophysical tuning curves obtained in our

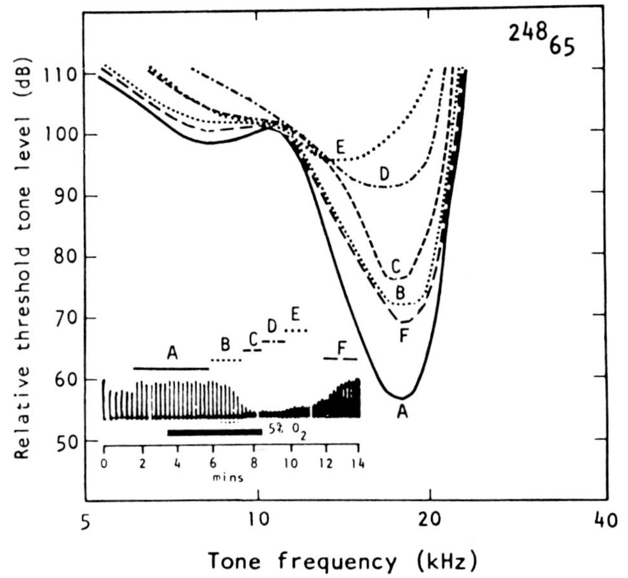

Fig. 3. Reversible effects of hypoxia on the tuning of a single cochlear fiber in the cat. (From Evans EF.[7] Reprinted with permission.)

laboratory recently using forward masking and a two interval, forced choice, adaptive procedure. They have all of the features noted in the physiological tuning curves shown in Figure 1. Although we cannot expect behavioral data to follow precisely the same pattern observed in physiological data for single neurons, recent studies indicate a number of similarities between tuning curves obtained at these two levels. The ability to obtain psychophysical data that are analogous in some respects to physiological tuning curves is particularly important in research involving impaired listeners. It allows us to make predictions concerning the nature of the impairment in physiological terms and to test those predictions in experiments with human subjects.

Much of the interest in tuning curve data for impaired listeners stems from demonstrations by Evans[7,22] and Evans and Wilson[23] of loss of tuning in eighth nerve tuning curves following various cochlear lesions. One example, from Evans,[22] is shown in Figure 3. The curve showing the poorest tuning has no finely tuned tip and has the shape we might expect to see based on the pattern of the traveling wave on the basilar membrane. Note that this loss of fine tuning is reversible. A number of investigators have obtained psychophysical tuning curve data for impaired listeners.[1-3,5,6,24] Examples of curves presented by Hoekstra and Ritsma,[2] Leshowitz and Lindstrom,[3] and Wightman et al[5] are shown in Figures 4, 5, and 6, respectively. In general, listeners with moderate sensorineural losses show broader tuning curves in the regions of the losses. This is true even when the data are compared with those for listeners with normal hearing tested at the same SPL. In tests using simultaneous masking, in regions where the loss is 50 dB or more, the tuning curves show an unusual W-shaped pattern first noted by Leshowitz et al.[25] The listeners apparently hear a roughness cue, not a combination tone, that makes the probe difficult to mask using maskers close to the probe tone in frequency. The majority of the tuning curves for impaired listeners continue to show some tuning, even at high levels. The tips of the tuning curves, however, are often missing.

Other parallels between physiological and psychophysical tuning curves have also been noted. Kiang and Moxon[26] have shown that eighth nerve fibers can also be "detuned" using a narrow band of noise a decade down in frequency from the characteristic frequency of the fiber. The noise causes a loss of sensitivity only at the tip of the tuning curve. A portion of their data is reproduced in Figure 7. O'Malley and Feth[27] have recently demonstrated the same effect in psychophysical tuning curves, using a probe at 3000 Hz and a narrow band noise at 300 Hz. A portion of their data is reproduced in Figure 8.

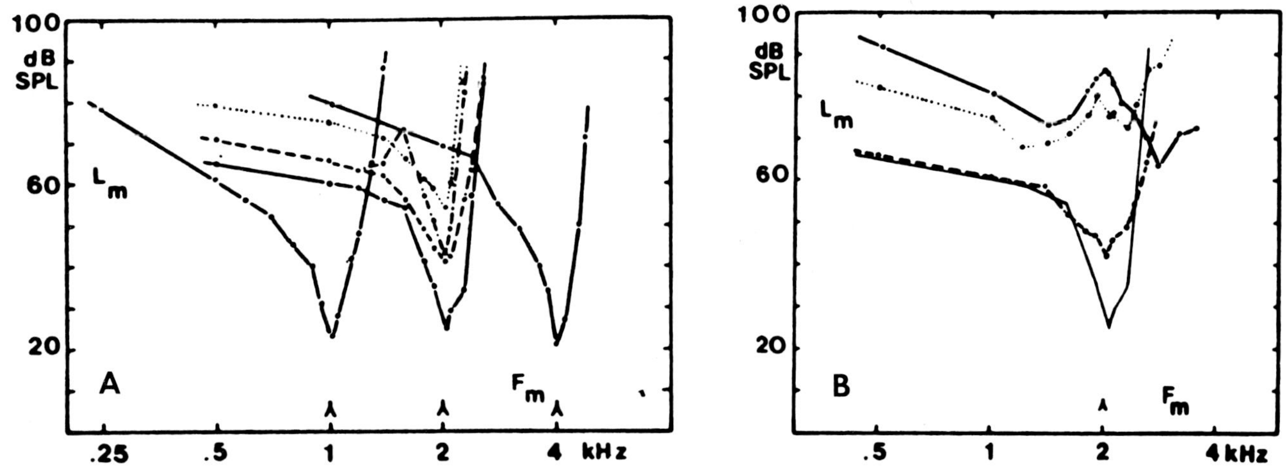

Fig. 4. Psychophysical tuning curves for A) one listener with normal hearing, and B) three listeners with sensorineural losses. The loss at the probe frequency is 30 dB for the dashed line, 50 dB for the dotted line, and 65 dB for the solid line. (From Hoekstra and Ritsma.[2] Reprinted with permission.)

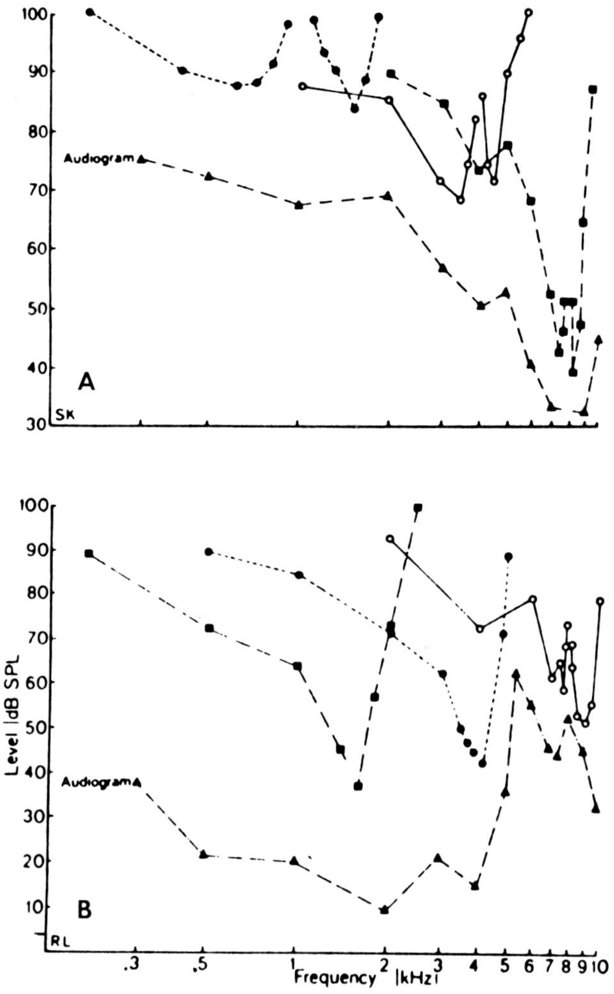

Fig. 5. Psychophysical tuning curves for two listeners with sensorineural losses. A) Sloping low frequency hereditary loss, B) High frequency loss due to acoustic trauma. (From Leshowitz and Lindstrom.[3] Reprinted with permission.)

A number of problems associated with psychophysical tuning curves should be noted. When the SPL of the probe tone is increased, as it is to maintain constant sensation level in tests of impaired listeners, combination tones begin to play an important role, the curves become broader, and the tip of the tuning curve moves away from the probe tone frequency.[1,20,28]

Some of these problems can be avoided by using a forward masking procedure but at least two of them remain. The first is that forward masking decays more rapidly over time as the difference in frequency between the masker and probe increases.[29,30] This means that the width or sharpness of tuning curves measured with a forward masking procedure is a function of the interval between masker and probe. The second problem is that as the probe intensity is increased in either simultaneous or forward masking, a wider region of the basilar membrane is stimulated and the subject has the option of listening in a frequency region away from the masker. This should cause the tuning curve to be sharper than it would otherwise be. Johnson-Davies and Patterson[31] have recently verified this hypothesis, using a band of noise in addition to the sinusoidal masker to prevent the subject from listening off frequency. There may well be other factors that influence the shape of psychophysical tuning curves. Until we understand all of these factors and the ways in which they interact with probe tone frequency and level, we will be unable to make comparisons in absolute terms with physiological data.

Although there are a number of problems in interpreting psychophysical tuning curves, we have no other measure that yields psychophysical data that so closely parallel physiological data under a number of conditions, including cochlear impairment and low frequency masking. The recent high level of activity in this area will no doubt continue, and it is quite possible that a simplified form of the tuning curve procedure, such as the one Zwicker and Schorn[6] have developed, will become a standard audiometric measure.

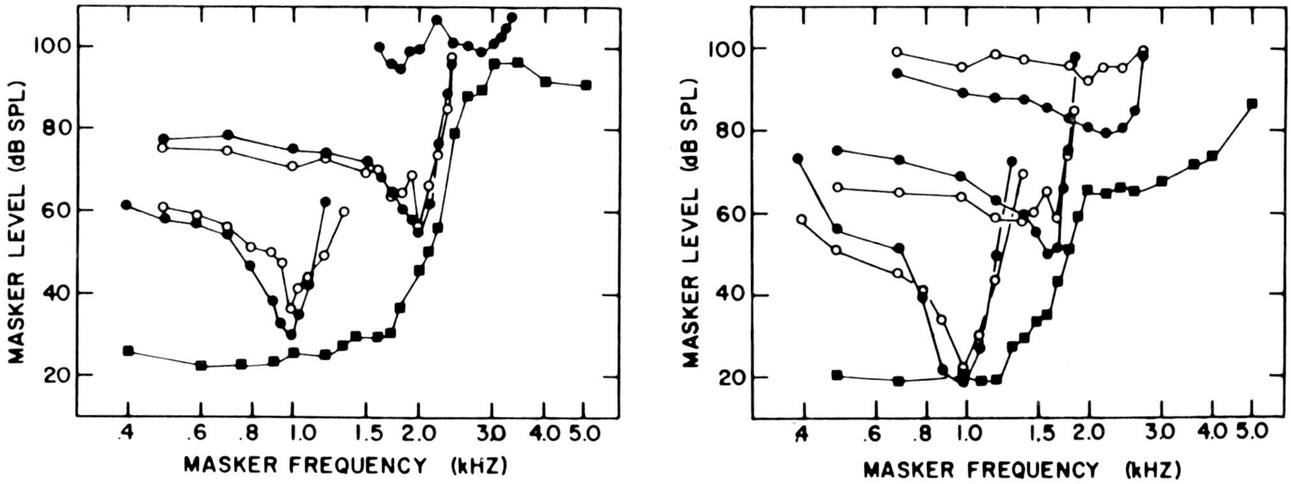

Fig. 6. Psychophysical tuning curves for two listeners with sensorineural losses. Open circles are for simultaneous masking, filled circles are for forward masking, and the squares show thresholds for the 20 msec probe. (From Wightman et al.[5] Reprinted with permission.)

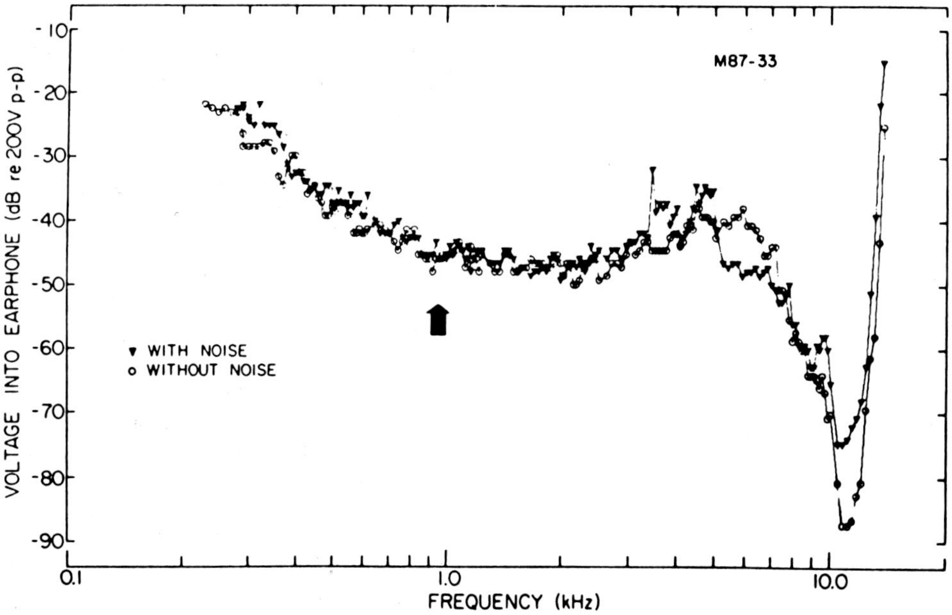

Fig. 7. Effect of a low frequency continuous noise on the tuning of an eighth nerve fiber with high characteristic frequency. (From Kiang and Moxon.[26] Reprinted with permission.)

PSYCHOPHYSICAL MEASURES OF SUPPRESSION

The second group of studies to be discussed deal with the suppression of masking. This area of research contains the fewest studies of impaired listeners but may eventually have the greatest impact on our understanding of the nature of sensorineural hearing loss and on future hearing aid design. As we noted above, a number of authors have speculated on the role of lateral inhibition in the frequency selectivity exhibited in masking experiments. Lateral inhibition or suppression has been clearly demonstrated in responses of single eighth nerve fibers by Sachs and Kiang[32] and in psychophysical masking studies by Houtgast.[33-35]

In physiological studies, suppression is defined as the reduction in the response to an excitatory tone at frequency f(1) that accompanies the addition of a suppressor tone at f(2). Maximum suppression is observed in conditions where f(2) is above f(1) in frequency. Javel et al[36] have shown that given these conditions, the amount of suppression in dB depends only on the level of f(2) and the distance on the basilar membrane between the traveling wave maxima for f(1) and f(2). This suggests that suppression is due to interactions between the spatial patterns on the basilar membrane at either a mechanical or a neural level.

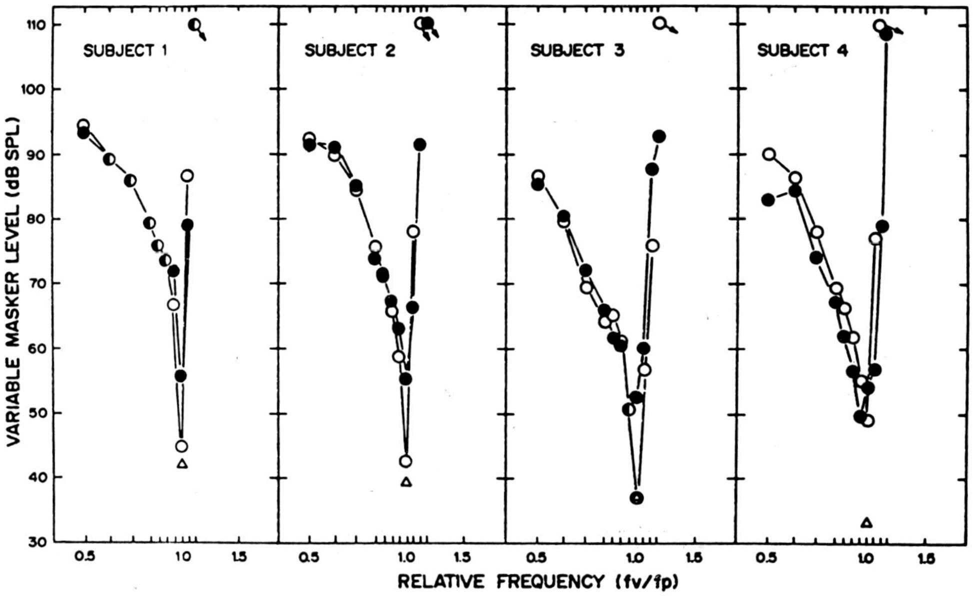

Fig. 8. Effect of a low frequency noise on the tips of psychophysical tuning curves. (From O'Malley and Feth.[27] Reprinted with permission.)

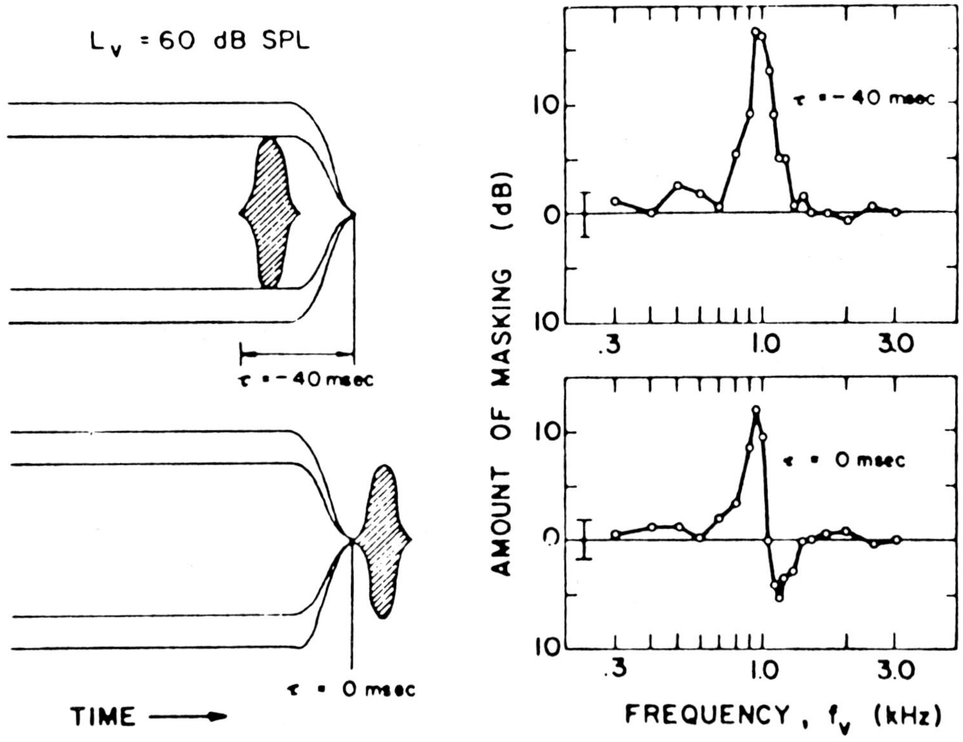

Fig. 9. Two tone suppression measured in a forward masking paradigm. The probe tone and one component of the masker are at 1000 Hz. The second component of the masker, called the suppressor, takes one of several values, some of which result in less masking than when the suppressor is not present at all. (From Shannon.[37] Reprinted with permission.)

In psychophysical studies, suppression is defined as a reduction in the effective level of a stimulus that accompanies the addition of a second stimulus. It has been studied most frequently in a forward masking procedure where the addition of a tone or noise to a masker causes a decrease in forward masking. The procedure and the resulting data are shown in Figure 9, from Shannon.[37] The frequen-

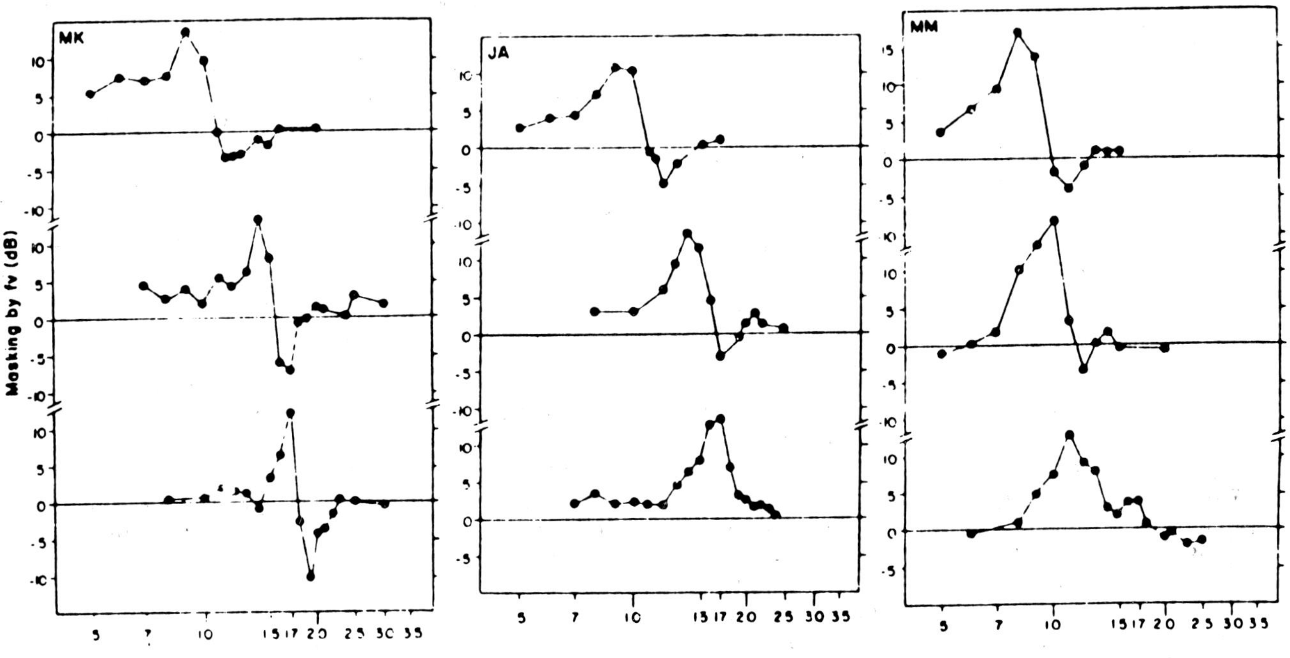

Fig. 10. Two tone suppression measurements from one listener (listener 1) with normal hearing and two listeners (listeners 2 and 3) with sensorineural losses. For listeners 1 and 2, probe frequencies from top to bottom were 1000 Hz, 1500 Hz and 2000 Hz. For listener 3, they were 900 Hz, 1000 Hz and 1200 Hz. Listeners 2 and 3 show no suppression in the two bottom panels, where the suppressors are located on the slopes of the losses. Tuning curves and audiograms for listeners 2 and 3 are shown in Figure 6. (From Wightman et al.[5] Reprinted with permission.)

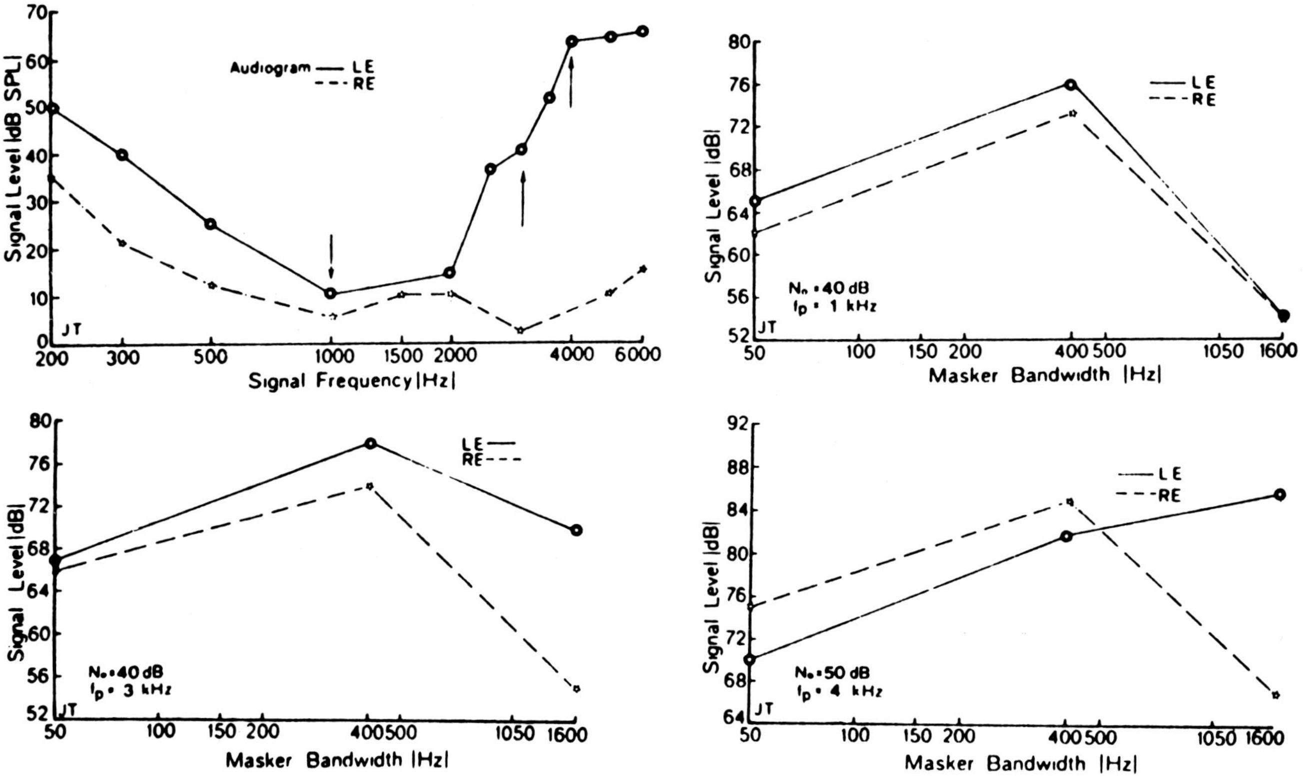

Fig. 11. Suppression measured in a band widening experiment for a listener with a unilateral sensorineural loss. In the normal ear, the threshold always improves as the masker bandwidth increases from 400 to 1600 Hz in a forward-masking procedure. This does not occur for the impaired ear at 4000 Hz (lower right panel). (From Leshowitz and Lindstrom.[3] Reprinted with permission.)

cies of the probe tone and one component of the masker are fixed while the frequency of the second component of the masker is varied. Note the dip in the function in the region of 1,200 Hz, indicating less forward masking when a 1,200 Hz component is added to the masker than when the masker consists of a single component at 1000 Hz.

Similar data obtained for one listener with normal hearing and two listeners with sensorineural losses are shown in Figure 10, from Wightman et al.[5] There is no suppression when the suppressor is in the frequency region on the slope of a high frequency loss. These results must be treated with caution, however, because there are also subjects with otherwise normal hearing who fail to show suppression.[37]

Leshowitz and Lindstrom[3] have also published data for an impaired listener who failed to show suppression in the region of the loss. These data are shown in Figure 11. The authors used noise as the suppressor of a sinusoidal masker in a forward masking paradigm. As the noise bandwidth is increased for a constant spectrum level noise, the noise outside the region of the critical band around the sinusoidal masker suppresses the masker and results in less forward masking. This does not occur, however, for the impaired ear at high frequencies. Weber[38] has reported detailed data for similar conditions for subjects with normal hearing. The large suppression effects normally observed with this procedure make it a good candidate for use in future work with impaired listeners.

Relations between psychophysical tuning curve data and suppression data in both the study by Leshowitz and Lindstrom[3] and the study by Wightman et al[5] led both groups of authors to suggest that the same mechanism was responsible for the finely tuned tips of tuning curves and for suppression. O'Malley and Feth[27] reached a similar conclusion. The large suppression effects observed in listeners with normal hearing for noise stimuli suggest that the suppression mechanism plays an important role in the perception of broadband stimuli such as speech. Suppression reflects a nonlinear transformation of the stimulus[39,40] that is very different from the transformations currently being investigated in hearing aid research. It is possible that aided speech perception could be improved by introducing transformations of the kind suggested by the data from studies of suppression, although we must recognize that only some of the components that normally produce these transformations are actually missing.

The recent research in frequency analysis summarized here suggests that it is now possible to obtain psychophysical measures of hearing that correspond to physiological measures of peripheral processing and, therefore, to interpret psychophysical data in terms of physiological mechanisms.

With additional research, it may be possible to obtain sufficient understanding of the peripheral processing of complex stimuli to specify the transformations of those stimuli that would be required to compensate for abnormal frequency analysis in impaired listeners.

ACKNOWLEDGMENTS — The help of Kevin Guthrie, Robert Guthrie, Doug Mellen, and Donna Neff in the preparation of this manuscript is gratefully acknowledged.

REFERENCES

1. Carney AE. An analysis of psychophysical tuning curves in normal and pathological ears. Dissertation, University of Minnesota, 1977.

2. Hoekstra A, Ritsma RJ. Perceptive hearing loss and frequency selectivity. In: Evans EF, Wilson JP, eds. Psychophysics and physiology of hearing. London: Academic Press, 1977.

3. Leshowitz B, Lindstrom R. Measurement of nonlinearities in listeners with sensorineural hearing loss. In: Evans EF, Wilson JP, eds. Psychophysics and physiology of hearing. London: Academic Press, 1977.

4. Pick G, Evans EF, Wilson JP. Frequency resolution in patients with hearing loss of cochlear origin. In: Evans EF, Wilson JP, eds. Psychophysics and physiology of hearing. London: Academic Press, 1977.

5. Wightman FL, McGee T, Kramer M. Factors influencing frequency selectivity in normal and hearing-impaired listeners. In: Evans EF, Wilson JP, eds. Psychophysics and physiology of hearing. London: Academic Press, 1977.

6. Zwicker E, Schorn K. Psychoacoustical tuning curves in audiology. Audiology 1978; 17:120-40.

7. Evans EF. Auditory frequency selectivity and the cochlear nerve. In: Zwicker E, Terhardt E, eds. Facts and models in hearing. New York: Springer-Verlag, 1974.

8. Festen JM, Houtgast T, Plomp R, Smoorenburg GF. Relations between individual differences of auditory functions. In: Evans EF, Wilson JP, eds. Psychophysics and physiology of hearing. London: Academic Press, 1977.

9. Garner WR, Hake HW, Eriksen CW. Operationism and the concept of perception. Psychol Rev 1956; 63:149-59.

10. Wegel RL, Lane CE. The auditory masking of one pure tone by another and its probable relation to the dynamics of the inner ear. Physiol Rev 1924; 23:266-85.

11. Jerger J, Tillman TW, Peterson JL. Masking by octave bands of noise in normal and impaired ears. J Acoust Soc Am 1960; 32:385-90.

12. Keith RW, Anderson CV. Remote masking for listeners with cochlear impairment. J Acoust Soc Am 1969; 46:393-8.

13. Martin MC. Critical bands in sensorineural hearing loss. Scand Audiol 1974; 3:133-40.

14. Martin EM, Pickett JM. Sensorineural hearing loss and upward spread of masking. J Speech Hear Res 1970; 13:426-37.

15. DeBoer E, Bowmeester J. Critical bands and sensorineural hearing loss. Audiology 1974; 13:236-59.

16. Rittmanic PA. Pure-tone masking by narrow-noise bands in normal and impaired ears. J Audiol Res 1962; 2:287-304.

17. Zwicker E. Masking and physiological excitation as consequences of the ear's frequency analysis. In: Plomp R, Smoorenburg GF, eds. Frequency analysis and periodicity detection in hearing. Leiden: Sijthoff, 1970.

18. Kiang NYS, Watanabe T, Thomas EC, Clark LF. Discharge patterns of single fibers in the cat's auditory nerve. Cambridge: MIT Press, 1965.

19. Small AM. Pure tone masking. J Acoust Soc Am 1959; 31:1619-25.

20. Vogten LLM. Pure-tone masking: a new result from a new method. In: Zwicker E, Terhardt E, eds. Facts and models in hearing. New York: Springer-Verlag, 1974.

21. Zwicker E. On a psychoacoustical equivalent of tuning curves. In: Zwicker E. Terhardt E, eds. Facts and models in hearing. New York: Springer-Verlag, 1977.

22. Evans EF. Temporary sensorineural hearing losses and 8th nerve changes. In: Henderson D, Hamernik RD, Dosanjh DS, Mills JH, eds. Effects of noise on hearing. New York: Raven Press, 1976.

23. Evans EF, Wilson J. The frequency selectivity of the cochlea. In: Moller A, ed. Basic mechanisms in hearing. New York: Academic Press, 1973.

24. Florentine M. Psychoacoustical tuning curves and narrowband masking in normal and impaired hearing. J Acoust Soc Am 1978; 63:S44A.

25. Leshowitz B, Lindstrom R, Zurek P. Measurements of frequency selectivity in listeners with sensorineural hearing loss. J Acoust Soc Am 1976; 59:52-3A.

26. Kiang NYS, Moxon EC. Tails of tuning curves of auditory-nerve fibers. J Acoust Soc Am 1974; 55:620-30.

27. O'Malley H, Feth LL. Relationship between auditory frequency selectivity and two-tone suppression. J Acoust Soc Am 1978; 63:530A.

28. Rodenburg M, Verschuure JV, Brocaar MP. Comparison of two masking methods. Acustica 1974; 31:99-106.

29. Rodenburg M, Verschuure JV, Brocaar MP. Comment on Wightman et al (1977). In: Evans EF, Wilson JP, eds. Psychophysics and physiology of hearing. London: Academic Press, 1977.

30. Widin GP, Viemeister NF. Intensity effects in forward masking: implications for psychophysical tuning curves. J Acoust Soc Am 1978; 63:S44A.

31. Johnson-Davies D, Patterson R. Psychophysical tuning curves: the width of the signal's excitation pattern. J Acoust Soc Am 1978; 63:S29A.

32. Sachs MB, Kiang NYS. Two-tone inhibition in auditory nerve fibers. J Acoust Soc Am 1968; 43:1120-8.

33. Houtgast T. Psychophysical evidence for lateral inhibition in hearing. J Acoust Soc Am 1972; 51:1885-94.

34. Houtgast T. Psychophysical experiments on 'Tuning Curves' and 'Two-Tone Inhibition.' Acustica 1973; 29:168-79.

35. Houtgast T. Lateral suppression in hearing. Dissertation, Institute for Perception, Soesterberg, The Netherlands, 1974.

36. Javel E, Geisler CD, Ravindran A. Two-tone suppression in auditory nerve of the cat: rate-intensity and temporal analyses. J Acoust Soc Am 1977; 63:1093-1104.

37. Shannon RV. Two-tone unmasking and suppression in a forward masking situation. J Acoust Soc Am 1976; 59:1460-70.

38. Weber DL. Suppression and critical bands in band-limiting experiments. J Acoust Soc Am 1978; 64:141-50.

39. Duifhuis H. Cochlear nonlinearity and second filter: possible mechanism and implications. J Acoust Soc Am 1976; 59:408-23.

40. Duifhuis H. Cochlear nonlinearity and second filter — a psychophysical evaluation. In: Evans EF, Wilson JP, eds. Psychophysics and physiology of hearing. London: Academic Press, 1977.

TIME COURSE OF AUDITORY PERCEPTUAL LEARNING

CHARLES S. WATSON PhD

OMAHA, NEBRASKA

The time course of auditory perceptual learning can vary from one hour to more than a year, depending on the task, the complexity of the sounds, and the level of stimulus uncertainty under which the tasks are learned. Previous studies are reviewed which show that longer training is required to identify sounds than to discriminate between them, while the least time-consuming task is to learn to detect a sound's presence. The time course of each of these tasks is greatly extended for complex sounds compared to those for single tones. The learning of a speech-like code would thus be expected to require longer training than that employed in previous psychoacoustic research. The consequences of this fact for the exploitation of residual hearing are briefly discussed.

This talk will depart somewhat from the direction of the preceding discussions of auditory research, which were primarily aimed at the properties of the peripheral auditory system. We do know, of course, that perception is explained at both the receptor organ level and at various stages upstream from the cochlea. Figure 1 is simply a reminder that our colleagues in vision have long been aware that visual perception must be understood in terms of much more than the mere physical properties of stimuli displayed on the retinal mosaic. In one of the earliest demonstrations, Necker,[1] in 1832, showed us the cube that bears his name (Fig. 1A). Viewers persist in seeing this two-dimensional stimulus as a three-dimensional object, either on a plane surface sloping down, or they reorganize it to be seen on a plane surface sloping up, but of course cannot see it both ways at once. In the so-called "birdbath illusion," Rubin[2] emphasized the role of assumed distance (Fig. 1B). If you look at the faces, the white area recedes into the distance, but when you focus on the birdbath the black area recedes. In the demonstration by Leeper[3] (Fig. 1C) one can see either, in his terms, a mother-in-law or a young wife and, of course, there are many reasons that you may be biased to initially see one or the other. Many studies have shown that your probability of seeing one or the other version of such ambiguous figures can be modified by various kinds of prior experience.

Many people do not see what's wrong with Kendler's poster[4] (Fig. 1D). The fact is that you *don't* see what's wrong with it until you look at it quite a long time, and Kendler's point was that processing of certain types of visual information depends enormously on expectancy and the psychological set that you bring to task.

Personal subjective experiences like those with visual illusions can provide compelling demonstrations that the same stimulus can result in more than one percept, and that prior experience is a major determinant of perception. But to convince ourselves that perception really changes in someone else, someone we are studying in an experimental context, we usually have to rely on demonstrations that that person can do one of several things in response to the stimulus. Most simply, if our concern is perception by another person, then he or she must demonstrate the ability to either detect, discriminate, or identify an uncertain stimulus. If a listener can do all three of these for a given set of stimuli, then we feel comfortable in claiming that they have adequate sensitivity, resolving power, and the channel capacity and storage required to process those stimuli. Over the course of time, a listener's ability to detect or discriminate or identify sounds may improve or change, and in a number of experiments in the literature it is rather clear that the time course of these changes varies enormously, depending on the tasks, on the stimuli, and on the way that those tasks are taught.

While visual perception has been clearly shown to change with experience, it has been convenient to assume that auditory perception is a less dynamic process, as though we simply "hear" whatever acoustic waveforms enter our ear canals, so long as they are within our range of frequency sensitivity. Although there have been only a few studies of auditory perceptual learning, compared to the hundreds in vision, those studies clearly show that we do learn to hear selected properties of sounds. To my knowledge there has been no attempt in recent years to summarize the facts of auditory perceptual learning, and that is what I'll try to do here.

Figure 2 is from one of the most widely cited studies of auditory detection learning for simple tones in a noise background. Gundy[5] trained groups of 30 listeners in about one hour to detect a tone. The dependent variable, d_s, reflects the listeners' abilities to distinguish between the tonal signals and

From the Human Communication Research Laboratories, Boys Town Institute, and the Department of Otolaryngology and Human Communication, Creighton University School of Medicine, Omaha, Nebraska. Supported in part by grants from the National Institute of Neurological and Communicative Disorders and Stroke and the Division of Research Resources of the National Institutes of Health.

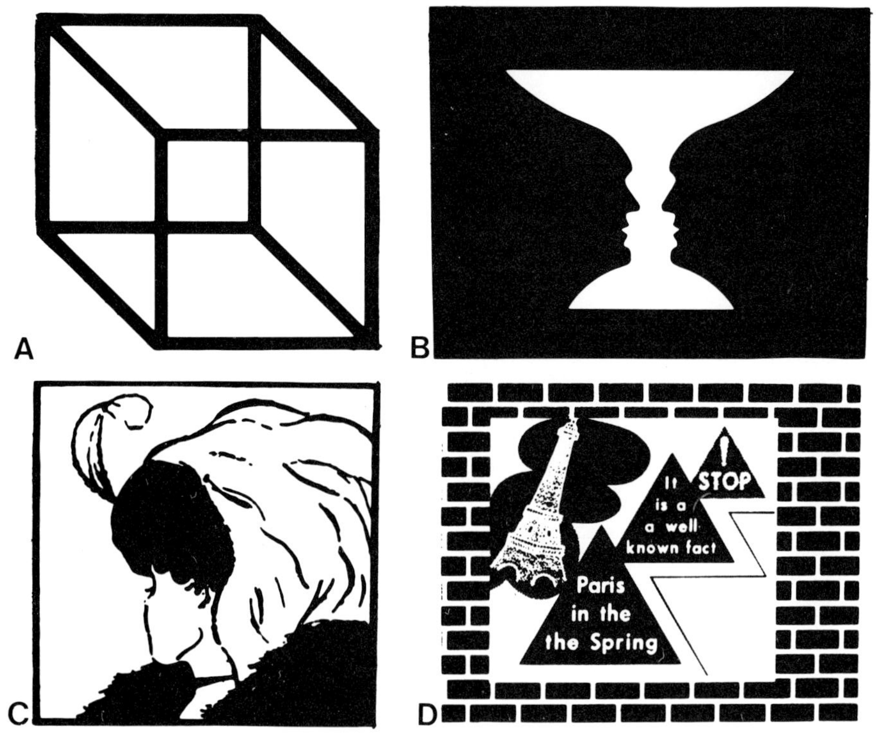

Fig. 1 A-D. Examples of some common stimuli used in the study of psychological factors in visual perception. (C - From Leeper.[3] D - From Kendler.[4] Reprinted with permission.)

the background noise, and is relatively unaffected by changes in their decision strategies.[6] He found that whether he gave the subjects feedback (F) after every trial, or not, and whether or not they were given a demonstration of the stimulus (S) before the experiment began, learning was complete in about an hour. At the break between the 6th and 7th blocks of trials, he gave a demonstration to all groups of subjects. Table 1 summarizes a few studies of this type, some done in our laboratory at CID, some by Gundy, and some by Zwislocki et al.[7] We find that they seem to agree that most simple detection learning is over in about an hour. That's a useful fact, because it says that the audiological endeavor is a reasonable one. Parenthetically, our data and those of Zwislocki et al suggest that it's not quite so reasonable at very low frequencies, where learning may go on for a bit longer.

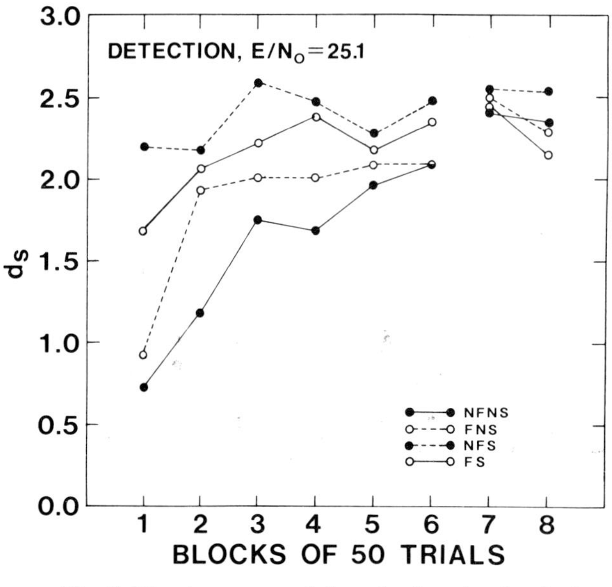

Fig. 2. The time course of detection learning for single tones presented in a broadband noise as reported by Gundy.[5] The four conditions are average data for listeners tested with and without trial-by-trial feedback (F) and with and without demonstrations of the signal to be detected (S). (Reprinted with permission.)

Next, let's turn to discrimination. Figure 3 shows the time course for learning the discrimination of two tonal frequencies, as studied by Auerbach.[8] He reported his data for several blocks of trials in each of four one-hour training sessions. Learning oc-

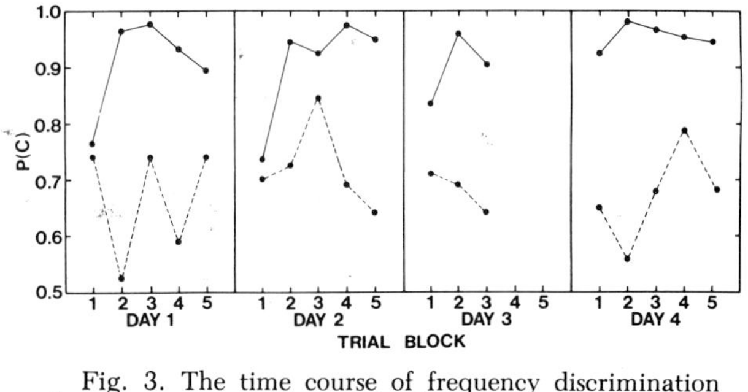

Fig. 3. The time course of frequency discrimination learning as reported by Auerbach.[8] (● —— ● - feedback; ● - - - ● - no feedback.) The major learning effect was seen in the first trial block of each one-hour session. The use of percent correct as the dependent variable may give a misleading picture of the course of learning. (Reprinted with permission.)

TABLE 1. TIME COURSE OF PERCEPTUAL LEARNING: AUDITORY DETECTION

	Task (Method)	*Stimulus*	*Est. Trials to Asymptote*	*Est. Time to Asymptote*
Zwislocki, Maire, Feldman and Rubin[7]	Fixed frequency Bekesy	100 Hz tone in quiet	20 Bekesy runs (5 mm/run)	1⅔ hours
	Fixed frequency Bekesy	1 kHz tone in quiet	20 Bekesy runs (5 mm/run)	1⅔ hours
Gundy[5]	Single interval rating (NFS)	1 kHz tone	300	<1 hour
Watson, Franks and Hood[18]	Sweep frequency Bekesy and 2AFC	125 Hz tone in quiet	NA	<1 week
	Sweep frequency Bekesy and 2AFC	1 kHz tone in quiet	NA	<1 week

curred mainly in the first trial block, in the data shown by the solid lines (the feedback conditions). What was happening in the later blocks isn't at all obvious. That is one of the shortcomings of many experiments that persist in using percent correct as the measure of performance. It's very hard to interpret percent correct judgments that are in the vicinity of 100%. We are quite sure from later experiments that further learning occurs beyond the time at which 100% correct discrimination is first approached. Nevertheless, the first-block data suggest a somewhat longer time course for discrimination learning than for detection. If we look at some other discrimination experiments the time to reach asymptotic discrimination performance is typically at least double that for the detection of simple stimuli. Table 2 summarizes the results of several studies of the learning of frequency discrimination.

The task that we are ultimately concerned with in auditory information processing is identification, not detection or discrimination. Figure 4 shows data for a simple identification task studied by Tanner and Rivette.[9] The stimulus was a pip (a very brief amplitude increment) that could occur at one of four positions on a tonal ramp. The ramp rose in one ear and, simultaneously, fell in the other, and the task was to identify the time at which the pip occurred on the ramp carrier. The special feature of these stimuli was that they were unlike any sounds in the listener's experience. As shown in the figure, their abilities to correctly identify the four sounds rose systematically over a period of at least 25 hours.

Figure 5 shows one of the oldest but best documented studies of the learning of an auditory identification task. Bryan and Harter[10] in 1899 studied the time required for railroad telegraphers to learn Morse code. The important point for us is that the time course to learn to correctly identify coded letters was systematic, but extremely long compared to other auditory tasks. These people worked four to six hours a day, for forty weeks, but were still far from asymptotic performance. Mainline performance for excellent operators was up to 180 to 200 letters per minute. In information theory terms, those operators were processing information at a rate of five to nine bits per second. That rivals the bit rate of information transmission in slow-paced connected discourse. This remarkable auditory performance is appreciated even more in light of the fact that the operators "chatted" with each other when not otherwise occupied, and laughed at each others' jokes! Table 3 shows the results of the Bryan and Harter study, plus several other experiments on the learning of simpler auditory identification tasks. Max Meyer[11] taught himself "perfect" pitch in 24 to 48 weeks; other people working with lower numbers of stimuli accomplished that same task somewhat more rapidly. One of the most recent and frequently cited studies of auditory identification is by Warren,[12] using sequences of three sounds. When he trained listeners until they mastered his task, requiring approximately six hours, the duration of the sequences that could be correctly identified dropped from more than 600 to less than 60 milliseconds.

In our own work,[13-17] we have been studying the discrimination of tonal sequences that are designed to have a similar frequency range and temporal complexity to those of spoken words. Figure 6 shows data collected when we used a forced choice task, and asked listeners to make what we call a minimal uncertainty discrimination; the tonal sequence or

TABLE 2. TIME COURSE OF PERCEPTUAL LEARNING: AUDITORY DISCRIMINATION

	Task (Method)	*Stimulus*	*Est. Trials to Asymptote*	*Est. Time to Asymptote*
Campbell and Small[19]	Frequency discrimination (2AFC)	800 msec-2 kHz tones in quiet	2600	4 hours
Loeb and Holding[20]	Frequency discrimination (2AFC)	770 or 870 Hz tones with noise or tonal backward masker	1600	4 hours
Watson and Kelly[16]	Frequency discrimination (3AFC)	40 msec-1 kHz tones in quiet	4200	7 hours
	Duration discrimination (3AFC)	40 msec-1 kHz tones in quiet	3000	5 hours

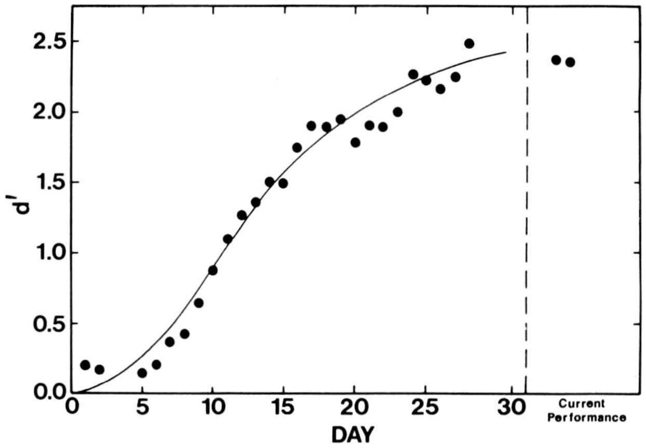

Fig. 4. The time course of learning for a simple auditory identification task as reported by Tanner and Rivette.[9] The stimuli are described in the text. (Adapted from Tanner WP, Sorkin RD. The theory of signal detectability. In: Tovias JV, ed. Foundation of modern auditory theory II. New York: Academic Press, 1972. Used with permission.)

pattern is the same on every trial and only one component of it is subject to variation. The dependent variable is the frequency change of a single component required for about 75% correct discrimination performance. The target here was 920 Hz, which means that the listeners were discriminating about a 60-Hz change in the beginning, but were down to 10 to 12 Hz after 14 days of training. In the midst of this experiment we shifted to an alternative procedure, to see whether we could speed up the training. Individual listener's data show that the new procedure helped some but not others, but the point is that the typical time course of auditory discrimination learning for this task, with a complex stimulus, was on the order of 10-14 hours. Figure 7 shows data from one of our current pattern discrimination experiments. In this case a new, word-length tonal pattern was presented on each trial. The listener's task on each trial was to decide which of three repetitions of a pattern was different from the other two. The differences were a change of the

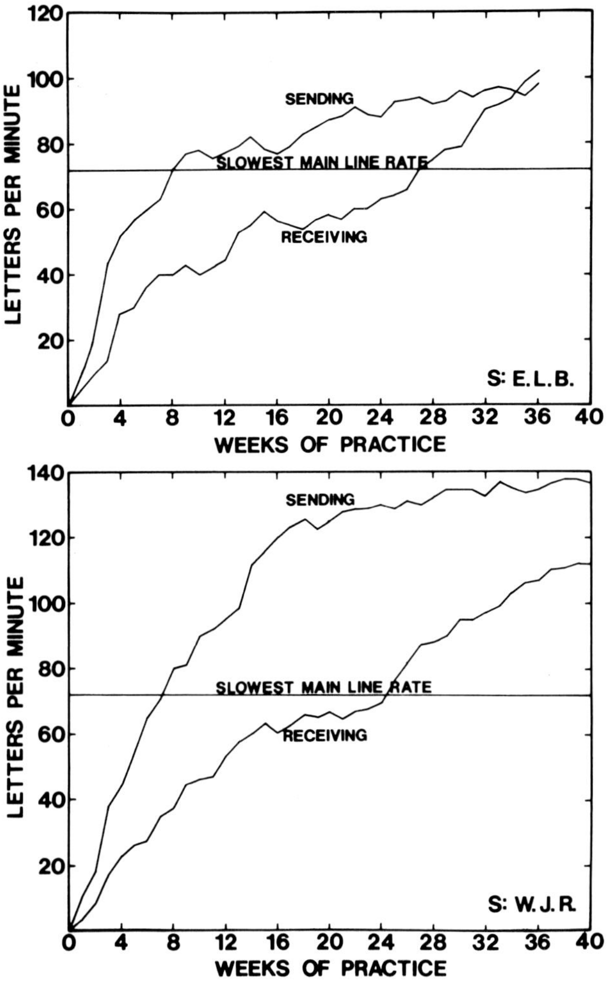

Fig. 5. The time course of learning the complex auditory identification tack represented by Morse code, as reported by Bryan and Harter.[10]

frequency, intensity, or duration of a single tonal component of a pattern. An automatic tracking system continuously adjusted the size of the stimulus differences (△F, △I, or △T) to maintain the

TABLE 3. TIME COURSE OF PERCEPTUAL LEARNING: AUDITORY IDENTIFICATION

	Task (Method)	*Stimulus*	*Est. Trials to Asymptote*	*Est. Time to Asymptote*
Bryan and Harter[10]	Morse code reception	Morse code	?	>40 weeks
Meyer[11]	Musical pitch identification	39 tones	?	24-28 weeks
Wedell[21]	Musical pitch identification	25 tones	600	2 weeks
Hartman[22]	Musical pitch identification	9 tones (300 mel spacing)	576	4 weeks
	Musical pitch identification	9 tones (100 mel spacing)	1,008	7 weeks
Tanner and Rivette[9]	Indicate in which of 4 temporal positions signal occurred	10 msec amplitude increments added to dichotic carrier	25,000	20 hours
Neisser and Hirst[23]	Temporal order identification	500 and 3400 Hz tones, broadband noise, and "scratch"	1,750	7 hours
Warren[12]	Temporal order identification	2500 Hz tone, filtered 1000 Hz square wave, 500-4000 Hz band noise	?	6 hours

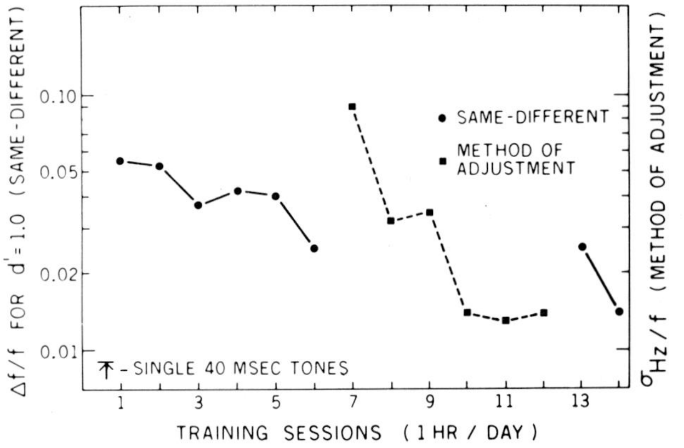

Fig. 6. Time course of discrimination learning, for word-length auditory patterns. Just-detectable changes in component frequency (△f/f) were reduced from 0.10 to approximately 0.015 over 14 hours of minimal-uncertainty training (after Watson, Kelly, and Wroton[14]). (Reprinted with permission.)

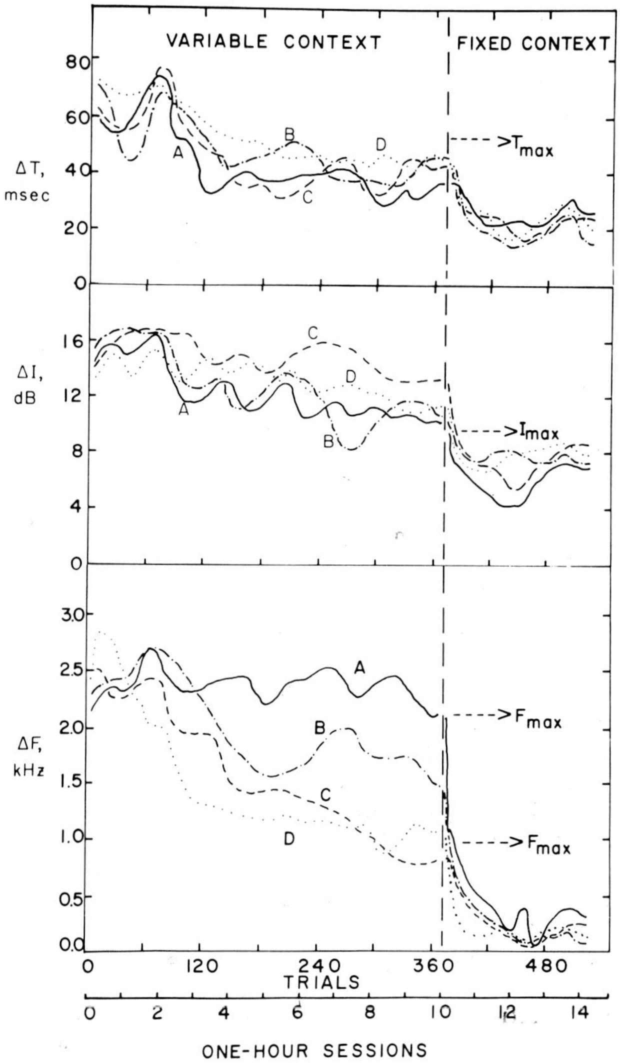

Fig. 7. The time course of learning a complex auditory discrimination task, in a study by Watson and Kelly.[17] The stimuli were word-length tonal patterns, and the task was to discriminate changes of the frequency, intensity, or duration of single tonal components.

listener's performance at 62% correct. The data tracks labeled A, B, C, and D are for four different target components within the patterns, for each of which discrimination improved over the course of ten one-hour training sessions, with 600 trials per session. After the initial ten hours of training the task was changed to one in which the same pattern was presented on each trial, although the listeners still did not know which component was subject to change. Under the new condition additional learning occurred, although its time course was somewhat shorter than in the first section of the experiment. Table 4 shows the estimated amount of training, in numbers of trials and in one-hour sessions, that we have found necessary to learn to discriminate between complex tonal patterns under various psychophysical methods and with different levels of stimulus uncertainty. By stimulus uncertainty is meant the predictability of the pattern to be heard

TABLE 4. TIME COURSE OF PERCEPTUAL LEARNING: DISCRIMINATION OF WORD-LENGTH TONAL PATTERNS

Task (Method)	*Stimulus* Number of Patterns	*Stimulus* Target Tones	Est. Trials to Asymptote	Est. Time to Asymptote
Frequency discrimination (method of adjustment)	1	Position 10; 815 Hz	5	½ hour
Frequency discrimination (method of adjustment)	1	Position 3; 815 Hz	10	1 hour
Frequency discrimination (same-different)	1	Position 2; 920 Hz	3,600	6 hours
Frequency discrimination (same-different)	50	Temporal positions (2, 4, 7, and 10); five frequencies (565-1327 Hz) at each position	6,000	10-15 hours
Intensity discrimination (3AFC)	New pattern on each trial	Temporal positions (2, 4, 7, and 10); five frequencies (565-1327 Hz) at each position	11,000	18 hours
Duration discrimination (same-different)	New pattern on each trial	Temporal positions (2, 4, 7, and 10); five frequencies (565-1327 Hz) at each position	13,000	20-25 hours
Random series of frequency duration, and intensity discrimination (3AFC)	New pattern on each trial	Temporal positions 3 and 8; two frequencies (534 and 1688 Hz) at each position	15,000	25-30 hours

on the next trial, typically scaled by the number of patterns in a catalog from which a sample is drawn on each trial. Additional uncertainty variation is accomplished by changes of the number of temporal or spectral components subject to change in a given pattern. The time to asymptotic discrimination performance in these experiments can be seen in the table to vary greatly with the level of uncertainty.

Previous studies of auditory perceptual learning, plus our own work on the discrimination of word-length tonal patterns, support the following general conclusion. For simple sounds, including especially single tones or notes played on a musical instrument, asymptotic detection performance is approached in 1-2 hours, discrimination in 2-6 hours, and identification in 10-100 hours, depending on the size of the stimulus catalogs. With more complex stimuli these times may be greatly extended, to several hours for detection, 4-12 hours for discrimination, and 20 to many hundreds of hours for identification, depending on the complexity of the stimuli and, again, on the size of the stimulus catalogs.

There are important messages in these facts of auditory learning for the measurement of auditory capability in general. For our purposes here, however, the message is somewhat different and more specific. The slowest form of auditory learning is always involved when we attempt to learn an auditory code, as in the case of drastic recoding of speech information for impaired listeners. We have rejected, time and again, auditory recoding schemes because of one of two reasons: either they were not successfully learned after a few weeks, or even a month or two of practice (an hour a day), or we reject them a priori because the transformed speech doesn't sound like anything that could be produced by a human vocal tract. The learning data reviewed here, especially the increases in the time course of learning as you go from detection to discrimination to identification tasks, as you go from simple to complex stimuli, and as you go from tasks in which you have a few stimuli in a catalog to many, clearly show that we shouldn't expect to learn to identify the sounds of human speech as we do, even if we didn't know anything about human speech at all, in less than two or three years. So to assume that a drastic auditory recoding scheme is a failure with a shorter trial than that is totally at odds with established fact.

The exploitation of residual hearing through drastic acoustic recoding of speech thus may require periods of learning as long as those required by children in learning the normal speech code. The data reviewed here suggest that such efforts should be made in two stages. Recoding schemes should be initially analyzed by measuring the discriminability of individual recoded phonemic elements. There is obviously no sense in proceeding to the high-uncertainty identification task represented by actual *use* of the new code, if its elementary components cannot be resolved. Thus the time-consuming part of code learning should be deferred until it is established that the listeners can cope with the reduced task. This strategy would allow us to make a valid selection from among alternative candidate codes, by means of the relatively speedy discrimination experiments. The extremely long training period to be devoted to a single new auditory code could thus be entered with reasonable expectation of success.

ACKNOWLEDGMENTS — The author gratefully acknowledges the many contributions of William J. Kelly to the pattern discrimination research described in this article, and the helpful suggestions of his colleagues Walt Jesteadt and Richard Lippmann.

REFERENCES

1. Necker LA. Observations on some remarkable phaenomena seen in Switzerland; and an optical phaenomenon which occurs on viewing of a crystal or a geometrical solid. Phil Mag 1832; 3:329-37.

2. Rubin E. Figure and ground. In: Beardslee DC, Wertheimer M, eds. Readings in perception. New York: D. Van Nostrand, 1958.

3. Leeper R. A study of a neglected portion of the field of learning: the development of sensory organization. J Genet Psychol 1935; 46:41-75.

4. Kendler HH. Basic psychology. New York: Appleton-Century-Crofts, 1963:209.

5. Gundy RF. Auditory detection of an unspecified signal. J Acoust Soc Am 1961; 33:1008-12.

6. Green DM, Swets JA. Signal detection theory and psychophysics. New York: Wiley, 1966.

7. Zwislocki J, Maire F, Feldman AS, Rubin A. On the effect of practice and motivation on the threshold of audibility. J Acoust Soc Am 1958; 30:254-62.

8. Auerbach CF. Improvement of frequency discrimination with practice: an attentional model. Organizational Behav Hum Perf 1971; 6:316-35.

9. Tanner WP, Rivette CL. Learning in psychophysical experiments. J Acoust Soc Am 1963; 35:1896(A).

10. Bryan WL, Harter N. Studies in the physiology and psychology of the telegraphic language. The acquisition of a hierarchy of habits. Psychol Rev 1899; 6:345-75.

11. Meyer ML. Is the memory of absolute pitch capable of development by training? Psychol Rev 1899; 6:514-16.

12. Warren RM. Auditory temporal discrimination by trained listeners. Cognitive Psychol 1974; 6:237-56.

13. Watson CS, Wroton HW, Kelly WJ, Benbassat CA. Factors in the discrimination of tonal patterns. I. Component frequency, temporal position, and silent intervals. J Acoust Soc Am 1975; 57:1175-85.

14. Watson CS, Kelly WJ, Wroton HW. Factors in the discrimination of tonal patterns. II. Selective attention and learning under various levels of stimulus uncertainty. J Acoust Soc Am 1976; 60:1176-86.

15. Watson CS. Factors in the discrimination of word-length auditory patterns. In: Hirsh SK, Eldredge DH, Hirsh IJ, Silverman SR, eds. Hearing and Davis: essays honoring Hallowell Davis. St. Louis: Washington University Press, 1976.

16. Watson CS, Kelly WJ. Discrimination of tonal patterns

with several levels of stimulus uncertainty. J Acoust Soc Am 1978(A); 64:S39.

17. Watson CS, Kelly WJ. Informational masking in word-length tonal patterns. J Acoust Soc Am 1978(A); 64:S39.

18. Watson CS, Franks JR, Hood DC. Detection of tones in the absence of external masking noise. I. Effects of signal intensity and signal frequency. J Acoust Soc Am 1972; 52:633-43.

19. Campbell RA, Small AM Jr. Effect of practice and feedback on frequency discrimination. J Acoust Soc Am 1963; 35:1511-4.

20. Loeb M, Holding DH. Backward interference by tones or noise in pitch perception as a function of practice. Percept Psychophys 1975; 18:205-8.

21. Wedell CH. The nature of the absolute judgments of pitch. J Exp Psychol 1934; 17:485-503.

22. Hartman EB. The influence of practice and pitch-distance between tones on the absolute identification of pitch. Am J Psychol 1954; 67:1-14.

23. Neisser U, Hirst W. Effect of practice on the identification of auditory sequences. Percept Psychophys 1974; 15:391-8.

NEUROPHYSIOLOGICAL CORRELATES OF AUDITORY MATURATION

ERIC JAVEL, PhD
OMAHA, NEBRASKA

At the time of its birth, the auditory system of the cat is not completely developed. Anatomic maturity of the peripheral auditory system, ie, the cochlea, auditory nerve and cochlear nucleus, is attained at about two or three weeks of age. Physiological response properties of neural elements of the peripheral auditory system change radically during the first few weeks of life, with most measures of responsiveness to acoustic stimuli reaching adult status by the end of the third or fourth postnatal week. The physiological maturation of neural responses correlates well with the anatomic maturation of the auditory structures. At least one physiological response property, namely the ability of cochlear nucleus neurons to time their discharges in response to low-frequency tones, is not fully achieved until the sixth postnatal week or later. Although considerably less is known about the development of the central auditory system, it appears that it is in part dependent upon the maturation of more peripheral elements. Auditory evoked responses, for example, follow roughly the same developmental time course as do the majority of response properties of peripheral neurons. This implies that the central system is ready to function at birth, but that it must await the maturation of more peripheral elements before it can function properly. In contrast to that of the cat and other mammals, the auditory system of the human is relatively well advanced at birth. Certain aspects of brain development, such as dendritic aborization and axonal myelination, undergo considerable change postnatally. How these factors influence hearing is not known.

INTRODUCTION

The early assessment of auditory function is of obvious clinical importance in identifying what may become problem areas in later life. The auditory system is typically presumed by clinicians to be fully functional at birth; however, in actuality not much is known about either the *degree* of performance the neonatal auditory system can attain, the *rate* of development of auditory function, or the *time* when the entire system is functionally mature.

A necesssary precursor to the development of adequate tests of neonatal auditory function is the understanding of the neonatal system's capabilities. It is not possible, however, to investigate directly many physiological aspects of human auditory function. Most of the information currently available regarding the auditory capabilities of neonates deals either with gross potentials recorded extracranially or with reflex activity.[1] Both of these measures entail complicated anatomical and physiological mechanisms, and they provide little insight into the precise nature of the developmental sequence. With other animals, however, aspects of maturation may be investigated directly, both on the gross and the cellular level. Assuming that human auditory development follows the same course of events as in lower animals, one may infer information about human auditory function by scaling aspects of the anatomic development of auditory structures of animals to those of man.

For several reasons, the cat is an appropriate choice of animals with which one may compare auditory development to that of man. Neuroanatomically, the two systems are similar, and cochlear function in the cat is virtually identical to that of man, albeit on a smaller scale.[2,3] Several anatomic and physiological studies of postnatal auditory maturation in the cat have been undertaken, most notably by the French groups headed by Pujol and Marty.[4-10] Likewise, the embryonic and neonatal development of the human auditory system has been studied,[11-16] as has auditory development in other animals such as the rabbit,[17] the oppossum,[18-20] and the mouse.[21-23] Even with this sizeable amount of work, however, the picture regarding auditory development is by no means complete. What is particularly weak is the state of knowledge regarding physiological development, although some ground is being gained. Studies of evoked potentials have been performed[4,24-26] as have studies of responses of single auditory neurons[4,8,27,28] and of cochlear potentials.[5,23,29-31] These works, taken together, suggest that at birth the ear is relatively insensitive to sound, but auditory function develops rapidly and reaches near-adult status by the age of three weeks.

In this presentation, we will review the major aspects of anatomic and physiological development in the neonatal cat. We will show that physiological maturation as measured by cochlear potentials, by responses of single neurons and by evoked potentials, proceeds in a rapid manner following birth, and that the time course of physiological development correlates well with the completion of neuroanatomic development. Also, we will show that even though most aspects of physiological responsiveness in the cat auditory system are complete by three or four weeks of age, there still remains at least one element, namely the temporal ordering of discharges, which attains adult status at a yet later time. Finally, we will identify directions future reseach might consider taking.

From the Department of Otolaryngology and Human Communication, Boys Town Institute and Creighton University School of Medicine, Omaha, Nebraska. This work supported by a Biomedical Research Development Grant from NIH.

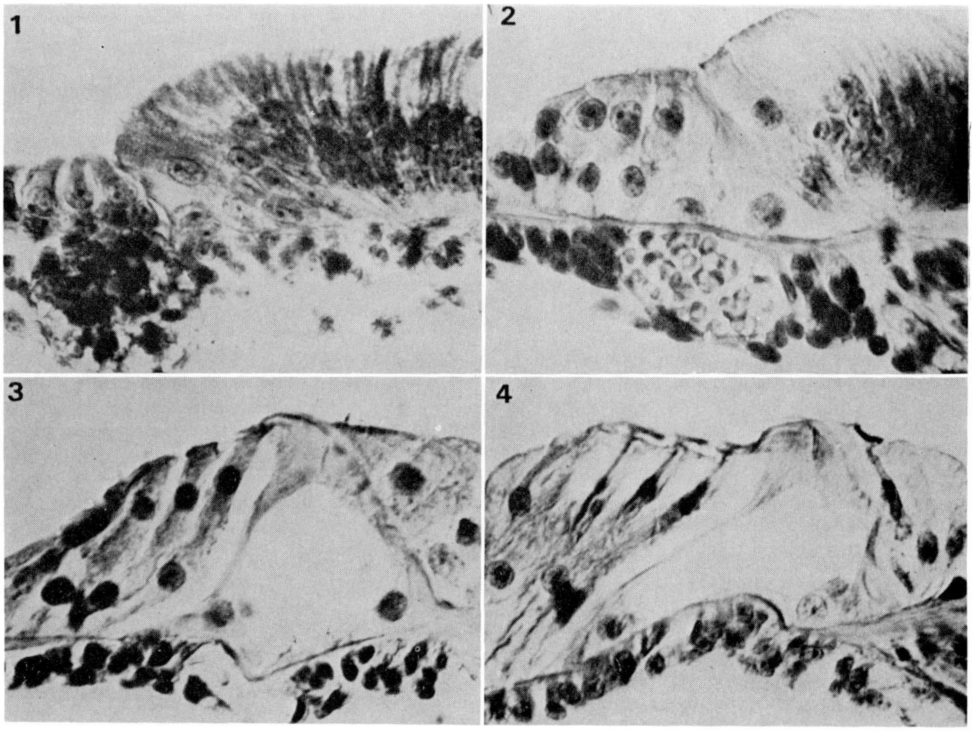

Fig. 1. Organ of Corti in cat at various time periods surrounding birth. 1) Basal turn of cochlea at 55 days gestation. Hair cells are recognizable, but the structure is markedly immature. 2) Basal turn at birth. Tunnel of Corti is not yet differentiated. 3) Basal turn at three days of age. Tunnel of Corti is open, and Nuel's space is visible. 4) Basal turn at 12 days of age. Adult conformation has been attained. (From Pujol and Marty.[6] Reprinted with permission.)

ANATOMIC CONSIDERATIONS

At the time of its birth, the auditory apparatus of the cat has not yet reached maturity. The external auditory meatus is closed, and the middle ear is filled with a gelatinous mesenchyme. The ossicles are not fully ossified, and the cochlear structures (particularly in the apex) are markedly underdeveloped. The auditory nerve is poorly myelinated, and axon diameters are small. Likewise, the cochlear nuclei are small and possess immature cells, some of which do not exist in the adult animal.

The external ear canal opens at about seven days of age, which coincides in time with resorption of the mesenchyme in the middle ear. By three weeks of age, the mesenchyme is fully resorbed, and the external and middle ears are fully functional.

The cat cochlea apparently develops in a base-to-apex sequence. At birth, the otic capsule has reached its final dimensions, but only the basal turn is fully ossified. The hair cells are recognizable, but they (particularly the outer hair cells) appear immature; the tunnel of Corti is not differentiated, and the supporting cells are poorly formed[6] (Fig. 1). The apex of the cochlea is structurally more immature than is the base: the hair cells are barely differentiated and the basilar membrane is thick. The stria vascularis is distinguishable, more so in the basal turn than the apical turn. The fact that the basal turn of the cochlea matures more rapidly than does the cochlear apex is curious, for it has been shown that in the mouse it is the basal turn cells which are "older."[32] Thus, while the adult cells of the cochlear apex appear earlier, they apparently mature later.

Compared with the organ of Corti, the spiral ganglion and auditory nerve appear to be more developed at birth. The neurons possess a myelin sheath, but the sheath is poorly developed. The neurons themselves are small and are arranged in dense masses. Neurons connected to inner hair cells apparently mature earlier than do neurons connected to outer hair cells.[7] The axons of the auditory nerve are relatively small and are poorly myelinated.[9] In the mouse, the neurons innervating the basal cochlear turn undergo final mitoses earlier than the neurons innervating the apex.

Following birth, the cochlea and auditory nerve develop rapidly. By the 12th day of age, the basal turn of the cochlea is anatomically mature: the tunnel of Corti and Nuel's space are open, the supporting cells are fully grown, the hair cells and their synapses are fully differentiated, and the stria vascularis is anatomically developed. The apical turn is not fully mature at 12 days, but it completes its development before the end of the third postnatal week.[6] At the same time that the cochlea is completing its maturational sequence, the auditory nerve is becoming better myelinated and axonal diameters are increasing. Even so, final dimensions for auditory nerve fibers are not reached until two months of age or later.[9]

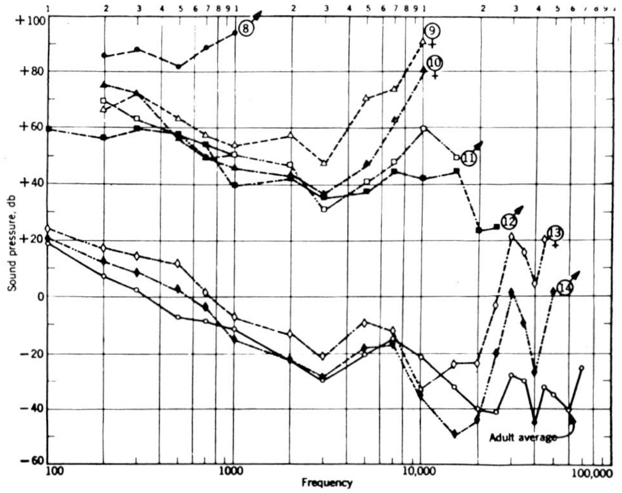

Fig. 2. Sensitivity curves showing development of cochlear microphonic threshold and frequency range in the mouse. Numbers on the curves indicate the age of each animal in days. All animals were born on the same day. Note the increase in frequency bandwidth and the decrease in threshold with increasing age. (From Crowley and Hepp-Reymond.[30] Reprinted with permission. Copyright 1966, Am Psych Assoc.)

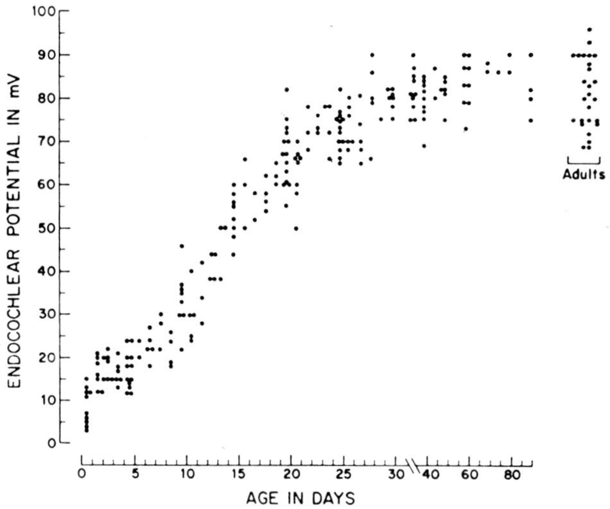

Fig. 3. Development of endocochlear potential in the cat. Adult values are attained during the fourth postnatal week. (From Fernandez and Hinojosa.[31] Reprinted with permission.)

The development of the cochlear nuclei coincides roughly with the development of the auditory nerve. At birth, the cochlear nuclei possess small, darkly-staining neurons which are densely packed. These neurons are apparently still in an active migratory phase, and considerably more neurons exist in the newborn kitten than in the adult.[33] In the anteroventral cochlear nucleus (AVCN), the dendritic trees of the neurons attain adult conformation by the end of the second postnatal month. By this time, the nucleus is of adult size and structure.

In summary, in the cat the cochlea and the structures peripheral to the cochlea are structurally mature by the end of the third postnatal week. The neural elements of the central auditory system, however, lag behind the cochlea in their structural development, taking two months or more to reach maturity.

PHYSIOLOGICAL CONSIDERATIONS

Cochlear Potentials. As might be expected, given the structural immaturity of the cochlea at birth, the electrophysiological potentials of the inner ear of the cat are also immature in the time period immediately following birth. In accordance with the rapid anatomic development of the cochlea, however, these potentials attain adult status by the end of the first postnatal month.

At birth, the cochlear microphonic (CM) is reduced in amplitude and is restricted to a relatively narrow band of frequencies. When recorded with an electrode placed on the round window (mesenchymal tissue having been aspirated), responses to frequencies less than 500 Hz are difficult to elicit, even at the highest signal levels. Likewise, responses above 5 kHz show grossly elevated thresholds. By five days of age, CM may be observed at all frequencies but thresholds are elevated and the input-output curve possesses a lower slope than that seen in adults. Studies of CM in the rat and mouse[23,30] present the same overall picture, except that onset of CM functioning occurs at a later date (Fig. 2).

The endocochlear potential is of very small amplitude at birth and increases steadily in magnitude with age, reaching adult amplitude during the fourth postnatal week[31] (Fig. 3). This is in apparent accord with the rate of development of the stria vascularis.

The whole-nerve action potential (WNAP) is not seen in the first few days of life and is not seen until CM has been established. Pujol and Hilding[5] could not elicit WNAP until seven or eight days following birth, but we* could observe WNAP on the third day using very intense clicks. The onset of WNAP may be correlated with the rapid myelination of auditory nerve fibers in the days following birth, with concomitant synchronization of afferent impulses in the auditory nerve.

Responses of Single Neurons. Despite the structural immaturity of the cochlea, auditory nerve and cochlear nuclei, responses to tones may be elicited from both the ventral and dorsal divisions of the cochlear nuclei at birth.[8] These responses are weak, however, with neurons possessing high thresholds, low discharge rates and curious temporal discharge cadences. Anteroventral cochlear nucleus neurons are tuned somewhat more broadly than those observed in adults.[28] These findings indicate that traveling waves are supported in the neonatal cochlea, but that they may undergo refinements in the weeks following birth.

*Javel E, Brugge JF, Kitzes LM. Unpublished data.

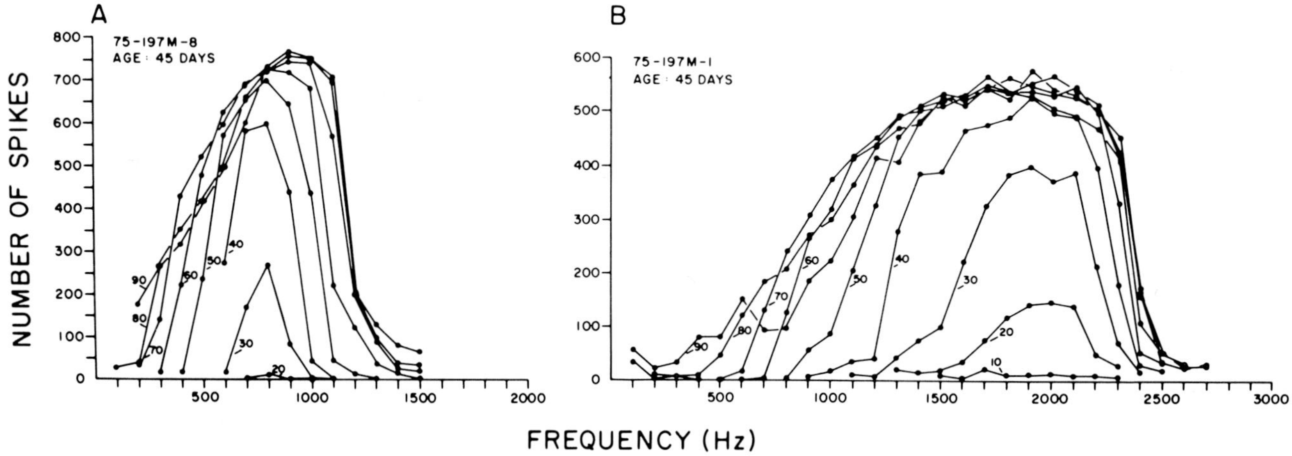

Fig. 4. A,B) Response areas of two anteroventral cochlear nuclei (AVCN) neurons taken from a 45-day-old kitten. The response areas are indistinguishable from those obtained in adult animals, in terms of shape, extent, threshold, and discharge rate. (From Brugge et al.[28] Reprinted with permission.)

During the first postnatal week, all AVCN neurons contacted possess exceedingly high thresholds, even more so than can be expected on the basis of the poorly functioning middle ear. Response areas taken from AVCN neurons at this time (Figs. 4-6) indicate the functional immaturity of these cells. In addition to the elevated thresholds and low discharge rate, the latent period to the first spike (Fig. 7) is lengthened considerably.[27,28] The long latent period cannot be accounted for on the basis of decreased conduction velocity in poorly myelinated fibers. All of the aforementioned response characteristics develop rapidly in the first few weeks following birth, and most aspects of AVCN neuron discharge patterns attain adult status by the end of the first postnatal month.

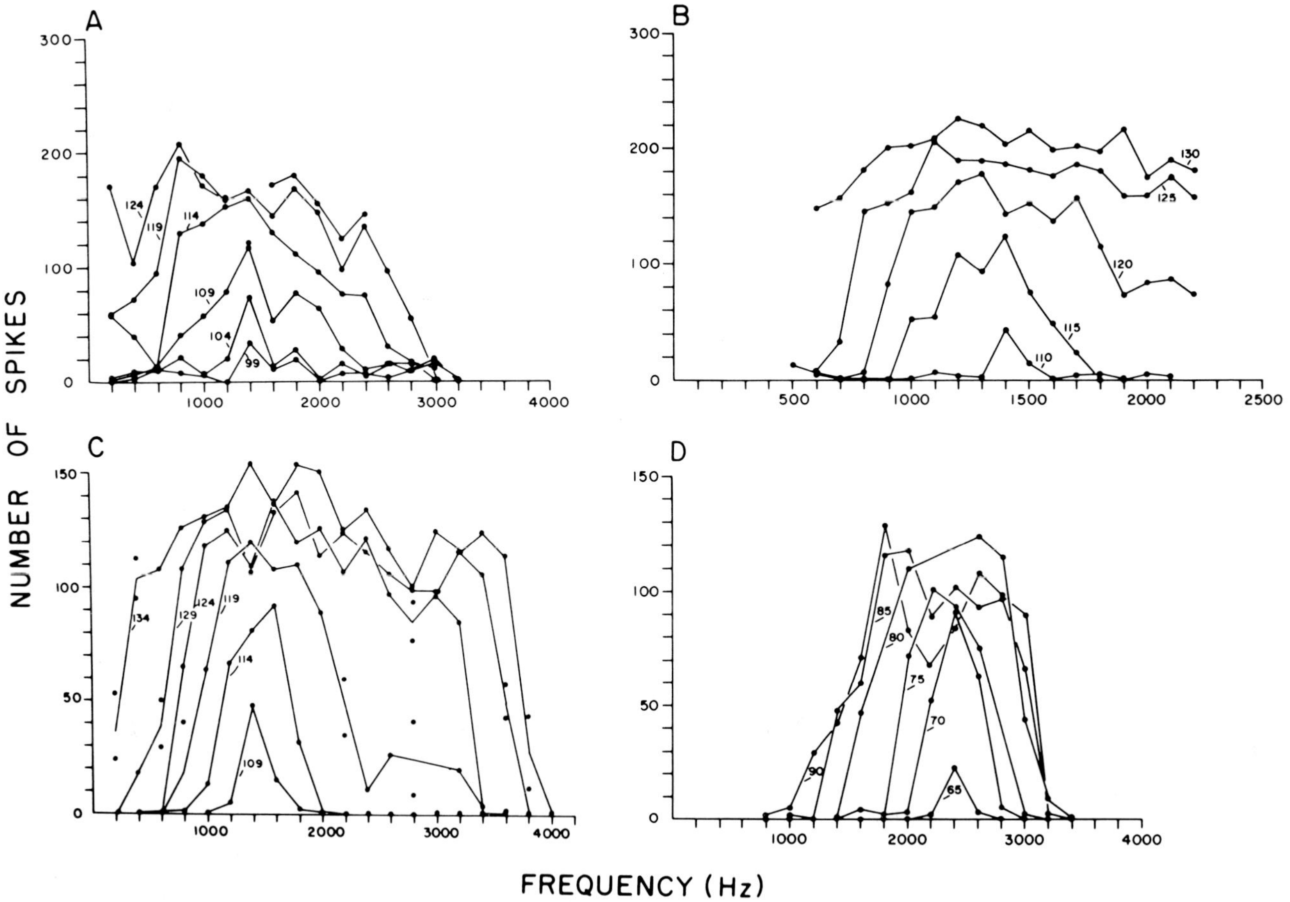

Fig. 5. Response areas of AVCN neurons taken from kittens of age A) four days, B and C) five days, D) seven days. While the neurons are tuned, the extent of the response areas is greater than that observed in adult cats, the thresholds for tones are greatly elevated, and the discharge rate is low. (From Brugge et al.[28] Reprinted with permission.)

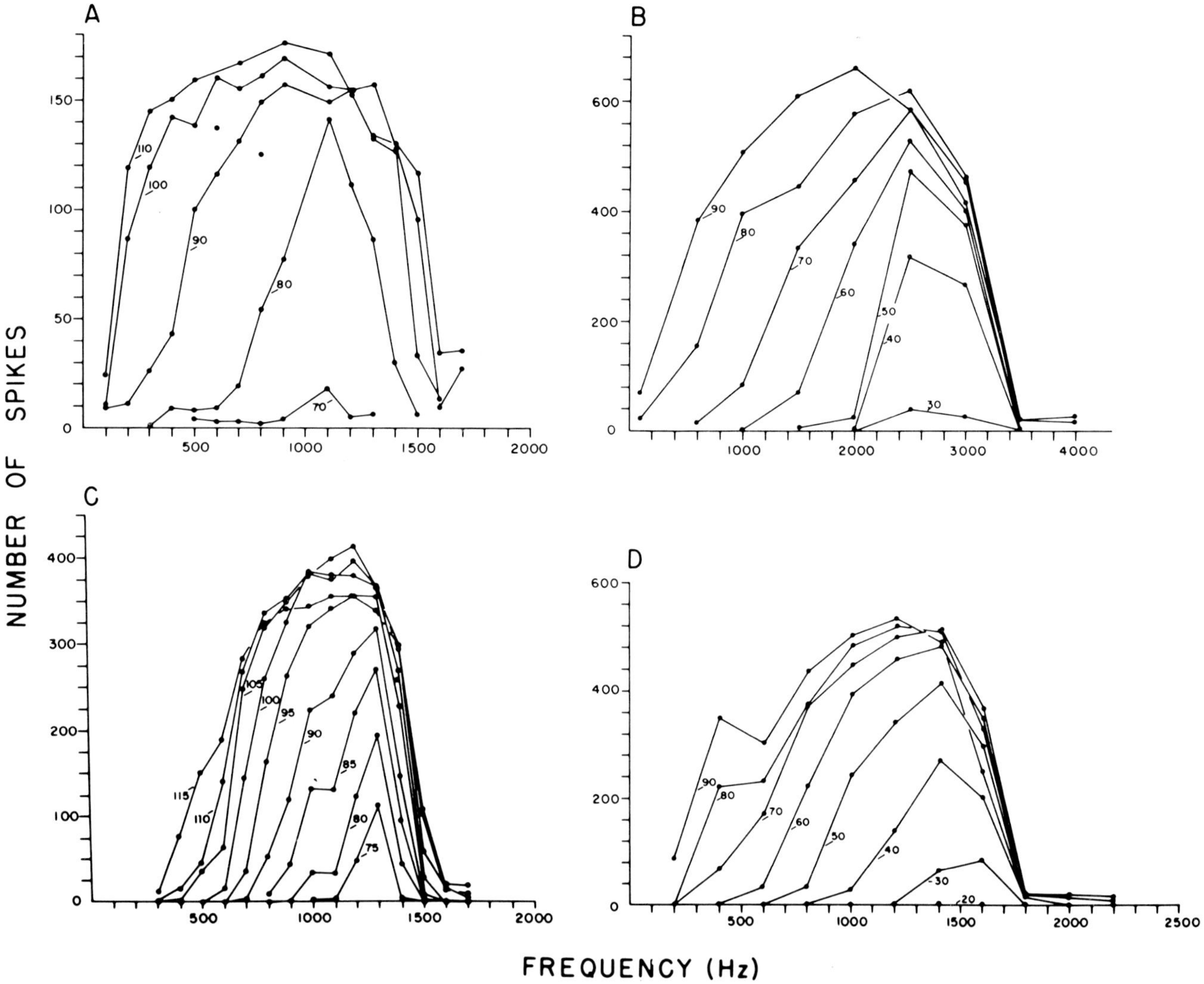

Fig. 6. Response areas of AVCN neurons taken from kittens of age A) 10 days, B) 18 days, C) 20 days, D) 29 days. As time passes and the neural and mechanical elements of the auditory system attain anatomic maturity, physiological responses also become more reminiscent of those seen in adults. By the fourth postnatal week, the majority of AVCN neurons have attained "adult" status with regard to threshold, frequency selectivity, and discharge rate. A minority of cells possess elevated thresholds interspersed with low-threshold neurons. (From Brugge et al.[28] Reprinted with permission.)

One characteristic, namely the ability of AVCN neurons to synchronize or "phase-lock" their discharges to the cycle of a low-frequency tone, is not fully developed even at six weeks postpartum.[27,28] Prior to the second postnatal week, AVCN neurons are unable to follow frequencies to the extent seen in adult animals, even though the stimuli may be strongly excitatory (Fig. 8). During the second postnatal week and continuing thereafter, an increasing proportion of neurons attain the adult ability to phase-lock to frequencies as high as 3000 Hz, although a significant number of neurons still do not possess this characteristic. Ultimately, the neurons separate into the two populations observable in AVCN of adult cats, ie, one group which phase-locks as well as auditory nerve fibers and another group which does not phase-lock above 1000 Hz (Fig. 9). Thus, the ability to phase-lock to pure tones is one of the last response characteristics to develop, and this development occurs in accord with the previously mentioned completion of myelination and growth of auditory nerve fibers.

Very few studies have been concerned with the development of discharge characteristics of neurons in auditory nuclei more central than the cochlear nucleus. What work has been done, however, seems to indicate that responses may be elicited at birth, although thresholds are high and tuning is broad.[34,35] It has been argued[4,36] that the central auditory pathway is ready to function at birth, but that a crucial peripheral element, namely the synapse between the hair cell and the spiral ganglion neuron, is not mature at birth, and this immaturity degrades the more central response. This maturation occurs over a three-to-four-week period following birth.

Evoked Potentials. The brainstem evoked response (BER) has been studied in kittens.[26,37] The results of these studies indicate that the BER is not

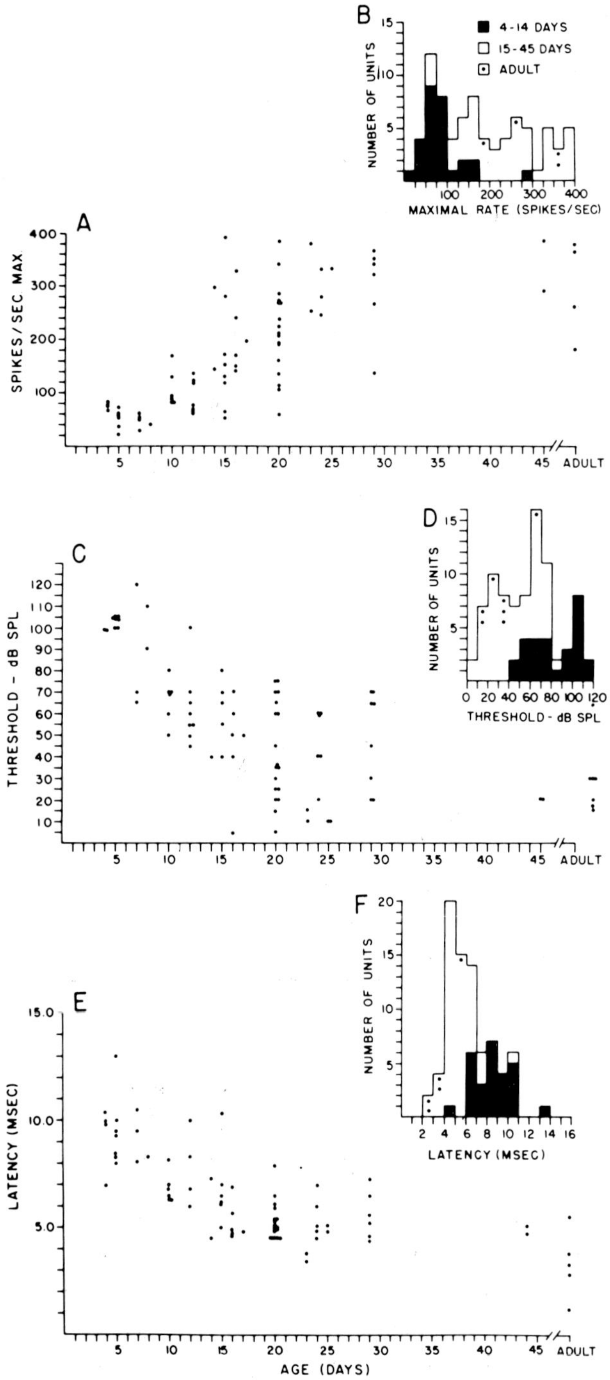

Fig. 7. A) Maturation of maximum discharge rate, C) threshold at characteristic frequency (CF), and E) first-spike latency, all as a function of age. By the third or fourth postnatal week, all indicators have attained essentially adult-like values. Inserts in the figure (B, D, F) indicate distribution of these measures by age. (From Brugge et al.[28] Reprinted with permission.)

easily elicited during the first postnatal week. By the end of the second week of life, however, it is present although the latencies of the individual peaks in the BER waveform are lengthened. Also, the waveform is of a different shape in newborns, with earlier waves showing double peaks and later waves being absent in younger animals. By the sixth postnatal week, the waveform and latency discrepancies are resolved and an adult-like response is observed (Fig. 10). Many of the aspects of the immature BER may be resolved when one considers that a) the time course of BER development follows the time course of myelination in the peripheral system, b) the thresholds for auditory responses decline drastically in the first two or three weeks of life, and c) the degree of phase-locked activity in the peripheral auditory nuclei grows substantially in the first postnatal month.

Several studies have traced the development of the cortical evoked response in kittens from the time of birth.[4,24,25] These have shown that the auditory evoked response (AER) possesses a low amplitude and increased latency in the first postnatal week, as well as an immature waveform and a high threshold. By four weeks of age, however, the AER is adult-like in amplitude and waveshape, and is near-adult in threshold and latency (Fig. 11).

DISCUSSION

The auditory system of the kitten, both anatomically and physiologically, is in a dynamic state of change during the first postnatal weeks. Coincident with attainment of structural maturity is the rapid development of physiological responsiveness at all levels of the system, with most measures of physiological responsiveness being indistinguishable from those of the adult cat at four weeks of age. At least one measure, ie, phase-locking, requires more time to develop.

For reasons cited earlier, the cat is a reasonable model with which one may compare human development. There is reason to believe, however, that the rates of development of cat and human are different, and that the human is functionally more advanced at birth than is the cat. A problem, then, is to transform the time course of cat auditory development such that it fits the time course of human auditory development. This is not an easy task, for the measures of auditory responsiveness previously used for humans differ from the more precise measures described above for cats.

Clinically, it is generally assumed that the human neonate possesses auditory thresholds and processing capabilities which are reasonably mature. The evidence for this assumption, however, is shaky, being based largely upon conditioned heart rate changes in response to sound and upon orienting and other reflexes. Both of these entail complicated central mechanisms, and the responses are elicitable only at relatively high signal levels. Nonetheless, it is reasonable to presume that the newborn human possesses a greater auditory capability than does the newborn cat.

The state of the auditory system of the newborn cat may be similar to that of the third-trimester

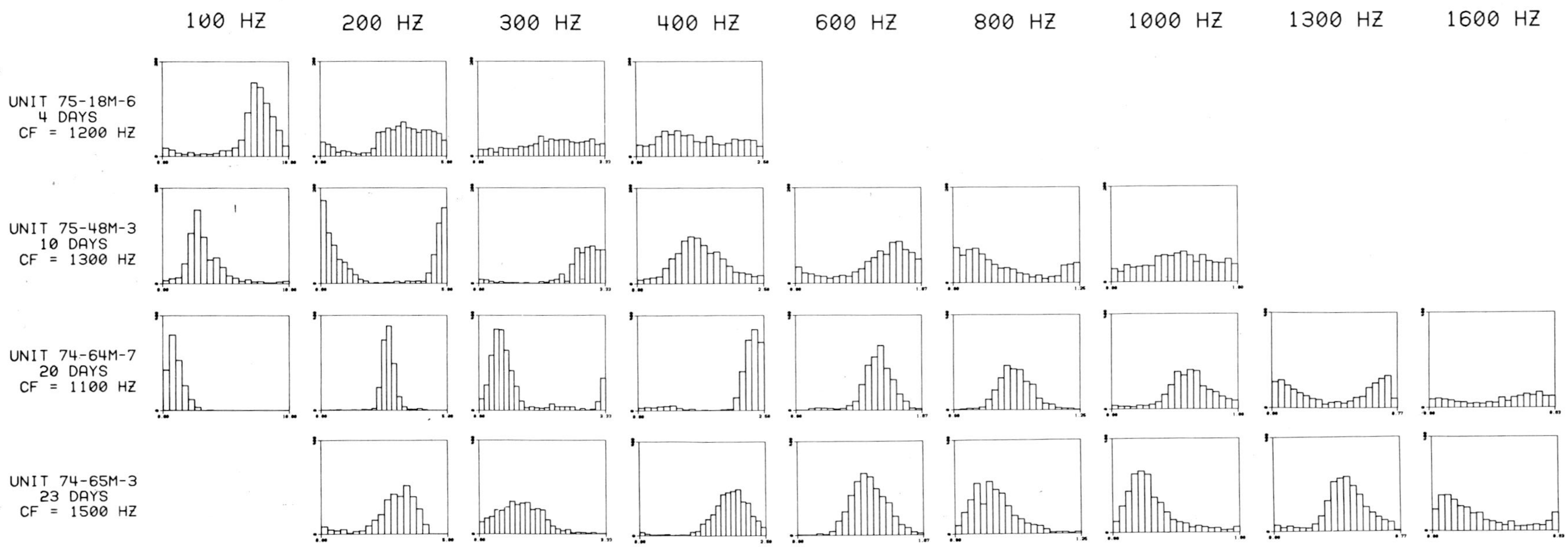

Fig. 8. Ability of AVCN neurons to time their discharges with regard to stimulus frequency (phase-locking) as a function of kitten's age. In the first postnatal week, no neurons are able to phase-lock to frequencies greater than 1000 Hz, even though stimuli may be strongly excitatory. Upper frequency limit for phase-locking increases with increasing age.

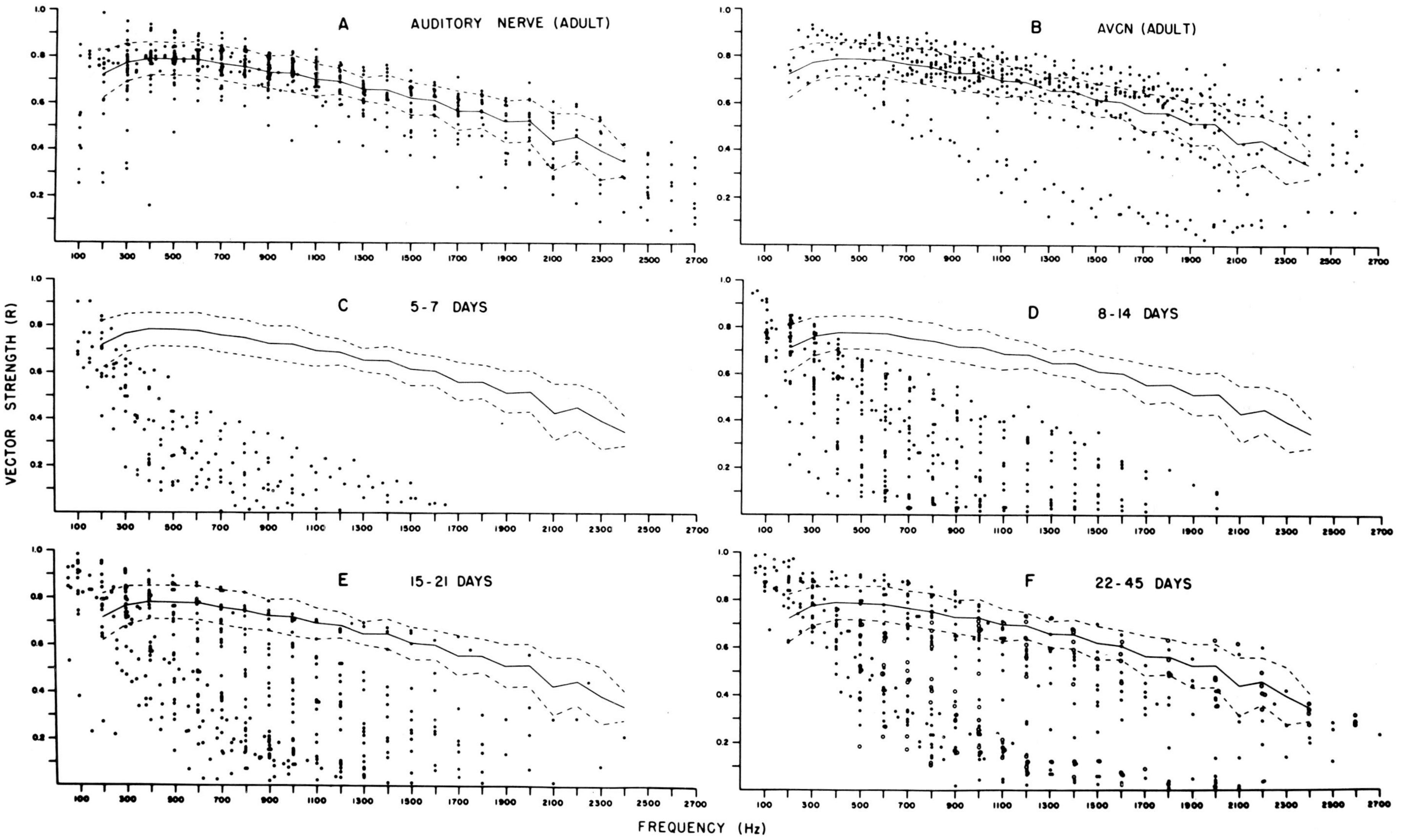

Fig. 9. A) Vector strength (R) as a function of frequency for adult cat auditory nerve fibers. The ribbon in each graph represents the mean ± one standard deviation of adult cats' vector strength values. B) Vector strength (R) in adult cats' AVCN neurons. Phase-locking in AVCN is as good or better than that in the auditory nerve. C-F) (R) as a function of frequency for AVCN neurons of kittens, grouped by age. During the first two postnatal weeks, no AVCN neuron was capable of phase-locking to the degree seen in adult cats. After that, the data separate into two populations, similar to that seen in the adult cat AVCN. (From Brugge et al.[28] Reprinted with permission. B) From Rose et al. Unpublished data.)

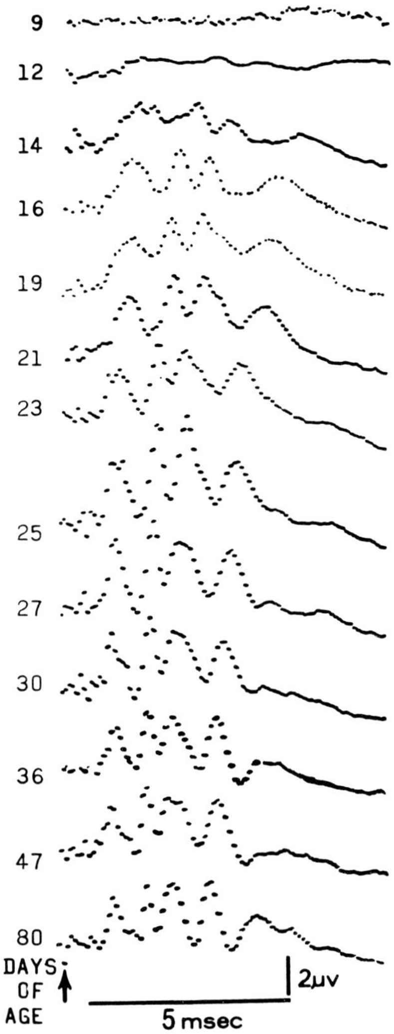

Fig. 10. Development of brainstem evoked response in kittens. Intensity was set to 60 dB re human audiometric threshold. This level is incapable of generating a response in kittens less than two weeks of age. Adult conformation and amplitude is attained after the fourth postnatal week. (From Jewett and Romano.[26] Reprinted with permission.)

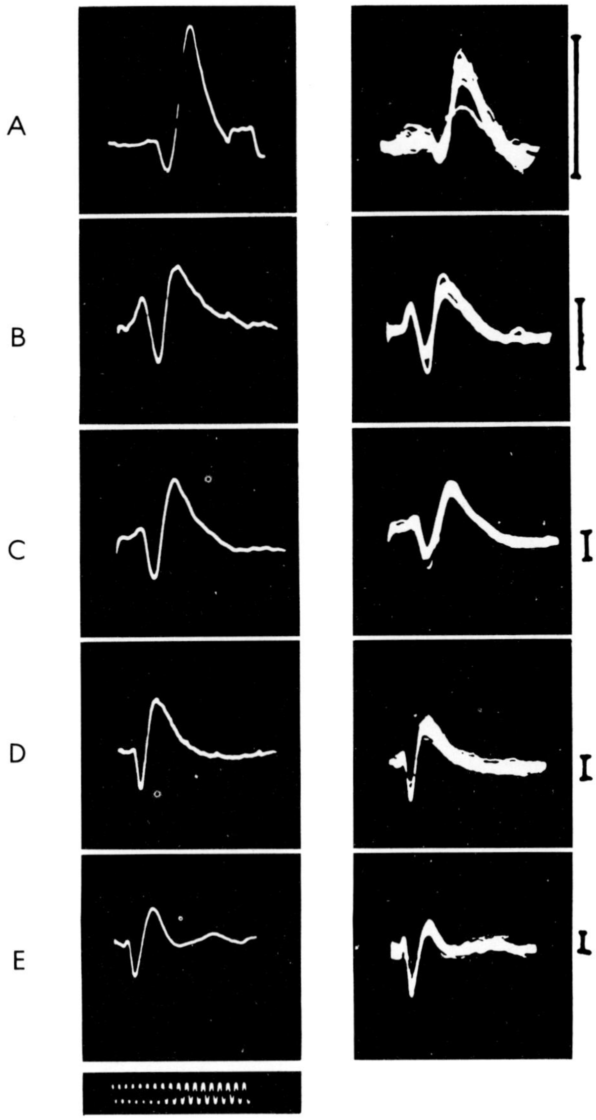

Fig. 11. Cortical evoked response in kittens, taken during the first weeks following birth. The response attains adult amplitude and waveshape near the end of the first postnatal month. Prior to this, amplitudes are reduced, latencies to the peaks are lengthened, and the waveshapes are atypical. The left-column represents single responses, and the right-hand column shows superimpositions of multiple responses. The vertical lines to the right indicate 100 uV. The sinusoid at the bottom indicates a time reference of 100 Hz. A) 9 days of age; B) 15 days; C) 22 days; D) 35 days; E) 91 days. (From Ellingson and Wilcott.[25] Reprinted with permission.)

human fetus. This does not mean, however, that upon emerging from the womb, the human is capable of mature auditory function. On the contrary, several studies have indicated that human auditory development, particularly the more central processing functions, proceeds for more than one year postpartum, even after all physiological indicators have attained adult status. Thus, while the cat is less mature at birth than the human, it catches up rapidly and passes the human. Owing to the greater degree of final development of the higher auditory centers, however, the human has a longer road to travel than does the cat.

If the physiological studies undertaken in the cat are any indicator, then human auditory performance in the time period following birth should be poor, especially with regard to tasks requiring central processing. For example, given the lack of frequency-processing ability in the neonatal cat, frequency discrimination should be poorly developed. How other aspects of human auditory performance are affected is not known, but it appears safe to presume that most aspects of auditory processing in the neonatal human are not fully developed at birth.

Of audiologic importance is human neonatal sensitivity to sound, ie, thresholds. Given the data available for the cat and the behavioral data on human infants, it is reasonable to assume that human auditory thresholds are elevated at birth. The precise extent of the elevation is not known, but extrapolation of the cat data would indicate that the threshold shift should not be great.

In conclusion, there is a growing understanding of the development of auditory capabilities in both cat and man. In spite of this, there exist several gaps in our knowledge. It is not known, for example, how development proceeds in auditory centers more central than the cochlear nuclei, nor is much known about the time course of "higher," ie, cortical, functions which influence perception and performance. These would include pattern or vocal discrimination and localization of sound in space, among others. Also, the effect on auditory performance of trauma or lesions at or before birth (such as anoxia, tumors, chemical imbalances, etc) is not known. As described above, the cat is a reasonable model upon which manipulations such as these may be performed. When these data are obtained for the cat, we may be in a position to develop better tests of human neonatal auditory function. In time, this would lead to an improved ability of the clinician to identify problem areas earlier in life than has thus far been practicable.

ACKNOWLEDGMENTS — The help of Edward J. Walsh and Jo Ann McGee is gratefully acknowledged. The manuscript was typed by Mrs. Carole Dugan and Mrs. Elizabeth Trimble.

REFERENCES

1. Graham FK, Jackson JC. Arousal systems and infant heart rate responses. In: Reese HW, Lipsitt LP, eds. Advances in child development. New York: Academic Press, 1970.

2. Bekesy GV. Experiments in hearing. New York: McGraw-Hill, 1960.

3. Greenwood DD. Critical bandwidth and the frequency coordinates of the basilar membrane. J Acoust Soc Am 1961; 33:1344-56.

4. Pujol R. Development of tone-burst responses along the auditory pathway in the cat. Acta Otolaryngol (Stockh) 1972; 74:383-91.

5. Pujol R, Hilding DA. Anatomy and physiology of the onset of auditory function. Acta Otolaryngol (Stockh) 1973; 76:1-10.

6. Pujol R, Marty R. Postnatal maturation in the cochlea of the cat. J Comp Neurol 1970; 139:115-26.

7. Pujol R, Carlier E, Devigne C. Different patterns of cochlear innervation during the development of the kitten. J Comp Neural 1978; 177:529-36.

8. Romand R, Marty R. Postnatal maturation of the cochlear nuclei in the cat: A neurophysiological study. Brain Res 1975; 83:225-33.

9. Romand R, Sans A, Romand MR, Marty R. The structural maturation of the stato-acoustic nerve in the cat. J Comp Neurol 1976; 170:1-16.

10. Köenig N, Pujol R, Marty R. A laminar study of evoked potentials and unit responses in the auditory cortex of the postnatal cat. Brain Res 1972; 36:469-73.

11. Kölliker A. Entwicklungsgeschichte des Menschen und der Hoheren Thiere. Leipzig: W Englemann, 1861.

12. Boettcher A. Über Entwicklung und Bau des Gebörlabyrinths. Dresden: Blockmann, Soba v Schultze, 1869.

13. Retzius MG. Das Gehörorgan des Wirbeltiere. Stockholm: Samson and Wallin, 1884.

14. Streeter GL. On the development of the membraneous labyrinth and the acoustic and facial nerve in the human embryo. Am J Anat 1906; 6:139-65.

15. Wada T. Anatomical and physiological studies on the growth of the inner ear of the albino rat. Am Anat Mem 1923; 10:1-174.

16. Bast T, Anson BJ. The temporal bone and the ear. Springfield: CC Thomas, 1949.

17. Anggard L. An electrophysiological study of the development of cochlear function in the rabbit. Acta Otolaryngol (Stockh) 1965; Suppl 203:1-64.

18. Larsell O, McCready E Jr, Zimmerman AA. Morphological and functional development of membranous labyrinth in the opossum. J Comp Neurol 1935; 63:95-118.

19. Larsell O, McCready E Jr, Larsell JF. Development of the organ of Corti in relation to the inception of hearing. Arch Otolaryngol 1944; 40:233-48.

20. McCready E Jr, Wever EG, Bray CW. The development of hearing in the opossum. J Exp Zool 1937; 75:503-17.

21. Kikuchi K, Hilding D. The development of the organ of Corti in the mouse. Acta Otolaryngol (Stockh) 1965; 60:207-22.

22. Ruben RJ. Development of the inner ear of the mouse: a radioautographic study of terminal mitoses. Acta Otolaryngol 1967; Suppl 220:1-44.

23. Alford BR, Ruben RJ. Physiological, behavioral, and anatomical correlates on the development of hearing in the mouse. Ann Otol Rhinol Laryngol 1963; 72:237-74.

24. Rose JE, Adrian H, Santibanez G. Electrical signs of maturation in the auditory system of the kitten. Acta Neurol Lat Am 1957; 3:133-43.

25. Ellingson RJ, Wilcott RC. Development of evoked responses in visual and auditory cortices of kittens. J Neurophysiol 1960; 23:363-75.

26. Jewett DL, Romano MN. Neonatal development of auditory system potentials averaged from the scalp of rat and cat. Brain Res 1972; 36:101-15.

27. Javel E, Brugge JF, Kitzes LM. Response properties of single neurons in anteroventral cochlear nucleus (AVCN) of the newborn cat: frequency selectivity and temporal ordering of discharges. J Acoust Soc Am 1975; Suppl 1:58:S64.

28. Brugge JF, Javel E, Kitzes LM. Signs of functional maturation of peripheral auditory system in discharge patterns of neurons in anteroventral cochlear nucleus of kitten. J Neurophysiol 1978; 41:1557-79.

29. McCready E Jr, Wever EG, Bray CW. A further investigation of the development of hearing in the opossum. J Comp Psychol 1940; 30:17-21.

30. Crowley DE, Hepp-Raymond MC. Development of cochlear function in the ear of the infant rat. J Comp Physiol Psychol 1966; 62:427-32.

31. Fernandez C, Hinojosa R. Postnatal development of endocochlear potential and stria vascularis in the cat. Acta Otolaryngol (Stockh) 1974; 78:173-86.

32. Lindermann HH, Ades HW, Bredberg G, Engstrom H. The sensory hairs and the tectorial membrane in the development of the cat's organ of Corti. Acta Otolaryngol (Stockh) 1971; 72:229-42.

33. Mlonyeni M. The late stages of the development of the primary cochlear nuclei in mice. Brain Res 1967; 4:334-44.

34. Romand R, Granier MR, Marty R. Development postnatal de l'activite par la stimulation sonore. J Physiol (Paris) 1973; 66:303-15.

35. Aitken LM, Moore DR. Inferior colliculus II. Development of turning characteristics and tonotopic organization in central nucleus of the neonatal cat. J Neurophysiol 1975; 38:1208-16.

36. Carlier E, Abonnenc M, Pujol R. Maturation des responses unitaires a la stimulation tonale dans le nerf cochleaire du chaton. J Physiol (Paris) 1975; 70:129-38.

37. Shipley C, Geary D, Norman R, Buchwald J. Development of brainstem auditory potentials in kittens. Neurosci Abst 1978; 4:10.

EFFERENT COMPONENTS OF THE AUDITORY SYSTEM

W. BRUCE WARR, PhD

OMAHA, NEBRASKA

The origins and terminations of the olivocochlear bundle, which provides an efferent innervation to the organ of Corti, are described on the basis of experiments using axonal transport of tracer substances and light microscopy in the cat. The cells of origin were labeled by the retrograde tracer horseradish peroxidase which was injected unilaterally into the cochlea. Labeled cells in the superior olivary complex could be dichotomized according to their location (lateral or medial), their size (small or large), and their preferred side of projection (uncrossed or crossed). All labeled olivocochlear neurons exhibited a positive reaction for acetylcholinesterase. To determine the cochlear projections of the neurons, injections of a radioactive amino acid were made into either the lateral or medial olivocochlear cell group. After allowing time for synthesis and axonal transport of radio-labeled protein to reach synaptic endings in the cochleas, the tissue sections of these specimens were processed for autoradiography. The results indicate that lateral olivocochlear neurons project to the region beneath the inner hair cells of both sides, whereas medial olivocochlear neurons project to the region beneath the outer hair cells of both sides. These findings are in substantial accord with previous experimental work but suggest that the organ of Corti receives a dual efferent innervation which is organized according to the location and morphology of its cells of origin. Accordingly, it is proposed that the two efferent components of the cochlear innervation described here be referred to as the *lateral* and *medial* olivocochlear systems, replacing the current designations of crossed and uncrossed olivocochlear bundles, the latter which are demonstrably heterogeneous in their origins and terminations and, probably, also in their functions.

INTRODUCTION

One of the most intriguing features of the auditory pathway is the existence of the recurrent projection to the organ of Corti known as the olivocochlear bundle (OCB). First described more than 30 years ago and known for a time as "the tract of Rasmussen" after its discoverer Grant Rasmussen,[1] this small group of nerve fibers has engaged the active research interest of anatomists, physiologists and psychologists alike. Emerging from these efforts are a number of findings which point toward an inhibitory role[2-8] for the OCB exerted both at the level of the outer hair cells[9-13] and upon the dendrites of cochlear nerve fibers with the organ of Corti.[14,15] Although the inhibitory action of the OCB has not been directly measured in behaving organisms, some workers have adduced evidence suggesting that these fibers may serve to improve the detection of signals in noise[16] or alternatively, may be engaged in the suppression of behaviorally irrelevant acoustic input.[17] A status report on our understanding of the OCB has been presented in an extensive 1974 review by Klinke and Galley.[18]

The purpose of this paper is to describe some recent experiments designed to clarify the origins and terminations of the OCB in the cat. These experiments have made use of some newly developed techniques for tracing axonal connections, and have produced some unexpected findings regarding the efferent innervation of the cochlea. It is hoped that these new data concerning the anatomical organization of the OCB will aid physiologists and psychologists in their pursuit of the ultimate functional significance of this fascinating fiber bundle.

METHODS

EXPERIMENT 1

Identification of the Cells of Origin of the OCB. The cells of origin of the OCB were identified by the method of retrograde transport of horseradish peroxidase (HRP).[19] The principle underlying this method is that HRP injected into a region containing synaptic terminals is taken up and rapidly transported intraaxonally in a retrograde direction to the neuronal cell body where it can be detected histochemically (Fig. 1).

Kittens ranging in age from newborn to three weeks were anesthetized and the round window of one side was exposed and injected with 1-20 μl of aqueous 10% HRP (Sigma Chemical Co, type VI). After 24 hours, the animals were reanesthetized and fixed by perfusion through the heart with a buffered aldehyde mixture. The brains were removed and frozen sections made at 40 μm through the brainstem. HRP was demonstrated by the procedures of Graham and Karnovsky using 0-dianisidine as the chromogen.[20] In some cases these same sections were further incubated for demonstration of acetylcholinesterase before being mounted on slides, counterstained with cresyl violet and coverslipped in Permount®.

EXPERIMENT 2*

Determination of the Projections of Olivocochlear Nerurons. The projections of olivocochlear neurons to the organ of Corti were identified by the method of autoradiography following

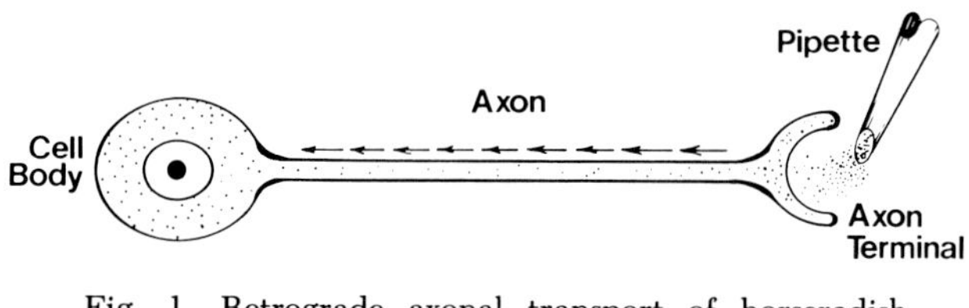

Fig. 1. Retrograde axonal transport of horseradish peroxidase.

*This work was performed in collaboration with Dr. John J. Guinan, Jr., Eaton-Peabody Laboratory of Auditory Physiology, Massachusetts Eye and Ear Infirmary, Boston, Massachusetts.

From the Boys Town Institute for Communication Disorders and Creighton University School of Medicine, Omaha, Nebraska. Supported by USPHS grants N007720: NS-14832; and BRDG No. 1 508 RR09003-01.

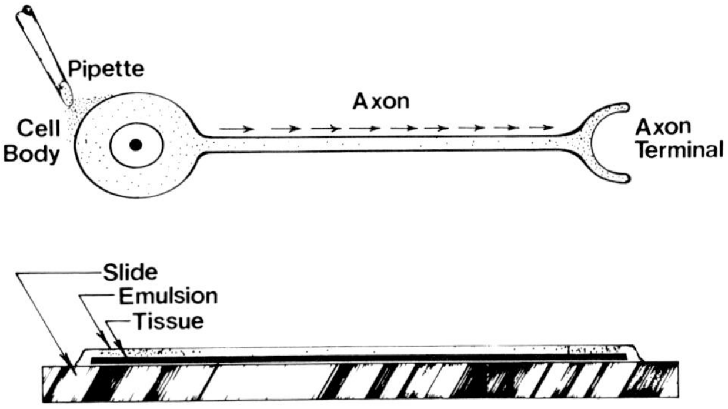

Fig. 2. Anterograde axonal transport of radio-labeled protein. Stippling over tissue in the microscope slide autoradiograph indicates silver grains.

anterograde axonal transport of radio-labeled protein (Fig. 2).[21] This method is basd on the fact that if a labeled amino is injected into the vicinity of neuronal cell bodies, it is taken up and incorporated into protein which are then rapidly transported to the axon terminal where they may be detected by autoradiography.

Twelve adult cats were anesthetized with Dial® -urethrane and prepared for bilateral acoustic stimulation. A gross recording electrode was advanced through the superior olivary complex via a ventral approach through the basioccipital bone.[22] Using evoked auditory responses as landmarks, the depths of various nuclei of the olivary complex were charted. The gross electrode was then withdrawn and an injection pipet affixed to a microliter syringe was inserted to an appropriate depth. An injection of 4-8μCi of ^{35}S-methionine (New England Nuclear Corp) was delivered continuously in a volume of 20-60 nanoliters of distilled water at a constant rate of 0.7 nanoliters per minute. The animal was maintained on anesthesia and kept at 37 C for 24 hours. Fixation was by perfusion through the heart with phosphate buffered (pH 7.4, 0.1M) 0.5% paraformaldehyde and 2% glutaraldehyde. The brain was removed and sectioned at 30μ on a freezing microtome. Every tenth section was mounted on slides, defatted in xylene and dried. The cochleas were also removed, decalcified in 10% buffered (pH 7.0) EDTA and embedded in araldite plastic to which 8% by volume of dibutylphthalate had been added as a softener. Sections were cut on a rotary microtome at 4-10μ in the plane of the modiolus. Serial sections were collected and mounted on slides. All slides were processed for autoradiography (AR) in Kodak NTB-2 liquid emulsion, boxed with dessicant and stored at 4 C until developed. Exposure times for the brain sections ranged from 7 to 42 days, and for the cochleas, from 14 to 120 days. Following development slides were usually counterstained with either neutral red (brain) or toluidine blue (cochleas), dehydrated, and covered in Permount. In assessing the autoradiographs of the cochleas, we used the criterion that four or more silver grains clustered within a 12 x 12 μ square constituted an autoradiographically (AR) positive finding. This criterion was set in order to reduce to a minimum the chance that randomly scattered "background" silver grains would be mistaken for grains caused by the disintegration of ^{35}S.

RESULTS

EXPERIMENT 1

Figure 3 shows the distribution of HRP-labeled olivocochlear neurons, as reconstructed from two newborn kittens, 24 hours after unilateral injections into the left cochlea. The counts shown in the figure are the larger of the values obtained in each locus in the two animals

Labeled neurons were scattered throughout the superior olivary complex, but appeared to form two fundamental groups on the basis of their size, location, and preferred side of projection. For example, there is a greater number of labeled cells in the lateral olivary zone on the injected side than in the same zone contralaterally. In the medial olivary zone, quite the opposite is true. Thus the projections to the cochlea from the lateral zone are predominantly ipsilateral, whereas from the medial zone they are predominantly crossed.

Rather obvious differences in neuronal size also were observed between the cells in the two groups (Fig. 4 A, B). Measurements length and width of cell bodies made on 50 labeled neurons in each locus

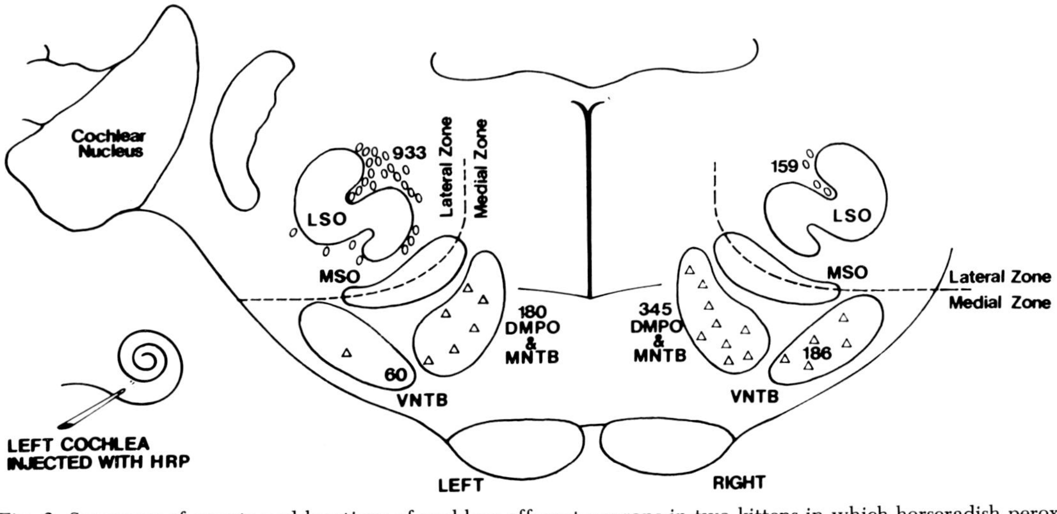

Fig. 3. Summary of counts and locations of cochlear efferent neurons in two kittens in which horseradish peroxidase (HRP) had access to only one labyrinth. Injected side is on the left. Total cochlear efferents: 1863; small cell - ○, large cell -△. Broken line passing through the medial superior olivary nucleus indicates the line of demarcation between the lateral and medial superior olivary zones. See text for further details. DMPO - Dorsomedial periolivary nucleus; LSO - Lateral superior olivary nucleus; MSO - Medial superior olivary nucleus; MNTB - Medial nucleus of the trapezoid body; VNTB - Ventral nucleus of the trapezoid body.

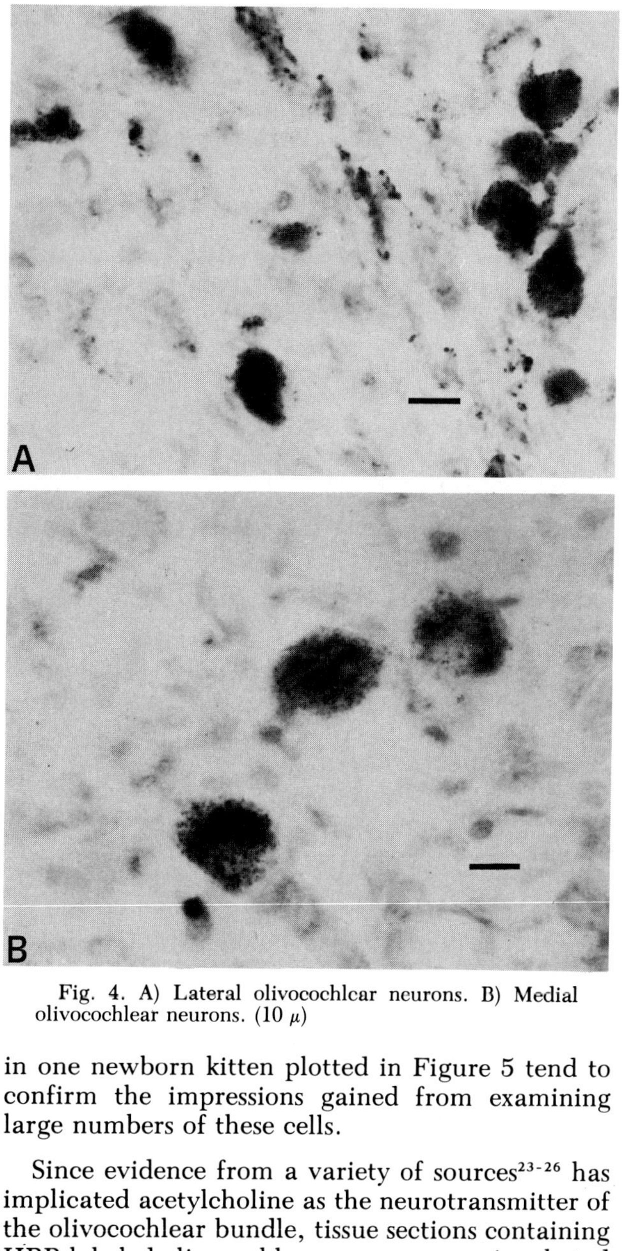

Fig. 4. A) Lateral olivocochlear neurons. B) Medial olivocochlear neurons. (10 μ)

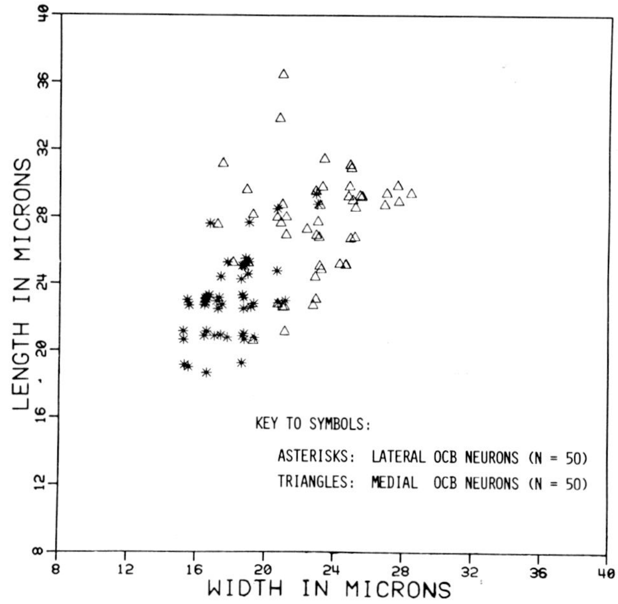

Fig. 5. Scatter plot of length versus width measurements of lateral and medial olivocochlear neurons.

in one newborn kitten plotted in Figure 5 tend to confirm the impressions gained from examining large numbers of these cells.

Since evidence from a variety of sources[23-26] has implicated acetylcholine as the neurotransmitter of the olivocochlear bundle, tissue sections containing HRP-labeled olivocochlear neurons were incubated for the demonstration of acetylcholinesterase, which is present in readily demonstrable amounts in cholinergic neurons. Virtually all HRP-labeled neurons were shown to contain acetylcholinesterase.[27]

EXPERIMENT 2

The difference between lateral and medial olivocochlear neurons with respect to their size and preferred side of projection prompted an investigation of the terminal distribution of their projections within the organ or Corti. The results from two typical animals, one with an injection of ^{35}S-methionine in the lateral zone, and one with an injection in the medial zone, will be presented. Figure 6 shows the results of an injection which was centered in the lateral zone, close to the dorsal hilus of the lateral superior olivary nucleus which is particularly heavily populated with small olivocochlear neurons. In the cochleas, clusters of silver grains, which are a reflection of radioactively labeled proteins in synaptic endings and their parent axons,[28] were located beneath inner hair cells (Fig. 7A) of both cochleas. The magnitude of labeling along the length of the organ of Corti was quantified by counting in each odd-numbered slide of a serial set, the silver grains which lay within a 12 x 12 μ grid square placed beneath the inner hair cell and beneath each of the three rows of outer hair cells. A count of seven or more silver grains was coded in the cochlear schematics in Figure 6 as filled symbols, four to six grains as half-filled symbols, and three grains or less as blank symbols. On the ipsilateral side, silver grains beneath inner hair cells were present throughout the length of the organ of Corti, but were somewhat sparse in the basal extremity, or "hook" region. Rarely, instances of weak or moderate accumulations of silver grains beneath outer hair cells were encountered. In the contralateral cochlea, the synaptic structures were generally somewhat more sparsely labeled than ipsilaterally, but were located predominantly beneath inner hair cells. Again, there were rare instances of labeled terminals beneath outer hair cells.

Much of the lower basal turn and hook regions were almost devoid of significant accumulations of silver grains. Thus, a marked bilateral asymmetry appears to exist in the projections of the lateral zone olivocochlear neurons.

In contrast to these findings, injections of ^{35}S-methionine into the medial zone of the superior olivary complex (Fig. 8) produced a distribution of silver grains which reflects a preponderance of syn-

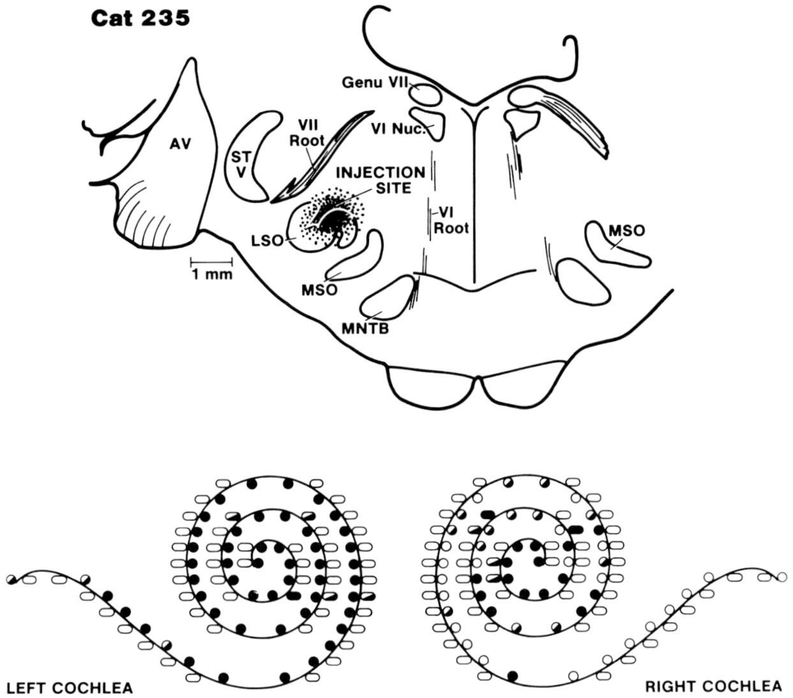

Fig. 6. Summary of autoradiograph observations in cat 235. In the upper portion of the figure is shown the center of the injection site located near the dorsal hilus of the left lateral superior olivary nucleus (LSO) where experiment 1 had revealed the presence of a particularly heavy concentration of small olivocochlear neurons. The lower two panels of the figure show the sites of silver grain clusters located on reconstruction of the organ of Corti. See text for key to symbols. AV - Anteroventral cochlear nucleus; LSO - Lateral superior olivary nucleus; MNTB - Medial nucleus of the trapezoid body; MSO - Medial superior olivary nucleus.

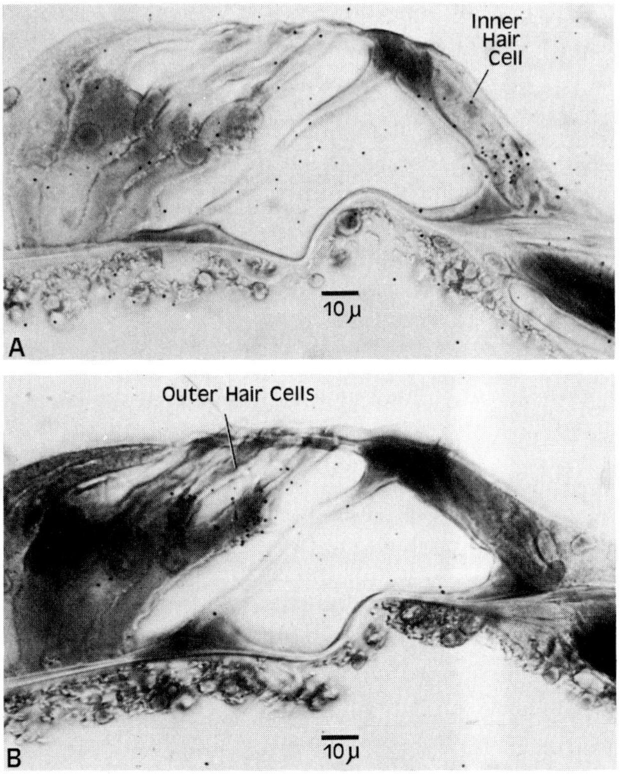

Fig. 7. A) Accumulations of silver grains beneath inner hair cell in cat 235, ipsilateral cochlea. B) Accumulations of silver grains beneath outer hair cells in cat 236, contralateral cochlea.

aptic labeling beneath the outer hair cells (Fig. 7B) of both cochleas. As also shown in Figure 8 a number of instances were encountered in which sparse accumulations of silver grains were present beneath the inner hair cells in both cochleas. This probably reflects, in large part, the presence of axons of passage which must traverse the region beneath the inner hair cells on their way to the outer hair cells. A more confident interpretation of these silver grains, however, can only be made with the electron microscope applied to autoradiographs. A comparison of the magnitude of labeling in the two cochleas, shows that the medial olivocochlear neurons project predominantly to the contralateral side, but the differences are not as marked as in the case of lateral olivocochlear neurons. In addition, the bilateral symmetry of projections from the medial zone is greater than that seen in the case of the lateral zone. While the generality of these observations must await further evidence, exceptions to the cases presented here have not been found in replications of injection sites similar to those presented here.

DISCUSSION

ORIGINS OF THE OLIVOCOCHLEAR BUNDLE

The distribution, density, and characteristic morphology of labeled neurons in the present study correspond closely to those of acetylcholinesterase-

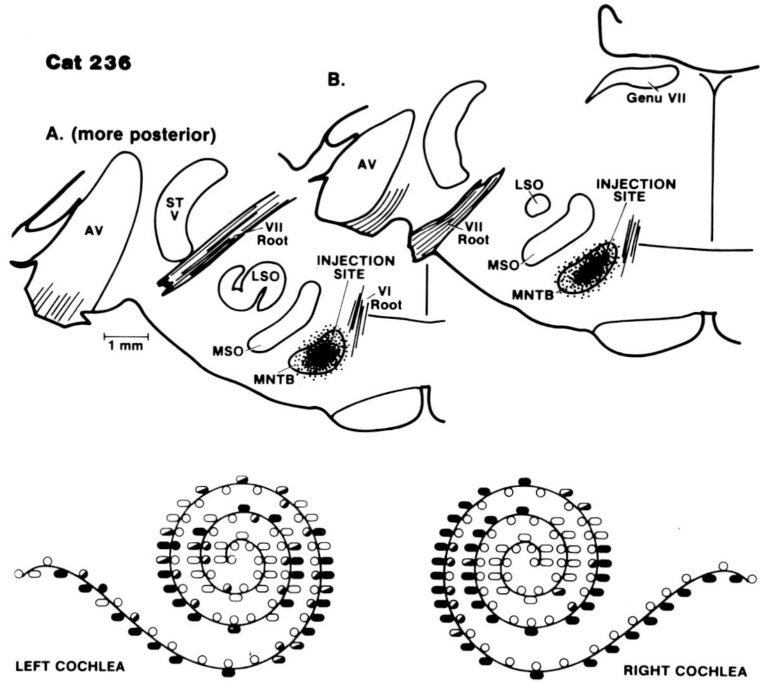

Fig. 8. Summary of autoradiographic observations in cat 236. In the upper portion of the figure is shown the centers of two injection sites located in the left medial nucleus of the trapezoid body (MNTB) where large olivocochlear neurons are distributed. The lower two panels of the figure show the sites of silver grains within the organ of Corti in the reconstructed cochleas. Symbols and abbreviations are the same as in Fig. 6.

positive neurons mapped by Osen and Roth[24] in the adult cat. The virtual identity of these two populations is further indicated by the simultaneous demonstrations of HRP and acetylcholinesterase in the same cells.[29] Thus, direct experimental evidence now supports the supposition that acetylcholinesterase-positive cells in the superior olivary complex constitute the cells of origin of the OCB.

It was entirely unexpected, however, that the areas containing olivocochlear neurons projecting to one side would exhibit such near perfect bilateral symmetry. Nor could it have been predicted that the majority of olivocochlear neurons are located ipsilateral to the cochlea to which they project, since the crossed OCB was believed to contain more axons than the uncrossed. In addition, the number of olivocochlear neurons labeled in our kittens (approximately 1,800) far exceeds the previous estimate (500) based on myelin studies in the adult cat.[30] It may be that many of the neurons labeled in the study have unmyelinated axons and further, that some olivocochlear neurons present in the kitten at birth ultimately disappear with the subsequent maturation of the organ of Corti. This question can be settled only by replication of this experiment on the adult cat.

PROJECTIONS OF OLIVOCOCHLEAR NEURONS

The application of the anterograde axonal transport technique in this study provides a demonstration of a direct axonal connection between the superior olive and the synaptic terminal fields beneath the hair cells of the organ of Corti. Previous approaches had used the technique of severing axons at the decussation of the OCB or in the vestibular nerve followed usually by electronmicroscopy study of degenerating endings.

DUAL EFFERENT INNERVATION

The findings of the two studies presented here are entirely consistent with each other regarding the origins of projections to each cochlea. For example, on the basis of the bilateral HRP-labeling of neurons in the lateral zone, one could predict (and we found) projections to both cochleas from an injection in this region. Accordingly, an integration of the two sets of experimental findings is presented in Figure 9. Two olivocochlear systems are emphasized in this schematic: 1) The small neurons of the lateral zone which project to the region beneath the inner hair cells[14] and, 2) the larger neurons of the medial zone which project predominantly, if not exclusively to the bases of outer hair cells.[10-13] The dichotomization of olivocochlear projections in this fashion largely complements most previous experimental work on the terminations of the crossed and uncrossed components of the OCB. Terminations beneath the inner hair cells were known to be mostly ipsilateral in origin,[15] and those beneath the outer hair cells mostly, but not exclusively, of contralateral origin.[12,13] In addition, developmental studies show that fine diameter axons destined for termination under the inner hair cells establish their synapses about the time of birth, whereas the synapses

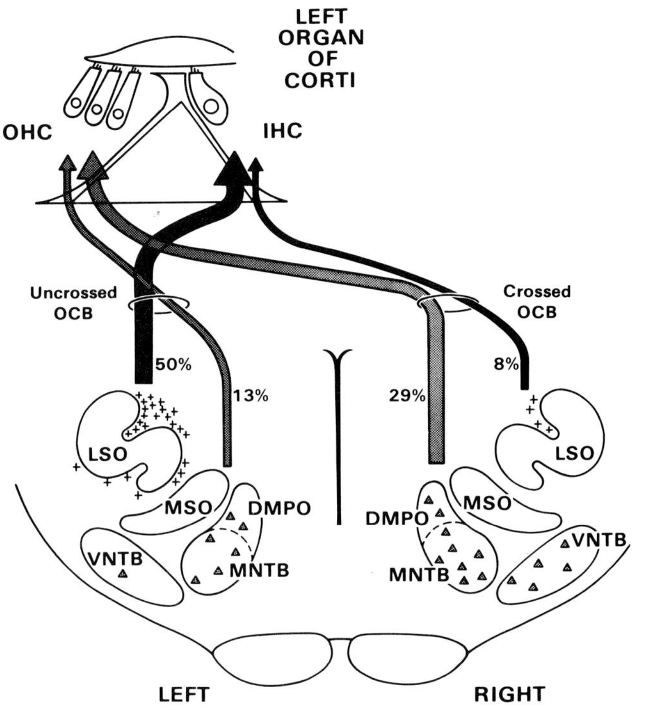

Fig. 9. Schema of the origins and terminations of the olivocochlear bundle in the cat, based upon HRP injections (origins and numerical estimates) and upon ^{35}S-methionine injections into the superior olivary complex (zones of termination). Crosses represent small OCB neurons; triangles represent large OCB neurons. The number of symbols of each kind and the widths of the lines originating from each region are proportional to neuronal contribution. It can be seen that a majority of OCB neurons to one cochlea originates on the ipsilateral side. Furthermore, the majority of OCB neurons are small, originate bilaterally, and do not innervate outer hair cells. DMPO - Dorsomedial periolivary nucleus; IHC - Inner hair cells; LSO - Lateral superior olivary nucleus; MNTB - Medial nucleus of the trapezoid body; MSO - Medial superior olivary nucleus; OCB - Olivocochlear bundle; OHC - Outer hair cells; VNTB - Ventral nucleus of the trapezoid body.

on the outer hair cells, provided by larger axons, do not develop until about seven days of age.[31] The rate of degeneration of these two fiber systems also differs.[32] Thus, the data presented here serve to integrate a substantial number of heterogeneous findings by showing that differences in olivocochlear connections appear to depend on their differential origins in the lateral and medial zones of the superior olivary complex. In light of this new evidence, the current terminology of "crossed" and "uncrossed" components of the OCB would appear to be no

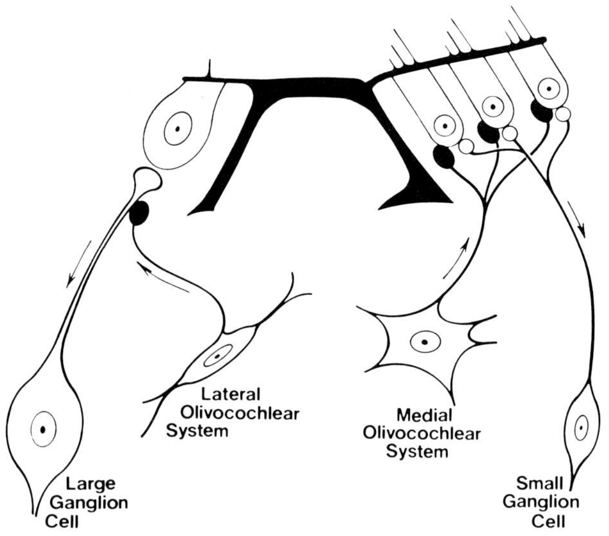

Fig. 10. Schematic diagram relating the afferent and efferent innervation of the organ of Corti.

longer appropriate, because both in terms of origins and terminations, these components are heterogeneous. Perhaps a more satisfactory designation for the olivocochlear system would be one which emphasizes the differential origins of projections to inner versus outer hair cells, and de-emphasizes whether they are crossed or uncrossed. To this end, I propose the terms *lateral* and *medial* olivocochlear systems, it being understood that at the level of the cochlea each contains ipsilateral and contralateral fiber contingents.

In summary, it may be permissible, purely on heuristic grounds, to present a tentative schematic that relates the efferent innervation to our present understanding of the afferent innervation of the organ of Corti. As illustrated in Figure 10, Spoendlin[33] has adduced evidence for the existence of two afferent systems, a larger and more populous one, consisting of large spiral ganglion cells, the peripheral processes of which are in postsynaptic relation to inner hair cells and, a smaller and less populus one, consisting of small spiral ganglion cells, the peripheral processes of which are in postsynaptic relation to outer hair cells. The lateral and medial olivocochlear systems may provide corresponding efferent pathways by which the central nervous system could separately influence these two afferent systems.

ACKNOWLEDGMENTS — I wish to acknowledge the collaboration of Dr. John J. Guinan, Jr., of the Eaton-Peabody Laboratory of Auditory Physiology, Massachusetts Eye and Ear Infirmary, Boston, Massachusetts, and the continual support and constructive advice of Dr. Nelson Y-s. Kiang, Director of that Laboratory. Further, I would like to thank Richard Short, David Baker and Phillip Somervell for their expert assistance.

REFERENCES

1. Rasmussen GL. The olivary peduncle and other fiber projections of the superior olivary complex. J Comp Neurol 1946; 83:141-219.

2. Galambos R. Suppression of auditory nerve activity by stimulation of efferent fibers to cochlea. J Neurophysiol 1956; 19:424-37.

3. Desmedt JE. Auditory-evoked potentials from cochlea to cortex as influenced by activation of the efferent olivocochlear bundle. J Acoust Soc Am 1962; 34:1478-96.

4. Desmedt JE, La Grutta V. Function of the uncrossed efferent olivocochlear fibers in the cat. Nature 1963; 200:472-4.

5. Fex J. Auditory activity in centrifugal and centripetal cochlear fibres in cat. Acta Physiol Scand 1962; 55 Suppl 189:5-68.

6. Sohmer HA. A comparison of the efferent effects of the homolateral and contralateral olivocochlear bundles. Acta Otolaryngol (Stockh) 1966; 62:74-87.

7. Wiederhold ML, Kiang NYS. Effects of electric stimulation of the crossed olivocochlear bundle on single auditory-nerve fibers in the cat. J Acoust Soc Am 1970; 48:950-65.

8. Murata K, Tanahashi T. Suppression of auditory nerve discharge by a contralateral stimulus. J Acoust Soc Am 1978; 64 Suppl 1:S136.

9. Engstrom H. On the double innervation of the sensory epithelia of the inner ear. Acta Otolaryngol (Stockh) 1958; 49:109-18.

10. Kimura RS, Wersall J. Termination of the olivocochlear bundle in relation to the outer hair cells of the organ of Corti in guinea pig. Acta Otolaryngol (Stockh) 1962; 55:11-32.

11. Spoendlin H. The organization of the cochlear receptor. Bibl Otorhinolaryngol 1966; 13:1-227.

12. Nakai Y, Igarashi M. Distribution of the crossed olivocochlear bundle terminals in the squirrel monkey cochea. Acta Otolaryngol (Stockh) 1974; 77:393-404.

13. Iurato S, Smith CA, Eldredge DH, et al. Distribuion of the crossed olivocochlear bundle in the chinchilla's cochlea. J Comp Neurol 1978; 182:57-76.

14. Smith CA. Innervation pattern of the cochlea. The internal hair cell. Ann Otol Rhinol Laryngol 1961; 70:504-27.

15. Smith CA, Rasmussen GL. Recent observations on the olivocochlear bundle. Ann Otol Rhinol Laryngol 1963; 72:489-505.

16. Dawson JH. Efferent olivocochlear bundle: some relationships to stimulus discrimination in noise. J Neurophysiol 1968; 31:122-30.

17. Oatman LC, Anderson BW. Effects of visual attention on tone burst evoked auditory potentials. Exp Neurol 1977; 57:200-11.

18. Klinke R, Galley N. Efferent innervation of vestibular and auditory receptors. Physiol Rev 1974; 54:316-57.

19. Lavail JH. The retrograde transport method. Fed Proc 1975; 34:1618-24.

20. Graham RC, Karnovsky MJ. The early stage of absorption of injected horseradish peroxidase in the proximal tubules of mouse kidney: ultrastructural cytochemistry by a new technique. J Histochem Cytochem 1966; 14:291-302.

21. Cowan WM, Gottleib DI, Hendrickson AE, Price JL, Woolsey TA. The autoradiographic demonstration of axonal connections in the central nervous system. Brain Res 1972; 37:21-51.

22. Guinan JJ, Guinan SS, Norris BE. Single auditory units in the superior olivary complex. Intern J Neuroscience 1972; 4:101-20.

23. Schuknecht HG, Churchill JA, Doran R. The localization of acetylcholinesterase in the cochlea. Arch Otolaryngol 1959; 69:549-59.

24. Osen KK, Roth K. Histochemical localization of cholinesterases in the cochlear nuclei of the cat, with notes on the origin of acetylcholinesterase-positive afferents and the superior olive. Brain Res 1969; 16:165-85.

25. Bobbin RP, Konishi T. Action of cholinergic and anticholinergic drugs at the crossed olivocochlear bundle-hair cell junction. Acta Otolaryngol (Stockh) 1974; 77:56-65.

26. Guth PS, Norris CH, Bobbin RP. The pharmacology of transmission in the peripheral auditory system. Pharm Review 1976; 28:95-125.

27. El-Badawi A, Schenk EA. Dual innervation of the mammalian urinary bladder. Am J Anat 1966; 119:405-28.

28. Jones EG, Hartman BK. Recent advances in neuroanatomical methodology. Ann Rev Neurosci 1978; 1:215-96.

29. Warr WB. Olivocochlear and vestibular efferent neurons of the feline brain stem: their location, morphology and number determined by retrograde axonal transport and acetylcholinesterase histochemistry. J Comp Neurol 1975; 161:159-82.

30. Rasmussen GL. Efferent fibers of the cochlear nerve and cochlear nucleus. In: Rasmussen GL, Windle WF, eds. Neural mechanisms of the auditory and vestibular systems. Springfield: Thomas, 1960; 105-15.

31. Pujol R, Carlier E, Devigne C. Differential patterns of cochlear innervation during the development of the kitten. J Comp Neurol 1978; 177:529-36.

32. Warr WB. Discussed by Spoendlin H. The olivocochlear bundle: its origins and terminations in the cat. In: Naunton RF, Fernandez C, eds. Evoked electrical activity in the auditory nervous system. New York: Academic Press, 1978; 64.

33. Spoendlin H. The afferent innervation of the cochlea. In: Naunton RF, Fernandez C, eds. Evoked electrical activity in the auditory nervous system. New York: Academic Press Inc, 1978; 21-41.

NEUROCHEMISTRY OF THE AUDITORY SYSTEM

ROBERT J. WENTHOLD, PhD

BETHESDA, MARYLAND

Two areas of auditory biochemistry are reviewed: the identification and characterization of neurotransmitters in the auditory system and the biochemical approach to the study of genetic hearing disorders. Studies to identify neurotransmitters at major auditory synapses are outlined. Evidence supporting glutamate or aspartate as the neurotransmitter for the auditory nerve is presented. The application of biochemistry to the study of genetic hearing disorders is discussed.

INTRODUCTION

In reviewing the literature on the auditory system, one is reminded how little research has been done in the area of auditory biochemistry. This is particularly disturbing since biochemistry has provided so much information to many other systems, and many of the problems facing auditory researchers today await a biochemical approach for solutions. Attempts have been made, and research is in progress, to investigate such areas as ototoxicity, cochlear metabolism, cochlear fluid composition and auditory neurotransmitters using biochemical techniques.[1-7] This article is not intended to be a review of auditory biochemistry since hardly enough material exists to make that appropriate. Rather, it will concentrate on two areas of auditory research: the chemistry of neurotransmitters in the cochlea and cochlear nucleus and the biochemical approach to the study of genetic hearing disorders. Both are relatively new to the study of the auditory system and rely heavily on the related disciplines of morphology, physiology, pharmacology and genetics. Therefore, some background information and data from the related fields will be presented. Since no serious biochemical study has been carried out in the area of genetic hearing disorders, this article will be limited to an introduction to the biochemistry of genetic hearing disorders.

CHEMISTRY OF NEUROTRANSMITTERS IN COCHLEA AND COCHLEAR NUCLEUS

A major objective of neurobiological research is to identify and characterize the neurotransmitter molecules that mediate synaptic transmission. A neurotransmitter is a substance which is released from the presynaptic terminal upon stimulation, moves across the synaptic cleft and interacts with receptor sites on the postsynaptic membrane causing excitation or inhibition in the postsynaptic neuron. Many substances have been suggested to function as neurotransmitters (Table 1), but few of these are proven neurotransmitters in the mammalian nervous system. Acetylcholine (ACh) is the neurotransmitter at the mammalian neuromuscular junction[8] and it is likely that ACh, γ-aminobutyric acid (GABA), norepinephrine, dopamine and serotonin are neurotransmitters in the mammalian CNS. The recently discovered class of putative neurotransmitters, neuropeptides, are present in discrete regions of the brain suggesting a possible neurotransmitter role.[9] However, more experimental work needs to be carried out on these substances and there is evidence that they may function as neuromodulators rather than as neurotransmitters.[10] To establish any substance as a neurotransmitter at a given synapse, it is generally agreed that several criteria must be satisfied.[11-13]

1. The substance must be present in the presynaptic terminal. It can be supplied by enzymatic synthesis within the terminal, by uptake through the terminal membrane or by transport from the cell body by way of axoplasmic transport.

2. The substance must be released from the presynaptic terminal upon stimulation.

3. The substance must interact with the postsynaptic receptor in a manner identical to that of the synaptically released neurotransmitter.

TABLE 1. LIST OF SUBSTANCES WITH CONFIRMED OR POSSIBLE NEUROTRANSMITTER ROLES

Acetylcholine	Carnosine
Dopamine	β-Endorphin
Noradrenaline	Leu-enkephalin
Adrenaline	Met-enkephalin
Serotonin	Luteinizing hormone-releasing hormone
Octopamine	Neurotensin
Histamine	Oxytocin
γ-Aminobutyric acid	Somatostatin
Glycine	Substance P
Glutamic acid	Thyrotropin-releasing hormone
Aspartic acid	Vasopressin
Taurine	

From the Laboratory of Neuro-otolaryngology, National Institute of Neurological and Communicative Disorders and Stroke, National Institutes of Health, Bethesda, Maryland.

REPRINTS — Robert J. Wenthold, PhD, Laboratory of Neuro-otolaryngology, National Institute of Neurological and Communicative Disorders and Stroke, National Institutes of Health, Bethesda, MD 20205.

4. Pharmacological agents which affect the interaction of the synaptically released neurotransmitter with the postsynaptic receptor, must affect the interaction of the applied substance and the postsynaptic receptor in an identical way.

5. A mechanism must exist for the inactivation of the substance after its release from the presynaptic terminal and interaction with the postsynaptic membrane. This is believed to involve either enzymatic inactivation, inactivation through uptake into neuronal or glial elements or diffusion of the neurotransmitter away from the receptor.

It is most convincing to establish presynaptic release (criterion 2) and identity of action (criterion 3). However, it is difficult to demonstrate these two points. Intracellular recording is required to show identity of action. In many neurons prolonged intracellular recording is not yet technically feasible and for dendritic synapses, the problem remains of how to investigate changes in membrane properties at dendritic sites far from the usual intrasomatic site of recording.[11] In the CNS it is unlikely that presynaptic release can be satisfactorily demonstrated because the site of collection is relatively far from the point of actual release and there are no known agents to selectively block the inactivating systems for many putative neurotransmitters. Although demonstration of the remaining three criteria is less convincing, these criteria are useful for screening several possible neurotransmitters to obtain likely candidates for neurotransmitter roles.

Establishing the presynaptic presence of a putative neurotransmitter provides a reasonable approach to the identification of the neurotransmitter at a given synapse. Neurotransmitter candidates can be quantitated by chemical assays or determined by histochemical methods. The metabolism of some of the better characterized putative neurotransmitters is known and it has been established that in many cases, the enzyme catalyzing the synthesis of the substance is a marker for the substance. These include choline acetyltransferase (ACh), glutamate decarboxylase (GABA), tyrosine hydroxylase (catecholamines), dopamine-β-hydroxylase (norepinephrine) and tryptophan hydroxylase (serotonin). The measurement of enzymes is preferable to that of small molecules because greater sensitivity is obtained with enzyme catalyzed reactions which can be maintained for up to several hours and because enzymes are less likely to show short-term fluctuations than are small molecules which can be rapidly metabolized. Furthermore, much progress has recently been made in neurotransmitter localization through immunohistochemistry. Although antibodies can be produced against some putative neurotransmitters, many are too small for the production of antibodies. However, antibodies can be made against their enzymes, and glutamate decarboxylase,[14-16] tyrosine hydroxylase,[17-20] dopamine-β-hydroxylase[21,22] and tryptophan hydroxylase[20,23] have been localized by immunohistochemistry.

The putative neurotransmitters, glutamic acid, aspartic acid and glycine, are common α amino acids and present in all cells. The general metabolism of these amino acids is known (Fig. 1), but has not been thoroughly investigated to determine if a specific metabolic pathway is used when these substances function as neurotransmitters. Although these amino acids are ubiquitous, some information on their possible neurotransmitter roles may be gained by studying their distribution in the nervous system. A study of the distribution of glycine in spinal cord first led to the suggestion that it may serve as a neurotransmitter.[24,25] The evidence is now strong that glycine is an inhibitory neurotransmitter in the spinal cord.[26] A more specific way of demonstrating the presynaptic presence of a substance, is to show a decrease in the substance when terminals degenerate, for example, after surgical or chemical destruction of a specific population of neurons. Under these conditions, levels of putative neurotransmitters, especially amino acids, can be altered due to metabolic changes or transneuronal effects and not as a direct result of terminal degeneration. It is important, therefore, to show the decrease in the substance occurs when terminals degenerate, that the decreased substance does not return to normal level later unless reinnervation occurs and that a general loss of all small molecules does not occur.

There are two major classes of synapses in the cochlea: afferent synapses between hair cells and afferent fibers, and efferent synapses between efferent fibers and hair cells or afferent fibers. With respect to identification of the neurotransmitter used, the efferent synapse is, by far, the best characterized synapse in the auditory system. Although it has not been proven, it is very likely that ACh is a neurotransmitter for the efferent fibers. Since there are at least two types of efferent endings in the cochlea,[27] those terminating on hair cells and those terminating on afferent endings, and since the efferent fibers originate from two sources, it is possible that more than one neurotransmitter is associated with the efferent system. Many of the criteria to establish ACh as an efferent neurotransmitter have been met. Although ACh has not been demonstrated in the efferent endings, experiments have been done showing choline acetyltransferase is associated with the efferent terminals.[28-30] The distribution of choline acetyltransferase in the cochlea follows that of efferent fibers and terminals and the enzyme decreases in the cochlea after the efferent fibers degenerate. Release of ACh to perilymph by stimulation of efferent fibers has been shown[31,32] and ACh antagonists block the synaptically released neurotransmitter.[31,33-36] Acetylcholinesterase, an enzyme which inactivates ACh,

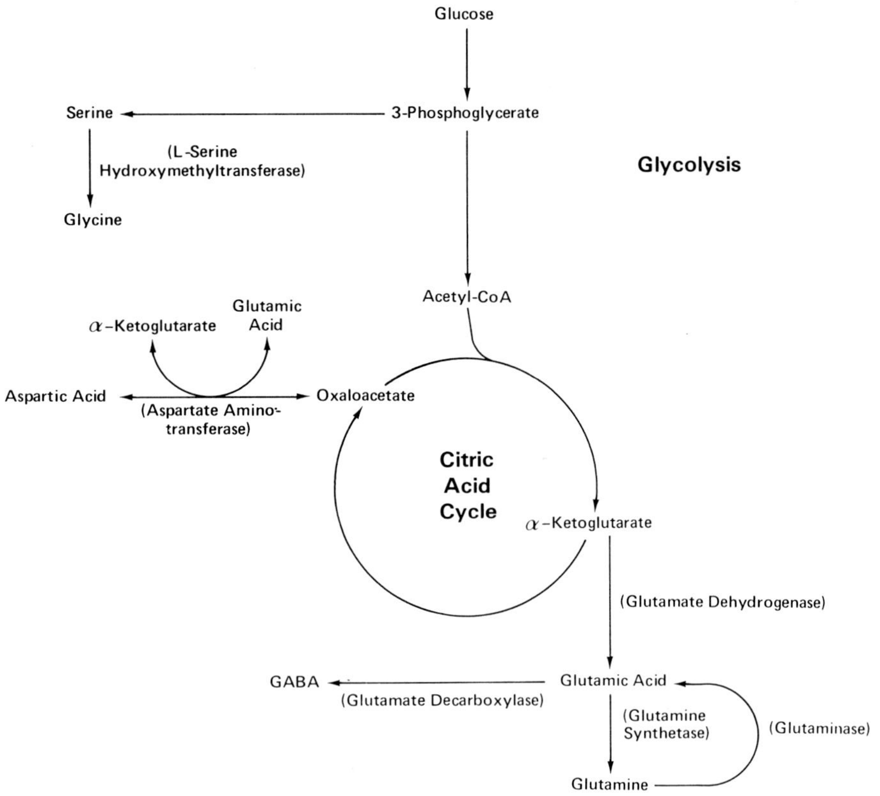

Fig. 1. Summary of the metabolism of glutamic acid, aspartic acid and glycine.

is present in the cochlea and appears to be associated with the efferent system.[27] Although it has been shown that locally applied ACh causes an increase in the cochlear microphonics and a decrease in the action potential of the auditory nerve,[37] it has not been demonstrated that locally applied ACh affects the postsynaptic membrane in a way identical to that of the synaptically released neurotransmitter. Since intracellular recording from mammalian hair cells has recently been accomplished,[38] this experiment can now be carried out.

There is very little information on the nature of the afferent neurotransmitter in the cochlea. The evidence is strong that it is not ACh,[28-30,33] GABA,[28,39-41] serotonin[42] or a catecholamine.[43-45] The observation that GABA is synthesized and stored by tissue preparations containing hair cells, led Flock and Lam[46] to suggest that GABA may serve as a hair cell afferent neurotransmitter. However, they failed to quantitate the GABA formed and studies have shown very low levels of GABA[39,41] and glutamate decarboxylase[28] in the organ of Corti, much lower than one would expect if GABA were a major hair cell neurotransmitter. The synthesis of GABA observed by Flock and Lam is likely due to low levels of glutamate decarboxylase found in many cells and not associated with a transmitter role for GABA.[47,48] Furthermore, physiological studies do not support GABA as a neurotransmitter in the cochlea.[49] Glutamic acid and aspartic acid are thought to be major excitatory neurotransmitters based on their high levels in neuronal tissue and their neuronal excitatory actions.[11,50-52] They have been suggested as neurotransmitters in the cochlea,[33,49,53] but the evidence is weak. Both amino acids are present at high concentrations in the organ of Corti,[39] but because of their general metabolic roles, their presence gives little information on their possible neurotransmitter status in the cochlea. Therefore, at this time glutamic acid and aspartic acid cannot be ruled out as candidates for the hair cell neurotransmitter. Since the afferent neutotransmitter is likely not one of the common neurotransmitters, eg, ACh, GABA, serotonin or a catecholamine, its identification may involve characterization of a compound of which there may be little information. The approach presently used by Sewell and Guth[54] involving perilymph collections during sound stimulation followed by analysis may provide some clues as to the nature of the afferent neurotransmitter.

There is evidence that the neurotransmitter for the terminals of the auditory nerve in the cochlear nucleus is not ACh,[28,55,56] GABA,[28,56-58] serotonin, a catecholamine,[28,59] taurine,[60] glycine,[57,60,61] met-enkephalin,[62,63] or leu-enkephalin.[62,63] This evidence is based on the distribution of the substance or its related enzyme in the cochlear nucleus and auditory nerve or the fact that the substance or related enzyme does not decrease in the cochlear

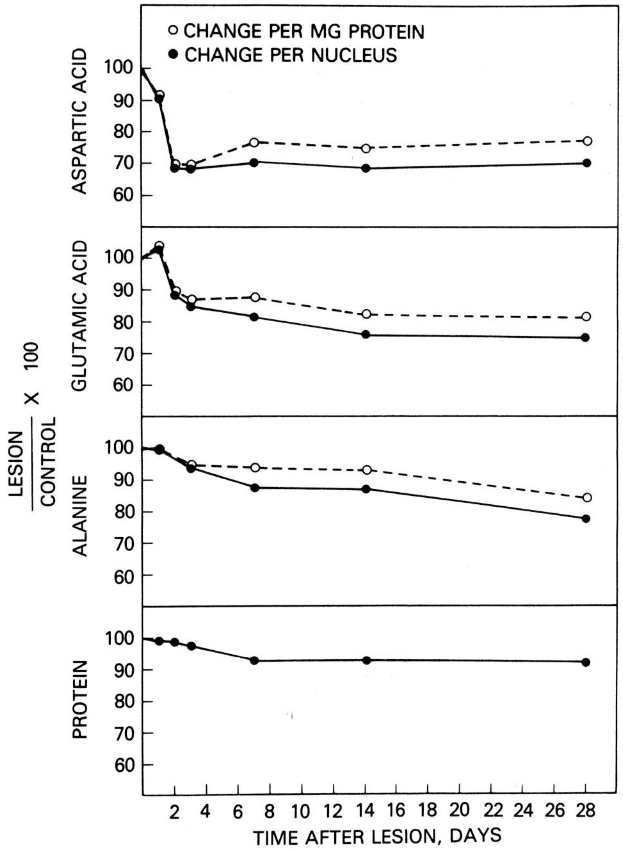

Fig. 2. Effect of unilateral cochlear ablation on the levels of aspartic acid, glutamic acid, alanine and protein in the ipsilateral cochlear nucleus of the guinea pig. Values are expressed as percent amino acid (either total amino acid in the nucleus or amino acid per milligram protein) remaining in the cochlear nucleus ipsilateral to the auditory nerve lesion relative to the amount in the contralateral, control cochlear nucleus. Each point represents the mean of 4-7 replications. Modified from reference 60.

nucleus after lesion of the auditory nerve. It should be emphasized that this data is not proof that these substances are not neurotransmitters for the auditory nerve. It may be at least as difficult to show definitively that a substance is not a neurotransmitter as it is to show a substance to be one. It must be considered that one of these substances could be a neurotransmitter for a small population of auditory nerve synapses, and that auditory nerve lesion would not cause a detectable change in the substance in the cochlear nucleus. This is especially important for substances which are present at high concentrations in the cochlear nucleus, for example amino acids, such that only a very small percent of the total would be associated with a population of terminals. Since two morphologically distinct populations of spiral ganglion cells give rise to auditory nerve fibers,[64] the possibility of two different auditory nerve neurotransmitters becomes more likely.

Recent findings suggest that the dicarboxylic acids, glutamic acid and aspartic acid, may function as neurotransmitters at primary auditory synapses. Three lines of evidence suggest one or both of these amino acids are concentrated in the presynaptic terminals: 1) Aspartic acid has a distribution in the cochlear nucleus similar to that of primary auditory teminals.[57,61] 2) Glutamic acid and aspartic acid decrease in the cochlear nucleus when primary auditory terminals degenerate.[60,65] 3) The decreases in both amino acids after lesion of the auditory nerve are greatest in areas of the cochlear nucleus that receive the greatest innervation by primary auditory fibers.[66] The first point has been demonstrated by Godfrey et al[57,61] who measured the levels of the putative neurotransmitters glutamic acid, aspartic acid, GABA and glycine in subdivisions of the cat and rat cochlear nucleus. Only the distribution of aspartic acid somewhat followed that of the primary auditory terminals.[67-69] Aspartic acid was not particularly high in the auditory nerve. These results, although suggestive, are difficult to interpret because aspartic acid like other amino acids is involved in many cellular functions not related to neurotransmission.

The decrease in glutamic acid and aspartic acid in the cochlear nucleus when primary auditory terminals degenerate provides stronger evidence that one or both of these amino acids is concentrated in auditory nerve terminals. Both amino acids decrease in the cochlear nucleus after the auditory nerve is surgically lesioned[60] (Fig. 2). The decrease in aspartic acid appears to occur somewhat earlier than that of glutamic acid but both decreased during the time period when primary auditory terminals were degenerating. Other amino acids measured did not decrease, except for alanine and its decrease was slight and did not coincide with degeneration of the primary terminals. Decreases in glutamic acid and aspartic acid in the cochlear nucleus of the genetically deaf waltzing guinea pig[70-72] also coincide with the morphological degeneration of spiral ganglion cells and corresponding primary auditory terminals.[65,73] Furthermore, the effect of auditory nerve lesion on glutamic acid and aspartic acid in the cochlear nucleus of the waltzing guinea pig is affected by loss of spiral ganglion cells with age (Fig. 3), suggesting the pools of these amino acids which are affected by auditory nerve lesion are also affected in the maturing waltzing guinea pig.

The final evidence showing that glutamic acid and aspartic acid are concentrated in primary auditory terminals is that the decrease in both amino acids after auditory nerve lesion[66] follows the distribution of primary auditory fibers[67-69] (Fig. 4).

In addition to the data suggesting that these amino acids are concentrated in primary terminals there is evidence that glutamic acid is released from auditory nerve terminals in the cochlear nucleus.[74] When cochlear nucleus slices are incubated in vitro, the major amino acids released in the presence of calcium and elevated potassium are glutamic acid,

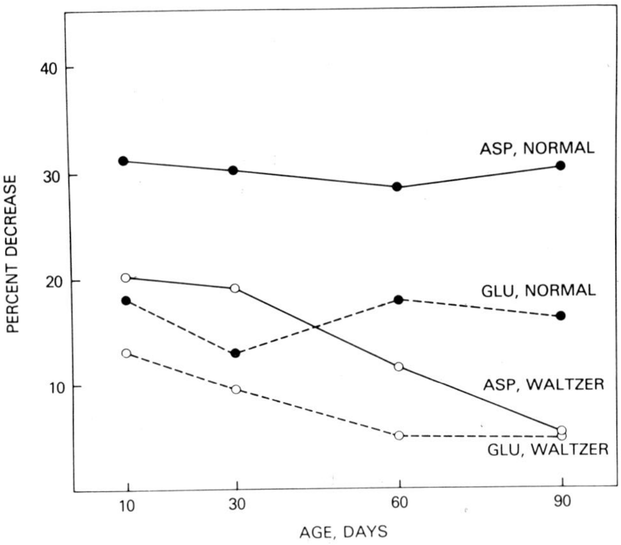

Fig. 3. Effect of unilateral cochlear ablation on the levels of aspartic acid and glytamic acid in the ipsilateral cochlear nucleus of the normal and waltzing guinea pig as a function of age. Data are expressed as the percent decrease in the amino acid (determined per milligram protein) in the ipsilateral cochlear nucleus relative to the amount in the contralateral control cochlear nucleus. Each point represents the mean of 4-6 replications. Modified from reference 65.

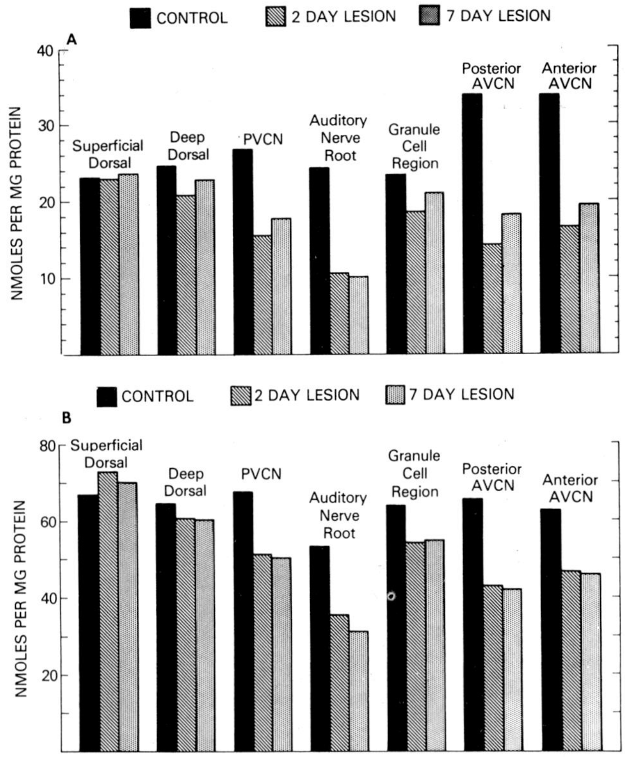

Fig. 4. A) Aspartic acid and B) glutamic acid in subdivisions of the cochlear nucleus of the guinea pig after auditory nerve lesion. Each value is the mean of 5 or 6 replications. Modified from reference 66.

GABA and glycine, all putative neurotransmitters. Furthermore, the calcium dependent, potassium evoked release of glutamic acid is decreased by 40% by auditory nerve lesion while the release of GABA and glycine are unaffected. Less aspartic acid than glutamic acid is released from the cochlear nucleus slices and auditory nerve lesion decreases the release of aspartic acid only by 26%. These experiments cannot replace in vivo demonstration of release after presynaptic stimulation for proving a substance is a neurotransmitter, but do suggest that the decrease in glutamic acid after auditory nerve lesion involves a pool of the amino acid that can be released in vitro under conditions known to cause release of other putative neurotransmitters.

Two lines of evidence suggest the presence of glutamic acid or aspartic acid receptors on cells in the cochlear nucleus which are innervated by primary auditory fibers. First, kainic acid, a structural analog of glutamic acid and suggested to cause selective degeneration of neurons having glutamic acid receptors,[75-77] selectively destroys neurons in the cochlear nucleus which are innervated by primary auditory fibers.[78] Second, there is evidence that both glutamic acid and aspartic acid excite neurons in the cochlear nucleus, and DL-α-aminoadipate, an antagonist of dicarboxylic amino acids,[79] blocks both the amino acid-induced and the synaptic excitations.[80]

All available data point to glutamic acid, aspartic acid or both as neurotransmitters for the auditory nerve, but two critical criteria, presynaptic release and identity of action, remain to be demonstrated for the synapse. It is interesting that both amino acids decrease when the primary auditory terminals degenerate and probably at slightly different times. Possibly both function as neurotransmitters, perhaps for different populations of synapses. It seems likely, however, that since glutamic acid and aspartic acid are closely related metabolically, one may decrease because it is an immediate metabolic precursor or product of the other.

The neurotransmitters for other inputs to the cochlear nucleus and its interneurons are poorly characterized. The high levels of glycine[57,61] and GABA[57,61] (as well as glutamate decarboxylase)[56] in the dorsal cochlear nucleus suggest they may function as neurotransmitters, but the sources and terminations of neurons containing them are unknown. Trapezoid body lesions do not cause a significant decrease in glutamate decarboxylase in the cochlear nucleus.[58] Choline acetyltransferase and acetylcholinesterase are found throughout the cochlear nucleus with highest levels in the dorsal cochlear nucleus and the granule cell area of the ventral cochlear nucleus.[55] Some of the enzyme activity may be associated with olivocochlear fibers which enter and terminate in the cochlear nucleus.[27,55,81] Comis and Guth[82] studied release of acetylcholine from the dorsal cochlear nucleus after stimulation of the olivocochlear fibers, but the results were ambiguous. Catecholamines[59,83] (mostly norepinephrine) and serotonin[59] are present in the cochlear nucleus. The presence of the peptides, met-enkephalin and leu-enkephalin,[62,63] suggests a possible neurotransmitter or neuromodulator role for them in the cochlear nucleus.

BIOCHEMICAL APPROACH TO THE STUDY OF GENETIC HEARING DISORDERS

The information contained in a gene is determined by the sequence of purine (adenine and guanine) and pyrimidine (cytosine and thymine) bases of the DNA. The DNA molecule forms a template on which other nucleic acid molecules of precise structure are synthesized. In gene replication complimentary molecules of DNA are synthesized. In the production of polypeptides, information is transferred from DNA to messenger RNA through the process of transcription and the information in the messenger RNA is transferred to the polypeptide through the process of translation. Although further changes may occur in the polypeptide to produce a functional protein, such as structural alterations and membrane incorporation, the basic amino acid backbone of the protein is formed at translation. Therefore, a change in the DNA sequence may result in an abnormal amino acid sequence in the protein product. Even a single nucleotide substitution may affect the growing polypeptide by insertion of an incorrect amino acid or by termination of the polypeptide's synthesis. Insertion of a single incorrect amino acid into the polypeptide may alter the properties of the protein so severely that it may be totally inactive, may function with limited efficiency, may function normally but have altered physical properties, or, if the substitution is in a noncritical region of the protein or involves an amino acid of similar hydrophobic and hydrophilic properties, may cause little or no functional or physical change. Termination of polypeptide synthesis by a base change in the DNA will likely lead to an inactive polypeptide. The effect this abnormality will have on the organism will depend on the normal role of the protein.

The ultimate objective of biochemical research on genetic disorders is to identify and characterize the protein that is either absent or defective in any one disease. Such a discovery is usually preceded by an understanding of the molecular events in which this protein is normally involved. In the study of the lipid storage disorders, for example, identification of the defective lysosomal enzyme was facilitated by the analysis of the accumulated lipid normally degraded by that particular enzyme.[84] Unfortunately extremely little is known about the biochemical defects involved in genetic hearing disorders, especially those in which only the auditory system is affected. Some disorders in which deafness is only one of several manifestations of the disease have been studied biochemically. For example, Hunter's and Hurler's syndromes, which in many cases lead to deafness, involve disorders of mucopolysaccharide metabolism with defective enzymes, sulfoiduronate sulfatase[85] and α-L-iduronidase,[86,87] respectively. Biochemical studies on the cochlea are limited by the small sizes of the cochlear structures, such that traditional biochemical techniques cannot be applied. In the guinea pig, the total dry weights of the organ of Corti and the stria vascularis are 16 μg and 12.5 μg, respectively.[88] Although cochlear enzymes can be studied through measurement of their enzymatic activities,[89] the amount of tissue essentially precludes extensive purification and characterization of most cochlear proteins. Only one cochlear protein has been purified, carbonic anhydrase, which is abundant in the spiral ligament, representing about 1% of the total protein.[90]

Several aspects of human genetic hearing disorders have been reviewed.[91-100] These disorders include all modes of inheritance, autosomal recessive, autosomal dominant and X-linked, with most examples being autosomal recessive. Morphological studies have been carried out on human temporal bones describing the degenerative processes for some genetic disorders.[99,100-102] From an experimental viewpoint, the several species of animals in which genetic deafness has been reported provides a promising area in which to investigate genetic hear-

TABLE 2. EXAMPLES OF GENETIC HEARING DISORDERS IN ANIMALS WITH PROGRESSIVE COCHLEAR DEGENERATION*

Animal	*References*	*Inheritance*	*Morphological Characteristics*
Waltzing guinea pig†	70-73	Dominant	Hair cell degeneration 10-60 days of age and spiral ganglion cell degeneration 30-90 days of age. No early strial abnormalities.
Deaf white cat	102-108	Dominant	Degeneration of both organ of Corti and stria vascularis begins shortly after birth. Later degeneration of spiral ganglion cells. May serve as animal model for Waardenburg's syndrome.
Hedlunk white mink	109-114	Recessive	Earliest degeneration occurs in the stria vascularis at 2 weeks of age. Later degeneration of organ of Corti.
Dalmation dog	115-119	X-linked	Both organ of Corti and stria vascularis degeneration present at 4 weeks of age. Spiral ganglion cell degeneration occurs later. Possible absence of efferent innervation.
Shaker — 1 mouse	120-123	Recessive	Hair cell degeneration occurs by 12 days of age. Virtual absence of efferent innervation.

*For other studies on genetically deaf animals see references 109, 120, 124-128.

†Two apparently distinct strains of waltzing guinea pig have been described. The first, described by Ibsen and Risty[129] in 1929 and Lurie[130] has degeneration of both the organ of Corti and stria vascularis apparent at birth and displays a recessive mode of inheritance. The waltzing guinea pig with dominant inheritance arose from NIH stock in 1953 and is currently maintained at the NIH.

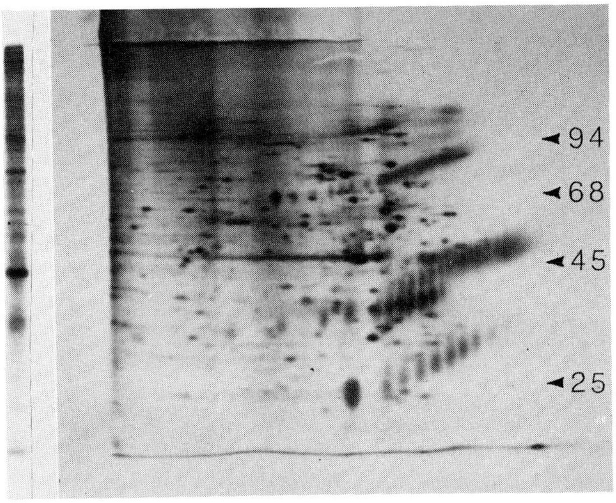

Fig. 5. One- and two-dimensional SDS gel electrophoresis analysis of proteins of the stria vascularis of the guinea pig. Cochlear proteins were labeled by exchanging perilymph with a solution containing 150 μCi of ^{35}S-methionine and animals were killed three hours later. One-dimensional electrophoresis was carried out following the method of Laemmli[135] and two-dimensional by the method of Ames and Nikaido,[131] both using 10% acrylamide. Molecular weight standards are phosphorylase b (94,000), bovine serum albumin (68,000), ovalbumin (45,000) and chymotrypsinogen (25,000). Proteins were detected using the method of Bonner and Laskey.[136]

ing disorders. In many cases the morphology of the degenerative processes have been described. Although the characteristics of many of these are similar to those occurring in humans, it remains to be determined if common molecular abnormalities are involved. It has been suggested, for example, that the deaf white cat may serve as a model for Waardenburg's syndrome.[103] Since a severely degenerated cochlea will almost certainly show abnormal biochemistry, the animals displaying progressive cochlear degeneration may be especially useful to the study of cochlear biochemistry (Table 2). These animals are born with a normal or near normal cochlea, determined morphologically, which then begins to degenerate shortly after birth. In some cases the animal may be able to hear for some time. Abnormal molecular events undoubtedly precede the morphological degeneration. The two possibilities that seem likely to occur are that either a defective protein is present earlier in development but does not cause cochlear degeneration, or a defective protein is synthesized only shortly before cochlear degeneration is observed. Although it may be statistically unlikely that a single abnormal protein can be detected among the several thousand different proteins in the cochlea, the analysis of proteins at critical times before morphological degeneration is observed may provide clues as to the molecular nature of the degeneration. Quantitation of the proteins such as the structural proteins, tubulin and actin; the enzymes involved in ionic maintenance, ATPase and carbonic anhydrase; citric acid cycle enzymes; and proteins associated with neurotransmission may give information as to the biochemical systems which are first affected. Quantitation of specific proteins is severely limited by the number of cochlear proteins which have been characterized. However, gel electrophoresis in combination with electrofocusing is capable of resolving 1,000 proteins.[131-134] Even small amounts of protein can be analyzed by labeling the proteins with radioactive amino acids. With this technique more than 200 proteins can be resolved from the guinea pig stria vascularis, a sample containing 3 to 6 μg of protein (Fig. 5).

In searching for the causes of genetic hearing disorders, it must be remembered that even in cases of genetic deafness in which only the cochlea is affected, the genetically defective protein may be elsewhere in the body and exert its toxic influence by production, or lack of production, of a diffusable substance. For example, in the case of phenylketonuria, the defective enzyme is phenylalanine hydroxylase located exclusively in the liver, but the disease causes abnormal brain development through the build-up of phenylalanine and the abnormal formation of its by-products.[137] The interesting study by Deol has shown that cochlear damage and deafness can be caused by induced hypothyroidism during development suggesting that in Pendred's syndrome and other similar conditions, the loss of hearing is secondary to hypothyroidism during fetal life.[138,139]

The analysis of cochlear proteins in genetically deaf animals represents only one of several approaches to the study of genetic hearing disorders. The recently developed technique of organ culture of the inner ear may be useful to the study of genetic deafness since conditions under which the cochlea develops can be controlled.[140,141] It has been reported that the development of the inner ear of the Kreisler mutant mouse in culture is similar to its in vivo development.[142] Metabolic abnormalities in the cochlea may be reflected in the composition of small molecules in cochlear fluids. Analysis of amino acids and sugars in perilymph of the normal and the deaf white cat showed no differences between the two animals; however, since an insensitive method of analysis was used, only large changes would be detected.[143]

REFERENCES

1. Brown RD, Feldman AM. Pharmacology of hearing and ototoxicity. Ann Rev Pharmacol Toxicol 1978; 18:233-52.

2. Drescher DG. A review of general cochlear biochemistry in normal and noise-exposed ears. In: Henderson D, Hamernik R, Dosanjh D, Mills J, eds. Effects of noise on hearing. New York: Raven Press, 1976:111-27.

3. Guth PS, Bobbin RP. The pharmacology of peripheral auditory processes; cochlear pharmacology. Adv Pharmacol Chemother 1971; 9:93-128.

4. Guth PS, Norris CH, Bobbin RP. The pharmacology of transmission in the peripheral auditory system. Pharmacol Rev 1976; 28:95-125.

5. Rauch S, Rauch I. Physico-chemical properties of the inner ear especially ionic transport. In: Keidel WD, Neff WD, eds. Handbook of sensory physiology, Berlin: Springer-Verlag, 1974:647-82.

6. Thalmann R. Biochemical studies of the auditory system. In: Tower DB, ed. The nervous system. Vol. 3. New York: Raven Press, 1975:31-44.

7. Thalmann R. Quantitative biochemical techniques for studying normal and noise-damaged ears. In: Henderson D, Hamernik RP, Dosanjh DS, Mills JH, eds. Effects of noise on hearing. New York: Raven Press, 1976:129-55.

8. Hubbard JI. Microphysiology of vertebrate neuromuscular transmission. Physiol Rev 1973; 53:674-723.

9. Brownstein MJ. Biologically active peptides in the mammalian central nervous system. In: Gainer H, ed. Peptides in neurobiology, New York: Plenum Press, 1977:145-70.

10. Barker JL. Physiological roles of peptides in the nervous system. In: Gainer H, ed. Peptides in neurobiology. New York: Plenum Press, 1977:295-343.

11. Curtis DR, Johnston GAR. Amino acid transmitters in the mammalian central nervous system. Rev Physiol Biochem Pharmacol (Berlin) 1974; 69:97-188.

12. Werman R. A review criteria for identification of a central nervous system transmitter. Comp Biochem Physiol 1966; 18:745-66.

13. Werman R. CNS cellular level: membranes. Annu Rev Physiol 1972; 34:337-74.

14. McLaughlin BJ, Barker R, Saita K, Roberts E, Wu JY. Immunocytochemical localization of glutamate decarboxylase in rat spinal cord. J Comp Neurol 1975; 164:305-22.

15. McLaughlin BJ, Wood JG, Saito K, et al. The fine structural localization of glutamate decarboxylase in synaptic terminals of rodent cerebellum. Brain Res 1974; 76:377-91.

16. Ribak CE, Vaughn JE, Saito K, Barker R, Roberts E. Immunocytochemical localization of glutamate decarboxylase in rat substantia nigra. Brain Res 1976; 116:287-98.

17. Pickel VM, Joh TH, Field PM, Becker CG, Reis DJ. Cellular localization of tyrosine hydroxylase by immunohistochemistry. J Histochem Cytochem 1975; 23:1-12.

18. Pickel VM, Joh TH, Reis DJ. Immunohistochemical localization of tyrosine hydroxylase in brain by light and electron microscopy. Brain Res 1975; 85:295-300.

19. Pickel VM, Joh TH, Reis DJ. Ultrastructural localization of tyrosine hydroxylase in noradrenergic neurons of brain. Proc Natl Acad Sci USA 1975; 72:659-63.

20. Pickel VM, Joh TH, Reis DJ. A serotonergic innervation of noradrenergic neurons in nucleus locus coeruleus: demonstration by immunocytochemical localization of the transmitter specific enzymes tyrosine and tryptophan hydroxylase. Brain Res 1977; 131:197-214.

21. Hartman BK. Immunofluorescence of dopamine-β-hydroxylase: application of improved methodology to the localization of the peripheral and central noradrenergic nervous system. J Histochem Cytochem 1973; 21:312-32.

22. Lundberg J, Bylock A, Goldstein M, Hansson H, Dahlström A. Ultrastructural localization of dopamine-β-hydroxylase in nerve terminals of the rat brain. Brain Res 1977; 120:549-52.

23. Joh TH, Shikimi T, Pickel VM, Reis DJ. Brain tryptophan hydroxylase: purification of, production of antibodies to, and cellular and ultrastructural localization in serotonergic neurons of rat midbrain. Proc Natl Acad Sci USA 1975; 72:3575-9.

24. Aprison MH, Werman R. The distribution of glycine in cat spinal cord and roots. Life Sci 1965; 4:2075-83.

25. Graham LT, Shank RP, Werman R, Aprison MH. Distribution of some synaptic transmitter suspects in cat spinal cord: glutamic acid, aspartic acid, γ-aminobutyric acid, glycine, and glutamine. J Neurochem 1967; 14:465-72.

26. Aprison MH, Daly EC, Shank RP, McBride WJ. Neurochemical evidence for glycine as a transmitter and a model for its intrasynaptosomal compartmentation. In: Berl S, Clarke DD, Schneider D, eds. Metabolic compartmentation and neurotransmission. New York: Plenum Press 1975:37-63.

27. Iurato S. Efferent innervation of the cochlea. In: Keidel WD, Neff WD, eds. Handbook of sensory physiology. Vol V/1. Berlin: Springer, 1974:261-82.

28. Fex J, Wenthold RJ. Choline acetytransferase, glutamate decarboxylase and tyrosine hydroxylase in the cochlea and cochlear nucleus of the guinea pig. Brain Res 1976; 109:575-85.

29. Godfrey DA, Krzanowski JJ, Matschinsky FM. Activities of enzymes of the cholinergic system in the guinea pig cochlea. J Histochem Cytochem 1976; 24:470-2.

30. Jasser A, Guth PS. The synthesis of acetylcholine by the olivocochlear bundle. J Neurochem 1973; 20:45-54.

31. Fex J. Neuropharmacology and potentials of the inner ear. In: Moller AR, ed. Basic mechanisms in hearing. New York: Academic Press, 1973:377-421.

32. Norris CH, Guth PS. The release of acetylcholine (ACh) by the crossed olivo-cochlear bundle (COCB). Acta Otolaryngol (Stockh) 1974; 77:318-26.

33. Bobbin RP, Konishi T. Action of cholinergic and anticholinergic drugs at the crossed olivo-cochlear bundle-hair cell junction. Acta Otolaryngol (Stockh) 1974; 77:56-65.

34. Fex J. Efferent inhibition in the cochlea by the olivocochlear bundle. In: de Reuch AVS, Knight J, eds. Ciba foundation symposium on hearing mechanisms in vertebrates. London: JA Churchill, 1968:169-81.

35. Fex J. Neural excitatory processes of the inner ear. In: Keidel WD, Neff WD, eds. Handbook of sensory physiology. Vol. V/1. Berlin: Springer, 1974:585-646.

36. Fex J, Adams JC. α-Bungarotoxin blocks reversibly cholinergic inhibition in the cochlea. Brain Res 1978; 159:440-4.

37. Bobbin RP, Konishi T. Acetylcholine mimics crossed olivocochlear bundle stimulation. Nature New Biol 1971; 231:222-3.

38. Russell IJ, Sellick PM. Tuning properties of cochlear hair cells. Nature 1977; 267:858-60.

39. Godfrey DA, Carter JA, Berger SJ, Matschinsky FM. Levels of putative transmitter amino acids in the guinea pig cochlea. J Histochem Cytochem 1976; 24:468-70.

40. Klinke R, Oertel W. Evidence that GABA is not the afferent transmitter in the cochlea. Exp Brain Res 1977; 28:311-4.

41. Tachibana M, Kuriyama K. Gamma-aminobutyric acid in the lower auditory pathway of the guinea pig. Brain Res 1974; 69:370-4.

42. Klinke R, Oertel W. Evidence that 5-HT is not the afferent transmitter in the cochlea. Exp Brain Res 1977; 30:141-3.

43. Densert O. Adrenergic innervation in the rabbit cochlea. Acta Otolaryngol (Stockh) 1974; 78:345-56.

44. Densert O. The effect of 6-hydroxydopamine on the rabbit cochlea. Acta Otolaryngol (Stockh) 1975; 79:339-51.

45. Klinke R, Evans EF. Evidence that catecholamines are not the afferent transmitter in the cochlea. Exp Brain Res 1977; 28:315-24.

46. Flock A, Lam DMK. Neurotransmitter synthesis in inner ear and lateral line sense organs. Nature 1974; 249:142-4.

47. Drummond RJ, Phillips AT. L-glutamic acid decarbox-

ylase in non-neural tissues of the mouse. J Neurochem 1974; 23:1207-13.

48. MacDonnell P, Greengard O. The distribution of glutamate decarboxylase in rat tissues; isotopic vs fluorimetric assays. J Neurochem 1975; 24:615-8.

49. Klinke R, Oertel W. Amino acids — putative afferent transmitter in the cochlea. Exp Brain Res 1977; 30:145-8.

50. Curtis DR. Gamma-aminobutyric and glutamic acids as mammalian central transmitters. In: Berl S, Clarke DD, Schneider D, eds. Metabolic compartmentation and neurotransmission: relation to brain structure and function. New York: Plenum Press, 1975:11-36.

51. De Feudis FV. Amino acids as central neurotransmitters. Annu Rev Pharmacol Toxicol 1975; 15:105-30.

52. Krnjévic K. Chemical nature of synaptic transmission in vertebrates. Physiol Rev 1974; 54:418-540.

53. Steinbach AB, Bennett MVL. Effects of divalent ions and drugs on synaptic transmission in phasic electroreceptors in a mormyrid fish. J Gen Physiol 1971; 58:580-98.

54. Sewell WF, Guth PS. Detection of the primary afferent auditory transmitter using biological assay. Neurosci Abst 1977; 3:11.

55. Godfrey DA, Williams AW, Matschinsky FM. Quantitative histochemical mapping of enzymes of the cholinergic system in cat cochlear nucleus. J Histochem Cytochem 1977; 25:397-416.

56. Wenthold RJ, Morest DK. Transmitter-related enzymes in the guinea pig cochlear nucleus. Neurosci Abst 1976; 2:28.

57. Godfrey DA, Carter JA, Lowry OH, Matschinsky FM. Distribution of gamma-aminobutyric acid, glycine, glutamate and aspartate in the cochlear nucleus of the rat. J Histochem Cytochem 1978; 26:118-26.

58. Fisher SK, Davis WE. GABA and its related enzymes in the lower auditory system of the guinea pig. J Neurochem 1976; 27:1145-55.

59. Fuxe K. Evidence for the existence of monoamine neurons in the central nervous system. IV. Distribution of monoamine terminals in the central nervous system. Acta Physiol Scand 1965; 64 Suppl 247:39-85.

60. Wenthold RJ, Gulley RL. Aspartic acid and glutamic acid levels in the cochlear nucleus after auditory nerve lesion. Brain Res 1977; 138:111-23.

61. Godfrey DA, Carter JA, Berger SJ, Lowry OH, Matschinsky FM. Quantitative histochemical mapping of candidate transmitter amino acids in cat cochlear nucleus. J Histochem Cytochem 1977; 25:417-31.

62. Altschuler RA. Met-enkephalin positivity in the small cells of the deep dorsal cochlear nucleus and posteroventral cochlear nucleus of the rat. Neurosci Abst 1979; 9:15.

63. Hökfelt T, Elde R, Johansson O, Terenius L, Stein L. The distribution of enkephalin-immunoreactive cell bodies in the rat central nervous system. Neurosci Lett 1977; 5:25-31.

64. Spoendlin H. The innervation of the cochlear receptor. In: Moller AR, ed. Basic mechanisms in hearing. New York: Academic Press, 1973:185-234.

65. Wenthold RJ, Gulley RL. Glutamic acid and aspartic acid in the cochlear nucleus of the waltzing guinea pig. Brain Res 1978; 158:295-302.

66. Wenthold RJ. Glutamic acid and aspartic acid in subdivisions of the cochlear nucleus after auditory nerve lesion. Brain Res 1978; 143:544-8.

67. Brawer JR, Morest DK, Kane EC. The neuronal architecture of the cochlear nucleus of the cat. J Comp Neurol 1974; 155:251-300.

68. Cohen ES, Brawer JR, Morest DK. Projections of the cochlea to the dorsal cochlear nucleus in the cat. Exp Neurol 1972; 35:470-9.

69. Olsen KK. Course and termination of the primary afferents in the cochlear nuclei of the cat. Arch Ital Biol 1970; 108:21-51.

70. Ernstson S. Heredity in a strain of the waltzing guinea pig. Acta Otolaryngol (Stockh) 1970; 69:358-62.

71. Ernstson S. Cochlear morphology in a strain of the waltzing guinea pig. Acta Otolaryngol (Stockh) 1971; 71:469-82.

72. Ernstson S. Cochlear physiology and hair cell population in a strain of the waltzing guinea pig. Acta Otolaryngol (Stockh) 1972 Suppl 297:1-24.

73. Gulley RL, Wenthold RJ, Neises GR. Changes in the synapses of spiral ganglion cells in the rostral anteroventral cochlear nucleus following hair cell loss. Brain Res 1978; 158:279-94.

74. Wenthold RJ. Release of endogenous glutamic acid, aspartic acid and GABA from cochlear nucleus slices. Brain Res 1979; 162:338-43.

75. Campochiaro P, Coyle JT. Ontogenetic development of kainate neurotoxicity: correlates with glutamatergic innervation. Proc Natl Acad Sci USA 1978; 75:2025-9.

76. Herndon RM, Coyle JT. Selective destruction of neurons by a transmitter agonist. Science 1977; 198:71-2.

77. McGeer EG, McGeer PL. Duplication of biochemical changes of Huntington's chorea by intrastriatal injections of glutamic and kainic acids. Nature 1976; 263:517-9.

78. Bird SJ, Gulley RL, Wenthold RJ, Fex J. Kainic acid injections result in degeneration of cochlear nucleus cells innervated by the auditory nerve. Science 1978; 202:1087-9.

79. Biscoe TJ, Evans RH, Francis AA, et al. D-α-aminoadipate as a selective antagonist of amino acid-induced and synaptic excitation of mammalian spinal neurons. Nature 1977; 270:743-5.

80. Martin MR, Adams JC. Effects of DL-α-aminoadipate on synaptically and chemically evoked excitation of anteroventral cochlear nucleus neurons of the cat. Neuroscience 1979; 4:1097-105.

81. McDonald DM, Rasmussen GL. Ultrastructural characteristics of synaptic endings in the cochlear nucleus having acetylcholinesterase activity. Brain Res 1971; 28:1-18.

82. Comis SD, Guth PS. The release of acetylcholine from the cochlear nucleus upon stimulation of the crossed olivo-cochlear bundle. Neuropharmacology 1974; 13:633-41.

83. Kromer LF, Moore RY. Cochlear nucleus innervation by central norepinephrine neurons in the rat. Brain Res 1976; 118:531-7.

84. Brady RO. Inborn errors of lipid metabolism. In: Meister A, ed. Advances in enzymology. Vol. 38. New York: J. Wiley and Sons Inc, 1973:293-315.

85. Bach G, Eisenberg F, Cantz M, Neufield E. The defect in the Hunter syndrome: deficiency of sulfoiduronate sulfatase. Proc Natl Acad Sci USA 1973; 70:2134-8.

86. Bach G, Friedman R, Weissmann B, Neufield EF. The defect in the Hurler and Scheie syndromes: deficiency of α-L-iduronidase. Proc Natl Acad Sci USA 1972; 69:2048-51.

87. Matalon R, Darfman A. Hurler's syndrome, an α-L-iduronidase deficiency. Biochem Biophys Res Comm 1972; 47:959-64.

88. Matschinsky FM, Thalmann R. Energy metabolism of the cochlear duct. In: Paparella MM, ed. Biochemical mechanisms in hearing and deafness. Springfield: Charles C. Thomas, 1970:265-94.

89. Thalmann R, Thalmann I, Comegys TH. Dissection and chemical analysis of substructures of the organ of Corti. Laryngoscope 1970; 80:1619-45.

90. Drescher DG. Purification of a carbonic anhydrase from the inner ear of the guinea pig. Proc Natl Acad Sci USA 1977; 74:892-6.

91. Brown KS. Genetic feature of deafness. J Acoust Soc Am 1973; 54:569-75.

92. Brown KS, Bergsma DR, Barrow MV. Animal models of pigment and hearing abnormalities in man. Birth Defects 1971; 7:102-9.

93. Fraser GR. Profound childhood deafness. J Med Genet 1964; 1:118-51.

94. Fraser GR. Genetic approaches to the nosology of deafness. Birth Defects 1971; 7:52-63.

95. Konigsmark BW, Gorlin RJ. Genetic and metabolic deafness. Philadelphia: WB Saunders, 1976.

96. Nance WE, McConnell FE. Status and prospects of research in hereditary deafness. Adv Hum Genet 1973; 4:173-250.

97. Paparella MM, Hanson DG, Rao KN, Ulvestad R. Genetic sensorineural deafness in adults. Ann Otol Rhinol Laryngol 1975; 84:459-72.

98. Proctor C. Diagnosis, prevention and treatment of hereditary sensorineural hearing loss. Laryngoscope 1977; 87 Suppl 7:1-60.

99. Schuknecht HR. Pathology of the ear. Cambridge: Harvard Univ Press, 1974.

100. Schuknecht H, Watanuki K, Takahashi T, et al. Atrophy of the stria vascularis, a common cause for hearing loss. Laryngoscope 1974; 84:1777-821.

101. Lindsay JR. Inner ear histopathology in genetically determined congenital deafness. Birth Defects 1971; 7:21-32.

102. Rebillard G, Rebillard M, Carlier E, Pujol R. Histophysiological relationships in the deaf white cat auditory system. Acta Otolaryngol (Stockh) 1976; 82:48-56.

103. Bergsma DR, Brown KS. White fur, blue eyes, and deafness in the domestic cat. J Hered 1971; 62:171-85.

104. Mair IWS. Hereditary deafness in the white cat. I. Hereditary and clinical aspects. Acta Otolaryngol (Stockh) 1973; Suppl 314:5-11.

105. Mair IWS. Hereditary deafness in the white cat. III. Cochlear histopathology. Acta Otolaryngol (Stockh) 1973; Suppl 314:23-35.

106. Mair IWS. Hereditary deafness in the white cat. IV. Primary auditory neuron histopathology. Acta Otolaryngol (Stockh) 1973; Suppl 314:36-48.

107. Mair IWS, Elverland HH. Hereditary deafness in the cat. An electron microscopic study of the stria vascularis and Reissner's membrane. Arch Otorhinolaryngol 1977; 217:199-217.

108. Pujol R, Rebillard M, Rebillard G. Primary neural disorders in the deaf white cat cochlea. Acta Otolaryngol (Stockh) 1977; 83:59-64.

109. Foss I. Stria vascularis and Reissner's membrane of hereditary deaf white mink. Exp Cell Res 1969; 58:452.

110. Hilding DA, Sugiura A, Nakai Y. Deaf white mink: electron microscopic study of the inner ear. Ann Otol Rhinol Laryngol 1967; 76:647-65.

111. Saunders LZ. The histopathology of hereditary congenital deafness in white mink. Pathol Vet (Basel) 1965; 2:256-63.

112. Shackelford RM, Moore WD. Genetic basis of some white phenotypes in the ranch mink. J Hered 1954; 45:173-6.

113. Sugiura A, Hilding DA. Cochleo-saccular degeneration in Hedlund white mink. Acta Otolaryngol (Stockh) 1970; 69:126-37.

114. Sugiura A, Hilding DA. Stria vascularis of deaf Hedlund mink. Acta Otolaryngol (Stockh) 1970; 69:160-71.

115. Anderson H, Henricson B, Lundquist PG, Wedenberg E, Wersäll J. Genetic hearing impairment in the Dalmatian dog. An audiometric, genetic and morphologic study in 53 dogs. Acta Otolaryngol (Stockh) 1968; 232:1-34.

116. Hudson WR, Ruben RJ. Hereditary deafness in the Dalmation dog. Arch Otolaryngol 1962; 75:213-9.

117. Igarashi M, Alford BR, Cohn AM, Saito R, Watanabe I. Inner ear anomalies in dogs. Ann Otol Rhinol Laryngol 1972; 81:249-55.

118. Lurie MH. The membranous labyrinth in the congenitally deaf collie and Dalmation dog. Laryngoscope 1948; 58:278-87.

119. Mair IWS. Hereditary deafness in the Dalmation dog. Arch Otorhinolaryngol 1976; 212:1-14.

120. Deol MS. Inherited diseases of the inner ear in man in the light of studies on the mouse. J Med Genet 1968; 5:137-58.

121. Kikuchi K, Hilding DA. The defective organ of Corti in Shaker-1 mice. Acta Otolaryngol (Stockh) 1965; 60:287-303.

122. Kikuchi K, Hilding DA. The spiral vessel and stria vascularis in Shaker-1 mice. Electron microscopic and histochemical observations. Acta Otolaryngol (Stockh) 1967; 63:395-410.

123. Mikaelian DO, Ruben RJ. Hearing degeneration in Shaker-1 mouse. Arch Otolaryngol 1964; 80:418-30.

124. Foss I. Stria vascularis and Reissner's membrane of the hereditary deaf white Norwegian Dunkerhound. J Ultrastruct Res 1968; 25:162-3.

125. Mikaelian DO, Warfield D, Norris O. Genetic progressive hearing loss in the C57/B16 mouse. Acta Otolaryngol (Stockh) 1974; 77:327-34.

126. Sidman RL, Green MC, Appel SH. Catalog of the neurological mutants of the mouse. Cambridge: Harvard Univ Press, 1965.

127. Sorsby A, Davey JB. Ocular associations of dappling (or merling) in the coat colour of dogs. I. Clinical and genetical data. J Genet 1954; 52:425-40.

128. Suga F, Hattler KW. Physiological and histopathological correlates of hereditary deafness in animals. Laryngoscope 1970; 80:81-104.

129. Ibsen H, Risty K. A new character in guinea pigs, waltzing. Anat Rec 1929; 44:294.

130. Lurie M. The waltzing (circling) guinea pig. Ann Otol Rhinol Laryngol 1941; 50:113-28.

131. Ames GFL, Nikaido K. Two-dimensional gel electrophoresis of membrane proteins. Biochemistry 1976; 15:616-23.

132. Anderson L, Anderson NG. High-resolution two dimensional electrophoresis of human plasma proteins. Proc Natl Acad Sci USA 1976; 12:5421-5.

133. Milman G, Lee E, Ghangas GS, McLaughlin JR, George M. Analysis of HeLa cell hypozanthine phosphoribosyltransferase mutants and revertants by two-dimensional polyacrylamide gel electrophoresis: evidence for silent gene activation. Proc Natl Acad Sci USA 1976; 73:4589-93.

134. O'Farrell PH. High resolution two-dimensional electrophoresis of proteins. J Biol Chem 1975; 250:4007-21.

135. Laemmli UK. Cleavage of structural proteins during the assembly of the head of bacteriophage T4. Nature 1970; 227:680-5.

136. Bonner WM, Laskey RA. A film detection method for tritium-labelled proteins and nuclei acids in the polyacrylamide gels. Eur J Biochem 1974; 46:83-8.

137. Knox WE. Phenylketonuria. In: Stanbury JB, Wyngaarden JB, Fredrickson DS, eds. The metabolic basis of inherited disease. New York: McGraw-Hill, 1972:266-95.

138. Deol MS. An experimental approach to the understanding and treatment of hereditary syndromes with congenital deafness and hypothyroidism. J Med Genet 1973; 10:235-42.

139. Deol MS. The role of thyroxin in the differentiation of the organ of Corti. Acta Otolaryngol (Stockh) 1976; 81:429-35.

140. Sobkowicz HM, Bereman B, Rose JE. Organotypic development of the organ of Corti in culture. J Neurocytol 1975; 4:543-72.

141. Van De Water TR, Ruben RJ. Organ culture of the mammalian inner ear. Acta Otolaryngol (Stockh) 1971; 71:303-12.

142. Van De Water TR, Ruben RJ. Symposium: new data for noise standards. III. Organ culture of the mammalian inner ear: a tool to study inner ear deafness. Laryngoscope 1974; 84:738-49.

143. Elverland HH, Mair IWS, Borud O. Hereditary deafness in the cat. Free amino acid and sugar content in the perilymph. ORL 1977; 39:241-6.

CHAIRMAN: MERLE LAWRENCE, PhD, ANN ARBOR, MICHIGAN

PANEL — RESEARCH PRIORITIES IN AUDITORY SCIENCE

THE OTOLOGIST'S VIEW

ROBERT RUBEN, MD

BRONX, NEW YORK

Physicians have always had three strategies in their approach to disease. These are prevention, care and cure. As we view communicative disorders from the perspective of these three principles, substantive deficits appear in our ability to meet the needs which this group of disorders present. Inspection of our knowledge and armamentarium quickly reveals that the overwhelming aspect of our activities is employed in caring for the patient. A certain amount of our knowledge has been developed in the area of prevention, eg, the rubella vaccine, the identification of toxic substances, genetic counselling, etc. Except in the area of otitis media, and this is debatable, there are no regimes which can effect cure. The question of why there are no cures must be asked as this will become the highest research priority in the development of our science. The answer to our rhetorical question is superficially easy. We do not have sufficient understanding of the basic mechanisms which underlie the disease states. The use of the word sufficient is significant for it implies a level of understanding of the disease which will allow for intervention which results in cure, either the restoration of function or the arrest of the disease process.

The knowledge of the pathological anatomy of the temporal bone has been, and continues to be, of the utmost importance in defining the histological end result of the disease processes of the inner ear. This knowledge does not afford a type of explanation of mechanisms for the inner ear which can be utilized to effect cure.

The history of the interface of medicine and science appears to be a continuous and gradual progression, apart from occasional dramatic advances by a few individuals. Indeed, when these sudden discoveries are closely analyzed it becomes apparent they are all based upon a massive body of technical and theoretical knowledge and also a set of social attitudes which have laid a foundation for the synthesis of the information and the creation of the new concept. Examples of this constant historical phenomena are Harvey's discovery of the circulation; Darwin's theory of evolution; Pasteur's discovery of the action of bacteria; Fleming's discovery of penicillin; or more recently, Watson and Crick's description of deoxyribonucleic acid (DNA). All of these advances and many more are really the synthesis of a large amount of available knowledge which in its totality creates a new concept. More directly stated, there must be an available store of information, techniques and attitudes before there can be significant advances.

Today there are at least two areas in which there can be advances made in our understanding of the disease processes of communicative disorders which should result in cure. The first of these is in the area of the molecular biology of sensorineural deafness. There has been and there continues to be assembled several sources of knowledge which must be integrated. These information banks are temporal bone pathology of various clinical entities; identification of the phenotypes of genetic disorders; elucidation of the embryonic mechanisms which control normal and abnormal inner ear development; phenotypic descriptions of the physiology of sensorineural deafness; the ultrastructure of the cells in the inner ear; and the beginning of the study of the molecular biology and biochemistry of the cells in the inner ear. All of the above information is directly concerned with the biology of the inner ear. There are large areas of information which exist outside of the present general knowledge of the inner ear. These consist of our massive contemporary fund of information of cell biology, molecular biology and biochemistry. The priority is to wed these two areas so that there may result a biochemical description of the various diseases which result in sensorineural deafness. This type of synthesis has successfully been carried out in a large number of neurological diseases, which have in some instances resulted in interventions which are curative in nature.

As the vast majority of sensorineural hearing loss,

From the Department of Otorhinolaryngology, Albert Einstein College of Medicine of Yeshiva University/Montefiore Hospital & Medical Center, Bronx, New York.

REPRINTS — R. J. Ruben, MD, Department of Otorhinolaryngology, Albert Einstein College of Medicine, 1300 Morris Park Avenue, Bronx, NY 10461.

especially in the young, is genetic in nature and as there is now a vast resource of information concerning the biochemistry of cells and its interaction with genetics, it is evident that this area should have our highest order of priority. The means for achieving these ends are easily stated but the execution requires effort. Fundamentally what is needed are people who can acquire knowledge in both the ear and cell biology who wish to work in this area. These individuals either singularly or collectively would need professional sophistication in the area of sensorineural deafness, pathology and pathophysiology of the ear, genetics, embryology, cell biology, molecular biology and biochemistry. They will require support both in terms of resources and career development so that they will have the freedom to carry out their work. It is felt that before the end of the century many of the diseases of the inner ear will have a chemical explanation which will result in the cure of some of the types of sensorineural deafness.

The second area in which there appears to be the opportunity for cure of a disease's effect in now being rapidly developed. This is the area of auditory deprivation. The information now available demonstrates that various types of auditory deprivation which occurs while the central nervous system is still plastic results in anatomic, physiological and behavioral alterations. The knowledge of what these differences are, what the meaning of the differences are in terms of adaptive behavior, eg, learning and language, and when they will occur will allow for the design of intervention strategies which can either ameliorate or circumvent the defect. Thus if we know what central nervous system change will be found in an infant born deaf our research questions become more direct. These are how to prevent the changes or how to construct an intervention program which will circumvent the anatomical, physiological difference. This area also needs individual workers who will have a depth of knowledge in several areas including developmental biology, anatomy, physiology, psychology, linguistics and education. Such individuals or groups need to be formed and they too will need support both in terms of resources and attitudes which will give them the opportunity to apply and build upon the resources of information and develop knowledge so that a significant amelioration of disease process can come about.

There are two areas of research priorities which would result in cure for some of the communicative disorders. These are molecular biology and biochemistry of the cell and the understanding of the total effects of auditory deprivation. Both of these areas already have a significant fund of information which needs to be applied and developed in the area of communicative disorders. The effecting of these priorities would change much of our present empirical intervention of care to a rational intervention for cure.

PANEL — RESEARCH PRIORITIES IN AUDITORY SCIENCE
THE AUDIOLOGIST'S VIEW

JAMES JERGER, PhD
HOUSTON, TEXAS

I would like to argue, in this brief presentation, that our most pressing research problem in auditory science is the development of new methods for measuring the ability of the hearing-impaired individual to cope with speech communication. With a few notable exceptions, the tools and techniques in use today are the tools and techniques invented just after World War II. If you are less than 34 years old, then speech audiometry, as we know it today, was invented before you were born.

These techniques, based largely on the correct repetition of phonemically balanced (PB) monosyllabic words, served us well in the early formative years of audiology, but advances in other areas of hearing science have long since demonstrated the limitations of PB words as the total edifice of speech audiometry.

In the area of hearing aids, for example, technological advances in the performance of the prosthetic device have so outdistanced our ability to measure them with speech audiometry that many frustrated but misguided investigators now argue for "nonlinguistic" evaluative techniques.

In diagnostic audiometry, the one area in which at least faltering steps toward the development of new techniques have been taken, dramatic advances in our understanding of central auditory disorders at both the brainstem and cortical level have taken place, but these have been isolated efforts by individuals without the benefit of a universally accepted set of research tools.

The most pressing need for better speech audiometric tools lies in the much neglected field of aural rehabilitation. We recommend hearing aids in the hope that they will help the user to understand what other people say to him, we teach speech reading so that he may exploit visual cues to the understanding of spoken language, and we institute auditory training procedures in order to improve his ability to recognize and differentiate the sounds of speech. Yet there is no satisfactory methodology for measuring success or failure in what we are trying to accomplish.

The situation is somewhat akin to the problem a physiologist would face if he wanted to measure the effect of a certain drug on blood pressure, but had no good way to measure changes in blood pressure, or to the problem a physicist might face if he wanted to study the effect of frictional resistance on the velocity of wave propagation, but had no way to measure velocity. Under these circumstances we would probably advise these gentlemen that it would be folly to undertake such experiments, and that their time and effort would be more effectively expended in the development of the essential tools.

A closely related issue is the problem of quantifying auditory handicap. We are in urgent need of a more refined scale of handicap that goes beyond "discrimination loss," the most obvious reason being that such a scale is the only validating criterion against which to assess proposed measures of speech understanding. Conversely, we cannot approach the refinement of a handicap scale until we have a firmer grasp of what is meant by loss in the ability to understand speech. The two concepts are inextricably interwoven and must be developed in parallel.

The interaction of speech perception with hearing loss is more complicated than most of us imagined 30 years ago. In that simpler era there were only two kinds of loss: conductive and perceptive. Conductives were thought to pose no problem in speech understanding, but perceptives were known to have two complications: a differential loss for high frequencies and loudness recruitment.

It was widely assumed that problems in speech understanding arose primarily from the fact that high-frequency consonant sounds were differentially attenuated by the high frequency loss. The problem was further conpounded by a certain inability to tolerate any excessively amplified sound due to the recruitment problem. Conventional speech audiometry, as we know it today, was conceived within this simple framework. But during the past 30 years two points have become increasingly clear. First, speech perception, especially in the hearing-impaired involves much more than "hearing all the sounds." Advances in speech science have shown that the simple phonemic structure of language does not fully describe a dynamic perceptual process in which a variety of temporal, even prosodic, cues play important roles. Secondly, there are more than two kinds of hearing loss, and their differential effect on speech understanding can be profound. Cochlear disorders are influenced not only by

From the Department of Otorhinolaryngology and Communicative Sciences, Baylor College of Medicine, and the Methodist Hospital, Houston, Texas.

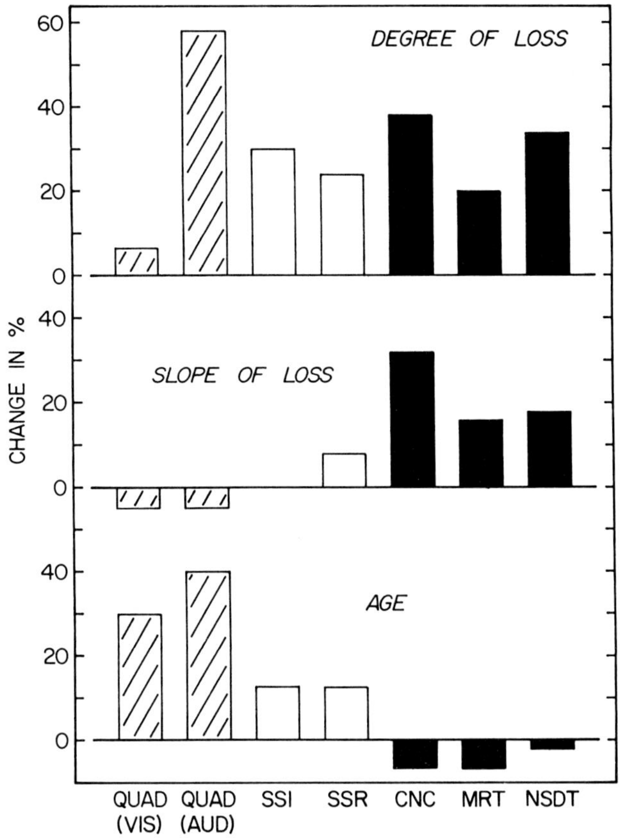

Fig. 1. Effects of three variables (degree of loss, slope of loss, and age) on a variety of tests of speech understanding in patients with sensorineural hearing loss.

audiometric configuration, but by distortion products, duration of loss, etiology, age of onset, and undoubtedly a variety of additional as yet undiscovered factors. All of these factors, especially in children, affect speech understanding in often poorly understood but surely complicated fashion.

Eighth nerve disorders, either alone or in combination with cochlear disorders, affect speech understanding by mechanisms that differ both quantitatively and qualitatively from their purely cochlear counterparts. Here the intensity and temporal features of speech seem to override the frequency dimension, and speech understanding may be devastated.

Central auditory disorders, either at the brainstem or higher levels, further complicate the picture. At this level complex perceptual disorders appear. The listener may hear all the individual sounds of speech in isolation, but he may be unable to cope with complex signal processing, especially in the presence of competing speech signals. Selective attention, a problem scarcely anticipated by conventional approaches to the measurement of speech understanding, is a dominant feature of central disorders.

In a sense every hearing impairment represents a combination of all the above-cited factors in some unknown mix. Usually the purely peripheral cochlear factors dominate, but in two important populations, young children and the elderly, the confounding effects of concomitant eighth nerve and central disorders can be quite substantial. It is in these two populations, especially, that the complex interactions of speech perception and auditory disorder are becoming increasingly manifest.

Figure 1 illustrates a case in point. We see the interactions of just three variables on a variety of speech intelligibility tasks administered to a sample of 97 patients with sensorineural hearing loss. The various tests fall into three general categories: 1) QUAD (auditory and visual) is a rather lengthy procedure designed as a validating criterion for measures of "practical hearing in everyday life." 2) SSI and SSR are tests of sentence recognition and identification, and represent a relatively synthetic approach to speech understanding. 3) CNC, MRT, and NSDT are tests of monosyllabic word repetition, consonant recognition, and nonsense syllable detection, respectively. They represent a relatively more analytic approach to speech understanding. We see, in Figure 1, the overall effects of three variables: 1) degree of sensitivity loss, 2) slope of audiometric configuration, and 3) chronological age. Note that degree of loss affects all measures except, of course, testing in the visual mode. Slope of loss, however, affects only the analytic tests, especially CNC. Age, on the other hand affects only the synthetic measures, SSI and SSR. The analytic measures are remarkably resistant to the effect of age. Yet aging is perhaps the single most important source of difficulty in speech understanding.

This simple analysis of only three variables and a limited number of tests illustrates the point that the present techniques of speech audiometry in widespread clinical use today are inadequate to cope with even the first order interactions between speech perception and hearing impairment.

A more adequate set of tools is urgently needed. The task is formidable, but not insurmountable. In order to bring speech audiometry up to date we must assign high priority to research in two areas: 1) defining more fully the nature of the speech-understanding problems of the hearing impaired, and 2) developing test instruments suitable to these problems.

We are, at the moment, becalmed in a windless sea of monosyllables. We can sail further only on the fresh winds of imagination.

PANEL — RESEARCH PRIORITIES IN AUDITORY SCIENCE
THE PHYSIOLOGIST'S VIEW

J. E. HIND, PhD
MADISON, WISCONSIN

After the diet of meat and potatoes we have enjoyed in the form of the solid research accomplishments described in the preceding papers, I must now ask you to focus your appetite on pie in the sky. I trust you will receive my comments with the skepticism appropriately reserved for those foolish enough to predict the future, especially the future course of science. Partly out of respect for the territorial interests of my fellow panelists but primarily because of the limitations of my own background and perspective I shall restrict my remarks to basic auditory physiology. However, it is obvious from the presentations at this conference that the otological and audiological clinics offer abundant opportunity for physiological research as well as for the application of tests and methods derived from the basic science laboratory. It is necessary to extend my subject to include anatomical considerations since most of the important problems in contemporary auditory physiology involve the correlation of structure with function. Time permits only a cursory listing of some problems and approaches that I consider likely to prove fruitful areas for investigation over the next few years; no implication of relative importance is implied by the order of presentation.

The past decade has witnessed great progress in our understanding of the mechanical vibratory properties of the middle ear and cochlea. The current controversy as to whether or not the motion of the basilar membrane is appreciably nonlinear is almost certain to be settled in the near future through improved measurement methods, including the laser interferometer. Determination of the mechanical parameters of the cochlear partition is a related and worthy goal in order that mathematical models may be solidly based upon directly measured physical parameters. However, even after a relatively complete picture of basilar membrane motion is achieved there will remain the challenging task of describing the effective mechanical stimulus to the individual hair cell, the problem of hair cell micromechanics. A frontal attack involving direct visualization of events seems remote, but important insight into micromechanical input are beginning to emerge through intracellular recordings from single hair cells, supplemented by data on the mechanical properties of the stereocilia, the latter considerably enlivened by Ake Flock's suggestion of the possibility of contractile activity in the sensory hairs. Lest success in these ventures lead to smugness on the part of mammalian physiologists, humility may be restored, at least for a spell, by the need to explain mechanical tuning in the simpler inner ears of lower forms.

Although Dr. Warr's presentation beautifully illustrated the substantial progress that has been made recently in our understanding of the innervation of the organ of Corti, complete specification of the synaptic relationships between receptor cells and afferent and efferent nerve fibers remains a very important objective. Similarly, Dr. Javel convincingly demonstrated that continuing attention may profitably be directed toward developmental processes, including abnormalities. Additional valuable insights into the structural basis of hearing loss may also confidently be predicted to result from the continuation of studies on animal ears that have been exposed to intense sound and ototoxic drugs.

Major advances in understanding of the excitatory process in the hair cell/nerve fiber transducer are assured as the growing repertory of techniques from cellular neurobiology is brought to bear on such problems as the ultrastructural and neurochemical bases of synaptic transmission, the electrical properties of hair cells vis-à-vis supporting cells, the site of origin of the nerve impulse, and the longstanding debates over the functional roles of inner vs outer hair cells and afferent vs efferent fiber systems. Dr. Wenthold's excellent presentation depicted the encouraging progress that has been made in identification of neural transmitters in the peripheral auditory system and at the same time gave us a vision of the vast territory in the field of neurochemistry that demands exploration. Continuing studies of metabolic and circulatory factors in the cochlea are certain to generate information useful not only for understanding of normal function but with significant implications for the clinic. Dr. Merzenich's paper clearly illustrated how carefully controlled animal studies on cochlear electrical prostheses are an essential adjunct to clinical development of this technique.

Neurobiological methods are also beginning to shed

From the Department of Neurophysiology, University of Wisconsin School of Medicine, Madison, Wisconsin.

light on the information processing capabilities of single neurons within the central nervous system as the input-output transformation of temporal discharge patterns may be studied in neuronal types identified by intracellular dye injected via the recording electrode. Modern histochemical tract-tracing techniques promise continued rapid growth in our knowledge of the wiring diagram of the auditory nervous system, providing new opportunities to identify groups of functionally related neurons. Finally, when anatomical and microelectrode observations are combined with shrewd exploitation of behavioral specializations, striking progress can be made toward understanding the physiological substrate of auditory perception as demonstrated by the brilliant studies of Nobuo Suga and his colleagues on echolocation in the bat. Beginning with years of patient study of the relation between the acoustical parameters of the bat's emitted cry and the attributes of the target that can be discriminated, successful hypotheses were generated as to the unique combination of emitted signal and suitably delayed and attenuated component of the echo required to activate specialized classes of neurons in the auditory cortex. To someone like myself who has spent many a frustrated hour trying to interest the neurons in cat auditory cortex in my simple pure tone stimuli, Suga's findings stand as both an inspiration and as a profoundly important guide for further attempts to unravel the functional role of the structures of the central auditory system.

I hope I will not disappoint this audience and the organizers of this conference when I refuse to assign relative priorities to the problems and approaches I have outlined. However, it doesn't require a prophet to recognize that cellular neurobiology will increasingly yield new insights into the mechanisms by which individual neurons process auditory information. These new insights will add to and illuminate the rich dividends returned by the familiar systems approach as embodied in the work of the classic auditory physiologist, the acoustic physicist and the communications engineer. Nevertheless, our enthusiasm for novelty must not result in the abandonment of mines from which the gold has been only partly extracted; on the contrary, it is essential that mining continue in all those traditional veins which still hold promise for answering important questions. In this connection I enthusiastically endorse Dr. Jesteadt's prediction that the interaction between physiology and psychoacoustics will prove to be very fertile ground.

In these days of intense competition for research dollars any discussion of research priorities would be incomplete without some mention of the basis upon which funding is allocated. My philosophy on this matter can be summarized by stating that I strongly believe that "targeting" is a concept that does not belong in the minds of those responsible for deciding which projects in basic auditory science should receive support since the idea is wholly incompatible with the unpredictable essence of basic inquiry. In my judgment, the only rational basic science funding strategy is that of total flexibility, with the freedom to exploit the most promising leads as they arise in the normal course of research. As so eloquently expressed yesterday by Dr. Silverman, this plea for unfettered funds must be accompanied by urgent and earnest effort on the part of the basic scientist to communicate to funding agencies and the public an appreciation of why such a policy is vital. The only known method to ensure long-term productivity in basic auditory science is to nurture our most precious resource, the future research investigators, to whom we must offer training in an ever-expanding array of disciplines, followed by reasonable assurance of support for their initial research endeavors. In this regard it is indeed gratifying to participate in the dedication of this superbly equipped new institute with its impressive complement of well-trained and enthusiastic young investigators, working in a setting calculated to promote as fully as possible the benefits of interdisciplinary interaction.

OROFACIAL EMBRYOLOGY, ANATOMY AND PHYSIOLOGY

DAVID P. KUEHN, PhD
DENVER, COLORADO

The orofacial region is intricately involved in shaping the speech signal that emerges from the speaker. Without this shaping, speech would be largely a communicatively indistinct blur. It is not surprising, therefore, that there is considerable interest in the embryology, anatomy, and physiology of this extremely important region of the body.

EMBRYOLOGY

Normal and Abnormal Facial Development. The topographical changes that occur in molding the undifferentiated primitive embryo to the distinctly human configuration of the fetus are fairly well understood. Figure 1 illustrates the development of the face at six stages from embryonic age four weeks to age eight weeks. The human embryo is a highly dynamic organism, and the formation of structures such as the nose and lips must obey a fairly rigid time schedule. During the fifth week, all the major structures that will eventually form the face are clearly distinguishable,[1] and in general except for further growth and shaping, the formation of the face is complete by about the seventh week of embryonic life. At this time, the entire embryo is only about 1.9 cm long.

One important aspect of development at this stage is the fusion of the nasolateral, nasomedial, and maxillary processes to form the upper lip. Failure of that fusion process results in cleft lip, a major birth defect that occurs with an incidence of approximately 1 in 700 live births. The exact mechanisms by which these facial processes are formed and fuse are not well understood in either the pathological or the normal embryo, but certainly considerable progress is being made.[2] Investigations for this purpose usually by necessity involve laboratory experiments with animals, especially the chick, because of easy access and manipulation of the embryo. It is known that certain cells, referred to as neural crest cells, migrate within the embryo to eventually form most of the facial structures. Clefts of the midfacial region have been induced in laboratory animals by removing segments of neural crest cells very early in embryonic life before cell migration has begun.[3] Therefore, studying the formation and migration of these very primitive embryonic cells appears to be an important area of future basic research.

Normal and Abnormal Palatal Development. The underlying mechanisms and embryonic failures involved in formation of the hard palate are somewhat better understood than those of the lip area.[4] However, many important questions still remain unanswered.[5] Figure 2 illustrates two stages in the development of the hard palate. Figure 2A is a section through the head of a seven-week human embryo. At this stage, the shelves which eventually form the hard palate are directed downward on each side of the tongue. During the next stages of development the tongue descends to a lower position, and the palatal shelves reorient to a horizontal position (Fig. 2B). The palatal shelves then fuse with each other and with the primitive nasal septum. Thus the oral and nasal cavities are separated. Not much more is known about the process beyond this general description; however, it appears that the timing of palatal shelf movement is of major importance and is the object of a considerable amount of current research. If the palatal shelves are slowed in their normal horizontal positioning for whatever reason, it may eventually be too late for them to make contact and fuse due to continued growth of the surrounding regions.[2] It is known that fusion of the palatal shelves and the nasal septum is normally complete by the 12th week of embryonic life. Failure of palatal fusion will of course result in cleft palate.

Etiology of Cleft Lip and Palate. There are clearly underlying genetic factors involved in producing clefts as indicated by studies dealing with families in which more than one member are affected. Factors that may be considered environmental probably also are important. These have possible adverse effects during prenatal development and have been identified mainly in research projects using laboratory animals. It is fairly easy to induce cleft palate in animals by the administration of teratogens at certain times in the embryonic period.[6] However, analogous environmental cause-effect relationships in the human remain elusive.[5]

Most authorities agree that except in rare instances, cleft lip and palate in the human are not caused by a single gene or single environmental

From the Department of Otolaryngology and Maxillofacial Surgery, University of Iowa, School of Medicine, Iowa City, Iowa. This report was supported in part by PHS Research Grant DE-00853, the National Institute of Dental Research.
REPRINTS — David P. Kuehn, PhD, Department of Speech Pathology and Audiology, University of Denver, Denver, CO 80208.

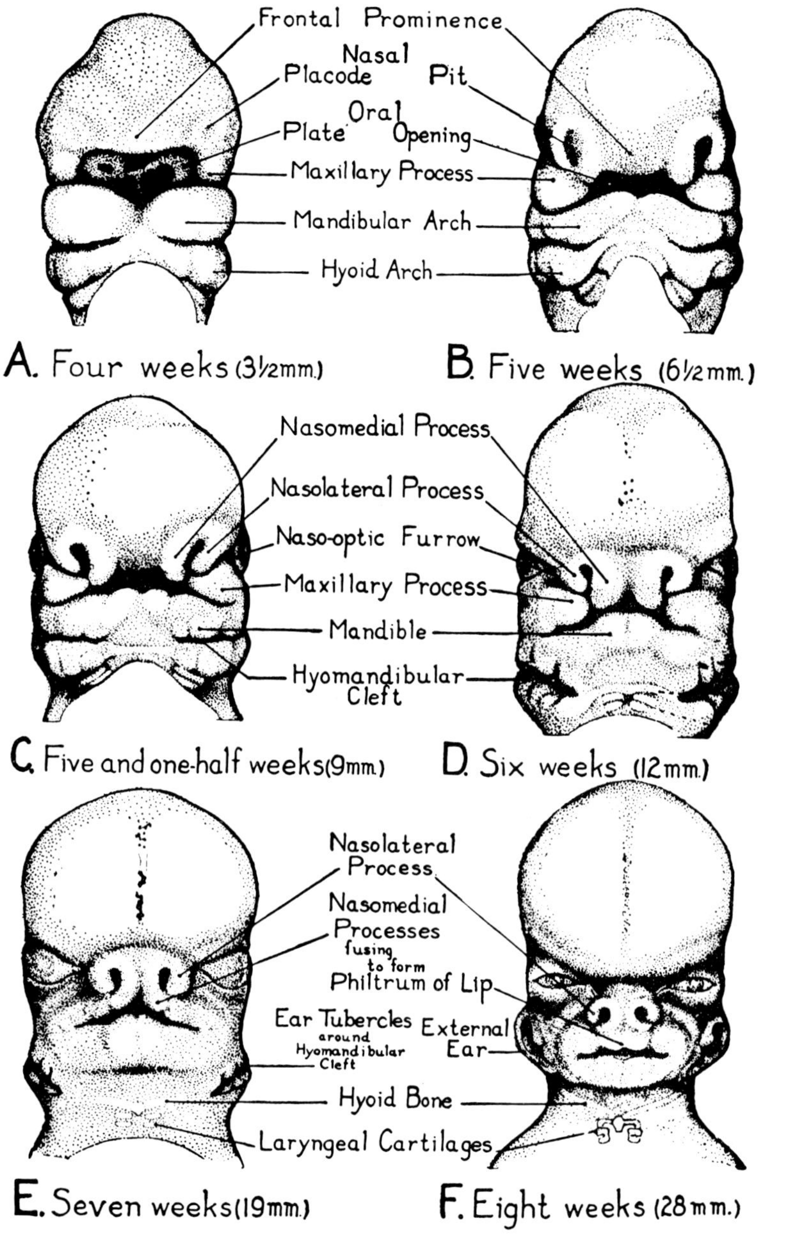

Fig. 1. A-F) Development of the face. (From Patten B. Human embryology. Philadelphia: Blakiston Co, 1946, after an original figure by W. Patten. Used with permission of McGraw-Hill Book Co.)

agent. Instead it seems more likely that clefts are the result of the interaction of genetic and environmental factors. This is called the multifactorial theory and has been described mainly by Fraser et al.[7] A threshold effect has been suggested, whereby given the proper combination of genetic and/or environmental factors, a cleft will result in certain individuals.

Prevention of Cleft Lip and Palate. Prevention of cleft lip and palate is limited at the present time to genetic counseling in cases where at least one family member is already affected. Prenatal diagnostic procedures such as direct visualization of the embryo are currently available.[8] Moreover, surgical procedures of an experimental nature have been accomplished in living rabbit embryos within the uterus.[9] However, such manipulation of the human embryo in utero appears extremely difficult and definitely does not warrant the risk at the present time. One reason is that the facial region is rather inaccessible, since in the young human embryo the face is pressed against the thorax. In short, prevention and diagnosis of clefts in the fetus and treatment of clefts before birth appear to be in the far distant future, if possible at all.

Future Research. In the meantime, researchers must continue the study of animal models in the laboratory since basic mechanisms underlying normal and abnormal orofacial development are still not well understood. A shift should gradually be made

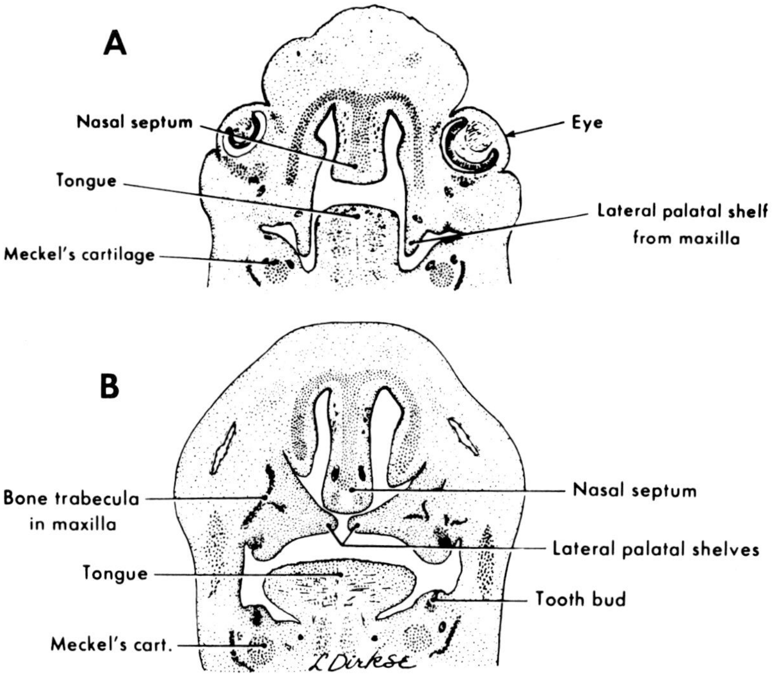

Fig. 2. Development of the palate. A) Section through the head of a seven-week embryo. B) Section through the head of an eight-week embryo. (From Patten.[1] Reprinted with permission.)

from lower animals to primate models which are closer to the human form. In addition, the search for environmental factors in humans should also be continued, especially among women with a family member already affected by a cleft.

ANATOMY AND PHYSIOLOGY

For those born with a cleft, the best surgical, dental, and speech pathology practices must be utilized in management regimes. This is often a long and very expensive process that involves a large team of professional practitioners with extensive experience treating the malformation. An important factor in expediting the management process is a thorough understanding of normal and abnormal anatomy and physiology.

Fetal and Infant Anatomy. It is known on the basis of studies of the fetus and infant that muscle origins are fairly normal in the cleft individual, but muscle insertions in the palate are grossly abnormal.[10,11] It is the objective of the surgeon to transpose these misaligned muscle fibers and other tissues into a more normal position which presumably will lead to a properly functioning mechanism.

Adult Anatomy and Physiology. Most of our current knowledge concerning orofacial anatomy and physiology has been derived from the normal adult. While important gains have been made in understanding the gross anatomy and physiology of the speech production mechanism, much is yet to be learned.[12]

The biomechanics of the orofacial region are very difficult to study because several different muscles insert into soft tissue structures from different directions. Most of the orofacial structures are *not* simple lever systems but rather involve potential force vectors that are varied and complex. These soft tissue structures, especially the tongue, are capable of changing shape while being moved because of activity of the muscles within them. To make matters even more complicated, activity of the orofacial structures must be coordinated with that of other regions crucial for the production of speech, such as the larynx and respiratory structures. Since speech is a highly dynamic process, the timing of all individual gestures must be coordinated accurately. Moreover, individual speakers may adopt different strategies in their physiological control mechanisms. In this regard, the variability among normal speakers is not well understood, since most studies to date have used very small numbers of subjects.

Neuromuscular Control Mechanisms. Neuromuscular control mechanisms are of current and great interest among speech scientists. It has been known for a long time that most regions of the body are endowed with a rich supply of sensory receptors. These receptors supply ongoing feedback information concerning a structure being moved and its immediate environment. However, neither the availability nor the possible functional significance of such sensory receptors in speech structures has been well specified. Future research should be aimed at elucidating these potentially important basic mechanisms and determining whether the abnormal individual uses them in the same fashion.

Compensatory Activity. In speakers with structural abnormalities, compensatory activity is sometimes observed. For example, the back wall of the throat may bulge forward to meet the soft palate in some individuals for whom palatal length and/or mobility is not sufficient. In other individuals such compensatory strategies appear to be neither learned nor, perhaps, possible. In these individuals, surgical, prosthetic, or therapeutic techniques must be utilized.

Future Research. Future research should focus on refining management techniques using updated anatomical and physiological data obtained from parallel laboratory experiments. It is in this fashion that clinical laboratory research may complement each other in advancing our knowledge.

A final note concerns the extremely important and relatively unexplored area of postnatal developmental anatomy and physiology, and their interaction with learning factors, especially in the neonatal period. How do normal infants learn to speak? Why do some infants born with a cleft lip and/or palate develop compensatory patterns while others do not? Can appropriate compensatory patterns be taught? Can we predict the need for intensive therapy in addition to initial surgery in problem cases? Are there growth patterns that contraindicate certain types of surgical manipulations? The list of such questions is virtually endless.

FILM DEMONSTRATION

A short film clip of a normal adult female taken from the film library at the University of Iowa was shown to underscore the complexity of the process of speech production and interaction among anatomical, physiological and learning factors. This x-ray film demonstrates movement of the tongue, soft palate, and other structures normally hidden from view. Such films have provided valuable information pertaining to orofacial activity during speech production. The rapidity of tongue tip movement is especially noteworthy. While viewing this film it is important to think of the infant learning to speak and to ask the following questions: How does the infant learn to position his speech structures appropriately while moving them independently and at rapid speeds? How can we help the disadvantaged child accomplish the same result in the most efficient manner?

REFERENCES

1. Patten BM. Embryology of the palate and the maxillofacial region. In: Grabb WC, Rosenstein SW, Bzoch KR, eds. Cleft lip and palate. Boston: Little Brown, 1971.

2. Fraser FC. Etiology of cleft lip and cleft palate. In: Grabb WC, Rosenstein SW, Bzoch KR, eds. Cleft lip and palate. Boston: Little Brown, 1971.

3. Johnston MC. Facial malformations in chick embryos resulting from removal of neural crest. J Dent Res 1964; 43:822.

4. Fraser FC. Cleft lip and cleft palate. Science 1967; 158:1603-6.

5. Burdi AR. Epidemiology etiology and pathogenesis of cleft lip and palate. Cleft Palate J 1977; 14:262-9.

6. Cahen RL. Evaluation of the teratogenicity of drugs. Clin Pharmacol Ther 1964; 5:480-514.

7. Fraser FC, Walker BE, Trasler WG. Experimental production of congenital cleft palate; genetic and environmental factors. Pediatrics 1957; 19:782-7.

8. Kaback MN, Valenti C, eds. Intrauterine fetal visualization: a multidisciplinary approach. New York: American Elsevier, 1976.

9. Horder TJ. Surgery of the mammalian embryo in utero. J Physiol (Lond) 1972; 225:3P-4P.

10. Dickson DR. Normal and cleft palate anatomy. Cleft Palate J 1972; 9:280-93.

11. Latham RA, Long RE, Latham EA. Cleft palate velopharyngeal musculature in a five-month-old infant: a three dimensional histological reconstruction. Cleft Palate J 1980; 17:1-16.

12. Maue-Dickson W. Anatomy and physiology. Cleft Palate J 1977; 14:270-87.

LARYNGEAL DEVELOPMENT AND CONGENITAL LESIONS

GABRIEL F. TUCKER, JR., MD

CHICAGO, ILLINOIS

In considering laryngeal development, functional development and the comparative anatomical approach of Sir Victor Negus must be included in addition to classical morphological development; postnatal questions are considered in addition to embryological and fetal development.

Negus' classic text *The Mechanism of the Larynx* was first published in 1929.[1] Figure 1 summarizes the evolution of the larynx from its first appearance in amphibians to its more elaborate structure in mammals. Its prime function in each case has been described as that of preventing the entrance into the lower respiratory tract of any substance except air. Thus, it is appropriate to point out at this time of dedication of a communication disorders center that the "voice box" function is only incidental to the primary function of the human larynx; a switch-valve mechanism, which allows us to breathe or swallow without inundating our bronchial tree.

During the act of swallowing the larynx must simultaneously close and be lifted away from the cervical spine to open the cricopharyngeal sphincter. Failure of this protective mechanism is seen in the neonate as pharyngolaryngeal discoordination or oral and pharyngeal dysphagia.[2]

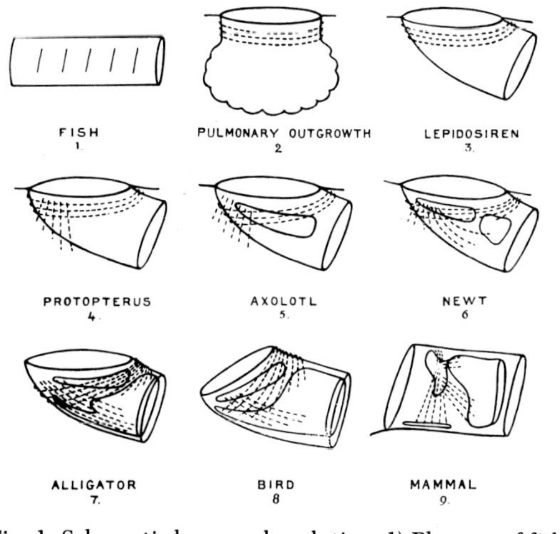

Fig. 1. Schematic laryngeal evolution. 1) Pharynx of fish with gill slits. 2) Commencing outgrowth from floor of pharynx. 3) Elongated trachea turning off towards thorax. 4) Primitive dilator mechanism. 5) Appearance of lateral cartilages. 6) Separation of cartilage into arytenoid and half of cricoid. 7, 8) Fusion of thyroid elements with cricoid. 9) Separation of thyroid from cricoid. Shortening of arytenoid; tilting of laryngeal aperture; division of sphincteric muscle into components. Interrupted lines: sphincteric muscle and dilator muscle. (From Negus.[1])

Failure of the larynx to open actively on inspiration leaves the vocal cords in a position to be caught in the inspiratory air stream thus producing a high-pitched inspiratory stridor. The relationship of bilateral vocal cord paralysis to associated central nervous system abnormalities in infants and children (Table 1) was recently reviewed by the Holingers.[3] A similar mechanism applies when a unilateral peripheral nerve lesion (ie, the inadvertent ligation of the left recurrent nerve in the surgery of patent ductus arteriosis) will produce stridor which is also inspiratory but which is associated with a lesser degree of obstruction.

The embryology of the human infant larynx has recently been reviewed.[4-8] Figure 2 differentiates the early embryonic period from the fetal period. Growth in the embryonic period is characterized by the establishment of organ systems; during the fetal period the embryonic organogenesis matures, physiological activity is established, and organ systems are integrated. In the embryonic period, the ex-

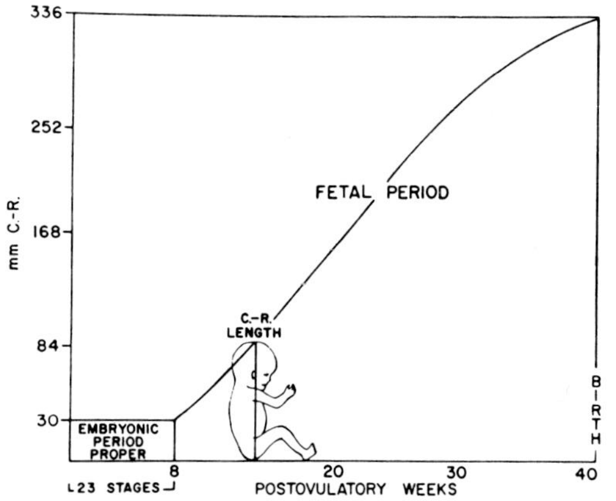

Fig. 2. The embryonic period proper, the first eight postovulatory weeks of development, is shown in relationship to the fetal period. Fetuses, as well as older embryos, are measured by their crown-rump length, which corresponds to the sitting height postnatally.

From the Laryngeal Development Laboratory, Division of Bronchoesophagology-Otolaryngology and Department of Communicative Disorders, Children's Memorial Hospital, Chicago, Illinois. Support from the Edward Shedd Wells Fund is gratefully acknowledged.

REPRINTS — Gabriel F. Tucker, Jr., MD, Division of Bronchoesophagology-Otolaryngology and Department of Communicative Disorders, 2300 Children's Plaza, Chicago, IL 60614.

TABLE 1. ETIOLOGY OF BILATERAL ABDUCTOR VOCAL CORD PARALYSIS IN INFANTS AND CHILDREN

Congenital			
Without associated anomalies		39	
With associated anomalies			
Neurologic	21		
Laryngeal	10		
Cardiac	8		
Other	4		
		43	
Total congenital			82 (55%)
Acquired			
Secondary to congenital anomalies			
Meningomyelocele, A-CM, hydrocephalus	24		
Hydrocephalus unrelated to A-CM	6		
Postoperative for congenital lesion	11		
		41	
Secondary to acquired conditions			
Infectious	7		
Neoplasm	7		
Birth trauma	2		
Guillain-Barré syndrome	2		
		18	
Total acquired			59 (40%)
Undetermined		8	8 (5%)
Total			149 (100%)

tremities develop in proximodistal sequence, first the limb buds, then the finger rays, then the hands. As we follow into the fetal period one finds functional bending of limbs, approximations of fingers and thumb sucking movements. Table 2 schematizes the developments of some of the main features of the respiratory system in relation to staging between three and six postovulatory weeks. By the end of the first trimester the larynx is completely formed, has identifiable vocal cords and a patent lumen. During the second trimester of pregnancy continuing laryngeal development is marked primarily by the development of glandular submucosal elements.[9]

In 1932, Tucker[10] reported the length of the living infant's vocal cord as being between 6 and 8 mm in the well-developed neonate. The subglottic anterior/posterior diameter, which is the critical dimension in the infant larynx, is approximately 5 to 7 mm at birth. This is a nonexpansible tract, as the cricoid cartilage represents the only complete ring in the entire laryngotracheobronchial tree. The average dimension is stated to be 6 mm; 5 mm is on the small side. A subglottic stenosis is defined as 4 mm or less. A more recent study[11] from our laboratory confirms this clinical measurement and also points out the soft tissue lumen (ie, the air column) may be less than the insinuated endotracheal tube, the passage of which is limited by the larger but firmer cartilaginous lumen (Table 3).

In a recent paper from our institution, Holinger et al[12] pointed out the age incidence of symptomatology and treatment in congenital subglottic stenosis. Figure 3 from that article dramatically points out that delay in diagnosis which is often seen. They also noted the increased incidence of tracheotomy in acquired stenosis. Early intubation of the dyspneic child may obscure forever whether a later diagnosis was, indeed, congenital, acquired or mixed. The tracheotomy required by acquired stenosis may, indeed, be thought of as a complication of intubation.

Ongoing studies in our laboratory wherein serial

TABLE 2. DEVELOPMENT OF SOME MAIN FEATURES OF RESPIRATORY SYSTEM IN RELATION TO STAGING FROM THREE TO SIX POSTOVULATORY WEEKS

Stage 9	*10*	*11*	*12*	*13*	*14*	*15*	*16*	*17*	*18*
Foregut Groove	Pharynx Laryngotrach. sulcus				Hypophar. eminence Arytenoid swellings Epithelial lamina	Larynx		Vestib. outgrowth Cricoid condens.	Hyoid chondrif. Thyroid condens. Muscular condens.
Pharyngeal			Tracheo-esoph. septum		Trachea				
Median	Pulmonary primordium		Lung bud	R + L Lung buds	R + L Lung buds	Lobar buds		Segmental buds	Some subseq. buds

*Modified from O'Rahilly and Boyden.[8]

Esoph. - Esophageal; Laryngotrach. - Laryngotracheal; Hypophar. - Hypopharyngeal; Vestib. - Vestibular; Condens. - Condensation; Condrif. - Condrification; Subseq. - Sebsequent.

TABLE 3. VARIATIONS IN LARYNGEAL DIMENSIONS WITH FETAL AGE

Age	Plane of Section	Cricoid Diameter (mm) Lumen-Air A-P	Lumen-Air Trans	Lumen-Cartilage A-P	Lumen-Cartilage Trans	Glottis Length (mm)
12 wk (f)	C		.58		1.45	
14	S	1.02		1.82		
15	S	1.09		2.18		2.9
16	S	1.45		2.9		2.5
18	S	1.45		2.45		2.5
19	C		1.8		3.6	
20	H	2.2	2.2	3.6	4.7	4.0
22	S	2.4		3.6		
23	C		1.8		4.1	4.4
25	S	2.2		3.6		
26	C		3.1		4.9	4.0
27 (t)	H	3.3	2.9	4.1	4.5	3.3
	C		3.3		5.8	3.6
30 (intub)	H	3.5	3.2	4.2	4.9	5.2
30	C		3.9		5.8	5.5
34	C		1.4		3.6	
37	C		3.7		4.6	
40	S	2.7		4.7		
41	C		4.1		5.9	
16 mo	C		5.7		6.8	7.7
40 mo	C		6.0		10.0	7.2
48 mo	C		5.9		7.0	

C - Coronal; S - Sagittal; H - Horizontal; Trans - Transverse.

horizontal sections are made of the larynges of those infants who do not survive their respiratory problems have revealed that subglottic stenosis is a clinical, not a histological entity.[13] There are, indeed, a number of histological patterns which can explain the clinical narrowing of the subglottic lumen. The relationship to intubation trauma is confirmed; cartilaginous distortions can be seen. Newer information is the presence of an excessive amount of glandular tissue in some larynges and in others the entrapment of the first tracheal ring within the cricoid arch.

The cricoid arch may well be the most prominent midline structure in the midpediatric neck below the hyoid. In the neonate, the body of the hyoid overrides the thyroid notch; appreciation of this fact is critical in determining by palpation the level of placement of a pediatric tracheotomy. Table 4 lists collected experiences with a number of congenital laryngeal anomalies.[14] It can be seen here that the most common cause of infant stridor, laryngomalacia, is not thought due to anatomical or physiological deficit but rather to a loss of tissue consistency in which the epiglottis and/or aryepiglottic folds and/or arytenoids tend to be caught in the inspiratory air stream. These symptoms are usually position dependent, ie, improved when the patient is prone; aggravated when the patient is recumbent; they seldom are a serious threat to the infant airway. To *assume* that any given patient's congenital stridor is due to laryngomalacia is to ignore such differential diagnoses as vocal cord paralysis, subglotic stenosis and the wide variety of less common alternatives enumerated above. It should be further noted that even if one can make the diagnosis of laryngomalacia endoscopically, there is a 20% likelihood of associated subglottic laryngotracheal problems which require not only that the laryngeal inlet be inspected but also that

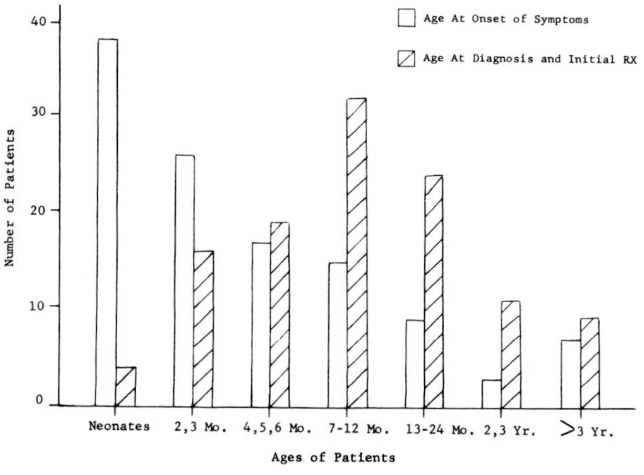

Fig. 3. Congenital subglottic stenosis (115 cases).

TABLE 4. CONGENITAL LARYNGEAL ANOMALIES

Type	No. of Cases
Laryngomalacia	1415
Bifid epiglottis	8
Absence of epiglottis	2
Webs	224
Atresia	43
Cysts	52
Laryngocele	6
Subglottic stenosis	278
Clefts	56
Hemangioma	95
Total	2179

TABLE 5. ANATOMICAL DISTRIBUTION OF CONGENITAL LARYNGEAL ANOMALIES*

Supraglottic		Congenital laryngomalacia	Congenital flaccid larynx Overdeveloped elongated epiglottis with broad base Excessive tubular short epiglottis Cri du chat
	Epiglottic	Bifid epiglottis Absence of epiglottis	
	Ventricular band	Webs	
	Aryepiglottic fold	Atresia. "Congenital cyst" Hemangioma	
	Ventricle	Laryngocele	
Glottic	True vocal cords	Webs. Atresia Vocal cord sulcus	
Subglottic	Infraglottic and cricoid	Stenosis. Webs Atresia. Cleft Hemangioma	

*Laryngeal cysts, paralysis and papilloma are excluded as they are not truly defects of laryngeal organogenesis.

the subglottic larynx be seen. Other lesions, such as atresia of the cricoid and posterior laryngeal cleft, are much more rare. A recent publication[14] systematizes anatomical distribution of congenital laryngeal anomalies (Table 5). There are, of course, many unanswered questions as to the exact embryogenesis of these lesions. Indeed, we still have only a vague outline of the calendaring of laryngeal development, the exact ages at which growth accelerates or plateaus, and the specific dimensions which one would expect at a given age. As one follows the child into adolescence, we do, of course, realize that the male larynx grows more quickly than the female but have yet to spell out the specific mechanism of sex differentiation and hormonal action.

We sincerely trust that the establishment of the Institute for Communication Disorders, here at Boys' Town, will indeed contribute to the welfare of all children with laryngeal problems by providing for us a better understanding and hopefully, therefore, more effective treatment.

REFERENCES

1. Negus VE. The mechanism of the larynx. St. Louis: CV Mosby, 1929.

2. Logan WJ, Bosma JF. Oral and pharyngeal dysphagia in infancy. Pediatr Clin North Am 1967; 14:47.

3. Holinger LD, Holinger PC, Holinger PH. Etiology of bilateral abductor vocal paralysis. Ann Otol Rhinol Laryngol 1976: 85:428-36.

4. Tucker JA, O'Rahilly R. Observations on the embryology of the human larynx. Ann Otol Rhinol Laryngol 1972; 81:520-3.

5. O'Rahilly R, Boyden EA. The timing and sequence of events in the development of the human respiratory system during the embryonic period proper. Z Anat Entwicklungsgesch 1973; 141:237-50.

6. O'Rahilly R, Tucker JA. The early development of the larynx in staged human embryos. Ann Otol Rhinol Laryngol 1973; 82 Suppl 7:1-27.

7. Tucker JA, Tucker GF. Some aspects of fetal laryngeal development. Ann Otol Rhinol Laryngol 1975; 84:49-56.

8. Tucker AJ, Vidic B, Tucker GF, Stead J. Survey of the development of laryngeal epithelium. Ann Otol Rhinol Laryngol 1976; 85 Suppl 30.

9. Tucker GF, Smith HR. A histological demonstration of the development of laryngeal connective tissue compartments. Trans Am Acad Ophthalmol Otolaryngol 1962; 66:308-18.

10. Tucker G. The infant larynx; direct laryngoscopic observations. JAMA 1932; 99:1899-902.

11. Tucker GF, Tucker JA, Vidic B. Anatomy and development of the cricoid serial section whole organ study of perinatal larynges. Ann Otol Rhinol Laryngol 1977; 86:766-9.

12. Holinger PH, Schild JA, Kutnick SL, Holinger LD. Subglottic stenosis in infants and children. Ann Otol Rhinol Laryngol 1976; 85:591-9.

13. Tucker GF, Osoff RH, Newman AN, Holinger LD. Histopathology of congenital subglottic stenosis. Laryngoscope 1979; 84:866-76.

14. Tucker JA, Tucker GF, Vidic B. Clinical correlation of anomalies of the supraglottic larynx with the staged sequence of normal human laryngeal development. Ann Otol Rhinol Laryngol 1978; 87:636-44.

LARYNGEAL SURGERY IN THE PEDIATRIC PATIENT

BLAIR FEARON, MD
TORONTO, ONTARIO, CANADA

The primary concern in laryngeal surgery in the infant and child is to relieve airway obstruction, rather than phonation. Because airway obstruction above the larynx may simulate or be confused with laryngeal pathology, these are described as the signs and symptoms of laryngeal disease. Although tracheotomy in the infant is frequently said to be a cause of a long-term problem, the procedure can be carried out in the smallest premature quite safely and without an extubation problem. The author's method of performing the operation is described. Most laryngeal surgery in the child is performed by the endoscopic approach, special scopes being used for special purposes. In addition to conventional instrumentation the cryoprobe and CO_2 laser are employed. The author's method of treating glottic and subglottic stenosis is outlined.

It must be remembered, in contrast to laryngeal surgery in the adult in which the function of the voice is one of the commonest concerns, in the child the primary problem is that of establishing or maintaining an adequate airway. Not only is the larynx in the child smaller than in the adult, but there are differences in characteristics such as were described by Dr. Tucker[1] earlier, but specifically in the dimensions of the triangular glottis. In the newborn, the average anteroposterior diameter is 7 mm and the posterior commissure is 4 mm across. The surface area of the glottic aperture with the vocal cords abducted is thus approximately 14 sq mm. Furthermore, the arytenoids in the infant are large and in fact remain roughly the same size throughout the individual's growth until maturity. Time does not permit description of all of the differences, but suffice it to say the position of the larynx from the neck changes with age; in the newborn it lies at the fourth cervical vertebra; in the six-year-old the fifth cervical vertebra; and in the adult at the lower border of the sixth, and technically the seventh cervical vertebra. The basic function of the larynx is to allow respiration and in doing so, to protect the airway from foreign material. Another protective mechanism of the larynx is to assist in expelling foreign material that may otherwise, in most cases at least, proceed further down the tracheobronchial tree. This mechanism is the "bechic blast" that Dr. Chevalier Jackson[2] described many years ago.

The first and foremost important signs and symptoms associated with respiratory obstruction are manifested by stridor, dyspnea, total blockage of one or more parts of the lung, and finally, apnea. The type of stridor gives some indication as to the position of the obstructing lesion. For example, inspiratory stridor is usually associated with obstruction at or above the level of the vocal cords. Obstructive lesions below the vocal cords are manifested by an expiratory component to the stridor primarily, although we can get a biphasic, to-and-fro stridor in glottic and subglottic lesions, as well as lesions in the trachea.

The second group of symptoms involves abnormalities of phonation in which the cry or voice is either abnormal or absent. The character of the cry is often indicative of laryngeal abnormality. A muffled sound is often related to supraglottic obstruction, as a supraglottic growth, swelling of the supraglottic tissue due to inflammation, or even a foreign body in the upper esophagus; a high-pitched or absent cry may be apparent in infants with laryngeal webs or cysts in the glottic area, vocal cord paralysis, or spasm of the vocal cords as is seen sometimes in hydrocephalus or certain brainstem lesions. A croupy type of cough is associated with edema of the subglottic space or partial tracheal obstruction. In older children abnormalities of formation are caused by neoplasms, episodes of specific or nonspecific infections of the larynx, vocal abuse or even functional dysphonias.

In establishing a diagnosis, observation of the patient is very important and it is surprising to me how often airway obstruction above the laryngeal level is confused with obstruction of the larynx or tracheobronchial tree. It is often not realized that nasal obstruction in the newborn will cause severe respiratory distress. Even simple adenoid hypertrophy can cause such severe obstruction that adenoidectomy may be necessary in the neonate. The author has removed adenoid in patients as young as two days of age with complete relief of respiratory distress. Bilateral choanal atresia in the newborn is another not uncommon cause of severe respiratory distress, although the temporary solution is simple — namely that of using an oral airway in the mouth until the obstruction can be corrected.[3] Craniofacial abnormalities such as the Pierre Robin syndrome, Crouzon's disease, etc, are abnormalities of development which can affect the nasopharyngeal

From the Departments of Otolaryngology of the Hospital for Sick Children and the University of Toronto.
REPRINTS — Blair Fearon, MD, Suite 308, Medical Arts Building, 170 St. George Street, Toronto, Canada M5R 2M8.

airway. Cystic hygroma involving the floor of the mouth and neck is a very difficult problem to manage in respect to the airway, and even with tracheotomy, management of the problem is difficult. Innominate artery compression of the trachea can give signs and symptoms almost identical at times with those of acute laryngotracheitis. This possibility must always be taken into account in the differential diagnosis of respiratory distress and I would emphasize the only certain way of making a diagnosis is by bronchoscopy.[4] A rather rare lesion causing respiratory distress is congenital stenosis of the lower trachea and this is another problem that only can be diagnosed by bronchoscopy.[5] X-rays are most important in studying lesions of the larynx but also at times they can be misleading. A radiologist unfamiliar with the larynx of the infant may quite readily diagnose pathology where in fact the picture is a variation of the normal and the true cause of the problem goes unrecognized.

TRACHEOTOMY

There is generally great fear in doing tracheotomies in a small child, but there is no reason that a tracheotomy, if done properly, should result in any serious problems for the child in the future. In 1964 we published a report on a group of premature infants with the idiopathic respiratory distress syndrome who could not be managed by intubation and mechanical ventilation and the lives of some of these patients were saved, literally, by performing a tracheotomy.[6] The gratifying aspect to this problem was that all of the infants who survived a disease were not a problem in extubation and, indeed, the tracheotomy was discontinued as soon as the disease was controlled. Because there had been nothing designed to connect the Bird respirator to the tracheotomy for intermittent positive pressure respirations (IPPR), it was necessary to improvise a means for the first patient, but this led to the Fearon modification of the Holinger tracheotomy tube in which the standard inner tube is replaced by one with a 15 mm adaptor to which the respirator could be attached. This series also led to the modification of a bronchoscope so that positive pressure ventilation could be carried on in patients with respiratory failure. This bronchoscope was in turn improved by Paul H. Holinger when the fiberoptic lighting system for the bronchoscope became available. The respiratory adaptor for the tracheotomy tube is also useful for carrying on anesthesia in tracheotomy patients of any age. In those children who have rather a fat neck or double chin, the extension on the inner cannula prevents the open end of the tracheotomy tube from being obstructed by soft tissues.

We have had made for us a series of scopes which we term laryngotracheoscopes,* which are 20 cm in length and in graduated sizes from 3 to 5 mm.[7] Besides being effective for doing tracheotomies on patients who require positive pressure ventilation, we also use them for serial dilatation of laryngeal stenosis. They may also be used for dilating tracheal stenosis and even some esophageal strictures. In any stricture or stenosis, it is imperative not to carry the dilatation to the point of undue trauma — tearing cicatrix will only worsen the stenosis so that constant, but firm pressure must be used as the laryngotracheoscope is advanced with a rotary movement. Another difference from the standard bronchoscope is that the laryngotracheoscope has no fenesters, making closed-circuit anesthesia or ventilation possible regardless of the position of the scope in the trachea.

In performing a tracheotomy on a small child, and in particular the newborn, it is most important to make the tracheotomy incision relatively low in the trachea rather than through the second and third tracheal rings, the classic position in the adult. In fact, in patients of approximately 1,200 gm or less we make the tracheal opening at the level of the seventh tracheal ring, thus avoiding the problem of extubation which is normally expected.[6]

In performing tracheotomies, whenever possible we do the tracheotomy with a broncoscope or a laryngotracheoscope in position.[8] This makes the trachea in the small child much easier to locate and makes the placing of the tracheotomy tube much more accurate. We have designed a chart showing the different sizes of bronchoscopes and tracheotomy tubes that we use in patients according to their age.[5] Indeed, the tracheal size correlates more accurately with the age than with the weight of the patient. In an emergency when one does not have an airway established either with an endotracheal tube or a bronchoscope, a "stab" tracheotomy can be performed. Under these circumstances it is most important that the head be hyperextended to reach the tracheal lumen as quickly as possible.[8]

LARYNGEAL SURGERY

In general there are two ways of carrying out surgery on the larynx either in children or in adults, namely, the peroral or the external neck approach. Although not many are familiar with the old Lynch suspension laryngoscope, it is most useful in selected patients for peroral surgery of the hypopharynx or larynx. Although it is awkward to use it may provide much greater exposure than the other types of laryngoscopes we use and, incidentally, this is truly a suspension laryngoscope. It does not have a self-contained light system, but this is no problem since we usually use the operating microscope with its own light system.

Because we did not find the Jako laryngoscope completely satisfactory for our needs, we had one

*Pilling Co, Philadelphia, Pa.

specially made* which, indeed, is a modification of the Jako, but differs in that it has the standard anterior commissure tip, a slot on the side to facilitate instrumentation, and an 11 mm extension on the proximal end of the scope, through which an inhalation anesthetic may be delivered. This makes visualization and instrumentation of the larynx very satisfactory. It comes in two lengths, 12.5 cm and 17.5 cm. Actually the latter laryngoscope can be used in any patient from one year onwards. It is retained in position with the Lewy holder and we use a foam headrest designed for eye surgery to serve as a head-holder for microlaryngoscopy.

One of the modalities for microlaryngoscopy treatment is a cryoprobe and we have found this in particular suitable for supraglottic hemangiomas. A more recent and more versatile modality of treatment is the CO_2 laser which has many uses, but in particular, to eradicate papillomata of the larynx as well as subglottic hemangiomas and certain laryngeal stenosis.

Although the CO_2 laser has no miracle properties, we find it preferable to other modalities for treatment of laryngeal papillomata. With it certainly there is less bleeding and the resection can be carried out with more precision and with less postoperative reaction than with conventional methods. The laryngoscope described previously is especially useful for laser surgery in the larynx since the anesthetist with whom we work can achieve excellent anesthesia without an endotracheal tube and at any age. In fact, we have one patient with massive tracheal papillomatosis in whom laser surgery to the papillomata would be virtually impossible to manage with an endotracheal tube.

As Dr. Tucker[1] has already mentioned, laryngomalacia is the commonest cause of stridor in the infant, although rarely a threat to life. Nonetheless, there are a few patients in whom the airway is compromised to the degree that a life-threatening situation may develop. In such patients we have been able to suture the epiglottis to the base of the tongue after denuding the mucous membrane from the adjacent surfaces. Congenital webs between the ventricular bands are very rare and in the one patient we have managed, although the cry was weak, the airway was not significantly compromised.

Mucus-containing cysts in the aryepiglottic folds or ventricular bands may be present at birth, and when large, cause a degree of obstruction to the glottic aperture on inspiration. Inspiratory stridor, weak, muffled or absent cry, suggests this possibility and easily can be seen on direct laryngoscopy. To relieve the airway obstruction the cysts can be aspirated with a long, large-bore needle without a general anesthetic, but definitive treatment is the resection of the walls of the cyst using biting forceps or the CO_2 laser, leaving the base open. Some congenital supraglottic cysts can be silent until they become infected, thus resulting in an abscess which will increase in size and thus obstruct the airway. The same method of surgery can be applied to these as with the noninfected cysts.

*Pilling Co.

Supraglottic hemangioma can cause a gradually increasing obstruction to inspiration. They may not be present at birth but symptoms usually develop in the first few months of life. In contrast to the subglottic hemangioma, the blood vessels are relatively large and, therefore, bleeding can be profuse from a biopsy. In our opinion, the cryoprobe is the safest and most effective method of management of this particular lesion.

Supraglottic lymphangiomas are much more diffuse and often involve a large area of the supraglottic structure. These can be removed by biting forceps, but we find the CO_2 laser more effective.

Laryngoesophageal clefts usually present in the newborn with symptoms similar to that of a tracheoesophageal fistula. There is choking with feeding and aspiration of feeding. The diagnosis is best made by direct laryngoscopy and bronchoscopy, although unless one is thinking of the possibility, the lesion may readily be missed. These patients present a challenge in management and the great danger is that of a chemical pneumonitis due to aspiration of gastric secretions, as well as from any food given orally. The first steps in the definitive management is to do a tracheotomy and at the same time, a gastrostomy. Small laryngeal clefts that do not involve the whole cricoid plate and the upper trachea may be corrected by a transoral approach, but a true laryngoesophageal cleft must be managed by open neck surgery. Surgery of the cleft should be carried out as soon as possible, because the longer the problem remains, the greater is the likelihood of irreversible pulmonary damage.

Glottic webs can vary from a small subclinical lesion between the cords at the anterior commissure to a total glottic involvement. Obviously in the latter, unless steps are taken immediately at birth, the child cannot survive and therefore a "stab" tracheotomy may be the only way of keeping the child alive. On occasion the glottic web may be very thin and one dilatation with the bronchoscope may solve the problem. More often the web is dense, and when the airway is severely limited tracheotomy should be carried out and definitive surgery can be accomplished later. Glottic webs can occur from prolonged endotracheal intubation and usually the subglottic space is involved as well. Some glottic webs can be correctred with the CO_2 laser but if this fails one can resort to a laryngofissure approach using a keel.[9]

Congenital or acquired subglottic webs or stenoses are much more common than the above and when the airway is severely compromised, tracheotomy may be necessary. If the cicatricial fibers creating the subglottic stenosis are not too dense, repeated transoral dilatations of the stenoses may correct the airway problem.[10] We occasionally use the laser for this purpose and have had some satisfactory results with this modality of treatment. When the response to dilatation or to the laser resection is unsatisfactory, then an external neck approach may be the answer. If the stenosis is confined to the cricoid area and the upper one or two tracheal rings, the Fearon-Cotton operation can provide a satisfactory airway.[11-14] If the stenosis involves the glottic area, the subglottic space and two or more tracheal rings, then a more extensive operation, such as described by Grahne[15] and Crysdale and Blatt[16] may be employed.

In our experience, subglottic hemangiomas are totally different in characteristics from hemangiomas elsewhere in the respiratory tract. The endoscopic appearance is an irregular, dull, red mass, partially circumferential in the subglottic space. It is quite firm and not friable and, in fact, it is difficult to get a good punch biopsy because of its density. Contrary to what one would expect, there is relatively little bleeding from the biopsy. When the airway is compromised severely, tracheotomy is necessary before definitive treatment can be established. In the past, we have had good results with high voltage external irradiation therapy, but recently we have used the CO_2 laser successfully and we have hopes that this may be the most satisfactory method of dealing with the problem.

Vocal nodules, often known as screamers' nodes, are a common cause of dysphonia in the child and our policy is to advise speech therapy where the motivation is great enough for the patient to follow the treatment faithfully. It is important to reassure the parents that this is a harmless lesion. Certainly there is no urgency for surgical correction once the diagnosis has been clearly established. Surgical removal with forceps or with the CO_2 laser can be carried out if the voice is affected so badly that the speech is unintelligible.

The commonest benign neoplastic disease in the child is juvenile papillomatosis, which is a very capricious disease and the main objective is that of maintaining an adequate airway. We avoid tracheotomy almost at all costs because we believe there is a danger of seeding the papilloma in the trachea if a tracheotomy is performed. Resection of the papillomata is carried out as often as necessary to maintain the airway. Although the CO_2 laser for this purpose has no magical qualities, we believe resection can be carried out with less trauma and more precision than one can accomplish with the conventional instrumental resection.

Primary and latent neoplastic disease of the larynx is rare in the child and most cases reported have followed earlier radiation therapy in the head and neck for benign conditions. However, we have one patient, a male of 12 years of age, with supraglottic squamous cell carcinoma large enough to cause respiratory embarrassment. In this instance, since there were no obvious secondaries, we elected to resect the growth with the CO_2 laser and this was followed by conventional radiation therapy. So far, after two years, there is no sign of recurrence.

In our experience with children, fractures of the larynx from external blunt trauma are relatively uncommon. However, if there is extensive damage to the laryngeal cartilages from either blunt or penetrating injuries, tracheotomy is mandatory even though the patient has no significant airway distress when first seen. Reconstruction of the laryngeal complex should be performed as soon as feasible with an external approach.

REFERENCES

1. Tucker GF Jr. Laryngeal development and congenital lesions. Ann Otol Rhinol Laryngol 1980; 89 Suppl 74:142-5.

2. Jackson C, Jackson C. Bronchoesophagology. Philadelphia: WB Saunders, 1950:152.

3. Fearon B, Dickson J. Bilateral choanal atresia in the newborn: plan of action. Laryngoscope 1968; 78:1487-99.

4. Fearon B, Shortreed R. Tracheobronchial compression by congenital cardiovascular anomalies in children. Ann Otol Rhinol Laryngol 1963; 72:949-69.

5. Fearon B, Ellis D. The management of long term airway problems in children. Ann Otol Rhinol Laryngol 1971; 80:669-77.

6. Fearon B, Smith C, Delivoria-Papadopoulos M, Levison H, Swyer PR. The idiopathic respiratory distress syndrome in the newborn: management by tracheotomy and intermittent positive pressure respiration. Ann Otol Rhinol Laryngol 1964; 73:1082-94.

7. Fearon B. Laryngotracheoscopes for diagnosis and treatment. Ann Otol Rhinol Laryngol 1977; 86:628.

8. Fearon B. Acute airway obstruction. In: Ferguson CF, Kendig EL Jr, eds. Disorders of the respiratory tract in children. Vol 2. Philadelphia: WB Saunders, 1972:1183-213.

9. Fearon B. Pediatric endoscopy. In: English G, ed. Otolaryngology. New York: Harper & Row, 1979; chap 55.

10. Fearon B. Management of subglottic stenosis of the larynx in the infant and children. Adv Otorhinolaryngol 1978; 23:97-103.

11. Fearon B, Cotton R. Surgical correction of subglottic stenosis of the larynx. Ann Otol Rhinol Laryngol 1972; 81:508-13.

12. Fearon B, Cotton R. Subglottic stenosis in infants and children: the clinical problem and experimental surgical correction. Can J Otolaryngol 1972; 1:281-9.

13. Fearon B, Cotton R. Surgical correction of subglottic stenosis of the larynx in infants and children: progress report. Ann Otol Rhinol Laryngol 1974; 83:428-31.

14. Fearon B, Crysdale W, Bird R. Subglottic stenosis in the infant and child: methods of management. Ann Otol Rhinol Laryngol 1978; 87:645-8.

15. Grahne B. Operative treatment of severe chronic traumatic laryngeal stenosis in infants up to three years. Acta Otolaryngol (Stockh) 1971; 72:134-7.

16. Crysdale W, Blatt J. Division of posterior cricoid plate in young children with subglottic stenosis. Laryngoscope 1976; 86:1451-8.

PREVENTION AND TREATMENT OF STUTTERING

WILLIAM H. PERKINS, PhD
LOS ANGELES, CALIFORNIA

Evidence is reviewed that forms the basis for prevention and treatment of stuttering as a problem of motor speech coordination. Simplification of phonatory complexity and retardation of phone rate have been demonstrated experimentally to virtually eliminate stuttering. These invariant relationships are used in rate control and breath stream management procedures to facilitate fluency.

Historically, the only lawful thing that could be said about stuttering is that it seems to be unlawful. So many exceptions have existed to every proposed rule that theorists have been free to speculate widely, and sometimes wildly, about the nature and appropriate treatment of this problem. Lacking compelling evidence for one view over another, there are probably about as many theories and therapies of stuttering as there are clinicians treating it.

For the development of maximally effective prevention and treatment strategies, a foundation is needed of some lawful characteristics of this disorder. We need some invariant relationships to which we can anchor our scientific and therapeutic hypotheses. Fortunately, such characteristics have begun to emerge. Not that they are particularly new: they've been under our noses for years, but have been largely ignored as part of the folklore of stuttering, or have been explained away as "distraction effects," a hypothetical explanation dependent entirely upon the validity of anticipatory-struggle theories and for which a growing body of negative evidence is accumulating.

In a nutshell, two methods of eliminating stuttering without exception have already been demonstrated. These involve the time-honored dictum to slow down, and an extension of the well known effect of whispering. Waiting in the wings to be demonstrated is rhythm, a technique that will likely prove equally as effective. Now let us look at the nature of these lawful effects, some inferences which can be drawn from them, and the clinical significance of them for the prevention and treatment of stuttering.

An adequate explanation of fluency and stuttering must account for inexplicable periods of fluency as well as for loss of fluency. For this intriguing problem, answers have been sought in every conceivable nook and cranny of the stutterer's soma and psyche. The big game hunters on these expeditions have more often than not returned, however, with little more to show than field mice. For years, the adaptation effect and consistency effect have been regarded as the most lawful characteristics of stuttering, but there have always been stutterers who did not show these effects. As Dean Williams and his associates[1-3] have been especially instrumental in demonstrating, these effects are also found in normal disfluency.

Having been raised on the premise that stuttering is learned, I found operant theory persuasive at first, and I still see the uses to which stuttering can be put as examples of operant learning. But our experience with manipulation of operant contingencies does not persuade me that nuclei of stuttered disfluencies are explained adequately as examples of learning.

The possibility that much stuttering may not evolve by learning from normal disfluency began to open with our use of delayed auditory feedback (DAF). In our experience with several hundred stutterers, DAF has been effective only as a means of enforcing syllable prolongation. By modeling the behavior we seek, the same release from stuttering can be obtained with or without DAF provided the same technique of syllable prolongation is used.

Doubt about the effect of rate retardation on stuttering was raised in recent studies that showed that slow word rates tend to reduce stuttering, but the effect is relatively weak.[4,5] These results puzzled us because they were so discrepant from our clinical experience. We suspected, though, that the reason for such small effects was that these investigators retarded word rate, which offered no assurance that phonetic rate was also retarded. It is prolongation of phones that we thought essential to reduction of stuttering.

To find out if our suspicion was correct, we devised an experiment in which we used sentences of monosyllabic words that were read normally, at two-second intervals without prolongation, and at two-second intervals with prolongation. Two-second intervals were used to simulate the 30-word-per-minute pace we used clinically to establish fluency. We reasoned that rate could be reduced by articulating rapidly at normal phonetic speeds and then pausing between syllables, or by articulating

From the Center for the Study of Communicative Disorders, University of Southern California, Los Angeles, California.
REPRINTS — William H. Perkins, PhD, 734 West Adams Blvd., Los Angeles, CA 90007.

slowly with syllable prolongation. Clinical experience led us to expect much more reduction of stuttering with the latter technique for retarding rate than with the former. The 19 subjects who met experimental requirements confirmed this expectation. Most showed some decrease in stuttering with syllable rate retarded with prolongation. All showed considerable decrease with phonetic rate retarded by means of syllable prolongation which practically eliminated stuttering.

Why is a slow phonetic rate so powerful a method of obtaining fluency? We have gathered considerable evidence that simplification of phonatory coordinations with respiration and articulation is universally effective in reducing stuttering.[6] One technique for facilitating these coordinations is to slow the phonetic rate at which they must be made; another is to simplify their complexity. Our rationale for simplification is progressively to reduce phonatory complexity from voiced to whispered to lipped speech. In this way, the number of physiological adjustments, especially phonatory adjustments, is sharply reduced from the voiced to whispered condition and is minimal under the lipped condition in which articulatory movements need not be coordinated with either phonatory or respiratory movements. Moreover, the rate at which phonatory coordinations must occur drops from the high-speed phone rate of about 14 phones per second (about twice the speed at which one can control the articulatory mechanism) to the much slower syllable rate of about six syllables per second.

The effects of simplifying these coordinations has been so stable that the procedure has become a diagnostic tool for us. Of the 30 subjects in the formal experiment, stuttering was considerably reduced when whispering, and invariably was all but eliminated when articulating silently. The only exception to this pattern in over 100 stutterers tested clinically was a woman with a motor speech disorder. When she did not show the expected pattern, we became suspicious that her disfluencies involved something other than typical stuttering. A neurological evaluation revealed that she was suffering from a rare myoclonic seizure disorder.

Admittedly, alternative explanations of these results are possible. We have tested articulatory and grammatic complexity in some unpublished experiments and have found their effects to be slight. We looked at the distraction effect, but it does not explain why lipping is more effective than whispering, unless one is willing to argue that lipping is more distracting than whispering. We considered communicative responsibility, but it requires the assumption that every subject had the same uncontrolled psychological reaction to each experimental condition, which hardly seems credible. Another possibility is that the effects are due to reduction in the levels of subglottal pressure required for whispering and lipping. Indeed, this factor does operate and may account in part for the effects, but it does not explain why a retarded phonetic rate using normal voice (with its higher subglottal pressure requirements) is equally as effective as is lipping in consistently reducing syllable disfluency.

We favor a discoordination hypothesis because it encompasses these known strong effects which eliminate stuttering: both retarded phonetic rate and simplification of phonatory complexity facilitate speech coordinations, hence contribute to fluency. This has become a cornerstone in our rationale for treatment. We view stuttering as discoordination of phonation with articulation and respiration. Therefore, we select shaping procedures for their power in facilitating these coordinations.

Although a variety of techniques can accomplish this purpose, our original experience was with syllable prolongation so we have continued with it as our initial facilitating technique. Next we include management of the breath stream to initiate voice with a soft breathy onset and then to help maintain airflow throughout the phrase without any breaks or stoppages in it. We explicitly avoid having stutterers monitor voice onset syllable by syllable and certainly not sound by sound. Speech sounds spoken at normal rates flow by twice as fast as one can control movement — high-speed speech is produced with low-speed equipment — and even syllables flow normally at one's upper limits of control. If it is possible to monitor individual sounds and syllables at normal rates without abandoning controls, we have not found the method. Our objective is to teach controls which can be used at normal speech rates so we concentrate on dimensions of the phrase which can be monitored, controlled and still preserve normal rates and expressiveness. In effect, what we seek are controls which, when mastered, will not be apparent when used. In a sense, our most successful graduates become skillful actors whose technique does not show when they sound like normal speakers.

A shift in our emphasis has occurred, however, in the last few years. Increasingly, we have stressed rhythm as the dimension that more than any other facilitates speech coordinations. Not that this is a startling direction to take; historically, stuttering is defined as a disorder of rhythm. Nor are we alone in pointing to it afresh; Wingate[7] has implicated it as the central element of stuttering. The reasons why we have shifted derive from both the research and clinical laboratory. The lead from our own work turned up in the discoordination experiment. One of the alternate explanations for the effect of whispering and lipping was that reduced stuttering was a consequence of increased effort and deliberate articulation. We reasoned that if this were the basis for improvement, then articulatory rate should have been retarded. What we found, instead, was that rate accelerated as fluency improved, suggesting that rhythm of speech had been facilitated.

This result gave impetus to the clinical impression that rhythm was the key to shaping normal rate and normal expressiveness without loss of control. We concluded that without control of prosody (the patterning of the elements of which make rhythm) we could not systematically produce normal-sounding speech. Admittedly, this is the most subtle and difficult of the dimensions of speech to make explicit. Of the elements of prosody — pitch, loudness, and duration — only the latter has proven clinically profitable. Attention to pitch and loudness yields artificial inflections worse than a beginning actor emoting Hamlet's soliloquy. Therefore, we avoid teaching how to stress syllables. Instead, we concentrate on how to shorten unstressed syllables.

Interestingly, a trade-off seems to exist between rhythm and the other dimensions with which fluency can be maintained. The stronger the rhythmic pattern, the more the speaker can, without disruption, survive hard vocal attacks, rapid rate, breaks in the breath stream, and any other condition conducive to stuttering. Conversely, the poorer the rhythm the more reliance must be placed on slow rate and smooth airflow to maintain fluency.

Our rationale for prevention of stuttering is twofold. It derives squarely from our conception of the nature of stuttering as having two facets: physiologically stuttering is a discoordination of speech, and psychologically it becomes useful and is reinforced as operant behavior. As you might suspect, some of our recommendations for children seem iconoclastic for those who hold traditional views. First, we attempt to facilitate the child's coordination of speech. One of our hypotheses is that preschool children showing early signs of stuttering are vulnerable to speech discoordination. When they attempt to speak at rates in excess of those they can manage, disfluency results. Accordingly, our first objective is to reduce pressure on the child for fast or jerky responses.

The other hypothesis related to facilitating coordination is that these young incipient stutterers are entering the social communication contest in a family of fast competitive talkers. If they are to make themselves heard, they must hurry to get a word in edgewise. Obviously, expecting them to slow down and speak smoothly while everyone else is whizzing along is hopeless. Thus we concentrate on the family and teach them to instruct by example rather than by direction. We try to turn the speaking contest around so that the objective is for everyone in the family to speak slowly and smoothly, and be a good listener. This program begins on a limited basis at first and is expanded as rapidly as possible to all speech at home. In this way the incipient stutterer is not singled out for special attention, favorable or unfavorable.

Our second objective is to help prevent these children from discovering payoffs in stuttering, especially the discovery that stuttering grabs attention. Another of our hypotheses is that children who are particularly vulnerable to having disfluencies enlarge into a full-blown problem of stuttering are the insecure ones who have had little success gaining attention when they speak. Undoubtedly, to attempt to participate in a conversation and have no one listen is as painful for children as it is for adults. Such children are probably candidates for strong reinforcement of disfluencies that the parents respond to with alarm. Even a negative reaction can be preferable to none.

Here is where our approach becomes controversial. Instead of the admonition to listen attentively to stuttered as well as nonstuttered speech, we instruct the parents in discriminative listening. They learn to attend selectively to their children when they speak smoothly and easily, and to be less attentive when speech becomes choppy and stuttered. Not that they are to punish stuttering or to call attention to it. Quite the contrary. The objective is to call attention to what the child is talking about when speaking effortlessly. It is the content of speech, not the speech itself that we encourage to be the focus of interest.

We have had only limited experiences so far with this prevention program, so it should be viewed as experimental until far more results have accumulated. Such experience as we have had, however, has been very encouraging and has given us increased confidence in the hypotheses from which we work.

REFERENCES

1. Williams D, Silverman F, Kools J. Disfluency behavior of elementary school stutterers and non-stutterers: the adaptation effect. J Speech Hear Res 1968; 11:622-30.

2. Williams D. Silverman F, Kools J. Disfluency behavior of elementary school stutterers and non-stutterers: loci of instances of disfluency. J Speech Hear Res 1969; 12:308-18.

3. Williams D, Silverman F, Kools J. Disfluency behavior of elementary school stutterers and non-stutterers: the consistency effect. J Speech Hear Res 1969; 12:301-7.

4. Ingham R, Martin R, Kuhl P. Modification and control of rate of speaking by stutterers. J Speech Hear Res 1974; 17:489-96.

5. Adams M, Lewis J, Besozzi T. The effect of reducing rate on stuttering frequency. J Speech Hear Res 1973: 16:671-5.

6. Perkins W, Rudas J, Johnson L, Bell J. Stuttering: discoordination of phonation with articulation and respiration. J Speech Hear Res 1976; 19:509-22.

7. Wingate M. Stuttering: theory and treatment. New York: Irvington Publishers, 1976.

PERCEPTUAL EVALUATION OF VELOPHARYNGEAL COMPETENCY

BETTY JANE PHILIPS, EdD

OMAHA, NEBRASKA

Eight public school speech/language pathologists estimated velopharyngeal competence on the basis of perceptual evaluation of speech characteristics of 24 subjects. These evaluations were made from tape-recorded speech samples. After orientation to a system for scoring speech characteristics associated with velopharyngeal incompetence they reevaluated the same 24 subjects. The evaluations were found to improve significantly with orientation and to correlate well with experts' live evaluations as well as evaluations based on instrumentation which included telefluorography, manometric and pressure-flow data. It was concluded that speech/language pathologists, who by nature of their education and training have expertise in identification of speech deviations, can apply their skills effectively in identifying velopharyngeal incompetence. Further it was suggested that orientation to a system for weighing speech characteristics related to velopharyngeal competency can improve their estimates.

A competent velopharyngeal valve is necessary to control air pressure and air flow for speech. Inability to uncouple the oral and nasal cavities will adversely influence both articulation and resonation. Speech characteristics such as hypernasal resonance, loss of oral air pressure for production of sibilants and plosives and inappropriate nasal air escape reflect the presence and the degree of incompetence of the velopharyngeal valving system.[1-5] Additionally, relatively unique compensatory speech behaviors such as glottal stops, pharyngeal fricatives, and nasal grimace may be demonstrated when the velopharyngeal valve is incompetent.[6-8] Speech/language pathologists must be able to recognize the symptoms of an inadequate velar mechanism so that they can refer for appropriate management.

Frequently, the speech/language pathologist who must assume this responsibility for identification and assessment of speech characteristics related to velopharyngeal incompetence is a person working in the field without benefit of extensive experience with velopharyngeal disorders, and without the assistance of instrumentation available in well-equipped clinical centers. Clinicians cannot rely on either a history of clefting or surgical repair as a basis for assessment of the adequacy of the valve. Anatomical and physiological constraints prohibit assessment of valving competence solely on the basis of visual examination of the oropharyngeal structures.[9] Thus, speech/language pathologists must develop, use, and depend on their skills in perceptual evaluation of speech characteristics to assess competency of the velopharyngeal mechanism. Experience suggests that many clinicians are uncomfortable in making such judgments and further, frequently are discouraged by physicians who sometimes refuse even to consider the clinician's concern for inadequate palatal valving. Thus, a question is posed, "How proficient are speech/language pathologists in assessing velopharyngeal competence on the basis of perceptual judgments of speech characteristics?" And, an additional question is, "Is there potential for improving the level of confidence and if necessary, the skill of speech/language pathologists by providing them orientation to the speech characteristics which serve as indicators of velopharyngeal incompetence?" The following is a report of a pilot study which has initiated an investigation into these questions.

Eight speech/language pathologists employed in the Omaha public schools were asked by their supervisor to participate in this study. All had master's degrees and held the Certificate of Clinical Competence in Speech/Language Pathology, but like other professionals, they had relatively little specific training in work with velopharyngeal disorders. The eight represented two different universities in terms of their graduate degrees. Two of the clinicians had neither taken a class nor received supervised clinical practicum in cleft palate. Each reported field experience in work with from one to four children with velopharyngeal disorders. All of the clinicians indicated that they lacked self-confidence in evaluation of velopharyngeal incompetence. Only three had taken a specific class in cleft palate and only three, but not the ones who had taken the class, had received supervised clinical practice with a cleft palate client.

These eight clinicians were asked to listen to randomly ordered audiotape recordings of the speech of 24 children. The children had been subjects in a research project at the University of Pittsburgh Cleft Palate Center. Some had repaired clefts, some unrepaired clefts, and some had no overt clefting. All had been suspected at some time of having velopharyngeal disorders. Subsequent judgments made by the University of Pittsburgh staff indicated that the children at the time of the project demonstrated a range representing competent to severely in-

From the Boys Town Institute for Communication Disorders and Creighton University School of Medicine, Omaha, Nebraska.

TABLE 1. A system for scoring speech symptoms associated with velopharyngeal incompetence

	Weighted Value 1	2	3
Resonance			
Mild to moderate hypernasality		____	
Severe hypernasality			____
Nasal Emission			
Visible (describe nostril evidencing poorest performance)			
Mild or moderate inconsistent[3]	+		
Mild to moderate consistent[3]		+	
Severe, consistent or inconsistent[3]			+
Audible nasal emission			+
Nasal turbulence			+
Facial grimace		____	
Phonation			
Mild hoarseness[1]	+		
Moderate to severe hoarseness[1]		+	
Reduced loudness		____	
Articulation			
Omission of fricatives or plosives	____		
Anterior sibilant distortions	____		
Reduced intra-oral pressure on fricatives		____	
Lingual-palatal sibilants		____	
Omission of fricatives plus hard glottal attack for vowels		____	
Reduced intra-oral pressure for plosives			____
Compensatory articulation such as glottal stops, velar or pharyngeal fricatives, inhalation or exhalation substitutions[2]			+
Column Total	____	____	____
Cumulative Total			____

[1]Add one point if consistent visible or audible nasal emission is present.
[2]Add three points if visible or audible nasal emission is present.
[3]Add one point if hyponasality is present.

Classification of velopharyngeal valving using cumulative score: 1-2 Borderline Competent, 3-6 Borderline, 7-9 Mild, 10-14 Moderate, 15 and Up Severe.

competent velopharyngeal mechanisms. Speech samples which were approximately one minute in length were recorded for each child. These recordings included counting from one to ten, production of sentences which contained nasals, plosives, sibilants, and affricates in prevocalic, intervocalic, and postvocalic contexts and blends and also a short sample of speech elicited in response to a picture. The evaluators heard each recording three times. They estimated the velopharyngeal competence, or conversely, incompetence of each child on the basis of their auditory perception of the speech characteristics supplemented by information given them, which included the child's age and sex, and the results of visual observations of nasal air escape on mirror examination and/or nasal grimace. They classified their estimates using the following descriptions: competent, borderline competent, borderline, mildly, moderately, or severely incompetent.

After the evaluators had completed their initial task, they were given a listing of speech characteristics associated with velopharyngeal disorders, a

TABLE 2. COMPARISON OF SPEECH/LANGUAGE PATHOLOGISTS' ESTIMATES OF VELOPHARYNGEAL COMPETENCY BASED ON PERCEPTUAL EVALUATIONS OF SPEECH COMPARED WITH ESTIMATES MADE BY EXPERTS AND ESTIMATES BASED ON INSTRUMENTATION

	Preorientation		*Postorientation*
Experts live speech evaluations	.63	$t = -4.89$ $P < .001$	.79
Telefluorographic data	.65	$t = -3.85$ $P < .01$	.81
Composite instrumentation data	.60	$t = -4.38$ $P < .001$	.76

method for scoring these characteristics and a system for estimating velopharyngeal competence or degree of incompetence from the total score derived (Table 1). The speech characteristics which were to be scored included attributes of resonation, nasal air escape or nasal emission, phonation, and articulation. The author developed this scoring system with Dr. Betty Jane McWilliams. Prior observations had indicated that estimates of velopharyngeal competence made when using the scoring system were in good agreement with evaluations of velopharyngeal competency assessed by instrumentation, eg, telefluoroscopy, manometric and pressure-flow studies. During the brief 30-minute orientation, in which the rating scale was described, the evaluators also heard tape-recorded demonstrations of the speech characteristics listed in the scale, and practiced scoring two speech samples which had not been included in the original 24.

The evaluators then listened to the same 24 tape-recorded speech samples they had heard previously. They identified the speech characteristics heard, and used the scoring system to arrive at an estimate of velopharyngeal valving competency.

The adequacy of the preorientation and postorientation ratings was measured against three criteria: 1) experienced speech/language pathologists' judgments of the live speech of the children, 2) telefluoroscopic evaluations of velopharyngeal competency based on data available for 14 of the 24 children, and 3) derived judgments of velopharyngeal competency based on various combinations of data available from instrumentation which included Hunter manometric, RD oral manometric, air pressure-flow, and telefluoroscopic studies. The judgments of live speech, telefluoroscopic, manometic, and air pressure-flow data were obtained on the same day as the audiotape recordings. The expert's live evaluations, the telefluoroscopic evaluations, and the composite instrumentation evaluations had resulted in estimates of velopharyngeal incompetence using the same rating scale the evaluators used.

Pearson product moment correlations were utilized to measure the relationship among the evaluators' ratings and the various criteria. In Table 2 the evaluators' judgments are compared with the experts' live judgments. The preorientation correlation between the evaluators and the experts was .63. Postorientation the correlation rose to .79. This improvement in the correlation proved to be significant at the .001 level of confidence.

The preorientation and postorientation evaluations were compared with those derived from the composite instrumentation data available for the 24 subjects. The correlation between the evaluators' ratings and the composite ratings based on video, manometric, and pressure-flow studies was .60 preorientation and rose to .76 postorientation. The difference between the preorientation and postorientation correlations was significant at the .001 level of confidence.

Similarly, the preorientation correlations with the 14 telefluoroscopic ratings was .65 while the postorientation correlation rose to .81. The difference was significant at the .01 level of confidence. Videofluoroscopic ratings were available for only 14 of the 24 subjects because for those with normal speech, exposure to radiation could not be justified, and because for some the videofluoroscopic findings were inconclusive.

There is no infallible measure of the competency of the velopharyngeal mechanism, each has limitations. There are no absolute criteria. The correlations between the clinician's evaluations and instrumentation were about the same level as correlations that can be expected when videofluoroscopy is compared with pressure-flow data, or with experts' live speech evaluations.[10] Thus, the correlations the evaluators achieved were considered a reasonably high or satisfactory level. The evaluators were found to be performing far below the experts before orientation but close to the level of the experts after the orientation. The improvement with the orientation may seem surprising in view of the clinician's lack of specific education and training. The findings suggest that the basic education and training of the speech/language pathologists had provided them necessary background information and skills so that a brief orientation, rather than a more lengthy form of continuing education, was productive in improving their evaluations of velopharyngeal competency.

The task the evaluators was given, rating the *degree* of incompetence of the velar mechanism, was unusual for them and particularly demanding. Speech/language pathologists usually simply indicate either that there is or isn't concern for velopharyngeal incompetence rather than estimate the degee.

To determine how these evaluators might have done on a concern/no concern decision, it seems likely that a decision to refer for evaluation and management to allied professionals would have

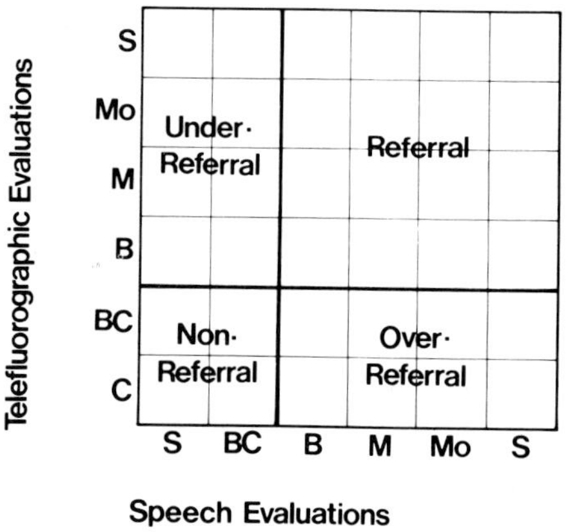

Fig. 1. Criteria for determining appropriateness of referrals when speech evaluations are used as the basis for referral. S - Severe; Mo - Moderate; M - Mild; B -Borderline; BC - Borderline competent; C - Competent.

been made when the speech characteristics indicative of velopharyngeal incompetence were present. Figure 1 illustrates criteria by which appropriateness of possible referral action might be studied. Although there are limitations to telefluorographic evaluations, it was arbitrarily assumed that subjects who were evaluated as competent or borderline competent would have been *under*referred if discovered to be incompetent on the basis of telefluoroscopy. Similarly, the assumption was made that subjects would have been *over*referred when a clinician's speech evaluation indicated incompetence but telefluorography indicated competence. The change in number of inappropriate referrals from preorientation to postorientation is demonstrated in Table 3. Clearly, the number of inappropriate referrals decreases. Observe that as shown in Table 3 that preorientation the inappropriate action would usually have been underreferral. At preorientation the clinicians would rarely have referred patients for whom there was no reason for concern. In fact, they would have missed some who should have been referred. These findings suggest that even at preorientation the speech clinicians' concerns for inadequate velopharyngeal valve for speech production deserved careful attention by the physician and follow-up through comprehensive evaluation by a cleft palate team. The field clinician should seek further evidence which will assist in determining the competency of

TABLE 3. THEORETICAL REFERRALS BASED ON PERCEPTUAL JUDGMENTS OF THE SPEECH OF 14 SUBJECTS BY EIGHT SPEECH PATHOLOGISTS WHEN TELEFLUOROSCOPY WAS USED AS THE CRITERIA FOR INDICATING APPROPRIATENESS OF REFERRAL

Referral for Comprehensive Evaluation of Velopharyngeal Competency	*Preorientation*	*Postorientation*
Appropriate action	53	99
Inappropriate action	59	13
Overreferral	4	4
Underreferral	55	9

TABLE 4. EXAMPLE OF INFORMATION WHICH CAN BE OBTAINED TO EVALUATE ONE SPEECH/LANGUAGE PATHOLOGIST'S ABILITY TO ESTIMATE VELOPHARYNGEAL COMPETENCE BY USE OF PERCEPTUALLY BASED JUDGMENTS OF SPEECH CHARACTERISTICS

Evaluator's Performance	*Preorientation*	*Postorientation*
Correlation with experts	.6058	.7171
Correlation with instrumentation	.5346	.7144
Underreferrals	7	1
Overreferrals	3	4

velopharyngeal valving for speech when there is doubt of a competent valve. The findings suggest that at postorientation they would have had greater awareness of speech characteristics which serve as the basis for concern. They probably have decreased their tendency to *under*refer and increased the number of appropriate referrals.

Speech/language pathologists who work within cleft palate centers have the advantage of feedback received from evaluations based on instrumentation such as telefluoroscopy. This helps them develop their skill in evaluating velopharyngeal incompetence and develops their confidence in the validity of these perceptually based judgements. Clinicians in the field typically do not have opportunity for feedback. The scoring system permits observation of the performance of individuals and makes it possible to give each evaluator feedback related to each of the evaluations made. Tables 4 and 5 illustrate feedback information which was developed for a single evaluator. In this instance, Table 5 suggests that for the specific child being evaluated, the clinician was having difficulty distinguishing compensatory articulation errors and had incorrectly

TABLE 5. COMPARISON OF ONE EVALUATOR'S RATINGS OF TAPE-RECORDED SPEECH CHARACTERISTICS ASSOCIATED WITH VELOPHARYNGEAL INCOMPETENCE AND RATINGS BASED ON EXPERTS' EVALUATIONS OF LIVE SPEECH

Speech Characteristics Evaluated	*Evaluator's Ratings*	*Experts' Ratings*
Hypernasality	0	0
Nasal emission (consistent visible)	1	1
Plus hyponasality	1	1
Nasal emission (audible)	0	0
Nasal grimace	0	0
Hoarseness	0	0
Articulation		
Omission of fricatives or plosives	1	1
Anterior sibilants (lateralized)	1	1
Reduced pressure (fricatives)	2	0
Lingual palatal sibilants	2	1
Compensatory articulation	3 (+3)	0
Glottal stops, pharyngeal fricatives		
Total	14	5
Classification	Moderate	Borderline

classified some as atypical patterns, eg, pharyngeal fricatives and glottals. When evaluations of each subject were studied, the problem in recognizing compensatory articulatory substitutions was observed several times. Feedback of this type can assist the individual evaluator in developing awareness of areas of weakness. By giving the evaluator opportunity to study the tape recordings with knowledge of the experts' judgments, the evaluator's performance probably can be improved.

In summary, the results of this study suggest that speech/language pathologists, who by nature of their education and training do have expertise in identification of speech deviations, can effectively apply their skills to evaluation of velopharyngeal problems. With orientation to a system for making perceptually based judgments of speech, their evaluations can improve. Their evaluations, as judged by comparisons with data from instrumentation, have validity and deserve careful consideration by those professionals to whom the clinician refers for in-depth evaluation of the velopharyngeal mechanism. Additionally, opportunity for comparison of the speech/language pathologists' perceptually based judgments with various criteria such as ratings by experts and from instrumentation, can be utilized to provide feedback which may further improve their evaluations and also provide them some indication of the validity of their evaluations.

ACKNOWLEDGMENT — The tape-recorded speech samples and criteria data were developed by the Cleft Palate Center at the University of Pittsburgh under NIH Grant No. D.E. 01697. Appreciation is expressed to Dr. Betty Jane McWilliams who gave permission for the use of the tapes and criteria data.

REFERENCES

1. House AS, Stevens KH. Analog studies of the nasalization of vowels. J Speech Hear Dis 1956; 21:218-32.

2. Dickson DR. An acoustic study of nasality. J Speech Hear Res 1962; 5:103-11.

3. Warren DW. Nsal emission of air and velopharyngeal function. Cleft Palate J 1967; 4:148-56.

4. Isshiki N, Honjou I, Morimoto M. Effects of velopharyngeal incompetence upon speech. Cleft Palate J 1968; 5:297-310.

5. Curtis JF. The acoustics of nasalized speech. Cleft Palate J 1970; 7:380-96.

6. Brooks AR, Shelton RL, Youngstrom KA. Compensatory tongue-palate-posterior pharyngeal wall relationships in cleft palate. J Speech Hear Dis 1965; 30:166-73.

7. Bzoch KR. Articulation proficiency and error patterns of preschool cleft palate and normal children. Cleft Palate J 1965; 2:340-9.

8. Spriestersback DC. The effects of oral facial anomalies on the speech process. Proceedings of the Conference: Communicative Problems in Cleft Palate 1965: 111-29.

9. Litzow T, Darley FL. Evaluation of velopharyngeal competence after primary repair of the palate. Mayo Clin Proc 1966; 41:524-35.

10. McWilliams BJ, Philips BJ. Velopharyngeal incompetence. Philadelphia: WB Saunders Co, 1979.

MORPHOPHONEMIC PROCESSES IN CHILDREN

JOHN LYBOLT, PhD
OMAHA, NEBRASKA

Classification of preschool children as language-delayed or articulation-impaired, as though these deficit areas were independent, has seldom been challenged. Three groups of ten preschool children were selected to represent normally developing, articulation-impaired, and language-delayed subjects. Their productions of /s/, /z/, /t/, and /d/ were assessed in tasks requiring application of articulatory and grammatical rules. Each group had difficulty applying both articulatory and grammatical rules, normal-speaking children performing best and language-delayed children applying the rules least consistently. Each group evidenced similar response patterns which conformed to developmental expectations.

A speech-language pathologist is asked to evaluate children with a wide range of communication deficits. Often, the parents' initial concern is that their child's speech is not intelligible. The reduction in speech intelligibility cannot be considered solely as an articulation deficit. On further testing, in addition to a presenting problem of impaired articulation, many children exhibit delays in specific aspects of oral expressive language ability. A growing body of literature suggests that children with functional articulation disorders have generalized linguistic deficits which involve speech sound, grammatical, and word-meaning areas.[1-3] The phonological analyses of these children's speech should not be carried out without reference to their syntactical and word-meaning systems. We do not know whether this apparent relationship can be mapped in clinical children, as it has not been fully mapped for normally developing children.

Normally developing children do learn rules for the speech sound, grammar, and word-meaning systems of their language conjointly. Ingram[4] reviewed literature concerning acquisition of the speech sound or phonemic repertoire, the development of sequential rules governing combination of phonemes into more or less complex syllable shapes, and rules in which phonemic markers are used to signal tense, number, or possession. The relative paucity of present research on the interrelationship of this developmental sequence was noted.

Articulation-delayed children may well show a specific impairment of grammatical markers, or of morphophonemic aspects of language development.[5] It would be of interest to compare the phonemic and morphophonemic productions of normal-speaking and clinical children across discrete production tasks. A phoneme at the end of a word signalling a grammatical morpheme would contribute, in most cases, more to word meaning than the same phoneme or speech sound, functioning to terminate the word. Articulation-impaired children have been found to change the degree of deviance of their phonemic output depending on the information value of the phoneme in question.[6] Whether articulation-impaired children alter their phonemic output in response to morphological demands, and those children's strategies in doing so, are questions that are presently of interest.

One discrete production task would involve a comparison of the same speech sounds articulated at the end of words and as grammatical morphemes. As an example, look at one instance of phonologically conditioned morphophonemic change, (Table 1). The voiceless phoneme /-p/ terminates a lexical stem, *jump*. The past tense morpheme /-t/ is then appended to the lexical stem. The choice between the allomorphs /-t/ and /-d/ is phonologically conditioned so similarity in voicelessness is maintained across the final phoneme of the stem and the allomorph. The allomorphs of the plural, possessive, third person present tense, and regular past tense include the consonant singletons /-s/, /-z/, /-t/, and /-d/, and are similarly phonologically conditioned. The addition of one of these allomorphs to a lexical stem creates a more complex syllable shape. For example, cow /kav/, a consonant-vowel sequence, is changed to a consonant-vowel-consonant sequence when /-z/ is added for the plural; mom /mam/, a consonant-vowel-consonant, is altered to a consonant-vowel-consonant-consonant sequence when changed to the possessive form, /mamz/. The developmental evolution of syllabic complexity in children was explored by Moskowitz.[7] Difficulty in maintaining more complex syllable shapes is a characteristic which has been noted for linguistically impaired children.[8,9] Children classed as articu-

TABLE 1. SOME MORPHOPHONEMIC CHANGES FOR REGULAR PAST TENSE

A phoneme /p/ ending a *lexical stem*	*jump*
A morpheme /t/ ending a *lexical stem*	*jumped*
Allomorph /t/ ending a lexical stem or /d/ is phonologically conditioned to	*jumped* /t/ not *jumped* /d/

From the Speech Pathology Services, Boys Town Institute, Omaha, Nebraska.

TABLE 2. MORPHOPHONEMIC AND PHONEMIC USAGE BY NORMAL-SPEAKING, ARTICULATION-IMPAIRED, AND SYNTACTICALLY DELAYED CHILDREN ACROSS THE THREE ELICITATION TASKS

	*Percentage of Scores in Morphophonemic Contexts**				*Percentage of Scores in Phonemic Contexts**			
	/-s/	/-z/	/-t/	/-d/	/-s/	/-z/	/-t/	/-d/
Normal-Speaking								
Correct	65.5	51.2	85.4	88.8	67.7	58.7	83.6	90.2
Distorted	16.3	17.1	0.1	0.1	12.9	13.9	0.6	0.2
Substituted	13.0	26.9	2.7	3.3	18.2	23.1	7.4	2.0
Omitted	4.6	4.8	10.0	7.8	0.7	2.3	7.4	6.3
Articulation-Impaired								
Correct	28.6	21.8	47.9	70.1	31.1	24.1	71.7	76.2
Distorted	13.9	17.9	3.9	0.6	20.1	16.2	3.0	1.4
Substituted	22.9	35.9	7.0	4.4	36.1	39.9	14.2	4.6
Omitted	29.5	20.7	39.3	23.1	12.6	16.5	11.1	14.2
Syntactically Delayed								
Correct	24.0	16.5	20.8	28.8	29.1	30.6	58.9	51.4
Distorted	2.6	1.3	1.2	0.7	9.3	3.8	2.0	0.8
Substituted	23.0	33.6	11.0	12.1	29.4	34.8	15.6	6.9
Omitted	50.4	47.4	63.9	57.3	26.8	30.4	19.6	36.3

*Attempts scored as "no response" have not been included.

lation-delayed and children classed as syntactically delayed might be expected to deal differently with tasks requiring that a consonant-vowel syllable be terminated with a grammatical morpheme.

METHODS

Subject Definition. Three groups of ten children were given speech production tasks. Each child was 4½ to 5½ years of age. All children scored within the range of normal on measures of hearing sensitivity, auditory speech sound discrimination, oral-motor abilities, comprehension of oral syntax and morphology, and a performance test of visual-motor ability. They demonstrated comprehension of the four morphemes which were elicited: the plural, the possessive, the third person verb tense, and the regular past tense.

The normal-speaking group included children above the 25th percentile for their age on the receptive and expressive portions of the Northwestern Syntax Screening Test[10] and the 50-item screening subtest of the Templin-Darley Tests of Articulation.[11] The articulation-impaired group of children scored above the 25th percentile on the receptive and expressive portions of the Northwestern Syntax Screening Test but scored below the 10th percentile on the articulation test (mn = -2.27 z-score units). The group of syntactically delayed children scored above the 25th percentile on the receptive portion of the Northwestern Syntax Screening Test, but scored below the 10th percentile on the expressive portion of the Northwestern Syntax Screening Test and the articulation test. In this way, three distinct groups of children were formed.

Task Definition. At least 20 productions of the speech sounds /-s/, /-z/, -t/, and /-d/ as word final phonemes and as grammatical morphemes were collected in counter-balanced word repetition, sentence repetition, and structured conversational tasks. Balanced elicitations of the phonemes as singletons and as consonant clusters were maintained, as was frequency of occurrence of the elicited words and length of sentences. The target speech sounds were produced 20 or more times on different vocabulary items across three tasks. Table 2 shows that the normal-speaking children, as expected, provided the most correct productions in each target context. The articulation-impaired children provided fewer, and the syntactically delayed children fewest correct productions. Moreover, each group provided the sound correctly more often when the target was not a grammatical morpheme. These differences were, in all cases, more clearly obtained for the plosives /-t/ and /-d/ than for /-s/ and /-z/. Differences across lexical function were significant at the $P<0.01$ level for correct and omitted tallies of /-t/ and /-d/ but not for tallies of /-s/ and /-z/.

None of the normal-speaking or articulation-impaired children omitted 100% of the 20 elicitations for any one speech sound in any of the various target contexts, whether or not it formed a grammatical morpheme. Surprisingly, in only four of the target contexts were 100% of the 20 tokens omitted by a child in the syntactically delayed group. For example, one syntactically delayed child did not supply a possessive /-z/ morpheme when it followed a vowel, another when plural /-z/ followed a vowel. The word final speech sound was supplied in correct, distorted, or substituted form at least once in 356 of 360 series of 20 elicitations of the speech sounds.

In further analyses, the percentage of responses scored as correct or omitted on each grammatical task were ranked across subject groups in Table 3. The ranking was compared with that proposed by Brown[12] as the expected order of emergence for these grammatical morphemes. For the grammatical morphemes requiring the /-s/ and /-z/ allomorphs, correct productions decreased with each later emerging morpheme. Brown found that the regular past tense, signalled by the allomorphs /-t/ and /-d/, emerged after the possessive but before the third person present verb tense. It was clear that each group of our children evidenced more consistent productions of the stop consonant allomorphs /-t/ and /-d/. Omitted tokens may be examined as instances in which children did not mark the word terminal grammatical slot by providing a correct, substituted, or distorted production. When the ranked omission tallies were examined, the expected developmental order was closely adhered to.

DISCUSSION

It was expected that the speech sound error rate

TABLE 3. RANKED PERCENTAGES OF PRODUCTIONS OF FOUR GRAMMATICAL MORPHEMES[12]

Grammatical Morphemes in Order of Mastery	*Normal-Speaking Percentage*		*Articulation-Impaired Percentage*		*Syntactically Delayed Percentage*	
	Correct	*Omitted*	*Correct*	*Omitted*	*Correct*	*Omitted*
Plural	56.6	4.1	27.3	18.4	20.5	42.2
Possessive	56.1	5.5	24.5	21.6	19.6	49.9
Regular past tense	85.8	8.9	58.4	31.2	25.9	60.6
Third person	56.1	6.2	21.9	29.8	19.1	65.1

of the articulation-impaired group would be greater than that of the normal-speaking group. The articulation-impaired children had been selected so their receptive and expressive language performance would be comparable to that of the normal-speaking group of children. It was not expected that the articulation-impaired children would evidence the reduced mastery of the grammatical morphemes assessed here. The percentage of omitted speech sounds would indicate that they did evidence difficulty with the morphophonemic component of their grammar. It was, of course, clear that the syntactically delayed children had reduced mastery of these grammatical morphemes. Children in each group were treating these phonologically conditioned allomorphs with more or less success. Even the most speech-impaired and language-impaired children, however, changed their production of speech sounds to accommodate phonologically conditioned grammatical morpheme markers.

The normal-speaking children would often inflect by substituting in their attempt to produce a grammatical morpheme. They would produce the word final speech sound correctly. The grammatical morpheme would be provided, but as a substitution for the correct phoneme. The articulation-impaired children very consistently evidenced this type of contrast in producing grammatical morphemes versus word final phonemes. This could be evidence of their difficulty in applying adult form sequential morphophonemic rules which have been derived from an incompletely formed set of phonological rules. The articulation-impaired children should have been expected, if they supplied a correct or distorted phoneme, to do so similarly for the grammatical morpheme. Instead, they substituted or omitted more often in morphological contexts.

Additional difficulty was noted in maintenance of C_n VC_n syllabic shapes. Panagos[3] and Ingram[4] interpreted reduced syllable complexity, or an open syllable pattern, as a kind of general language delay. The articulation-impaired children and certainly the syntactically delayed children evidenced this pattern. The syntactically delayed children had difficulty with the articulatory programming of the grammatical morphemes and with the maintenance of phonemes in more complex syllabic patterns. It was evident in the ranking of correct and omitted productions for plural, possessive, past, and present tense forms that the syntactically delayed children observed appropriate sequential morphological and phonological forms inconsistently.

Preschool children should be viewed as imperfect masters of their system for marking tense, number, possession and other grammatical categories; it was an unexpected finding that the articulation-impaired children showed as much difficulty with morphological forms as they did. It was unexpected that the contrast between productions for word final environments and grammatical morpheme environments was as great as it was. The gradual developmental pattern demonstrated for normal children in acquisition of speech sound and oral expressive language systems demonstrated by Moskowitz,[7] Brown,[12] Oller et al,[13] and others, apparently extends to linguistically delayed children, and to their acquisition of morphophonemic systems.

SUMMARY

It becomes obvious that the context in which an utterance is programmed becomes important in assessing the degree of alteration of the expected adult form. It is probable that children's perception of the communication context, the semantic or informational load of the phoneme, the perceived intelligibility of their utterance, and the reaction of the listener both verbal and nonverbal, affect children's phonological and morphophonemic output.

REFERENCES

1. Whitacre JD, Luper HL, Pollio HR. General language deficits in children with articulation problems. Lang Speech 1970; 13:231-9.

2. Menyuk P, Looney PL. Relationships among components of the grammar in language disorder. J Speech Hear Res 1972; 15:395-406.

3. Panagos JM. Persistence of the open syllable reinterpreted as a symptom of language disorder. J Speech Hear Disord 1974; 39:23-31.

4. Ingram D. Phonological disability in children. New York: Elsevier, 1976.

5. Menyuk P. The acquisition and development of language. Englewood Cliffs: Prentice-Hall, 1971.

6. Leonard LB. A preliminary view of information theory and articulatory omissions. J Speech Hear Disord 1971; 36:511-7.

7. Moskowitz AL. The acquisition of phonology. Working paper No. 4, Language Behavior Research Laboratory. University of California, Berkeley, July 1971.

8. Gallagher TM, Shriner TH. Articulatory inconsistencies in the speech of normal children. J Speech Hear Res 1975; 18:168-75.

9. MacIvimey GP. The development of English morphology: an acquisition model. Lang Speech 1975; 18:120-44.

10. Lee LL. Northwestern syntax screening test. Evanston: Northwestern University Press, 1971.

11. Templin MC, Darley FL. The Templin-Darley tests of articulation. Iowa City: University of Iowa Bureau of Educational Research and Service, 1969.

12. Brown R. A first language: the early stages, Cambridge: Harvard University Press, 1973.

13. Oller DK, Wieman LA, Doyle WJ, Ross C. Infant babbling and speech. J Child Lang 1975; 3:1-11.

RESEARCH PRIORITIES IN SPEECH

ROLLAND J. VAN HATTUM, PhD
BUFFALO, NEW YORK

The need for increased research activity in speech and its disorders is reviewed. Increasing interest in language and its disorders appears to have lessened research activity in areas commonly identified as speech disorders: articulation, voice and rhythm. Yet these areas, as well as all aspects of the total communication function, are little understood and some current understandings are even likely to be inaccurate. Thus, not only is additional new research needed but reinvestigation of current beliefs is also essential. Goals for communication research can be classified under five areas: better understanding of the speech mechanism, the communication processes, the individual as a communicator, disorders of speech, and prevention and remediation. Specific research needs are discussed in each of these five broad categories.

The recent explosion of interest in language and its disorders has seemed to lessen interest in the continuing problems of individuals with communication deficits labelled "speech." While philosophical discussion continues regarding the relationship between these basic aspects of communiation,[1] it is not difficult to recognize the need for continued and in fact increased study of disorders of articulation, voice, and rhythm. Evidence for this need can be found by comparing a 1979 NINCDS document[2] with one published in 1969.[3] Over ten years research needs do not seem to have changed markedly, suggesting that our progress in understanding speech processes and disorders through deliberate inquiry has not been adequate.

Further, we are becoming increasingly aware of the critical nature of communication to each individual. In fact, after breathing, communication is the next most important human activity. Each individual attempts to communicate with every available resource, to an extent that we are only now beginning to fully appreciate. It has been relatively recently that we have begun to attend to the nonverbal, behavioral aspects of communication and we still have not satisfactorily integrated the study of the many communication processes which in their totality include even such aspects as the odors we emit and the psychic messages we attempt to transmit, apparently sometimes successfully.

In its broadest sense, the word "language" represents the sum of our communication system. The oral-verbal portion, speaking and hearing, is the most understood. Yet, by comparison with our knowledge of purely physical phenomena, we are functioning at the very beginning. As Denes and Pinson[4] point out, our present understanding is at best incomplete and at worst incorrect. They add that some of what we now believe to be true will someday be as outdated as Helmholtz's resonance theory of hearing is today. They note, "This is as it should be, for science is a vital, dynamic activity, not a static body of established truths." Contrast our advances in the area of communication with that in other areas as described by the National Research Council in 1976.[5] Their report states, "Three decades since World War II have been a time when monumental leaps of understanding were achieved in all scientific disciplines. Profound insights, hard won by disciplined minds, illuminated the nature of the cosmos and revealed the forces that shape the earth's surface, the molecular nature of cellular life, and the wondrous subtleties and complexities of life in higher plants and animals. Lively imagination and rigorous treatment of evidence have permitted reconstruction, at least in outline, of the historical evolution of the universe, of planet Earth, and of life." How ironic that they later state, "The most important economic resource — perhaps the only indispensable resource — is 'human capital' . . . the nation that gets the most out of its people, ie, the nation in which human development flourishes, will be the richest nation in the twenty-first century, regardless of mineral resources or climate." If only financial commitment to speech research mirrored those accurate thoughts and stirring words!

It would be impossible to explore adequately the priorities in research in the confines of available time and to also develop the hypothesis that much that we hold as basic truth in speech needs reinvestigation. Thus, no pretense can be made to establish research priorities here but only to highlight some matters of special interest to me and hopefully reflect concerns of fellow professionals. In so doing, as a clinician, it should be noted that my interests lie in what von Bekesy referred to as "strategic problems." I would like to consider this matter by exploring five goals aimed at developing better understanding of 1) the speech mechanism; 2) the communication processes; 3) the individual as a

From the Department of Communication Disorders, State University College at Buffalo, Buffalo, New York.

communicator; 4) disorders of speech; and 5) prevention and remediation.

1. *Better Understanding of the Speech Mechanism.* Information regarding pathological conditions and resultant effects can only be interpreted by comparison to data concerning the normal system. Improvements in instrumentation and research methodology have advanced our knowledge but we still need much more definite information regarding anatomy. The need exists to develop our relatively general perceptions of the relationship between vibratory activity in the larynx and the acoustic output of the glottal vibration, particularly for such variables as glottal air flow, effective thickness of the vibrating folds, effective vibrating lengths of the folds, and shaping of the laryngeal tube in relation to components of laryngeal resistance. We need better understanding of the larynx as an aerodynamic system and of biochemical aspects such as the cytochemical features of laryngeal epithelium and the neurochemical aspects of the superior or recurrent laryngeal nerves.[6] Even less is known about the tongue, in spite of the fact that it is considered the principal articulator. Information regarding the dimensions of movement for the tongue and how they are executed by the muscles remains meager at best.

In respiration, needed expansion includes the area of respiratory muscle activity during speech, particularly in regard to which muscles function most importantly and under what conditions. Also, data are needed pertaining to the timing of muscle activity in relation to variables of the speech utterance and respiratory characteristics such as lung volume. For clinical use, we need research which seeks to relate pathological states of the respiratory mechanism to disorders of speech.

In all anatomical areas better understanding is needed of the growth of the facial structures which form the oral, pharyngeal and nasal passages and the laryngeal structures in embryological stages through childhood and adolescence, and the relationship of such growth to significantly associated variables such as general bodily growth and possible endocrine factors.

Many problems remain unsolved regarding details of the development, function, control, and structure of the mechanism used for speech production and the relationship with the identified disorders.[2]

2. *Better Understanding of the Communication Processes.* Much of the information currently available regarding communication has been obtained from research using relatively static states. Comprehensive study is needed to explore continuous speech which relates the acoustic signal to what is happening in all parts of the speech mechanism.

To understand speech production "as a skilled motor performance which can be learned, practiced, and perfected and which can be disrupted and interfered with as a result of structural changes due to disease or injury, a much better understanding of the habit system which constitutes our learned motor skills is needed."[3] We need to determine the smallest movement pattern constituting a unitary speech gesture and whether speech gestures maintain a discrete or independent unity in the rapid flow of continuous speech, or become reorganized into larger automatisms or synergisms[6] which in themselves constitute learned habit patterns. Also, we need to know the relationships among such habit patterns, and, when these patterns are deficient or defective, how they can be modified most effectively.[3]

The use of computers and improved vocal tract models has been helpful and continued improvement in these areas is certain. However, even if a model were created which completely and accurately duplicated the human speech mechanism it would be lacking in factors such as intellect and motivation that play important roles in comunication processes.

3. *Better Understanding of the Individual as a Communicator.* Many statements have been made regarding the importance of communication. No one is more convinced of the vital nature of this process than I am. Yet we have little hard data. Data from the 1950 White House Conference[7] is still frequently presented, attesting to the paucity of more recent scientific information. What are the many and varied specific effects of communication disorders on individuals?

This has particular significance for young children. We have followed a cyclic path in terms of early intervention and "waiting for maturation." No one has been more cyclical than I have.[8,9] At one time I believed that therapeutic intervention should be delayed until maturation had run its course. However, after viewing the impact of communication differences on young children I have come to the conclusion that delay, even though speech may eventually be within normal limits without therapy, can cause social, psychological and educational problems. Again, data are needed to support this contention as well as to document when such differences actually become damaging to children. I suspect it is some time around the fourth birthday. If so, we must make every effort to speed the maturation of those maturing more slowing in communication through prevention and/or early intervention. The nature of this intervention needs exploration as well.

4. *Better Understanding of Disorders of Speech.* The extent to which we have been unable to define speech disorders scientifically, even by 1978, is surprising. How many dysfluencies a minute constitute

stuttering? How frequently must a sound be produced incorrectly before it can be considered an articulation error? How different must voice be to be considered defective? We have relied on an intuitive model too long. We must develop objective descriptions of defectiveness which are consistent and measurable.

We must also establish the relative roles of brain injury, other physical injury, genetic factors and faulty learning in the various disorders. That is, global consideration of speech symptomatologies has been largely inadequate.

Specific speech disorders require individual study. In misarticulations, what is the relationship between differences in the speech mechanism and the phonemic errors? Why are some individuals with deviant structures still able to produce normal to near normal articulation? We need to identify subgroups of misarticulation types. For example, are there misarticulation subgroups which are primarily peceptual and others which are primarily motor? More precise descriptions of dysarthria and apraxia, with emphasis on normal reference data and identification of possible subtypes, are indicated. In stuttering, after years of relatively unrewarding research regarding psychological and sociological characteristics, there appears to be as much disagreement as ever as to the cause and appropriate therapeutic handling. Considerable work is needed in identifying possible subgroups within the stuttering population.

In voice, we must quantify and identify the vocal parameters affected by vocal abuse and structural deviation and investigate the relationships between surgical techniques and success in habilitation of such speech disorders as those associated with cleft palate and laryngectomy, as well as improving prosthetic devices.

In addition to the more common types of speech disorders, our studies must be expanded in less frequently occurring problems which result from such things as ablative surgery and various low prevalence syndromes and similar conditions. Much more research is needed on specific populations such as the mentally retarded, behaviorally disordered, and learning-disabled.

5. *Better Understanding of Prevention and Remediation.* For some reasons, the Sabans and Salks in this discipline are difficult to find. There is still little emphasis on prevention. There appears to be much greater valence provided "curing" even though prevention will ultimately prove to be more productive. This cannot be delayed prevention such as speech improvement in schools. Some day children will undergo periodic checks for communication development as they now do for physical development.[9] Predictive formulations which can lead to early detection and prevention need considerable study as do efficient delivery systems.

Greater study of the therapeutic process is needed. In all areas, clinicians with vastly differing philosophies and seemingly significant disparities in methodology demonstrate success. There must be aspects of commonalities that we have not discovered. This could prove to be very fruitful investigation.

In a 1959 special report on *Research Needs in Speech Pathology and Audiology*,[10] it was pointed out that much research has been performed in the area of speech and hearing but that a limited number of contributions have come from the profession. It is further noted that speech and hearing have not been reduced to disciplines which are rigorous in nature. It is unfortunate that twenty years later almost identical statements could be made. This is not to fault those professionals who have been attempting to establish a scientific discipline with little outside assistance or cooperation — sometimes, in fact, in the face of opposition. Funding, particularly from the Federal government, has been ridiculously low and grossly inadequate when the importance of the problem is viewed. The irony of the previously reported National Research Council statement[5] is evident.

There is need for vastly expanded research facilities with proper funding and with interdisciplinary involvement. There are almost no existing "truths." In many ways, we must begin again, reinvestigating what has been accepted as basic tenets and intensifying our efforts to enlarge our body of knowledge and the clinical application of scientific facts. The researcher, the clinician and, the educator must work hand in hand in developing strategies for improving our scientific base and function. Communication disorders specialists, as a group, must move farther away from being technicians and closer to being scientists. Only then can we serve the communicatively handicapped in a manner and to the extent that our commitment demands.

ACKNOWLEDGMENTS — Appreciation is due Dr. Kenneth Perrin, American Speech and Hearing Association, Dr. Christy Ludlow, National Institute of Neurological and Communicative Disorders and Stroke, and Dr. Katherine Harris, City University of New York, for their assistance.

REFERENCES

1. Kavanagh JF, Cutting JE, eds. The role of speech in language. Cambridge: The MIT Press, 1975.

2. National Institute of Neurological and Communicative Disorders and Stroke. Report of the panel on communicative disorders. Bethesda, Md: National Institute of Neurological and Communication Disorders and Stroke, 1979.

3. National Institute of Neurological Diseases and Stroke. Human communication and its disorders: an overview. Bethesda, Md: National Institute of Neurological Diseases and Stroke, 1969 (NINDS Monograph No. 10)

4. Denes PB, Pinson EN. The speech chain. Garden City, NY: Anchor Books, 1973.

5. National Academy of Sciences. The National Research Council in 1976: current issues and studies. Washington, DC: National of Academy of Sciences, 1976: 3.

6. Jenkins JJ, Shaw RE. In: Kavanagh JF, Cutting JE, eds. The role of speech in language. Cambridge: The MIT Press, 1975.

7. American Speech and Hearing Association, Committee on the Midcentury White House Conference. Speech disorders and speech correction. J Speech Hear Disord 1952; 17:129-37.

8. Van Hattum RJ. Evaluating elementary school speech therapy. Except Child 1959; 25:326-31.

9. Van Hattum RJ. Services of speech clinicians in schools: progress and prospects. ASHA 1976; 18:59-63.

10. American Speech and Hearing Association. Research needs in speech pathology and audiology. Washington, DC: American Speech and Hearing Association, 1959.

LANGUAGE DEFICIENCY IN CHILDREN

DONALD M. MOREHEAD, PhD
KERSTIN E. MOREHEAD
WILLIAM A. MOREHEAD
SAN FRANCISCO, CALIFORNIA

Research in cognition and language has provided useful constructs which suggest that specific deficits underlie language deficiencies in children. In addition, this research has provided procedures that determine what a child knows about language at a particular level of development and has established a sequence of linguistic development that maps the specific content and structure of training programs. Two new areas of research offer additional approaches to assessment and remediation. One approacch focuses on the actual principles and strategies that normal children use to learn language, making it possible to determine which methods are most efficient. The second research approach looks at the contextual conditions adults and children provide the first language learner. Preliminary work suggests that the natural conditions found universally in first language learning may be the best indicators of how to proceed with language-deficient children.

Recent theories in linguistics and psychology have followed the tradition of Freud, using the study of the child to describe and explain the origin and development of behavior. Both Chomsky[1] and Piaget[2] have made the child central in their theories of general linguistics and epistemology. The effect of this emphasis has been to stimulate more research in language and cognitive development than in other areas of behavior.[3] Children with language disorders are now able to benefit from these efforts, because we now have a great deal of information about language acquisition and because many highly trained linguists and psycholinguists are now working in this area.[4-9]

Even though there is considerable variation in the rate that normal children learn language, it is generally expected that by a child's third birthday, he will have the beginnings of a productive system of communication. There is no hard evidence for the degree of acceptable variation beyond what generations of children have led us to expect. Precocity in linguistic development generally correlates with high levels of intelligence, but there are striking exceptions. For example, Einstein reportedly did not speak until he was three. There are also less notable exceptions of children who possess normal and sometimes superior operative intelligence but who are considerably delayed in the beginnings of language as well as in the time they require to learn language. This group of children is best described by the clinical syndrome of childhood dysphasia.[10,11] Because many children with language disorders represent unique cases, dysphasic children, who are generally free of multiple deficits, are frequently used as the experimental group in comparative research. The study of these children has also helped to clarify theoretical and clinical issues in other populations of language-deficient children.[12]

One of the controversies that has surrounded this particular group has been the issue of simple delay versus unconventional difference. The early work of Menyuk[13] and Lee[14] suggested that dysphasic children develop some linguistic rules that are nonconventional and seldom found in the productions of normal children. Their findings have often been misinterpreted to mean that the linguistic systems developed by these children are "bizarre," an unfortunate word choice because it implies that their language is exotic rather than merely a variation of normal child language.

When we began our research at Stanford in the late 1960s we decided to replicate the earlier comparative research, using different methods and controls because there was reason to suspect that some of the differences found by Menyuk[13] and Lee[14] could be accounted for by the way they had matched their subjects. Much of cognitive and linguistic development evolves according to similar general rules or organizational principles, with subsets of rules defining sequential levels of complexity in highly diverse groups of children. If two groups of children are matched on standard criteria such as chronological age and the experimental group is delayed in their linguistic development, then it is reasonable to predict that their linguistic systems will show different levels of complexity. Since we had no standardized language test such as the Leiter Performance Scale, which had been used successfully in matching deaf and normal subjects according to mental age, we used mean length of utterance (MLU). A number of researchers had previously shown MLU to be a reliable indicator of linguistic level since everything a child does in organizing an early linguistic system increases length of utterance.[15] After selecting and matching 15 normal with 15 dysphasic children, we wrote grammars which describe the format that children use in organizing aspects of the adult language. The results showed the dysphasic and normal children to have highly similar linguistic systems at each of five lev-

REPRINTS — Donald M. Morehead, PhD, 50 Mallorca Way, San Francisco, CA 94123.

els of early development and further that both groups followed the same developmental sequence.[16,17] Similarities like those we found for syntax, morphology, and transformational development have also been demonstrated in phonology,[18,19] morphology,[20] semantics[21,22] and pragmatics.[23]

Since dysphasic children are clearly inefficient in constructing linguistic rule systems, it is not unreasonable to suspect that they would more often than normal children derive an inadequate or false hypothesis about the ways in which the adult language is structured. What needs to be demonstrated to support the claim of qualitative difference is that the variation in their rule formation and use exceeds the variation found in normal children. To determine variation differences, Bloom et al[24] have suggested that variable rules developed by Labov[25] to study regional dialect and Black English be used. Very little deviation in the surface constraints of language can make an utterance ill-formed or unintelligible, as demonstrated by a simple transposing rule used in pig Latin or word order changes in second language learning.

In the past, language clinicians have generally relied on their own clinical experience and intuition, buttressed by a battery of standardized tests and relevant medical data. However, much of this information, though important in the overall management of the child, does not give specific direction in assessing linguistic level or in providing linguistic data for training. In fact, even those tests that were developed to assess specific abilities, such as the Illinois Test of Psycholinguistic Abilities, have not been demonstrated to be very effective guides to training.[26]

Since the developmental sequence is similar in dysphasic and normal children, a number of researchers have used the extensive data on normal children to develop new assessment techniques and training programs. These programs can now establish from the analysis of a free speech sample the level of linguistic functioning and determine the set of utterances to be used first in training. Moreover, the same analytic techniques for determining level and training materials can be used to evaluate both the child's progress and the training program itself.[27] Most of the programs focus on syntax and morphology[28-30] or semantics.[31] A recent detailed effort by Bloom and Lahey[7] coordinates not only the structure and content of an utterance, but also its use in developing assessment and training procedures.

Most dysphasic children show not only a lag in acquisition time but also significant delays in the actual onset of understanding and speaking language.[16] With the current emphasis on early detection and increased attempts to train very low level children, there is now a large population for whom knowledge of linguistic structures and their developmental sequence has no immediate clinical use. Fortunately, since Piaget's work[32,33] on cognitive development, there has been a substantial amount of research on the cognitive and social factors leading to symbolism and language. As a result, we now have a useful account of potential precursor behaviors that precede the onset of two-word utterances. Since early linguistic behavior evolves within the context of sensorimotor development, once the substage of sensorimotor development has been established, it is possible to determine the approximate level of early linguistic functioning, using the behavioral and linguistic studies of this period.[34-43]

Several tests are available for determining sensorimotor substages by scaling a number of developments that occur within the first two years, such as imitations, means-end relations, and object permanence.[44] Included in these developments are early forms of representation which presumedly lead to the expression of early propositions that allow the child to designate or semantically mark what he knows in single word forms and early syntax. Several researchers have used aspects of these developments in training studies as they appear to have considerable utility in inducing the child to label objects.[45-47]

From the study of the origins and development of cognition, Piaget[33] postulated that language is only one part of a larger system of representation. This larger system also includes deferred imitation, imagery, symbolic play, dreams, and art. Inhelder[48] was the first to test the hypothesis that children with delayed language also have a delay in other representational behaviors. Though Inhelder[48] reported the data from only one child, her results indicated that there may be a general representational deficit in dysphasic children. Similar results were also reported by deAjuriaguerra and his associates[11] on a larger population of 17 dysphasic children, along with a detailed case study of one child. Recent research has continued to support the results of Inhelder and deAjuriaguerra et al in the areas of imagery,[49] symbolic play,[50] and early representations related to language use.[23] (See Morehead and Morehead,[51] Morehead,[17] and Leonard[52] for reviews.)

If representational behaviors turn out to be interdependent and the representational deficit hypothesis is correct, then it is likely that language and other representational behaviors have a common or shared base that needs to evolve before any of them can appear. There is preliminary evidence that certain sensorimotor behaviors such as means-end relations, imitation, and prelinguistic communications may be important for the onset of gestures and language in normal children.[53] Related to these observations is Snyder's report[23] that sixth stage means-end relations are the only sensorimotor development measured by the Uzgiris and Hunt[44] scales that differentiate young normal and language-delayed children. It is entirely possible that a general representational deficit is simply a higher level manifestation of an earlier occurring impairment in certain but essential precursors to symbolic behaviors. In fact, temporal auditory processing deficits may be another, lower level example, which reflects the inability to reconstruct one level of processing at a different level.[54,55]

It appears that at least a basic symbolic system, with or without intelligible speech, is crucial to the formation of propositional or adult thinking. For example, deaf children who have adequate symbolism though deficient language do not appear to have the same degree of difficulty in formal operation tasks as children with general symbolic deficits and low level language such as dysphasics.[56,57] The cost of not being able to develop an adequate symbolic system may well be adult thinking. If this is the case, then early detection, long-term treatment, and occupation planning are essential in the management of these children.[11,58]

As we have seen, cognitive and linguistic research has provided valuable information on possible deficits underlying language in dysphasic children, procedures to determine what the child knows at a particular level of development, and a sequence of linguistic behaviors that reflect the directions which training must take. What this or any other research has not provided is much information about the actual conditions necessary for learning a first language. This is the information we now need to direct intervention with any degree of confidence.

Two areas of research seem to have the most promise for understanding language learning. The first is derived from the way children approach language, based on the sequence and organization of the systems they develop. A number of researchers have found that children use different approaches or strategies to arrive at the same point in an evolving grammar.[15,41,59] In surveying the literature on children learning a number of different languages, Slobin[60] postulated a series of universal operating principles and their corresponding strategies. For example, children pay close attention to word order and avoid interruption or rearrangement of linguistic units regardless of language being learned. In addition, he also described very general principles for learning any complex system, such as the principle that children seldom work on form and function at the same time. Rather, they use new forms to express what they already know or, if the information is new, it is first expressed in a known form.

Knowledge of operating principles and strategies has clearly indicated that the child is an active rather than a passive participant in language learning and that he probably uses something akin to hypothesis-testing or a best guess method to determine the organization or reorganization of his system based on additional linguistic interaction.[41] The study of strategies will be useful in understanding the degree of efficiency and the particular methods used by delayed children in learning language. In addition, it can also provide a clear focus for training efforts; for example, programs should not introduce a new structure without its content being already known. In spite of these recent efforts, we still know very little about the way normal children learn language and almost nothing about the approach used by language-deficient children, except to say that it is obviously inefficient (see MacNamara[61] for a review of language learning research).

A more promising area of research for language training has looked not at how children approach language learning but rather at the contextual conditions adults provide as a setting for that task.[62-64] The importance of social interaction for language learning is clearly demonstrated in a study of a child with normal hearing raised by deaf parents; this child's primary linguistic input consisted of television, a few hearing friends, and young children at a nursery school. The child's language was severely delayed even though he had passively heard considerable language. With broad interactional exposure, the child's language soon progressed rapidly.[65]

Reciprocal interactions begin very early, even before the infant uses single words. Rhythmical motor patterns, dyadic vocal exchanges, and mutual gaze are behaviors that are operative by three months of age.[66-68] As children begin to use more conventional forms of exchange, adults continue to accommodate their speech and language productions according to the general linguistic level of the child.[69] For example, Snow[70] has reported that the semantic terms which so aptly characterize early syntax, such as negation and recurrence, can also be used to describe the language spoken to children at this level.

Adults accommodate more than just the content of their language when talking to children. Recent research has shown that adults speak at a slower rate[71] with changes in both pitch and intonational contours.[72,73] Adult forms are simpler and easier to say, shorter and highly repetitive.[74] Moreover, adults cue the child on turn-taking and seldom interrupt,[75] talk mostly about what the child already knows[76] and generally about objects and events in the immediate context.[38,77] Adults are not only sensitive to the linguistic level of the child but they also seldom correct the errors children make except for pronunciation and "naughty" words.[15] They seem primarily concerned with the truth value and whether or not the child has successfully communicated his intention.[78] It is apparent from this research that adults not only adjust specific behaviors to the linguistic needs of the child but also that their general social interactions provide an optimal setting for language learning. Children as young as four years also adjust their speech when talking to younger children.[79] (See Snow and Ferguson[64] for a review.)

There is some evidence that parents of language-delayed children have difficulty interacting with these children, showing less accommodation to their general developmental status, including linguistic development. Significantly, this lack of accommodation is not found in parents of children with other kinds of handicaps such as mental retardation.[80] These findings indicate that the inability to communicate in the absence of an intellectual deficit may severely affect the dynamics of social interaction. Of course this conclusion assumes that the child's liability causes the disruption rather than the reverse. It is undoubtedly the case that both combinations can be found.[81]

This new line of research, which focuses on the contextual functions of language, is already having a significant impact on the methods studied in training research. Training studies are now attending to the importance of contextual information,[82] modeling as defined in social learning theory rather than imitation[83] and the kind of discourse used in a clinical setting.[84] More significantly, the view that children learn language by using it in a variety of contexts and that the people around them are the primary facilitators of language calls into serious question the utility of many traditional training methods.[85] It appears that the natural conditions in which normal children learn language are going to be the best indicators of how to proceed in language training.

REFERENCES

1. Chomsky N. Aspects of the theory of syntax. Cambridge: MIT Press, 1965.

2. Piaget J. Genetic epistemology. New York: Columbia University Press, 1970.

3. Blumenthal A. Language and psychology: historical aspects of psycholinguistics. New York: John Wiley, 1970.

4. Lenneberg E, Lenneberg E, eds. Foundations of language development: a multidisciplinary approach, vol II. New York: Academic Press, 1975

5. Aaronson D, Rieber R, eds. Developmental psycholinguistics and communication disorders. Ann NY Acad Sci 1975;263.

6. Morehead D, Morehead A, eds. Normal and deficient child language. Baltimore: University Park Press, 1976.

7. Bloom L, Lahey M. Language development and language disorders. New York: John Wiley, 1978.

8. DeVilliers J, DeVilliers P. Language acquisition. Cambridge: Harvard University Press, 1978.

9. Caramazza A, Zurif E, eds. Language acquisition and language breakdown. Baltimore: The Johns Hopkins University Press, 1978.

10. Luchsinger R, Arnold G, eds. Voice-speech-language. Belmont: Wadsworth Publishing, 1965.

11. DeAjuriaguerra J, Jaeggi F, Guignard F, et al. The development and prognosis of dysphasia in children. In: Morehead D, Morehead A, eds. Normal and deficient child language. Baltimore: University Park Press, 1976:345-86.

12. Miller J, Chapman R, Bedrosian J. Defining developmentally disabled subjects for research. N Z Speech Therapist's J 1978; 33:2-17.

13. Menyuk P. Comparison of grammar of children with functionally deviant and normal speech. J Speech Hear Res 1964; 7:109-21.

14. Lee L. Developmental sentence types: a method for comparing normal and deviant syntactic development. J Speech Hear Disord 1966; 31:311-30.

15. Brown R. A first language. Cambridge: Harvard University Press, 1973.

16. Morehead D, Ingram D. The development of base syntax in normal and linguistically deviant children. J Speech Hear Res 1973; 16:330-52.

17. Morehead D. The study of linguistically deficient children. In: Singh S, ed. Measure procedures in speech, hearing and language. Baltimore: University Park Press, 1975: 19-53.

18. Ingram D. Current issues in child phonology. In: Morehead D, Morehead A, eds. Normal and deficient child language. Baltimore: University Park Press, 1976: 3-28.

19. Ingram D. Phonological disability in children. London: Arnold, 1976.

20. Johnston J, Schery T. The use of grammatical morphemes by children with communication disorders. In: Morehead D, Morehead A, eds. Normal and deficient child language. Baltimore: University Park Press, 1976: 239-58.

21. Leonard L, Bolders J, Miller J. An examination of the semantic relations reflected in the language usage of normal and language-disordered children. J Speech Hear Res 1976; 19:371-92.

22. Freedman P, Carpenter R. Semantic relations used by normal and language impaired children at stage 1. J Speech Hear Res 1976; 19:784-95.

23. Snyder L. Pragmatics in language disabled children: their prelinguistic and early verbal performatives and presuppositions. Dissertation, University of Colorado, Boulder, 1975.

24. Bloom L, Lightbown P, Hood L. Structure and variation in child language. Monogr Soc Res Child Dev 1975; 40.

25. Labov W. The logic of nonstandard English. In: Williams F, ed. Language and poverty. Chicago: Markam, 1970.

26. Hammill D, Larsen S. The effectiveness of psycholinguistic training. Except Child 1974; 41:5-14.

27. Rees N. Bases of decision in language training. J Speech Hear Disord 1972; 37:283-305.

28. Tyack D, Gottsleben R. Language sampling, analysis and training: a handbook for teachers and clinicians. Palo Alto: Consulting Psychological Press, 1974.

29. Lee L. Developmental sentence analysis. Evanston: Northwestern University Press, 1974.

30. Crystal D, Fletcher P, Garman M. The grammatical analysis of language disability: a procedure for assessment and remediation. London: Arnold, 1976.

31. Miller J, Yoder D. An ontogenetic language teaching strategy for retarded children. In: Schiefelbusch R, Lloyd L, eds. Language perspectives — acquisition, retardation, and intervention. Baltimore: University Park Press, 1974:505-28.

32. Piaget J. The origins of intelligence in children. New York: Humanities, 1952.

33. Piaget J. Play, dreams, and imitation in childhood. New York: Norton, 1962.

34. Sinclair H. Language acquisition and cognitive development. In: Moore T, ed. Cognitive development and the acquisition of language. New York: Academic Press, 1973:9-25.

35. Lezine I. The transition from sensorimotor to earliest symbolic function in early development. In: Early development. Research publication of Association for Research in Nervous and Mental Disease 1973; 51:221-32.

36. Bloom L. One word at a time: the use of single-word utterances. The Hague: Mouton, 1973.

37. Edwards D. Sensory motor intelligence and semantic relations in early child grammar. Cognition 1973; 2:395-434.

38. Nelson K. Structure and strategy in learning to talk. Monogr Soc Res Child Dev 1973:38.

39. Clark E. What's in a word? On the child's acquisition of semantics in his first language. In: Moore T, ed. Cognitive development and the acquisition of language. New York: Academic Press, 1973:65-110.

40. Carter A. The transformation of sensorimotor morphemes into words: a case study of the development of "more" and "mine." J Child Lang 1975; 2:233-50.

41. Bowerman M. Semantic factors in the acquisition of rules for word use and sentence construction, In: Morehead D, Morehead A, eds. Normal and deficient child language. Baltimore: University Park Press, 1976:99-180.

42. Greenfield P, Smith J. The structure of communication in early language development. New York: Academic Press, 1976.

43. Bates E. Language in context. New York: Academic Press, 1976.

44. Uzgiris I, Hunt J. Assessmant in infancy. Urbana: University of Illinois Press, 1975.

45. Morehead D. Early grammatical and semantic relations: some implications for a general representational deficit in linguistically deficient children. In: Ingram I, ed. Papers and reports on child language development. Stanford: Committee on Linguistics, 1972:1-12.

46. Bricker D. Imitative sign training as a facilitator of word-object association with low-functioning children. Am J Ment Defic 1972; 76:509-16.

47. Bricker W, Bricker D. An early language training strategy. In: Schiefelbusch R, Lloyd L, eds. Language perspectives: acquisition, retardation, and intervention. Baltimore: University Park Press, 1974:431-68.

48. Inhelder B. Observations on the operational and figurative aspects of thought in dysphasic children. In: Morehead D, Morehead A, eds. Normal and deficient child language. Baltimore: University Park Press, 1976:335-44.

49. Johnston J, Ramstad V. Cognitive development in preadolescent language-impaired children. Paper presented to American Speech and Hearing Association. Chicago, 1977.

50. Lovell K, Hoyle H, Siddall M. A study of some aspects of the play and language of young children with delayed speech. J Child Psychol Psychiatry 1968; 9:41-50.

51. Morehead D, Morehead A. From signal to sign: a Piagetian view of thought and language during the first two years. In: Schiefelbusch R, Lloyd L, eds. Language perspectives — acquisition, retardation, and intervention. Baltimore: University Park Press, 1974:153-90.

52. Leonard L. Language impairment in children. Merrill-Palmer Quarterly 1980; 25:205-32.

53. Bates E, Camaioni L, Volterra V. The acquisition of performatives prior to speech. Merrill-Palmer Quarterly 1975; 21:205-26.

54. Rees N. Auditory processing factors in language disorders: the view from Procrustes' bed. J Speech Hear Disord 1973; 38:304-15.

55. Tallal P. An experimental investigation of the role of auditory temporal processing in normal and disordered language development. In: Caramazza A, Zurif E, eds. Language acquisition and language breakdown. Baltimore: The Johns Hopkins University Press, 1978.

56. Robertson A, Youniss J. Anticipatory visual imagery in deaf and hearing children. Child Dev 1969; 40:123-35.

57. Furth H, Youniss J. Formal operations and language: a comparison of deaf and hearing adolescents. Int J Psychol 1971; 6:49-64.

58. Weiner P. A language-delayed child at adolescence. J Speech Hear Disord 1974; 39:202-12.

59. Bloom L. Language development: form and function in emerging grammars. Cambridge: MIT Press, 1970.

60. Slobin D. Cognitive prerequisites for the development of grammar. In: Ferguson D, Slobin D, eds. Studies in child language development. New York: Holt, Rinehart and Winston, 1973:175-208.

61. MacNamara J. Language learning and thought. New York: Academic Press, 1977.

62. Schaffer H. Studies in mother-infant interaction. London: Academic Press, 1977.

63. Lewis M, Rosenblum L. Interaction, conversation, and the development of language. New York: John Wiley, 1977.

64. Snow C, Ferguson C, eds. Talking to children: language input and acquisition. Cambridge: Cambridge University Press, 1978.

65. Sachs J, Johnson M. Language development in a hearing child of deaf parents. In: von Raffler-Engel W, LeBrun Y, eds. Baby talk and infant speech. Amsterdam: Swets and Zeitlinger, 1976.

66. Freedle R, Lewis M. Prelinguistic conversations. In: Lewis M, Rosenblum L, eds. Interaction, conversation and the development of language. New York: John Wiley, 1977:157-86.

67. Stern D. Mother and infant at play: the dyadic interaction involving facial, vocal and gaze behaviors. In: Lewis M, Rosenblum L, eds. The effect of the infant on its caregiver. New York: John Wiley, 1974.

68. Bruner J. The ontogenesis of speech acts. J Child Lang 1975; 2:1-19.

69. Phillips J. Syntax and vocabulary of mothers' speech to young children: age and sex comparisons. Child Dev 1973; 44:182-5.

70. Snow C. Mothers' speech research: from input to interaction. In: Snow C, Ferguson C, eds. Talking to children: language input and acquisition. Cambridge: Cambridge University Press, 1978.

71. Blount B, Padgug E. Prosodic, paralinguistic, and interactional features in parent-child speech: English and Spanish. J Child Lang 1977; 4:67-86.

72. Garnica O. Some characteristics of prosodic input to young children. In: Snow C, Ferguson C, eds. Talking to children: language input and acquisition. Cambridge: Cambridge University Press, 1978:63-88.

73. Ferguson C. Baby talk as a simplified register. In: Snow C, Ferguson C, eds. Talking to children: language input and acquisition. Cambridge: Cambridge University Press, 1978:219-35.

74. Snow C. Mothers' speech to children learning language. Child Dev 1977; 43:549-65.

75. Snow C. The development of conversation between mothers and babies. Child Lang 1977; 4:1-22.

76. Brown R. Words and things. New York: Free Press, 1958.

77. Brown R, Cazden C, Bellugi U. The child's grammar from I to III. In: Hill JP, ed. Minnesota symposia on child psychology. Minneapolis: University of Minnesota Press, 1969; 92:79-92.

78. Brown R, Hanlon C. Derivational complexity and order of acquisition in child speech. In: Hayes J, ed. Cognition and the development of language. New York: John Wiley, 1970:155-207.

79. Shatz M, Gelman R. The development of communication skills: modifications in the speech of young children as a function of listener. Monogr Soc Res Child Dev 1973; 38:1-37.

80. Wulbert M, Inglis S, Kriegsman E, Mills B. Language delay and associated mother-child interactions. Develop Psychol 1975; 11:61-70.

81. Cramblit N, Siegel G. The verbal environment of a language-impaired child. J Speech Hear Disord 1977; 42:474-82.

82. Leonard L. Relational meaning and the facilitation of slow-learning children's language. Am J Ment Defic 1975; 80:180-5.

83. Courtright J, Courtright I. Imitative modeling as a theoretical base for instructing language-disordered children. J Speech Hear Res 1976; 19:655-63.

84. Prutting C, Bagshaw N, Goldstein H, Juskowitz S, Umen I. Clinician-child discourse: some preliminary questions. J Speech Hear Disord 1978; 43:123-39.

85. Hubbell R. On facilitating spontaneous talking in young children. J Speech Hear Disord 1977; 42:216-31.

ASPECTS OF MOTHER-CHILD INTERACTION AS RELATED TO THE REMEDIATION PROCESS

SANDY FRIEL-PATTI, PhD

DALLAS, TEXAS

Selected aspects of mother-child interaction are discussed with initial consideration given to the evidence regarding the emergence of conversational exchanges between normally developing language-learning children and their mothers. The results of a preliminary investigation in the area of mother-child interaction involving the clinical population of language-disordered children are presented. The research results are discussed in terms of the remediation process.

INTRODUCTION

The recent theoretical focus on semantic intention and the pragmatics of an utterance have broadened the perspective of child language research to include the whole of communicative competence. All facets of the speech act are now of interest, although the focus remains on children's acquisition of linguistic skills in conversational exchanges.[1] The concerns of the special subset of investigators interested in the atypical population of language-disordered children have mirrored the current emphases of child language researchers so that the recent thrust of the investigation of language-disordered children has included a consideration of broader communicative behaviors. Consequently, in an attempt to discuss selected aspects of mother-child interaction and the remediation process, initial considerations must be given to the evidence regarding the emergence of conversational exchanges between normal language-learning children and their mothers.

EMERGENCE OF CONVERSATIONAL EXCHANGES

Early interaction patterns between mothers and their infants have been the focus of researchers attempting to delineate the behavioral components and specific interactant strategies for the participants. Two very early bidirectional strategies are smiling and eye gazing between a mother and her baby. These two behaviors are vital determiners of socialization and attachment with the caregiver.[2]

The early periods of mutual gazing and smiling have been described as rudimentary forms of communication in that each partner is acknowledging the presence of the other and establishing a sense of interactant exchange.[3,4] Mutual gaze and smiling behaviors are thus significant factors in the establishment of early mother-infant bonding patterns.[5-7] It is therefore not accidental that the emergence of eye gaze coupled with smiling coincides with the time that mothers most often report that their babies have become "real persons."[8] Interactive smiling emerges approximately one and one-half to two weeks before a marked increase in the infant's production of comfort sounds. Smiling and vocalization are then produced together in social, interactive context.[9] Thus, in addition to being a crucial aspect of mother-child bonding, the synchronous interaction of gazing, smiling and vocalization in face-to-face interaction also appears to be critical in establishing the foundations for communicative exchanges. The mutual regulation of behavior between mothers and their babies is impressive. Mothers consistently are said to approach their newborns with the expectation that the infant will participate in the interaction. Similarly, mothers tend to respond to the infant's actions as if they are intentional and highly meaningful.[10-12] An interesting feature of these exchanges is that they appear to be already based in a mutual awareness of the rhythmic ebb and flow of gaze and gaze aversion, proximal and distal physical cues, vocal turn-taking and smiling.

The adult model of communicative exchange proposed by Kendon[13] posits that the occurrence of gaze aversion acts as a regulator to avoid overstimulation and/or emotional overload on the interaction. It would seem that the rudimentary beginnings of such regulation is apparent in these early mother-child dyadic exchanges.[14] Indeed, the infant and mother are a constant cycle of behavior alternating between attention and withdrawal of attention. Brazelton and his colleagues report[10] that the strength of the dyadic exchange dominates the individual meaning of the participants' behaviors and that no behavior can really be considered separately from the cluster displayed. Initially, the needs of the baby take precedence and serve to shape the mother's response. However, the mother's assessment of the baby's needs and her sensitivity to the dynamic pacing of the interaction appear to be vital for the development of a successful communi-

From the Department of Audiology and Speech Sciences, Purdue University, West Lafayette, Indiana.

REPRINTS — Sandy Friel-Patti, PhD, UTD/Callier Center, 1966 Inwood Road, Dallas, TX 75235.

cative style. Mothers typically have been described as quite flexible in their ability to employ a variety of strategies which serve to focus and maintain the infant's interest. Mothers also learn to establish a pace of stimulation which includes sufficient time for the child to respond.[10,15-17] Lewis and Freedle[18] conclude that such mother-infant interaction ". . . reflects what we believe to be a rather finely tuned and potentially meaning-laden system wherein each allows the other to act."

This quality of maternal sensitivity for pacing the interaction so as to avoid overstimulation and provide time for the infant's response has thus far eluded quantitative measurement or even careful definition of the behavioral components. There have been just a few studies in which reports are made of mothers who have not established such a pattern and the interactive pace is clearly disrupted.[19,12] In these instances, the mother is typically described as "controlling" the interaction or "overstimulating" the infant. Furthermore, there appears to be mutual dissatisfaction in which both the mother and child attempt to control one another.[19]

Within the framework of mothers who are successful in establishing and maintaining a mutually satisfactory dynamic pace, the mode of vocalization has been examined. Between mothers and their three- to four-month-old infants, two modes of vocalization have been observed: the alternating mode includes instances of vocal turn-taking whereas during the coactional mode of vocalization both mother and infant perform the same or similar behavior simultaneously. Bateson[15] has observed a behavioral pattern which results in the alternating mode of vocalization between a mother and her child. Thus, a dialogue exchange is sustained for the two participants. The alternation mode of vocalization seems to be the medium for interactive dialogue in addition to those periods of play when the mother assumes an instructional or teaching role. On the other hand, when the play seems to be highly charged, the coaction system is more likely to dominate.[20]

It is tempting to assume that the mother is in fact "teaching" the baby nuances of eye gaze patterns for a successful dialogue. However, the evidence is quite contrary to such a simplistic interpretation. Mothers in fact violate the "rules" of adult interaction for gazing when they interact with their infants. They maintain a very intimate distance and engage in prolonged periods of gazing at their baby, possibly to monitor the child's arousal level.[16,17,20] This rule violation also holds for mothers' patterns of vocalized exchanges with their infants. That is, a mother tends to assume both roles of speaker and listener: she describes, asks questions and provides the appropriate response to her own question.[21]

While mothers may violate the "rules" of adult discourse, at the same time they also provide a very rich forum for the unfolding of the infant's communication skills. These alternating vocal exchanges between mother and infant have typically been reported as early as 8 to 12 weeks after birth.[15,18] The joint performance of the two participants seems to prefigure adult conversational exchanges:[15]

> Here we see infants and mothers gazing at each other, as each smiles and vocalizes, apparently with pleasure and a sort of delighted courtesy. As with adult conversation, there is near-constant communication in one modality (visual) and intermittent, alternating communication in another.

True interaction can be seen to exist in that behavioral influences are bidirectional for the dyad.[15-17] The communication network is composed of both maternal and infant behaviors and each of the participants can, and does, initiate the exchange. The caregiver-infant communication matrix is made up of more than the vocalizations of each member. Looking and smiling for either infant or mother also serves as an elicitor or response to a vocalization.[18]

The phenomenon of mutual regard (ie, the regulation of a joint focus of attention) has been found operative within the mother-child dyad as early as four months of age.[3] Mutual regard is heightened when the mother verbally draws the child's attention to the shared point of reference. Bruner describes this process as the emergence of semanticity for the child. He believes that through this cycle of behavior the child learns that things have labels and saying the label becomes a way of establishing joint reference, especially in the context of joint action. The simultaneous occurrence of the two events of visual regard and verbalization may serve to single out the object for special attention. This "here and now" referential aspect of speech for describing objects or events to which the child is already attending appears to play a significant role in early language experiences.[22] In this way, the mother serves to identify and organize early forms of communicative interaction. The infant's behavioral response is elaborated, contained or shaped by the mother's interpretation of the child's communicative intent. Eventually, the child assumes a more active role and the mother becomes the recipient of action. That is, the child learns to shift from the recipient to the agent of the act with the previous agent (the mother) assuming the complementary role of receiver.

The special features of attention and the infant's (or the mother's) success in achieving joint action appear to permit the child to enter into a linguistic community rather quickly.[3] Exposure to selected samples of utterances associated with action enhances the child's comprehension and eventual production of utterances based on action.[23]

Another aspect of mother-child interaction which has been closely examined is mother's child-directed speech. It is well known that maternal speech addressed to children has conspicuous stylistic changes. Mothers use fewer words per minute, fewer disfluencies, smaller type-token ratios and fewer fragmented sentences when compared to the speech they address to older children and adults.[24] Therefore, mothers' speech to young children about two years of age is generally simpler and more redundant with a higher rate of repetition of utterances.[25] Research findings support the notion that mothers are very sensitive to their children's developing linguistic competence and reflect this sensitivity in the speech they use with their children.[26]

It can generally be said that mothers perceive their children's ease or difficulty in comprehension and tend to modulate their verbal input accordingly. The most dramatic changes in maternal speech occur between the time the child is 18 to 30 months of age; this period also coincides with the time that most children make tremendous linguistic leaps from one word and/or two word combinations to comparatively sophisticated conversational abilities at 30 months. Maternal speech mirrors these changes in children's language performance.

PRESENTATION OF CLINICAL RESEARCH

This evidence regarding the early establishment of mother-infant communication matrices at 8 to 12 weeks of age and the further refinement of the interactive exchange in later infancy and early childhood has been culled from a variety of investigations with a focus on the language-proficient child. It seems reasonable to presume that children who are experiencing difficulty in the acquisition of language are delayed in all aspects of the communicative process. Since language is clearly one determiner of socialization and interaction strategies, language-disordered children can be suspected to be deficient in these as well.

In an effort to better understand the nature of conversational exchanges between mothers and their language-learning children, a preliminary investigation was conducted to probe the interactions of both language-proficient and language-deficient children.[27] The specific clinical population of language-deficient children all displayed a primary language disorder in that they had no obvious sensory or intellectual deficits to warrant the delay in language acquisition. The objectives of the pilot investigation were twofold: 1) to examine patterns of verbal and nonverbal behaviors exhibited by normal and language-deficient children, and 2) to develop a methodology for recording, measuring, and analyzing the particular nonverbal behavior of eye gaze.

The results of the mother-child interactive sessions revealed clear differences for the two groups of children while the mothers of both groups tended to behave similarly on the measures employed. One of the most interesting findings was that the normal language-learning children initiated significantly more interactive episodes than did the language-disordered child. Furthermore, the results of a descriptive analysis of selected mother-child dyads[28] suggested that mothers and their normal language-learning children have well-developed mutual interaction patterns based on previous experience with successful dialogue. Communication for these dyads was clearly a shared experience. However, the mothers and their language-disordered children had a much slower interactive pace than the normal dyads, possibly due to the nature of the linguistic limitations of the language-disordered children. Some of the mothers of the language-disordered children were found to be extremely sensitive to their children's difficulties in communication. These mothers were flexible in their use of other means for keeping the pace of interaction moving. Not all mothers of language-disordered children were able to tolerate limitations on the dyadic interaction. In such cases, it was apparent that effective communication was not achieved. These results were intriguing and invited further clarification and substantiation in a larger sample size. A follow-up study is currently in progress.

IMPLICATIONS FOR THE REMEDIATION PROCESS

It would be premature at this point to suggest that clear behavioral patterns have been identified with communicative exchange and communicative breakdown. Further specification of these phenomena is warranted. However, there are several trends which can be discerned which offer insight into the process of remediation.

The mutual regulation of behavior within the mother-child dyad is a relatively robust phenomenon. The synchrony of the behavioral repertoire of the two participants is extremely impressive. This mutual regulation can apparently serve the establishment of interaction or it can serve to disrupt the interactive flow. Stern[19] describes a disrupted interactive pattern as also being mutually regulating in that the behavior of the one participant was influenced by the other and vice-versa. It would seem appropriate, then, to focus on the dyad as the unit of study for the evaluation of conversational competence rather than trying to scrutinize behaviors in isolation. That is, it may be necessary to examine a cluster of behaviors since isolation of individual elements often obscures the interpretation of the behavior in question.

The fact that the mothers of the two groups of children were found to behave similarly on the measures employed bears thoughtful consideration. It seems, therefore, that some mothers of language-disordered children are sensitive to their children's needs. These mothers are also flexible in trying to accommodate to their children's needs. In contrast to mothers of normal language-learning children, mothers of language-disordered children are frequently described as more "directive" in their interactions with their children. This may result from maternal attempts to assist the child in organizing play behavior, for example, or attempts to structure the setting to facilitate the child's participation in the interaction. Mothers of normal language-learning children most often operate in response to what their child had said; the mothers of the language-disordered children do not often have that opportunity and so they assume the role of initiator of the interaction more often. This observation that mothers of language-disordered children are more directive in the interaction dovetails rather nicely with the finding that the normal language-learning children initiated significantly more interactive episodes than the language-disordered children did. This seems to substantiate the impression that normal language-learning children are indeed more spontaneous in an interaction and their mothers do have the choice of following the lead of the children. The language-disordered, on the other hand, did not initiate interactive episodes with the same frequency as the normal children. Hence, the mothers of the language-disordered children were themselves classified as initiator or maintainer of the interaction. It is useful to recognize the mutual regulation of the behavior of both interactants in this case. That is, it would seem likely that such an interactive style for language-disordered children and their mothers has evolved from past experience. These mothers may have discovered the need to direct the interaction based on a long interactive history of unsuccessful attempts and/or frustration on the part of the child to direct or maintain the dialogue.

These results are as yet inconclusive and follow-up research is currently in progress to substantiate the findings of the preliminary study. However, it is hoped that these observations will suggest a reconsideration of the role played by mothers with their language-deficient children.

REFERENCES

1. Ervin-Tripp SM, Mitchell-Kernan C. Child discourse. New York: Academic Press, 1977.

2. Eveloff HH. Some cognitive and affective aspects of early language development. Child Dev 1971; 40:1895-907.

3. Bruner JS. The ontogenesis of speech acts. J Child Lang 1975; 2:1-19.

4. Richards MPM. The development of psychological communication in the first year of life. In: Conolly K, Bruner J, eds. The growth of competence. New York: Academic Press, 1974:119-32.

5. Klaus MH, Kennell JH, Plumb N, Zuehlke S. Human maternal behavior at the first contact with her young. Pediatrics 1970; 44:187-92.

6. Moss HA, Robson KS. Maternal influences in early social visual behavior. Child Dev 1968; 37:404-8.

7. Robson KS. The role of eye-to-eye contact in maternal-infant attachment. J Child Psychol Psychiatry 1967; 8:13-25.

8. Wolff PH. Observations on the early development of smiling. In: Foss BM, ed. Determinants of infant behavior, vol 2. New York: John Wiley, 1963:113-38.

9. Stark RE. Features of infant sounds: the emergence of cooing. J Child Lang 1978; 5:379-90.

10. Brazelton TB, Koslowski B, Main M. The origins of reciprocity: the early mother-infant interaction. In: Lewis M, Rosenblum LA, eds. The effect of the infant on its caregiver. New York: John Wiley, 1974:49-76.

11. Sherrod KB, Friedman S, Crawley S, Drake D, Devieux J. Maternal language to prelinguistic infants: syntactic aspects. Child Dev 1977; 48:1662-5.

12. Snow CE. The development of conversation between mothers and their babies. J Child Lang 1977; 4:1-22.

13. Kendon A. Some functions of gaze-direction in social interaction. Acta Psychol 1967; 26:22-63.

14. Field TM. Effects of early separation, interactive deficits and experimental manipulations on infant-mother face-to-face interaction. Child Dev 1977; 48:763-71.

15. Bateson MC. Mother-infant exchanges: the epigenesis of conversational interaction. In: Aaronson D, Rieber RN, eds. Developmental psycholinguistics and communication disorders. Ann NY Acad Sci 1975; 263:101-13.

16. Stern DN. Mother and infant at play: the dyadic interaction involving facial, vocal and gaze behaviors. In: Lewis M, Rosenblum LA, eds. The effect of the infant on its caregiver. New York: John Wiley, 1974:187-213.

17. Stern DN. The goal and structure of mother-infant play. J Am Acad Child Psychiatry 1974; 13:402-21.

18. Lewis M, Freedle R. Mother-infant dyad: the cradle of meaning. In: Pliner R, Krames L, Alloway T, eds. Communication and affect: language and thought. New York: Academic Press 1973:127-55.

19. Stern DN. A micro-analysis of mother-infant interaction: behavior regulating social contact between a mother and her 3½ month-old twins. J Am Acad Child Psychiatry 1971; 10:501-17.

20. Stern DN, Jaffe J, Beebe B, Bennett SL. Vocalizing in unison and in alternation: two modes of communication within the mother-infant dyad. In: Aaronson D, Rieber RN, eds. Developmental psycholoinguistics and communication disorders. Ann NY Acad Sci 1975; 263:88-99.

21. Zlatin MA, Horii Y. Final report of grant no. NE-G-00-3-0077. U.S. Department of Health, Education, and Welfare. National Institute of Education, 1976.

22. Ervin-Tripp SM. Language acquisition and communicative choice. Stanford: Stanford University Press, 1973.

23. Berko J, Brown R. Psycholinguistic research methods. In: Mussen PH, ed. Handbook of research methods in child development. New York: John Wiley, 1960:517-57.

24. Broen PA. The verbal environment of the language-learning child. ASHA Monograph No. 17. Washington: American Speech & Hearing Association, 1972.

25. Snow CE. Mothers' speech to children learning language. Child Dev 1972; 41:549-65.

26. Phillips JR. Syntax and vocabulary of mothers' speech to young children: age and sex comparisons. Child Dev 1973; 42:182-5.

27. Patti SF. Good looking: an analysis of verbal and nonverbal behaviors in a group of language-disordered children. Paper presented at Annual Convention of American Speech & Hearing Association, 1976.

28. Patti SF. Nonverbal/verbal relationships in mother-child dyads with normal and language disordered children. Paper presented at Annual Convention of American Speech & Hearing Association, 1977.

LANGUAGE STIMULATION GROUP
HABILITATION MODEL

PETER K. HIXSON, PhD
OMAHA, NEBRASKA

Bloom's model of normal language development is reviewed in relation to clinical practice and is then expanded to account for disordered development. Four primary and four secondary assessment areas are then considered: language, cognition, motor, and affective development and nonverbal symbolic skills, attentional skills, social development, and physical-medical integrity. Finally, a way of integrating this evaluative information into the model of normal development is discussed and a sample curriculum is outlined.

In childhood language research, it has been the tradition to study children who demonstrate essentially normal patterns of language development in order to isolate and define those factors essential for the acquisition of a specific language system, as well as those factors which appear to be universal to the acquisition of languages in general. By understanding the way in which the normal child acquires and eventually controls his native language system, we can develop models and procedures which allow us to compare the child having difficulty acquiring language with his normally developing peers. Conversely, when this type of testing isolates those areas of a pathological language system which are deficient or absent, their relative contribution to the normal language acquisition process can be inferred and used to test the adequacy of present language-learning models.

As a result of her early research with normally developing children, Bloom[1] proposed a three-part model in which she isolated those factors which she believed contributed in important ways to normal language development. These factors are schematized in Figure 1. The first of the factors from this model to be considered relates to a child's cognitive/perceptual development. It refers to children's ability to perceive their environment through a variety of sensory modes such as audition, vision, and taction, and then to organize this information in such a way that they eventually are able to operate on their environment to consistently produce and predict desired outcomes. This aspect of the child's development has been studied in depth by Piaget[2-4] who has delineated different stages of cognitive development where children first interact with their environment by using trial and error strategies, later begin to apply consistent but perceptually-bound strategies, and eventually move into a period of adult-like, logical-operational thought where their interactions with the environment are controlled by highly structured rules and operating principles which allow them to not only consider actual observed events, but to hypothesize about possible events and outcomes.

A second factor is the child's linguistic experience. In order to acquire language, children must not only be consistently exposed to a particular linguistic system, but also must have certain linguistic skills which allow them to explore and organize their perceptions of language, much in the same way that they explore and organize perceptions of their environment. The important thing to remember, however, is that language presents a very different kind of information to be schematized than does the environment, and thus may require different learning strategies.

The third element in Bloom's model is the child's nonlinguistic experiences. It is not sufficient for children to be exposed to a language system and to develop cognitive and linguistic schema if their opportunity to apply this information is overly lim-

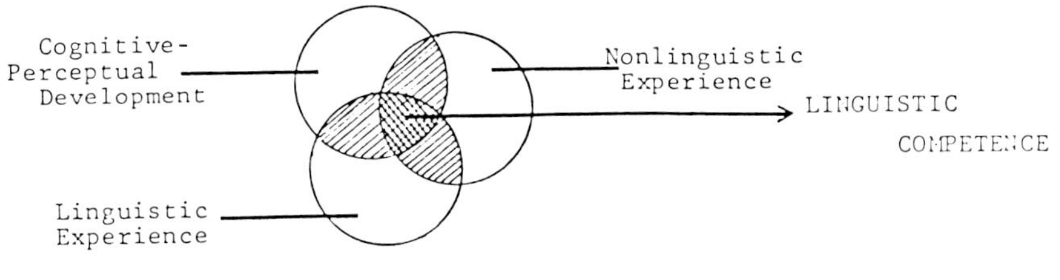

Fig. 1. Interrelationships of hypothetical components in language development. (From Bloom.[1] Reprinted with permission)

From the Department of Otolaryngology and Human Communication, Boys Town Institute/Creighton University School of Medicine, Omaha, Nebraska.

TABLE 1. PRIMARY DEVELOPMENTAL ASSESSMENT AREAS

Language
Cognitive
Motor
Affective

ited, since without a sufficiently broad base of experience, the way children organize and interact with their environment and the conclusions they draw from these interactions may not readily generalize to new information and novel situations.

After considering a large number of studies related to these various aspects of the child's development, Cromer[5] concluded that:

> Our cognitive abilities at different stages of development make certain meanings available for expression. But, in addition, we must also possess specifically linguistic capabilities in order to come to express these meanings in language, and these linguistic capabilities may indeed be lacking in other species or in certain pathological conditions.

The particular program model then, which I am suggesting at this time considers cognitive perceptual development, nonlinguistic experience, and linguistic experience as essential factors for developing linguistic competence. Competence in this context relates to internalized knowledge about our language system which allows us to utilize it effectively in a wide variety of communication situations. For many of the children at Boys Town Institute, however, possessing knowledge about language is not sufficient, for as Cromer suggests, many of these children demonstrate what we might term as performance deficits. While these children are able to comprehend a wide variety of language stimuli, they are not able to produce language in a consistent or intelligible manner. These children demonstrate problems in oral motor competency, application of rules, retrieval of information, etc, which significantly affects the quantity and quality of their linguistic output. Other children may demonstrate similar deficits in utilizing strategies and information essential for language comprehension. Thus, we must consider a language intervention program that not only allows these children to develop linguistic competence as shown in the model in Figure 1, but also must provide specific intervention experiences to develop and improve linguistic performance which can then become part of the linguistic experience.

LANGUAGE ASSESSMENT

Now that we have reviewed several critical aspects of language acquisition which we are assuming are crucial for normal language development, it is important to ask how we can apply this information to a clinical population. In doing so, we can focus the four primary assessment areas listed in Table 1.

One area to be considered is the child's developing linguistic system. Several components can be isolated within this general area of language development. The first of these relates to the way children order and structure their output according to grammatical rules: the syntax of their language. Secondly, we can consider the content of this language output: the complexity of its semantics and the range of meanings expressed. Thirdly, we need to consider the way children articulate or produce the various speech sounds of their language system, since these sounds not only form the basis for the words of their language, but also allow them to differentiate meanings at the morphological level, such as changes in tense and number. Finally, we must not only measure the ways in which children are able to use language, their pragmatic language skills in producing questions, directing others, describing and reporting information, etc, but also the way children are able to combine these pragmatic functions in different discourse situations. This last aspect of language involves testing the way the child is able to adapt his communication system to meet the demands of different situations, such as those posed by talking with an adult or other children, responding to questions on a test, responding to hypothetical questions, statements, etc.

A second major assessment area is the area of cognitive development. Here we are looking at general intellectual functioning both in terms of verbal and nonverbal intellectual skills. This area also includes the child's ability to perceive, process, and retain information through a variety of sensory modalities. Further, it considers his ability to utilize this information in solving problems, as well as the degree of complexity of the problems he is able to solve.

A third area to be considered is the child's motor development. Here we are looking at his play patterns, his exploratory behavior, as well as his specific motor skills. In addition, by studying the child's motor development, we are provided with opportunities to see how he interacts with other children, since much of the child's interaction with his peers during the preschool and early school years is through play activities which require a wide variety of motor skills. In addition, we are able to see how the child utilizes language during his play, and how he problem-solves when the problem requires basic motor abilities for its solution.*

Finally, it is important to look at the child's affective development. In this instance we are interested in parent/child relationships, child/child relationships, the child's concept of self, and his play and exploratory behaviors, as well as his general behavior.

*Bruya L. Unpublished data, 1977.

TABLE 2. SECONDARY ASSESSMENT AREAS

Nonverbal symbolic
Attentional
Social
Physical-medical

In addition to these primary assessment areas, when considering a child for a language intervention program, we also look at several secondary assessment areas. These are listed in Table 2. First, we are interested in measuring the child's nonverbal symbolic skills. These skills generally relate to the child's ability to represent and symbolize information through other means than oral language, such as drawing, modeling, role play, dance, music, etc. Secondly, we are interested in attentional skills. In this case, we observe how well he can delay reinforcement, how well he is able to ignore distractions, his ability to consistently plan and execute motor sequences without trial and error behavior, and his ability to separate essential auditory and visual information from nonessential information. Thirdly, we are interested in whether or not the child is relating to his peers at an age-appropriate level, how he socializes with other children and adults, as well as how he is able to adapt to new situations and demands. And finally, we are interested in the child's physical-medical integrity. How well does his basic physical system function? Are there specific physiological or medical disorders which can account for the difficulties the child is having in learning language, or with learning in general?

PROGRAM CURRICULUM

After we have isolated those factors important for normal language development, and have tested the child with a suspected language disorder in order to delineate deficit areas, we must next determine the type of program we are going to utilize. In this particular instance, we are only considering one type of program, and only a limited aspect of this program. The purpose here is to demonstrate how certain of the factors we have considered thus far can be integrated into a therapy program. It is important when developing such a program to consider that all of the above factors interact throughout the child's development. It is not sufficient to consider these factors in isolation, since providing remediation for each of them separately and then hoping that they somehow combine is not an effective strategy for therapy. Thus, if we only consider children's linguistic systems without considering the other factors of cognitive development and nonlinguistic experience, we will probably be able to improve their language output, but will fail because we have given them nothing to talk about.

If we just limit ourselves to language remediation, we can break the complexities of language learning into three basic factors of form, content, and use, or in more linguistic terms we can break language down into syntax, semantics, and pragmatics. This breakdown is shown in Table 3. Our goal, as Bloom[6] has suggested is to facilitate the child's ability "to use conventional forms of language to represent content for some purpose or use." Thus, we not only want to give the child something to talk about but also to provide a means of structuring this information, and the ability to use this structured information in a variety of contexts. In considering these aspects of form, content, and use, we are also forced to consider the other factors we have mentioned earlier; that is, the child's cognitive development, his linguistic experience, his motor development, and his affective development, since all of these various realms of experience contribute information which facilitates language learning.

TABLE 3. CURRICULUM OUTLINE

- General cognitive area
  - Specific concept
    - Content-vocabulary
    - Form-linguistic structures
    - Use-language functions

In practice then, we choose an area of cognitive development, a specific concept which occurs within this general cognitive realm, and vocabulary, linguistic structures, and language functions useful in expressing this concept. For example, if in developing a language curriculum at Boys Town Institute, as shown in Table 4, we were to choose the general cognitive area of seriation, or the child's ability to organize information into specific hierarchies, we could then break down this general cognitive realm into several more specific areas. We could next decide to focus on a particular concept area such as *time*. Then, by choosing specific vocabulary items such as *first*, *middle*, *last*, *next*,

TABLE 4. LANGUAGE CURRICULUM

- Seriation
  - Concept area: time
    - Vocabulary:
      - First
      - Middle
      - Last
      - Next
      - Before
      - After
    - Linguistic structure:
      - Aux. verbs - is, are, am (was, were)
      - Models - can, will, obligatory do
      - Negatives, not
      - Conjunctions - and, but, because
    - Function:
      - Commands, imperatives, directives: self and others
      - Request information
      - Give information
      - Describe

before and *after*, we could determine for the child specific content related to this concept area. Since one of our primary goals is to further language growth, we then would select linguistic structures which the child both requires in order to develop his language competence and also are appropriate to express this particular vocabulary. In this instance, we might choose words such as: *is, are, am, can, will, not,* and *but*. These words allow the child to say such things as, "He is in the middle" or "Can you stand in the middle" or "He is not the first, but he is the next one." Finally, we need to allow the child to experience this language in a variety of situations, so that he learns to use the structures and vocabulary he has developed to communicate effectively with others. In this instance, we might provide activities which allow the child to request information, give information, and describe events.

In summary then, it is important in developing an habilitation model for the preschool child to consider several realms of experience including nonlinguistic experience, linguistic experience, and cognitive-perceptual development, as well as those factors necessary for developing linguistic performance in the child. Secondly, the child must be tested in order to determine which of these areas are deficient. Finally, we must combine these different areas of experience into a well-integrated program, so that the child is able to see the relationship between one realm of experience and another one, and thus develop a functional, broad based communication system, rather than specific isolated cognitive, linguistic, or perceptual skills. Any habilitation model must consider that children need to learn to communicate with others, not just to demonstrate specific isolated skills.

REFERENCES

1. Bloom L. Language development: form and function in emerging grammars. Cambridge: MIT Press, 1970.

2. Piaget J. The origins of intelligence in children. New York: Norton Press, 1962.

3. Piaget J. The psychology of intelligence. Totowa NJ: Littlefield, Adams, 1960.

4. Piaget J. Piaget's theory. In: Mussen PH, ed. Carmichael's manual of child psychology. 3rd ed. New York: John Wiley and Sons, 1970.

5. Cromer RF. The development of language and cognition: the cognition hypothesis. In: Foss B, ed. New perspectives in child development. Hammondsworths: Penguin Books Ltd, 1974.

6. Bloom L. An integrative perspective on language development. In: Papers and reports on child language developement. Department of Linguistics. Stanford University, No. 12, Dec, 1976.

LANGUAGE-BASED LEARNING DISABILITIES

PAMELA E. HOOK, PhD

NEW HAVEN, CONNECTICUT

The purpose of this paper is to highlight the complexity of the relationship between oral language development and the acquisition of reading skills. As background information, a hierarchy of language development including factors related to both oral and written language is discussed. Case studies of two learning-disabled males are presented to illustrate the differences in reading skills between two children with similar language comprehension abilities. Discussion of the underlying processing deficits responsible for these differences is also included.

The recognition of the importance of oral language and auditory processing in learning to read is relatively recent. In the field of learning disabilities, initial emphasis was on the visual-perceptual difficulties of children with reading problems. Historically, the field of learning disabilities grew out of investigations in the late 19th century by neurologists who were studying brain-damaged adults with language deficits and reading disorders. At that time, awareness developed among neurologists and ophthalmologists that children existed who seemingly had normal intelligence and had not experienced any obvious brain damage, but were having difficulty in acquiring language or in learning to read. The children with language disorders were referred to as having "developmental aphasia" while those with reading disorders were referred to as having "developmental dyslexia." Early descriptions of these developmental disorders tended to separate oral language deficits from reading disabilities. Gradually, however, the relationship between language disorders and reading disorders became recognized, and generic terms were developed to include both disorders. Presently, the most commonly accepted term is "specific learning disability."

The importance of the comprehension of oral language in the evaluation and remediation of specific learning disabilities has become increasingly apparent. The following excerpt from the definition of specific learning disability formulated by the National Advisory Committee on Handicapped Children in 1968 and incorporated into congressional legislation in 1969 highlights the emphasis on language problems as the basis for many learning disabilities:[1]

> Children with special learning disabilities exhibit a disorder in one or more of the basic psychological processes involved in understanding or using spoken or written languages. These may be manifested in disorders of listening, thinking, talking, reading, writing, spelling or arithmetic.

To appreciate the effect of language disorders on achievement in reading and written language formulation, it is essential to understand the following hierarchy of language development adapted from Myklebust:[2]

Hierarchy of Language Development

Visual Language Expression (Writing)

↑

Visual Language Comprehension (Reading)

↑

Oral Language Expression

↑

Oral Language Reception

↑

Inner Language

↑

Alerting and Attention

↑

(Hearing Sensitivity)

In discussing the levels of language development on this hierarchy, normal hearing sensitivity will be assumed. This does not imply, however, that children with hearing losses cannot have specific learning disabilities in addition to their hearing impairment. In fact, according to the Office of Demographic studies at Gallaudet College, Washington, DC, as many as one third of all children with sensorineural losses are felt to have additional handicapping conditions which may include specific learning disabilities.[3] Also, one might speculate that the effects of so-called mild bilateral conductive hearing loss in the presence of preexisting learning disability may result in a marked problem in language and learning. In other words, the combined effects may be far greater than one would assume.

The above hierarchy of language development illustrates the close relationship between oral lan-

From the Department of Otolaryngology and Human Communication, Boys Town Institute and Creighton University School of Medicine, Omaha, Nebraska.

guage and reading. Each level builds on skills acquired at previous levels; thus, difficulty at one level affects development at all higher levels. The first level, alerting and attention, is the basis for language learning. Although information may be transmitted adequately to the brain, it will not be processed meaningfully if the child is not attending to it appropriately. Through attention and interaction with his environment, the child develops an inner language system or preverbal organization of the world. It is upon this inner language system or nonverbal cognitive organization that the comprehension of language is based. In other words, it is necessary to understand the concepts before it is possible to understand the auditory symbols associated with them. As the child develops some control over language comprehension skills, he begins to increase his ability to express his ideas verbally. Thus, reception precedes expression or, in other words, language comprehension skills precede and affect language production skills. By the age of five or six, most children have developed control over the most important elements of their oral language, both receptively and expressively. Reading and writing, which represent visual receptive and expressive language, are built on the existing oral language system. To explain, reading is a visual symbol system superimposed on an existing auditory symbol system, and therefore deficits in oral language development will affect the acquisition of reading and written language skills.

Although this hierarchy can serve as a framework for understanding relationships between language and reading in normal children, it is important to recognize that both oral language and reading acquisition are complex processes and the relationship between acquiring skills in each area is complicated. Hierarchies of processing and memory skills necessary for both oral language and reading acquisition have been developed. Time does not allow an in-depth discussion of the factors involved in information processing and storage, but certain key points will be highlighted. Evaluation of these processes is necessary, since planning and implementing an appropriate remedial program in large part is dependent on identifying a child's specific pattern of strengths and weaknesses in storing, processing, and associating auditory and visual information.

To illustrate the complex relationship between language disorders and reading, two severely language-delayed children, one 12-year-old and one 14-year-old, with different patterns of strengths and weaknesses in reading and information processing, will be described. Their scores are representative of patterns seen in a number of children at our clinic. As can be seen in Table 1, the language deficits are apparent in each case on tests of intelligence where scores on language-based tasks are found to be over 50 points below scores on performance tasks involving nonverbal intelligence. In both children, the language scores indicate disorders affecting comprehension of abstract or relational terms as well as connected language. Relative to their chronological age, child A has slightly better language comprehension abilities than child B, but his scores are significantly below average. Both children exhibit even more significant problems in expressive language than in receptive language. Scores in expressive language are around the five-to-six year level.

TABLE 1. RESULTS OF INTELLIGENCE, LANGUAGE, READING, MEMORY, AUDITORY AND VISUAL PROCESSING TESTS

	Case Studies	
	Child A (Age 12)	*Child B (Age 14)*
Intelligence	Quotient	Quotient
Verbal	62	51
Performance	114	102
Language	Age (yr)	Age (yr)
Comprehension	8 to 10	6 to 8
Use	5 to 6	6 to 7
Reading	Grade	Grade
General	1.6	3.7
Comprehension	1.4	2.5
Word Identification	1.4	5.0
Phonics	1.9	6.0
Memory	Age (yr)	Age (yr)
Auditory	5 to 6	5 to 8
Visual	6 to 11	9 to 13
Auditory processing	7 to 8	17
Visual processing	6 to 7	10 to 17

With the similarity of the language disorders in these children, and in light of the hierarchy of language development discussed above, one might expect to find the children to have similar disorders in reading. In examining reading performance, shown in Table 1, however, one begins to see significant differences. General reading scores for child B fall at a high third-grade level while for child A they are at a low first or preprimer level. Analyzing the different skills involved in reading, one notes that child A exhibits a relatively flat profile with similar scores in word identification, word attack or phonics and passage comprehension. Child B on the other hand shows very significant differences between his ability to identify words or apply phonic word attack skills and his ability to understand what he is reading. As would be expected with severe deficits in oral language comprehension, reading comprehension for both children is very delayed with scores falling at a high first to low second grade level. In child B, word identification skills, on the other hand, do not appear to correlate well with reading comprehension skills since scores on word identification are at a fifth-grade level and scores on phonic word attack are at a sixth-grade level. Thus, severe language deficits do not necessarily affect a child's ability to learn word identification skills. Children such as child B with poor oral language and reading comprehension but average to above average word identification skills are often referred to as "hyperlexic." They can identify many more words in reading than they can understand.

Further examination of each child's strengths and weaknesses in storing, processing and retrieving both auditory and visual information, illustrated in Table 1, helps to explain the difference between these children in their reading skills. In the area of memory, both children show significant deficits in auditory memory which have almost certainly interfered with language learning. Child B, however, shows important strengths in visual memory while child A has specific deficits in this area. Child B also shows strengths in all areas of auditory and visual processing which do not involve meaningful integration and interpretation. In other words, in addition to good visual memory, the ability to discriminate, analyze, and synthesize nonmeaningful, rote kinds of auditory and visual information are areas of particular strength for child B. In contrast, child A shows deficits in all areas involving auditory and visual memory, auditory processing, and some areas of visual processing.

In summary, I would like to emphasize the importance of the hierarchy of language acquisition in evaluating children suspected of having specific learning disabilities, but, at the same time, caution against oversimplification. As discussed above, the acquisition of both oral language and written language skills is quite complex and involves abilities not only in the comprehension of verbal materials, but also in the storage, processing, association and retrieval of both auditory and visual information. Differentiating between patterns of strengths and weaknesses as illustrated by child A and child B is essential in that the remedial program for each of these children would be quite different. Therapy should be based on the child's specific pattern of strengths and weaknesses. Child B has many skills in the mechanics of reading which may be quite useful in his remedial program, while child A has yet to acquire even basic reading mechanics.

REFERENCES

1. National Advisory Committee on Handicapped Children. Special education for handicapped children, first annual report. Washington, DC: US Department of Health, Education and Welfare, Jan 31, 1968:4.

2. Myklebust H. The psychology of deafness. 2nd ed. New York: Grune and Stratton, 1964.

3. Office of Demographic Studies. Annual survey of hearing impaired children and youth: additional handicapping conditions, age at onset of hearing loss, and other characteristics of hearing impaired students-United States: 1968-69. Series D, No. 3.

RESEARCH PRIORITIES IN LANGUAGE AND LEARNING

PAUL FLETCHER, PhD

READING, ENGLAND

The paper reviews recent work in the area of linguistics applied to abnormal language development, specifically in the area of grammar. Particular attention is paid to the notion of linguistic profiling as a procedure for assessment and remediation, using information from normal language development research as a guide. It is suggested that in addition to the potential benefit of the continuing advance in knowledge of normal language acquistion for studies of language disorders, the study of the language of mothers to children could prove of considerable value to the speech and language pathologist.

Stimulated originally by the success of transformational grammar, linguists and psychologists working on children's development have made considerable advances over the last fifteen years in characterizing the course of the language development of normal children, particularly in the area of grammar. It would be impossible here to attempt a summary of this research, but there are two important findings that are relevant. First, the order of acquisition of the syntactic pattern of a language is 'approximately invariant.'[1] That is, although there are considerable differences in the rate of acquisition (children proceed through the language-learning process at different speeds) all normal children generally share a common developmental course. The second finding is that children systematically make mistakes in their language as they learn it, and the existence of such systematic error has given us some evidence as to how they learn. The most often quoted example in this area is that of past tense acquisition. In English there are regular and irregular verbs, and while the regular verbs mark past simply by adding *-ed* (orthographically speaking), irregular verbs mark past tense in a variety of ways (eg, ***break** - **broke**, **sleep** -**slept**, **hit** - **hit***). Children's acquisition of the past tense forms appears to proceed in three stages. First they use sporadic irregular forms, and second they use regular forms exclusively, even for irregular verbs (eg, ***breaked**, **sleeped**, **hitted***). Only after some considerable time do they manage to differentiate between the regular and irregular forms. The existence of systematic error is not however limited to past tenses. Question forms, plurals, determiners, pronouns, various other verb forms, coordinating and subordinating sentences are other examples of areas of the grammar where systematic error has been noted.

The success of syntactic investigation into normal children's language has led to the application of this knowledge to the language-disabled child. There are currently available a number of approaches to grammatical disability which ally linguistic descriptions and information on normal language acquisition[2,3] but here I want to concentrate on that developed by Crystal and his associates.[4,5] This procedure involves using a syntactic profile chart of development, constructed on the basis of research into normal child language acquisition, and applying this to a sample of data from language-disordered children to determine the extent of their language delay or deviance.* The comparison effected in this way with normal syntax development for assessment purposes can be carried further and the normal scale used as a specification of the aims of a remediation program. This thoroughgoing application of a normal developmental scale to the area of language abnormality is justified by the absence of any other satisfactory basis for assessing what language-disabled children say or understand, by its proven usefulness in clinical practice and as a research tool (see Crystal[5] for a wide range of reports on clinical and research applications), and because it is primarily a descriptive procedure allowing the user to characterize the *what* of the language he is interested in, but making no claims about the *how*.† We have already outlined some evidence which suggests that the language learning of normal children may involve rule learning, as in the case of past tense. The syntactic profile, which does rely on the 'relative invariance' hypothesis and so predicts the occurrence of past tense before, say, past participles, has nothing directly to say about the *way* in which the child learns forms. Nevertheless the occurrence of systematic error in the language-disabled child's output will similarly inform investigators about the processes (whether like or unlike the normal ones) which he may be following.

The present, then, sees us engaged in the widespread clinical use of syntactic assessment proce-

*Deviance here is defined as the appearance in the language sample of syntactic structures which (a) would not be used by adults and (b) do not appear as part of normal child language development.[4]

†That is, the syntactic framework is regarded as a useful heuristic, and explanations for acquisition are sought elsewhere.

From the Department of Linguistic Science, University of Reading, Reading, England.

dures and the provision of remediation programs, with the background to the whole enterprise being normal language development. This situation would lead us to expect the delineation of research priorities from those sources: (a) gaps in current knowledge of normal development which are thrown into relief by their importance in the area of disability, and (b) advances in knowledge, in this relatively new and still rapidly-growing field, which add new information either about the course of development, or about the process of learning and variables which affect this. I will outline some examples of how both the gaps and the advances could affect our research planning.

The Verb Phrase. One of the major single problems which appears to affect children with specific language disability (a notoriously heterogeneous group) is the mastery of the verb phrase system.[6] Verb forms in English signal an important set of meanings. They refer to time (present, past and future), they refer to the temporal aspects of actions (whether or not they are continuous, for example), and via the modal auxiliaries like *can, may, must,* etc., they refer to such notions as possibility, necessity, ability and volition. The child has to master the syntax of verb forms — how to get the right parts in the right order. This is not so easy to do, presumably, with a form like *could have broken it*, and is even more complex when one considers question forms (*could George have broken?*). At the same time he has to be able to use the forms appropriate to the situation: when exactly does one use present tense forms, or the modal auxiliary *could*? In order to begin to consider the problem of remediating deficiencies in the area of the verb phrase in language-disabled children it is necessary to know the order in which the forms are acquired by normal children. Unfortunately by comparison with other topics the verb phrase has been approached unsystematically and it has only proved possible to piece together some information about the earliest stages of verb phrase acquisition from a variety of sources.[7,8] Much remains to be done, both in specifying the order of acquisition of forms, and in providing appropriate remediation procedures for teaching them. As we have already indicated, the meaning contrasts signalled by verb phrase forms are diverse and complex, and the general functional complexity of verb forms ensures that the period of their acquisition in normals extends from just after the second birthday into the school years. Detailed assessment information, particularly about the later acquired forms, would be of considerable help.

Another somewhat neglected research area can also be touched on in this context: the detailed study of remediation. I think it can safely be said that in both phonology (as applied to articulation disorders) and in syntax, the linguistic approach has been a valuable addition to the clinician's armory as far as assessment is concerned, and to some extent in the specification, on the basis of the assessment, of remediation goals. But to my knowledge there are only a handful of studies which follow up linguistic assessments with detailed investigation of the progress of subsequent remediation. Such work would be designed to provide information about the ways in which various subgroups of the language-disabled population go about learning language, or, to put it another way, go about using the structured input that the clinicians give them. Let us take one part of the verb phrase as a concrete example, the contrast between present and past progressive:

He is running.

He was running.

Let us suppose that the clinician has a number of ways of demonstrating this contrast to the child or children she is dealing with. A number of questions arise. Which is the most satisfactory remediation procedure? How many trials (to whatever criterion is adopted) does the child need before he can use the forms being taught? Can he generalize the form contrast across a number of verbs, or is he restricted to verbs which have been used in his training? How long does it take for the contrast, once established in training, to be used by the child spontaneously? The comparison of answers to questions such as these across different children and distinct subgroups could place remediation on a sounder footing.

RECENT ADVANCES

I will now turn to recent work in normal language development research which could shed light on abnormal development.

'Motherese.' In the 1970s much research energy has been devoted to the topic of the language addressed to children, which has concentrated particularly on the language of mothers.[9] One major success of this research has been the information provided about the nature of the 'primary linguistic data,' the kind of language the mother addressed to the child. Mother language appears to constitute a distinct language variety: it has quite specific phonetic, syntactic and semantic characteristics which set it apart from other varieties of language the mother uses. At present the relationship between this primary linguistic data and the linguistic progression of the child is not clear; we do not know how children use the modifications. There is disagreement concerning the formal and functional correlation between the mother's modified language and the language of the child, and it is not clear whether when we try to consider the relationship between mother language and child language we should be concerned about measuring syntactic or semantic complexity. What help is this in considering language disorders? The application, as often, is descriptive. As I have said, linguists and others have been successful in describing a variety

of language that is used to normal children. Two interesting lines of inquiry are suggested: (a) if as has been suggested[10] it is the mother's conversational competence which makes for successful language development, is it the case that mothers of children with language difficulty but not specific organic impairment are poor at constructing the appropriate language input? (b) does the nature of motherese provide us with any guidelines concerning the organization of language input in the clinic? To return to this area of the verb phrase, does an examination of the ways in which mothers of normal children refer to and make explicit, say, notions of time in their everyday conversation with the child assist our organization of structured input for children who are language-disabled? The expression of time in normal children's language begins with references to the immediate past, and only later do forms refer to remote past, and to future time. To what extent is this a function of the way mothers use the forms in their input, or is the behavior a function of the child's stage of conceptual development? Another more general question which could usefully be asked concerns the structure of normal mother-child conversations. A feature of the protocols of spontaneous speech recorded by Roger Brown and his associates[1] was the way in which mothers would respond to a child's utterance by expanding, paraphrasing or supplementing it. Rarely this feature of conversation might draw attention only to the form of a child's utterance, as in this exchange with a three-year old:

D. Who did found something?

Father. Who did *found* something?

D. What did you find?

The child has heard his mother talking about some money that was lost and uses an incorrect form; the father explicitly draws attention to this. More commonly there is expansion of form and of meaning, as this example with a two-year old shows:

D. Me blow.

Father. You're blowing the candles out, are you?

Here the parent has extended the grammatical form of the verb phrase and included the object of the action the child is engaged in. Once again we could envisage an extension of this area of inquiry, from the structure of conversations[11] to the structure of therapeutic interaction.

CONCLUSIONS

I have briefly ranged over a number of topics, but I hope the overall intention is clear. Potentially useful information for language disorders is accumulating in the field of normal language development research. As far as assessment is concerned, if the model of normal language development is used as a descriptive framework in the assessment of language disability, then clearly any information about the course of that development is potentially useful; priorities in this area may well be dictated by specific problems of language-disabled children. Also there are recent advances in research into the factors, particularly the mother's language, that affect the course of acquisition, which may shed light on remediation and the way in which the language-disabled child processes the structured input provided for him. This area — the process of acquisition by the language-disabled child in clinical contexts — is perhaps the most neglected area of study, and there is a need here for basic research into the construction and evaluation of remediation procedures, which again can either draw on work already available from the normal field, or provide the stimulus for the appropriate research.

REFERENCES

1. Brown R. A first language. Cambridge, Mass: Harvard University Press, 1973.

2. Lee L. Developmental sentence analysis: a grammatical assessment procedure for speech and language disorders. Evanston: Northwestern University Press, 1974.

3. Dever R. T.A.L.K.: Teaching the American language to kids. Columbus: Charles E. Merrill, 1978.

4. Crystal D, Fletcher P, Garman M. The grammatical analysis of language disability. London: Edward Arnold, 1976.

5. Crystal D, ed. Working with LARSP. London: Edward Arnold, 1979.

6. Crystal D, Fletcher P. Syntactic profiles. In: Fillmore C, Kempler D, Wang WS-Y, eds. Individual differences in language ability and language behavior. New York: Academic Press, 1979.

7. Fletcher P. A microprofile of the verb phrase. In: Crystal D, ed. Working with LARSP. London: Edward Arnold, 1979.

8. Fletcher P. The verb phrase. In: Fletcher P, Garman M, eds. Language acquisition. Cambridge: Cambridge University Press, 1979.

9. Snow C, Ferguson C, eds. Talking to children. Cambridge: Cambridge University Press, 1977.

10. Wells G. Variation in child language. In: Fletcher P, Garman M, eds. Studies in language acquisition. Cambridge: Cambridge University Press, 1979.

11. Dore J. Conversation and preschool language development. In: Fletcher P, Garman M, eds. Studies in language acquisition. Cambridge: Cambridge University Press, 1979.

ELECTROCOCHLEOGRAPHY AND AUDITORY BRAINSTEM ELECTRIC RESPONSES IN PATIENTS WITH PONTINE ANGLE TUMORS

J. J. Eggermont, PhD

M. Don, PhD

D. E. Brackmann, MD

Supplement 75 — Vol. 89, November-December, 1980, No. 6, Part 2

THE ANNALS OF OTOLOGY, RHINOLOGY & LARYNGOLOGY

THE ANNALS PUBLISHING COMPANY
4949 FOREST PARK BLVD.
ST. LOUIS, MISSOURI 63108

ELECTROCOCHLEOGRAPHY AND AUDITORY BRAINSTEM ELECTRIC RESPONSES IN PATIENTS WITH PONTINE ANGLE TUMORS

J. J. EGGERMONT, PhD
NIJMEGEN, THE NETHERLANDS

M. DON, PhD
LOS ANGELES, CALIFORNIA

D. E. BRACKMANN, MD
LOS ANGELES, CALIFORNIA

In 45 patients with surgically proven pontine angle tumors, compound action potential (AP) and summating potential (SP) were recorded with transtympanic electrocochleography (ECochG) together with brainstem electric responses (BSER). The aims were to quantify the mechanism by which tumors cause hearing loss and to evaluate the diagnostic potentials of ECochG and BSER for detecting eighth nerve and brainstem tumors. Except for AP latency and narrow band AP waveform, response parameters recorded by ECochG are uncorrelated. Four uncorrelated parameters were abnormal in only 10% of the cases, three in 25%, two in 40%, and one in 90%.

The BSER criterion was the latency delay between waves I and V and resulted in about 90% detection, improving to 95% when used in combination with the interaural wave V delay criterion.

ECochG results provide evidence that, for hearing losses up to 60 dB HL, the origin is cochlear, resembling that caused by Menière's disease. Evidence is presented that the increase in I-V delay in the BSERs is caused by differential action of the tumor upon low and high frequency fibers in the auditory nerve and that desynchronization of the firings of the nerve fibers is of more importance than an increase in neural conduction time.

ECochG as the sole test for detection of pontine angle tumors appears to be of limited value. Brainstem response on its own has great merits; however, it should be emphasized that no wave I was detected in about 30% of the cases. The 95% detection score obtained with BSER depends on specifying the latency of wave I. For these cases, we substituted the latency of the AP recorded by ECochG.

INTRODUCTION

The ultimate goal of all diagnostic procedures for eighth nerve tumors is early detection. Of the available new screening methods with minimal discomfort for the patient, electroaudiometric tests seem most promising. Some potentially important claims have been made about the diagnostic value of electrocochleography (ECochG) and auditory brainstem electric responses (BSER). In particular, Gibson and Beagley,[1,2] studying transtympanic ECochG in 89 patients with proven retrocochlear lesions and later Morrison et al[3] studying more of these patients, claim detection scores as high as 89% (11% false negatives), with about 20% false positives. Their criteria were broadening of the compound action potential (AP) waveform, preservation of a clear cochlear microphonic (CM) potential, and observation of APs for stimulus levels below the hearing threshold of the patient. The authors admit that broad AP waveforms also occur in Menière's disease and that the CM preservation also occurs in pure cochlear hearing loss. They also acknowledge that in only 27% of patients in their series was the peripheral "hearing" threshold more than 15 dB lower than the subjective one. The authors reached their high scores by combining evidence from all three criteria.

Brackmann and Selters[4] were less optimistic about the usefulness of ECochG in the diagnosis of eighth nerve tumors. They also encountered problems with the similarity of AP waveforms in eighth nerve tumors to those in Menière's disease.

In a series of 23 confirmed acoustic neuromas, Clemis and Mitchell[5] considered the diagnostic merits of latency, amplitude, and waveform of the click-evoked AP and concluded that ECochG is of little value in the differential diagnosis of the tumors. Odenthal and Eggermont[6] studied additional parameters, including latency-intensity and amplitude-latency relationships, that in eighth nerve tumors were frequently found outside the range for normal ears and for ears with Menière's disease. In further studies of a series of 14 patients with various types of pontine angle tumors, they found that the ECochG thresholds were considerably better than the subjective ones in 50%.[7,8] These studies also revealed evidence that the narrow band contributions to the compound AP in tumor ears were monophasic in shape, as opposed to diphasic and N1, N2-type responses found in Menière's disease.[8] These findings appeared potentially useful in the detection of pontine angle neurinoma.

However, a subsequent report by Innitzer[9] demonstrated that the presumed abnormalities for the amplitude-latency relationship did not apply to his series of tumors. Thus, whether Innitzer's findings are representative of eighth nerve tumors or whether the claims made for diagnostic criteria are useful in practice remains unanswered.

Since the advent of BSER, the usefulness of this

From the Ear Research Institute, Los Angeles, California.

technique in differentiating eighth nerve tumors from other conditions, such as Menière's disease, has been tested in several series of patients. Reports of Starr and Hamilton,[10] Thornton and Hawkes,[11] and Terkildsen et al,[12] on small series were followed by reports on larger series: Rosenhammer[13] described findings in 29 patients, Clemis and Mitchell[5] discussed results obtained in 23 patients with acoustic neuromas, and Selters and Brackmann[14] reported the results of BSER in 46 tumor cases. While Rosenhammer considered the general morphology and the ability to reproduce the response, Selters and Brackmann elaborated on the quantitative, ie, numerical detection criteria based on the latency differences for waves V recorded from the tumor ear and the other ear. An experimentally obtained correction factor for differences in the audiograms was found to be necessary. A corrected interaural wave V latency difference of 0.2 msec was established, resulting in a 91% (9% false negatives) detection score and also allowing about 10% false positives to be tested subsequently. In these 10% false positives, an abnormally long interaural latency difference for waves V was found but contrast x-ray techniques could not demonstrate a tumor. Clemis and McGee[15] used the interaural latency difference as a diagnostic criterion and reported two false negative cases in 27 surgically proven tumor cases.

The correction criterion of Selters and Brackmann[14] was arbitrarily drawn for good balance between undetected and falsely detected tumors. Ideally, a correction criterion should depend only on the validity of the brainstem potential generation and should not be influenced by cochlear or middle ear pathology. The I-V delay, which appears to be independent of stimulus levels[16] and site of generation along the cochlea,[17] may be an ideal criterion if it can be shown to be independent of cochlear pathology. Another recently proposed criterion does not require the actual identification of the various waves, which in eighth nerve tumors can be a particularly difficult problem, but is based on the deconvolution of the BSER with the AP to yield a compound impulse response of the brainstem.[18]

This study presents a complete report of the ECochG and BSER findings in a group of 45 surgically confirmed pontine angle tumors, 42 of which were eighth nerve tumors. Effects of the tumor on the auditory periphery will be compared to those thought to be of pure cochlear origin. Whether ECochG offers cues to the detection of a tumor (cues which cannot be explained by the amount and type of cochlear hearing loss, ie, the loss found by ECochG) will be discussed. The usefulness of the I-V delay in the BSER for tumor detection will be evaluated against and in combination with the interaural wave V latency difference.

TABLE 1. DISTRIBUTION OF TUMOR SIZES

Size (cm)	*Number*	*SRT (dB)**		*Speech Discrimination (%)*	
		Mean	SD	Mean	SD
<1	4	31	21	67	45
1 to 2	14	42	16	55	35
2 to 3	15	48	26	52	35
>3	12	45	27	65	38

*SRT value is the average pure tone threshold for the three speech frequencies (0.5, 1 and 2 kHz).

The combination of results of brainstem responses with results of ECochG should yield a precise description of the type of hearing loss produced by the tumor. Correlations of these results with size and type of the tumor will be noted. Finally, an estimate of the smallest tumors detectable by electroaudiometry will be given to answer the question, "Is early detection of eighth nerve tumors possible after all?"

METHODS

Survey of Patient Material. All patients were studied at the Ear Research Institute (ERI) in Los Angeles, California, from January 1977 to May 1978, and were referred by the Otologic Medical Group, Inc. (OMG), in Los Angeles. Prior to the investigations at ERI, the diagnosis of a pontine angle tumor had been established at OMG and surgery had been scheduled. The patients were asked to participate in this study if their general condition allowed it. They were informed that the results of this investigation would not affect their surgery. About 40% of the patients who underwent surgery participated in this research program.

The tests conducted at OMG which led to the final diagnosis of a tumor were audiometry, speech discrimination, impedance and stapedius reflex, including the reflex decay,[19] BSER,[14] electronystagmography with particular attention to saccadic eye movements, x-rays, and/or computerized tomography of the temporal bones. When results of diagnostic tests and general otologic and neurologic examinations raised suspicion of a tumor, a myelogram was obtained. It should be emphasized, therefore, that we had full knowledge of the presence of the tumor and of the audiogram and BSER test results obtained at OMG when we examined the patients at ERI with our ECochG and BSER tests.

The 45 tumors consisted of 42 eighth nerve tumors with the final pathological diagnosis of neurilemmoma, 1 subarachnoid cyst (0.5 cm), one petrosal meningioma (3 cm), and one pontine glioma (2.5 cm) protruding into the pontine angle with the microscopic diagnosis of astrocytoma, grade 1-2. One eighth nerve tumor occurred in a patient with von Recklinghausen's neurofibromatosis whose tumor in the other ear was not included in this series. All tumors were considered as a group and any deviation in the four typical cases is mentioned.

A survey of the sizes of the tumors (Table 1) indicates that about half were large (above 2.5 cm) and only four, including the subarachnoid cyst, were small.

The tumor size determined at surgery was correlated with the audiometrical profile drawn about a week prior to surgery. For a general impression of the hearing, the speech reception threshold (SRT), which is defined here as the mean value of the pure tone thresholds at 0.5, 1 and 2 kHz, and the speech discrimination score at the level 30 dB above the SRT were considered. One foreign patient with no comprehension of English was excluded from this survey. Figures 1 and 2 show the relation between tumor size and both indices of hearing. It is obvious that no correlation exists. Thus, a prediction of the size of the tumor based on conventional audiometric data seems pointless.

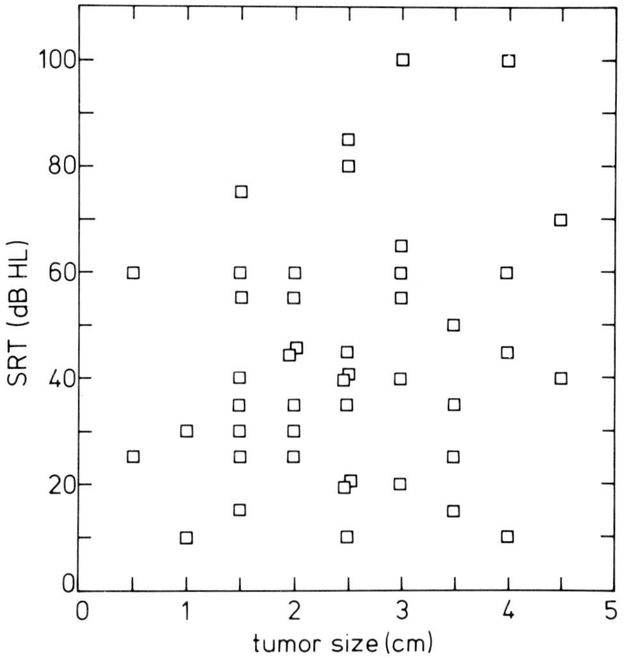

Fig. 1. Relationship between speech reception threshold and tumor size; no correlation exists.

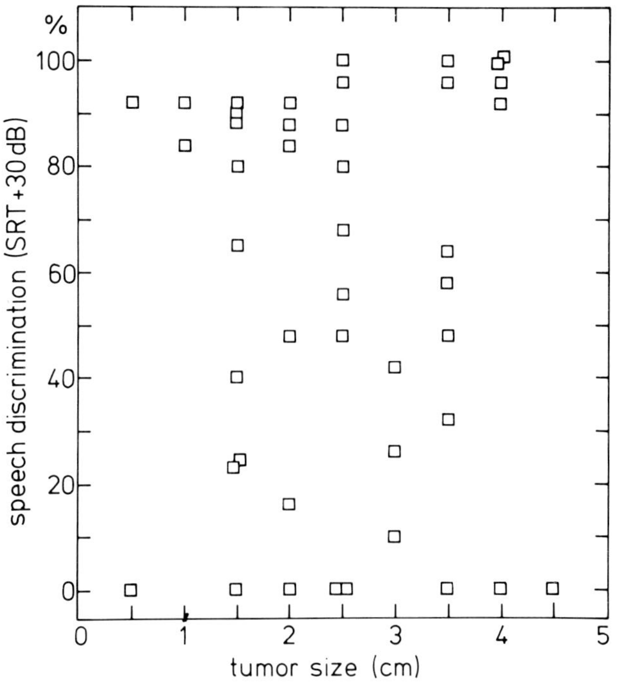

Fig. 2. Relationship between speech discrimination and tumor size. High speech discrimination or no speech discrimination can be obtained regardless of tumor size.

Table 1, which lists the mean and standard deviation for each tumor-size group, further illustrates that the size of the tumor is not related to hearing ability. The consistency of the substance of the tumor and the site of the tumor may, however, relate to hearing ability. The very hard material of the 0.5 cm arachnoid cyst resulted in a complete absence of speech discrimination. On the other hand, some 4 cm eighth nerve tumors produced only minor hearing losses with speech discrimination intact. These findings may relate to the fact that very large tumors that do not affect hearing may be undetected for some time, but small tumors that produce serious hearing problems are likely to be diagnosed early. Selters and Brackmann[14] show that the magnitude of the interaural wave V latency difference is linearly related to the size of the tumor, and that, in very large tumors that press against the brainstem, an increase in the wave III-V delay is found upon stimulation of the nontumor ear. This III-V delay, though a good indicator for brainstem involvement, would also decrease the actual interaural wave V delay, thereby altering the linear relationship between tumor size and interaural wave V delay.

Electroaudiometric Methods. The ECochG procedure with transtympanically placed electrodes is described by Eggermont et al,[20] and recording of the BSER is described by Don and Eggermont.[17] We used the same recording equipment and parameters for the ECochG as for BSER with the exception of filtering: 10 Hz - 10 kHz for ECochG and 100 Hz - 3 kHz for BSER.

Patients lay in a comfortable supine position on a bed in an acoustically treated soundroom (IAC). The ear to be examined by ECochG was anesthetized with an iontophoretic application of lidocaine and epinephrine for 11 minutes. After the ear canal was dried, EEG disc electrodes were applied to the vertex, the forehead, and both mastoids. A sterilized, Teflon® -insulated (except at the tip) needle electrode was placed on the promontory and kept in place by an elastic band.

Stimuli were tone bursts of 2, 4, and 8 kHz and clicks delivered by an electromagnetically shielded loudspeaker (Amplaid, Type V) placed 1 m from the patient's ear. APs were recorded at levels up to 110 dB HL if necessary for well-determined input-output curves and AP thresholds. Subsequently, if the amount of hearing loss permitted, narrow band APs were derived with high-pass noise masking[21] for clicks of 90 dB peak equivalent (pe) SPL (about 70 dB SL for normal ears). The needle electrode was then removed and the recording of BSER potentials began. Stimuli were delivered by TDH-49 headphones with MX-41 circumaural cushions.

Calibration of the intensity levels for tone bursts delivered by the loudspeaker was done with a General Radio sound level meter (GR 1933). Subjective thresholds for normals in the same position as the patient were determined according to the procedure of Spoor and Eggermont,[22] ie, with the same tone bursts used in the ECochG but presented at 30/sec. The level at which the AP amplitude equals 0.1 μV was, in general, 10 dB above the subjective hearing threshold.[22] All data presented are corrected to accommodate this difference. The correction factor is frequency independent and applies only to a threshold set at 0.1 μV for 500 averages. Any other combinations would require a different correction (eg, 0.05 μV and 2000 averages require a few decibels). The clicks for the BSER recordings were set at a convenient level, usually 70 dB above the normal hearing threshold. If no response was obtained, the level was increased.

RESULTS

ELECTROCOCHLEOGRAPHY

AP Waveforms. Various types of AP waveforms are encountered in pathological ears[23] depending on the frequency of the tone bursts, the shape of the audiogram, and the pathology. That eighth nerve tumors cause AP waveforms to be abnormally broad was reported as early as 1972.[24]

Figure 3 shows AP waveforms for 2 kHz tone burst stimulation at various stimulus levels in three eighth nerve tumor ears. The left series represents the typical broad waveform, which somewhat resembles that of Menière's disease,[25] with an unusually large jump in the AP latency between 75 and 85 dB HL. The middle series represents a case in which the AP waveform is normal at high intensities and abnormal at lower intensities. The right

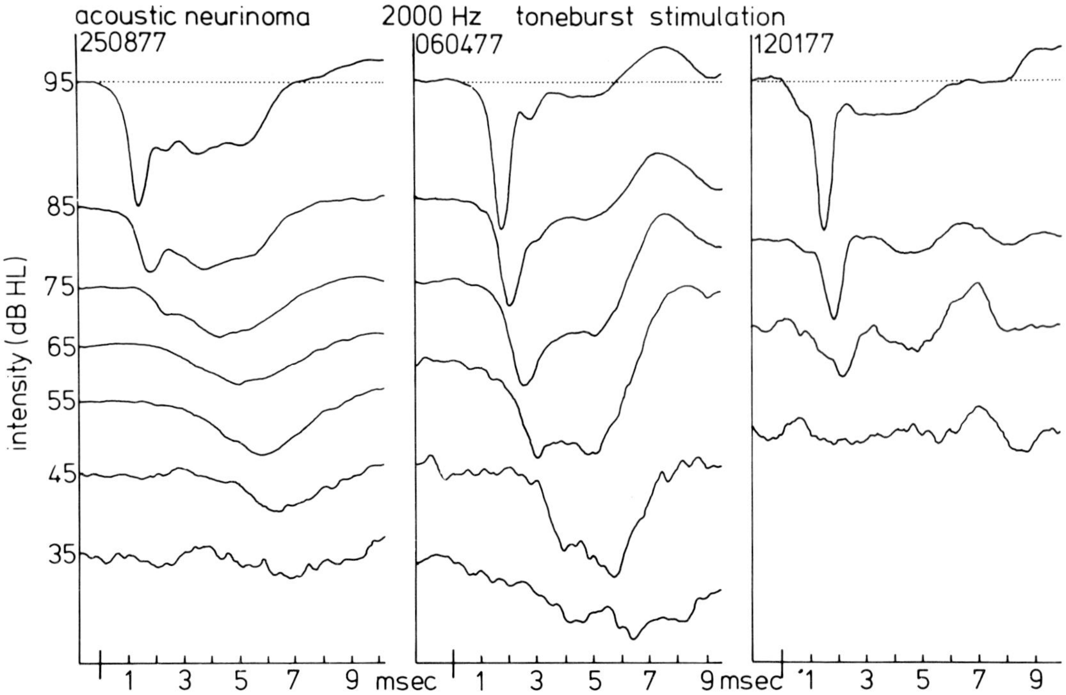

Fig. 3. Compound AP waveforms in response to 2 kHz tone burst stimulation in three ears with acoustic neurinoma. Depending on the individual case as well as on stimulus intensity, broad characteristic waveforms or nearly mormal APs can be found. It appears that the AP waveform is not consistently abnormal in acoustic neurinoma ears.

series shows normal AP waveforms at all intensities tested. Of the 33 ears tested, only 10 showed abnormally broad AP waveforms, while the waveforms of the remaining 23 were as expected according to the audiogram.

AP Stimulus-Response Relationships. For the ears represented in Figure 3, the amplitude-intensity and latency-intensity functions have been plotted in Figure 4. Amplitude and latency are plotted on a logarithmic scale. In the example with the typical broad waveform (250877) represented by the open squares, the amplitude-intensity function looks normal, with an AP threshold of 20 dB HL. The audiogram (see insert) shows a moderate high frequency hearing loss.

The amplitude-intensity function (Fig. 4, open triangles) for the waveforms of patient 120177 (Fig. 3, right) shows an elevated AP threshold at 2 kHz of 55 dB HL and nearly normal AP amplitude at high intensities. The amplitude-intensity function has, therefore, a very steep rise, resembling the findings in recruiting ears.[25] The audiogram shows a flat 60 dB loss for frequencies of 1 kHz and above.

The other example, indicated by filled circles, shows a slightly elevated threshold at 2 kHz (30 dB) and a moderately steep, rising amplitude-intensity function. The audiogram showed a moderate hearing loss for the low and middle frequencies and steeply increasing thresholds for the higher frequencies.

The latency-intensity functions for these three

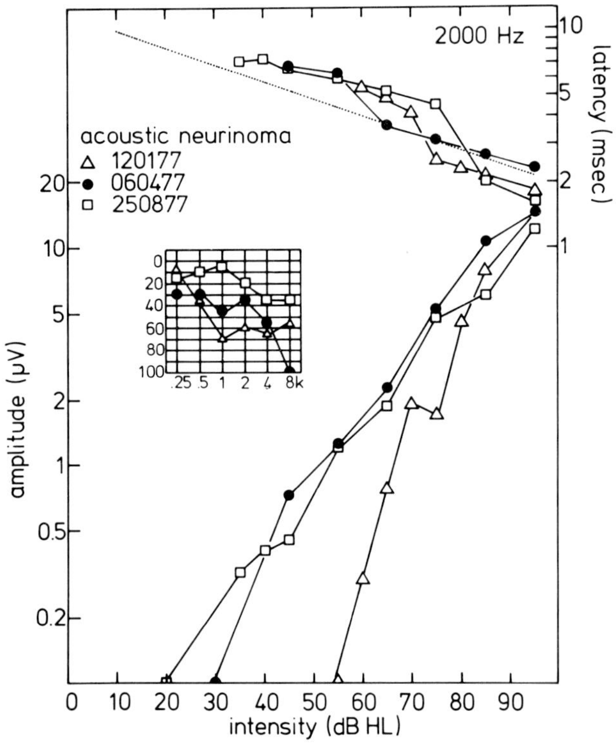

Fig. 4. Input-output curves for the ears represented in Fig. 3. Despite threshold differences of 35 dB, the output at high intensity (90 dB) is virtually identical. This phenomenon is thought to be characteristic of recruiting ears. The latency functions (upper part of Figure) tend to reach values that are larger than normal for a particular intensity level. The audiograms for the three ears are also shown.

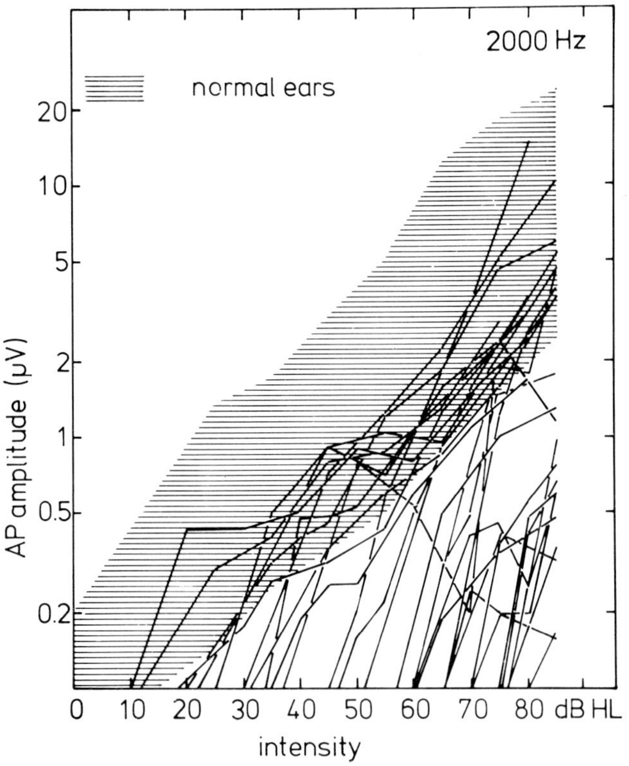

Fig. 5. AP amplitude-intensity relationships for all tumor cases in which ECochG was performed. A large number of curves lie completely within the actual normal range, including curves that at high stimulus levels reach normal. This indicates that the slope of the curves increases with increasing AP threshold.

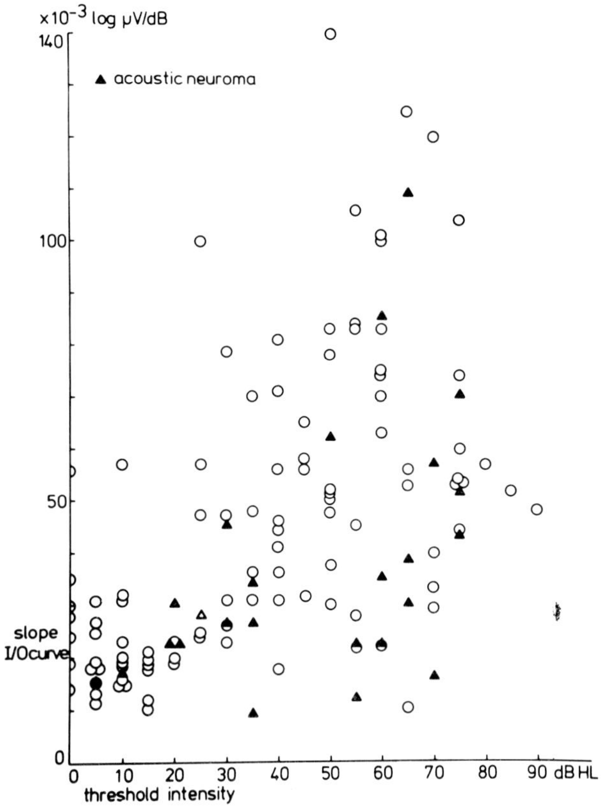

Fig. 6. Quantitative relationship between the slope of the amplitude-intensity function and the AP threshold intensity for normal and pure cochlear hearing loss ears (open circles) and acoustic neurinoma ear (filled triangles).

ears are abnormal in that they lie above the upper boundary of normal ears (dotted line) for intensities less than 70 dB HL. However, they fall within the range for ears with Menière's disease.[25]

Twenty-eight of 32 ears tested by ECochG yielded measurable APs at 2, 4, and 8 kHz. Figure 5 shows their amplitude-intensity functions for 2 kHz tone burst stimulation. The shaded area represents the range of absolute amplitude values found in 27 normal ears. The majority of tumor ears with thresholds up to 65 dB HL reach normal AP amplitude values at high tone burst intensities. In cases with AP thresholds exceeding 60 dB HL, steeply rising amplitude-intensity curves are found, but even at 85 dB HL the normal output level is not reached.

The slope of the amplitude-intensity function has been used previously as an indication for the presence of recruitment,[26] and it was noted that the higher the AP threshold for tone burst stimulation, the steeper the input-output function.[25] To quantify this for the eighth nerve tumor ears, the values of the slopes of the AP amplitude-intensity functions (calculated for the AP amplitude range of 0.1-1.5 μV) are plotted in Figure 6 for normal ears (thresholds up to and including 15 dB), recruiting ears, and eighth nerve tumor ears (filled triangles). Nearly all the slope values found in eighth nerve tumors are within the range of those for normal ears and pure cochlear hearing losses. The conclusion might therefore be drawn that the hearing loss produced by a tumor of the eighth nerve is, on the cochlear level, indistinguishable from that of recruiting ears.

As noted in the three ears in Figures 3 and 4, the latency-intensity function tends to become abnormal. This is substantiated in group data in Figure 7. About two thirds of the individual functions are clearly outside the normal range (shaded). This abnormality also occurs in ears with Menière's disease, but to a lesser degree.[25] Therefore, a highly abnormal latency-intensity function may remain a useful indication of an eighth nerve tumor.

AP Parameter Interrelationships. AP parameters as a function of stimulus intensity indicate that, in eighth nerve tumor ears, most relationships depend upon the audiogram, as in recruiting ears.[25] This is also illustrated by AP parameter interdependency, such as amplitude-latency and width-latency functions.[20] As previously shown for ears with Menière's disease,[27] nearly all amplitude-latency points, each representing one single AP, fall within the normal group (2 SD) boundaries. A previous report[7] shows that, for eighth nerve tumor ears, some points tend to lie above the normal range. This report shows all individually recorded APs as open circles (Fig. 8) compared to the shaded normal range. Some points

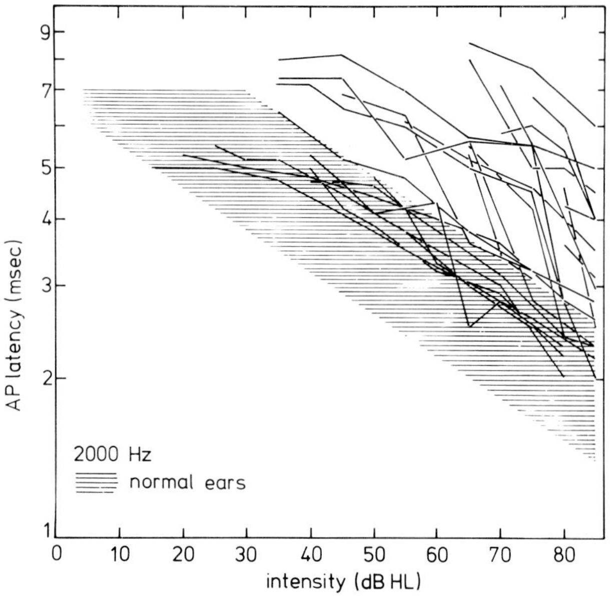

Fig. 7. AP latency-intensity functions for the acoustic neurinoma ears. A large number of curves lie above the actual range of latency values found in normal ears.

are above the normal range, but most are within the normal range. This demonstrates that the amplitude-latency function is not a useful diagnostic criterion.

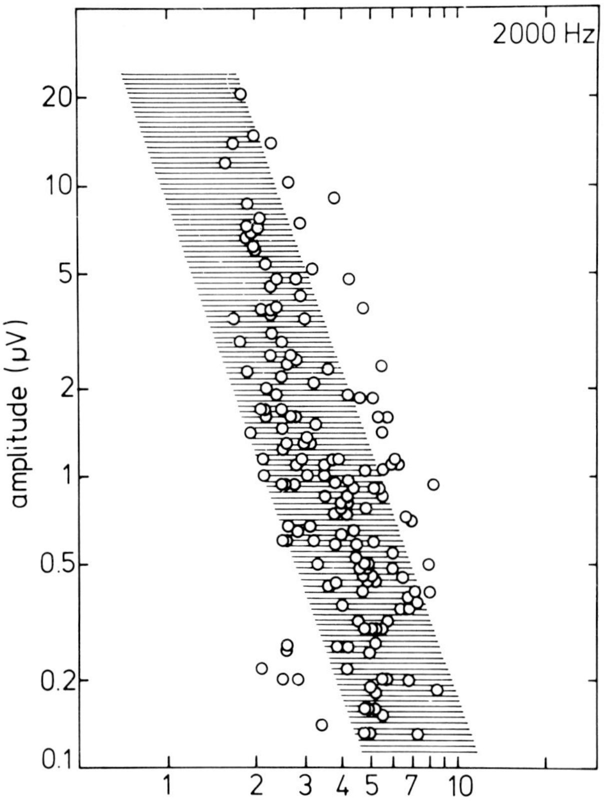

Fig. 8. AP amplitude-latency data for 2 kHz tone burst stimulation for acoustic neurinoma ears compared to the range found for normal ears. The shaded area represents the normal range between 2 SD boundaries.

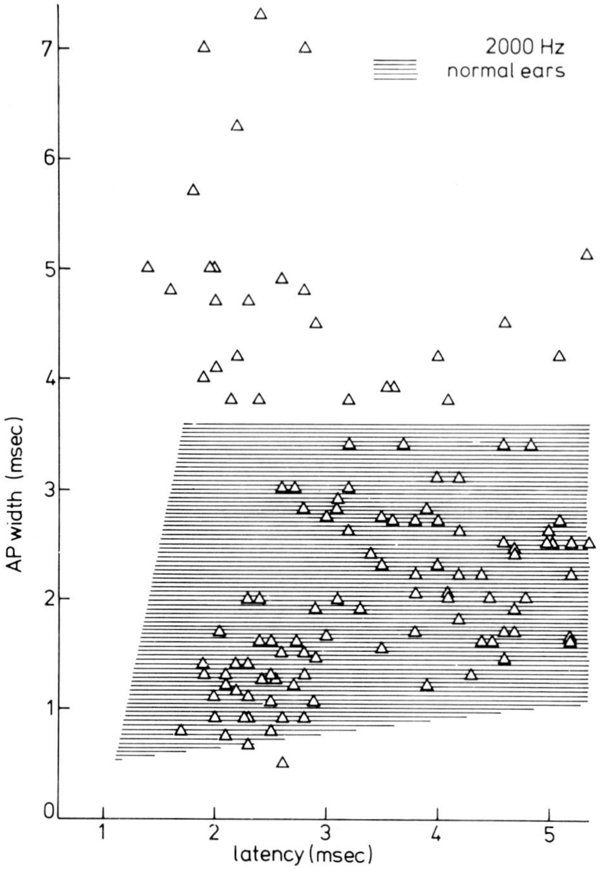

Fig. 9. AP width-latency data for 2 kHz tone burst stimulation for the tumor ears. About 20% of the points are well outside the actual normal range.

Reports about very broad click-evoked APs and their uniqueness in acoustic neurinomas have been published.[1-3,24] Gibson and Beagley,[1] considering a width of the AP at the baseline extending beyond 4 msec as abnormal, found that a very large number of ears with Menière's disease, as well as ears with acoustic neurinoma, qualified. Especially for tone burst stimulation, the width of the AP at the baseline is likely to be influenced by a summating potential (SP). Since reference data for the width of APs evoked by 4 msec tone bursts were obtained at about one third of the AP amplitude value for normal and recruiting ears[20] and plotted as a function of AP latency, the procedure was repeated here. It was found that, in high frequency cochlear losses, the group data formed a subset of the range for normal values. In Figure 9, the width, plotted as a function of latency for all APs with latencies up to 5 msec evoked by 2 kHz tone bursts, is compared to the shaded normal range. About 25% of the latency points of eighth nerve tumor patients fall outside the normal range. However, as a practical diagnostic indicator, this parameter must also be considered insufficient.

Narrow Band Action Potentials. Waveforms of compound APs may differ widely due to either the ratio of the SP to AP amplitude, as with Menière's

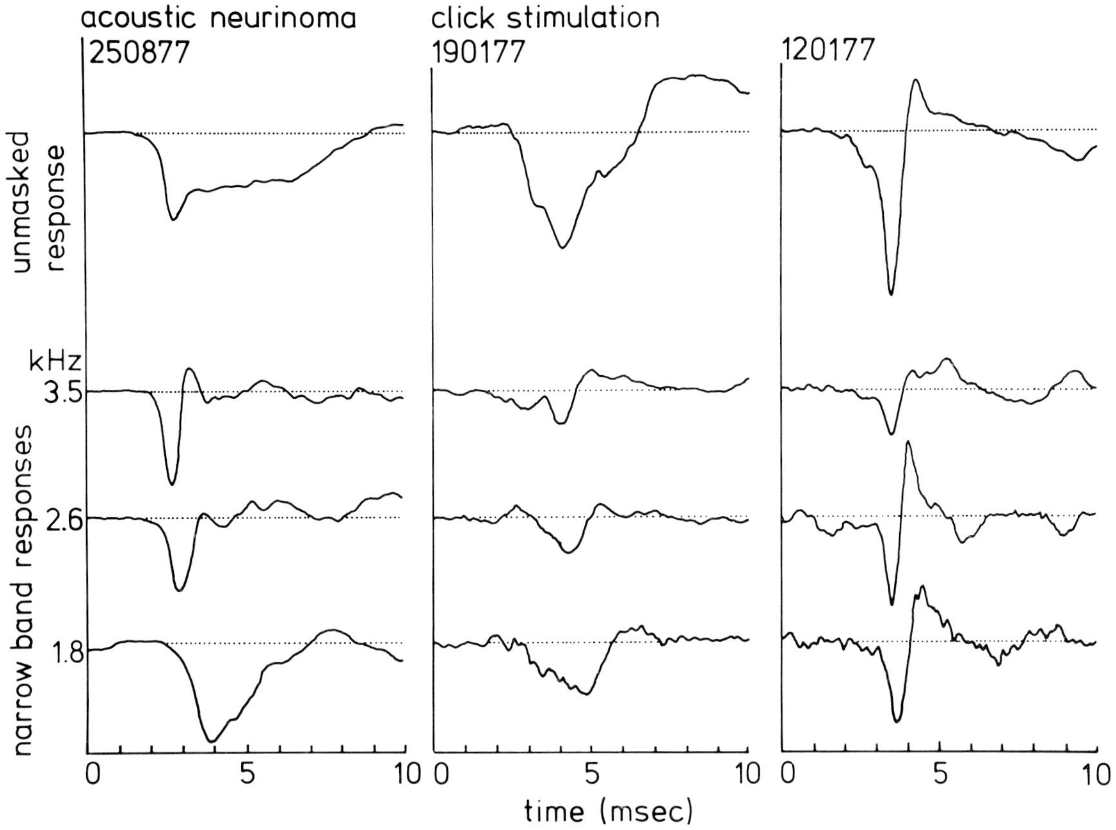

Fig. 10. Narrow band AP waveforms in acoustic neurinoma ears. From dominantly monophasic narrow band APs in the left series to strictly biphasic narrow band responses in the right series, the relationship to the compound AP waveform is clear.

disease,[7] or a representation of cochlear activity different from that of normals, as with high frequency hearing loss.[7] Another explanation might be that the unit contributions to the compound AP can have different waveforms for different types of hearing loss. Other studies[7,8] show that three different unit shapes can be considered: the normal biphasic shape, a W-shaped N1, N2-type found predominantly in Menière's disease, and a monophasic type observed only in eighth nerve or other pontine angle tumors. Broad compound APs can be produced by a dominantly negative SP, by monophasic unit contributions, and/or by severe high frequency hearing loss. Which is most pronounced in eighth nerve tumors and whether a monophasic narrow band response can be used as a diagnostic criterion have to be investigated.

The technique of narrow band AP derivation can yield an estimate of the unit contribution waveform. Teas et al[28] originated the technique which was modified for compound AP evaluation in man[21,29] and for the BSERs.[17] A narrow band response is a compound AP or BSER originating from the excitation of a restricted area along the cochlear partition. It is obtained by high-pass noise masking of click-evoked APs or BSERs and subtracting responses obtained in the presence of maskers with cut-off frequencies differing by a given fraction of an octave. With one half octave, this yields contributions of 3 mm-wide regions on the cochlear partition, innervated by about 2,000 to 2,500 nerve fibers. Because the population contributing to a narrow band AP is more uniform than that to a whole nerve AP, interpretation of single nerve fiber contributions is more straightforward. For three tumor ears, Figure 10 shows the click-evoked compound AP waveforms together with the narrow band APs originating from regions around 3.5, 2.6, and 1.8 kHz (conversion of place along the cochlea in equivalent frequency according to von Békésy's map[30]). The first example (left), showing a very broad compound AP waveform, apparently is built from dominantly monophasic contributions, especially at the lower central frequencies (CFs). The waveform of the compound AP (middle) is still broad, but the narrow band responses are more biphasic. A normal biphasic type of compound AP (right) more clearly shows narrow band contributions. In fact, only about half of the 17 patients for whom a narrow band analysis was possible (hearing loss not exceeding 60 dB at most frequencies) showed dominantly monophasic narrow band responses. The mere presence of monophasic responses is a promising detection criterion, but since it is not present in the majority of tumor cases, its general diagnostic value is limited.

To obtain more quantitative information, the latency-dependence and amplitude-dependence of

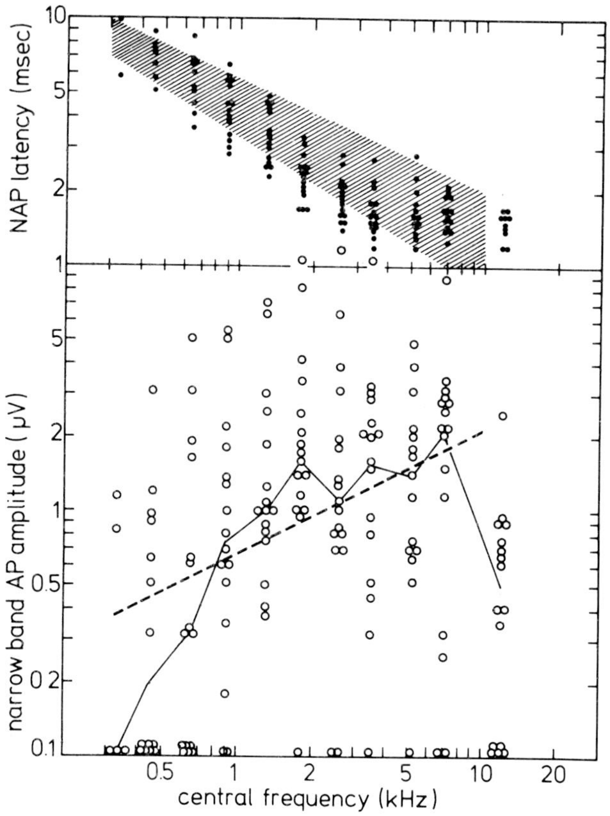

Fig. 11. Narrow band action potential (NAP) amplitude and latency distributions. The upper part of the Figure shows that the latency increases as central frequency decreases. Comparison with the range for normal ears shows that shorter-than-normal latencies occur in the 2-4 kHz range. The amplitude distribution shows relatively large ranges of values at any given central frequency; a factor of ten is quite common. The solid line connects the median values; the broken line with a slope of −3 dB/octave represents the median value for a group of normal ears. Except for the high and low frequency ends of the distribution, this −3 dB/octave slope is also found for the tumor ears.

the narrow band responses on the CF of the narrow bands have been evaluated. The narrow band AP latency in eighth nerve tumor ears and in all other ears investigated gradually increases with decreasing CF (Fig. 11, top). The range of absolute values in normal ears is shaded. Latencies in the 2-4 kHz area in eighth nerve tumor ears are lower than normal. This phenomenon, which also occurs in some ears with Menière's disease, seems related to a greatly deteriorated frequency selectivity of the ear.[31] Again, eighth nerve tumors can produce the same effects as those in (presumed) pure cochlear hearing loss.

That the narrow band response latencies do not fall above the normal range indicates that the increased latencies, as observed for the compound AP (Fig. 7), depend on the relative contributions of the various narrow bands to the compound AP and not on changes at the single fiber level. It is, therefore, likely that abnormal latency-intensity relationships reflect the shape of the audiogram (relative contributions) and the manner in which narrow band responses sum (cancellation occurs for diphasic narrow band contributions and not for monophasic contributions[7]).

The amplitude of the narrow band responses reflects the number of responding nerve fibers and the amount of synchronization between their firings. The latter depends on cochlear mechanics[21] and decreases when the narrow band AP latency increases. For normal ears, the average decrease in narrow band AP amplitude is about 3 dB/octave toward lower CFs at a click level 90 dB pe SPL. This intensity is well within the range where all narrow band outputs are saturated, which means that all fibers respond.[32] The narrow band AP amplitude then becomes a measure for the number of nerve fibers innervating the narrow bands. Under the presumption that the synchronization conditions along the cochlea do not differ in eighth nerve tumor ears and normal ears (a presumption supported by the narrow band latency data) the amplitude distribution can be used to investigate the amount of loss of neural elements in addition to the amount of cochlear loss.

Figure 11, bottom, shows that this −3 dB/octave change in amplitude applies except to the extreme high and low frequency ends of the distribution. In addition, all amplitudes are within the normal range.[32] Comparing the presently obtained amplitude distribution with those obtained in cochlear hearing loss ears[31] shows that the scatter in the data is the same for tumor ear data and cochlear loss data but slightly larger than for the normal data. The drop in amplitude at the high and low frequency ends mirrors the results obtained in pure cochlear losses.[31] Thus, at the effective recording site, which is generally considered the internal auditory meatus (IAM),[33] there is no reason to assume a loss of responding nerve fibers. Most of the hearing loss produced seems to be of pure cochlear origin.

Summating Potentials. The SP recorded from the human promontory[20] is assumed to represent the status of the (outer) hair cells in the basal-most 10 mm of the cochlea.[34] The hair cells near the electrode produce the larger contributions, and it is estimated that the decrease in amplitude will be about 1-2 dB/mm[35] from the promontory. Normal ears therefore have larger SP amplitudes for a given stimulus level when the tone burst frequency increases.[7] On the other hand, ears with high frequency hearing losses are expected to show a rapid decrease in SP amplitude. In ears with Menière's disease,[36] the SP amplitude at 85 dB HL stimulation was independent of the amount of hearing loss up to 50 dB HL; for larger hearing losses, the SP decreased more markedly the higher the tone burst frequency. Figure 12 shows the SP values obtained for 2, 4, and 8 kHz tone burst stimulation at 85 dB HL and plotted as a function of AP threshold. The median value

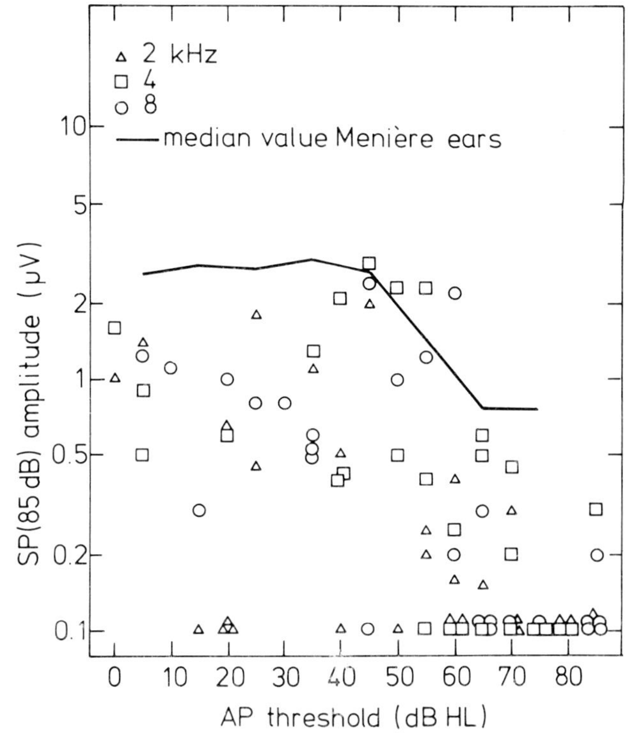

Fig. 12. Summating potential (SP) amplitudes for 85 dB HL tone bursts as a function of the AP threshold. Up to 50 dB HL thresholds, the SP amplitude appears stable; for higher hearing losses, the SP amplitude decreases. This trend is also observed in a large group of ears with Menière's disease whose median value is indicated. However, the median values of tumor ears are smaller by a factor of at least two.

curve for SP to 2 kHz tone burst stimulation (85 dB HL) in a group of 112 ears with Menière's disease is added for comparison. At low hearing loss levels, the median value for the ears with Menière's disease is about twice that for normal ears[7,36] and, as Figure 12 shows, also twice that for the ears with acoustic neurinoma. The trend is that the SP in ears with acoustic neurinoma is below the median value for that in ears with Menière's disease but also stays relatively constant up to AP thresholds of about 50 dB HL and then decreases. The SP at 85 dB HL stimulation in eighth nerve tumor ears is smaller than the SP found in ears with Menière's disease by at least a factor of two. Because of the exponential nature of the SP amplitude distributions in ears with Menière's disease[36] and with acoustic tumor, the SP amplitude is not a useful diagnostic parameter.

Subjective vs Objective Thresholds. As previously stated, the presumed recording site of the AP is at the level of the IAM. By comparing AP thresholds with subjective (audiometric) ones, the status of the auditory system at two very remote points, the auditory periphery and the cortical level, is evaluated. It has been demonstrated that, for normal ears and ears with a pure peripheral hearing loss, ie, conductive and cochlear hearing losses, the correspondence between the two methods of threshold estimation is

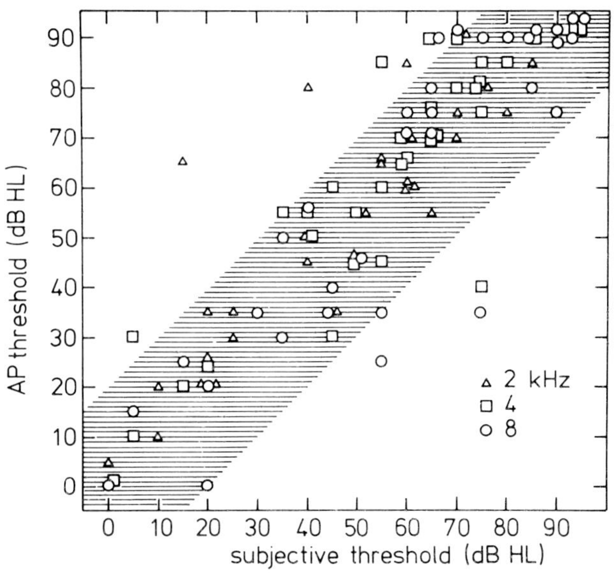

Fig. 13. Relationship between objective and subjective hearing thresholds. Peripheral and central (subjective) measurements are similar except for a few ears with a lower peripheral than central threshold or with the reverse. This similarity indicates that eighth nerve tumors usually produce a peripheral hearing loss.

good.[7,22] In fact, the values of 95% of about 100 ears were found within the shaded area of Figure 13. This comparison was performed at five frequencies, ie, the AP threshold for 500 Hz tone burst stimulation was compared with the subjective threshold obtained audiometrically at 500 Hz and the same was done for 1, 2, 4, and 8 kHz. For individual frequencies, especially 1, 2, and 4 kHz, the normal range was even narrower. The data obtained from pontine angle tumor cases are compared only for 2, 4, and 8 kHz and are mostly within normal range. A few ears had much higher subjective than AP thresholds. One was the meningioma, with much better ECochG thresholds for 4 and 8 kHz. Three eighth nerve tumor cases showed an abnormally large difference at 8 kHz only. In these cases, therefore, an additional retrocochlear component in the hearing loss exists. Also, a few ears had AP thresholds larger by far than subjective ones. For example, one case had a subjective threshold (2 kHz) of only 15 dB and an AP threshold of 65 dB. Such discrepancies have been found before and have been attributed to a general loss of synchrony in the firings of the individual nerve fibers. There may be an auditory sensation due to the processing of irregular firings in the auditory nerve but the firings are not sufficiently time-locked to the tone bursts to give rise to a measurable compound AP. The cases mentioned are exceptions for this series of pontine angle tumors and especially for eighth nerve tumors. Therefore, the presumed criterion of better AP thresholds than audiometric ones fails to have practical diagnostic value.

Diagnostic Value of Combining ECochG Parameters. Table 2 shows results of ECochG in all tumor

TABLE 2. SURVEY OF ECochG PARAMETER WITH RESPECT TO ITS DIAGNOSTIC VALUE IN INDIVIDUAL PATIENTS (DATA FOR 2 kHz TONE BURSTS)

Case	*ECochG Threshold-Subj Threshold*	*Amplitude-Latency Function*	*Width-Latency-* (△)	*Latency-Intensity* (τ)	*Amplitude-Intensity* (*A*)	*SP-Amplitude* (*SP*)	*NAP-wform* (*NAP*)	*Tumor Size* (*cm*)
1	—	—	—	+	—	+	+	3.0
2	—	—	—	—	—	—	+	4+
3	—	—	—	+	—	+	—	3.0
4	—	—	+	+	—	—	+	3.5
5	—	—	+	—	—	+	+	2.5
6	—	—	—	+	+	+	—	1.5
7	—	—	+	—	+	+	—	1.5
8	—	—	—	—	—	○	—	3.0
9	—	—	—	+	—	+	○	2.5
10	—	—	—	+	—	+	—	4+
11	—	—	—	—	—	—	—	1.5
12	—	—	+	+	+	+	—	1.5
13	—	—	+	+	+	+	○	2.5
14	—	—	—	+	+	+	○	1.5
15	—	—	—	—	—	+	—	0.5
16	—	—	—	—	+	—	—	3.5
17	—	—	+	+	—	—	—	1.5
18	—	○	+	○	○	+	○	3.5
19	—	—	—	—	—	+	—	2.5
20	—	○	○	○	—	—	—	3.0
21	—	—	+	—	—	—	—	1.5
22	—	—	—	+	—	+	+	1.0
23	—	—	—	+	+	—	—	2.5
24	—	—	+	+	—	+	+	3.5
25	—	—	+	+	—	—	+	1.5
26	—	—	—	+	+	—	○	0.5
27	—	—	—	+	+	+	○	0.5
28	—	—	—	+	—	—	○	1.0
29	—	—	—	—	—	—	—	1.5
30	—	—	—	—	—	—	—	2.0
31	—	—	—	—	—	+	—	4+
32	—	—	—	—	—	—	—	2.5

A - Amplitude; SP - Summating potential; NAP - Narrow band action potential; wform - Waveform; + - Abnormal finding; — - Normal finding; ○ - Could not be measured.

cases. An abnormal finding is indicated by "+;" "−" indicates normalcy; and "○" indicates parameters that could not be measured (eg, in the narrow band AP analysis). From these data, correlation coefficients for grouped data were calculated[37] and are shown in the correlation matrix in Table 3. The results indicate that most parameters are uncorrelated, that a very weak positive correlation exists between the monophasic narrow band AP waveform and the width-latency and latency-intensity function, and that abnormalities in the amplitude-intensity function are related to abnormalities in the latency-intensity function. However, only the correlation $r = 0.39$ is significantly different from zero. Therefore, we conclude that abnormalities indicated by the various parameters are independent and may be combined to improve their

TABLE 3. CORRELATION COEFFICIENT MATRIX FOR ECochG PARAMETERS

	△	τ	A	SP	NAP
△	1	0.14	0.07	−0.02	0.27
τ		1	0.29	0.18	0.39
A			1	0.17	−0.14
SP				1	0.10
NAP					1

diagnostic value. Considering three abnormal parameter values as a strong indication of the presence of a tumor, we would detect only 25% of these eighth nerve tumors. A looser criterion of any two abnormal findings scores 70%, and one abnormal finding might be encountered in 90% of the cases. It must be mentioned that, eg, in Menière's disease, an increase in AP width is a common finding. However, it always is associated with an increased or normal SP,[27] while in acoustic neuroma cases the combination which leads to diagnosis is broad APs with abnormally small SP. In high frequency cochlear loss, the common finding is loss of SP accompanied by steep input-output curves[20] while small SP and more shallow input-output curves is a diagnostic for acoustic neuromas. This underlines the value of combining at least two independent parameters.

BRAINSTEM ELECTRIC RESPONSES

Normal BSER. Recording of field potentials from the auditory nervous system by scalp electrodes results in a series of five to seven waves in the latency range from 1 to 10 msec. The waves are denoted by Roman numerals.[38] These waves, the first of which

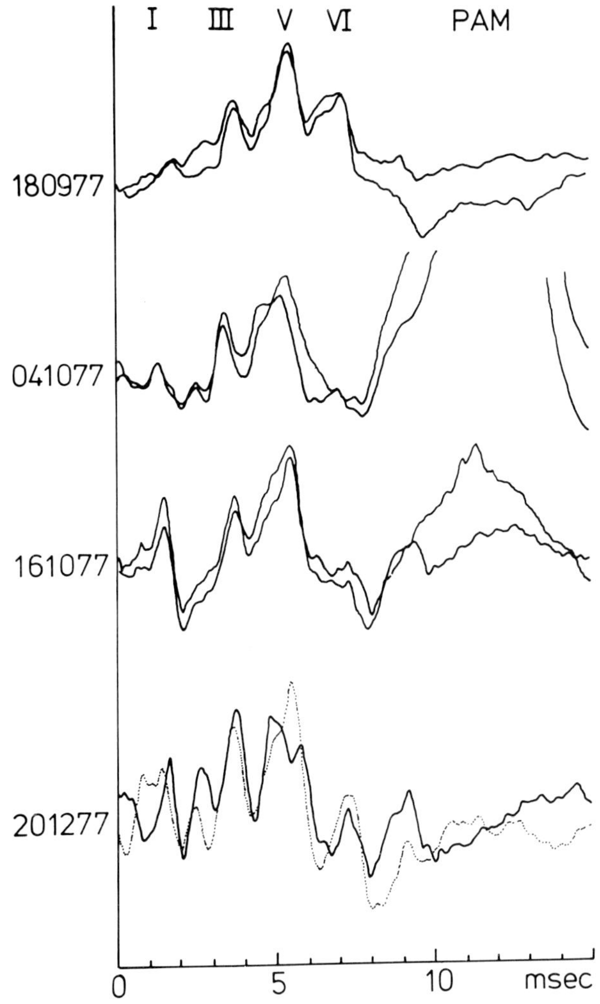

Fig. 14. Waveforms of brainstem responses in normal subjects. Waves I, III, and V are usually easily identifiable despite some variability in shape. The last trace compares the responses obtained for rarefaction (dotted line) and condensation clicks (solid line), particularly the wave IV/V complex changes. PAM - Postauricular muscle.

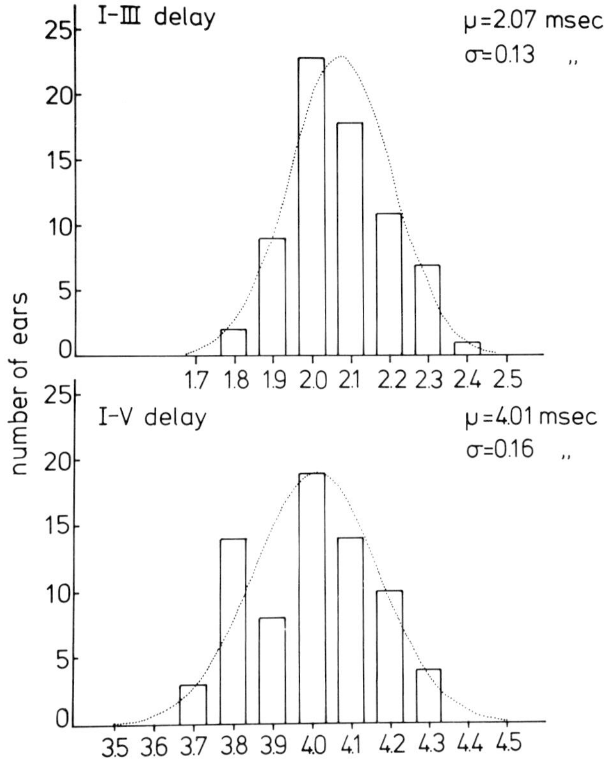

Fig. 15. Distributions for the I-III delay and I-V delay in normal ears appear to be gaussian. The mean values (μ) and standard deviations (σ) for the fitted normal distributions are indicated.

is the same as the AP recorded in ECochG, have been attributed to the sequential activation of various nerve tracts or auditory nuclei in the brainstem.[10,39] The smallness of these potentials, together with an unfavorable signal-to-noise ratio in the case of muscle activity (eg, postauricular muscle, neck muscles), require repetition of the averaging series and comparison of two subsequent recorded waveforms. Figure 14 shows four examples (from normal ears) demonstrating the repeatability in each case and the variation in morphology among cases. The last example compares rarefaction clicks (dotted response) with condensation clicks (solid response); the others and all subsequent material are for alternating condensation and rarefaction clicks. Despite differences which might occur in the morphology of the BSER, a few parameters are remarkably stable, not only among subjects in a particular laboratory but also among investigations in different laboratories. This stability applies particularly to delays between waves I and III, and waves I and V. To obtain a reference point for abnormality of the BSER, data from about 75 normal ears have been represented in histogram form (Fig. 15). This histogram representation of the number of ears with a particular delay between waves I and III, and between I and V suggests that the delays are normally distributed with mean values of 2.07 and 4.01 respectively. Standard deviations were 0.13 and 0.16 msec respectively.

For further understanding of the effect of a pure cochlear hearing loss, Figure 16 plots differences in the I-V delay between the normal ear and the pathological ear in cases (mostly Menière's disease patients) of unilateral hearing loss. This distribution is definitely peaked, centered around a 0.02 msec longer delay for the pathological ear (SD = 0.19 msec). Differences exceeding 0.4 msec are suspect for brainstem abnormality, ie, the problem is not likely of pure cochlear origin. This 0.4 msec is related to the Selters and Brackmann[14] criterion of the interaural wave V latency differences. The present criteria for interwave delays have the advantage of not requiring a correction for audiogram differences.

BSER Waveforms in Pontine Angle Tumor Cases. Figure 17 presents waveforms representative of patients with eighth nerve tumors. The upper trace shows a normal BSER with a I-V delay of 4.0 msec, equal to the mean value for the group of normal

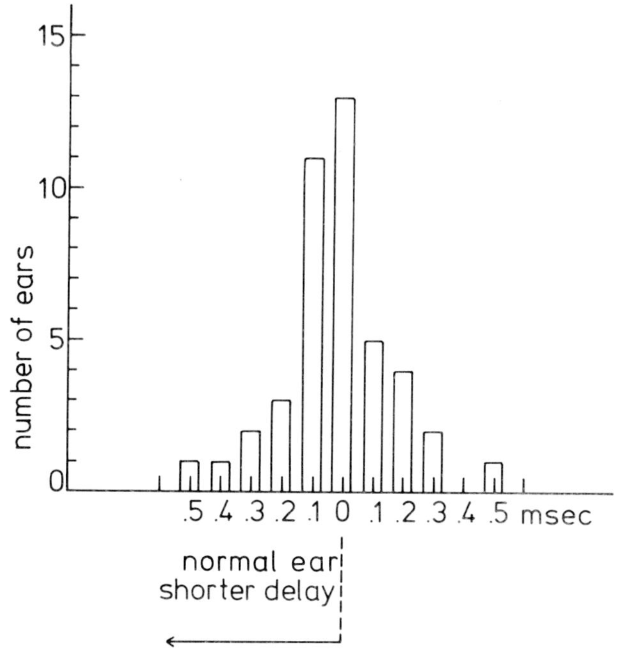

Fig. 16. The distribution of the difference in the I-V delays between both ears in patients with unilateral hearing loss of pure cochlear origin appears to be markedly peaked. The dominantly occurring differences are 0 or 0.1 msec, with the normal ear having the shorter latency.

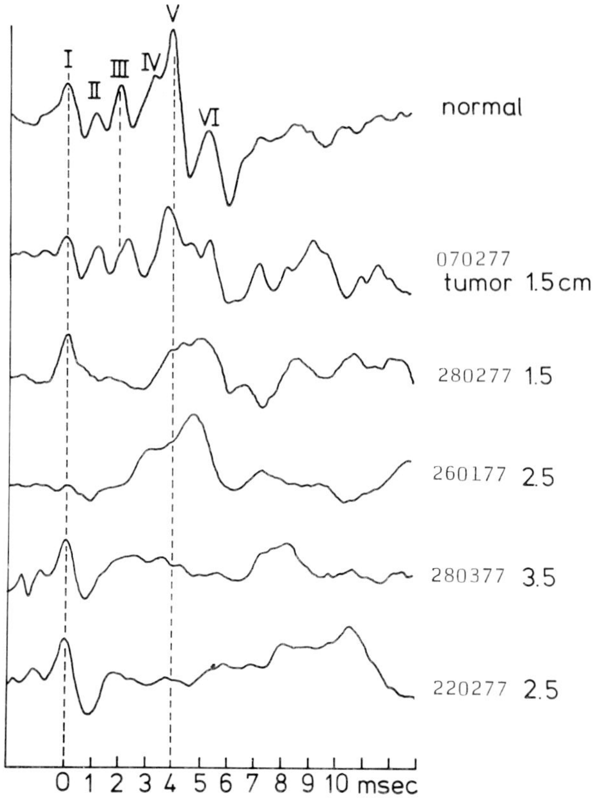

Fig. 17. Waveforms of brainstem electric responses in acoustic neurinoma cases. The normal morphology indicated in the upper trace is only rarely observed in tumor cases. However, the second trace is an example of prolonged I-III and I-V delays. In most cases, identification of the waves, except I, becomes difficult.

ears, in which all waves are clearly present and indicated. The second trace, at first glance, shows a normal pattern, with all waves clearly visible. Closer inspection reveals that the I-III delay was prolonged beyond normal limits. The usual prominence of wave V seems to have been usurped by wave IV, making wave V seen as the small inflection after wave IV. In this case a tumor of 1.5 cm in diameter was found. Merely assuming the largest wave to be wave V and comparing it with wave V of the other ear would not reveal any abnormality.

It is illustrative to compare this case with the brainstem glioma case. Although the glioma protruded into the pontine angle and partially filled the IAM, the I-III delay was 1.8 msec, which is normal, and the I-V delay was 4.7 msec, which is abnormal. The main increase in delay, therefore, occurred after wave III.

The third trace presents a clear wave I (all waves I, which may have different absolute latencies, are aligned for comparison) followed by a broad diffuse wave about 4 msec later. The largest peak of this broad wave, together with what appears to be wave VI, ie, the general morphology of the decreasing part of this broad wave, point to its being wave V. Thus, the I-V delay is increased by about 1.5 msec. Comparison of the second and third trace waveforms, both representing 1.5 cm tumors, indicates that peak identification is a major problem in the validation of most BSER-based diagnostic techniques.

The fourth trace represents a 2.5 cm tumor case. The general morphology is clear: a small, hardly visible wave I followed by a broad, partly fused, wave III-V complex. Although this is a larger tumor than in the former case, the wave I-V delay is somewhat smaller. The next trace shows a response with a clear wave I, but no further waves can be identified. Whether the bump around 8 msec represents any synchronized activity attributable to a given wave remains unclear. This situation, found often, was also seen in the last trace: a clear wave I and the inclination to interpret the wave at 10-11 msec latency as wave V. As shown, when wave I is present it is usually easily identified, especially when ECochG is also performed. The identification of wave V for delays exceeding 7 msec is often difficult and the result is usually ambiguous. This problematic identification must be kept in mind when quantitatively assessing tumor size and delays in the BSER. For the normal ear or the pure cochlear hearing loss ear, wave V remains visible longer than the other waves when stimulus intensity is lowered than for eighth nerve tumors. The absence of wave V in the presence of wave I might indicate a tumor. This is the interpretation in the following material. For clarification, let us note that in the meningioma case, only wave I was clearly visible and there was no sign of any later wave.

Wave I-V Delay in Pontine Angle Tumors. As

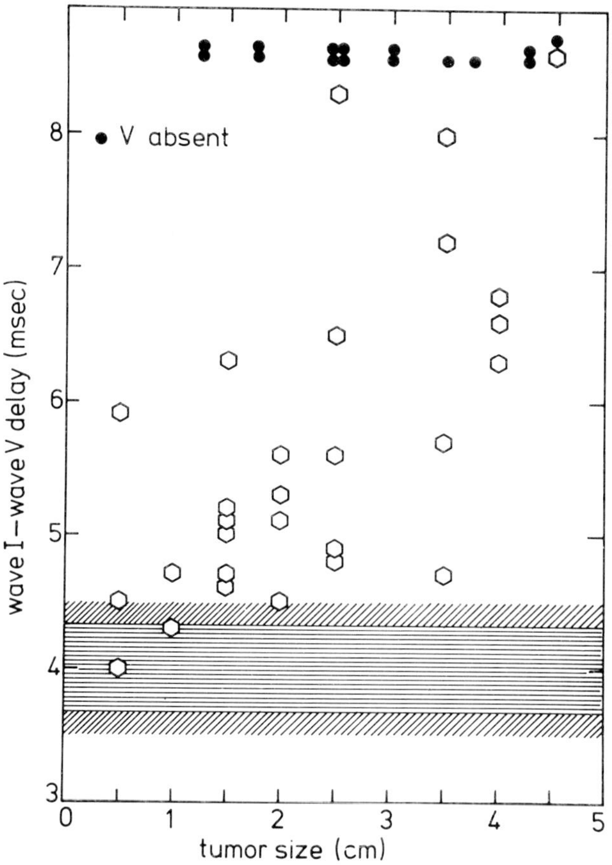

Fig. 18. The wave I-V delay in acoustic neurinoma cases appears related to tumor size. The shaded areas represent the 95 and 99.7% boundary lines respectively for a group of normal ears. Two tumor ears are definitely within the normal range; two others are borderline normal. Wave V is frequently absent in almost all tumor sizes except the smallest.

shown previously, the mean I-V delay for a group of normal ears and pure cochlear hearing loss ears is about 4 msec. In tumor cases wave V is identifiable more often than wave III. Therefore, we will compare the I-V delay of the tumor ears with the nontumor ears. Interpreting delays outside the range indicated by the mean plus 2 SD (including 95% of the normal ears) as suspicious and those outside the 3 SD range as a definitive indication of abnormality, we obtain the hatched areas in Figure 18. The horizontally hatched area represents the 95% area and the extended regions include 99.7% of the normal ears. Any value outside this range is unlikely to belong to a normal ear or pure cochlear loss ear. And because the I-V delay is considered, it is also unlikely that a conductive hearing loss is affecting the criterion, as might be the case when only the absolute wave V latency is considered. For the tumor ears, the wave I-V delay was estimated and plotted as a function of tumor size. Cases without an identifiable wave V are indicated with black dots. In 14 cases (32%) with wave I absent, the criterion was the AP wave V delay based on the recorded transtympanic ECochG. Two cases with relatively small tumors fall within the 95% boundary for normal ears. An additional two were on the borderline of normality.

The impression is that increasing tumor size results in larger I-V delays. It is possible to fit an exponential curve through the data:

$$\text{(I-V) delay} = 4.2 \exp (0.13 \times \text{tumor size in cm})$$

with a correlation coefficient of 0.7. A power curve fit yielded a lower correlation coefficient. A fitted exponential curve, however, depends heavily upon points such as the 8.5 msec delay for the 4.5 cm tumor case, and for these large delays all restrictions outlined previously hold.

Thus, any quantitative relationships must be regarded cautiously. From a diagnostic perspective, the I-V criterion yields a score (based on results of tumor ears only) of 39 of 43 (about 90%) based on the strict criterion. The advantage in these tumor cases was, however, that wave I could be estimated from the ECochG and that the I-V delay could be computed. Moreover, the presence of wave I in ECochG and the absence of a BSER is highly indicative of a pontine angle tumor or other brainstem pathology. If ECochG is not performed and no BSER can be detected, a tumor or other brainstem pathology are indicated only when the hearing loss in the pure tone audiogram does not exceed 70 dB for frequencies of 1 kHz and up.

If the interaural time differences for waves V (IT5) are also considered, another criterion (one that supplements the former criterion) is available. As in Figure 16, it is unlikely in the case of a normal or a cochlear hearing loss that the I-V delays for both ears differ by more than 0.4 msec. Consider a case in which the I-V delay in the nontumor ear of a patient is 3.7 msec and that of the tumor ear is 4.3 msec. Because both delays are within the normal range, use of only the I-V delay criterion would result in a false negative. Comparison of both ears shows the abnormality.

On the other hand, an interaural wave V latency difference of 0.3 msec may occur in cases in which both ears show a considerable hearing loss without a recordable wave I. One must say that no abnormalities can be found. According to our present criterion of 0.4 msec, ECochG or improved recording techniques in BSER may yield the wave I-V delays which, on the tumor ear, may be outside the normal range.

It is therefore advantageous to combine both the I-V and the interaural difference criteria, as shown in Figure 19. For all tumor cases in which both measures could be taken (21 of 43), the strict rule that at least one of the two criteria shows abnormalities may now be applied.

Two cases with borderline I-V criterion have definitely abnormal interaural (IT5) criterion. Another two cases with normal IT5 criterion have definitely

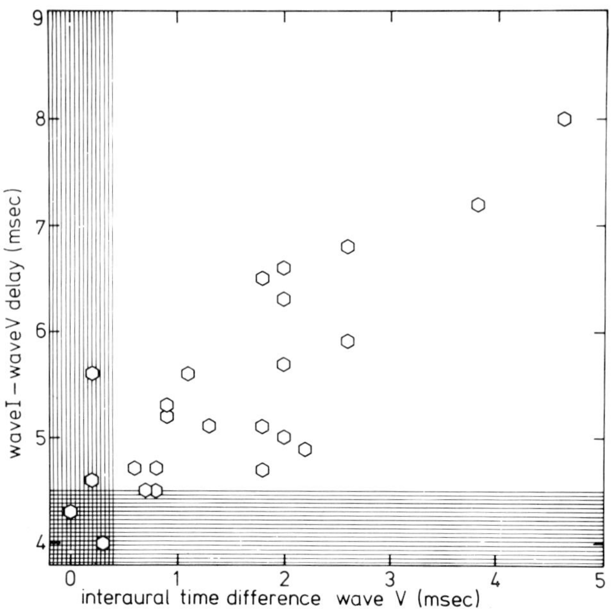

Fig. 19. The relation between the wave I-V delay and the interaural latency difference between waves V is shown with the criteria for normal. The longer the I-V delay, the longer the interaural time difference; however, because audiograms differed for each ear, this relation is not simple. The responses may be normal for one criterion but abnormal for the other. The combination of both criteria may augment the detection score.

abnormal I-V criterion. And finally, in two cases both criteria fall in the normal range. Thus, when at least one of the two criteria was abnormal, the tumor was detected in 19 of the 21 cases. We also found that in 15 additional cases, wave I could be measured but wave V could not, a situation strongly indicative of a tumor or brainstem pathology. If we add these 15 to the 19 detected by either the I-V or the IT5 criterion, we arrive at a tumor detection score of 34 of 36 (approximately 95%). An additional seven cases with no BSER detected and no ECochG available were beyond our estimation of the usefulness of BSER in detecting eighth nerve tumors. The high score of 95% must be regarded as optimum. It is not likely to occur in the real diagnostic situation in which one does not know if a pontine angle tumor is present.

COMBINED RESULTS OF ECochG AND BSER ON OPTIMUM DIAGNOSIS

With the high diagnostic score based on the BSER and the AP latency, ECochG supplies additional information only when it indicates a tumor and the BSER does not. One of the two cases with a normal BSER (where the I-V delay was 4.0 msec) had a normal ECochG; in the other case, the latency-intensity function, the amplitude-latency function, and the monophasic narrow band responses were strongly indicative of an eighth nerve tumor (case 22, Table 2). Therefore, for cases with strong clinical indications of a tumor but with normal or borderline normal BSER, we suggest that the test battery be supplemented with ECochG. In practice, replacing the mastoid electrode with an ear canal electrode[40] may be sufficient to detect a clear wave I. However, this solution may not be adequate when additional evidence regarding the other ECochG tests is needed; thus, one must consider the use of an ear canal-mastoid recording configuration.[18]

DISCUSSION

Site of Eighth Nerve Tumors. In all eighth nerve tumor cases studied, the amount of "objective" hearing loss was identical to the amount of subjective hearing loss. This finding argues against additional effects of the tumor on the central side of the IAM upon the hearing threshold. For the meningioma case, which was a medially situated tumor, ECochG thresholds were better than subjective thresholds by 35-40 dB at 4 and 8 kHz. For the brainstem glioma case, the ECochG thresholds were 20 dB better than subjective thresholds at 8 kHz and equal for 2 and 4 kHz.

The slopes of the AP amplitude-intensity functions of tumor cases appear to be in the same range and show the same dependency upon the AP threshold as those in Menière's disease and other hearing losses with recruitment. The behavior of the SP amplitude as a function of AP threshold is also similar, apart from a scale factor, to that in Menière's disease. Additional information from a narrow band analysis in 17 of the 45 eighth nerve tumors shows that the number of viable neurons in a narrow band is in the same range as in normal or recruiting ears, thereby ruling out neural degeneration at the site of the IAM. Thus, there is abundant evidence, especially for milder hearing losses (up to 60 dB) caused by eighth nerve tumors, that the hearing loss is purely cochlear. For more severe hearing losses, all the evidence (slope of the AP amplitude-intensity curve, SP amplitude) again indicates a cochlear site of action, but additional degeneration of the nerve fibers cannot be ruled out. The fact that cochlear hearing loss with relatively good preservation of the SP amplitude up to 50 dB hearing loss is comparable to that found in Menière's disease indicates a common interference pattern. The origin and growth of eighth nerve tumors will probably involve the cochlear blood supply by slowly reducing it. This would cause a metabolic dysfunction on the cochlear level, followed by hair cell degeneration.

The best quantifiable effect of eighth nerve tumors on the BSER is the increase in the delay between waves I and III and accordingly between waves I and V.

Selters and Brackmann[14] postulate that pressure of the tumor against the auditory nerve causes a reduction in neural conduction velocity, leading to longer delays. It is more likely, however, that the major effect of the tumor is to abolish synchronized

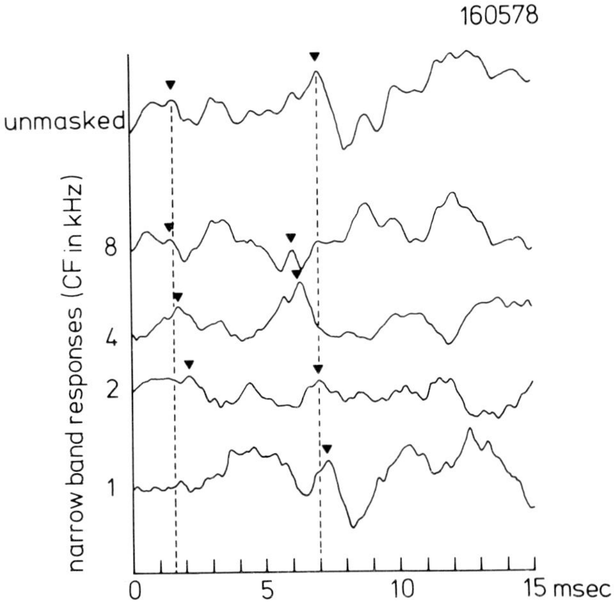

Fig. 20. A possible explanation for the increase in I-V delay as a result of the action of the tumor. For the click-evoked BSER, a I-V delay of nearly 5.5 msec was estimated. It appears that in the individual octave narrow bands, the I-V delay does not exceed 4.5 msec (borderline normal). Wave I from the unmasked response originates from the region above 4 kHz, while the largest contributions to wave V come from the 1-4 kHz range. The pressure of the tumor at a site central from where wave I is generated prevents basal contributions to wave V, resulting in a prolonged I-V delay.

firings for the high frequency fibers which run along the outside of the auditory nerve. This would cause an increase in the I-III and I-V delay of the BSER. Wave I, originating from the intact peripheral part of the nerve, would primarily represent high frequency fiber activity; the dominant contribution to waves III and especially V would be from the middle frequency fibers which respond with a longer latency (travelling wave delay), as demonstrated by Don and Eggermont.[17] As the effect of the tumor increased, the I-V delay would approach 8-10 msec, the approximate theoretical maximum. A simple test of this hypothesis is comparison of the I-V delay in each narrow band of a derived BSER analysis with that for the unmasked response. We conducted this test in a patient with the original I-V delay estimated as 5.4 msec (Fig. 20). Between waves I and V were multiple peaks that were of low amplitude and not likely to be wave V. The octave narrow band analysis shows a I-V delay of 4.5 msec for the region above 8 kHz and for the 4-8 kHz region. The lower the frequency band, the more indistinguishable wave I, but the latency of wave V in the unmasked response corresponds with the contribution from the 1-4 kHz range, while the latency from wave I corresponds with the above 8 kHz range. Thus, although the I-V delays in the narrow bands are borderline normal, the overall I-V delay is definitely abnormal.

Since the peripheral and subjective thresholds are identical in nearly all eighth nerve tumor cases, the action of the tumor will produce not a real conduction block but a desynchronizing effect on the high frequency nerve fibers and probably a minor increase in conduction delay.

Abnormal Findings in the ECochG. Although most ECochG findings indicate a cochlear type of hearing loss, they also include some abnormal tumor-specific properties.

First, the latencies as a function of intensity generally fall above the normal range, as do the AP latencies in ears with Menière's disease.[25] However, in 30% of the studied cases, the latencies are longer than those of Menière's disease. Since long duration occurs with use of tone burst stimulation, especially for 2 kHz, and does not occur in the narrow band AP derivation (compare Figs. 7 and 11), the abnormal course of the latency-intensity function may be related to the manner in which the narrow band contributions add up to the compound AP. Most cases with abnormally long AP latencies also had monophasic narrow band contributions (note the correlation coefficient of 0.39 between τ and NAP in Table 3). In this situation, the usual cancelling of positive and negative deflections leading to sharply peaked APs is lacking. The result is broad APs and abnormally long AP latencies in the middle intensity range. At high tone burst levels, the basal part of the cochlea still dominates the AP response; at low levels (ie, in ears with little hearing loss) only one or two more apically situated narrow bands contribute to the AP. Thus, at both ends of the intensity scale, latencies tend to be normal.[7]

The abnormally broad APs, especially those with short latencies (Fig. 8), are due to this same interaction and not to a pronounced negative SP,[8] as in Menière's disease. Gibson and Beagley[1] suggest that in acoustic neurinomas a "slow-wave" is superimposed upon the AP similar to that found in denervated cat cochleas by Kiang and Peake.[41] This potential was not considered an SP. If this slow wave really is an entity different from the AP, it nevertheless is separable in narrow band contributions and therefore has a distributed origin. At the moment, we prefer the explanation of broad APs on the basis of monophasic narrow band contributions.

How can one explain the occurrence of monophasic narrow band contributions? On the basis of the normal narrow band responses,[21,29] one interprets its waveform as reflecting those of the contributing neural units. Recording a negative monophasic unit response in an extracellular recording situation requires an anatomical conduction block at the central side of the IAM.[42] Kiang et al[43] were able to demonstrate in the cat that the unit contribution at the round window had a biphasic shape, which is similar to that found for narrow band APs at high CFs in normal human ears.[21] When a gross response is recorded, an anatomical conduction block is not necessary to obtain a mono-

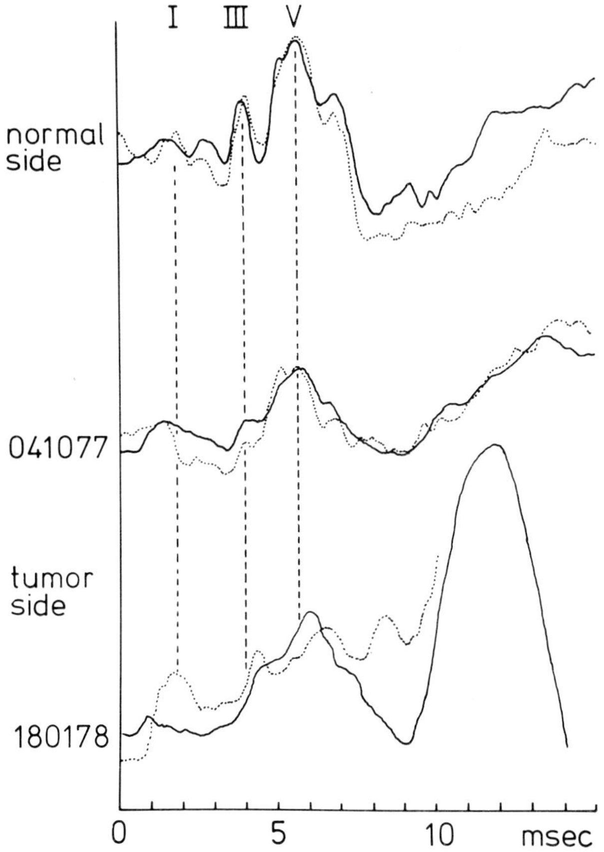

Fig. 21. Difficulties in the detection of acoustic neurinoma. In the first BSER session of this case, the interaural latency difference appeared to be zero; the second time, three months later, a clear increase beyond the normal range was seen. Because wave I was difficult to identify in the second session, ECochG was also performed. Use of the wave I latency from ECochG demonstrated that the I-V delay was also abnormal. Thus, in only three months, dramatic changes in the BSER occurred.

phasic narrow band contribution. The action of the tumor on the nerve might result in differences in neural conduction times leading to desynchronized spike transmission along the auditory nerve. Although all fibers (in the narrow band) at the beginning of the nerve fire simultaneously (incident negative deflection), the synchronous firing pattern across the auditory nerve is already destroyed at the central side of the IAM. Thus, no positive deflection (indicating synchronous activity at the central part of the IAM) can be detected with the promontory electrode.

Whether this mechanism is the real cause for the abnormalities in the AP waveform is difficult to assess. Large tumors are likely to produce this effect, although no relation between a monophasic narrow band response and tumor size could be demonstrated. The arachnoid cyst (0.5 cm), the brainstem glioma (1.5 cm), and eighth nerve tumors from 1 to 3.5 cm produced monophasic responses.

Glazenburg's work[44] on production of broad APs and monophasic narrow band responses should be noted. Reversible changes in the waveform of the click and tone burst evoked AP recorded from the guinea pig could be produced by gently stretching the vestibular nerve at the IAM. In this situation, broad APs and monophasic narrow band responses could be produced. Direct involvement of auditory nerve was ruled out. If stretching of the vestibular nerve results in APs of the same shape as those in acoustic neurinoma cases, the occurrence of these abnormal APs in very small tumors can be traced to the origin of most eighth nerve tumors, the superior or inferior vestibular nerve.

Limits of Electroaudiometry in Eighth Nerve Tumor Detection. Figure 18, with the I-V delay in the BSER related to the tumor size, demonstrates that tumors that will remain undetected are small (< 1 cm). A survey of ECochG results generally leads to findings explainable on the basis of the amount and type of hearing loss; however, a monophasic narrow band response may occasionally give a definite indication. It is therefore realistic to base early detection of eighth nerve tumors on the BSER.

In this context, it is helpful to discuss recordings performed by one of the authors (JJE) at the ENT Department of the Leiden University Hospital in a series of patients with surgically proven medium-sized acoustic neurinomas. In two representative cases, the first BSER recordings were borderline normal, as was the ENG and the stapedius reflex decay. X-rays of the temporal bones did not show abnormalities. All tests were repeated three months later. Figure 21 shows the BSER recordings from the first patient. The upper tracings show the responses from the normal side recorded on the first test session (solid line) and on the second test session (dotted line) three months later. Repeatability was considered excellent for the normal ear.

The second set of tracings in Figure 21 show two recordings from the tumor ear obtained in the first test session. These responses show a diffuse wave I with a shorter latency than that of the normal ear. Waves III and V have the same latency values as the normal ear. The wave I-V delay seemed prolonged. However, because repeatability for wave I was poor, no definite conclusion could be drawn.

The third set of tracings in Figure 21 show two recordings from the tumor ear taken on the second test session three months later. These tracings show now a definite shift in waves III and V. Again, wave I was not clear. A simultaneously performed ECochG showed broad APs with a latency comparable to the dotted curve wave I. X-ray tomography of the petrous bone taken during the interval between the two test sessions indicated the presence of a tumor. At surgery, the patient had a 1.5 cm eighth nerve tumor removed.

The second case (Fig. 22) is more dramatic because only six weeks elapsed between the two BSER

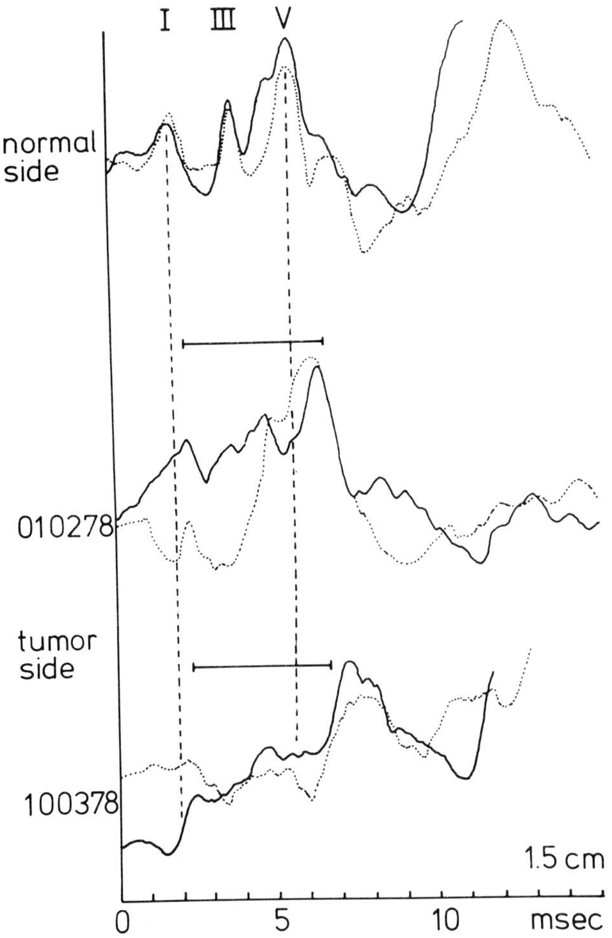

Fig. 22. Difficulties in the detection of acoustic neurinoma. In this case the I-V delay could be measured. The first time it was within the 99.7% range of normalcy and borderline with respect to the 95% range. The I-V delay of the normal ear appeared to be relatively short, so that the difference between the I-V delays of both ears was also borderline normal. After only six weeks, all criteria (the I-V delay, the interaural latency difference, and the differences in I-V delays) were definitely abnormal. In an actual diagnostic situation, findings of borderline normal require reassessment after six weeks to three months.

recording sessions. The first set of tracings shows the normal ear response at the first recording session (solid line) and six weeks later at the second session (dotted line). The responses are comparable.

The second set of tracings shows the first session recordings from the tumor ear. These responses showed well-defined various waves and a borderline normal I-III delay. The difference between the I-V delay for both ears was also borderline normal.

Recordings shown in the third set are taken from the tumor ear six weeks later and now show marked abnormalities. The definition of wave I became less clear although its latency remained the same. The wave I-V delay was clearly abnormal. The patient was operated upon and a 1.5 cm eighth nerve tumor was removed. Although eighth nerve tumors increase slowly in size,[45] these examples show that small changes in tumor size may not cause measurable changes in the patient's hearing but may markedly affect the BSER. Tumors in these cases probably had reached a critical size in terms of their involvement with the auditory nerve. In particular, small changes in the tumor size have marked effects on the later waves of the BSER but do not noticeably affect wave I or the audiogram. The explanation is not an effect upon the brainstem, but rather the gradual change in the effect of the tumor upon nerve fibers with different characteristic frequencies (Fig. 20). In addition, the larger tumor series demonstrates that tumors smaller than 1.5 cm may produce a marked abnormality in the BSER. Thus, the critical size of the tumor varies from patient to patient.

In conclusion, early diagnosis of eighth nerve tumors is possible. It largely depends upon the completeness of the test battery and strong suspicion. It appears that electroaudiometric methods are among those which show the presence of a tumor the earliest.

CONCLUSIONS

1. The dominant effect of eighth nerve tumors causing a hearing loss is on the cochlea, probably by interference with the blood supply.

2. There is some evidence that an additional disturbance at the neural level, probably by direct effect on the auditory nerve, occurs. This does not further increase the amount of hearing loss.

3. Tumor size can be correlated with only certain BSER parameters, notably the I-V delay. No correlation with the amount of hearing loss or the speech discrimination was found.

4. Because most ECochG parameters indicate a pure cochlear hearing loss without neural involvement, assessing the state of hearing at the peripheral site of the IAM therefore has limited value in the differential diagnosis.

5. BSER yields high detection scores: up to 90%. The larger the tumor, the easier its detection. It is likely that small tumors (< 1 cm) will be missed.

SUMMARY

For a series of 45 surgically proven pontine angle tumors including 42 acoustic neurinomas, the compound AP and SP were recorded with transtympanic ECochG together with the BSER. The aims of this study were to quantify the mechanism by which pontine angle tumors cause hearing loss, and to evaluate the diagnostic potentials of ECochG and BSER with respect to the detection of auditory nerve and brainstem tumors.

By ECochG we evaluated the width of the AP response (abnormal in 30% of the cases), the slope of the AP amplitude-intensity curve (abnormal in 9%), the amplitude of the SP (abnormal in 50%), the waveform of the narrow band AP (abnormal in

40%), and the difference between the ECochG thresholds and the subjective hearing thresholds (abnormal in 8%) on their diagnostic merits. Except for the AP latency and narrow band AP waveform, these parameters appear to be uncorrelated, and a combination of individual scores can be used. Four uncorrelated parameters were found abnormal in only 10% of the cases, three in 25%, two in 40%, and one in 90%.

To eliminate effects of the middle and inner ear upon the brainstem response criterion used to differentiate cochlear from retrocochlear pathology, the delay in latency between waves I and V (Jewett nomenclature) was tested as a criterion. From a group of about 70 normal-hearing subjects and 43 subjects with unilateral hearing loss of cochlear origin, evidence was obtained that the I-V delay is not affected by cochlear hearing loss. Based on a mean I-V delay of 4.01 msec for the normal ears and a standard deviation of 0.16 msec, together with the apparent normal distribution of the delays, a I-V delay exceeding 4.33 msec was considered suspect and, for delays above 4.49 msec, as conclusive evidence for the presence of a pontine angle tumor. Based on the 4.49 msec criterion, the test missed 10% of the tumors but included no false positives. The 4.33 msec criterion resulted in 5% missed tumors but included 5% false positives. The combination of the I-V delay criterion with the interaural wave V delay resulted in about 5% improvement on the basis of the strict criterion and no change in the less strict criterion results.

Electrocochleographic results provide substantial evidence that, for hearing losses up to 60 dB HL, the origin is purely cochlear, resembling in many ways that caused by Menière's disease. A peripheral (from the IAM) neural loss can be ruled out in these cases. Evidence is presented that the increase in I-V delay is caused by the selective action of the tumor upon low and high frequency fibers in the auditory nerve and that desynchronization of the firings of the nerve fibers is of more importance than an increase in neural conduction time. ECochG as the sole test for detection of pontine angle tumors appears to be of limited value. BSER on its own has great merits; however, it should be emphasized that in about 30% of the cases in this study, no wave I was detected in the recordings. For these cases, we substituted the latency of the AP recorded by ECochG. Thus, the 95% score obtained on the basis of BSER depends on the ability to identify the latency of wave I.

ACKNOWLEDGMENTS — We acknowledge Dr. Claus Elberling and Dr. Roger Thornton for their helpful comments on an earlier version of this paper. We thank Janet Lewis for her help in testing the patients and with data processing, and the Otologic Medical Group in Los Angeles for recruiting the patients. We also thank Diane Foster for editing the manuscript.

REFERENCES

1. Gibson WPR, Beagley HA. Transtympanic electrocochleography in the investigation of the retrolabyrinthine disorders. Rev Laryngol Otol Rhinol (Bord) 1976; Suppl 97:507-17.

2. Gibson WPR, Beagley HA. Electrocochleography in the diagnosis of acoustic neuroma. J Laryngol Otol 1976; 90:127-40.

3. Morrison AS, Gibson WPR. Beagley HA. Transtympanic electrocochleography in the diagnosis of retrocochlear tumors. Clin Otolaryngol 1976; 1:153-7.

4. Brackmann DE, Selters WA. Electrocochleography in Meniere's disease and acoustic neuromas. In: Ruben RM, Elberling C, Salomon G, eds. Electrocochleography. Baltimore: University Park Press, 1976:315-9.

5. Clemis JD, Mitchell C. Electrocochleography and brainstem responses used in the diagnosis of acoustic tumors. J Otolaryngol 1977; 6:447-59.

6. Odenthal DW, Eggermont JJ. Electrocochleographic study of Meniere's disease and pontine angle neurinoma. In: Ruben RM, Elberling C, Salomon G, eds. Electrocochleography. Baltimore: University Park Press, 1976:215-46.

7. Eggermont JJ. Electrocochleography. In: Keidel WD, Neff WD, eds. Handbook of sensory physiology, vol V, pt 3. New York: Springer-Verlag, 1976:625-705.

8. Eggermont JJ, Odenthal DW. Potentialities of clinical electrocochleography. Clin Otolaryngol 1977; 2:275-86.

9. Innitzer J. Die Elektrokochleographie als neuro otologische Untersuchungs methode. Laryngol Rhinol Otol (Stuttg) 1976; 55:349-58.

10. Starr A, Hamilton AE. Correlation between confirmed sites of neurological lesions and abnormalities of far-field auditory brainstem responses. Electroencephalogr Clin Neurophysiol 1976; 41:595-608.

11. Thornton ARD, Hawkes CH. Neurological applications of surface-recorded electrocochleography. J Neurol Neurosurg Psychiatry 1976; 39:586-92.

12. Terkildsen K, Huis in't Veld F, Osterhammel P. Auditory brainstem responses in the diagnosis of cerebro-pontine angle tumors. Scand Audiol 1977; 6:43-7.

13. Rosenhammer HJ. Observations on electric brainstem responses in retrocochlear hearing loss. Scand Audiol 1977; 6:179-96.

14. Selters WA, Brackmann DE. Acoustic tumor detection with brainstem electric response audiometry. Arch Otolaryngol 1977; 103:181-7.

15. Clemis JD, McGee T. Brainstem electric response audiometry in the differential diagnosis of acoustic tumors. Laryngoscope 1979; 89:31-42.

16. Starr A, Achor J. Auditory brainstem responses in neurological disease. Arch Neurol 1975; 32:761-8.

17. Don M, Eggermont JJ. Analysis of the click evoked brainstem potentials in man using high-pass noise masking. J Acoust Soc Am 1978; 63:1084-92.

18. Elberling C. Compound impulse response for the brainstem derived through combinations of cochlear and brainstem recordings. Scand Audiol 1978; 7:147-57.

19. Sheehy JL, Inzer BE. Acoustic reflex test in neuro-otologic diagnosis. Arch Otolaryngol 1976; 102:647-53.

20. Eggermont JJ, Odenthal DW, Schmidt PH, Spoor A. Electrocochleography: basic principles and clinical applications. Acta Otolaryngol (Stockh) 1974; Suppl 316:1-84.

21. Eggermont JJ. Analysis of compound action potential responses to toneburst in the human and guinea pig cochlea. J Acoust Soc Am 1976; 60:1132-9.

22. Spoor A, Eggermont JJ. Electrocochleography as a method

for objective audiogram determination, In: Hirsh SK, Eldredge DH, Hirsh IJ, Silverman SR, eds. Hearing and Davis: essays honoring Hallowell Davis. St. Louis: Washington University Press, 1976:411-8.

23. Aran JM, Pelerin J, Lenoir J, Portmann CL, Darrouzet J. Aspects theoretiques et pratiques des enregistrements electrocochleographiques selon la methode etablie à Bordeaux. Rev Laryngol Otol Rhinol (Bord) 1971; Suppl 92:601-44.

24. Portmann M, Aran JM. Relations entre pattern cochleographique et pathologie retrolabyrinthique. Acta Otolaryngol (Stockh) 1972; 73:190-6.

25. Eggermont JJ. Electrocochleography and recruitment. Ann Otol Rhinol Laryngol 1976; 86:138-49.

26. Portmann M, Aran JM, Lagourgue P. Testing for recruitment by electrocochleography. Ann Otol Rhinol Laryngol 1973; 82:36-43.

27. Schmidt PH, Eggermont JJ, Odenthal DW. Study of Meniere's disease by electrocochleography. Acta Otolaryngol (Stockh) 1974; Suppl 316:75-84.

28. Teas DC, Eldredge DH, Davis H. Cochlear responses to acoustic transients: an interpretation of whole nerve action potentials. J Acoust Soc Am 1962; 34:1438-89.

29. Elberling C. Action potentials along the cochlear partition recorded from the ear canal in man. Scand Audiol 1974; 3:13-9.

30. von Békésy G. Hearing theories and complex sounds. J Acoust Soc Am 1963; 35:588-601.

31. Eggermont JJ. Narrow band AP latencies in normal and recruiting ears. J Acoust Soc Am 1979; 65:463-70.

32. Eggermont JJ. Stimulus-response relations for promontory recorded compound action potentials in normal and recruiting ears. In: Naunton RF, Fernandez C, eds. Evoked electrical activity in the auditory nervous system. New York: Academic Press, 1978:209-19.

33. Davis H. Principles of electric response audiometry. Ann Otol Rhinol Laryngol 1976; Suppl 28.

34. Eggermont JJ. Human electrocochleography. In: Beagley HA, ed. The technological basis of auditory investigations. Oxford: Clarendon Press, 1979:283-301.

35. Eggermont JJ. Electrocochleography and brainstem audiometry in audiological disorders. In: Moore E, ed. Handbook of electrocochleography and brainstem audiometry. (In press.)

36. Eggermont JJ. Summating potentials in Meniere's disease. Arch Otorhinolaryngol 1979; 222:63-75.

37. Spiegel M. Statistics. Schaum's outline series. New York: McGraw-Hill, 1961.

38. Jewett DL, Romano MN, Williston JS. Human auditory evoked potentials: possible brainstem components detected on the scalp. Science 1970; 167:1517-8.

39. Buchwald JS, Huang CM. Far-field acoustic response: origins in the cat. Science 1975; 189:382-4.

40. Coats AC. On electrocochleographic electrode design. J Acoust Soc Am 1974; 56:708-11.

41. Kiang NYS, Peake WT. Components of electrical responses recorded from the cochlea. Ann Otol Rhinol Laryngol 1960; 69:448-58.

42. Beagley HA, Legouix JP, Teas DC, Remond MC. Electrocochleographic changes in acoustic neuroma: some experimental findings. Clin Otolaryngol 1977; 2:213-9.

43. Kiang NYS, Moxon EC, Kahn AR. The relationship of gross potentials recorded from the cochlea to single unit activity in the auditory nerve. In: Ruben RH, Elberling C, Salomon G, eds. Electrocochleography. Baltimore: University Park Press, 1976; 95-116.

44. Glazenburg BE. On the simulation of effects produced by acoustic nerve tumors. Thesis, Leiden University, Leiden, The Netherlands, 1979.

45. Gussen R. Pathology of eighth nerve tumors and petrosal meningiomas. In: Tower DB, ed. The nervous system, vol 3. New York: Raven Press, 1975.

MENIÈRE'S DISEASE AND ENDOLYMPHATIC HYDROPS

CLINICAL-HISTOPATHOLOGICAL CORRELATIONS

Bernard G. Fraysse, MD
Antonio Alonso, MD
William F. House, MD

COMPUTER-AIDED AND GRAPHIC RECONSTRUCTION OF THE HUMAN ENDOLYMPHATIC DUCT AND SAC

A METHOD FOR COMPARING MENIÈRE'S AND NON-MENIÈRE'S DISEASE CASES

Juan-Carlos M. Antunez, MD
Frank R. Galey, PhD
Fred H. Linthicum, MD
Gilbert D. McCann, PhD

Supplement 76 — Vol. 89, November-December, 1980, No. 6, Part 3

THE ANNALS OF OTOLOGY, RHINOLOGY & LARYNGOLOGY

THE ANNALS PUBLISHING COMPANY
4949 FOREST PARK BLVD.
ST. LOUIS, MISSOURI 63108

CONTENTS

Menière's Disease and Endolymphatic Hydrops: Clinical-Histopathological Correlations.
B. G. Fraysse, MD, A. Alonso, MD, W. F. House, MD 2

Computer-Aided and Graphic Reconstruction of the Human Endolymphatic Duct and Sac: A Method for Comparing Menière's and Non-Menière's Disease Cases.
J. C. M. Antunez, MD, F. R. Galey, PhD, F. H. Linthicum, MD, G. D. McCann, PhD 23

MENIÈRE'S DISEASE AND ENDOLYMPHATIC HYDROPS
CLINICAL-HISTOPATHOLOGICAL CORRELATIONS

BERNARD G. FRAYSSE, MD
TOULOUSE, FRANCE

ANTONIO ALONSO, MD
MADRID, SPAIN

WILLIAM F. HOUSE, MD
LOS ANGELES, CALIFORNIA

The clinical-histopathological correlation between Menière's disease and endolymphatic hydrops was done to explain, as much as possible, causes of symptoms of Menière's disease. Twenty-three temporal bones with endolymphatic hydrops from 17 patients were reviewed and clinical and histopathological findings were correlated. Histopathological examination revealed frequent, severe deformities in the labyrinthine walls and permanent changes in Reissner's membranes. Evidence of rupture was difficult to assess. Of 21 ears of patients with the clinical diagnosis of Menière's disease, 93% had endolymphatic hydrops. A statistical correlation between increased area of the cochlear duct and hearing loss was found. Some correlation was also found between frequency of vertigo and results of electronystagmography with histopathological findings. Consequently, the mechanical effect of endolymphatic hydrops seems to have greater significance in the production of symptoms of Menière's disease than the biochemical effect of ruptures. In a review of ten unusual cases from this series of 17 patients, traumatic neuromas or remnants of vestibular structures were found after an incomplete labyrinthectomy. Histopathological findings of four patients who had undergone endolymphatic subarachnoid shunt surgery are described.

The history of Menière's disease can be roughly divided into two eras. The first began in 1861, when Prospere Menière[1] described an association of vertigo and sensorineural hearing loss as a clinical entity caused by a labyrinthine disorder. Hallpike and Cairns'[2] histopathological finding of endolymphatic hydrops in Menière's disease marked the second era. However, endolymphatic hydrops can be found in diseases other than Menière's,[3] conversely, clinical symptoms of Menière's disease could be present without histopathological evidence of endolymphatic hydrops.[4]

These two factors pose problems in an attempt to correlate clinical diagnosis with histopathological findings. Other factors also complicate this correlation. One is that the main symptoms of Menière's disease are subjective; another is that morphological changes found after death represent only one stage in the evolution of the disease. Therefore, selection of a homogeneous group of cases to study both clinically and histopathologically is difficult and sometimes arbitrary.

For these reasons, cases presented were chosen from two groups of patients: one with a clinical history compatible with the diagnosis of Menière's disease, one with definite histopathological evidence of endolymphatic hydrops.

This study: 1) reviews 23 temporal bones with the histopathological finding of endolymphatic hydrops; 2) correlates cochlear and vestibular symptoms with histopathological findings; and 3) with ten case reports illustrates responses to medical and surgical treatments.

HISTOPATHOLOGICAL FINDINGS

All temporal bones were removed between 6 and 24 hours after death, placed in formaldehyde, decalcified in Versene®, and embedded in celloidin. Specimens were sectioned in the horizontal plane at a thickness of 20 μm, and every tenth section was stained with hematoxylin and eosin.

Study of the middle ear sought evidence of chronic otitis media because of the possible cause-effect relationship between chronic otitis media and endolymphatic hydrops.[5] Presence of chronic otitis media was found in four temporal bones from three patients; however, severity and location of the hydrops varied in these bones.

In the inner ear, the labyrinthine membranes, vestibular aqueduct and endolymphatic sac, and sensorineural elements were examined.

LABYRINTHINE MEMBRANES

The cochlear duct and the vestibular membranes were studied separately.

Cochlear Duct. In cases of endolymphatic hydrops, Reissner's membrane presented two main modifications: dilation and morphological changes. Dilation was studied in the apical, middle, basal, and hook areas of the cochlea and was classified as slight, moderate, or severe (Fig. 1).

Dilation was present in the apical turn in all cases and affected only this turn in three cases. Prolapse of Reissner's membrane through the helicotrema or filling the whole scala vestibuli appeared in four

From the Otologic Medical Group, Inc., and the University of Southern California, Los Angeles; the Service d'ORL, Hopital Universitaire de Toulouse, France; and the ENT Department of the Special Center "Ramon y Cajal," Madrid, Spain. This work was supported by funds from the Ear Research Institute, Los Angeles.

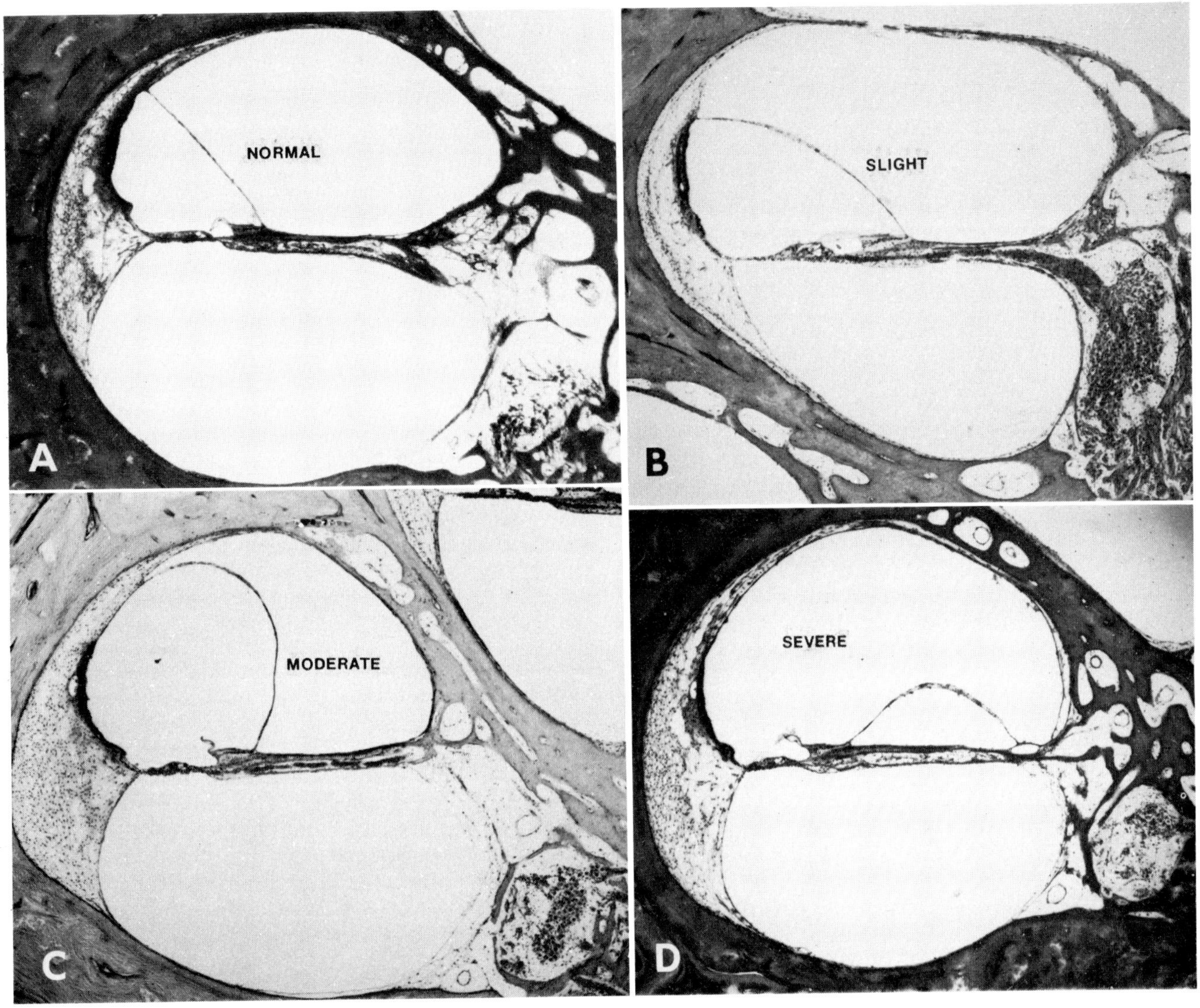

Fig. 1. Different degrees of dilation of the cochlear duct. A) Normal; B) Slight; C) Moderate; D) Severe.

cases (Fig. 2). In 16 cases, Reissner's membrane bulged severely or moderately in all turns (Fig. 3). In eight cases, moderate or severe dilation appeared in the hook area (Fig. 4), in three cases Reissner's membrane was prolapsed into the vestibule (Fig. 5), and in two cases reached the footplate (Fig. 5).

From these observations, the first area of Reissner's membrane to be involved seems to be in the apical turn. In later stages, distention is greater in the middle and basal turns. The cochlear duct has the capacity for high dilation, filling the whole scala vestibuli and even herniating through into the helicotrema and into the scala tympani.

Many authors[6-9] have described morphological changes of Reissner's membrane and indicated the association of endolymphatic hydrops with collapse, fibrosis, and ruptures. In three temporal bones Reissner's membrane was found collapsed[10,11] (Fig. 6). In cases with severe bulging, fibrous tissue

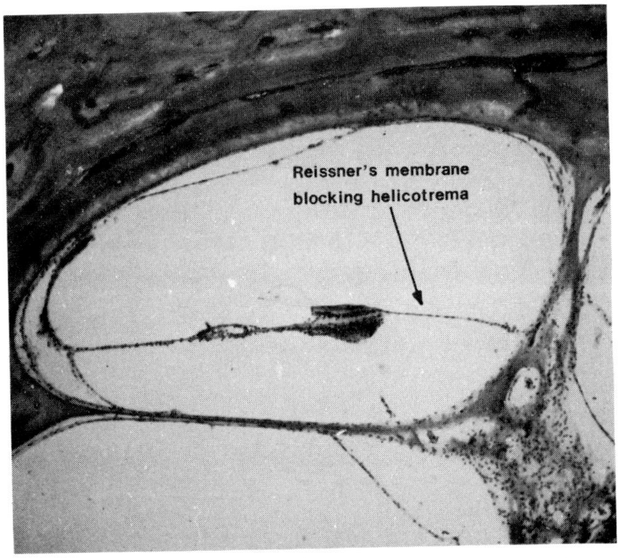

Fig. 2. Dilated Reissner's membrane obliterating the scala vestibuli and blocking the helicotrema.

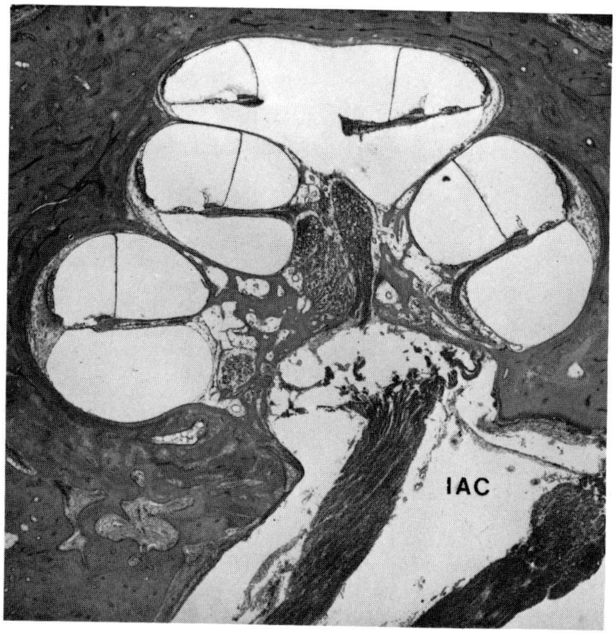

Fig. 3. Midmodiolar section showing a moderate dilation of Reissner's membrane in all turns.

between Reissner's membrane and the endosteum of the scala vestibuli was observed. In cases with an abnormally high attachment of Reissner's membrane to the outer wall of the scala vestibuli, this fibrous tissue or the condition of Reissner's membrane pressed against the wall of the scala vestibuli prevented an attempt to follow the course of the membrane from the top of the stria to the abnormal attachment.

The theory that rupture and healing of Reissner's membrane are a result of overdilation was first postulated by Lawrence and McCabe in 1959[6] and later described by others.[7,12,13] Evidence of ruptures in Reissner's membrane that occurred antemortem was difficult to assess in five cases in this series because histopathological evidence of a reparative

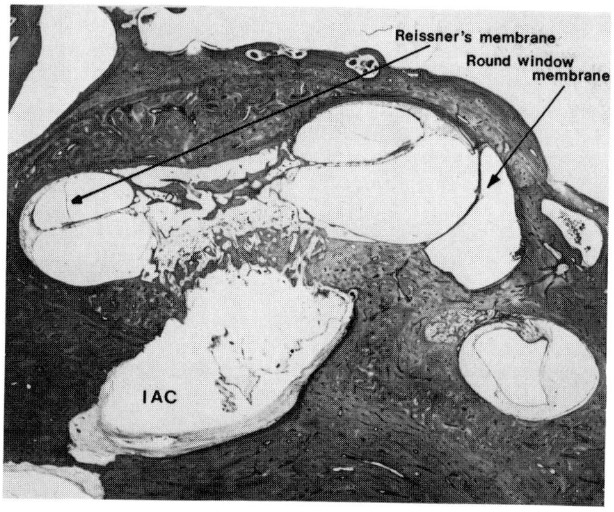

Fig. 4. Moderate dilation of Reissner's membrane in the hook area.

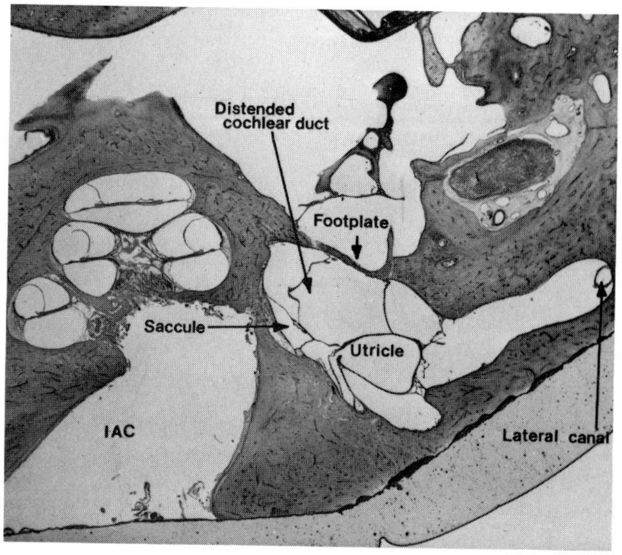

Fig. 5. Reissner's membrane from the hook area prolapsed to the vestibule and reaching the footplate.

process or of scar tissue at the edges of the rupture was not clearly shown. Therefore, the possibility of artifacts introduced during manipulation cannot be excluded.[14] In addition, no rupture or evidence of healing was found in 11 cases with severe bulging of Reissner's membrane, in four cases of herniation through the helicotrema (Fig. 7), nor in three cases of collapse. If ruptures did occur, they would have been small tears, less than 200 μm or 0.2 mm (the distance between two stained sections), or they would have occurred only rarely. Either situation would account for their going undetected. If ruptures occurred only rarely, correlating them with the frequency of recurrent symptoms would be difficult.

On the other hand, cross sections of Reissner's membrane in cases of longstanding hydrops showed

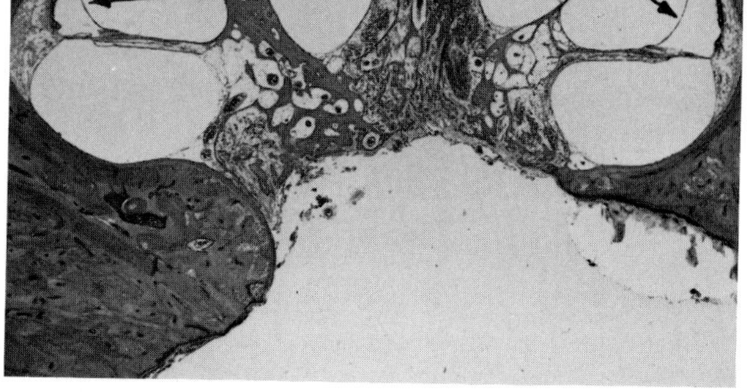

Fig. 6. Midmodiolar section showing a collapse of Reissner's membrane.

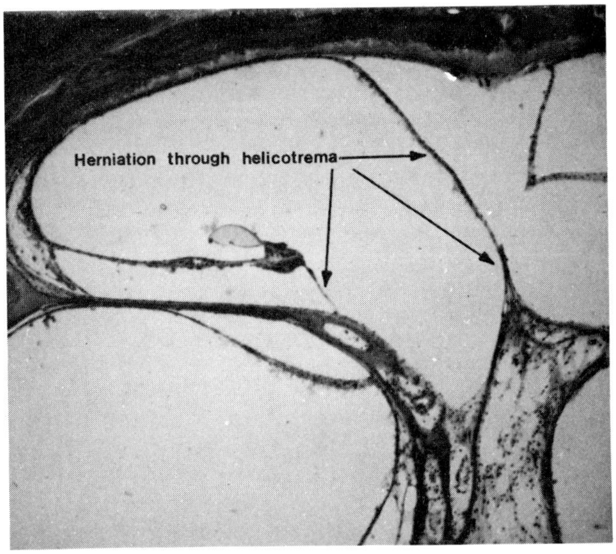

Fig. 7. Herniation of Reissner's membrane through the helicotrema.

approximately the same number of cells per area and the same distance between them as in a normal

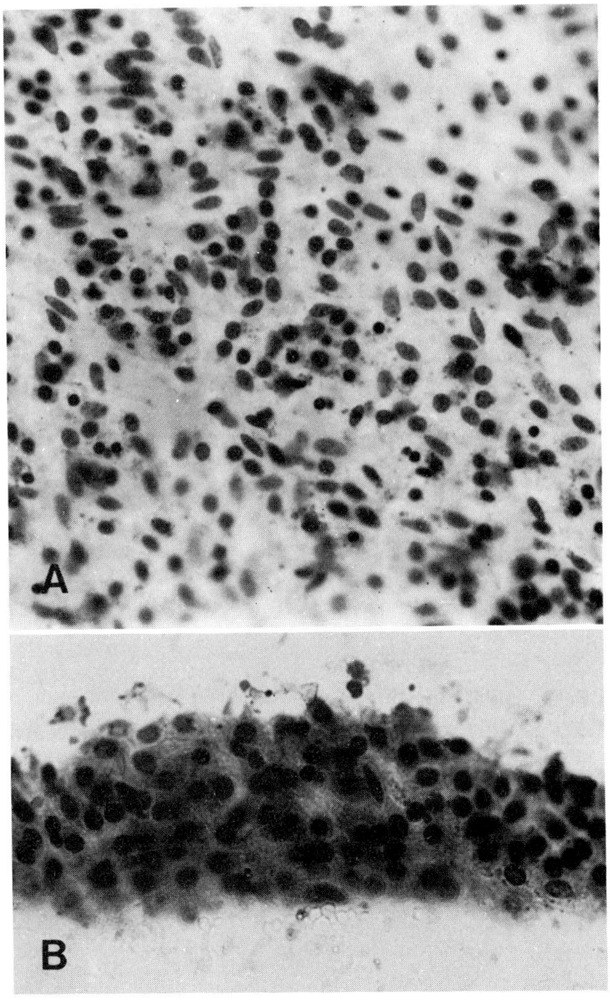

Fig. 8. Cross section of distended Reissner's membrane showing A) approximately the same number of cells per area (x325); and B) the same distance between them as in a normal membrane (x325).

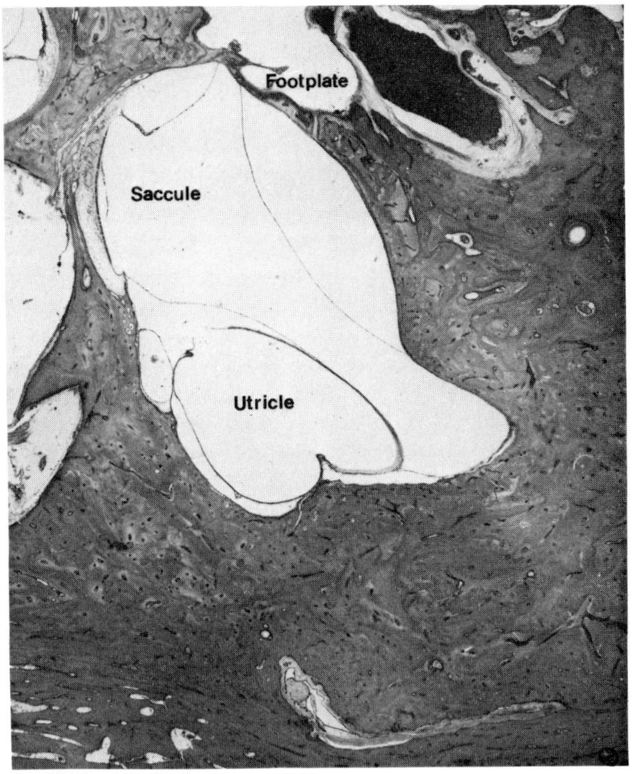

Fig. 9. Distended saccule pressed against the footplate and bulging into the nonampullated end of the lateral semicircular canal.

membrane (Fig. 8A, B). This finding could indicate a proliferation of cells in response to stretching.*

From these observations it seems probable that in the early stages of the disease, or "compensated" Menière's disease,[15] Reissner's membrane conserves its elasticity, expanding and relaxing after each attack. In chronic conditions, or "decompensated" Menière's disease, Reissner's membrane may permanently lose its elasticity.[16,17]

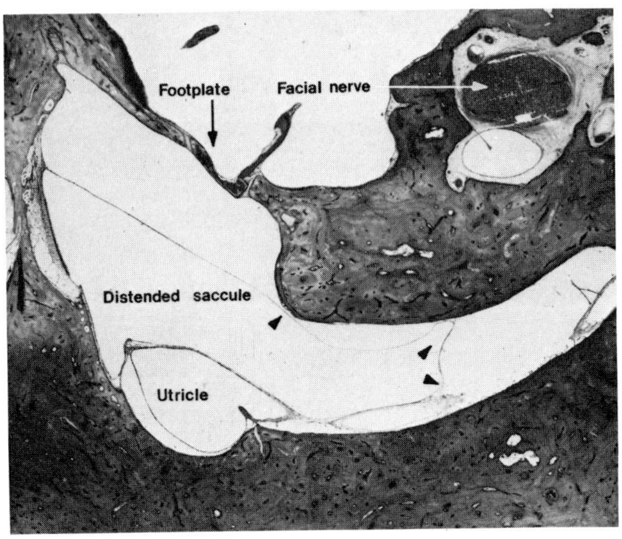

Fig. 10. Distended saccule bulging into the nonampullated end of the lateral semicircular canal.

*Johnsson L-G. Personal communication.

TABLE 1. CASE MATERIAL, CLINICAL DIAGNOSIS, AND HISTOPATHOLOGICAL FINDINGS OF ENDOLYMPHATIC HYDROPS

Case	Sex	Age at Death	Duration of Disease	Diagnosis	Presence of Hydrops
1	M	53	12	Probable Menière's rt.	Rt. yes; Lt. no
2	F	77	28	Probable Menière's bilateral	Rt. yes; Lt. no
3	F	71	29	Definite Menière's rt.	Rt. yes; Lt. no
4	F	75	10	Probable Menière's rt.	Rt. yes; Lt. no
5	F	67	11	Definite Menière's rt.	Rt. yes; Lt. no
6	F	85	15	Probable Menière's lt.	Rt. yes; Lt. yes
7	F	84	15	Sensorineural hearing loss rt.	Rt. —; Lt. yes
8	M	58	9	Definite Menière's rt.	Rt. yes; Lt. no
9	F	29	—	Sensorineural hearing loss bilateral	Rt. yes; Lt. no
10	M	85	25	Probable Menière's lt.	Rt. no; Lt. no
11	M	64	29	Congenital syphilis	Rt. yes; Lt. yes
12	M	68	27	Probable Menière's bilateral	Rt. yes; Lt. no
13	F	59	18	Definite Menière's bilateral	Rt. yes; Lt. yes
14	M	84	53	Definite Menière's bilateral	Rt. yes; Lt. no
15	F	55	4	Probable Menière's rt.	Rt. yes; Lt. no
16	M	82	—	Probable Menière's bilateral	Rt. yes; Lt. no
17	F	48	2	Probable Menière's rt.	Rt. yes; Lt. no

Therefore, we found no correlation between ganglion cell loss and hydrops.

Stria Vascularis. The stria vascularis was atrophic in most cases with hydrops, but this condition did not correlate with hearing loss.

As previously described by many authors,[10,21,22] hearing loss and abnormal vestibular response in endolymphatic hydrops did not seem to result from degenerative changes in the sensorineural elements or in the ganglion cell population.

MATERIAL

Case material (Table 1) is based on seven males and ten females. Mean value of duration of disease was 19 years, with extremes of 2 and 53 years. Mean age of death was 67 years, with the youngest 29 and the oldest 85.

Of the 24 ears of these 17 patients, 7 ears from 5 patients were clinically categorized as definite Menière's disease,* ie, with documented fluctuating sensorineural hearing loss, and with an association of episodic vertigo, tinnitus, and pressure in most cases. Eleven ears from nine patients were clinically categorized as probable Menière's disease, ie, with episodic vertigo and a history of fluctuating hearing loss that was not documented on the hearing tests. One of these 11 ears showed no hydrops on histopathological examination. Two ears were from one patient with the diagnosis of congenital syphilis. Four ears were from four patients with nontypical history.

CLINICAL-HISTOPATHOLOGICAL CORRELATIONS

These four clinical categories were correlated with the presence or absence of endolymphatic hydrops. Table 2 shows that in all cases of definite clinical Menière's disease, endolymphatic hydrops was present. In cases of probable Menière's disease, all but one case showed the presence of endolymphatic hydrops. The patient with congenital syphilis and severe bilateral hydrops had a clear history of episodic vertigo and fluctuating hearing loss in both ears. Of the four patients with an unclear history, but with endolymphatic hydrops, two with the clinical diagnosis of unilateral Menière's disease showed bilateral endolymphatic hydrops; the other two patients, with unilateral endolymphatic hydrops (on the cochlear duct and also in the vestibule), were diagnosed as having sensorineural hearing loss.

These criteria for classification of Menière's disease appear to be accurate. Of 18 ears classified as definite or probable Menière's disease, only 1 did not show a hydrops. This could either be an error in diagnosis or Menière's disease without hydrops. Of the six cases of bilateral hydrops, two were diagnosed as unilateral Menière's disease. These may be examples of conservative diagnostic criteria. Of the two patients with endolymphatic hydrops who were diagnosed as having a sensorineural hearing loss, one diagnosis could be explained by the fact that the long duration of the disease could change the symptomatology to that of inactive Menière's disease, with no fluctuating symptoms. In the other case, the clinical history was poor.

Hearing loss, vestibular symptoms, and evolution of the disease were correlated with histopathological findings. Studied were correlations between the hearing test and the increased area of the cochlear duct, between the vestibular symptoms and electronystagmography and the histopathological findings in the vestibule, and between the duration of the disease and the increased volume of the endolymphatic system.

TABLE 2. CORRELATION BETWEEN THE CLINICAL DIAGNOSIS AND THE PRESENCE OR ABSENCE OF ENDOLYMPHATIC HYDROPS

Presence of Hydrops	Definite Menière's	Probable Menière's	Congenital Syphilis	Other Diagnosis
No	—	1	—	—
Yes	7	10	2	4

*Denia A, Jenkins H, Baloh R. Menière's disease: a workable classification. Unpublished data.

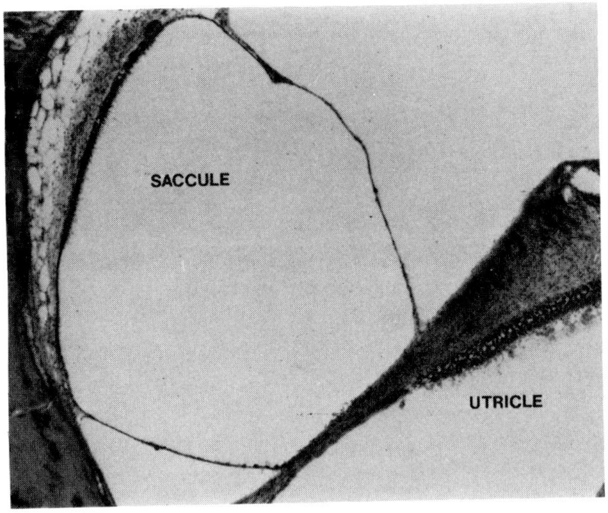

Fig. 11. Dilated saccule in contact with the utricle.

Vestibular Membranes. Dilation of the saccular membrane can extend towards the footplate, the utricle, and the nonampullated end of the lateral canal. The saccule was pressed against the footplate (Fig. 9) in ten cases; bulged inside the nonampullated end of the lateral canal (Fig. 10) in five cases; dilated but not in contact with any structure in four cases; dilated and in contact with the utricle (Fig. 11) in two cases; found with fibrotic adhesions on the wall on the vestibule (anterior or posterior to the footplate) in five cases; collapsed (Fig. 12) in three cases. In contrast to the frequent dilation of the saccule, the utricle appeared normal or slightly dilated in five cases.

These observations led to the following findings. 1) When the saccule was pressed against the footplate or bulging into the nonampullated end of the lateral canal, there was a moderate or severe dilation of the cochlear duct. 2) In cases with only a slight bulge in the apical turn, the saccular membrane was not dilated. 3) In cases of bilateral Menière's disease, the saccule was dilated more on the side with greater dilation of the cochlear duct. Therefore, we conclude that a correlation exists between dilation of the cochlear duct and of the saccular membranes.

VESTIBULAR AQUEDUCT AND ENDOLYMPHATIC SAC

Correlation between vestibular disorders and the endolymphatic system was first demonstrated in fish.[18] Later animal experiments have shown that destruction of the endolymphatic sac leads sooner or later to endolymphatic hydrops.[19] Accordingly, we searched for morphological changes in the vestibular aqueduct and in the endolymphatic sac that might identify a possible cause of endolymphatic hydrops. An irregularity of the osseous canal wall[20] was found in six cases (Fig. 13). In one case, the beginning of the vestibular aqueduct was blocked by abnormal bone in all serial sections (Fig. 32A, C). In another case, the orifice of the vestibule was

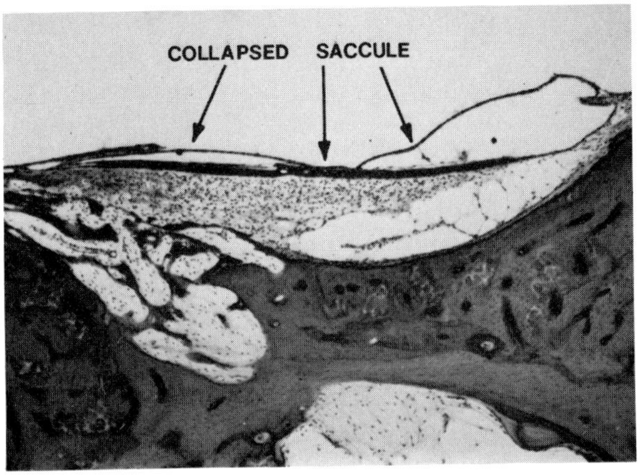

Fig. 12. Collapse of the wall of the saccular membrane.

blocked by ossification inside the vestibule (postlabyrinthectomy) (Fig. 27A), but it appeared normal as it traversed the posterior face of the temporal bone toward the sac. In one case of congenital syphilis and bilateral severe hydrops, the vestibular aqueduct was blocked by microgummate consisting of perivascular round cell accumulation. In seven temporal bones with endolymphatic hydrops the vestibular aqueduct and endolymphatic duct did not show any significant morphological change. In four temporal bones with previous surgery, visualization of the vestibular duct and endolymphatic sac was difficult. In conclusion, our study of the endolymphatic sac showed no consistent morphological changes.

SENSORINEURAL ELEMENTS

Hair Cells. Considering the ages of the patients, autolysis postmortem, and artifacts introduced during the processing, no direct correlation was found between endolymphatic hydrops and hair cell loss. In unilateral cases of hydrops, there were no significant differences between the neural elements of the two ears.

Ganglion Cells. The ganglion cell population was decreased in some cases with severe endolymphatic hydrops, but in other severe cases it was normal.

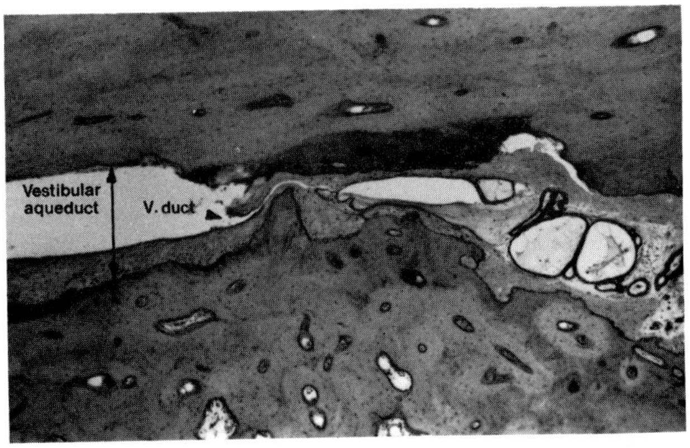

Fig. 13. Irregularity of the osseous canal wall of the vestibular aqueduct.

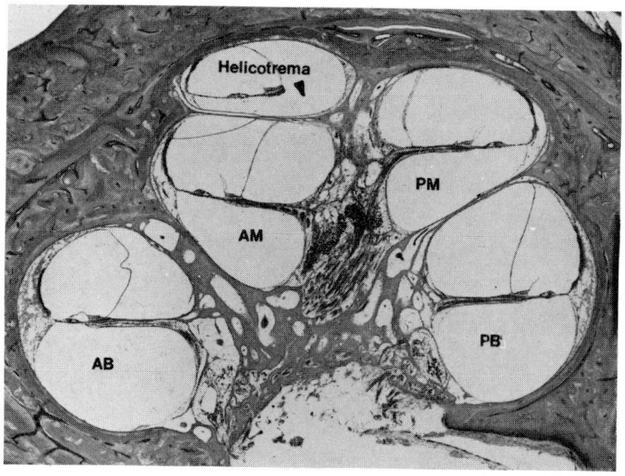

Fig. 14. Horizontal midmodiolar section of the temporal bone. The five areas of the cochlea examined are the anterior and posterior basal turns (AB and PB), anterior and posterior middle turns (AM and PM), and the apical turn (▼).

Increased Area of the Cochlear Duct and Hearing Loss. Fifteen temporal bones, chosen from a group of 23, provided data necessary to permit a correlation between the increased volume and hearing loss. Excluded from study were cases with audiometric results not available, with artifacts in the midmodiolar sections, and with a surgical procedure that had modified one of these parameters.

A variant of a method described by Antoli-Candela[13] was used. A midmodiolar section from each temporal bone was used to estimate the increased area of the cochlear duct. To provide a reference for each temporal bone, the five areas of the cochlea examined in horizontal midmodiolar sections were labeled (Fig. 14). To measure the increased volume of the cochlear duct, the horizontal midmodiolar sections were projected with a Bausch and Lomb trisimplex microprojector, and the area of the distended scala media was calculated by outlining this area with a compensating polar planimeter.*

The percent increase in volume was estimated by measuring each area of the scala media in a midmodiolar section and calculated by using a mean value from ten normal temporal bones. In cases of unilateral hydrops, the normal contralateral side was used when available. A computer system† performed the statistical analysis of these data. Mean value, standard deviation, correlation coefficient (r), and level of significance (P) were calculated and used to perform statistical tests.[23]

Purposes of this study were : 1) to correlate the total volume increase of the cochlear duct in the midmodiolar sections with the average hearing loss for pure tones, 2) to correlate the volume increase in each area and the hearing loss for the corresponding frequency,[24,25] and 3) to correlate the relative increased volume and hearing loss in each temporal bone. The third correlation was done to determine whether a larger volume increase in the cochlear areas of a given ear correspond to the frequencies of the audiogram with a greater hearing loss.

TABLE 3. RESULTS SHOWING THE CORRELATION BETWEEN THE INCREASED VOLUME OF THE SCALA MEDIA IN EACH AREA AND THE HEARING LOSS TO THE FREQUENCY CORRESPONDENT

Area of Cochlea in Midmodiolar Section	*Frequency of Maximum Sensitivity (kHz)*	*Correlation Coefficient (r) Between Increased Volume and Hearing Loss*	*Level of Significance (P) of Correlation Coefficient (r)*
Anterior basal	0.4	0.463	0.05
Posterior basal	1, 2	0.569	0.01
Anterior middle	0.5	0.482	0.05
Posterior middle	0.25	0.315	—

In the sample of 15 temporal bones, statistical analysis indicates a significant correlation ($P = 0.01$) between the total increased volume of the cochlear duct and the average hearing loss ($r = 0.638$) (Fig. 15). A clear correlation between the increased volume of the scala media in each area and the hearing loss in the frequency corresponding to that area is apparent for every turn except the posterior middle turn (Fig. 16A-D). No reason to explain this fact was found. Results are shown in Table 3.

To determine whether a relationship exists between relative increased volume and hearing loss in each temporal bone, a correlation was done be-

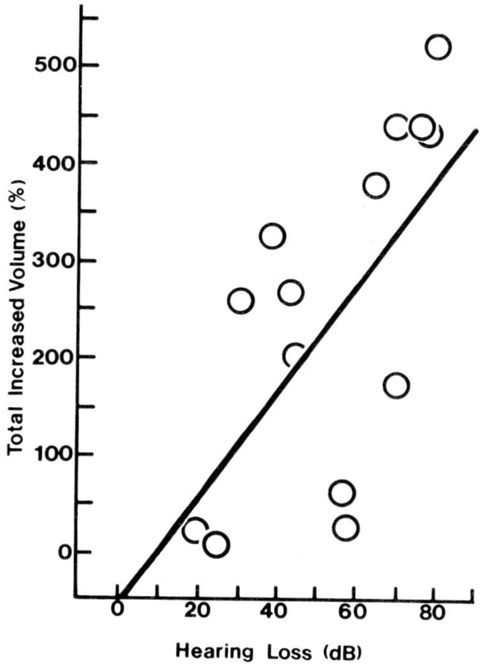

Fig. 15. Total increased volume of the cochlear duct versus average hearing loss.

---

*Kueffel and Esser Co. II, 62.0022.

†Nicolete Med 80.

tween the relative volume of each area and the relative hearing loss of the tone corresponding to that area. To measure the relative increase of volume and hearing loss, the difference between the actual value corresponding to the area and the average value for the whole cochlea was used. The test of independence did not show a significant correlation. Furthermore, the estimated value of the correlation coefficient was close to zero (Fig. 17). This lack of correlation indicates that results of the audiogram of a patient with Menière's disease do not aid in predicting in which area the increased volume of the scala media will be greater in relation to the frequency correspondent.

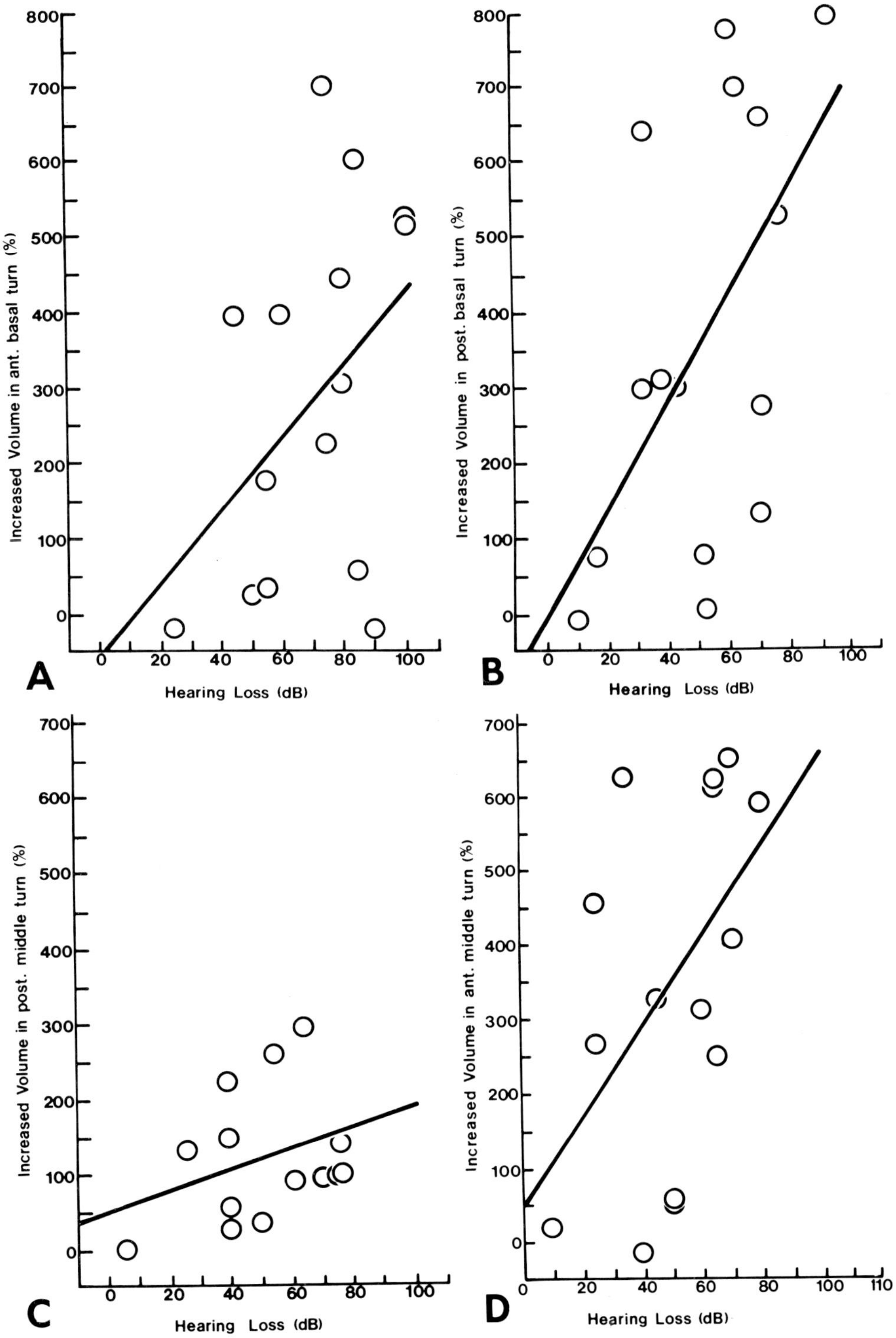

Fig. 16. A) Increased volume in the anterior basal turn versus hearing loss in the frequency 4 kHz. B) Increased volume in the posterior basal turn versus hearing loss in the frequencies 1 and 2 kHz. C) Increased volume in the posterior middle turn versus hearing loss in the frequency 0.25 kHz. D) Increased volume in the anterior middle turn versus hearing loss in the frequency 0.5 kHz.

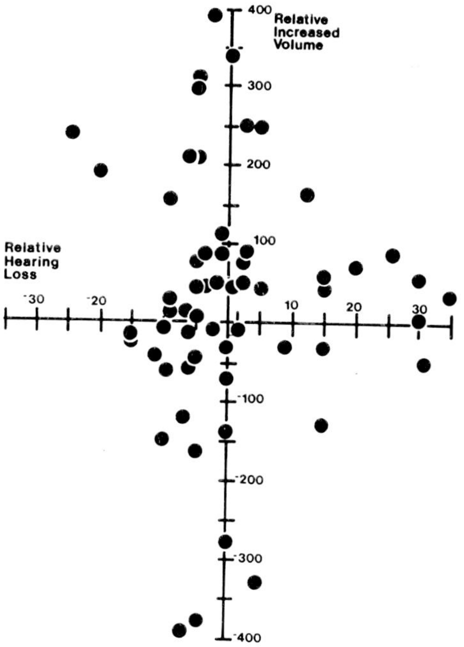

Fig. 17. Relative increased volume versus relative hearing loss in each turn of 15 temporal bones.

These observations demonstrate a correlation between total increased volume of the cochlear duct and average hearing loss. This correlation is strengthened by the finding in unilateral cases of hydrops of no significant differences between the neural elements of the diseased ear and those of the normal ear.

Vestibular Symptoms and Electronystagmography with Histopathological Findings in the Vestibule. The purpose was to correlate the frequency of vertigo and results of electronystagmography (ENG) with dilation of the saccule and utricle and with particular features of the semicircular canals. Frequency of vertigo was classified into three groups: more than two attacks per week, from one to four attacks per month, and fewer than one attack a month. The amount of dilation of the saccular membranes was arbitrarily classified as severe, moderate, or slight.

TABLE 4. CORRELATION BETWEEN FREQUENCY OF VERTIGO AND DILATION OF THE SACCULAR MEMBRANE

Dilation of Saccule	Frequency of Attacks 2-3X Per Week	1-4X Per Month	Fewer Than Once a Month
Severe	4	1	4
Moderate	0	1	0
Slight	0	0	1
Normal	0	1	1

Correlation between the frequency of vertigo and the dilation of the vestibular contents can be seen in Table 4. Except for the fact that all patients with frequent attacks of vertigo had severe dilation of the vestibular contents, there was no significant relationship between these two parameters. This is emphasized in three patients with few attacks of vertigo whose saccule was found dilated against the footplate.

The correspondence between results of ENG (spontaneous nystagmus, positional testing, and caloric tests) and the vestibular contents was studied. In four patients with normal ENGs, the membranes of the saccule and utricle were normal or slightly dilated but never in contact with the footplate. In three patients whose ENGs showed no response to caloric testing, the saccular membrane was greatly dilated. Of them, two with no caloric response had the saccule against the footplate (Fig. 18); the other patient, whose ENG showed no response bilaterally, had the saccule against the footplate on one side and extending eight tenths of the distance to the footplate on the other side. Two patients who showed maximal positional nystagmus in the supine position had the saccule against the footplate, one with bulging of the saccule into the nonampullated end of the lateral semicircular canal. In addition,

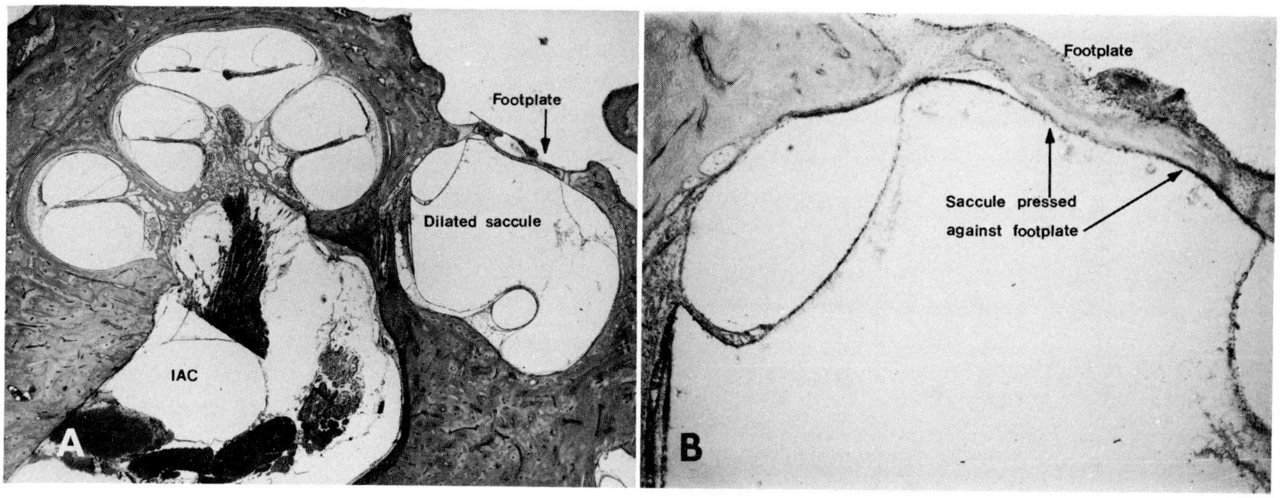

Fig. 18. A) Dilation of the saccular membrane pressed against the footplate. B) Magnification of area with saccule pressed against footplate.

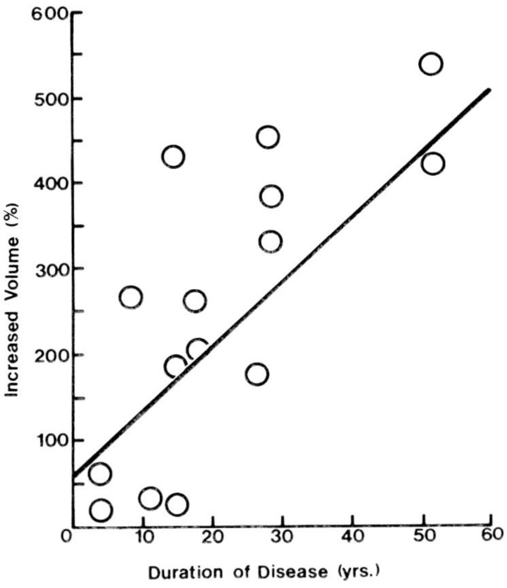

Fig. 19. Duration of disease versus increased volume of the cochlear duct.

the posterior canal showed fibrous tissue and giant cells in one of these cases and ossified tissue in the other.

From these observations, the following are apparent: 1) A correlation exists between the amount of dilation of the vestibular contents and the response to caloric tests. 2) In cases of positional nystagmus, some abnormalities were found in the semicircular canals.

Duration of the Disease and Histopathology. The purpose was to correlate the duration of the disease with increased volume of the cochlear duct and hearing loss, and the duration of the disease with increased volume of the vestibular contents.

To correlate the duration of the disease with the increased volume of the cochlear duct and also with the average hearing loss, statistical methods described previously were used.

A statistically significant relationship was found ($r = 0.767$; $P = 0.0005$) between the duration of the disease and the increased volume of the cochlear duct (Fig. 19). A statistically significant relationship was also found ($r = 0.661$; $P = 0.005$) between the duration of the disease and the average hearing loss (Fig. 20). Patients with longer durations of the disease had greater volume increases of the cochlear duct and greater hearing losses.

There was some correlation between the duration of the disease and the behavior of the vestibular content (saccule): patients whose disease lasted less than ten years had slight or no dilation of the saccule, while patients whose disease lasted more than ten years showed severe distention of the saccule.

CASE REPORTS

Through ten case reports, this section illustrates

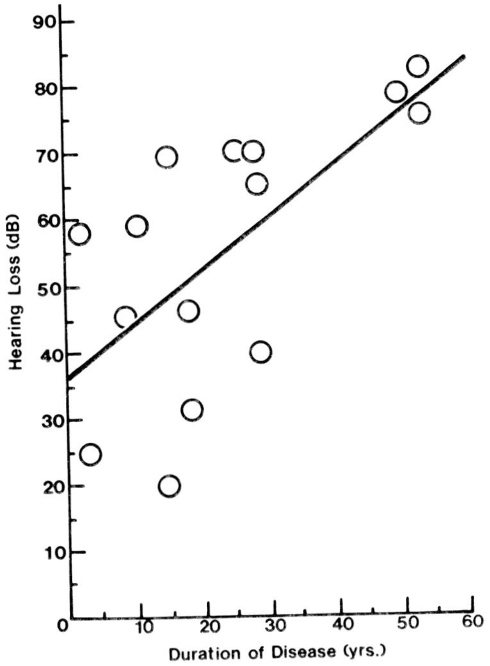

Fig. 20. Duration of the disease versus average hearing loss.

the response to medical and surgical treatment and describes some unusual histopathological findings.

In this group of cases, seven patients underwent

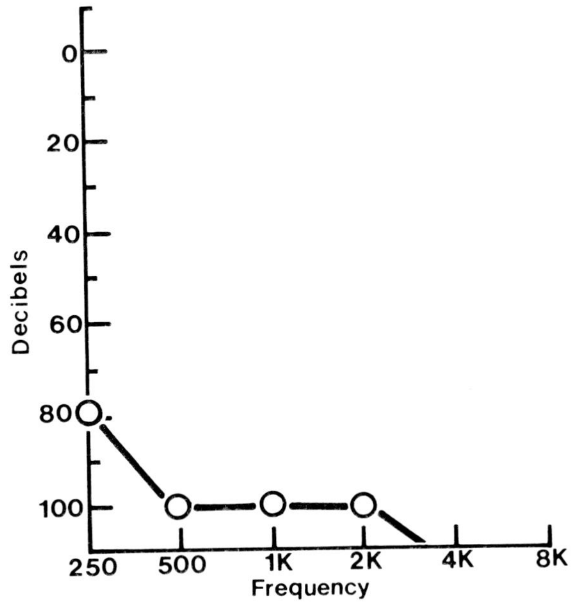

Spontaneous		Yes
Positional		Supine
Caloric Test		No Response on right, or right paresis
		Right Preponderance

Fig. 21. (Case 1) Audiogram and ENG results.

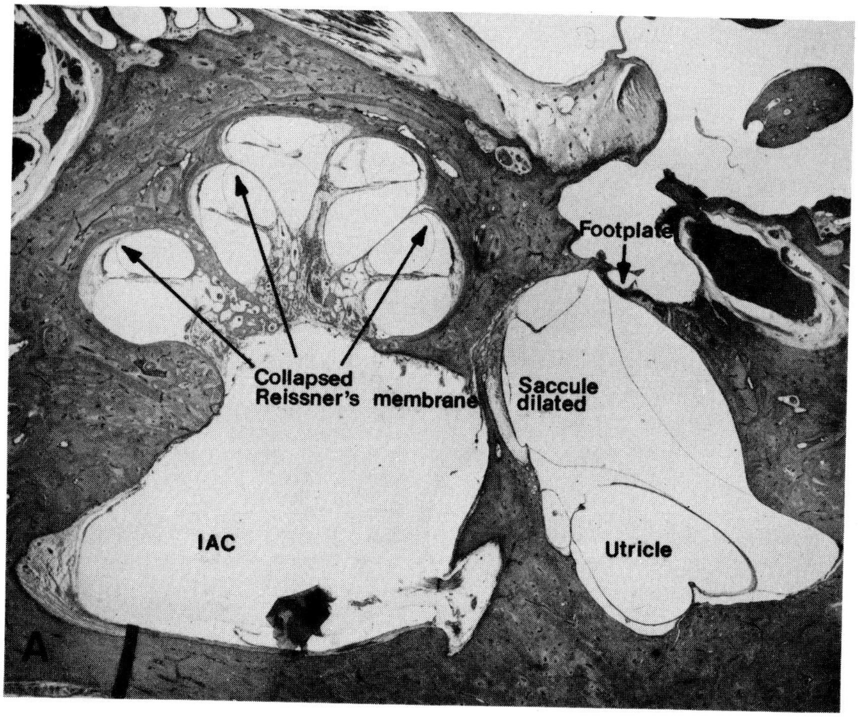

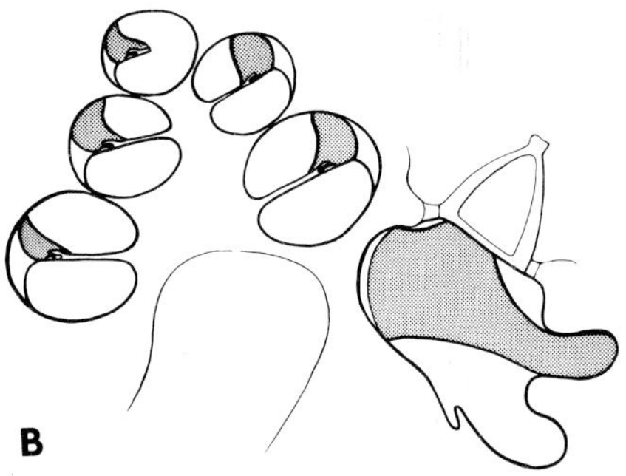

Fig. 22. (Case 1) A) Temporal bone section and B) line drawing showing collapsed Reissner's membrane with dilation of the saccule against the footplate and extending into the nonampullated end of the lateral semicircular canal.

one or more of the following surgeries: transcanal labyrinthectomy, endolymphatic subarachnoid shunt, otic-perotic shunt, and middle fossa eighth nerve section. A summary of the clinical history and histological findings is given for each case. Results of electronystagmography and of the last audiometric test before death are illustrated. The increased area of the endolymphatic system is shown by a shadowed area in a schematic diagram of the cochlea and vestibule. Also, a photograph of the main histopathological findings is presented.

Case 1. This white male was first seen at the age of 51 years with symptomatology of right Menière's disease of six years' duration. He was previously treated medically and by ultrasound therapy without improvement. He had severe sensorineural hearing loss on the right side. ENG showed a spontaneous and positional nystagmus; the bithermal caloric test revealed no response on the right side (Fig. 21). Petrous pyramid x-rays were normal. Because of the failure of medical treatment, the patient underwent an endolymphatic subarachnoid shunt in May 1964, and was free of vertigo for 18 months. Then vertigo recurred. The patient died in December 1966 of an unrelated cause.

The temporal bone showed a collapsed Reissner's membrane in all of the turns and an important dilation of the saccular membrane against the footplate and extending into the nonampullated end of the lateral semicircular canal (Fig. 22A,B). The macula of the saccule presented spaces in the sensory epithelium, suggesting some degeneration in this area. Unfortunately, the medial walls of the sac and shunt tube were lacking in this specimen.

COMMENT. The presence of empty spaces in the sensory epithelium of the saccule suggests degeneration in this area, probably produced by ultrasound therapy.

Case 2. This 68-year-old white female had a history of recurrent vertigo, right tinnitus, and fluctuating hearing loss of ten years' duration. Vertigo attacks became debilitating and her hearing in the affected ear unserviceable. There was total sensorineural hearing loss on the right side (Fig. 23). Petrous pyramid x-rays revealed no evidence of dilation of the internal auditory canal. Accordingly, a labyrinthectomy was performed through a transcanal oval window approach. Following surgery, she was constantly unsteady and had persistent tinnitus. ENG showed complete inactivity of the right ear, as expected after surgery. The patient died at age 77 of an unrelated cause.

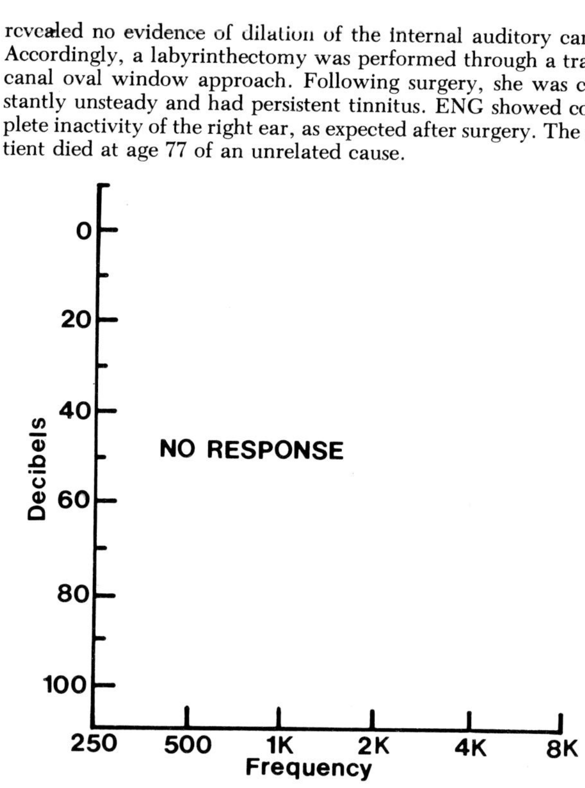

Spontaneous	Yes
Positional	L.L. 7
Caloric Test	No Response on right No Preponderance

Fig. 23. (Case 2) Audiogram and ENG results.

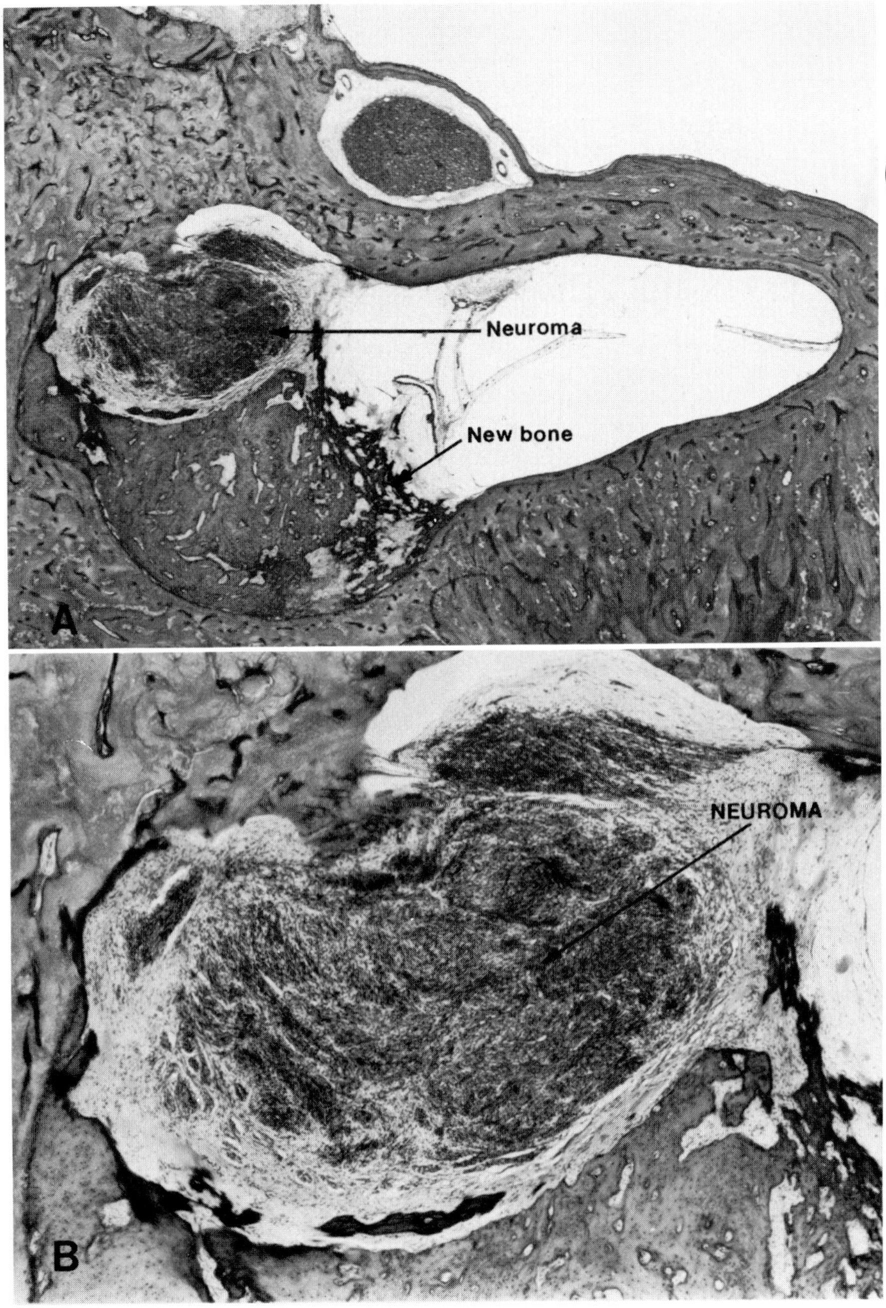

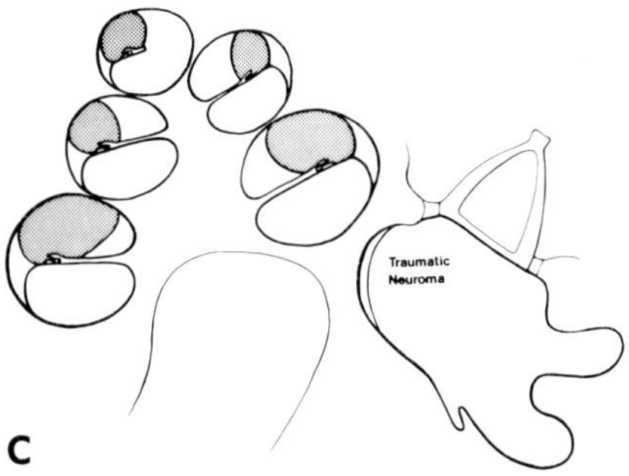

Fig. 24. (Case 2) A) Temporal bone section, B) magnification, and C) line drawing of vestibule filled by a traumatic neuroma on the saccular nerve and partially surrounded by new bone formation in the vestibule.

The temporal bone showed a severe dilation of the cochlear duct (Fig. 24C). Inside the vestibule was a traumatic neuroma on the superior vestibular nerve, partially surrounded by new bone formation in the vestibule (Fig. 24A,B). The crista of the posterior canal was intact and some cupula was attached. A few neurons were seen.

COMMENT. The limited area of destruction, persistence of the posterior canal, and the traumatic neuroma of the superior vestibular nerve probably explain her disability and recurrent dizziness following surgery.

Case 3. This 65-year-old female was first seen in June 1960, complaining of dizziness, nausea, and vomiting for several years. Each attack was preceded by buzzing and fullness of the right ear, characteristic of Menière's disease. Hearing was normal on the left side, with fluctuating hearing loss on the right. The ice water caloric test revealed no response on the right side (Fig. 25). She was treated by vasodilators without benefit. A subarachnoid endolymphatic shunt operation was performed in October 1961. From then to the last follow-up three years later, the patient had no vertigo, no pressure, only slight tinnitus, and her hearing remained the same, continuing to fluctuate. The patient died at age 71 of an unknown cause.

The temporal bone showed a severe dilation of the cochlear duct; the saccular membrane was pressed against the footplate (Fig. 26B). Figure 26A shows the cerebellum and the area where the shunt tube was placed. There is no fibrotic reaction around the cerebellum, the pia, or the arachnoid where the opening for the shunt was performed. Unfortunately, in this section the opening from the end of the endolymphatic duct to the subarachnoid space cannot be traced.

COMMENT. This patient underwent a shunt operation that was successful, with complete control of vertigo and slight improvement of hearing follow-

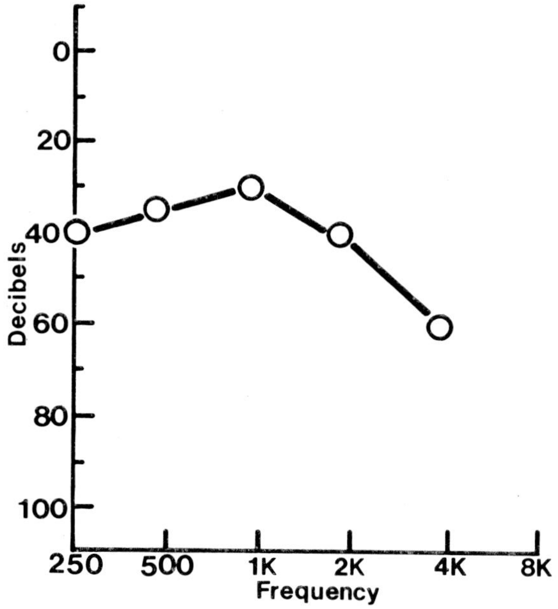

Spontaneous	– –
Positional	– –
Caloric Test	No Response, right, to 30° ice water
	– –

Fig. 25. (Case 3) Audiogram and ENG results.

ing surgery. In the various histopathological sections examined, communication between the endolymphatic sac and the subarachnoid space can be seen, but communication between the end of the endolymphatic duct and the subarachnoid spaces cannot be seen clearly.

Case 4. This 70-year-old female had severe attacks of vertigo and total hearing loss in the right ear following stapes surgery one year before. A transcanal right labyrinthectomy was performed in March 1964. Following surgery, this patient was slightly unsteady, but free of vertigo. The patient died of an accident four years later.

The right temporal bone presented severe dilation of the cochlear duct with herniation through the helicotrema (Fig. 27B). The labyrinth was filled with new bone extending into the semicircular canals and the beginning of the endolymphatic duct, which was blocked by the ossification of the vestibule (Fig. 27A). However, a few fibers can be seen in the area where the macula of the saccule would normally be found.

COMMENT. Ossification of the vestibule is probably secondary to the transcanal labyrinthectomy. The endolymphatic hydrops could have been present before the first surgery; if so, that would explain why the stapedectomy was followed by a total hearing loss. Or, hydrops could have been secondary to either of the surgeries. Slight unsteadiness postsurgically could be related to partially remaining structures of the vestibular content.

Case 5. This 62-year-old female had a typical history of Menière's disease of six years' duration: attacks of vertigo two or three times a week, fluctuating hearing loss, tinnitus, and pressure in the right ear. There was bilateral sensorineural hearing loss. The ENG was normal (Fig. 28D). After failure of a medical treatment (vasodilation and histamines), she underwent an endolymphatic subarachnoid shunt operation in July 1971, with temporary relief for one year. A year later her problem returned and a revision was done. The evaluation was favorable for almost a year, but because symptoms recurred anew, a middle fossa vestibular nerve section was performed after one year. Following this surgery, the patient was free of vertigo and hearing stabilized at the same level as before the nerve section. She developed facial nerve paralysis postoperatively. The patient died in June 1976, of an unrelated cause.

The histopathologic report showed that the cochlear duct was almost normal except in the hook area where Reissner's membrane was prolapsed into the vestibule and applied to the underside of the footplate (Fig. 28F). The saccular membrane was somewhat collapsed (Fig. 28A). The posterior and superior canals were filled with fibrous and osteoid tissue. The left temporal bone was normal.

COMMENT. Although the posterior and superior canals were filled with fibrous and osteoid tissue (Fig. 28C), probably secondary to the first operation, the hearing remained stable. After the vestibular nerve section, the superior and inferior vestibular nerves had degenerated (Fig. 28E), but the hair cells in the utricle and the ampulla of the posterior canal appeared almost intact. Although the patient had a facial nerve paralysis postoperatively, no surgical damage or degeneration of the nerve was seen (Fig. 28B).

Case 6. This 75-year-old female complained of recurrent episodic vertigo and unsteadiness of six years' duration, associated with a fluctuating hearing loss, tinnitus, and pressure in the left ear for the last six months. There was a severe sensorineural hearing loss on the same side. The ENG showed maximum positional nystagmus in the supine position, but the caloric test was normal (Fig. 29B). Petrous pyramid x-rays were normal. Medication was of no benefit and the patient underwent an otic-perotic shunt in April 1964. (This operation consists of the insertion of a platinum tube through the round window membrane and through the basilar membrane.) Following this procedure the hearing remained stable and the pressure and vertigo subsided, but the patient suffered constant unsteadiness and continued tinnitus. Because these symptoms persisted, she underwent a transcanal labyrinthectomy on the left side six months later. In the follow-up unsteadiness continued and tinnitus became progressively worse, constant, and bilateral, but more severe in the left and changing with position. The patient died at age 85 of unknown causes.

The temporal bone showed Reissner's membrane greatly distended in all turns of the cochlea (Fig. 29D). The utricle and ampulla of the semicircular canals appeared normal. The membrane of the saccule was collapsed upon the sensory epithelium. There was a defect in the bone of the promontory, just at the round window. The basal turn was filled with fibrous tissue, part of which was ossified, but with no involvement of the labyrinth (Fig. 29A,C). A large artery extended into the internal auditory canal as far as Scarpa's ganglion (Fig. 29E).

COMMENT. The fact that all the labyrinthine membranes stayed in place could explain the constant unsteadiness after a labyrinthectomy with only "suction" of the vestibular contents. Growth of new bone into the cochlea or vestibule is common after any surgery that violates these spaces, such as insertion of a platinum tube in the hook area in this case. The constant and severe tinnitus in the left ear, which was relieved by changes in position, could be

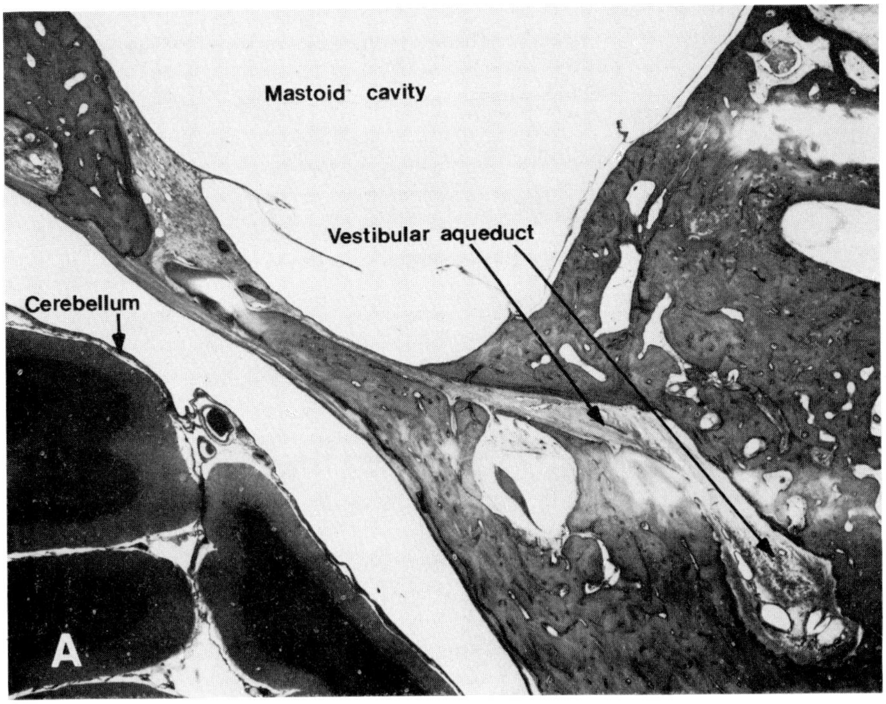

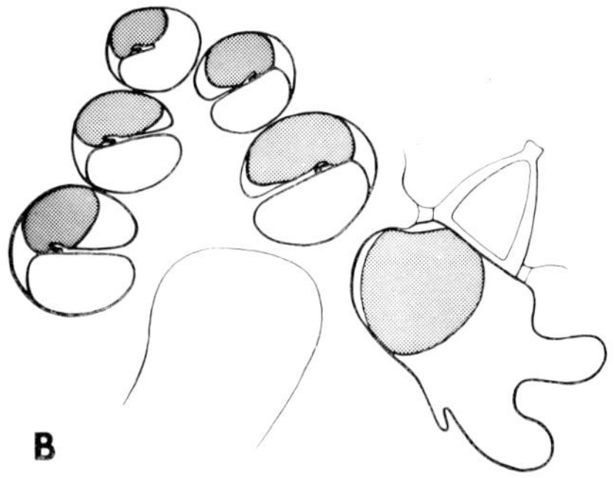

Fig. 26. (Case 3) A) Temporal bone section and B) line drawing showing cerebellum, vestibular aqueduct, and the mastoid cavity after endolymphatic subarachnoid shunt surgery.

explained by the presence of the large artery in the internal auditory canal.

Case 7. This 81-year-old female complained of total hearing loss on the right side after a stapes mobilization performed 20 years before, a progressive hearing loss in the left ear for 12 years, and moderate tinnitus in the left. She also related some unsteadiness, but no vertigo. Audiometric findings showed no response on the right and a sensorineural hearing loss on the left (Fig. 30). Petrous pyramid x-rays were reported as "presumptive evidence of labyrinthine otosclerosis, bilateral." Surgery was not recommended. The patient died at age 84 of unknown causes.

The left ear showed a moderate to severe bulging of Reissner's membrane and a severe dilation of the saccule in contact with the footplate and bulging into the nonampullated end of the lateral semicircular canal (Fig. 31B). The entire cochlea and the superior and lateral canals were ossified in the right temporal bone (Fig. 31A). The labyrinth was filled with fibrous tissue and with bundles of fibers from the superior vestibular nerve.

COMMENT. The right ear could have had hydrops prior to surgery, and apparently an infection developed when the vestibule was opened. In spite of the severe bulging of the cochlear duct and saccule in the left ear, the patient complained only of "balance trouble."

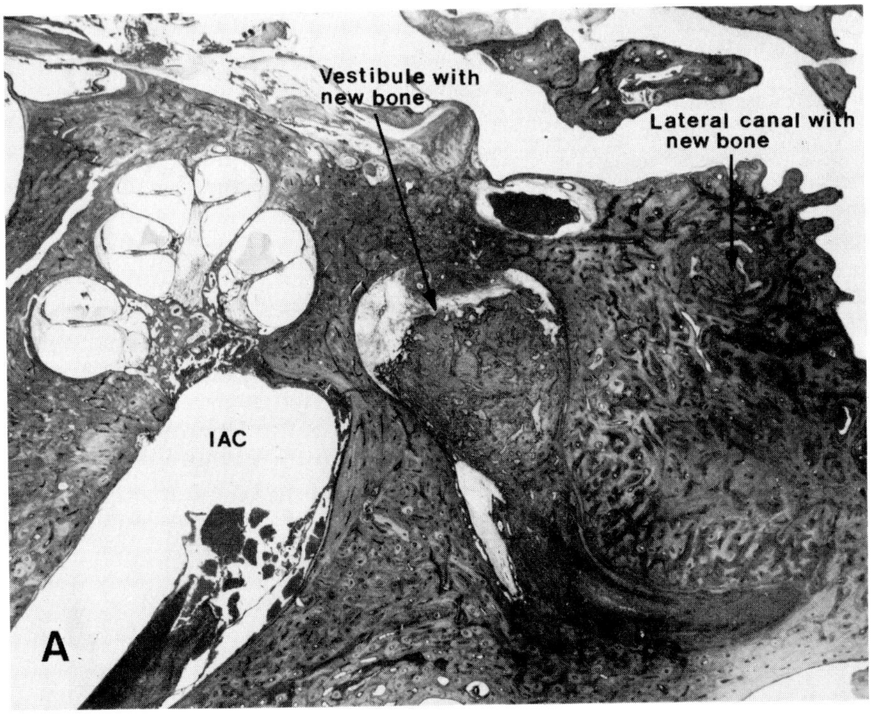

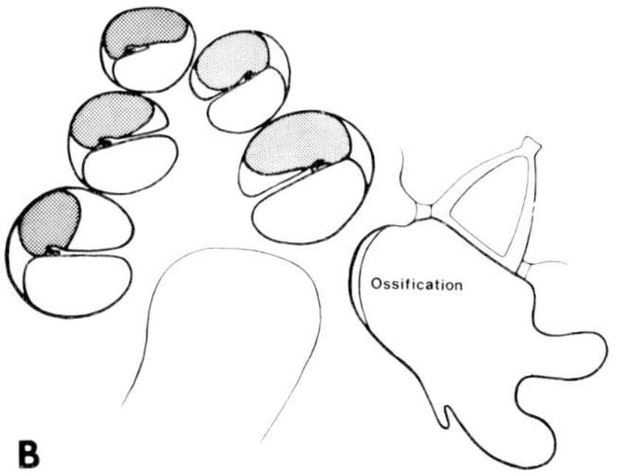

Fig. 27. (Case 4) A) Temporal bone section and B) line drawing showing the labyrinth filled with new bone extending into the semicircular canals and the beginning of the endolymphatic duct.

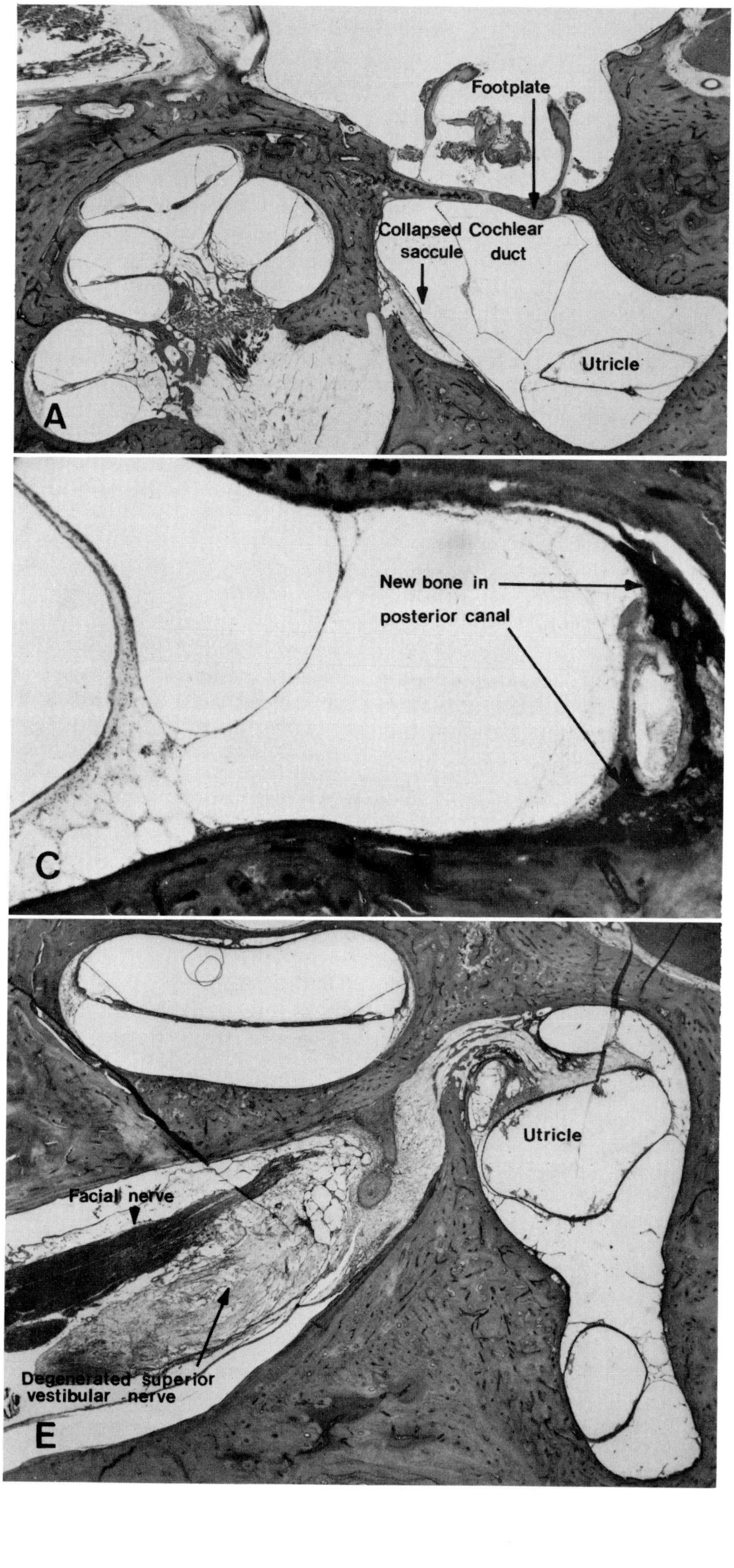

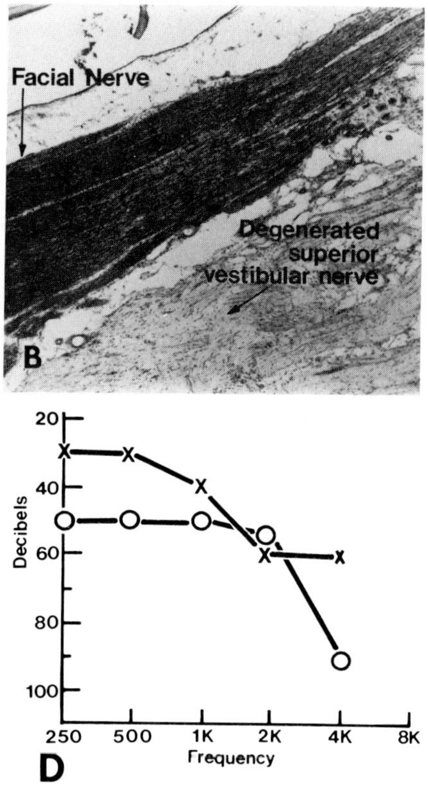

Spontaneous	No	
Positional	No	
Caloric Test	No RVR	No Preponderance

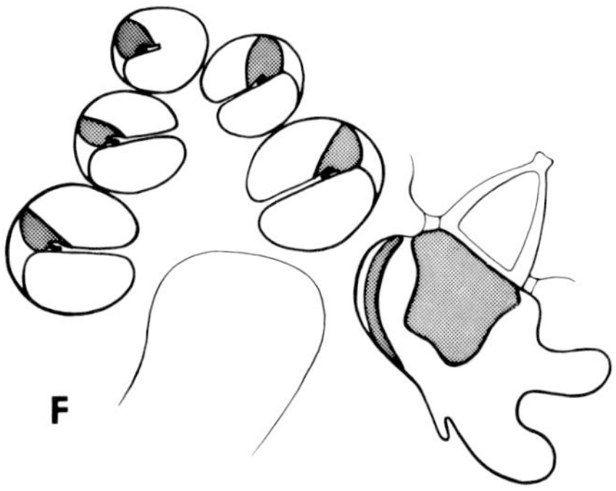

Fig. 28. (Case 5) A) Horizontal midmodiolar section showing a normal cochlear duct except for the hook area, where Reissner's membrane is prolapsed into the vestibule and pressed against the footplate. The saccular membrane is collapsed. B) Although the patient suffered postoperative facial nerve paralysis, no surgical damage or degeneration of the nerve is seen. C) Posterior semicircular canal filled with fibrous and osteoid tissue. D) Audiogram. E) Degeneration of the vestibular nerve after vestibular nerve section. F) Line drawing of area shown in A.

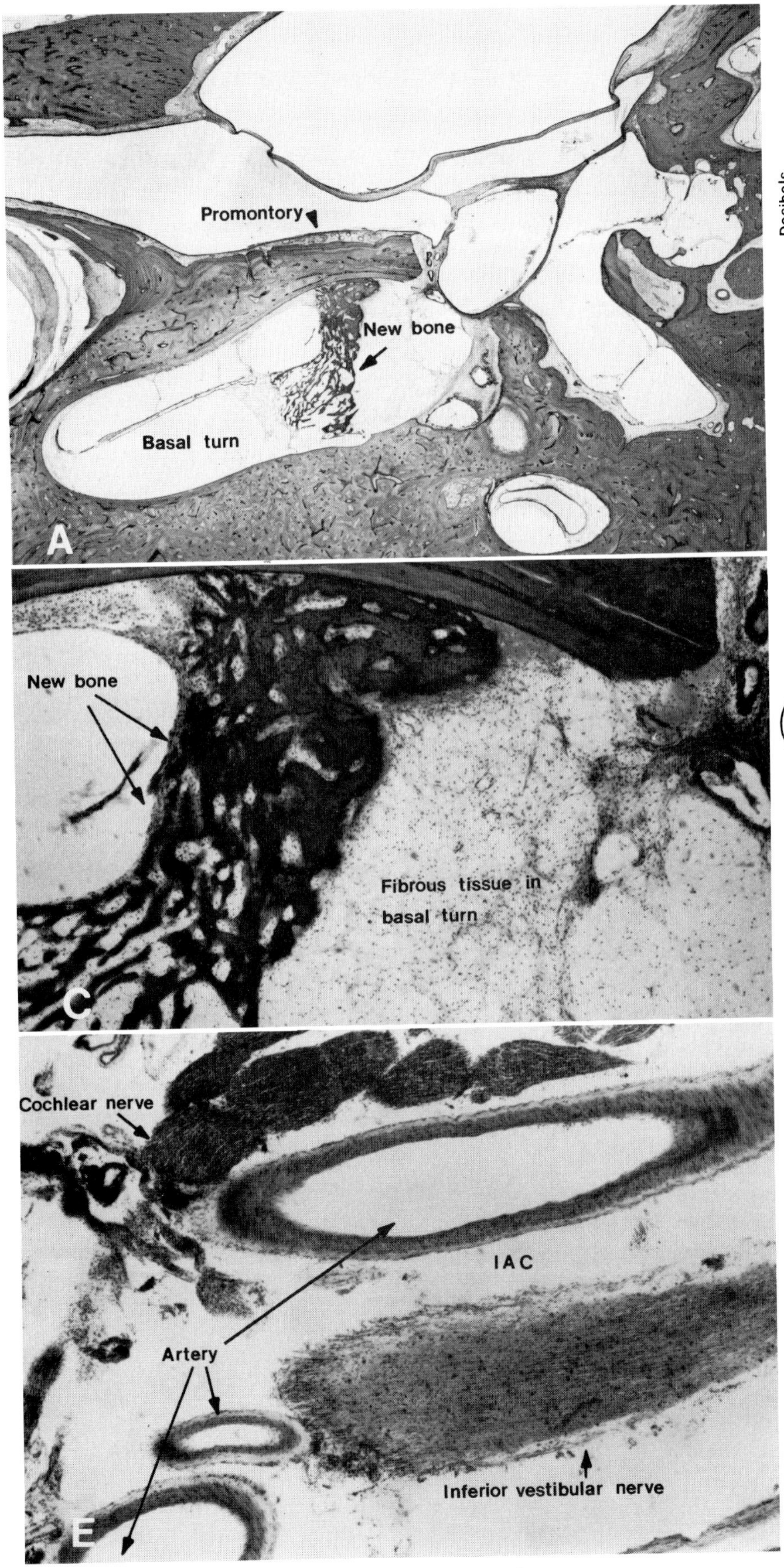

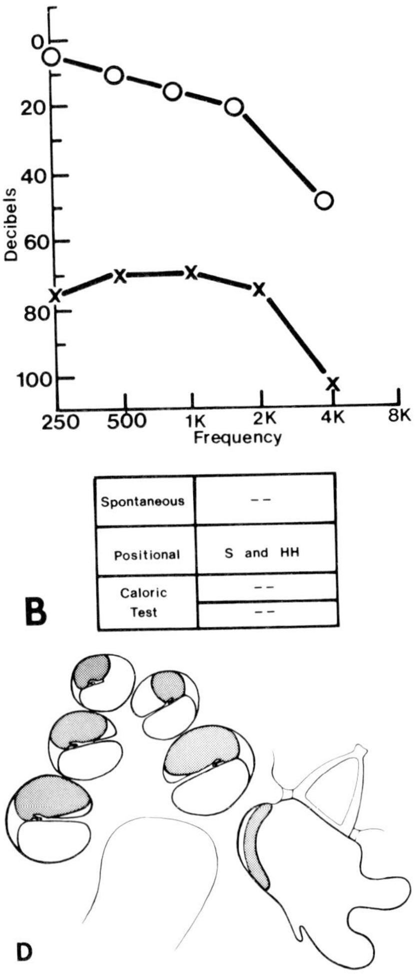

Fig. 29. (Case 6) A) Basal turn filled with fibrous and osseous tissue. B) Audiogram and ENG results. C) Magnification, and D) line drawing of area shown in A. E) Large artery extending into the internal auditory canal as far as Scarpa's ganglion.

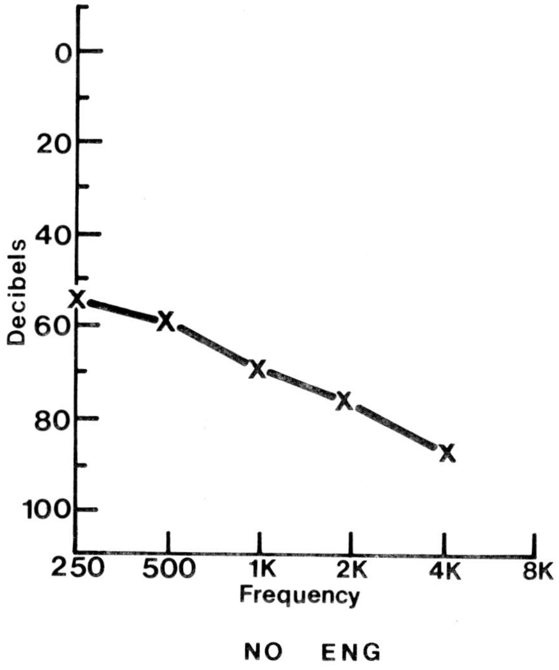

Fig. 30. (Case 7) Audiogram.

Case 8. This 29-year old female, hospitalized for treatment of diabetes, was seen seven days after the onset of buzzing in both ears and a severe hearing loss. Dizziness and fluctuating hearing did not occur previously. Because she was confused when seen, a complete history was not obtained. Examination of her ears, nose, and throat revealed no significant abnormalities. Clinical and audiometric examination revealed no response in either ear. She died during hospitalization from diabetic complications three days later.

Histopathological sections revealed a normal right temporal bone. The left showed moderate to severe bulging of Reissner's membrane in the cochlea and a severe dilation of the saccule in contact with the footplate (Fig. 32A,B). Interestingly, this temporal bone showed abnormal bone obstructing the beginning of the endolymphatic duct (Fig. 32C), which was seen in all serial sections.

COMMENT. Histopathological findings were consistent with those of unilateral endolymphatic hydrops. In this case there were two factors that could have influenced the development of hydrops: abnormal bone growing and obstructing the beginning of the endolymphatic duct, and clinical evidence of a severe metabolic disorder. However, a definite assessment cannot be made.

Case 9. This 77-year-old male suffered attacks of vertigo once or twice a month, pressure, tinnitus, and an undocumented fluctuating hearing loss in the left of 16 years' duration. Neurological evaluation, petrous pyramid x-rays, and ENG were normal. There was a bilateral sensorineural hearing loss (Fig. 33B). The clinical diagnosis was unilateral left Menière's disease. Vasodilators and sublingual histamines were prescribed. In spite of medical treatment, episodic vertigo and hearing loss persisted. The patient died at age 85 of unknown causes.

The temporal bone showed no dilation of the endolymphatic duct system (Fig. 33A).

COMMENT. Although the clinical study was compatible with the diagnosis of Menière's disease, there was no hydrops in the endolymphatic system.

Case 10. This 60-year-old male was examined for progressive hearing impairment of 25 years' duration, with a sudden decrease in hearing four weeks previously. He also complained of episodic rotary vertigo, unsteadiness worsened by walking in the dark, bilateral tinnitus, and pressure in the ears. This patient had been treated for congenital syphilis that was first diagnosed when he was 16, when interstitial keratitis set in. There was bilateral sensorineural hearing loss. ENG revealed no response on either side to the caloric test (Fig. 34F). The patient died of a heart attack three years after the first visit.

The temporal bone showed an important dilation of both cochlear ducts (Fig. 34A,B,D). The vestibular membranes also presented severe distortion: the saccular membrane was pressed against the footplate on the left side and on the right side the saccule extended eight tenths of the distance to the footplate. An in-

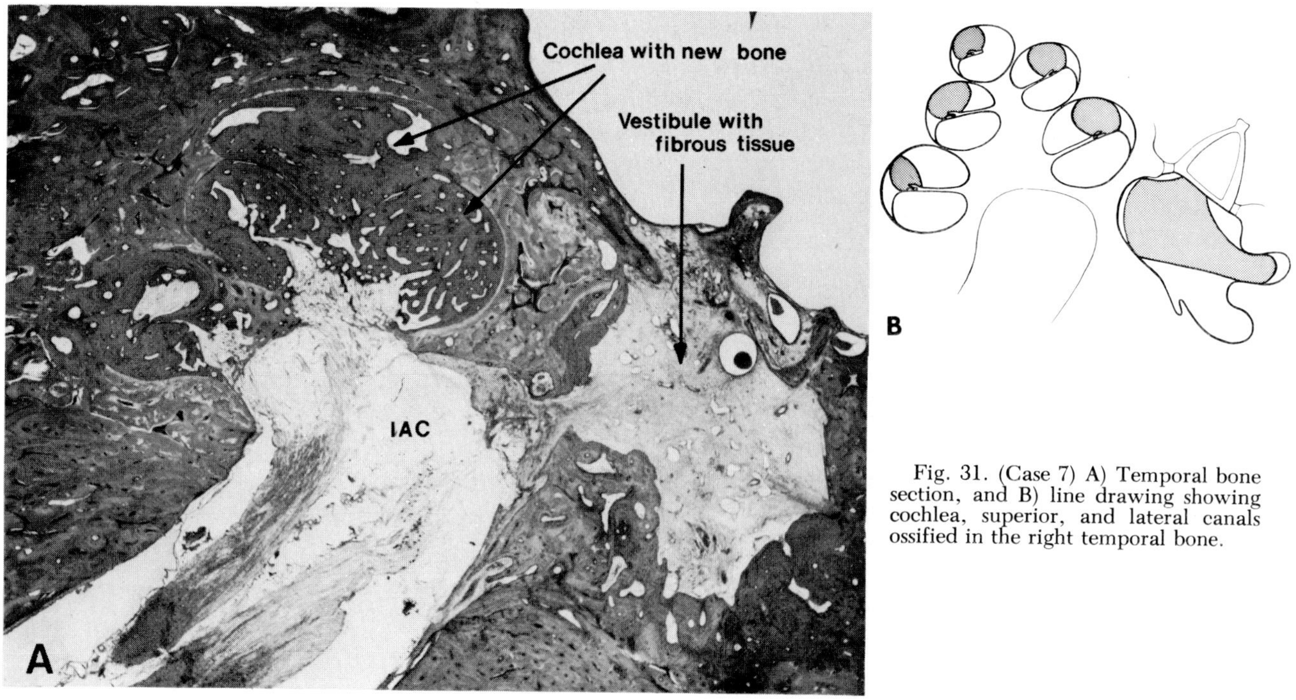

Fig. 31. (Case 7) A) Temporal bone section, and B) line drawing showing cochlea, superior, and lateral canals ossified in the right temporal bone.

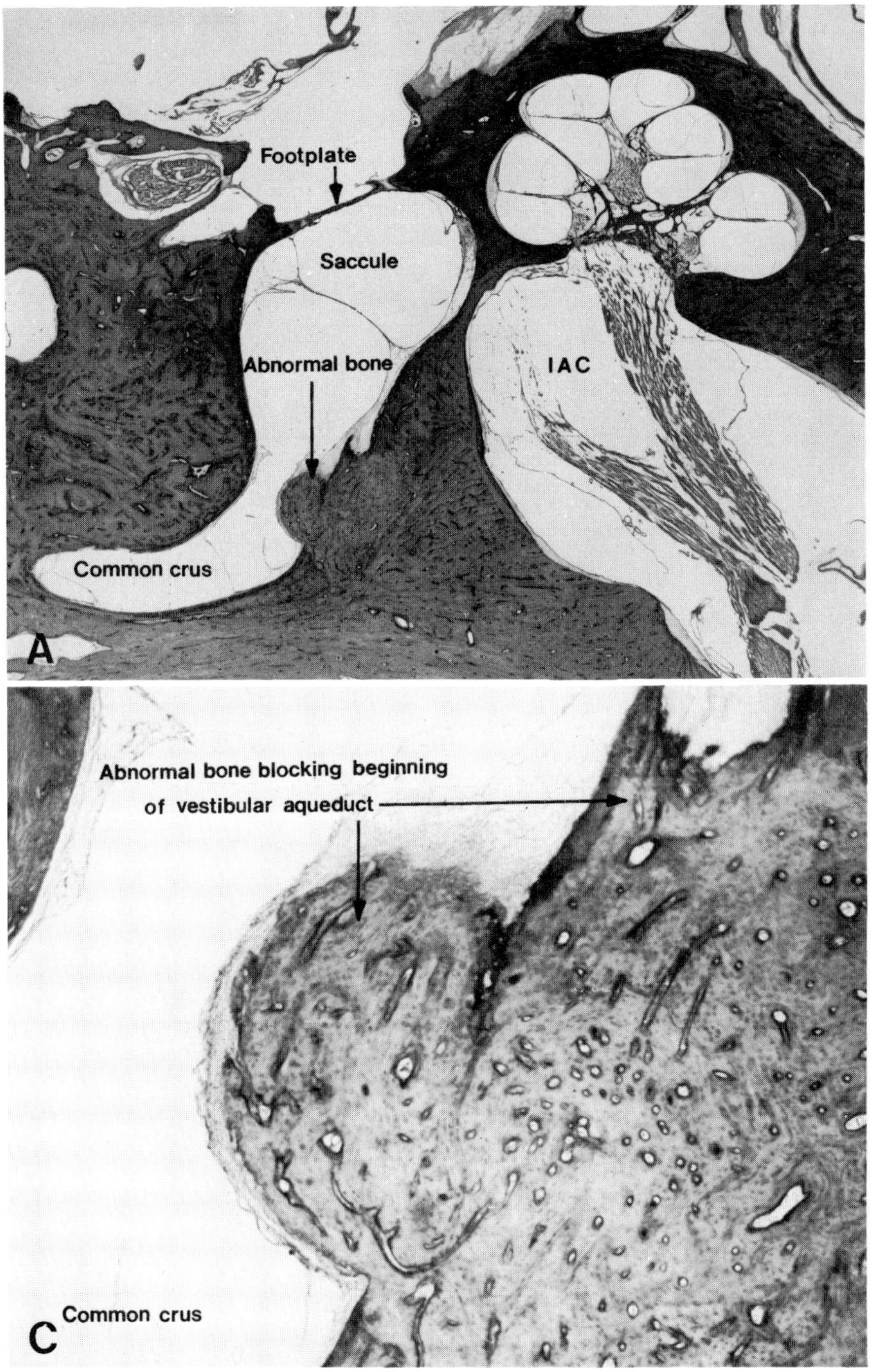

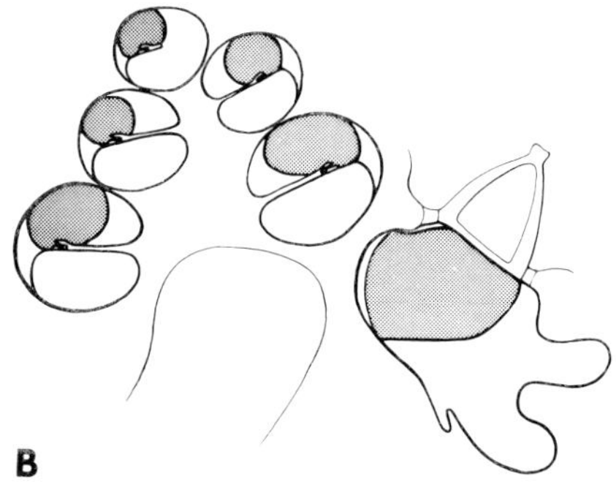

Fig. 32. (Case 8) A) Horizontal midmodiolar section, and B) line drawing showing severe dilation of the endolymphatic system and abnormal bone. C) Magnification of the abnormal bone obstructing the beginning of the endolymphatic duct.

flammatory process obliterated the vestibular aqueduct on both sides. The vestibular aqueduct disappeared into a microgumma consisting of perivascular round cell infiltration and foreign body giant cells. This lesion extended into the posterior canal. On the eighth nerve on the left side, Schwann cells, lymphocytes, and giant cells proliferated (Fig. 34C). These lesions were also found in the osseous wall and labyrinthine membranes (Fig. 34E).

COMMENT. It appears that the hydrops was secondary to an obliteration of the vestibular aqueduct by a luetic process in both ears. The reason for the vestibular symptoms could be the hydrops or it could be traced to the gummata on the eighth nerve and the invasion of the posterior canal by the luetic process.

SUMMARY

This study is based on 17 patients chosen because of either their histopathological evidence of hydrops or their clinical history of Menière's disease. Aims of the study were to describe the histopathological findings of 23 temporal bones with endolymphatic hydrops and to correlate, if possible, these findings with clinical histories.

Histopathological Findings. In all temporal bones the cochlear duct in the apical turn was dilated. In cases of severe hydrops the greatest bulging of Reissner's membrane was in the middle and

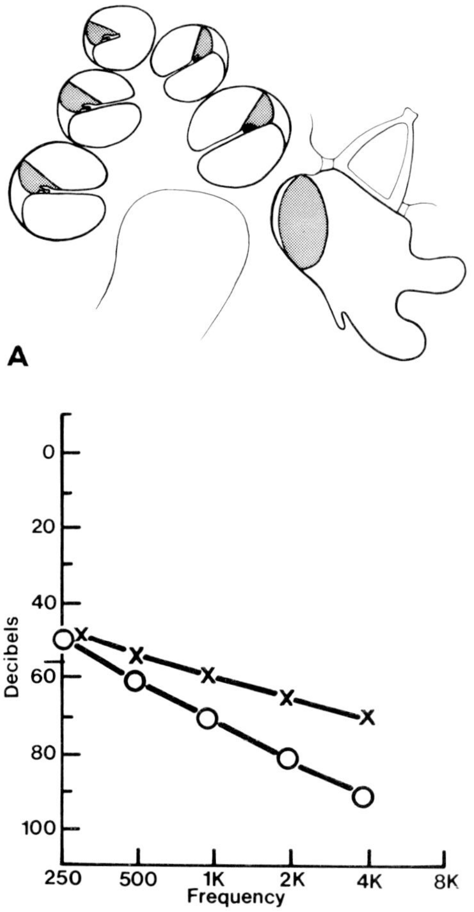

Spontaneous	No	
Positional	No	
Caloric Test	No - RVR	No Preponderance

B

Fig. 33. (Case 9) A) Line drawing of temporal bone showing no dilation of the endolymphatic duct system. B) Audiogram.

basal turns. In cases of severe hydrops the amount of dilation of the cochlear duct corresponded with the amount of dilation of the saccule. In contrast, dilation of the utricle was absent or slight. Morphological changes in the labyrinthine membrane consisted of collapsed Reissner's membrane, proliferation of cells in the distended Reissner's membrane, and fibrosis between the labyrinthine wall and endosteal layers. Presence of antemortem ruptures and healing was not demonstrated.

No major abnormalities were found in the vestibular aqueduct or endolymphatic sac, except in two cases with a blocked vestibular aqueduct. No specific degenerative changes in sensorineural elements or stria vascularis were observed.

Clinical-Histopathological Correlations. Clinical diagnosis of Menière's disease was classified as follows: definite Menière's disease (episodic vertigo and documented fluctuating hearing loss) and probable Menière's disease (episodic vertigo, but no documentation of fluctuating hearing loss). Correlation between clinical diagnosis of Menière's disease, as defined above, and the presence of endolymphatic hydrops was valid in 80% of the cases. Of the remaining 20%, 10% had bilateral endolymphatic hydrops and were diagnosed clinically as unilateral Menière's disease. Of the other 10%, half were clinically diagnosed as Menière's disease with no findings of hydrops; half were not diagnosed as Menière's disease, but evidence of hydrops was found.

The increased area of the cochlear duct showed statistical correlation with the duration of the disease and with the total average hearing loss. A correlation was also found between the increased area in each turn of the cochlea and its corresponding frequency, except for the posterior middle area. For a given cochlea, these two parameters were distributed as independent events.

In the vestibular system a correlation was found between the severity of the symptom and the dilation of the saccular wall.

Case Reports. Histopathological findings of effects of surgery are reported. Of three patients who underwent transcanal labyrinthectomies, one had a traumatic neuroma in the labyrinth; two showed only partial removal of the labyrinthine structures, with remnants left in contact with neural fibers. Of four patients who underwent endolymphatic subarachnoid shunts, two had total control of vertigo; histopathological findings were severe endolymphatic hydrops in one case and moderate in the other. The other two had temporary relief of vertigo; histopathological findings were collapse of the cochlear duct in one case and collapse of the saccule in the other.

CONCLUSION

Two factors, the frequency of deformity in the labyrinthine membranes and the clear statistical correlation between dilation of the labyrinthine membranes and clinical symptoms, suggest that endolymphatic hydrops has a direct effect on the symptoms of Menière's disease. Assuming this is true, two conclusions can be drawn: 1) The mechanical effect of this endolymphatic hydrops in the production of symptoms of Menière's disease seems significant. In this study no ruptures were seen, and a biochemical effect of possible ruptures seems unlikely. 2) Any therapy that aims to reduce the excess accumulation of endolymph is theoretically valid.

During the course of Menière's disease Reissner's membrane may be permanently impaired, with no capacity to recuperate its physical properties. Therefore, treatment should be directed towards minimizing the possibility of permanent change.

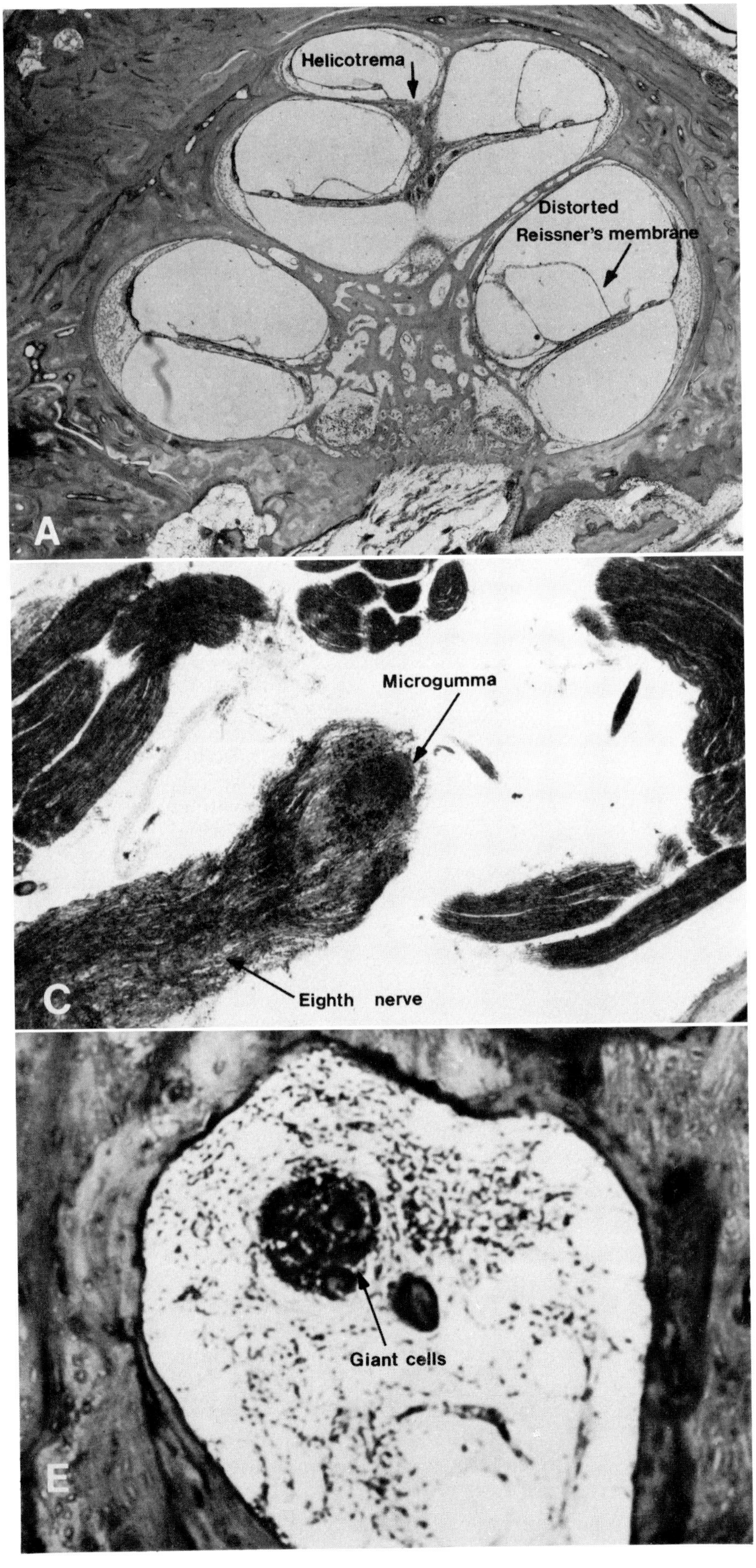

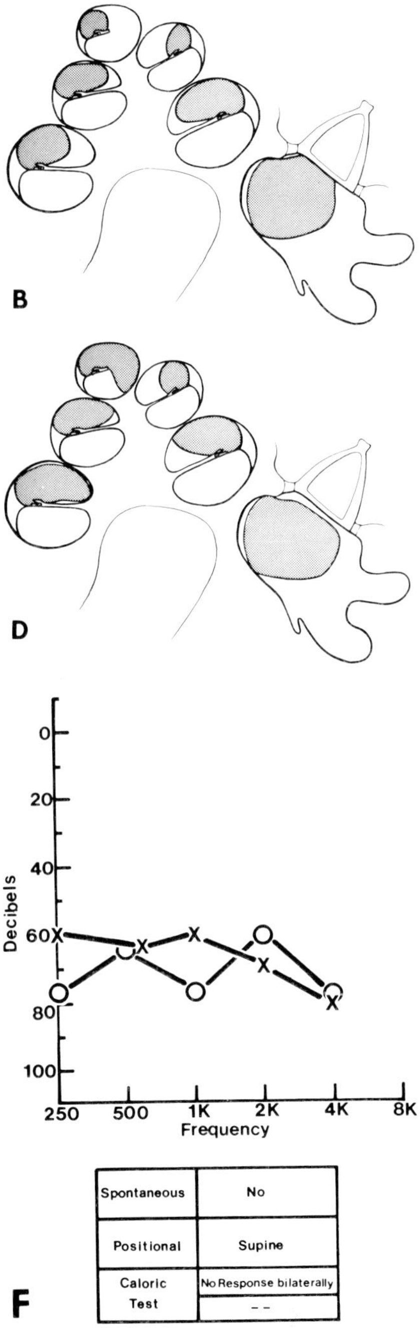

Fig. 34. (Case 10) A) Midmodiolar section, and B) line drawing showing a severe distortion of Reissner's membrane. C) Lymphocytes and giant cells on the eighth nerve on the left side. D) Line drawing showing dilation of cochlear duct. E) Microgumma consisting of perivascular round cell infiltration and foreign body giant cells found in the osseous wall and labyrinthine membranes. F) Audiogram and ENG results.

From the correlation found between clinical symptoms and histopathological evidence of hydrops, it can be assumed that episodic vertigo and a history of fluctuating hearing loss, even if undocumented, are sufficient for the diagnosis of Menière's disease after other possibilities have been eliminated.

Histopathological findings of patients who remained unsteady after labyrinthectomy by transcanal approach showed a traumatic neuroma or remnants of vestibular structures. Therefore, when a destructive procedure is indicated, an eighth nerve section may prove more successful than a transcanal labyrinthectomy.

ACKNOWLEDGMENTS — The authors are indebted to the Ear Research Institute for the use of its facilities. This study was performed in the Institute's Eccles Temporal Bone Pathology Laboratory, directed by Dr. Fred H. Linthicum, Jr.

The authors gratefully express their deep appreciation to the following persons for their contributions to this article: Dr. Fred H. Linthicum, Jr., Dr. George Kelemen, Dr. James Sheehy, and Prof. Imrich Friedmann for their extremely valuable scientific advice; Dr. Ruben Budelli for his technical advice regarding computerized data; Diane Foster for her editorial assistance; Debra Adams for her illustrations; and Cynthia A. Smith and Janetta Paladini for their invaluable assistance in preparing the manuscript.

REFERENCES

1. Menière P. Memoire sur des lesions de l'oreille interne donnant lieu a des symptomes de congestion cerebrale apoplectiforme. Gaz Med Paris 1861; 16:597-601.

2. Hallpike C, Cairns H. Observations on the pathology of Meniere's disease. J Laryngol Otol 1938; 53:625-54.

3. Friedmann I. Pathology of the ear. London: Blackwell Scientific Publications, 1974:479.

4. Wustrow F, Borkowsky B. Results after conservative and surgical methods of therapy as well as critical observations on the pathogenesis of Meniere's disease. Z Laryngol Rhinol Otol 1960; 39:133-52.

5. Paparella M, Goycoolea H, Meyerhoff W, Shea D. Endolymphatic hydrops and otitis media. Presented at the Middle Section Meeting of the American Laryngological, Rhinological, and Otological Society, Inc., New Orleans, January 22, 1978.

6. Lawrence M, McCabe BF. Inner ear mechanics and deafness. (Meniere's syndrome.) JAMA 1959; 171:1927-32.

7. Schuknecht H, Benitez J, Beekhuis F. Further observations on the pathology of Menière's disease. Ann Otol Rhinol Laryngol 1962; 71:1039-53.

8. Altmann F, Kornfeld M. Histological studies of Menière's disease. Ann Otol Rhinol Laryngol 1965; 74:915-43.

9. Lindsay J. Labyrinthine dropsy and Meniere's disease. Arch Otolaryngol 1942; 35:853-67.

10. Lindsay J, Kohut R, Sciarra P. Menière's disease: pathology and manifestations. Ann Otol Rhinol Laryngol 1967; 76:1-22.

11. Schuknecht H. Correlation of pathology with symptoms of Meniere's disease. Otolaryngol Clin North Am 1968; 1:433-9.

12. Lindsay J. Hydrops of the labyrinth. Arch Otolaryngol 1960; 71:500-10.

13. Antoli-Candela F Jr. The histopathology of Meniere's disease. Acta Otolaryngol (Stockh) 1976; Suppl 340.

14. Linthicum FH Jr, Schwartzman JA. An atlas of micropathology of the temporal bone. Philadelphia: WB Saunders, 1974.

15. House WF. Meniere's disease: management and theory. Otolaryngol Clin North Am 1975; 8:515-35.

16. House WF. A theory of the production of symptoms of Meniere's disease. Otolaryngol Clin North Am 1968; 1:441-5.

17. Tonndorf J. Mechanical causes of fluctuant hearing loss. Otolaryngol Clin North Am 1975; 8:303-11.

18. Portmann G. Recherches sur la physiologie du sac et du canal endolymphatique des selaciens. C R Soc Biol 1921; 85: 1070-2.

19. Kimura R, Schuknecht H. Membranous hydrops in the inner ear of the guinea pig after obliteration of the endolymphatic sac. Pract Otorhinolaryngol (Basel) 1965; 27:343-54.

20. Kelemen G. Anatomical observations on the distal extremity of the vestibular aqueduct. J Laryngol Otol 1976; 90:1071-9.

21. Altmann F, Fowler EP Jr. Histological findings in Menière's symptom complex. Ann Otol Rhinol Laryngol 1943; 52: 52-80.

22. Kristensen H. Histopathology in Ménière's disease. Acta Otolaryngol (Stockh) 1961; 53:237-45.

23. Dixon WJ, Massey FJ. Introduction to statistical analysis. New York: McGraw Hill, 1957.

24. Fernandez C. Dimensions of the cochlea. J Acoust Soc Am 1952; 24:519-23.

25. Schuknecht H. Temporal bone removal at autopsy: preparation and uses. Arch Otolaryngol 1968; 87:33-49.

COMPUTER-AIDED AND GRAPHIC RECONSTRUCTION OF THE HUMAN ENDOLYMPHATIC DUCT AND SAC

A METHOD FOR COMPARING MENIÈRE'S AND NON-MENIÈRE'S DISEASE CASES

JUAN-CARLOS M. ANTUNEZ, MD
RIO DE JANEIRO, BRAZIL

FRANK R. GALEY, PhD
LOS ANGELES, CALIFORNIA

FRED H. LINTHICUM, MD
LOS ANGELES, CALIFORNIA

GILBERT D. MCCANN, PhD
PASADENA, CALIFORNIA

The anatomy of the human endolymphatic duct system of three cases — one with Menière's syndrome (with no histopathological evidence of endolymphatic hydrops), one with Menière's disease (with histopathological evidence of endolymphatic hydrops), and one with no evidence of disease — has been studied by means of computer-aided and graphic reconstruction from serial sections of temporal bones. The reconstructions have revealed a canalicular arrangement of the epithelial lining of the rugose portion of the human endolymphatic sac. Accordingly, new nomenclature, "pars canalicularis," is suggested for this portion. The computer produced lateral and medial views of the endolymphatic duct and sac of the patient with Menière's syndrome. The computer also calculated the luminal volume, the surface area of the epithelium, and the surface-to-volume ratio of the rugose portion of the sac.

In addition, the authors graphically reconstructed the rugose portion of the sac of all three cases. Measurements of the dimensions of these reconstructions were made, from which the luminal volume was estimated. The reconstructed images and the calculations allowed quantitative comparison of the microscopic anatomy of the rugose portion of the sac in the Menière's syndrome and Menière's disease ears with that in an ear without evidence of disease.

Significant differences were found in the volumes of the rugose portion of the sac of the three cases. The results suggest that the luminal volume of the rugose portion of the sac of Menière's disease patients may be significantly reduced. The authors speculate that endolymphatic hydrops may be the result of a loss of epithelial surface area in the canalicular portion, thus diminishing its resorptive function.

The computer and graphic reconstruction techniques in conjunction with their analytical capabilities provide a new method for studying inner ear structures. These techniques have the potential to expand the capabilities of quantitative morphology and provide the means for deriving clinically useful data from histopathological and ultrastructural material.

INTRODUCTION

The role of the endolymphatic duct and sac in the etiology of Menière's disease is of increasing interest. Knowledge of the anatomy and physiology of the endolymphatic duct and sac in normal and pathological conditions is essential for progress in the proper treatment of patients suffering from Menière's disease.

This study aims to demonstrate the potential of computer-aided and graphic reconstruction techniques and associated quantitative analytical techniques for increasing knowledge of Menière's disease and its pathological correlate, endolymphatic hydrops.

Findings are discussed in relation to the new anatomical information revealed by the study and in relation to details of anatomy and physiology of the endolymphatic duct system.

REVIEW OF THE LITERATURE

Anatomy of the Endolymphatic Duct and Sac. The endolymphatic sac was discovered by Cotugno[1] in 1774 and rediscovered by Boettcher[2] in 1869. Since then, many investigators have studied its anatomy and possible functions.

Guild,[3] in his classic study of the structure, normal contents, morphology, and histology of the ductus and saccus endolymphaticus in the guinea pig, defined the ductus endolymphaticus as that "elongated narrow portion of the membranous labyrinth extending from the sacculus to the saccus endolymphaticus proprius." The ductus endolymphaticus proprius, on the basis of the structure of its wall, was subdivided into three portions:

1. pars proximalis, lying entirely within the dilated portion of the vestibular aqueduct;

2. pars intermedia, lying partly within the vestibular aqueduct and partly between the layers of the dura mater near its external aperture;

3. pars distalis, lying in the dura mater. Its lumen may be patent or potentially patent.

Topographically, the saccus endolymphaticus proprius is covered partly by bone and partly by the dura mater. Accordingly, Guild,[3] Sterzi,[4] and Portmann[5] called these respective parts "subosteal" and "intradural."

From the University of Rio de Janeiro, Brazil; the Ear Research Institute, the Electron Microscopy Laboratory of the Ear Research Institute, the Department of Otolaryngology at the University of Southern California, and the Otologic Medical Group, Inc, Los Angeles; and the California Institute of Technology, Pasadena.

Bast and Anson,[6] studying reconstructions in correlation with serial sections, introduced new nomenclature for the various portions of the human endolymphatic duct and endolymphatic sac, referred to as the "endolymphatic duct system." The endolymphatic duct is divided into two parts, the "sinus" and the "isthmus," and the endolymphatic sac into three parts, the "proximal" or "rugose portion," the "sac proper" or "enlarged flattened portion," and the "distal projection."

Their reconstructions by the Born method[7] of the luminal space within the rugose portion of the endolymphatic sac showed the extent of the complicated folding of the lining epithelium seen in sections.

> The irregularly shaped excavations of the reconstructions represent hillocks of tissue in the sections which project into the lumen of the duct; conversely, the ridges of the reconstruction represent crypts in the tissue where the lining epithelium extends downward into the supporting connective tissue layer.[6]

The endolymphatic sac proper includes approximately two thirds of the sac and extends from the rugose portion to its distal projection.

Zechner and Altmann[8] authored the most recent anatomical and histological report on the human endolymphatic duct and sac, based on the study of 190 temporal bones. Three main portions were distinguishable in the adult:

1. The vestibular portion, or sinus, of the duct begins with the confluence of the utricular and saccular duct and ends where the duct enters the bony vestibular aqueduct.

2. The intraosseus portion, or isthmus, of the duct shows considerable variation in the width of the lumen. The duct widens as it goes into the endolymphatic sac.

3. The endolymphatic sac is partly contained within the wide dural portion of the bony canal (the vestibular aqueduct); the remainder lies between the periosteal portion of the dura and the dura proper.

The proximal third of the endolymphatic sac is within the periosteal layer of the bony capsule.

> The wall of this portion forms many true folds which protrude into the lumen and this part is therefore called *pars rugosa* . . . Sometimes villi originating from opposite sides of the wall meet and fuse thus subdividing the main lumen into numerous compartments . . . In this way a complicated canalicular system is formed which represents an enormous enlargement of the surface of the wall of the pars rugosa.[8]

The distal two thirds of the sac, "the pars intraduralis," lies between the two layers of the dura. In the adult the lumen of this pars is narrow and slit-like.

Labyrinthine Hydrops. The secretion of endolymph has been associated with the stria vascularis[9] and the plana semilunata within the ampullae, utricle, and saccule[10-13] due to their histological and ultrastructural features compatible with secretory activity.

Resorption has been associated with the external spiral sulcus of the cochlear duct[9] and the endolymphatic sac due to their histological, ultrastructural,[14] and physiological[15-16] features compatible with resorption.

Today there is general agreement that at least part of the endolymph circulates from the cochlear duct to the distal portion of the sac. This portion has been considered the place of collection of endolymph and/or the "pressure regulator"[17] of the system.

Recent studies have shown that endolymphatic hydrops, associated primarily with Menière's disease,[18] is also seen in several other conditions.[19-22]

Of the many theories on the cause of hydrops, almost all suggest either overproduction or faulty resorption of endolymph. Kimura and Schuknecht[23] proposed blockage of the endolymphatic duct and consequent excessive accumulation of endolymph as a cause of hydrops. Modern surgical procedures, such as otic-perotic shunt,[24,25] decompression of the endolymphatic sac,[26] otic-mastoid shunt,[27,28] and endolymphatic subarachnoid shunt,[29,30] are based on the assumption that these mechanical factors are the cause of the hydrops.

METHODS

Three temporal bones were selected from the Eccles Temporal Bone Laboratory of the Ear Research Institute for study: case 1, with Menière's syndrome (unilateral: episodic vertigo, fluctuating hearing loss, tinnitus, and fullness); case 2, with Menière's disease (the above symptoms plus histologically confirmed endolymphatic hydrops); and case 3, with no evidence of disease. All of these temporal bones contained the complete endolymphatic duct system from the vestibule to the distal portion of the sac.

All bones were removed from 6 to 24 hours after death, placed in formaldehyde, decalcified in Versene®, and embedded in celloidin. Specimens were sectioned in the horizontal plane at an average thickness of 25 μm, and stained with hematoxylin and eosin. Cases 1, 2, and 3 had a total of 170, 90, and 110 sections respectively, which were numbered consecutively.

Due to problems inherent in processing this many sections, some intersections were lost. However, in no case was the distance between two consecutive sections more than 100 μm, ie, equivalent to four missing sections. To compensate for missing sections, duplicates or triplicates (as necessary) of the section before and the section after the missing section were used. This method avoided alterations in the anatomical size of the structure to be reconstructed.

Pictures of each section were taken with the Zeiss photomicroscope with a 2.5x objective and a total optical magnification of 10x. Negatives were printed on Kodak® fine grain positive film at a photographic magnification of approximately 7.5 times.

Graphic Reconstruction. Graphic reconstruction of the rugose portion of the endolymphatic sac only was made in all three cases according to modifications of the method of Gaunt and Gaunt.[31]

The use of photographs of histological sections on transparent film to reconstruct microstructures is based on overlapping sections by matching features appearing in one photograph with the same features appearing in the following photograph according to the methods of Sjöstrand[32] and Fox et al.[33] Reference marks to insure accuracy of alignment were added to each photo.

Only epithelial structures were traced from the pictures onto tracing paper. Connective tissue with blood vessels and the bony vestibular aqueduct were not traced. Tracings were consolidated on one sheet of graph paper by translating each successive tracing along the ordinate at the distance proportionate to the thickness of the section. Reference marks were aligned with parallel lines along the ordinate.

Both the lateral and medial views were reconstructed. The line in the tracing represented the epithelium either on the lateral or medial side of the endolymphatic sac. This procedure yielded composite projections of the lateral or medial views of the three endolymphatic sacs studied. Shading was added to these projections for comparison to the computer-aided reconstruction.

Measurements of the dimensions of the reconstructions were taken. The length (superior-inferior) was calculated directly from the number of sections used and the average thickness of the sections. The width (anterior-posterior) was calculated as the average of the measurements of the chord in each tracing connecting the ends of the arc of the concavity formed on the lateral side of the sac. The thickness (medial-lateral) was calculated as the average of the measurements of the median of the maximum and minimum diameters of the lumen in each tracing.

Computer-Aided Reconstruction. The tracings of the epithelium of the endolymphatic duct, the rugose portion of the sac, and a truncated segment of the distal portion of the sac of case 1 were entered into a PDP 11/45 computer at California Institute of Technology. A magnetic pen was used to retrace the tracings onto a Tektronix® tablet. The computer programs of the image analysis system developed by Shantz[34] and Shantz and McCann[35] produced on a color video monitor, color-coded surface renderings of medial and lateral views of the duct and sac. These views were photographed with a 35 mm camera.

In addition, the image analysis system was used to calculate the luminal volume, epithelial surface area, and the surface-to-volume ratio of the rugose portion of the sac. The measurements from graphic reconstructions of case 1 were compared to the volume determined by the computer.

CASE HISTORIES

Case 1. A 76-year-old male consulted the Otologic Medical Group, Inc, complaining of tinnitus and progressive, fluctuating hearing loss in his left ear for 16 years. In the last three years he had dizziness and a sensation of fullness in the left ear. Hour-long attacks of vertigo occurred every two months. His general health was good. Otologic examination revealed normal ear canals and normal and mobile eardrums bilaterally. Audiograms during his first visit showed moderate bilateral sensorineural hearing loss averaging 42 dB in the right and 53 dB in the left ear with speech discrimination scores of 84 and 50% respectively. A complete neurotological evaluation showed normal polytome x-rays and a normal vestibular response. Clinical diagnosis of bilateral presbycusis and left Menière's syndrome was made. Medical treatment was begun, and the patient did not return for six years, at which time audiograms showed bilateral and moderate sensorineural hearing loss averaging 65 dB in the right ear and 63 dB in the left ear. These measurements were slightly worse than at the first visit. Discrimination scores were the same. Despite medical treatment, the patient did not notice improvement. The patient died at age 84 from unrelated causes.

The left temporal bone showed atrophy in 25% of the stria vascularis. The population of neuron and ganglion cells was normal. No endolymphatic hydrops was found. The right temporal bone showed a normal endolymphatic system and atrophy of 50% of the stria vascularis. The organ of Corti and spiral ganglia appeared normal.

Case 2. This 60-year-old female consulted the Otologic Medical Group, Inc, for tinnitus, dizziness, fullness, and hearing loss in her right ear. The audiogram showed a right sensorineural hearing loss of 50 dB. No discrimination scores were available in the chart. Petrous pyramid x-rays showed no abnormalities. Electronystagmography showed a slightly reduced vestibular response on the right side. Menière's syndrome was diagnosed. Medical treatment was instituted but proved ineffective. Because the attacks of dizziness occurred more frequently, the patient underwent a transcanal labyrinthectomy eight years later. The patient died at 78, 18 years after the surgery, still complaining of balance problems.

Histological study of the right temporal bone showed a small traumatic neuroma on the saccular nerve, bulging of Reissner's membrane, intact crista of the posterior canal, and endolymphatic hydrops. The left temporal bone showed normal contents of the endolymphatic system.

Case 3. A 53-year-old male consulted the Otologic Medical Group, Inc, because of a discharge in his right ear. Audiograms showed a slight conductive hearing loss in the right ear (air conduction 32 dB; bone conduction 25 dB) with normal hearing in the left ear (air conduction 6 dB; discrimination 100%). The patient died two years later. His left ear was selected for study. No abnormalities were found.

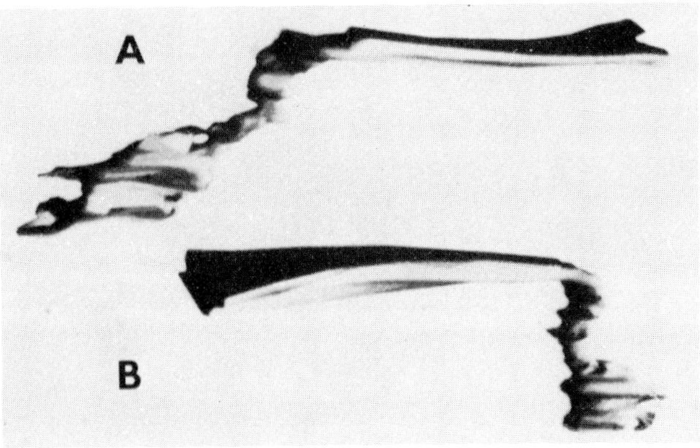

Fig. 1. Computer-aided reconstruction of the endolymphatic duct. A) Lateral view. B) Medial view.

RESULTS

COMPUTER-AIDED RECONSTRUCTION

Computer-aided reconstruction resulted in both lateral and medial views for each of the following portions of the endolymphatic duct system:

Endolymphatic Duct (Figs. 1 and 2). The computer-aided technique showed that the endolymphatic duct begins with confluence of the saccular and utricular ducts. Based on its direction, the endolymphatic duct can be divided into two portions:

1. The horizontal portion (Fig. 3A). From its origin, the endolymphatic duct runs parallel to the saccule in a horizontal direction for approximately 2 mm. It is a straight, elongated channel, the midway diameter of which is approximately 0.133 mm. The horizontal portion corresponds to the vestibular portion, or sinus, of the duct, as described by Zechner and Altmann.[8]

2. The vertical portion (Fig. 3B). The endolymphatic duct suddenly bends almost 90° inferiorly for approximately 0.2 mm. Its shape changes from

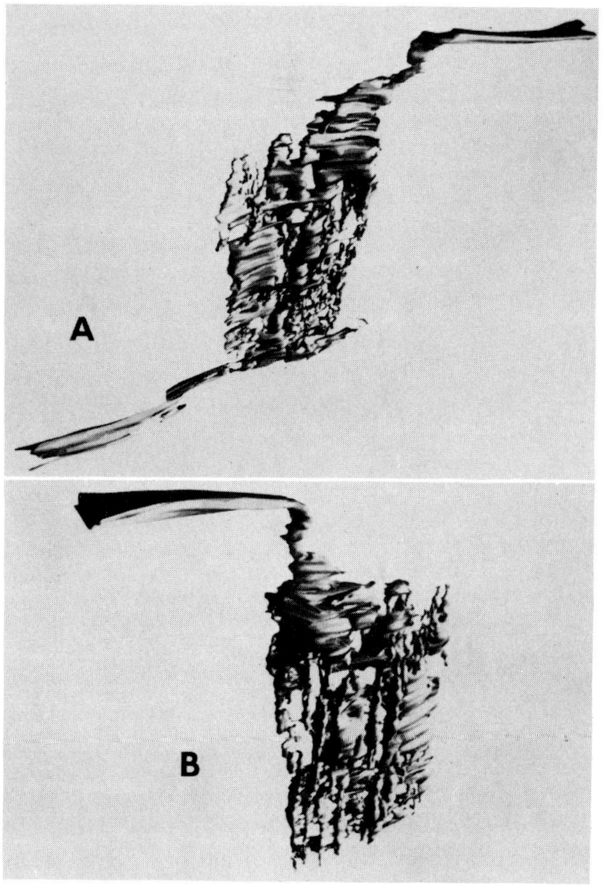

Fig. 2. A) Photomontage of the computer-aided lateral view of the endolymphatic duct, the pars rugosa, and a truncated segment of the distal portion of the sac. B) Photomontage of the computer-aided medial view of the endolymphatic duct and the pars rugosa.

wide to narrow to wide, with diameters of 0.26 mm, 0.13 mm, and 0.46 mm respectively. The vertical portion merges either as a single or a divided channel into the next portion of the sac. This vertical portion corresponds to the isthmus of the duct, as described by Zechner and Altmann.[8]

Rugose Portion of the Sac (Figs. 2, 4, and 5). The rugose portion of the sac is located between the vertical portion of the duct and the distal portion of the sac. The general course of this portion is vertical with a slight lateral concavity. It is composed of vertical canaliculi of various diameters running roughly parallel from the duct to the distal portion of the sac.

None of the canaliculi is of constant size; their diameters increase and decrease continuously over their length. Three different types of canaliculi can be distinguished, although precise classification can be difficult.

1. Primary. Primary canaliculi are the largest and thickest. Their shape is irregular. They are fully formed or are being formed by the confluence of smaller, thinner canaliculi. Primaries also give origin to smaller canaliculi. Primaries may divide

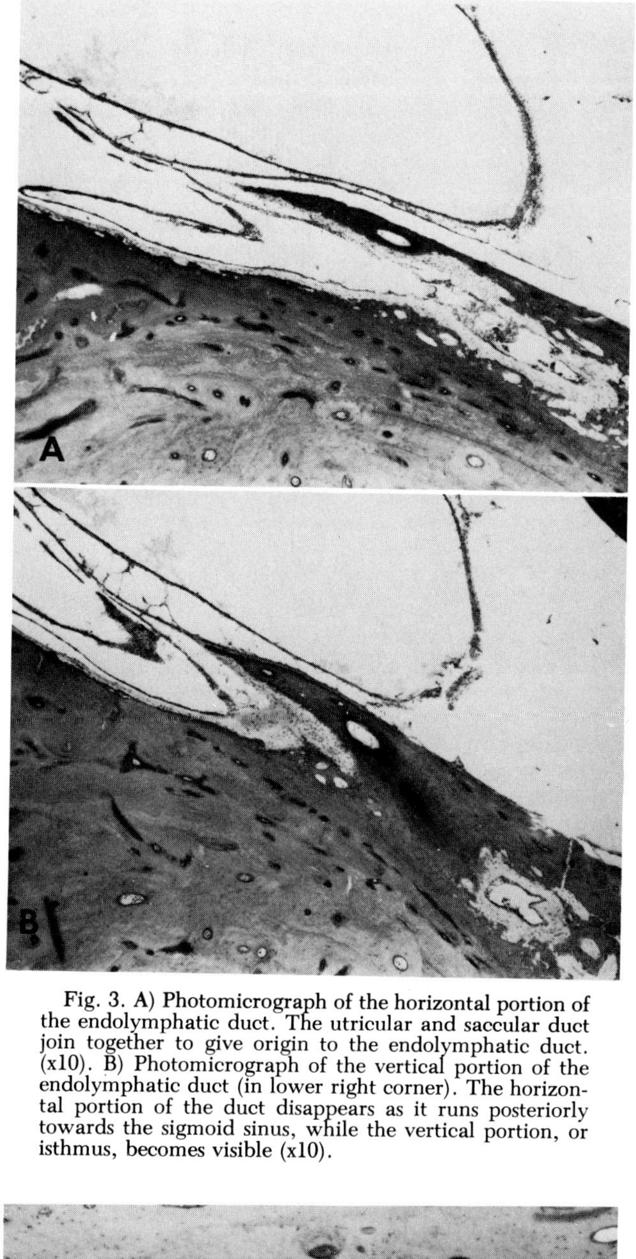

Fig. 3. A) Photomicrograph of the horizontal portion of the endolymphatic duct. The utricular and saccular duct join together to give origin to the endolymphatic duct. (x10). B) Photomicrograph of the vertical portion of the endolymphatic duct (in lower right corner). The horizontal portion of the duct disappears as it runs posteriorly towards the sigmoid sinus, while the vertical portion, or isthmus, becomes visible (x10).

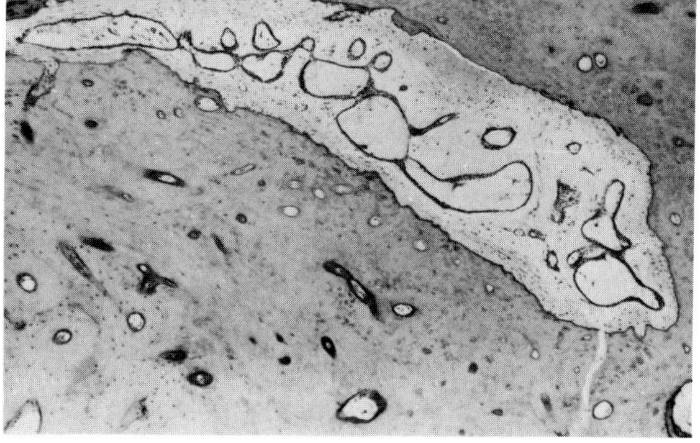

Fig. 4. Photomicrograph of the pars rugosa. Note that most of the epithelial outlines are closed circles, thus forming the walls of canaliculi in the reconstruction. (x10)

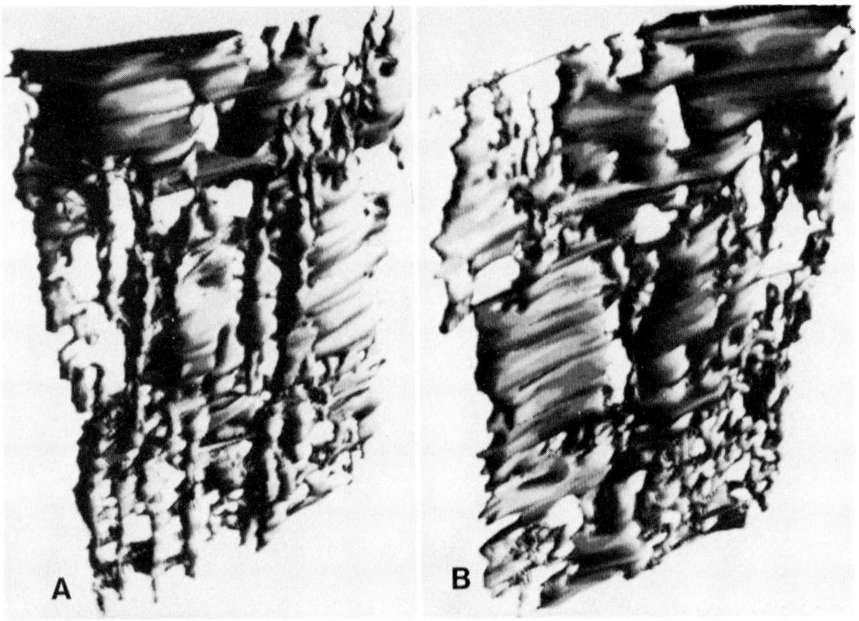

Fig. 5. A) Computer-aided image of the medial side of the pars rugosa. The surface of this portion is irregular because almost all its parallel canaliculi arise from this side. B) Computer-aided image of the lateral side of the pars rugosa. This side, with a smooth surface, shows primary canaliculi and blunt-ending canaliculi.

into two, three, four, or sometimes five branches, each one ending either as a cul-de-sac or connecting to another canaliculus.

2. Secondary. These are smaller and thinner than primaries, from which they originate. Secondaries are vertically parallel to primaries for various distances (0.25 to 0.8 mm). All secondaries end in other canaliculi. Secondaries may join directly with other canaliculi or divide into two or three branches that end in the primary canaliculus of origin, in other primaries, or in tertiary canaliculi.

3. Tertiary. All tertiary canaliculi end without connecting to other canaliculi. All tertiaries are smaller than primaries but may be the same size as secondaries. Tertiaries also run vertically parallel to primaries for various distances (0.25 to 0.5 mm) and also originate from primaries. Some tertiaries travel vertically downwards from their origin; others run vertically upwards. All end without connecting to others.

Invaginations of epithelium and subepithelial connective tissue into the luminal space are observable in sections. These invaginations are canalicular in nature and secondary or tertiary in character. These canaliculi do not show in the reconstruction due to the surface rendering performed by the computer.

Differences between the lateral and the medial views of the canalicular portion are apparent. Most secondary and tertiary canaliculi seem to arise from the medial side.

The shape of the canalicular portion is roughly that of a cylinder, the cross-section of which is crescent-shaped. The dimensions of this cylinder are represented in Table 1.

TABLE 1. DIMENSIONS OF THE ENDOLYMPHATIC DUCT AND SAC

	Length (mm)	*Width (mm)*	*Average Thickness (mm)*	*Volume* $(mm)^3$	*Surface* $(mm)^2$	*Surface-to-Volume Ratio*
E. Duct						
Horizontal	2.00		0.133			
Vertical	0.20		0.300 (0.13-0.46)*			
E. Sac						
Canalicular						
Case 1	2.47	1.91 ±0.02	0.110 ±0.003	0.516 0.641†	42.28†	65.9†
Case 2	2.22	1.78 ±0.04	0.070 ±0.002	0.276		
Case 3	2.75	2.76 ±0.05	0.150 ±0.004	1.062		

*Range of dimensions.

†Computer-determined values.

E. - Endolymphatic.

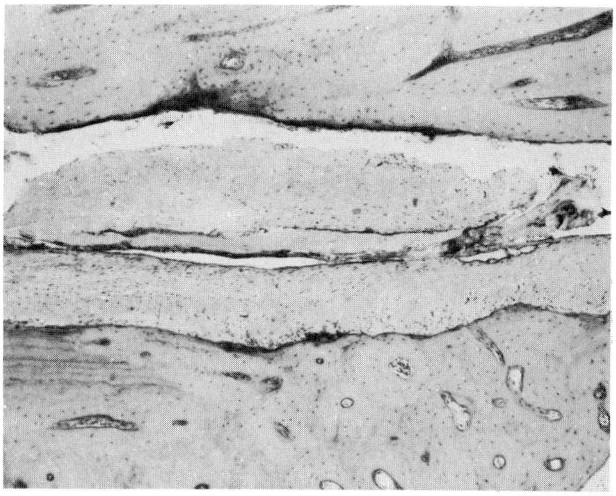

Fig. 6. Photomicrograph of the distal portion of the sac. In the adult, this portion is narrow and flat and surrounded by connective tissue. Note in this section that the distal portion and its surrounding connective tissue are intraosseous. (x10)

As calculated by the computer, the canalicular portion has an epithelial surface area of 42.28 mm^2 and a volume of 0.64 mm^3. The surface-to-volume ratio is 65.9/1. The surface-to-volume ratio of a hypothetical cube of the same volume is 7.2/1. Because of its canalicular nature, the sac has 9.4 times more surface area than a cube.

Distal Portion of the Sac (Figs. 2 A and 6). The intraosseous part of the distal portion of the endolymphatic sac is connected to the inferior end of the canalicular portion and extends posteriorly towards the sigmoid sinus. The layers of the wall of the sac are collapsed along all but the final end. Therefore, the collapsed layers indicate a potential cavity. The dimensions of this portion are shown in Table 1.

GRAPHIC RECONSTRUCTION

Graphic reconstruction offered lateral and medial views (Figs. 7-9). Most features seen through computer-aided reconstruction could also be seen in graphic reconstructions.

As in the computer-aided reconstruction, the course of the canalicular portion of the sac is generally vertical.

The general shape of the sacs reconstructed by the graphic method is roughly that of a crescent-shaped cylinder. The dimensions of the sac of each case are represented in Table 1. The volume calculated from measurements of the sac from case 1 is 19% different from the volume of the same sac as determined by the computer. The percent differences between cases 1 and 2, 2 and 3, and 1 and 3 are respectively 46%, 74%, and 51%.

The lateral and medial views show differences: the lateral wall has a relatively smooth surface; the medial surface appears irregular because of secondary and tertiary canaliculi that arise from this side.

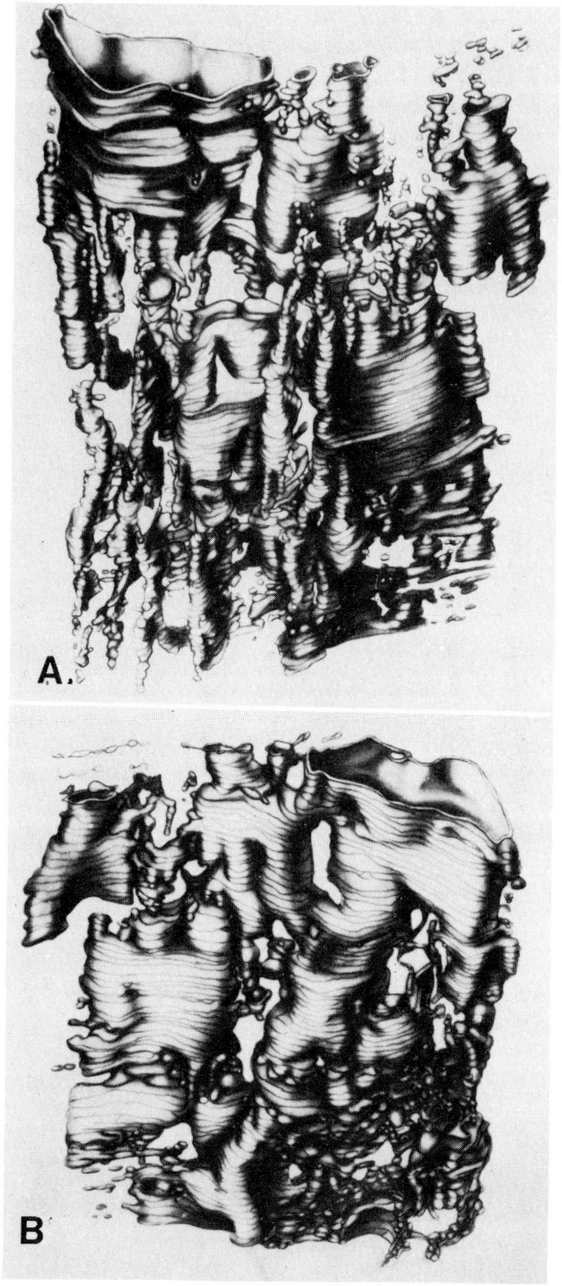

Fig. 7. (Case 1) Artist's drawings from graphic reconstruction of the medial (A) and lateral (B) sides of the pars rugosa. Each horizontal line within the canaliculi represents the outline of one section. The external surface of the structure was shaded to show contours. Figure 7 A and B are comparable to Figure 5 A and B respectively.

Invaginations of epithelial-lined canaliculi into the lumen are observable in sections of the three cases studied and are particularly apparent in the sections from case 3, the normal ear (Fig. 10). These canaliculi are not included in the graphic reconstruction illustrations because the method is intended to illustrate external surface features and not internal structural details.

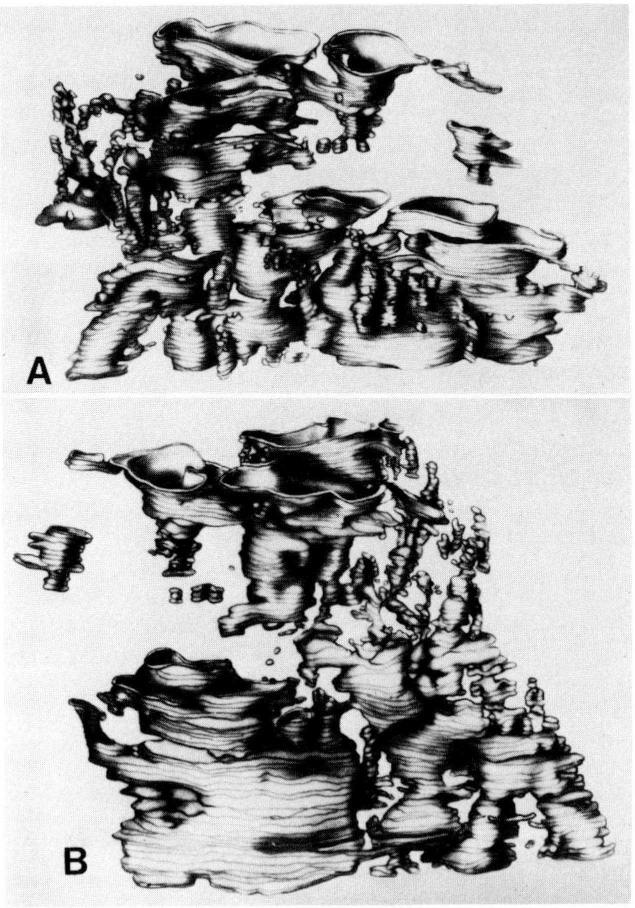

Fig. 8. (Case 2) Artist's drawing from graphic reconstruction of the medial (A) and lateral (B) sides of the pars rugosa. Because some canaliculi appear disjointed, the lumen of other canaliculi can be seen in different sections. Primary, secondary, and tertiary canaliculi can also be seen.

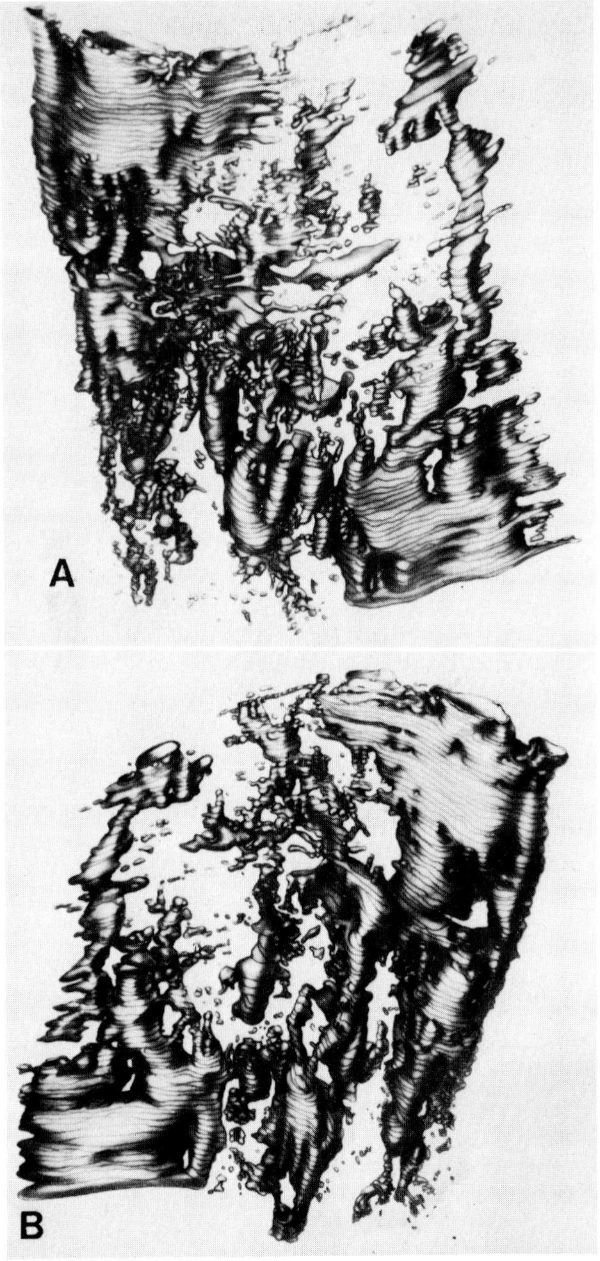

Fig. 9. (Case 3) Artist's drawing from graphic reconstruction of the medial (A) and lateral (B) sides of the pars rugosa. Primary, secondary, and tertiary canaliculi can be seen irregularly distributed.

DISCUSSION

General Anatomy. This study confirms the results of Bast and Anson[6] that the endolymphatic duct system is not a straight channel. It can be divided into three identifiable sections: the duct, the rugose portion of the sac, and the distal portion of the sac.

The term "rugose" for this portion of the sac arose from histological studies and reconstructions of Bast and Anson.[6] They used the Born reconstruction method which did not reveal the intricate canalicular system of this portion. Computer-aided and graphic reconstructions have revealed that this portion is not rugose, made by folds; instead, it is truly canalicular. Accordingly, the authors tentatively propose to rename this portion of the endolymphatic sac the "pars canalicularis."

The diversity of sizes and configurations of the canaliculi, the extensive invaginations, and the variation of these conditions among the three cases studied suggest that the pars canalicularis is not a static structure. Rather, it may be a dynamic structure. This concept warrants further investigation. Application of computer-aided reconstruction techniques in conjunction with morphometric analysis at the ultrastructural level as well as the histological level on many samples may yield information on the dynamic nature of the epithelium of the pars canalicularis.

Case Correlations. The canalicular nature of the sac was a common feature of the three cases studied. Primary, secondary, and tertiary canaliculi could be seen in all three cases. They seemed to originate from the medial side.

Qualitatively, no clear anatomical differences were seen in the three cases. However, the volumes

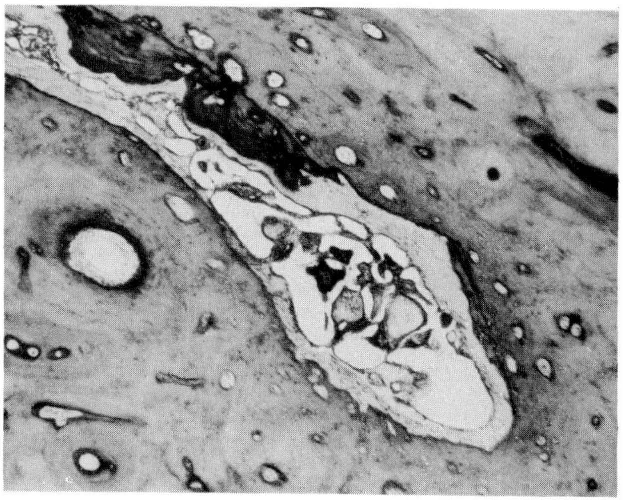

Fig. 10. (Case 3) Photomicrograph of the pars rugosa. The invaginations of epithelial-lined canaliculi are particularly evident in this section. (x10)

calculated by this technique appeared to be significantly different from each other. The computer measurement and manual measurement of the volume of the canalicular portion of case 1 differed by 19%. Case 3, without evidence of disease, had the largest calculated volume. Case 2, with Menière's disease, had the smallest calculated volume. The results may have been influenced by two conditions: 1) This patient underwent a surgical procedure (transcanal labyrinthectomy) that may have affected the canalicular portion of the sac. 2) This case had a well-pneumatized mastoid with the duct and the sac running posteriorly between air cells. These factors may have increased the possibility of section cut defects and, therefore, the possibility of technical artifacts. These possibilities, in turn, may account for the apparently small volume.

Other investigators have also reported differences in the pars rugosa of Menière's disease patients and patients with no evidence of disease. Arenberg and Andersen[36] reported that the more advanced the disease, the greater the changes. Yuen and Schuknecht[37] reported statistically significant differences between the diameter of the endolymphatic duct in normal patients and that in Menière's disease cases. Clemis and Valvassori[38] described radiological (and thus macroscopical[1]) differences in the vestibular aqueduct of Menière's disease patients and that of normal patients. Egami and Sando,[39] in a quantitative study of 11 temporal bones of ten patients with histological endolymphatic hydrops, found no statistically significant differences in widths of the vestibular aqueduct between ears with and those without hydrops. However, they did find statistically significant differences ($P<0.05$ by t-test) in widths of the endolymphatic sac in ears with and those without hydrops ($ES = 0.14 \pm 0.03$ mm in ears with hydrops and 0.29 ± 0.11 mm in cases without hydrops).

Based on clinical history, case 1 was correctly diagnosed as Menière's disease. However, the histological study showed no endolymphatic hydrops. According to the definition of Menière's disease by the Committee on Hearing and Equilibrium as

> a disease of the membranous inner ear characterized by deafness, vertigo, and usually tinnitus, and has as its pathologic correlate hydropic distention of the endolymphatic system,[40]

this case was not Menière's disease despite the clinical impression. Should it be considered idiopathic sensorineural hearing loss? Because this case had no hydrops, is the anatomy to be considered normal, that is, as far as "normal" can be determined?

Similarly, future studies that use computer-aided analysis and reconstruction will confront questions such as: Which endolymphatic sacs are to be considered Menière's disease samples? Can fresh tissue obtained from surgical biopsy be considered a Menière's disease sample if the presence of hydrops in the patient is unknown? Are there really histological, ultrastructural, or even macroscopical differences in the endolymphatic duct system of Menière's disease patients and that of normal cases? If so, do those changes occur only at an advanced stage of the disease? Are changes the cause or the consequence of the endolymphatic hydrops?

The application of computer-aided reconstruction from serial sections of temporal bones in conjunction with quantitative morphological analysis of many samples of both normal and Menière's disease cases are required before meaningful conclusions can be drawn. The influence of other factors such as age, duration and severity of disease, and range of normal variations should be included in the analysis. The authors are continuing these studies.

Computer-Aided and Graphic Techniques. This study demonstrates that the computer has potential as a valuable tool for increasing knowledge of anatomy and in providing clinically useful quantitative morphological data. These uses can be applied to otology and other fields.

At this time, the computer-aided reconstruction technique has limitations. One is the time required to enter the data. Another is the large amount of computer time required to generate each shaded picture. For each limitation, the more complicated the structure, the more time required. In this study, data entry took approximately eight hours and the computer took approximately two hours to produce each view.

The graphic method is a relatively simple procedure that requires no special equipment or special knowledge of computers. It can be readily used to compare the general shape of structures from any angle. In conjunction with morphometric techniques (which are anticipated in future studies), values as reliable as those obtained from the computer can probably be obtained (but not as quickly) for the volume, surface area, and surface-to-volume ratio.

SUMMARY AND CONCLUSIONS

The computer-aided and graphic reconstruction techniques applied in this study have revealed a new anatomical feature, canaliculi, in the intermediate portion, or pars rugosa, of the endolymphatic duct system in the three studied cases. This would not have been detected without these reconstruction methods. They can be a useful research tool by providing a broader and more accurate understanding of anatomy and pathology.

Lateral and medial views of the pars rugosa of the sac show that this portion is composed of many vertical canaliculi arising predominantly from the medial side. According to their size, point of origin, and manner of ending, the canaliculi are classified as primary, secondary, and tertiary. The authors, pending further investigation, tentatively propose to rename the pars rugosa the "pars canalicularis" to reflect this multichannel system.

The computer has also been used to make volume and surface area determinations of the pars canalicularis from one endolymphatic sac. Rough estimates of volume of the pars canalicularis by direct measurement manually from the sections were determined.

Considering the anatomy, topography, and surface-to-volume ratio of this portion, the authors agree with other investigators that this portion is probably involved in the resorption of endolymph. Qualitatively, the anatomical differences of the canalicular portion are not immediately apparent in the three cases studied. However, the volume determinations indicate that the pars canalicularis may be significantly smaller and less active in Menière's disease patients than in normal persons.

The authors speculate that the endolymphatic hydrops of Menière's disease patients may at least in part be either the cause or the effect of the loss of epithelial surface area of the canalicular portion of the sac. Further investigations applying the techniques employed in this study may help to confirm this hypothesis.

ACKNOWLEDGMENTS — The authors are indebted to William F. House, MD, for his invaluable scientific advice; Shannon Brunjes, MD, and Curt Welch, for assistance in use of the Ear Research Institute computer for manuscript preparation; Diane Foster for editorial assistance; Sheila Odnert and Cynthia Smith for photographic reproductions; Julianne Grieder for illustrations; Ruth Gruelach and Agnes Ward for preparation of temporal bone sections; Susan Jones, Janetta Paladini, and Ruth Crair for typing of the manuscript; Manuel Escobedo for help with tracings; and Dale Knudsen for assistance with using the computer programs at California Institute of Technology, Pasadena, California.

REFERENCES

1. Cotugno D. De aquaeductibus auris humanae internae. 1760.

2. Boettcher A. Uber den Aqueductus Vestibuli bei Katzen und Menchen. 1869.

3. Guild SR. Observations upon the structure and normal contents of the ductus and saccus endolymphaticus in the guinea pig. Am J Anat 1927; 39:1-56.

4. Sterzi G. Il sacco endolinfatico: Ricerche anatomiche ed embriologiche. Morphol Jahrb 1909; 39:446-96.

5. Portmann G. Recherches sur le sac et le canal endolymphatiques: Sac et canal endolymphatiques du cobaye. C R Soc Biol 1919; 82:1384-7.

6. Bast TH, Anson BJ. The temporal bone and the ear. Springfield: Charles C. Thomas, 1949:43-64.

7. Born G. Die plattenmodellirmethode. Arch Mikrosk Anat Entwicklungsmech 1883; 22:584-99.

8. Zechner G, Altmann F. Histological studies on the human endolymphatic duct and sac. Pract Otol Rhinol Laryngol 1969; 31:65-83.

9. Saxén A. Histological studies of endolymph secretion and resorption in the inner ear. Acta Otolaryngol (Stockh) 1951; 40:23-31.

10. Dohlman GF. The mechanism of secretion and absorption of endolymph in the vestibular apparatus. Acta Otolaryngol (Stockh) 1965; 59:275-88.

11. Bairati A, Iurato S. The ultrastructural organization of plana semilunata. Exp Cell Res 1960; 20:77-83.

12. Borgheson E. Glandular structures in the planum semilunatum. Acta Otolaryngol (Stockh) 1961; 53:585.

13. Kimura R, Lundquist PG, Wersäll J. Secretory epithelial linings in the ampullae of the guinea pig labyrinth. Acta Otolaryngol (Stockh) 1964; 57:517-30.

14. Lundquist PG, Kimura R, Wersäll J. Ultrastructural organization of the epithelial lining in the endolymphatic duct and sac in the guinea pig. Acta Otolaryngol (Stockh) 1964; 57:65-80.

15. Silverstein H. Biochemical and physiologic studies of the endolymphatic sac in the cat. Laryngoscope 1966; 76:498-512.

16. Ishii T, Silverstein H, Balogh K Jr. Metabolic activities of the endolymphatic sac: an enzyme histochemical and autoradiographic study. Acta Otolaryngol (Stockh) 1966; 62:61-73.

17. House WF. Menière's disease: management and theory. Otolaryngol Clin North Am 1975; 8:515-35.

18. Hallpike CS, Cairns H. Observations on the pathology of Menière's syndrome. J Laryngol Otol 1938; 53:625-55.

19. Wolff D. The pathology of Cogan's syndrome causing profound deafness. Ann Otol Rhinol Laryngol 1965; 74:507-20.

20. Kimura RS, Schuknecht HF, Ota CY, Jones DD. Obliteration of the ductus reuniens. Acta Otolaryngol (Stockh) 1980; 89:295-309.

21. Kimura RS. Experimental blockage of the endolymphatic duct and sac and its effects on the inner ear of the guinea pig: a study on endolymphatic hydrops. Ann Otol Rhinol Laryngol 1967; 76:664-87.

22. Schuknecht HF, Northrop C, Igarashi M. Cochlear pathology after destruction of the endolymphatic sac in the cat. Acta Otolaryngol (Stockh) 1968; 65:479-87.

23. Kimura RS, Schuknecht HF. Membranous hydrops in the inner ear of the guinea pig after obliteration of the endolymphatic sac. Pract Otorhinolaryngol (Basel) 1965; 27:343-54.

24. Fick IA van N. Sacculotomy for hydrops. Laryngoscope 1965; 75:1539-46.

25. Fick IA van N. Ménière's disease: aetiology and new surgical approach: sacculotomy. J Laryngol Otol 1966; 80:288-306.

26. Shambaugh GE Jr. Decompression of the endolymphatic sac. Otolaryngol Clin North Am 1968; 1:613-21.

27. Shea JJ. Teflon film drainage of the endolymphatic sac. Arch Otolaryngol 1966; 83:316-9.

28. Paparella MM, Hanson DG. Endolymphatic sac drainage for intractable vertigo: method and experiences. Laryngoscope 1976; 86:697-703.

29. House WF. Subarachnoid shunt for draining of hydrops: a preliminary report. Laryngoscope 1962; 72:713-29.

30. House WF. Subarachnoid shunt for draining of hydrops: a report of 146 cases. Laryngoscope 1965; 75:1547-51.

31. Gaunt WA, Gaunt PN. Three dimensional reconstruction in biology. Baltimore: University Park Press, 1978.

32. Sjöstrand FS. A search for the circuitry of directional selectivity and neural adaptation through three-dimensional analysis of the outer plexiform layer of the rabbit retina. J Ultrastruct Res 1974; 49:60-156.

33. Fox J, Galey F, Wayland H. Action of histamine on the mesenteric vasculature. Microvasc Res 1980; 19:108-26.

34. Shantz MJ. Description and classification of neuronal structures in the frog retina. Doctoral thesis, California Institute of Technology, Pasadena, 1976.

35. Shantz MJ, McCann GD. Computational morphology: three-dimensional computer graphics for electron microscopy. Trans Biomed Eng 25:99-103.

36. Arenberg KI, Andersen HR. The surgical anatomy of the endolymphatic sac. Arch Otolaryngol 1977; 103:1-11.

37. Yuen S, Schuknecht HF. Vestibular aqueduct and endolymphatic duct in Menière's disease. Arch Otolaryngol 1972; 96:553-5.

38. Clemis JD, Valvassori GE. Recent radiographic and clinical observations on the vestibular aqueduct. A preliminary report. Otolaryngol Clin North Am 1968; 1:339-46.

39. Egami T, Sando I. Pathology of the vestibular aqueduct and endolymphatic sac in temporal bones with endolymphatic hydrops. In: Hood JD, ed. Vestibular mechanisms in health and disease. London: Academic Press, 1978:122-8.

40. Alford BR. Menière's disease: criteria for diagnosis and evaluation of therapy for reporting. Trans Am Acad Ophthalmol Otolaryngol 1972; 76:1462-4.

AMINOGLYCOSIDE OTOTOXICITY FOLLOWING MIDDLE EAR INJECTION

Michael D. Rudnick, PhD

Irwin A. Ginsberg, MD

Pamela S. Huber, MS

Supplement 77 — Vol. 89, November-December, 1980, No. 6, Part 4

THE ANNALS OF OTOLOGY, RHINOLOGY & LARYNGOLOGY

ACKNOWLEDGMENTS

The authors would like to acknowledge the substantive advice given by Werner K. Noell, MD, Department of Physiology, Division of Neurobiology, and Robert G. Summers, Jr., PhD, Department of Anatomical Sciences at The State University of New York at Buffalo, School of Medicine. We are also indebted to Richard R. Gacek, MD, Chairman, Department of Otolaryngology, State University of New York at Syracuse, College of Medicine; members of The Buffalo Otological Group, Buffalo, New York; and James D. Sedwick for their technical guidance in the development of this project. A special thanks belongs to Mrs. Pamela Filipski for her editorial typing, her assistance in the composition of the illustrations and her sustaining good humor.

This work was made possible through grants provided by The Gebbie Foundation, The James H. Cummings Foundation, The Western New York Foundation, and The W.J. Connors Foundation. We sincerely wish to thank them for their support and patient understanding.

THE ANNALS PUBLISHING COMPANY
4949 FOREST PARK BLVD.
ST. LOUIS, MISSOURI 63108

AMINOGLYCOSIDE OTOTOXICITY FOLLOWING MIDDLE EAR INJECTION

MICHAEL D. RUDNICK, PhD

IRWIN A. GINSBERG, MD

PAMELA S. HUBER, MS

BUFFALO, NEW YORK

From The Hearing Foundation of Buffalo, 897 Delaware Avenue, Buffalo, NY 14209.

Presented as part of Dr. Rudnick's doctoral dissertation to the Department of Anatomical Sciences, State University of New York at Buffalo, New York.

PREFACE

The well-established vestibulotoxicity of streptomycin following systemic administration has been exploited toward vestibular ablation in patients with intractable bilateral recurrent vertigo. A more direct approach toward vestibular ablation is needed for the patient with unilateral disease. This four-part study examines the methodology for transtympanic drug injection; establishes an anatomical criterion and a quantitative analytical technique for measuring drug effects; documents the comparative ototoxicities of streptomycin, dihydrostreptomycin and neomycin; and finally, explores the effect of vestibular stimulation on selective ototoxicity. The results are compared to those reported following systemic administration and the implications of the results are discussed in regard to hypotheses of the mechanism of selective ototoxicity.

CONTENTS

AMINOGLYCOSIDE OTOTOXICITY FOLLOWING MIDDLE EAR INJECTION

I. Experimental Approach and Histological Criteria for Evaluating Drug Effects. Michael D. Rudnick, PhD, Irwin A. Ginsberg, MD, Pamela S. Huber, MS 1

II. Quantitative Analytical Procedure. Michael D. Rudnick, PhD, Irwin A. Ginsberg, MD, Pamela S. Huber, MS, in cooperation with Joel S. Rose, MA 10

III. Comparative Quantitative Analysis. Irwin A. Ginsberg, MD, Michael D. Rudnick, PhD, Pamela S. Huber, MS 17

IV. Influence of Vestibular Stimulation. Pamela S. Huber, MS, Irwin A. Ginsberg, MD, Michael D. Rudnick, PhD 25

AMINOGLYCOSIDE OTOTOXICITY FOLLOWING MIDDLE EAR INJECTION

I. EXPERIMENTAL APPROACH AND HISTOLOGICAL CRITERIA FOR EVALUATING DRUG EFFECTS

MICHAEL D. RUDNICK, PhD

IRWIN A. GINSBERG, MD

PAMELA S. HUBER, MS

BUFFALO, NEW YORK

The rationale and methodology for transtympanic drug injection have been established. By the use of phase contrast and Normarski differential interference contrast microscopy to study "surface preparations" of both cochlear and vestibular sensory structures, the degenerative cellular changes which resulted from the localized administration of aminoglycoside antibiotics have been examined toward the selection of an anatomical criterion for the measurement of ototoxicity. The "collapse" cell has been selected for this purpose because of its positive identification, persistence and inability to recover.

Recurrent vertigo is one of the more incapacitating symptoms resulting from inner ear disease for which effective therapy is not available. Eliminating vestibular function either bilaterally or unilaterally can very effectively control the symptoms of vertigo. Bilateral vestibular ablation can be accomplished by systemic streptomycin administration, although not without some risk to hearing. Unilateral vestibular ablation is more difficult to obtain when preservation of residual hearing is desired. Those procedures which are designed to preserve hearing are not uniformly successful and a more reliable approach to selective ablation of vestibular function is needed. It is this need which prompted the present study.

Streptomycin is more selectively toxic to the vestibular system, while dihydrostreptomycin is more toxic to the cochlea when administered systemically. It was hoped that a way could be found to exploit this difference in specificity, the ultimate goal being to find or develop a drug which would have absolute selectivity for the vestibular apparatus.

Aminoglycoside ototoxicity has been studied for over 30 years. The usual approach has been that of systemic injections followed by a morphological qualitative analysis of the effects on the sensory cells of the inner ear. The majority of such studies was limited to observations of the sensory cells of the organ of Corti, eg, those of Kohonen and Tarkkanen[1] and Kacker.[2] Other studies considered only the vestibular system, eg, those of Wersäll and Hawkins,[3] Spoendlin,[4] and Watanuki and Meyer zum Gottesberge,[5] while relatively few studies considered both compartments of the inner ear.[6-16] However, none of these studies can be considered both quantitative and comparative. Nonetheless, it is apparent that each member of the aminoglycoside family of drugs exerts a different effect on inner ear sensory structures — different in terms of degree and different in terms of topographical distribution. Although not without equivocal or contradictory results, the weight of these reports indicates that following systemic administration, dihydrostreptomycin, kanamycin, and neomycin are primarily cochleotoxic; streptomycin, vestibulotoxic; and gentamicin, toxic in both compartments.[8,17,18]

There are no comparative data available to document the specific ototoxicities of aminoglycoside antibiotics on sensory structures in the inner ear when administered transtympanically, that is, when applied directly into the middle ear space. However, several animal studies[12] and clinical trials[6,7] employed streptomycin via this approach to achieve unilateral vestibular ablation. The several reports in which other aminoglycoside antibiotics were locally administered either clinically[19] or experimentally[20-22] have produced few insights into the comparative effects of locally applied drugs. At best, these studies indicate that the effects of drugs may differ when applied locally versus systemically.[5-7,23] It is an important goal of this study to document the effects of transtympanically applied aminoglycoside antibiotics and to compare them with those reported for the systemic application.

The results of this investigation are reported in four parts. In part I, the standard procedure for transtympanic drug administration is presented and some of the histological findings discussed. The effects of streptomycin, dihydrostreptomycin and neomycin are evaluated toward the selection of an anatomical criterion with which ototoxicity can be measured. In part II, the method of data collection and the quantitative analytical procedure is established. In addition, factors contributing to skewed results are identified statistically and experimental animals are eliminated on a rational basis. The tools derived in parts I and II are applied in part III to a

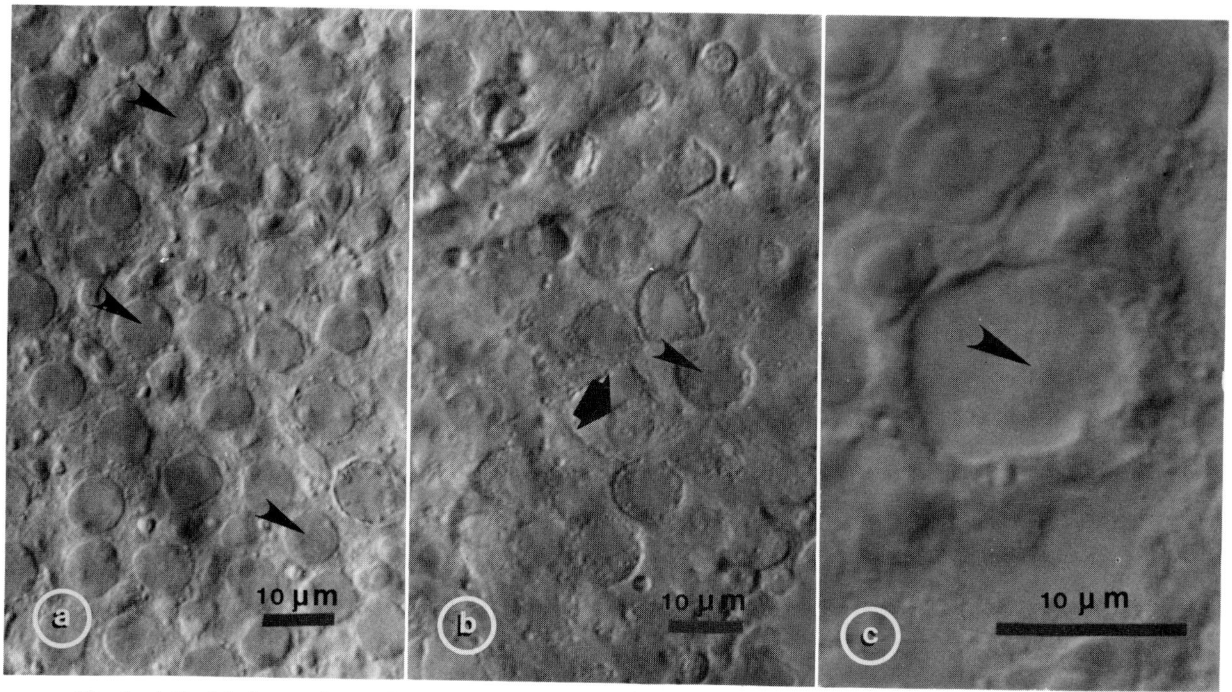

Fig. 1. a) Nuclei of normal macula sacculi sensory cells (arrowheads). b) Pyknotic nucleus (arrow) in a shrunken cell. Note the translucent cytoplasm under the arrow. The arrowhead identifies a normal sensory cell and nucleus. Lateral crista ampullaris, 10 mg dihydrostreptomycin. c) Cell at arrowhead is swollen and translucent. No nucleus can be distinguished in this cell. Macula sacculi, 50 mg streptomycin.

comparative quantitative analysis of the ototoxicities of streptomycin, dihydrostreptomycin and neomycin relative to each other and to the various regions within the inner ear. It has been reported that cochear stimulation enhances membrane permeability in that compartment.[24] We hypothesize that for this reason appropriate stimulation would potentiate the effects of aminoglycosides on sensory cells in the vestibular system. This hypothesis is tested in part IV. The experimental animals used in part I are included in part II. Those animals which survived the eliminations reported in part II appear for analysis in part III. Part IV reports on a subgroup of the neomycin-treated guinea pigs which are analyzed as one group in part III.

METHODS

Animals. Thirty-three pigmented guinea pigs of both sexes weighing between 300 and 500 gm were used in this study. Prior to treatment experimental animals were selected on the basis of a steady weight gain, otoscopic examination, Preyer's reflex and gait. Animals noted to have evidence of infection (pus, or squamous or fibrous metaplasia) in the middle or inner ear at the time of sacrifice were eliminated from the study. Animals were anesthetized by intraperitoneal injection of sodium pentobarbital,* 30 mg/kg diluted to 30% with Hanks' balanced salt solution.

Middle Ear Injection. The tympanic membrane was visualized by aligning the visual path of a Zeiss operating microscope with a speculum clamped into a Shea speculum holder† which also served to restrain the animals. A tuberculin syringe with a 30 gauge, 12 cm needle was attached to a micromanipulator. The needle was bent to a 45° angle near its base in order to displace the syringe and micromanipulator from the optical path. The syringe, needle and saline were sterilized before use.

The needle was adjusted for penetration of the posteroinferior quadrant of the tympanic membrane. The needle was then advanced to the medial wall of the middle ear. Over a period of 7-12 seconds, 0.1 cc of antibiotic in saline was injected. A successful injection was evidenced by the visualization of fluid approaching, but not reaching, the puncture in the tympanic membrane. In each case the right ear was approached first. Occasionally, the full 0.1 cc could not be injected into the middle ear. In these cases the injectant was removed and the left ear attempted. If the left ear injection was unsuccessful, that animal was deleted from the study. The animal was next supported, injected side up, for three hours in a cradle designed to elevate the snout 45° in order to minimize the escape of fluid through the auditory tube[25] and to insure that the injectant pooled over both the round and oval windows.

Tissue Preparation. One week after injection (with the exception of three animals which were allowed four weeks for recovery) the guinea pigs were sacrificed by decapitation and their temporal bones processed by the "surface specimen" technique[26] with the following modifications: prior to fixation the temporal bones were incubated for 20 minutes at 37 C in a buffer solution originally intended for succinic dehydrogenase histochemistry.[5] It consisted of 0.06M sodium succinate, 0.2M phosphate buffer (pH 7.4) and Ringer's solution in a 2:2:1 ratio. In preparation for this incubation the osseous labyrinth was opened widely, particularly over the ampullae. We discovered that this incubation facilitated

TABLE 1. INJECTION SCHEDULE

Drug and Recovery Period		*Number of Guinea Pigs Receiving Each Dosage*					
		Dosage in Mg					
		0	*10*	*25*	*50*	*100*	*Subtotal*
Streptomycin	1 wk	—	0	3	3	3	9
Streptomycin	4 wk	—	0	0	3	0	3
Dihydrostreptomycin	1 wk	—	0	3	3	3	9
Neomycin	1 wk	—	3	3	3	0	9
Saline	1 wk	3	—	—	—	—	3
Total animals in study							33

*Diabutal®, Diamond Laboratories, Des Moines, Iowa.

†V. Mueller, Chicago, Ill.

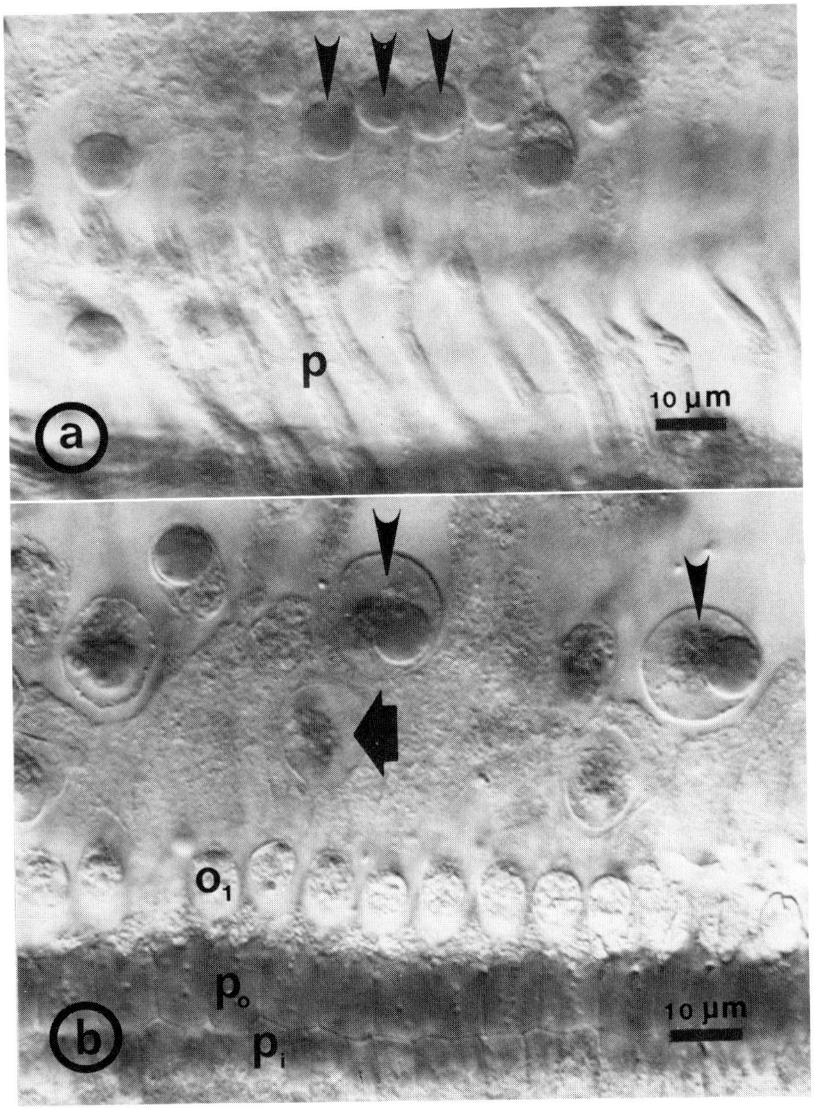

Fig. 2. a) Three normal first row outer hair cell nuclei are indicated (arrowheads). Compare the width of these cells to those in b (arrowheads). P - Bodies of outer pillar cells. b) Arrowheads identify swollen third row outer hair cells. A pyknotic nucleus is also included (arrow). Notice that the cytoplasm of the swollen and pyknotic cells contain areas deficient in internal structure. These cells are considered translucent unlike the normal cell bodies of first row outer hair cells (O_1). P_o - Head of outer pillar cell; P_i — Head of inner pillar cell. Organ of Corti, 3.5 turn, 25 mg dihydrostreptomycin.

the subsequent microdissection of vestibular structures by allowing the easier separation of sensory epithelia from the underlying connective tissue and nerve fibers.

Following incubation the temporal bones were immersed in 10% neutralized, buffered formalin and refrigerated for at least two days. Subsequent preparation proceeded as described by Hawkins and Johnsson.[26] All sensory structures of the 66 temporal bones were analyzed under dark phase contrast microscopy. Preparations were also studied and photographed with Nomarski differential interference contrast optics.[27,28]

Injection Schedule. The animals were divided into five experimental groups. One of the drugs (streptomycin,* dihydrostreptomycin* or neomycin†) or saline was administered once to each animal according to the schedule in Table 1. The opposite ears of the animals were not injected and, therefore, served as internal controls.

RESULTS

During microdissection certain sensory structures fragmented as if brittle, making it very difficult to obtain good preparations. The degree of fragility was evaluated subjectively and recorded for possible correlation with other morphological changes at the cellular level. It was found that fragmentation often occurred in areas of high cellular damage. This was easily demonstrated in the organ of Corti. The vestibular structures, being less regularly organized, fragmented along less well-defined lines.

All sensory cells considered abnormal had damaged nuclei. Pyknosis was usually encountered in these cells (compare Fig. 1a to 1b; 2a to 2b). Often, especially at low drug concentrations, this was the only apparent abnormality. In cells where other changes were noted the nuclear aberrations were more pronounced and included clumping of chromatin, deep invaginations of the nuclear membrane, fragmentation, or total loss of nuclear remnants

*Sigma Chemical Corp, St. Louis, Mo.

†Schwarz/Mann, Orangeberg, NY.

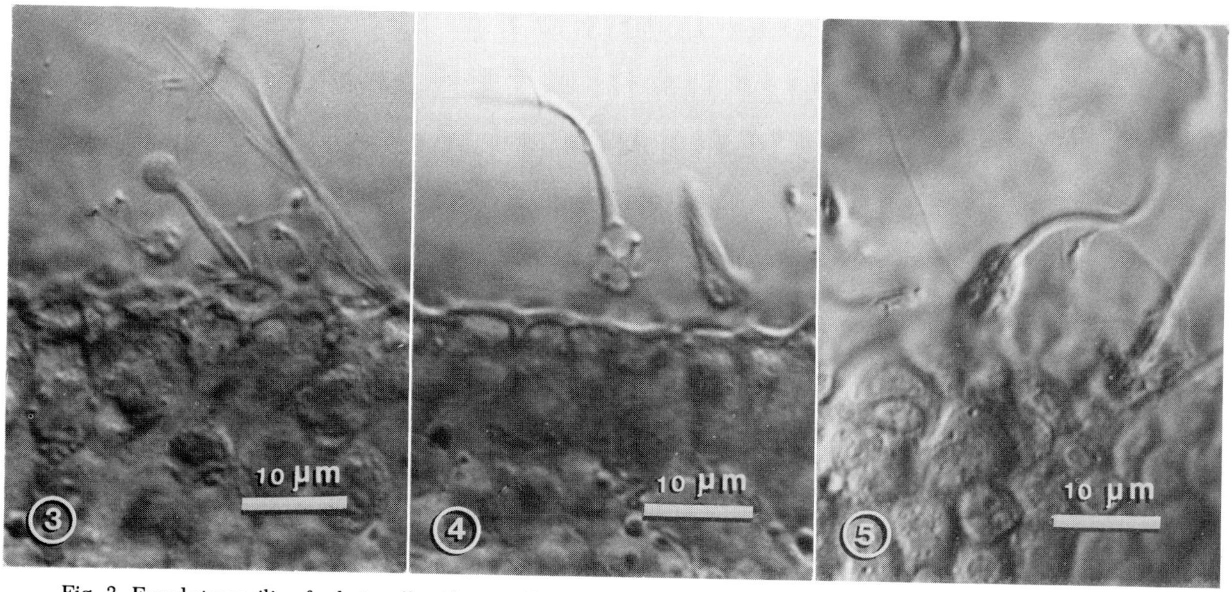

Fig. 3. Fused stereocilia of a hair cell with a swelling or bleb at the distal end. Macula utriculi, 50 mg streptomycin.

Figs. 4 and 5. Large blebs projecting into the endolymphatic space from the luminal surface of hair cells. Note the fused stereocilia projecting from the blebs. Optical sectioning confirms the continuity of stereocilia, blebs and sensory cells. Posterior crista ampullaris, 50 mg streptomycin.

(Fig. 1c). In this study the nucleus appeared to be the first organelle to show signs of ototoxic damage at the light microscopic level.

In drug-treated animals the stereocilia presented a variety of morphologies ranging from completely normal to total absence (Figs. 3-5). However, such changes could be related neither to the drug employed nor to its dosage. Even the presence or absence of stereocilia was an inconsistent finding in this investigation. It was found that cells in control specimens, anatomically sound in other respects, were sometimes devoid of stereocilia.

Concomitant with the profound nuclear changes were three phenomena which suggested a sequence

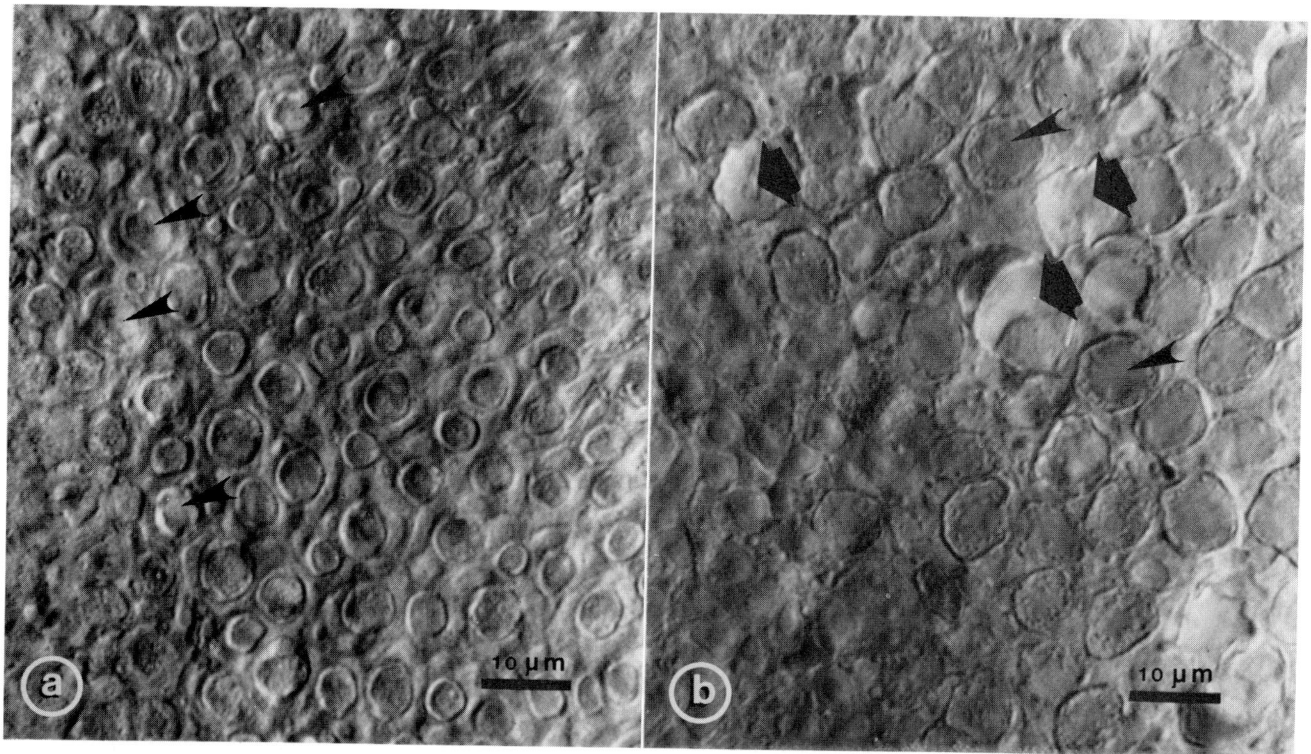

Fig. 6. a) Apical surface of the macula shows several translucent cells (arrowheads). b) At the level of sensory cell nuclei translucency is more apparent and the cells seem slightly swollen (arrows) compared to the adjacent normal cells (arrowheads). Macula utriculi, 50 mg streptomycin.

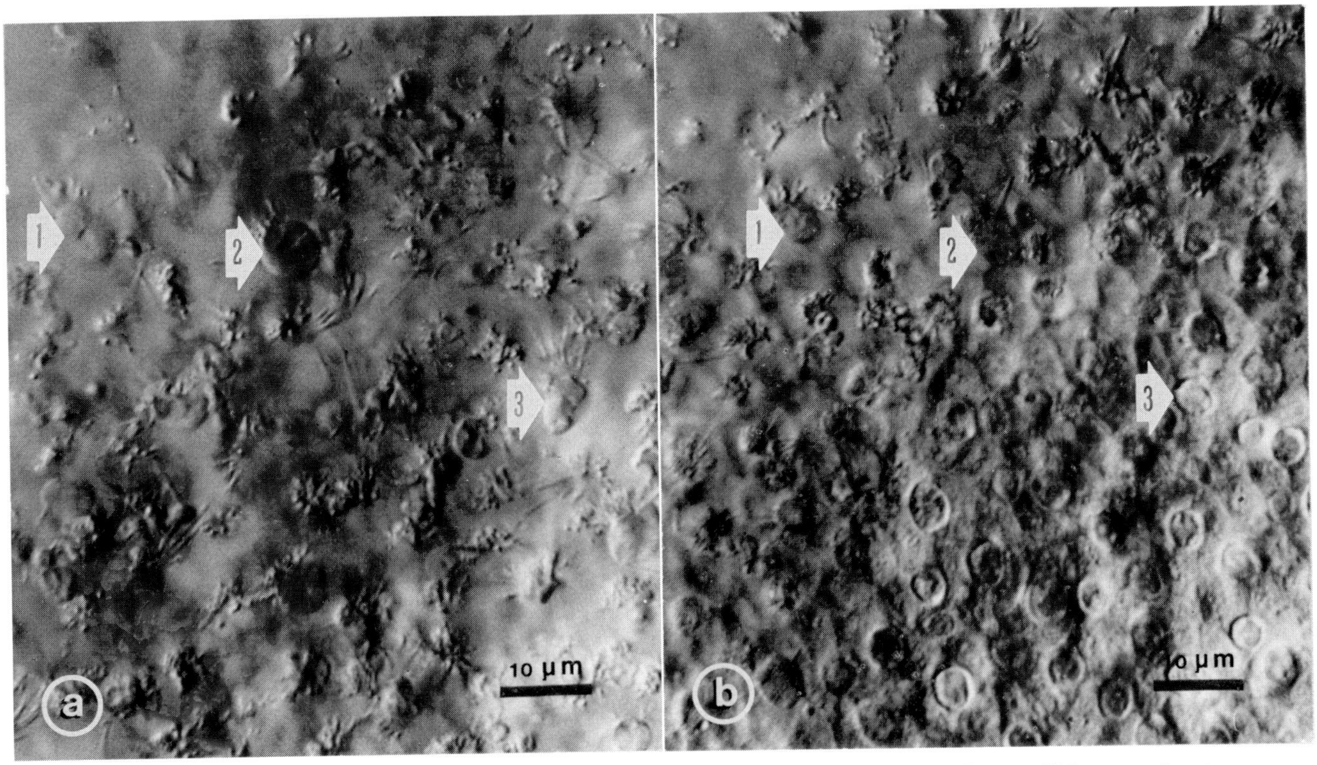

Fig. 7. a, b) Two focal levels of a macula treated with dihydrostreptomycin (50 mg) to illustrate blebs protruding into the endolymphatic space from the apical surfaces of sensory cells. Numbered arrows identify corresponding locations in a and b. Notice that the stereocilia of cells 1 and 2 are oriented at approximately 11 o'clock to the blebs. This orientation reflects the polarization of the free surface (see text). Cell 3 is translucent, which is a common association with blebs.

leading to cell death: a) cellular translucency, b) cellular swelling or "bleb" formation, and c) cellular lysis. In the cochlea, translucent cells were frequently swollen (Fig. 2b). However, in the vestibular system translucent cells did not appear to swell as greatly (Fig. 6) but, instead, gave rise to "blebs" or pouches of cell membrane which extended from the apical surface of sensory cells into the endolymphatic space (Fig. 7).[3,4,12,29,30] These may appear as a small bubble at the cell surface, a single drop-shaped evagination reaching several micrometers into the endolymphatic space (Fig. 7) or rarely, as a bag nearly equal in size to the cell from which its arises. It is interesting to note that these blebs almost always emerged from the noncuticular or kinociliary pole of the sensory cell surface.

The "stellate," "spider," "scar," or "collapse" cell was considered to be the final stage of degeneration wherein a cell could still be recognized as having been a sensory cell.[31] Viewed at the level of the apical membrane of the cell, its appearance resembled that of an unevenly tightened drumhead and might represent the collapsed surface of a ruptured sensory cell (Figs. 8-10).[2,29,31] The cell bodies of many of these cells had irregular outlines and appeared somewhat shrunken (Figs. 1b and 6b). The collapse cell stage is apparently the most persistent morphological stage that a damaged sensory cell dwells in before complete removal and replacement by expansion of the contiguous supporting cells (Figs. 8b and 10). By four weeks postinjection, the tissues have apparently stabilized. The remaining sensory cells appeared healthy as did the supporting cells, many of which were hypertrophied to fill in the spaces vacated by degenerated sensory cells (Fig. 11).

Generally, the severity of cell changes and the proportion of cells showing these changes increased with the increase in dosage of each drug. It is also to be noted that regardless of which drug was administered, the morphological alterations always appeared the same. In fact, the only way to distinguish the antibiotics on the basis of their morphological effects was by the specific topographical distribution of damaged cells. This finding is thoroughly investigated in part III of this study.[32]

All 36 control ears were within normal limits morphologically. That is, no more than 3% of the sensory cells in any region of the inner ear showed the structural aberrations just described. Previous experience with young guinea pigs has disclosed that this is the normal background level of "spontaneous" degeneration. The most basal segment of the organ of Corti, or "hook" region, showed rather high, though variable, damage which failed to correlate with drug dosage. In fact, control ears often showed pathology well in excess of 3% within this region.

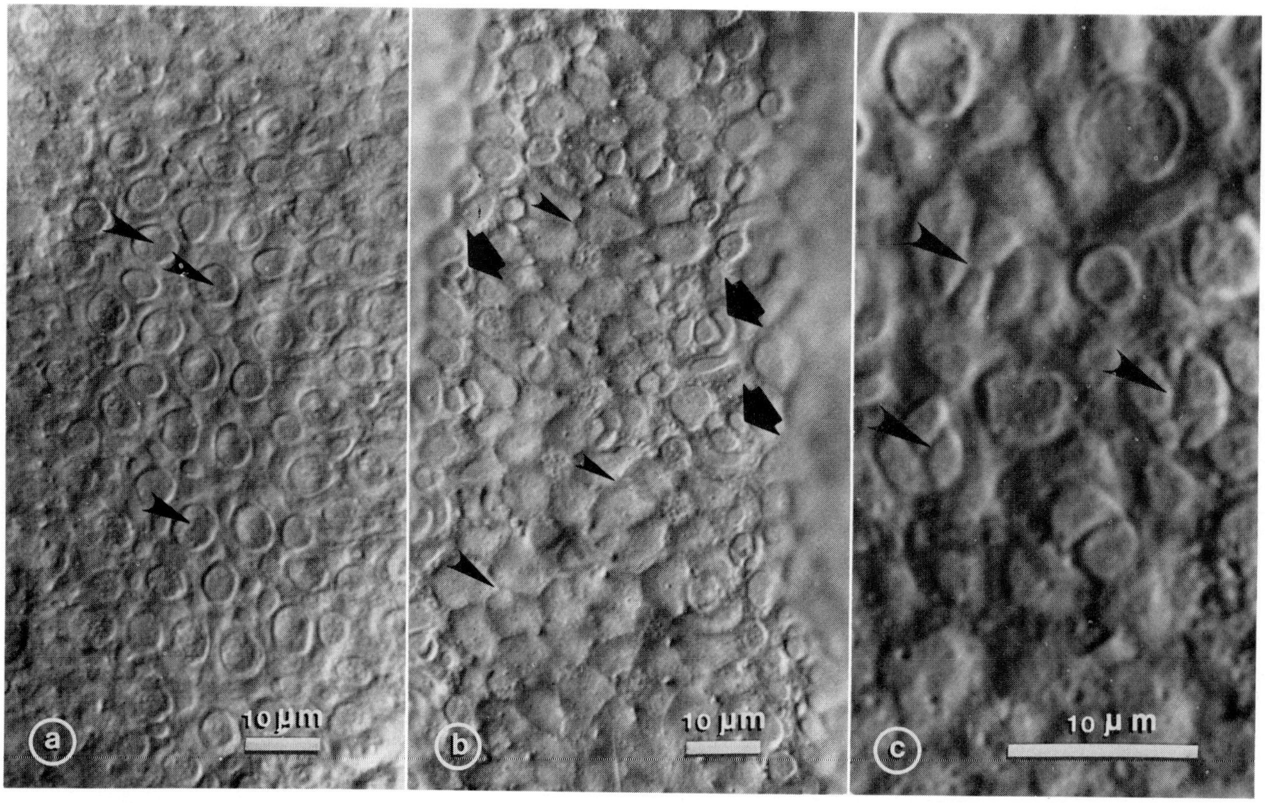

Fig. 8. a) Apical surface of normal macula sacculi sensory cells (arrowheads). b) Dihydrostreptomycin (100 mg)-treated lateral crista ampullaris, crest region. Arrows indicate collapse cells. Arrowheads denote areas where supporting cells have replaced degenerated sensory cells. c) Collapse cells (arrowheads) of dihydrostreptomycin (50 mg)-treated macula sacculi.

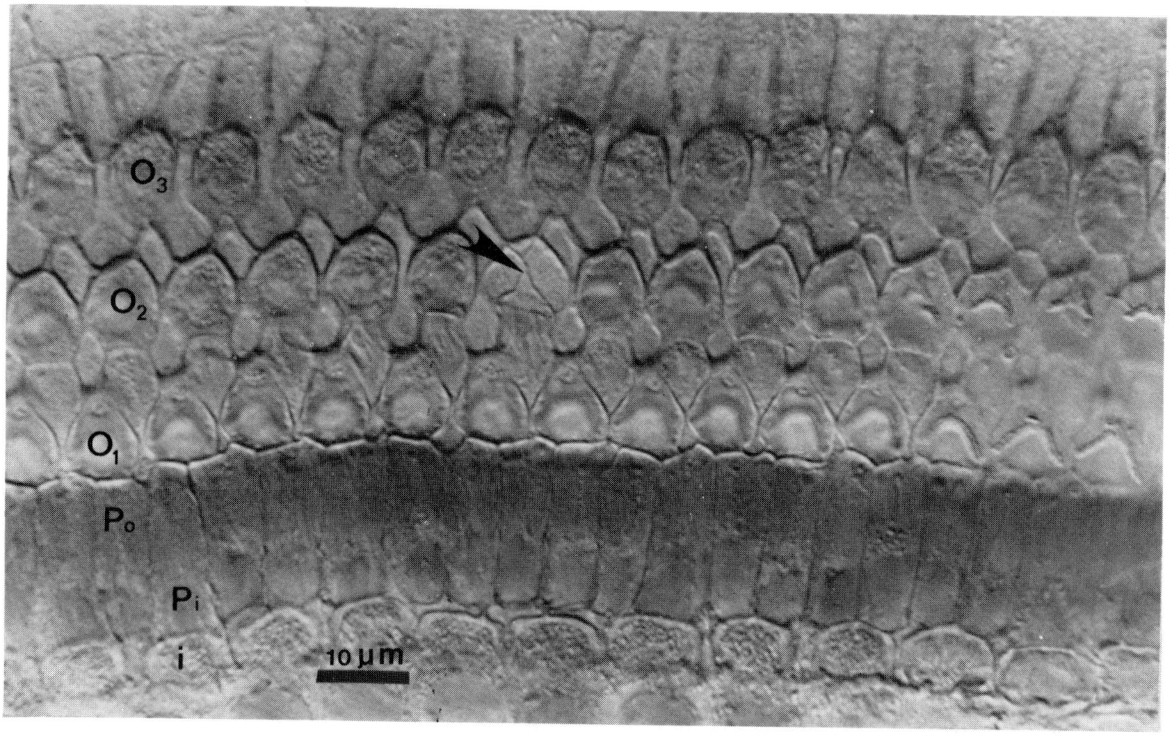

Fig. 9. Organ of Corti (3.5 turn) of a streptomycin (50 mg)-treated guinea pig. Arrowhead indicates a collapse cell. i - Inner hair cell row; O_1, O_2, O_3 - Rows of outer hair cells; P_i and P_o - Heads of inner and outer pillar cells.

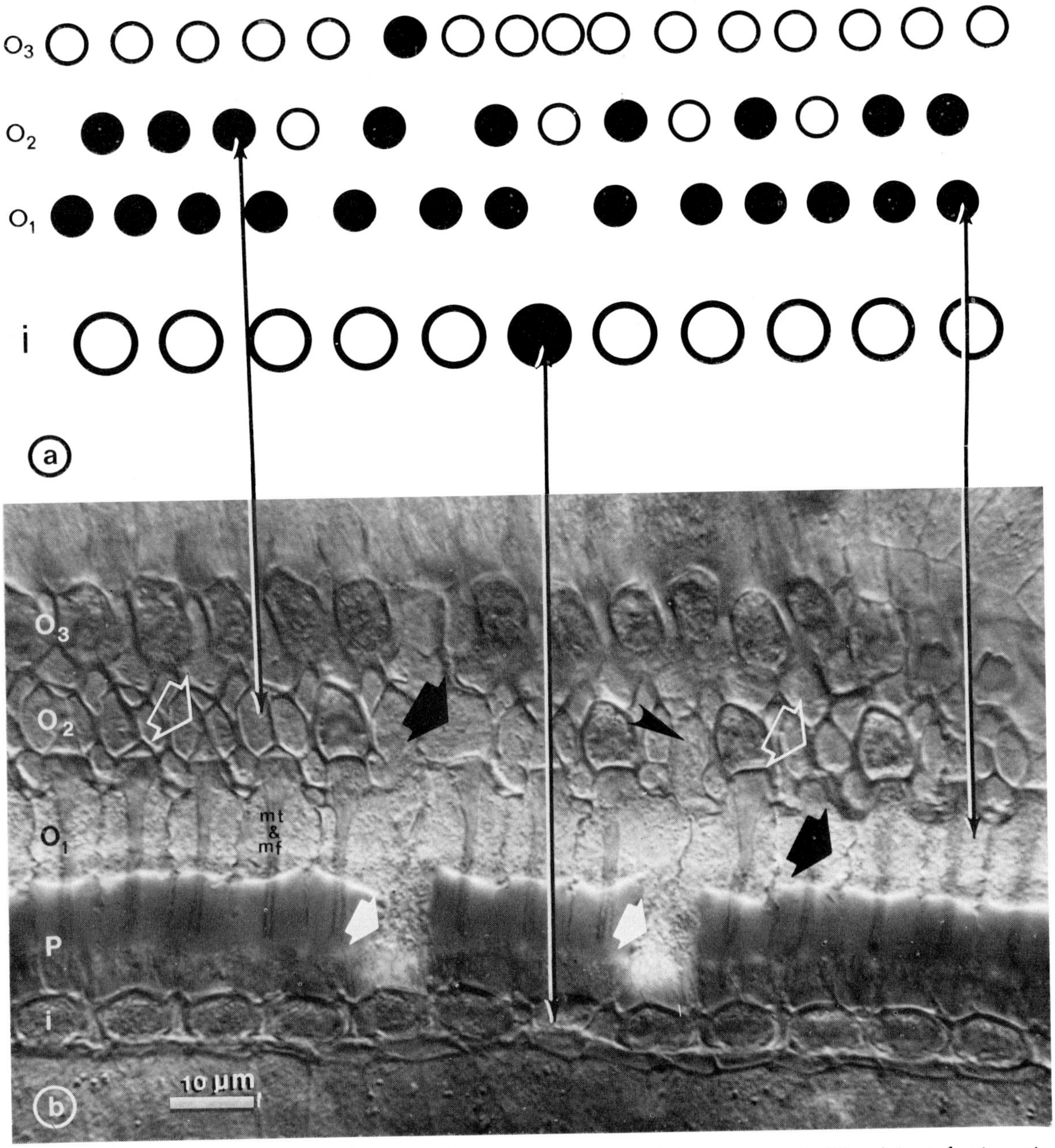

Fig. 10. Cochleogram and micrograph of the organ of Corti (2.5 turn) from a neomycin (10 mg)-treated guinea pig which illustrates the use of collapse cells (open white arrows) and phalangeal scars (solid black arrows) in mapping cellular damage. Observe the head of an outer pillar cell forming a scar at the site of a degenerating second row outer hair cell (arrowhead). All first row outer hair cells (O_1) have been replaced by phalangeal scars. Solid white arrows mark the positions of degenerated pillar cells. i - Inner hair cell row; O_1, O_2, and O_3 - Rows of outer hair cells; P - Heads of pillar cells; mt & mf - Microtubules and microfilaments.

DISCUSSION

The systemic administration of aminoglycoside antibiotics for the ablation of vestibular sensory cells has been suggested for the treatment of recurrent bilateral vertigo. However, vertigo usually presents unilaterally. In the case of streptomycin, only a slight proclivity for the afflicted side has been reported following systemic injections[33] and, therefore, systemic injections may compromise the normal ear. In addition, the possibility exists that other systems may be disturbed as, for example, the kidneys. An alternative approach is the application of these drugs directly into the labyrinth. However, this too is unacceptable since it carries with it significant surgical risk and expense.[34]

Transtympanic administration is a simple, low risk technique which restricts treatment to the diseased ear of patients with unilateral involvement. From the experimental point of view, the uninjected ear serves as an excellent internal control for determining whether pathology existed prior to treatment and for insuring that treatment is indeed restricted to the injected side.

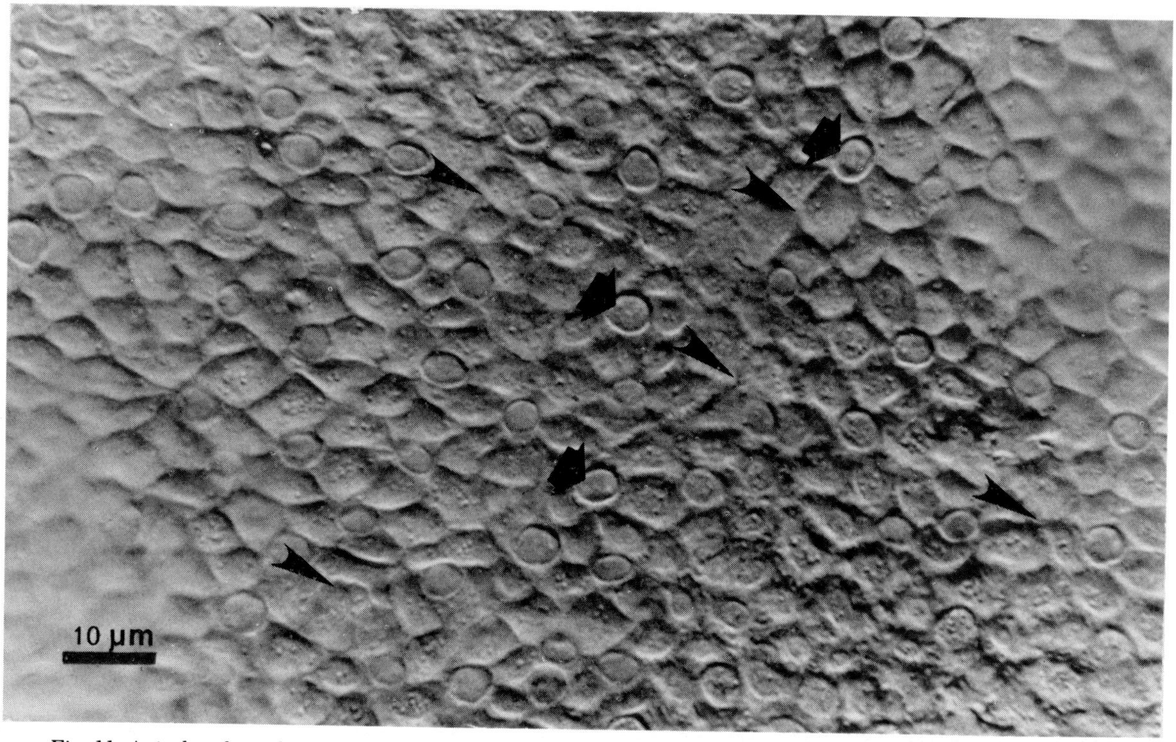

Fig. 11. Apical surface of a streptomycin (50 mg)-treated macula sacculi obtained four weeks postinjection. Although no collapse cells are observed, the density of hair cells (arrows) is diminished. Supporting cells have replaced degenerated hair cells whose positions may be assumed (arrowheads) from experience with the normal "pattern" of vestibular sensory and supporting cells.

If ototoxicity is measured by counting degenerated sensory cells, the vestibular sensory structures would be recorded as normal four weeks after treatment since all of the damaged cells had either recovered or been replaced by hypertrophied supporting cells.[12,35] With the exception of a lower sensory cell density (compare Fig. 8a to Fig. 11), the apparently normal appearance of the tissue at four weeks could give the false impression of low sensitivity to the drug. Although a regular pattern of sensory cells does not exist in the vestibular system, generally each sensory cell is surrounded by about four to six supporting cells and each supporting cell usually contacts at least one sensory cell. Observation of this "pattern" only suggests the position previously occupied by a sensory cell. At a one-week postinjection recovery time, supporting cell hypertrophy is minimized and the maximum number of damaged cells can be observed in the terminal stages of degeneration. For this reason, a one-week recovery period appears to be an optimum period for this type of study.[5] The organ of Corti presents no problem in this regard because the position of each sensory cell is preserved in its row following cell death and replacement by a "phalangeal scar."[35]

The incubation of temporal bone specimens following decapitation instead of their rapid fixation has undoubtedly led to qualitative effects on the tissues. The most positive of these is the facilitation of vestibular microdissection, so essential to this and future studies of this neuroepithelium. Differences in our observations of these sensory structures from those of earlier investigators were likely a result of this incubation. However, since our goal was to select a reliable morphological criterion for the measurement of ototoxicity, and not to document the effects of aminoglycoside antibiotics on hair cells per se, these differences were not of great importance to the present investigation.

The various morphologies of the stereocilia[2,29,31,36] and the fragility of tissue[2,37] were inconsistent from trial to trial, correlated poorly, if at all, with drug dosage, and were sometimes observed in control tissues. These observations may have resulted from mechanical trauma during tissue preparation and/or from an increased lability of these structures acquired during incubation. Whatever the cause, both the fragility of the tissues and the appearance of the stereocilia were considered unreliable measures of ototoxicity. The nucleus also presented an array of changes which, when arranged in a logical sequence, suggested a progression leading to cell death. However, when compared to concomitant alterations at the cell surface, it became uncertain as to what constituted a terminal nucleus. Collapse cells, which we judge to represent the end-stage of degeneration, were accompanied by nuclei representing the range of morphologies. Because of this uncertainty, the nucleus is also considered an unreliable structure for the evaluation of ototoxicity. The nuclear changes, cellular translucency, cellular swelling, bleb formation and the collapsed appearance of the apical surface of hair cells were all findings limited almost exclusively to the sensory cells of experimental ears. Since both experimental and control tissues underwent the same incubation, we feel confident that these observations were attributable to the drugs tested in this study.

The intact supporting elements constitute a stable matrix for the sensory cells.[2] Presumably, the hair cells undergo lysis and their ruptured corpses are witnessed as collapse cells. It is difficult to imagine such a cell regaining its vitality, and so, due to its relatively long persistence and easy identification, the collapse cell is adopted as the cell form best suited for the measurement of ototoxicity. In the following papers all observations of ototoxicity are based upon numerical comparisons of normal hair cells to collapse cells.

REFERENCES

1. Kohonen A, Tarkkanen J. Cochlear damage from ototoxic antibiotics by intratympanic application. Acta Otolaryngol (Stockh) 1969; 68:90-7.

2. Kacker SK. Neomycin-induced spiral organ degeneration in the guinea pig. Laryngoscope 1970; 80:391-9.

3. Wersäll J, Hawkins JE Jr. Vestibular sensory epithelia in the cat labyrinth and their reactions in chronic streptomycin intoxication. Acta Otolaryngol (Stockh) 1962; 54:1-23.

4. Spoendlin H. Ototoxizität des streptomyzins. Pract Oto-Rhino-Laryngol 1966; 28:305-22.

5. Watanuki K, Meyer zum Gottesberge A. Toxic effects of streptomycin and kanamycin upon the sensory epithelium of the crista ampullaris. Acta Otolaryngol (Stockh) 1971; 72:59-67.

6. Schuknecht HF. Ablation therapy for the relief of Meniere's disease. Laryngoscope 1950; 66:859-70.

7. Schuknecht HF. Ablation therapy in the management of Ménière's disease. Acta Otolaryngol (Stockh) 1957; Suppl 132.

8. McGee TM, Olszewski J. Streptomycin sulfate and dihydrostreptomycin toxicity. Arch Otolaryngol 1962; 75:295-311.

9. Farkashidy J, Black RG, Briant TDR. Effect of kanamycin on the internal ear: an electrophysiological and electron microscopic study. Laryngoscope 1963; 73:713-27.

10. Duvall AJ, Wersäll J. Site of action of streptomycin upon inner ear sensory cells. Acta Otolaryngol (Stockh) 1964; 57:581-98.

11. Hawkins JE Jr, Johnsson LG, Aran JM. Comparative tests of gentamicin ototoxicity. J Infect Dis 1969; 119:417-31.

12. Lindeman HH. Regional differences in sensitivity of the vestibular sensory epithelia to ototoxic antibiotics. Acta Otolaryngol (Stockh) 1969; 67:177-89.

13. Wersäll J, Lundquist PG, Björkroth B. Ototoxicity of gentamicin. J Infect Dis 1969; 119:410-6.

14. Webster JC, McGee TM, Carrol R, Benitez JT, Williams ML. Ototoxicity of gentamicin. Histopathologic and functional results in the cat. Trans Am Acad Ophthalmol Otolaryngol 1970; 74:1155-65.

15. Igarashi M, Lundquist PG, Alford BR, Miyata H. Experimental ototoxicity of gentamicin in squirrel monkeys. J Infect Dis 1971; 124 Suppl: S114-24.

16. Gonzalez G, Miller N, Wasilewski V. Progressive neuro-ototoxicity of kanamycin. Ann Otol Rhinol Laryngol 1972; 81:127-31.

17. Sheffield PA, Turner JS Jr. Ototoxic drugs: a review of clinical aspects, histopathologic changes and mechanisms of action. South Med J 1971; 64:359-63.

18. Hawkins JE Jr. Ototoxic mechanisms. Audiology 1973; 12:383-93.

19. Brummett RE, Harris RF, Lindgren JA. Detection of ototoxicity from drugs applied topically to the middle ear space. Laryngoscope 1976; 86:1177-87.

20. Ilberg Cv, Spoendlin H, Arnold W. Autoradiographical distribution of locally applied dihydrostreptomycin in the inner ear. Acta Otolaryngol (Stockh) 1971; 71:159-65.

21. Webster JC, Carroll R, Benitez JT, McGee TM. Ototoxicity of topical gentamicin in the cat. J Infect Dis 1971; 124 Suppl: S138-44.

22. Morizono T, Johnstone BM. Ototoxicity of topically applied gentamicin using a statistical analysis of electrophysiological measurement. Acta Otolaryngol (Stockh) 1975; 80:389-93.

23. Friedmann I, Bird ES. Effect of ototoxic antibiotics and of penicillin on the sensory areas of the isolated fowl embryo otocyst in organ cultures: an electron-microscope study. J Pathol Bacteriol 1961; 81:81-90.

24. Goldstein AJ. Permeability of the organ of Corti. Ann Otol Rhinol Laryngol 1973; 82:166-74.

25. Koide Y, Hata A, Hando R. Vulnerability of the organ of Corti in poisoning. Acta Otolaryngol (Stockh) 1966; 61:332-44.

26. Hawkins JE Jr, Johnsson LG. Microdissection and surface preparations of the inner ear. In: Smith CA, Vernon JA, eds. Handbook of auditory and vestibular research methods. Springfield: Charles C Thomas, 1976:5-52.

27. Kuhn FA, Thalmann R, Marovitz WF. Comparison of Normarski differential interference contrast and phase contrast microscopy of the guinea pig organ of Corti. Laryngoscope 1971; 81:1090-118.

28. Kuhn FA, Thalmann R, Marovitz WF. Normarski differential interference contrast of the normal and pathologic guinea pig organ of Corti. Laryngoscope 1971; 81:1787-801.

29. Hawkins JE Jr. Experimental pathology. In: Iurato S, ed. Submicroscopic structures of the inner ear. New York: Pergamon Press, 1967:278-89.

30. Wersäll J, Björkroth B, Flock A, Lundquist P-G. Sensory hair fusion in vestibular sensory cells after gentamicin exposure: a transmission and scanning electron microscope study. Arch Klin Exp Ohren Nasen Kehlkopfheilkd 1971; 200:1-14.

31. Engström H, Ades HW, Andersson A. Structural pattern of the organ of Corti. Stockholm: Almqvist and Wiksell, 1966.

32. Ginsberg IA, Rudnick MD, Huber PS. Aminoglycoside ototoxicity following middle ear injection. III. Comparative quantitative analysis. Ann Otol Rhinol Laryngol 1980; 89 Suppl 77:17-24.

33. Hanson HV. Treatment of endolymphatic hydrops (Ménière's disease) with streptomycin. Ann Otol Rhinol Laryngol 1951; 60:676-91.

34. Feinmesser M, Sohmer H. Influence of streptomycin and dihydrostreptomycin on the cochlear potentials of the guinea pig. Ann Otol Rhinol Laryngol 1965; 74:48-58.

35. Watanuki K, Kawamoto K, Katagiri S. Repair pattern in the reticular lamina of the organ of Corti after hair cell loss. Ann Otol Rhinol Laryngol 1969; 78:1210-9.

36. Jordan VM, Pinheiro ML, Chiba K, Jimenez A. Postmortem changes in surface preparations of the cochlea. Ann Otol Rhinol Laryngol 1973; 82:111-25.

37. Portmann M, Darrouzet J, Aran JM. Etude experimentale sur la cellule de l'organe de Corti conditions normales et pathologiques. Int Audiol 1967; 6:380-5.

AMINOGLYCOSIDE OTOTOXICITY FOLLOWING MIDDLE EAR INJECTION

II. QUANTITATIVE ANALYTICAL PROCEDURE

MICHAEL D. RUDNICK, PhD

IRWIN A. GINSBERG, MD

PAMELA S. HUBER, MS

In cooperation with

JOEL S. ROSE, MA

BUFFALO, NEW YORK

A statistical methodology has been established to describe and compare, quantitatively, the ototoxic effects of aminoglycoside antibiotics. Sampling techniques for obtaining reliable estimates of cell damage in the organ of Corti and the vestibular system are described in this paper. The relationship of drug dosage to the percentage of hair cell damage in each inner ear sensory region was expressed as the slope of the least-squares linear regression line and was tested to reject the null hypothesis ($slope_u = 0$) at the 0.05 level of significance. It was determined that, in each of the cases discussed, dosage and damage correlated positively and that by repeated computations, each time controlling for one observed or measured variable, guinea pigs contributing skewed results could be eliminated on a rational basis. By this method of careful selection, statistically significant relationships have been established from the data.

In the preceding paper a methodology for transtympanic drug administration was described and the collapse cell was selected as the histological criterion for the measurement of ototoxicity.[1] In the following papers the specific toxic effects of three aminoglycoside antibiotics are analyzed and their toxicities compared. To accomplish this goal quantitatively required not only the careful selection of subjects but also reliable methods of data collection and statistical analysis. This paper addresses these problems.

METHODS

Experimental Controls. One hundred two pigmented guinea pigs (53% male, 47% female) were selected, injected and evaluated as described in part I of this study.[1] At the time of sacrifice and during microdissection, the middle and inner ears were examined for evidence of infection. Animals showing bloody exudate, pus, or squamous or fibrous metaplasia were discarded. If, during histological analysis, significant damage was noted on the noninjected side (>3% collapse cells), the same damage was assumed to have preexisted on the injected side, and the animal was eliminated from the study.

Data Collection. The material to be analyzed consisted of flat mounts of each of the five vestibular sensory structures and the organ of Corti from both the left and right temporal bones. Under dark phase contrast microscopy, normal sensory cells and collapse cells in selected areas of each sensory structure were counted.

The organ of Corti was dissected into eight segments. Starting from the region of the promontory, the first one half to three fourths of the first turn was designated "0.5 turn." Alternating segments ending at the apex, called "3.5 turn," were selected to represent the entire organ of Corti.[2] The most basal segment, termed the "hook" region, was not counted owing to its high, though variable, damage in both experimental and control ears. In order to avoid unequal weighting of cell counts due to unequal segment lengths, 80 hair cells from the inner hair cell row and 100 hair cells from each of the three outer hair cell rows were counted in each of the four representative segments. Figure 1 is a reproduction of a typical cochleogram which shows the position of each collapse cell or phalangeal scar as a black circle. One cochleogram was prepared from each experimental cochlea, provided the noninjected side was found to be within normal limits. Two guinea pigs were selected at random for complete cell counts in order to evaluate the sampling technique.

Vestibulograms were obtained according to the following procedure: Using a net reticle to facilitate counting, three grid areas* were analyzed from each of the five vestibular sensory structures. Two peripheral areas and one central area† from each structure were selected for counting. Figure 2 is a typical example of a vestibulogram. The approximate location of each area counted is indicated for each structure. These locations were subjectively assigned either a peripheral or central status for the computer analysis. Thus, 15 grid areas were counted and were considered representative of the entire vestibular system in each animal. Complete cell counts were taken from two randomly selected guinea pigs in order to evaluate the efficiency of the sampling method.

In addition to recording physical data, subjective observations were included in a daily log. This information, along with the cell counts, was encoded on a data form (Fig. 3) from which computer cards were punched and analyzed.§

Experimental Protocol. One middle ear from each guinea pig was injected with a specific dosage of either streptomycin, dihydrostreptomycin, or neomycin.[1] One hundred two successful injections were performed with the subsequent exclusion of eight animals due to evidence of infection in the middle or inner ears, detected at sacrifice or during microdissection. Table 1 presents the schedule for injection of the 94 remaining animals.

RESULTS

The 94 control (noninjected) ears showed neither a collapse cell count greater than 3% nor the morphological changes described in part I[1] of this study. The nine sham-injected control ears were likewise free of pathology and were anatomically indistinguishable from their opposite ears.

----

*Each grid area equals 0.01 mm^2.

†A central area is defined as one which includes the regions termed "striola" of the macula or "crest" of the crista ampullaris.

§Control Data Corporation Cyber 173 computer programmed with *The Statistical Package for the Social Sciences* (SPSS-6000 version 7.0).[3,4]

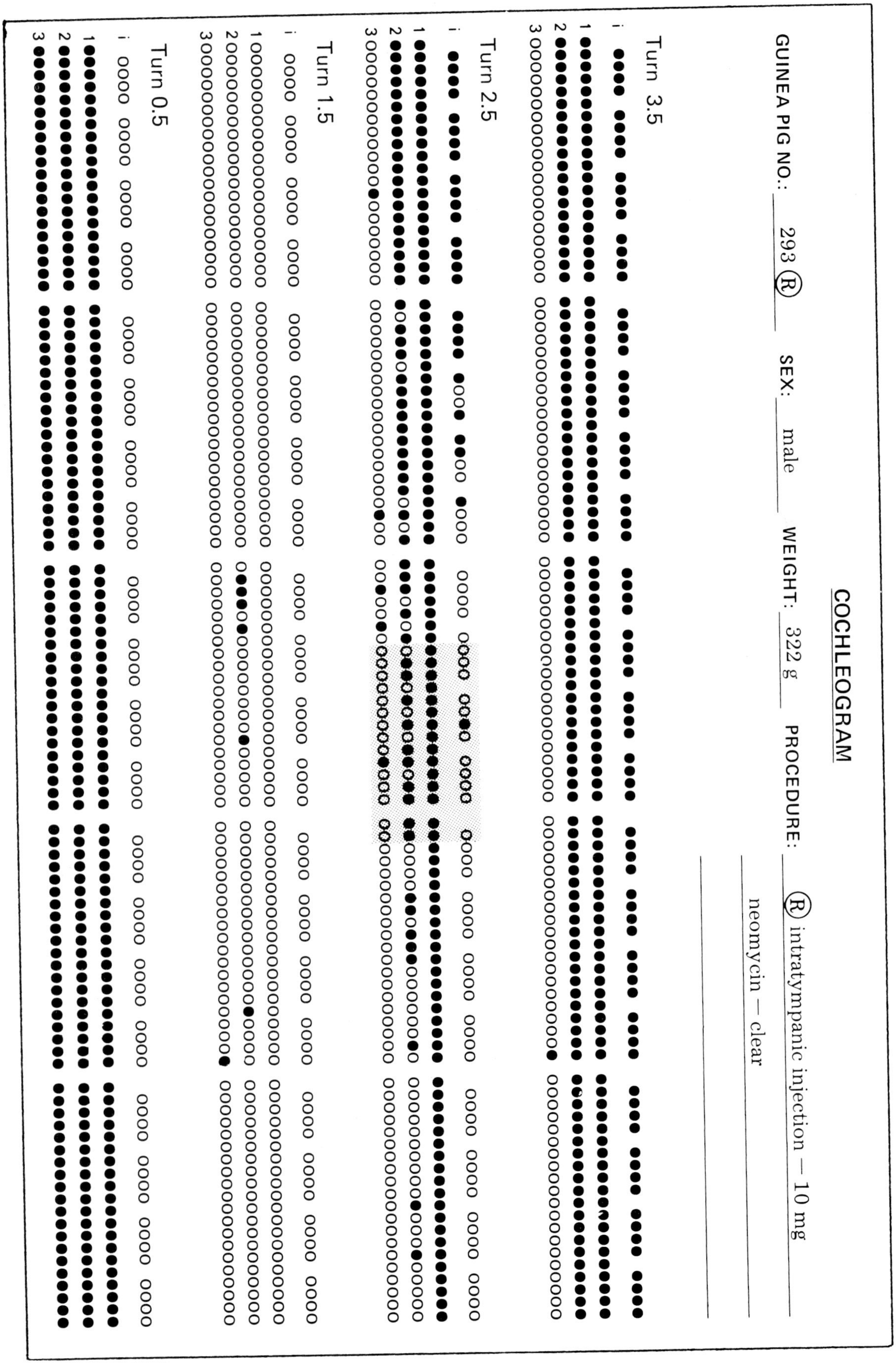

Fig. 1. Cochleogram. Shaded area corresponds to Fig. 10 of part I of this study. i - Inner hair cell row; 1, 2, and 3 - First, second and third rows of outer hair cells.

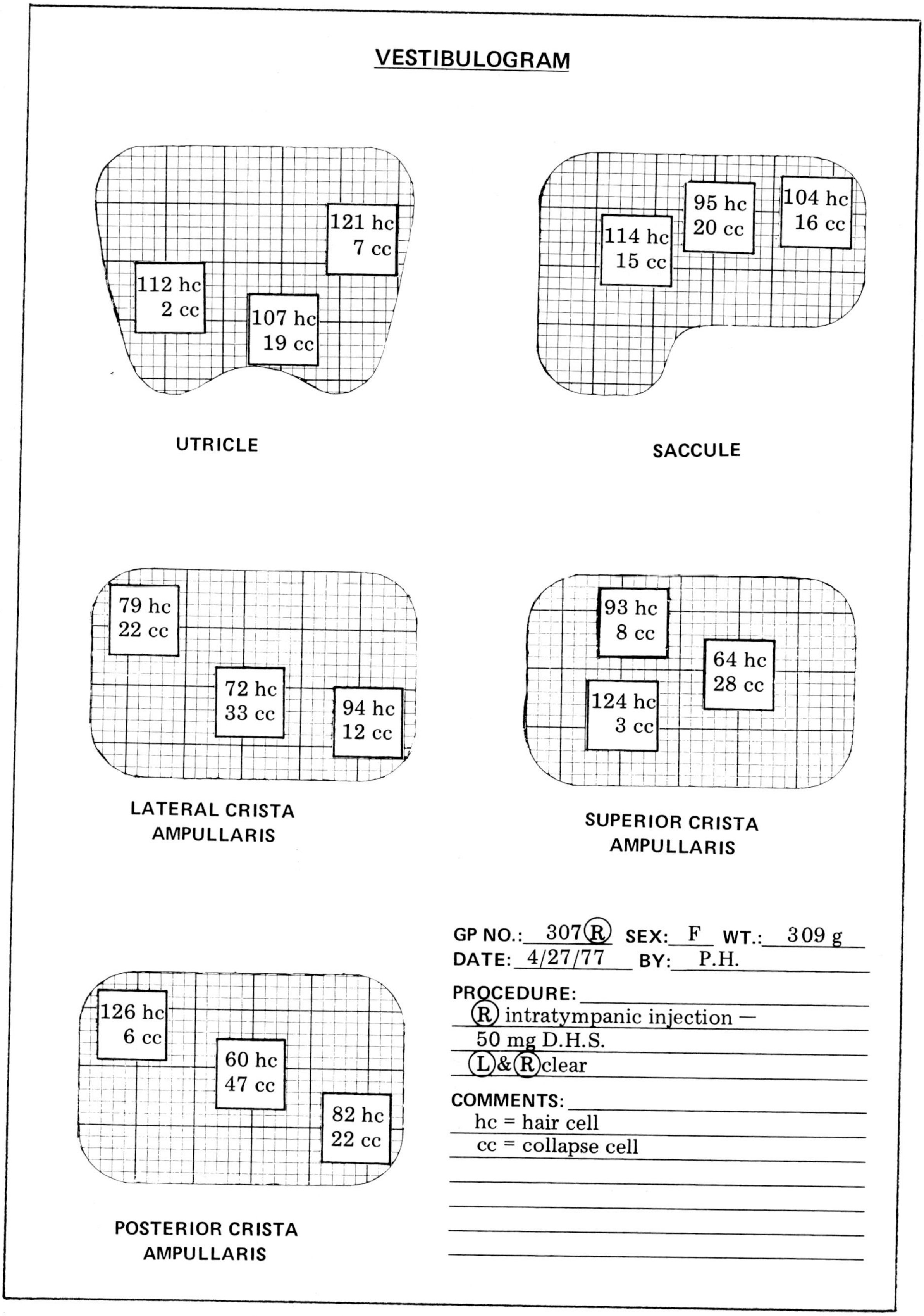

Fig. 2. Vestibulogram.

AMINOGLYCOSIDE ANTIBIOTIC OTOTOXICITY

1. Data set identification — HFB — 01-03
   Hearing Foundation of Buffalo
2. Guinea pig number — 04-06
3. Card number — 1 — 07
4. Sex — 08
   1 male
   2 female
   8 not ascertained
5. Weight prior to treatment (grams) — 09-12
   9998 not ascertained
6. Weight at sacrifice (grams) — 13-16
   9998 not ascertained
7. Ear injected — 17
   1 right
   2 left
8. Preyer reflex — 18
   1 positive reflex (+)
   2 weak reflex
   3 no reflex (-)
   8 not ascertained
9. Gait — 19
   1 normal (N)
   2 abnormal
   8 not ascertained
10. Drug injected — 20
    1 neomycin (Neo.)
    2 dihydrostreptomycin (DHS.)
    3 streptomycin (Strep.)
    4 kanamycin (Kan.)
    5 gentamicin (Gen.)
    6 saline
11. Dosage (miligrams) — 21-23
12. Otostimulation — 24
    1 rocked (R)
    2 immobilized (I)
13. Sound deadened environment — 25
    1 yes (S.D.)
    2 no
14. Infected or bloody – injected side — 26
    1 infected (I)
    2 not infected, but bloody
    3 clear (C)
15. Infected or bloody – non-injected side — 27
    1 infected (I)
    2 not infected, but bloody
    3 clear (C)

AMINOGLYCOSIDE ANTIBIOTIC OTOTOXICITY (CONT'D.)

GP NO.:________

16. Comments present in record book 5 a or b — 28
    1 yes
    2 no
17. Damage to vestibular system in numbers of cells
    998 not counted

	normal cells	collapse cells	
a. crista – superior – central area			29-34
b. crista – superior – peripheral area			35-40
c. crista – lateral – central area			41-46
d. crista – lateral – peripheral area			47-52
e. crista – posterior – central area			53-58
f. crista – posterior – peripheral area			59-64
	* * * * * * 2		01-07
g. macula – utricle – central area			08-13
h. macula – utricle – peripheral area			14-19
i. macula – saccule – central area			20-25
j. macula – saccule – peripheral area			26-31

18. Damage to Organ of Corti in numbers of cells

	Inner hair cells 98 not counted	Outer hair cells 998 not counted row 1	row 2	row 3	
a. turn 3.5					32-42
b. turn 2.5					43-53
c. turn 1.5					54-64
d. turn 0.5					65-75

Fig. 3. Data form.

TABLE 1. INJECTION SCHEDULE

	Number of Guinea Pigs Receiving Each Dosage						
	Dosage in Mg						
Drug	*0*	*5*	*10*	*25*	*50*	*100*	*Subtotal*
Streptomycin	—	0	8	9	16	4	37
Dihydrostreptomycin	—	0	4	6	10	5	25
Neomycin	—	4	9	7	3	0	23
Saline	9	—	—	—	—	—	9
Total animals in study							94

Items 17 and 18 of the data form (Fig. 3) contain all of the cell counts collected from each experimental ear. The counts in each region were analyzed separately or combined logically with other regions to allow for the analysis of each region, combination of regions, or the entire compartment. In this study 54 regions and their combinations were analyzed. These are listed in Table 2 of part III under "Region."[5] The analysis of each region was based upon all of the sampled cells in that region. For example, "Outer Hair Cells" refers to all three rows of outer hair cells in all four of the segments counted and implies that the values to the right describe the dosage-damage relationships of all outer hair cells in the organ of Corti.

The reliability of the sampling method was tested by performing complete cell counts of the organs of Corti and the vestibular sensory structures from the two randomly selected guinea pigs. For the organ of Corti it was found that the sampling method surveyed approximately 37% of the available sensory cells and that the estimates of cell damage were reliable within a 3% margin. It has also been determined that estimates of vestibular damage were based upon approximately 15% of the available sensory cells. This sampling method yielded data which were reliable within a 7% margin.

The primary question in this study was: Is there a positive dosage-damage relationship between aminoglycoside antibiotics and the various regions of the inner ear? And, if that positive relationship exists, is it statistically significant? Following affirmation, the pattern of susceptibility in those regions could be characterized and the relative toxicity of each drug compared. Graphs were prepared which relate drug dosage (abscissa) to the percentage of damage (ordinate) in each region of the inner ear for each drug tested. Each graph contained the least squares linear regression line which best fit the data. The regression line was characterized by its slope and y-intercept (see part III, Table 2, Slope_u and Intercept_u). All relationships reported in this study have been tested to reject the null hypothesis ($\text{slope}_u = 0$) at the 0.05 level of significance. Unless otherwise stated, all reported relationships are to be regarded as significant. Graphs used to illustrate the important relationships reported in parts III and IV of this study include broken lines indicating the 95% confidence intervals for the regression lines.[5,6]

These computations revealed that a positive relationship existed between the dosages of all three drugs and the damage to all 54 regions. However, many of these relationships, although positive, were not statistically significant. Three causes of this problem have been identified. First, a particular region was not counted in enough cases to allow a statistical analysis. A case in point is the peripheral regions of saccular maculae where the grid locations nearly always overlaid the central areas. Second, regardless of the dosage administered, no toxic effect was detected. Inner hair cells of dihydrostreptomycin-treated guinea pig cochleas illustrate this point. The term "Insufficient Data" listed in Table 2 of part III identifies these regions.

The third cause of statistically insignificant dosage-damage relationships was extraneous sources of variation in the amount of damage observed. Consequently, an attempt was made to identify the factor(s) contributing to this variance so that cases could be eliminated on a rational basis. To this end the data were reanalyzed to control for the effect of one variable at a time. If the significance of the relationships of interest increased, then a condition predisposing certain cases to variant results would have been identified, and those cases could be eliminated from the file.

Altogether 11 variables were tested. Ten of these were based on items 4 through 9, and 12 through 16 of the data form (Fig. 3). The 11th was considered in a test to determine if the potency of the antibiotics diminished over the three-year course of experimentation. Briefly, the guinea pigs receiving a particular drug were analyzed according to their sequence number to test if the dosage versus damage responses were lessened toward the end of the study. If so, a factor reflecting the rate of potency loss could be applied to the data, effectively compensating for this variable. No such diminished potency loss was detected, however.

This analysis has disclosed that by the elimination of experimental animals which had lost weight during the week following injection and by the elimination of guinea pigs for which the first attempt at transtympanic injection had failed, the significance of the dosage versus damage relationships was improved greatly. That these eliminations were important to the credibility of this study was borne out by the observation that despite a 39% loss in an already small population (37 guinea pigs were thus eliminated), the significance of 81% of the relationships of interest was improved markedly (10% remained substantially the same and 9% were diminished).

Having identified and eliminated the important sources of unreliable data, new statistics were generated and recorded in Table 2 of part III. All considerations to follow reflect relationships derived from this more highly selected population.

As previously defined, Table 2 of part III contains the slope and intercept of the least-squares linear regression line (identified as "Unconstrained" in the Table) which best fits the dosage versus damage data for each drug in each region. All of the values listed reflect not only a positive relationship of dosage to damage but also a statistically significant one. The actual relationships were not linear, as should be realized by noting the very diverse intercept$_u$ values (range, −14% to +55%). Logically, and from the controls, it is understood that at zero dosage of a drug, only a background level of hair cell damage (0 to 3% damage) was observed. Consequently, another regression line forced through the origin was calculated for each relationship. The slope of this line has been identified in Table 2 of part III as "Slope$_o$." From these values, comparisons can be made between drugs for each region (horizontally) and between regions for each drug (vertically) using the Table.

DISCUSSION

Care in the control of variables is a particularly important requirement in a quantitative study which measures subtle differences in effects. The use of internal controls has assured us that, as far as could be tested, the experimental (injected) ears were free of cell damage before the administration of antibiotics.

Variance in the data prior to the elimination of the 37 cases, though not extraordinary in comparison to other reports of inner ear toxicity,[2] initially prevented a meaningful statistical analysis in this study. By repeating the dosage versus damage analysis, each time deleting a group of animals which had an observed or measured variable in common, we were able to identify those variables which were the sources of much of the disparate data. The controls for good otologic health were apparently too gross to uncover subclinical pathological conditions. It was discovered that if guinea pigs lost weight following transtympanic injection or if an obstacle to receiving the entire dosage of injectant was encountered, the chances were greatly increased that the data derived from these animals would be skewed. It was thought originally that the loss of weight following injection was the result of vestibular discomfort and the pursuant loss of appetite. This may indeed be the case, but its connection to the unreliable drug effects remains unknown. An explanation may be that surgery caused an exacerbation of a previously subclinical infection. Voldrich suggested that an infection in the middle ear may increase the uptake of drugs into the labyrinth.[7]

The inability of some middle ears to accept the full 0.1 cc of injectant was assumed to have been the result of either individual anatomical variations in middle ear volume, or the pathological accumulation of fluid in the middle ear prior to surgery. Regardless of the source of this difficulty, switching to the opposite ear usually solved the volume problem. Analysis made it apparent, however, that a low middle ear volume, even unilaterally, was an indication of some bilateral abnormality predisposing the inner ear to an unreliable response to the injected drug. The underlying causes remain unresolved. However, the remarkable improvement in the data following the exclusion of these cases justified their elimination from the study.

The time required for microdissection and cell counting demanded that restrictions be made in selecting an experimental design. The range of dosages was selected to provide a range of damage from which the rate of toxic change could be determined. This rate, expressed as the regression coefficient in Table 2 of part III, is illustrated as the slope of a line in this study (part III, Figs. 1-6; part IV, Figs. 1-3). The necessity of standardizing the recovery period at one week has left to the future a study of the effect of "delayed" dihydrostreptomycin ototoxicity which has been reported following its systemic administration.[8,9]

Several trials at the same dosage level were required in order to provide a reliable estimate of each dosage-damage relationship. Because the dosages were grouped at intervals rather than being spread along the range, and, given the normal variance in the data, it was not feasible to present the dosage-damage relationships as true curves. The most reliable estimates of these relationships are provided by the least-squares linear regression lines. The constrained regression lines are very useful when estimating relative toxicities but are less reliable than the unconstrained regression lines when absolute figures are required. With these precautions in mind, one may interpret the slope of the regression line forced through the origin (slope$_o$ values) as the percent damage increment to be obtained for each additional milligram of drug. To illustrate, reference to Table 2 of part III indicates that the toxicity of dihydrostreptomycin on the vestibular system was 0.37% damaged hair cells per milligram; or, 3.7% damage/10 mg; or, 37% damage when 100 mg of dihydrostreptomycin was administered transtympanically. Instances where these lines might be misleading are identified as they occur in the subsequent papers.

An attempt was made to collect data separately from peripheral and central regions of each vestibular sensory structure since it has long been suspected that central regions are more susceptible to ototoxic agents than are peripheral regions.[10-14] However, the selection of grid areas for counting and their subsequent assignment to either a central or peripheral status for the computer analysis were subject to biasing. There was a tendency to select areas for counting in which the structures were intact. This favors the selection of the more central areas of maculae and the more peripheral areas of cristae. Nevertheless, clear trends in support of the theory of central susceptibility to ototoxic agents are demonstrated in part III of this study.

REFERENCES

1. Rudnick MD, Ginsberg IA, Huber PS. Aminoglycoside ototoxicity following middle ear injection. I. Experimental approach and histological criteria for evaluating drug effects. Ann Otol Rhinol Laryngol 1980; 89 Suppl 77:1-9.

2. Falk SA, Haseman JK, Klein R, Falk MK. Methyl mercury ototoxicity: a model for the surface preparation technique. Laryngoscope 1973; 83:1769-82.

3. Nie NH, Hull CH, Jenkins JG, Steinbrenner K, Bent DH. Statistical package for the social sciences. 2nd ed. New York: McGraw-Hill, 1975.

4. Hohlen M. Statistical package for the social sciences — 6000 version 7.0 update. Vogelback computing center document no. 437. Evanston: Northwestern University Press, 1977.

5. Ginsberg IA, Rudnick MD, Huber PS. Aminoglycoside ototoxicity following middle ear injection. III. Comparative quantitative analysis. Ann Otol Rhinol Laryngol 1980; 89 Suppl 77:17-24.

6. Huber PS, Ginsberg IA, Rudnick MD. Aminoglycoside ototoxicity following middle ear injection. IV. Influence of vestibular stimulation. Ann Otol Rhinol Laryngol 1980; 89 Suppl 77:25-28.

7. Voldrich L. Kinetics of streptomycin, kanamycin and neomycin in the inner ear. Acta Otolaryngol (Stockh) 1965; 60:243-8.

8. Glorig A. Effect of dihydrostreptomycin hydrochloride and sulfate on the auditory mechanism. Ann Otol Rhinol Laryngol 1951; 60:327-35.

9. Shambaugh GE Jr, Derlacki EL, Harrison WH, et al. Dihydrostreptomycin deafness. JAMA 1959; 170:1657-60.

10. Berg K. Toxic effect of streptomycin on the vestibular and cochlear apparatus. Acta Otolaryngol (Stockh) 1951: Suppl 97.

11. Neumann G, Neubert K. Sensularien des Innenohres unter der Einwirkung von Streptomycin. Arzneim Forsch 1958; 8:63-72.

12. Wersäll J, Hawkins JE Jr. Vestibular sensory epithelia in the cat labyrinth and their reactions in chronic streptomycin intoxication. Acta Otolaryngol (Stockh) 1962; 54:1-23.

13. McGee TM, Olszewski J. Streptomycin sulfate and dihydrostreptomycin toxicity. Arch Otolaryngol 1962; 75:295-311.

14. Lindeman HH. Regional differences in sensitivity of the vestibular sensory epithelia to ototoxic antibiotics. Acta Otolaryngol (Stockh) 1969; 67:177-89.

AMINOGLYCOSIDE OTOTOXICITY FOLLOWING MIDDLE EAR INJECTION

III. COMPARATIVE QUANTITATIVE ANALYSIS

IRWIN A. GINSBERG, MD

MICHAEL D. RUDNICK, PhD

PAMELA S. HUBER, MS

BUFFALO, NEW YORK

Hypotheses to explain the selective ototoxicity of aminoglycoside antibiotics may be grouped into two categories: 1) a partition effect and 2) innate hair cell selectivity. The results of this study give evidence that, in fact, both mechanisms may interplay. This conclusion is induced from the observations that following the transtympanic administration of streptomycin, dihydrostreptomycin and neomycin: 1) All three drugs elicited nearly the same topographic pattern and degree of damage in the vestibular compartment. 2) All three drugs elicited nearly the same topographic pattern but widely different degrees of damage in the cochlear compartment (neomycin> >streptomycin> dihydrostreptomycin). 3) Neomycin caused the same devastating cochlear hair cell damage as reported for its systemic administration. 4) Dihydrostreptomycin was significantly more vestibulotoxic than cochleotoxic, and streptomycin was both significantly more cochleotoxic than vestibulotoxic and significantly more cochleotoxic than was dihydrostreptomycin. The latter observations are discussed with regard to contrasts with the literature reporting the drug effects following systemic administration.

Hypotheses reported in the literature to explain selective ototoxicity may be classified into two categories. One is the partition effect, or the effect of different rates of drug transport to and from the cochlear and vestibular chambers of the inner ear.[1-7] The second is innate hair cell selectivity, or the ability of different drugs to bind preferentially to different hair cells[8-10] or to a particular substance in their immediate environment, eg, glycocalyx, tectorial membrane, statoconial membrane, or cupula.[11] The present study establishes the topographic pattern or specific distribution of toxic changes which results from the transtympanic administration of streptomycin, dihydrostreptomycin, and neomycin. Once a pattern has been established, a comparison of the relative toxicities of these drugs between inner ear compartments and between specific regions within each compartment is presented. The results, when compared to those of previous studies utilizing the systemic route of entry, will contribute to a clarification of the mechanism of selective ototoxicity.

METHODS

Fifty-seven pigmented guinea pigs of both sexes were selected, injected, and their inner ear tissues prepared for examination as described in parts I and II of this study.[12,13] Table 1 summarizes the injection schedule. Cell counts were performed and the data were analyzed according to the format established in part II of this study.[13]

RESULTS

The findings of this study are reported in two sections. Section 1 deals with the topographic distribution of cell damage which resulted from the administration of each drug. These results may be predicted by comparing regression coefficients vertically under the $Slope_o$ column of Table 2 for each drug. Before reporting on the differences in sensitivity between different regions for each drug, t tests were applied to assure that the differences were indeed significant. In section 2, the ototoxicities of the three drugs are compared. These results may be predicted by comparing the $Slope_o$ regression coefficients horizontally for each region listed in Table 2. As before, every stated relationship has been tested for significant differences using the two-tailed t test at the 0.05 level of significance.

PATTERN OF OTOTOXICITY

Streptomycin. The most significant result in terms of contrasts with the literature on systemic applications was that in this study streptomycin more profoundly affected the organ of Corti than the vestibular system. This was true not only in the basal turn, where it might have been expected on the basis of its predicted route of entry through the round window membrane, but also throughout the entire length of the organ of Corti. The constrained least-squares linear regression lines and their confidence intervals comparing the effects of streptomycin on the organ of Corti and the vestibular system are plotted in Figure 1.

In the organ of Corti, outer hair cells were more sensitive to streptomycin than were inner hair cells (Table 2). Damage to outer hair cells decreased from base to apex and, although the typical pattern of damage for successive rows of outer hair cells was upheld in this study, row 1 was not significantly more susceptible than row 2, nor was row 2 significantly more damaged than row 3 following treatment with streptomycin.

In the vestibular system a comparison of toxicity for central and peripheral regions, either for in-

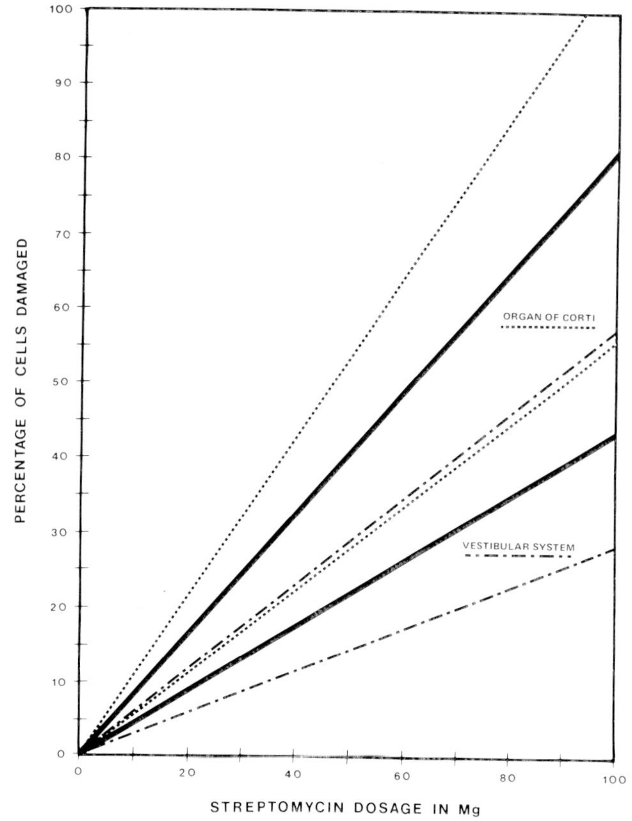

Fig. 1. Percentage of damaged sensory cells in the organ of Corti and in the vestibular system as a function of streptomycin dosage.

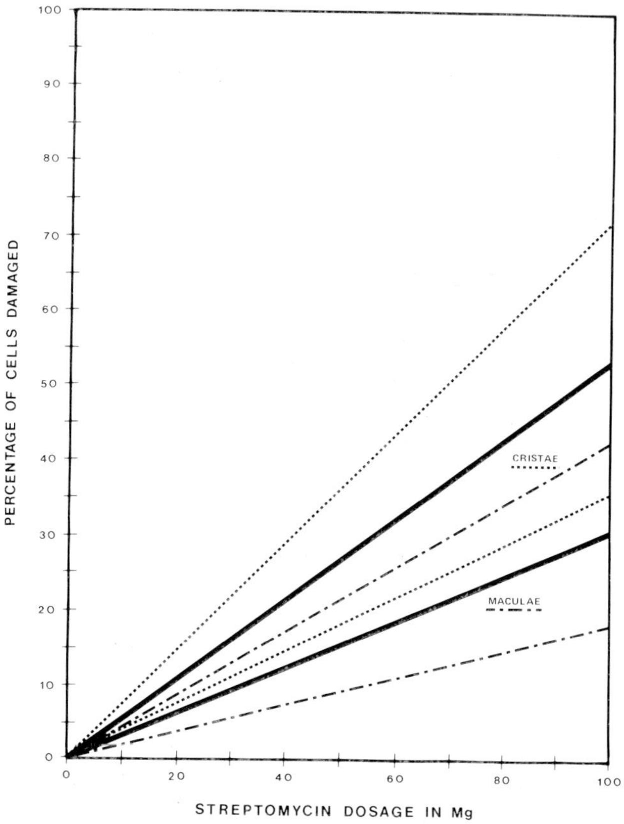

Fig. 2. Percentage of damaged sensory cells in the cristae and in the maculae as a function of streptomycin dosage.

dividual structures or for any combination of structures, always showed the central regions to be more dominantly affected. The cristae were significantly more damaged than the maculae as documented in Figure 2. The posterior cristae ampullares appeared to be more sensitive to streptomycin than the superior cristae ampullares, with the lateral cristae ampullares the least affected of the three. Finally, the utricular maculae were more susceptible to the toxic action of streptomycin than were the saccular maculae.

Table 3 provides a summary of mean percent damage values for selected regions which resulted from the transtympanic injection of streptomycin at the dosage levels indicated. This sample, derived directly from the cell counts, demonstrates the amount of damage that was observed at each dosage level. This Table is included here for comparison with the computer calculated slopes of these same relationships which are documented in Table

TABLE 1. INJECTION SCHEDULE

	Number of Guinea Pigs Receiving Each Dosage						
			Dosage in Mg				*Sub-*
Drug	*0*	*5*	*10*	*25*	*50*	*100*	*total*
Streptomycin	—	0	4	5	7	1	17
Dihydrostreptomycin	—	0	4	2	4	3	13
Neomycin	—	4	9	5	2	0	20
Saline	7	—	—	—	—	—	7
Total animals in study							57

2. Observe that the calculated slopes of the least-squares linear regression lines, even those forced through the origin, substantially reflect the actual observations.

Dihydrostreptomycin. Dihydrostreptomycin was significantly more vestibulotoxic than cochleotoxic when administered transtympanically. This is in contrast to the literature on the systemic application of this drug. This finding would not have been predicted from the relatively small differences in the calculated slopes of dosage versus damage relationships from the various regions in each compartment. However, *t* tests comparing the toxicity of dihydrostreptomycin observed in each compartment confirmed that any region within the vestibular system was significantly more vulnerable to dihydrostreptomycin than was any region in the organ of Corti (Fig. 3).

Inner hair cells, it would seem, were not susceptible to the toxic action of dihydrostreptomycin at the dosages tested. Only those inner hair cells of the most apical turn registered enough damage to allow a statistical analysis. Even so, the damage proved to be insignificant.

As with streptomycin, dihydrostreptomycin-treated ears showed the same overall pattern of outer hair cell degeneration. That is, within each segment, the three rows were nearly equally sensitive to antibi-

PERCENT DAMAGE PER Mg DRUG

REGION			[1]REGRESSION COEFFICIENTS								
			STREPTOMYCIN			DIHYDROSTREPTOMYCIN			NEOMYCIN		
			Unconstrained		Forced through Origin	Unconstrained		Forced through Origin	Unconstrained		Forced through Origin
			[2]Slope$_u$	[2]Intercept$_u$	[3]Slope$_o$	Slope$_u$	Intercept$_u$	Slope$_o$	Slope$_u$	Intercept$_u$	Slope$_o$
Crista Superior – Central Area			0.42	2.24	0.46	0.26	14.20	0.47	Insignificant		0.59
Crista Superior – Peripheral Area			0.44	- 2.80	0.30	0.51	- 0.84	0.35	0.34	0.18	0.30
Crista Superior			0.42	0.95	0.44	0.35	5.79	0.43	0.38	1.43	0.45
Crista Lateral – Central Area			Insignificant		0.40	Insignificant		0.37	0.51	3.88	0.65
Crista Lateral – Peripheral Area			Insignificant		0.35	0.48	0.89	0.42	0.25	- 0.86	0.15
Crista Lateral			0.43	2.58	0.39	0.27	7.21	0.36	0.52	- 0.45	0.48
Crista Posterior – Central Area			0.61	- 0.29	0.65	0.50	8.31	0.56	0.58	2.53	0.58
Crista Posterior – Peripheral Area			0.42	- 3.08	0.28	0.61	- 1.48	0.47	Insignificant		0.21
Crista Posterior			0.61	- 1.00	0.59	0.48	7.35	0.53	0.43	1.76	0.42
Macula Utriculi – Central Area			0.52	- 5.50	0.43	0.39	3.66	0.41	0.40	- 0.14	0.38
Macula Utriculi – Peripheral Area			Insignificant		0.22	Insignificant			0.13	0.15	0.13
Macula Utriculi			0.47	- 1.92	0.41	0.40	0.89	0.37	0.22	0.08	0.21
Macula Sacculi – Central Area			0.27	- 1.76	0.24	Insignificant		0.16	0.46	- 0.81	0.41
Macula Sacculi – Peripheral Area			Insufficient Data			Insufficient Data			Insufficient Data		
Macula Sacculi			0.25	- 1.79	0.22	Insignificant		0.16	0.46	- 0.81	0.41
Cristae Central Areas			0.54	2.30	0.57	0.30	11.46	0.47	0.51	3.20	0.64
Macular Central Areas			0.38	- 3.92	0.30	Insignificant		0.24	0.44	- 0.52	0.40
Vestibular Central Areas			0.45	- 1.02	0.42	0.24	8.95	0.37	0.41	3.08	0.53
Cristae Peripheral Areas			0.48	1.18	0.41	0.56	- 0.08	0.49	Insignificant		0.26
Macular Peripheral Areas			Insignificant		0.22	Insignificant			0.13	0.15	0.13
Vestibular Peripheral Areas			0.43	0.30	0.35	0.55	- 0.87	0.47	0.17	1.09	0.21
Cristae			0.51	1.58	0.53	0.33	7.67	0.44	0.41	0.96	0.45
Maculae			0.34	- 1.87	0.30	Insignificant		0.24	0.31	- 0.06	0.29
VESTIBULAR SYSTEM			0.45	- 0.76	0.43	0.27	6.52	0.37	0.34	1.21	0.38
+I.H.C.	3.5 Turn		0.79	- 7.32	0.64	Insignificant			1.61	54.04	3.81
I.H.C.	2.5 Turn		0.73	-13.98	0.46	Insufficient Data			2.20	31.20	3.47
I.H.C.	1.5 Turn		0.71	-13.99	0.43	Insufficient Data			2.88	3.97	3.04
I.H.C.	0.5 Turn		0.92	-13.78	0.65	Insufficient Data			3.05	- 2.99	2.93
†O.H.C.	3.5 Turn	Row 1	0.86	- 8.62	0.69	0.19	- 3.60	0.14	1.57	55.44	3.82
O.H.C.	3.5 Turn	Row 2	0.79	- 9.70	0.60	0.08	- 6.92	0.08	2.02	39.41	3.63
O.H.C.	3.5 Turn	Row 3	0.71	- 7.63	0.56	0.13	0.30	0.14	2.39	24.59	3.39
O.H.C.	2.5 Turn	Row 1	0.92	-11.77	0.69	0.09	- 1.42	0.07	1.61	54.04	3.81
O.H.C.	2.5 Turn	Row 2	0.87	-11.59	0.64	Insignificant			2.15	33.24	3.50
O.H.C.	2.5 Turn	Row 3	0.72	-11.41	0.50	0.04	- 0.46	0.03	2.50	19.53	3.30
O.H.C.	1.5 Turn	Row 1	1.21	- 5.72	1.10	0.33	- 6.14	0.24	2.47	18.32	3.22
O.H.C.	1.5 Turn	Row 2	1.09	- 2.71	1.04	0.15	- 2.88	0.11	2.46	18.76	3.22
O.H.C.	1.5 Turn	Row 3	1.02	- 5.82	0.91	0.04	- 0.47	0.03	2.60	14.04	3.17
O.H.C.	0.5 Turn	Row 1	1.42	- 4.72	1.33	1.04	- 8.12	0.92	1.90	41.18	3.57
O.H.C.	0.5 Turn	Row 2	1.41	- 4.85	1.31	1.05	- 9.52	0.91	2.03	35.93	3.50
O.H.C.	0.5 Turn	Row 3	1.40	- 4.88	1.30	1.05	-10.01	0.91	2.05	35.36	3.49
O.H.C.	3.5 Turn		0.79	- 8.65	0.62	0.13	- 1.33	0.12	1.99	39.81	3.61
O.H.C.	2.5 Turn		0.84	-11.59	0.61	0.05	- 0.55	0.04	2.09	35.60	3.54
O.H.C.	1.5 Turn		1.11	- 4.75	1.02	0.17	- 3.16	0.13	2.51	17.04	3.20
O.H.C.	0.5 Turn		1.41	- 4.82	1.31	1.05	- 9.22	0.91	1.99	37.49	3.52
O.H.C.	All Turns	Row 1	1.11	- 7.71	0.95	0.41	- 4.76	0.34	1.89	42.24	3.60
O.H.C.	All Turns	Row 2	1.04	- 7.21	0.90	0.32	- 3.22	0.28	2.17	31.83	3.46
O.H.C.	All Turns	Row 3	0.96	- 7.44	0.82	0.31	- 2.72	0.27	2.39	23.38	3.34
O.H.C. & I.H.C.	3.5 Turn		0.79	- 8.37	0.62	0.11	- 1.03	0.09	1.91	42.81	3.65
O.H.C. & I.H.C.	2.5 Turn		0.82	-12.09	0.58	0.04	- 0.43	0.03	2.11	34.68	3.52
O.H.C. & I.H.C.	1.5 Turn		1.03	- 6.70	0.89	0.14	- 2.50	0.10	2.59	14.29	3.17
O.H.C. & I.H.C.	0.5 Turn		1.31	- 6.70	1.17	0.83	- 7.28	0.72	2.22	28.97	3.39
Inner Hair Cells			0.79	-12.26	0.54	Insignificant			2.43	21.56	3.31
Outer Hair Cells			1.04	- 7.45	0.89	0.35	- 3.57	0.30	2.15	32.48	3.47
ORGAN OF CORTI			0.98	- 8.47	0.82	0.28	- 2.81	0.23	2.21	30.18	3.43

[1]**Regression Coefficients** relate % damage to mg of drug injected.

[2]**Slope$_u$** is interpreted as the % damage increment above the **Intercept$_u$** value obtained for each mg of drug injected.

[3]**Slope$_o$** is interpreted as the % damage increment obtained for each mg of drug injected with the values adjusted to comply with the finding that at zero dosage of a drug no damage is observed. These values are used in comparing drug sensitivity between regions for each drug (vertically) and between drugs for each region (horizontally).

+ Inner Hair Cells

† Outer Hair Cells

TABLE 2.

TABLE 3. STREPTOMYCIN OTOTOXICITY

Region	Mean Percent Damage at Each Dosage Level — Dosage in Mg: 10	25	50	100
Cristae central areas	7	30	28	50
Cristae	6	29	26	50
Maculae	5	8	12	42
Vestibular central areas	4	17	20	46
Vestibular peripheral areas	5	20	20	—
Vestibular system	4	18	19	46
Outer hair cells (0.5 turn)	0	33	79	100
Outer hair cells	3	17	44	100
Organ of Corti	3	13	38	100

otic and also, the damage was most marked in the basal turn (0.5 turn).

The values summarizing the relationships of dosage to damage for the vestibular regions under "Dihydrostreptomycin" in Table 2 indicate almost identically the same pattern and degree of damage as the corresponding values for streptomycin and neomycin. That is, the peripheral regions of all five vestibular sensory structures were less affected by dihydrostreptomycin than were the central regions. Further, the lateral cristae were less damaged than either the posterior or the superior cristae, with the posterior cristae significantly more vulnerable than the superior cristae. The cristae were significantly more damaged than the maculae and the utricular maculae appeared to respond more than the saccular maculae to dihydrostreptomycin treatment.

Table 4 indicates the mean percent damage that was obtained experimentally in selected regions of dihydrostreptomycin-treated animals at each dosage level. These values were derived directly from the cell counts and were included for comparison with the calculated overall dosage-damage relationships listed in Table 2. Unlike streptomycin, dihydrostreptomycin did not react precisely as the least-squares linear regression lines would predict: at lower dosage levels, experimental observations indicated that more damage resulted to vestibular structures and less to cochlear structures than would have been supposed from the $slope_0$ values. This is illustrated in the unconstrained regression lines of Figure 3.

Neomycin. Without question, the most profound reaction encountered in this study took place in the cochlea following the transtympanic administration of relatively small amounts of neomycin. The data demonstrated a threshold between 10 to 25 mg above which all inner and outer hair cells were destroyed. A comparison of the cochleotoxicity and vestibulotoxicity of neomycin need not be belabored since there was almost an order of magnitude difference in regression coefficient values between the two compartments (Fig. 4).

An analysis of cell counts following the administration of 5-10 mg of neomycin allowed the discrimination of relative toxicities in the organ of

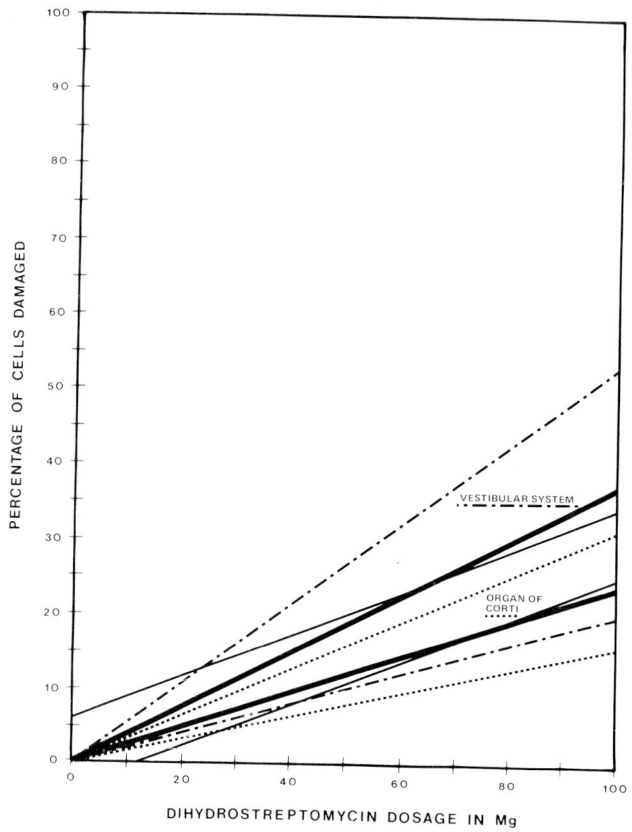

Fig. 3. Percentage of damaged sensory cells in the vestibular system and in the organ of Corti as a function of dihydrostreptomycin dosage (thick solid lines and their confidence intervals, broken lines). Unconstrained regression lines are also included (thin solid lines). See text for explanation.

Corti. *T* tests revealed significant differences in the sensitivity of each segment to neomycin in the following order: turn 3.5>0.5>2.5>1.5. It is of interest to note that both outer hair cells and inner hair cells of the apical turn were the most sensitive cells along the length of the organ of Corti.

An analysis of vestibular systems revealed nearly the same distribution of toxic changes and, on the average, nearly the same degree of toxicity to its structures as has been reported for the other aminoglycoside antibiotics. One exception was in the saccular maculae where there was more damage than in the utricular maculae over the dosages tested (Table 2).

It may be of interest for future studies to note that the differential sensitivities of central and peripheral regions of vestibular sensory structures were much greater for neomycin than they were for either streptomycin or dihydrostreptomycin. *T* tests of these differences were computed for all vestibular structures individually, and in combination, with the result that central regions were significantly more vulnerable to the toxic action of neomycin than were peripheral regions (Fig. 5).

Table 5 presents the mean percent damage values obtained directly from the cell counts of neomycin-

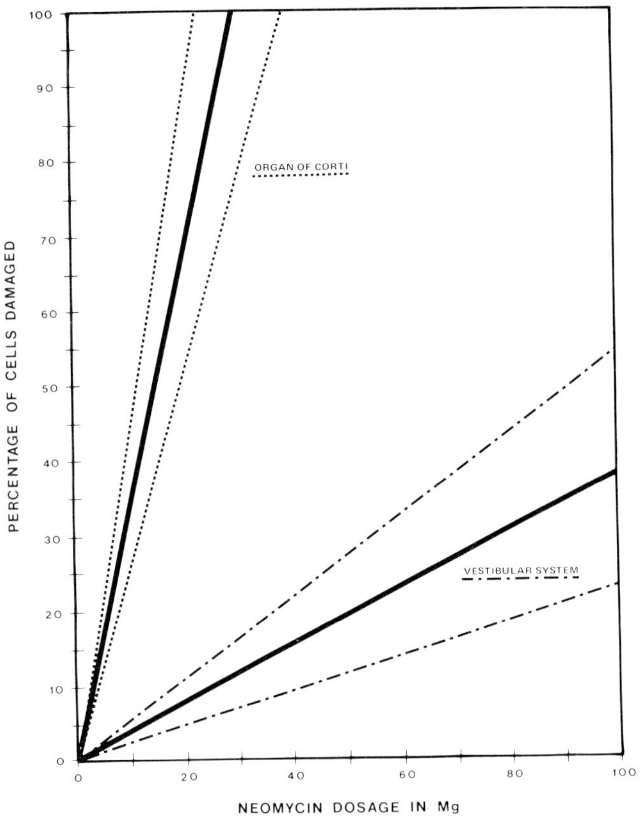

Fig. 4. Percentage of damaged sensory cells in the organ of Corti and in the vestibular system as a function of neomycin dosage.

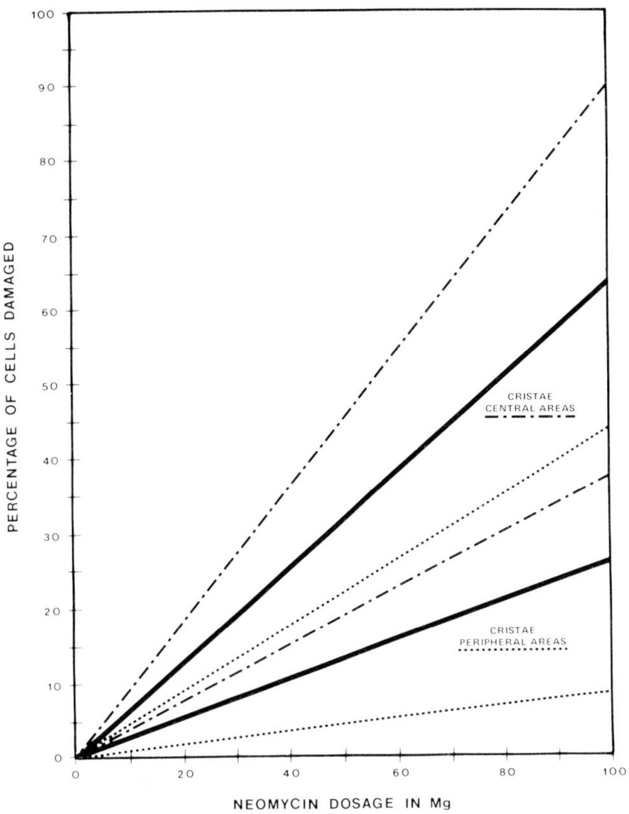

Fig. 5. Percentage of damaged sensory cells in the central areas of cristae and in the peripheral areas of cristae as a function of neomycin dosage.

treated inner ear structures at each dosage level. When the values for vestibular structures in Table 2 are compared to the values in Table 5, one finds a strikingly high correlation. This and the observation that intercept$_u$ values listed in Table 2 very nearly equal zero suggest that the response characteristics of vestibular structures to neomycin may be truly linear.

RELATIVE TOXICITY OF DRUGS

Streptomycin vs Neomycin. *T* tests were hardly necessary to demonstrate that for every region in the organ of Corti neomycin was significantly more toxic than streptomycin (Table 2, and Fig. 6). The *t* tests did tell us, however, that vestibular systems which received streptomycin responded too similarly to vestibular systems which received neomycin to be discerned statistically. The analysis also revealed that peripheral regions of vestibular structures tended toward less damage following neomycin than following streptomycin treatment.

Dihydrostreptomycin vs Neomycin. Here again, neomycin was extraordinarily cochleotoxic, making further comparisons to dihydrostreptomycin unnecessary in this compartment (Table 2 and Fig. 6). In the vestibular system dihydrostreptomycin and neomycin had essentially the same overall effect. A comparison of means disclosed that the peripheral areas of vestibular sensory structures were less vulnerable to neomycin than to dihydrostreptomycin treatment.

Streptomycin vs Dihydrostreptomycin. As re-

TABLE 4. DIHYDROSTREPTOMYCIN OTOTOXICITY

Mean Percent Damage at Each Dosage Level

Region	*Dosage in Mg* 10	25	50	100
Cristae central areas	9	42	27	37
Cristae	5	41	22	38
Maculae	3	14	15	20
Vestibular central areas	7	33	22	30
Vestibular peripheral areas	1	33	22	30
Vestibular system	4	32	19	33
Outer hair cells (0.5 turn)	0	18	25	100
Outer hair cells	0	5	7	32
Organ of Corti	0	4	6	26

TABLE 5. NEOMYCIN OTOTOXICITY

Mean Percent Damage at Each Dosage Level

Region	*Dosage in Mg* 5	10	25	50
Cristae central areas	6	8	20	22
Cristae	4	5	12	23
Maculae	0	3	9	12
Vestibular central areas	6	7	15	20
Vestibular peripheral areas	0.8	3	7	5
Vestibular system	3	5	11	17
Outer hair cells (0.5 turn)	46	63	100	100
Outer hair cells	32	63	100	100
Organ of Corti	29	61	100	100

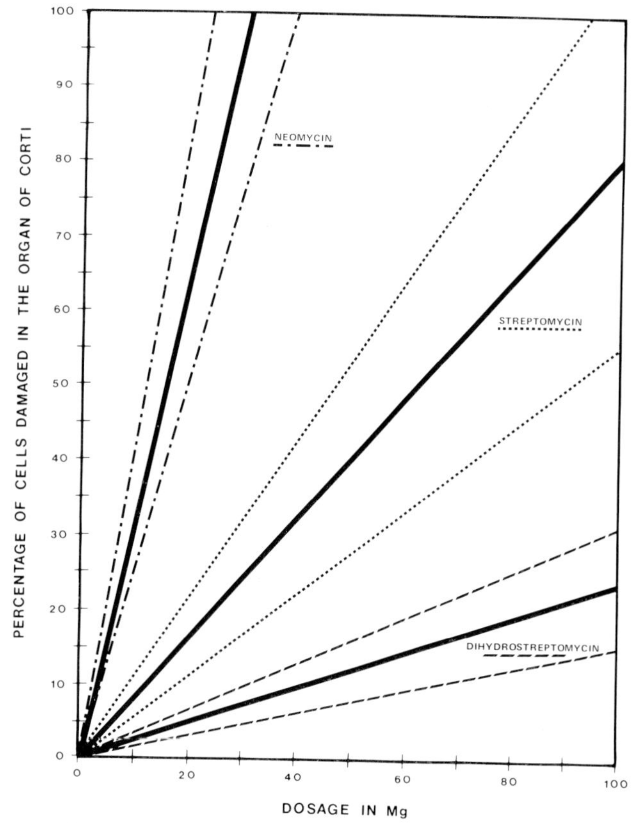

Fig. 6. Percentage of damaged sensory cells in the organ of Corti as a function of neomycin, streptomycin and dihydrostreptomycin dosage.

ported, streptomycin was significantly more cochleotoxic than vestibulotoxic and dihydrostreptomycin was significantly more vestibulotoxic than cochleotoxic when administered transtympanically in this study. *T* tests revealed that streptomycin was significantly more toxic in the cochlear compartment than was dihydrostreptomycin (Table 2 and Fig. 6). Not one of the vestibular sensory cell regions registered a statistically significant difference in its response to treatment with streptomycin or dihydrostreptomycin.

DISCUSSION

Lindeman[9] has established that, whether administered systemically or transtympanically, streptomycin is most toxic to type I hair cells in central vestibular regions, less so to type I hair cells in peripheral regions and least toxic to type II hair cells wherever encountered.[14,15] Spoendlin[15] asserted that the cause of this difference in sensitivity may relate to the higher metabolic rate for proteins in type I hair cells. Spoendlin,[15] Watanuki and Meyer zum Gottesberge,[16] and Watanuki et al[17] have suggested that type I hair cells are phylogenetically more recent and are more differentiated than type II hair cells, either condition making them, in principle, more vulnerable to environmental stresses such as the presence of toxic drugs. Although type I and type II hair cells were not differentially evaluated in this study, our finding of higher susceptibility in the central regions of vestibular sensory structures supports the observations of earlier investigators. The concept of regional selectivity is of great interest because as Lindeman[9] suggested, function may also differ in the central and peripheral regions of vestibular sensory structures.

There was one instance in this study in which less damage resulted to the phylogenetically newer part of the inner ear: in those animals which received dihydrostreptomycin there was less damage to their cochleas and saccules (pars inferior, the phylogenetically newer division of the inner ear[18]) than there was to their cristae and utricles. However, no conclusion should be drawn from this observation until the possibility of a "delayed" onset of ototoxicity has been examined following the transtympanic administration of dihydrostreptomycin. This phenomenon has long been recognized as a peculiar characteristic of systemically injected dihydrostreptomycin.[19,20]

As indicated in Table 4 and Figure 3, the actual responses to dihydrostreptomycin administered in low dosages may depart from the calculated overall relationships documented in Table 2 by causing greater vestibular damage and less cochlear damage. In an attempt to clarify the meaning of this observation, *t* tests were run comparing dihydrostreptomycin to streptomycin for the lowest dosage cases alone (0 to 25 mg). The population was so small (nine streptomycin, six dihydrostreptomycin) that predictions based upon our data must be, at best, guarded. Our data indicated that, for every region within the vestibular compartment, damage was greater following low dosage dihydrostreptomycin treatment (with the reverse being true for all regions within the cochlear compartment) than was indicated by the calculated overall relationships. The reliability of this observation could not be documented by tests for significance owing to the very small population and its usual variance. Indeed, this particular question demands a more thorough study because of its clinical importance. It may be found, for example, that dihydrostreptomycin is an effective agent for unilateral vestibular ablation, causing minimal high frequency hearing loss, when administered transtympanically in multiple, low dosages.

The selective ototoxicity of aminoglycoside antibiotics may be explained on the grounds of several hypotheses described in the literature. As previously suggested, these hypotheses may be divided into two categories: 1) the partition effect and 2) innate hair cell selectivity.

The former case has at its basis the pharmacological principle of compartmentalization.[5] Systemic application allows the drugs to disseminate throughout the body, reaching the inner ear via the circulatory system. The rate of selective transport to or from each inner ear compartment may vary depending upon inherent differences in the drugs being transported, in the secretory or excretory epithelia through which the drugs must pass to gain entrance into or exit from the endolymphatic spaces, or both.[2-4,6,21,22] In fact, the drugs may have their primary effect in altering the transport epithelia of the inner ear. In this case, hair cell damage would result secondarily.[10]

To further complicate this picture, the nephrotoxicity of certain aminoglycoside antibiotics has been reported.[3,23-25] Damage to kidneys reduces the rate of clearance of the drugs from the body which results in an increased titer in the blood and, therefore, in the inner ear fluids. Case reports of permanent deafness or vertigo following drug therapy for infection have been published.[26,27]

The transtympanic route of administration eliminates this synergistic nephrotoxic effect and may also reduce the variance in the actual drug dosage reaching inner ear hair cells which might otherwise have resulted from individual differences in systemic compartmentalization. In the case of middle ear administration, the drugs need only traverse the round window membrane and the membranous labyrinth to reach the sensory cells.[15,28,29] The rate of clearance of drugs from the inner ear still depends, however, upon compartmental factors just as it does following the systemic route of entry. For this reason the effects of differential rates of drug clearance from inner ear compartments should have no influence upon the interpretation of the findings reported in this study.

It has been suggested that the direct application of the drugs might elicit a different response than when injected systemically.[16,28] Schuknecht[30,31] tested streptomycin both systemically and transtympanically under both clinical and experimental conditions. He found that the high vestibulotoxicity and low cochleotoxicity which followed the systemic administration of streptomycin was lost when applied locally. In fact, he reported a functional loss occurring simultaneously in both compartments. Friedmann and Bird[1] exposed cultured organ of Corti to constant dosages of streptomycin. They found that the hair cells appeared to be less sensitive to dosages in the nutrient medium than to the same dosages applied systemically in vivo. This suggests that streptomycin may be concentrated in the cochlea following systemic injections. It is, therefore, logical to predict that a difference in selective ototoxicity might result from a difference in the mode of administration of the drugs.

Our results have shown that following transtympanic injection the pattern of ototoxicity *within* the cochlea or *within* the vestibular system was nearly identical to that following the systemic administration of these drugs.[9,14,15,32-34] These data favor the hypothesis that the mechanism of aminoglycoside ototoxicity involves innate hair cell selectivity.

An analysis of the relative ototoxicities of the antibiotics *between* compartments following transtympanic injection revealed several interesting relationships. First, all three drugs exerted nearly the same effect upon vestibular sensory structures — both in terms of topographic distribution and in terms of degree. Second, in the organ of Corti the three drugs tested differed greatly in their degree of damage (neomycin> >streptomycin>dihydrostreptomycin) though they did not differ appreciably in the pattern of that damage. Third, neomycin, whether applied systemically or locally, yielded the same effect. Fourth, streptomycin was significantly more cochleotoxic than vestibulotoxic while dihydrostreptomycin was significantly more vestibulotoxic than cochleotoxic. This is in contradistinction to the literature on the systemic application of these drugs and is attributable to the alternate route of entry tested in this study.

These relationships are offered as evidence that there exists a partitioning effect within the inner ear which acts in concert with innate hair cell selectivity to produce that pattern and degree of morphological change which are documented in this and other reports.

REFERENCES

1. Friedmann I, Bird ES. Effect of ototoxic antibiotics and of penicillin on the sensory areas of the isolated fowl embryo otocyst in organ cultures: an electron-microscope study. J Pathol Bacteriol 1961; 81:81-90.

2. Voldrich L. Kinetics of streptomycin, kanamycin and neomycin in the inner ear. Acta Otolaryngol (Stockh) 1965; 60:243-8.

3. Stupp H, Rauch S, Sous H, Brun JP, Lagler F. Kanamycin dosage and levels in ear and other organs. Arch Otolaryngol 1967; 86:515-21.

4. Meyer zum Gottesberge A, Stupp HF. Streptomycinspiegel in der Perilymphe des Menschen. Acta Otolaryngol (Stockh) 1969; 67:171-6.

5. Stupp H. Untersuchung der Antibiotikaspiegel in den Innenohrflüssigkeiten und ihre Bedeutung für die spezifische Ototoxizität der Aminoglykosidantibiotika. Acta Otolaryngol (Stockh) 1970; Suppl 262.

6. Ilberg Cv, Spoendlin H, Arnold W. Autoradiographical distribution of locally applied dihydrostreptomycin in the inner ear. Acta Otolaryngol (Stockh) 1971; 71:159-65.

7. Stupp H, Küpper K, Lagler F, Sous H, Quante M. Inner ear concentrations and ototoxicity of different antibiotics in local and systemic applications. Audiology 1973; 12:350-63.

8. El-Mofty A, El-Serafy S. Effect of ototoxic antibiotics on the oxygen uptake of the membranous cochlea. Ann Otol Rhinol Laryngol 1966; 75:216-24.

9. Lindeman HH. Regional differences in sensitivity of the vestibular sensory epithelia to ototoxic antibiotics. Acta Otolaryngol (Stockh) 1969; 67:177-89.

10. Hawkins JE Jr. Ototoxic mechanisms. Audiology 1973; 12:383-93.

11. Sedwick JD. Determination of the ability of ototoxic

aminoglycoside antibiotics to bind to acidic mucopolysaccharides. Prog Rep Hearing Found Buffalo 1973.

12. Rudnick MD, Ginsberg IA, Huber PS. Aminoglycoside ototoxicity following middle ear injection. I. Experimental approach and histological criteria for evaluating drug effects. Ann Otol Rhinol Laryngol 1980; 89 Suppl 77:1-9.

13. Rudnick MD, Ginsberg IA, Huber PS, Rose JS. Aminoglycoside ototoxicity following middle ear injection. II. Quantitative analytical procedure. Ann Otol Rhinol Laryngol 1980; 89 Suppl 77:10-16.

14. Wersäll J, Hawkins JE Jr. Vestibular sensory epithelia in the cat labyrinth and their reactions in chronic streptomycin intoxication. Acta Otolaryngol (Stockh) 1962; 54:1-23.

15. Spoendlin H. Zur Ototoxizität des Streptomyzins. Pract Oto-Rhino-Laryngol 1966; 28:305-22.

16. Watanuki K, Meyer zum Gottesberge A. Toxic effects of streptomycin and kanamycin upon the sensory epithelium of the crista ampullaris. Acta Otolaryngol (Stockh) 1971; 72:59-67.

17. Watanuki K, Stupp HF, Meyer zum Gottesberge A. Toxic effects of gentamycin upon the peripheral vestibular sensory organs. Laryngoscope 1972; 82:363-71.

18. Schuknecht HF, Igarashi M, Gacek RR. Pathological types of cochleo-saccular degeneration. Acta Otolaryngol (Stockh) 1965; 59:154-70.

19. Glorig A. Effect of dihydrostreptomycin hydrochloride and sulfate on the auditory mechanism. Ann Otol Rhinol Laryngol 1951; 60:327-35.

20. Shambaugh GE Jr, Derlacki EL, Harrison WH, et al. Dihydrostreptomycin deafness. JAMA 1959; 170:1657-60.

21. Balogh K Jr, Hiraide F, Ishii D. Distribution of radioactive dihydrostreptomycin in the cochlea. Ann Otol Rhinol Laryngol 1970; 79:641-52.

22. Muraveiskaya VS. Determination of streptomycin, dihydrostreptomycin, colimycin and monomycin concentration in labyrinth fluid of guinea pigs. Antibiotiki 1965; 10:245-50.

23. Igarashi M, Lundquist PG, Alford BR, Miyata H. Experimental ototoxicity of gentamicin in squirrel monkeys. J Infect Dis 1971; 124 Suppl S114-24.

24. Waitz JA, Moss EL Jr, Weinstein MJ. Aspects of the chronic toxicity of gentamicin sulfate in cats. J Infect Dis 1971; 124 Suppl S125-9.

25. Tachibana M, Mizukoshi O, Kuriyama K. Inhibitory effects of kanamycin on glycolysis in cochlea and kidney — possible involvement in the formation of oto- and nephrotoxicities. Biochem Pharmacol 1976; 25:2297-301.

26. Ruben RJ, Daly JF. Neomycin ototoxicity and nephrotoxicity. Laryngoscope 1968; 78:1734-7.

27. Jackson GG, Arcieri G. Ototoxicity of gentamicin in man: a survey and controlled analysis of clinical experience in the United States. J Infect Dis 1971; 124 Suppl S130-7.

28. Koide Y, Hata A, Hando R. Vulnerability of the organ of Corti in poisoning. Acta Otolaryngol (Stockh) 1966; 61:332-44.

29. Haug HP, Giebel W, Breuninger H. Ausbreitung von Tetracyclin im Innenohr nach unterschiedlicher Applikation im Mittelohr. Arch Otorhinolaryngol 1978; 218:229-38.

30. Schuknecht HF. Ablation therapy for the relief of Meniere's disease. Laryngoscope 1950; 66:859-70.

31. Schuknecht HF. Ablation therapy in the management of Ménière's disease. Acta Otolaryngol (Stockh) 1957; Suppl 132.

32. Berg K. Toxic effect of streptomycin on the vestibular and cochlear apparatus. Acta Otolaryngol (Stockh) 1951; Suppl 97.

33. Hawkins JE Jr, Lurie MH. Ototoxicity of streptomycin. Ann Otol Rhinol Laryngol 1952; 61:789-809.

34. McGee TM, Olszewski J. Streptomycin sulfate and dihydrostreptomycin toxicity. Arch Otolaryngol 1962; 75:295-311.

AMINOGLYCOSIDE OTOTOXICITY FOLLOWING MIDDLE EAR INJECTION

IV. INFLUENCE OF VESTIBULAR STIMULATION

PAMELA S. HUBER, MS

IRWIN A. GINSBERG, MD

MICHAEL D. RUDNICK, PhD

BUFFALO, NEW YORK

Guinea pigs were given transtympanic dosages of neomycin followed by three hours of either vestibular stimulation or immobilization to test the hypothesis that inner ear hair cell membrane permeability is increased for drugs as a consequence of the transduction process. It was found, however, that neither the topographic pattern nor the degree of hair cell damage differed between the two groups. It is concluded that if the transduction process is accompanied by cell membrane permeability changes, the effect is not an increased susceptibility to neomycin toxicity. A measurable effect of stimulation was the significant decrease in the standard deviation of the mean dosage-damage response at each dosage level. This increase in reliability probably resulted from mixing of the inner ear fluids (especially in the vestibular compartment) which encouraged consistent dosages to the hair cells with each repeated trial. Finally, the impact of these findings on hypotheses related to the mechanism of selective ototoxicity is discussed briefly.

In 1973, Goldstein reported that in vivo sound stimulation or mechanical trauma during tissue preparation caused an increase in outer and inner hair cell membrane permeability.[1] This suggested the possibility that the uptake of drugs by inner ear hair cells may be enhanced by mechanical stimulation.

In this study each guinea pig was given one transtympanic injection of neomycin. This was followed by either rocking or immobilizing each animal for a three-hour period. If the rocked group showed an increase in hair cell damage over the immobilized group, then the hypothesis would be supported.

Another effect of rocking may be a more even distribution of drugs in the labyrinth than that following the systemic or transtympanic route of entry alone. If mechanical stimulation alters the topographic pattern of inner ear hair cell damage reported in part III of this study,[2] then the credibility of the hypothesis of innate hair cell specificity as the basis for the mechanism of selective ototoxicity[3-6] would be diminished.

METHODS

Twenty-seven pigmented guinea pigs (60% male, 40% female) were selected and injected with neomycin as described in part I of this study.[7] Immediately following injection and while still anesthetized, the guinea pigs were fixed to cradles which elevated their snouts 45°. The animals were then either left immobilized or rocked for a period of three hours. Otostimulation was accomplished by fixing the cradles and guinea pigs to a rocking-type solution mixer which moved through a vertical 30° arc at a frequency of 30 cycles per minute (see Table 1 for the injection schedule).

The animals were returned to their cages for one week prior to decapitation, incubation, fixation and microdissection.[7] Cell counts were performed and the data were analyzed according to the format established in part II of this study.[8]

RESULTS

The behavioral responses to vestibular stimulation varied greatly but several generalizations could be made: those guinea pigs which received a dosage of neomycin followed by rocking for three hours demonstrated the greatest effect when released from their restraints. In several instances this consisted of uncontrolled rolling to the right, even after reaching the cage wall. This behavior persisted for only a few minutes. Thereafter, the guinea pigs sat quietly with their heads lowered and turned toward the right. When encouraged to walk, their gait was, at best, unstable and they tended to walk in a right-handed circle. Attempts to right themselves were initially frustrated until, with gradual improvement, all evidence of vestibular dysfunction disappeared. The group of guinea pigs which received saline followed by rocking had less severe ataxia which persisted for only a few minutes. Animals which received drugs and were immobilized usually appeared lethargic, and their heads were lowered and turned toward the injected side for a day or two after surgery. Some of these guinea pigs tended to walk in a circle during the initial recovery period. Saline-injected and immobilized animals were virtually free of vestibular disturbance. Their righting

TABLE 1. INJECTION SCHEDULE

Drug — Otostimulation	*Number of Guinea Pigs Receiving Each Dosage*					
	Dosage in Mg					
	0	*5*	*10*	*25*	*50*	*Subtotal*
Neomycin — rocked	—	4	5	3	0	12
Neomycin — immobilized	—	0	4	3	1	8
Saline — rocked	3	—	—	—	—	3
Saline — immobilized	4	—	—	—	—	4
Total animals in study						27

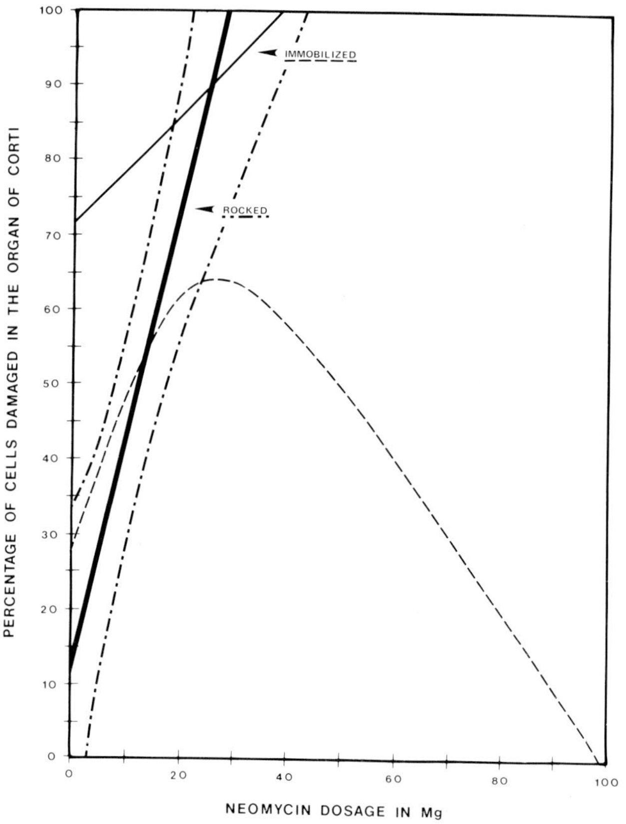

Fig. 1. Percentage of damaged sensory cells in organ of Corti as a function of neomycin dosage following immobilization and following rocking.

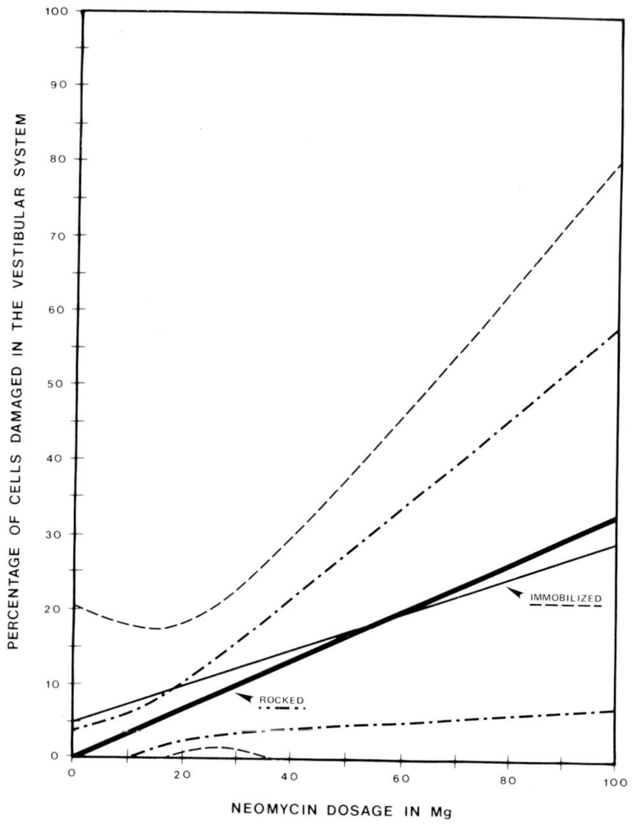

Fig. 2. Percentage of damaged sensory cells in the vestibular system as a function of neomycin dosage following immobilization and following rocking.

reflexes were normal, and they soon returned to normal activity.

At the time of sacrifice and during microdissection, no evidence of infection was detected in the 27 guinea pigs. Histological analysis showed that all 34 control ears were within the normal limits set previously.[7]

The effects of otostimulation were determined by *t* tests comparing the means of the dosage versus damage relationships in each region of the inner ear between rocked and immobilized groups. The results of this analysis were that no significant differences in the topographic pattern or degree of toxicity existed between the rocked and immobilized groups. In fact, no relationship differed significantly from those reported previously.[2]

However, an examination of the standard deviations of the means suggested an interesting phenomenon. It was found that within each region of the vestibular system the standard deviations of the means were less for the rocked group than for the immobilized group. This was also true within the organ of Corti, but to a smaller degree. An analysis of variance disclosed that vestibular stimulation produced significantly more consistent or reliable results than immobilization following the transtympanic administration of neomycin.

Figures 1 and 2 present the unconstrained least-squares linear regression lines and confidence intervals which describe the effects of transtympanically injected neomycin on the hair cells in the organ of Corti (Fig. 1) and the vestibular system (Fig. 2) following either rocking or immobilization. Note that the least-squares linear regression lines for the rocked group cross the ordinate closer to the origin than do the lines representing the immobilized group. This approaches the logical value of zero hair cell damage resulting from zero drug dosage as indeed was the finding among the controls. More dramatic, however, are the broken lines depicting the 95% confidence intervals for the regression lines. Clearly, making predictions based upon data from the rocked group would be much more reliable than making predictions based upon data from the immobilized group.

The data derived from the immobilized group were occasionally skewed to the extent that computing dosage-damage relationships would lead to the conclusion that increasing the dosage of neomycin would have no increased effect on inner ear hair cells. This effect is illustrated in Figure 3. By rocking the guinea pigs following the transtympanic administration of neomycin, the variance in the data was sufficiently decreased to reveal that a significant, positive dosage-damage relationship existed

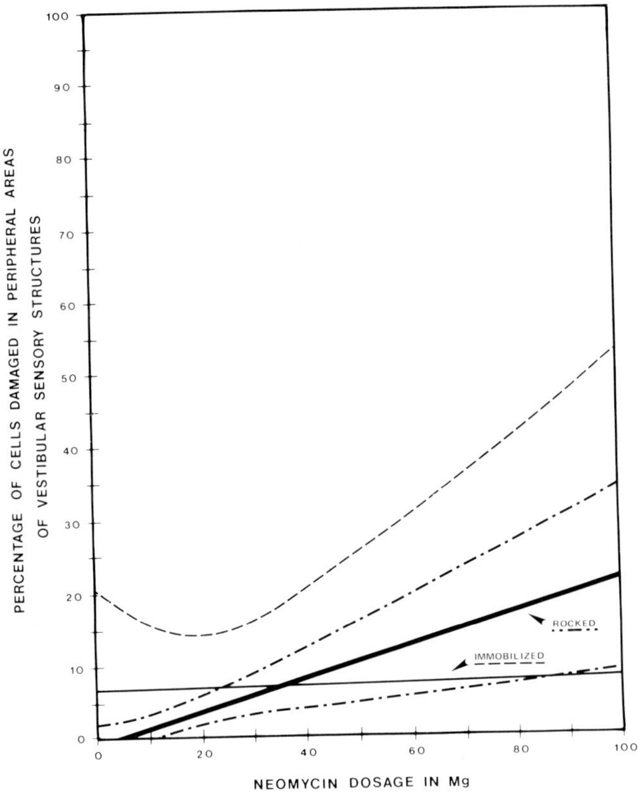

Fig. 3. Percentage of damaged sensory cells in the peripheral regions of vestibular sensory structures as a function of neomycin dosage following immobilization and following rocking.

in the peripheral regions of vestibular sensory structures.

DISCUSSION

The regimen of vestibular stimulation was apparently sufficient to elicit both a behavioral and a statistical effect. If this stimulation caused a change in sensory cell membrane permeability as Goldstein suggested,[1] its effect was not a facilitation of toxicity. No conclusion can be made relating stimulation to permeability changes, nor can it be concluded that stimulation enhances the uptake of drugs by hair cells.

In the immobilized group, antibiotic must reach each sensory structure through passive diffusion alone. The disparate data from this group may have resulted from individual differences which impede diffusion. For example, the middle ear mucosa was thickened in some animals, particularly over the round window membrane. Rocking may have physically mixed the inner ear fluids so that a concentration gradient was maintained between the middle and inner ears. The effect of this gradient may have been to drive antibiotic from the middle ear into the fluid spaces of the inner ear. By this mechanism, it is suggested that rocking encourages a uniform distribution of drugs within the inner ear and a consistent dosage to sensory cells with each repeated trial. The decreased variance in the data reported for the rocked animals may be thus explained. The observation of lower standard deviations within the vestibular compartment than within the cochlear compartment may simply reflect the different anatomical conformation of the fluid spaces which encourages gross fluid movement.

The hypothesis that selective drug ototoxicity results from the selective transport of drugs into each compartment within the inner ear following systemic administration (the partition effect)[6,9-16] cannot be the only mechanism involved in selective ototoxicity. In our study, the local application of aminoglycoside antibiotics bypassed the transport epithelia of the inner ear but nonetheless resulted in the same pattern of hair cell damage *within* each compartment as has been reported following the systemic administration of these drugs.[6,17-21] Further mixing of the inner ear fluids by rocking did not alter the pattern or degree of hair cell damage but merely stabilized the results. The comparative ototoxicity of drugs *between* compartments, however, *was* altered by changing their route of entry[2] so that selective transport must at least contribute to the understanding of selective ototoxicity. The mechanism of selective ototoxicity must also involve drug selectivity at, or immediately surrounding, the hair cells themselves (innate hair cell selectivity).[22] Only this would explain the consistent regional pattern of hair cell susceptibility to drugs regardless of the route of entry or extent of distribution in the inner ear fluid spaces.

REFERENCES

1. Goldstein AJ. Permeability of the organ of Corti. Ann Otol Rhinol Laryngol 1973; 82:166-74.

2. Ginsberg IA, Rudnick MD, Huber PS. Aminoglycoside ototoxicity following middle ear injection. III. Comparative quantitative analysis. Ann Otol Rhinol Laryngol 1980; 89 Suppl 77:17-24.

3. Moskowitz M, Kelker NE. Sensitivity of cultured mammalian cells to streptomycin and dihydrostreptomycin. Science 1963; 141:647-8.

4. El-Mofty A, El-Serafy S. Effect of ototoxic antibiotics on the oxygen uptake of the membranous cochlea. Ann Otol Rhinol Laryngol 1966; 75:216-24.

5. Lindeman HH. Regional differences in sensitivity of the vestibular sensory epithelia to ototoxic antibiotics. Acta Otolaryngol (Stockh) 1969; 67:177-89.

6. Hawkins JE Jr. Ototoxic mechanisms. Audiology 1973; 12:383-93.

7. Rudnick MD, Ginsberg IA, Huber PS. Aminoglycoside ototoxicity following middle ear injection. I. Experimental approach and histological criteria for evaluating drug effects. Ann Otol Rhinol Laryngol 1980; 89 Suppl 77:1-9.

8. Rudnick MD, Ginsberg IA, Huber PS, Rose JS. Aminoglycoside ototoxicity following middle ear injection. II. Quantitative analytical procedure. Ann Otol Rhinol Laryngol 1980; 89 Suppl 77:10-16.

9. Friedmann I, Bird ES. Effect of ototoxic antibiotics and of

penicillin on the sensory areas of the isolated fowl embryo otocyst in organ cultures: an electron-microscope study. J Pathol Bacteriol 1961; 81:81-90.

10. Muraveiskaya VS. Determination of streptomycin, dihydrostreptomycin, colimycin and monomycin concentration in labyrinth fluid of guinea pigs. Antibiotiki 1965; 10:245-50.

11. Voldrick L. Kinetics of streptomycin, kanamycin and neomycin in the inner ear. Acta Otolaryngol (Stockh) 1965; 60:243-8.

12. Stupp H, Rauch S, Sous H, Brun JP, Lagler F. Kanamycin dosage and levels in ear and other organs. Arch Otolaryngol 1967; 86:515-21.

13. Meyer zum Gottesberge A, Stupp HF. Streptomycinspiegel in der Perilymphe des Menschen. Acta Otolaryngol (Stockh) 1969; 67:171-6.

14. Balogh K Jr, Hiraide F, Ishii D. Distribution of radioactive dihydrostreptomycin in the cochlea. Ann Otol Rhinol Laryngol 1970; 79:641-52.

15. Stupp H. Untersuchung der Antibiotikaspiegel in den Innenohrflüssigkeiten und ihre Bedeutung für die spezifische Ototoxizität der Aminoglykosidantibiotika. Acta Otolaryngol (Stockh) 1970; Suppl 262.

16. Stupp H, Küpper K, Lagler F, Sous H, Quante M. Inner ear concentrations and ototoxicity of different antibiotics in local and systemic applications. Audiology 1973; 12:350-63.

17. Berg K. Toxic effect of streptomycin on the vestibular and cochlear apparatus. Acta Otolaryngol (Stockh) 1951; Suppl 97.

18. Hawkins JE Jr, Lurie MH. Ototoxicity of streptomycin. Ann Otol Rhinol Laryngol 1952; 61:789-809.

19. McGee TM, Olszewski J. Streptomycin sulfate and dihydrostreptomycin toxicity. Arch Otolaryngol 1962; 75:295-311.

20. Wersäll J, Hawkins JE Jr. Vestibular sensory epithelia in the cat labyrinth and their reactions in chronic streptomycin intoxication. Acta Otolaryngol (Stockh) 1962; 54:1-23.

21. Spoendlin H. Zur Ototoxizität des Streptomyzins. Pract Oto-Rhino-Laryngol 1966; 28:305-22.

22. Ilberg Cv, Spoendlin H, Arnold W. Autoradiographical distribution of locally applied dihydrostreptomycin in the inner ear. Acta Otolaryngol (Stockh) 1971; 71:159-65.